Dermatology in
Traditional Chinese Medicine

Biographical details

Professor **Xu Yihou** graduated in June 1963 from Hubei College of Traditional Chinese Medicine with a Bachelor of Medicine degree. He then began work as a doctor in the Dermatology Department of Wuhan Hospital of Traditional Chinese Medicine. During his years at the hospital, he specialized in the treatment of skin diseases, subsequently being appointed Deputy Chief Doctor of the department before assuming his present position of Chief Doctor and Professor.

A supervisor of Ph.D. students, Professor Xu is currently working by invitation at the China Association of Traditional Chinese Medicine Clinical Research Center in the IACH Hong Kong Baptist University as Professor and Chief Doctor in research and clinical practice.

Professor Xu has accumulated more than 40 years of clinical experience in the treatment of skin disorders and, thanks to this wealth of experience, he has published a number of books and dozens of articles in national and international journals. His books include *Diagnosis and Treatment of Skin Diseases in Traditional Chinese Medicine*, *Acupuncture in the Treatment of Skin Diseases*, *Treatment of Skin Disorders of the Hands and Feet*, *A Summary of Xu Yihou's Clinical Experiences in the Treatment of Skin Diseases*, *Treatment of Pruritus*, and *A Collection of Shan Canggui's Experiences in Treating External Diseases*.

Yi Sumei, a graduate of Nanjing University of Traditional Chinese Medicine and Nanjing Normal University, pursued a career as acupuncturist and physiotherapist before becoming a lecturer and vice-professor at Nanjing University of Traditional Chinese Medicine, where she teaches TCM to Chinese and foreign students. She has also been engaged in translation and interpreting for many years and has been a visiting lecturer in Italy and the Philippines. She has been involved in the compilation or translation of more than 20 books on TCM or English.

Trina Ward, with a background in anthropology, started studying Chinese medicine in Australia in 1988 and graduated in 1992 after completing an internship at the Shu Guang Hospital in Shanghai and studying Chinese at Feng Chia University, Taiwan. A member of the British Acupuncture Council (MBAcC) and the Register of Chinese Herbal Medicine (MRCHM), she has worked in the UK on the Council of the RCHM as Research Officer. In 2002, she completed an MPhil at Exeter University on safety aspects of Chinese herbal medicine. Practicing in London alongside Western doctors, she is keen to promote the integration of Chinese medicine with Western medicine.

Aruna Sahni is a practicing acupuncturist and Chinese herbalist. She has a previous degree in Biochemistry and Genetics, after which she worked as a production editor for three years on scientific and medical journals for Oxford University Press. She then trained in acupuncture at the London School of Acupuncture and did a postgraduate course in Nanjing, subsequently training in Chinese herbal medicine at the London College of Traditional Acupuncture. She has worked in the NHS in a GP's surgery and in various London hospitals in the field of HIV. Currently, she has a private practice at the Traditional Acupuncture Centre in Waterloo, is studying conventional medicine, and is a member of the editorial team of the European Journal of Oriental Medicine.

Dermatology in Traditional Chinese Medicine

Written by
Xu Yihou
Chief Doctor and Professor, Dermatology Department
Wuhan Hospital of Traditional Chinese Medicine

Translated by
Yi Sumei
Vice-Professor, Nanjing University of Traditional Chinese Medicine

Foreword by
Li Lin

Subject editors
Trina Ward MPhil, BSc (Hons), MBAcC, MRCHM
Aruna Sahni BSc (Hons), ClinAc (Nanjing), MBAcC, MRCHM

Medical consultant
Robert J Dickie FRCGP, DRCOG, BMedBiol

Donica Publishing Ltd

Note

Medical knowledge is constantly changing. As new information becomes available, changes in treatment, procedures, equipment, and the use of drugs and/or materia medica become necessary. The editors/authors/contributors and the publishers have, as far as it is possible, taken care to ensure that the information given in this text is accurate and up to date. However, readers are strongly advised to confirm that the information, especially with regard to the permitted usage of materia medica, complies with the latest legislation and standards of practice.

Although every effort has been made to indicate appropriate precautions with regard to the legal status and usage of materia medica and the other therapies discussed in this book, neither the publishers nor the authors can accept responsibility for any treatment advice or information offered, neither will they be liable for any loss or damage of any nature occasioned to or suffered by any person acting or refraining from acting as a result of reliance on the material contained in this publication.

First published 2004

ISBN 1 901149 03 X

British Library Cataloguing in Publication Data
A catalogue record for this book is available from the British Library

Commissioning editor Yanping Li
Managing editor Rodger Watts
TCM consultant Zhou Lei
Cover design Paul Pang
Photographs Xu Yihou and Yu Ruiyao
Illustrations Wang Wei

Printed in the United States of America by King Printing Co., Inc.
The publisher's policy is to use paper manufactured from sustainable forests.

Contents

Acknowledgments

This book could not have been written without the constant help and encouragement of my family, friends and colleagues. I am particularly indebted to my wife Cai Tiquan for her unwavering support throughout the five years it took to complete the work.

I am also very grateful to my esteemed colleague Dr. Li Lin for kindly agreeing to write a foreword to this volume; receiving recognition from one's peers is always a particular honor.

My particular thanks are also extended to Professor Zhang Zhili from Beijing Traditional Chinese Medicine Hospital for permission to include a number of his case studies and to Dr. Yu Ruiyao from the 301 Military Hospital in Beijing for allowing use of some of his photographs.

Hao Shengli from the People's Medical Publishing House in Beijing also deserves thanks for her invaluable assistance in the original Chinese edition.

In addition, this book could not have been compiled without the assistance of my translators Yi Sumei, Fu Zhiwen, Ding Xiaohong, and Zhu Meiwei. Zhou Lei and Zhong Yongtao provided invaluable help in adapting this book for English-language readers, and my colleagues in the UK, Trina Ward, Aruna Sahni and Dr. Robert Dickie, made a major contribution to the final version.

Last but certainly not least, without the unstinting energy, support, assistance, and insight of Yanping Li at Donica Publishing, this book could never have been completed in its present form.

To all of them, I express my heartfelt gratitude.

Foreword

Since coming to the United Kingdom to open my own busy Traditional Chinese Medicine practice ten years ago, I have come to realize the lack of a definitive English-language practical dermatology book specifically oriented toward the skin disorders more commonly seen by a TCM practitioner in Western countries. It is therefore with great pleasure that I strongly recommend this book as an essential clinical guide for practitioners and students alike, allowing them to develop and improve their diagnostic skills and expand their range of treatment for the skin disorders they meet in their daily practice.

I have known Professor Xu since we began working together 20 years ago on the editorial committee of *External Diseases in Traditional Chinese Medicine*, compiled by our mentor, Professor Zhu Renkang, one of the most eminent TCM dermatologists of the modern era. Along with a group of mature specialists with a wealth of clinical experience, we pooled our knowledge to help produce the book. At the time, I was constantly impressed by the insights he gave into the treatment of a variety of common and less common skin conditions and we forged a friendship based on mutual esteem that has lasted until the present day.

As the next generation, it is our duty to carry on the tradition established by our predecessors, collect our own personal experiences together and hand them on to future generations of doctors. The nature of diseases changes over time, with some being brought under control and new ones appearing. For this reason, medical knowledge needs constant updating. Modern life with its increased stress and dietary challenges manifests itself in a number of skin disorders according to Traditional Chinese Medicine theory; one only has to consider the increase in the number of patients in Western countries with atopic eczema or contact dermatitis to see evidence of this. Based on a thorough understanding of pattern identification, TCM practitioners can adapt their skills to treat all types of skin disorders whatever their origin and this book provides them with the tools for success.

It is worth underlining the four major features of *Dermatology in Traditional Chinese Medicine* – its comprehensive coverage of a wide range of skin disorders, its wealth of practical information presented in an exceptionally user-friendly fashion, the excellence of the translation into English, and the broad spectrum of case histories and up-to-date clinical experience reports, where the author has not been afraid to offer alternative approaches to those suggested by his 40 years of clinical experience. I have the highest esteem for Professor Xu's straightforward scientific approach and fully endorse his efforts to promote throughout the world the use of Chinese medicine in the treatment of skin disorders.

It is my opinion that by following the principles discussed in this book, practitioners will be helped to develop their skills with the ultimate aim of treating their patients competently and effectively. I have no hesitation in recommending this book to all those who treat patients with skin conditions.

Li Lin
London 2004

Author's preface

In China, as in other countries throughout the world, patients with skin disorders form a significant proportion of those who consult doctors practicing Chinese medicine. Working essentially in a hospital environment in China, Traditional Chinese Medicine (TCM) doctors will see a wide range of skin disorders and will have the opportunity to treat both everyday and difficult cases. In most Western countries, however, the trend still seems to be that many patients with skin conditions consulting TCM practitioners do so because they have not received a satisfactory response from other treatments, in many instances in relation to common conditions such as eczema, psoriasis or acne.

Whatever the case, a dermatologist must never forget that what a doctor may consider a common condition with a generally satisfactory prognosis may blight the patient's daily life and make him or her feel a social outcast. Every case must be treated seriously with a thorough and complete TCM diagnosis, and appropriate reassurance offered to the patient. TCM, with its emphasis on the individuality of the patient, has proven down the ages that treatment of the cause or root of the disorder can often bring about a more satisfactory and longer-lasting effect than focusing solely on the symptoms or manifestations.

After graduating in 1963, I chose dermatology as my specialty and the last 40 years have been an enriching and rewarding experience for me. It is my hope that some of my passion for this subject will communicate itself to readers in this book at the same time as offering them the opportunity to broaden their treatment options based on my clinical experiences.

Compilation principles

This book is aimed at all practitioners of Traditional Chinese Medicine including acupuncturists, whether they are just starting in the profession or whether they have already gathered a certain degree of experience; it can also be used by advanced students to see how theory can be turned into effective practice. Although this is essentially a TCM book, it is hoped that some

practitioners of Western medicine will also find much to think about as they seek to find the best referral options for treating their skin patients.

The book focuses essentially on commonly seen skin disorders, but also includes some examples of rarer conditions, for which in my experience TCM treatment has proven effective. The main emphasis has been placed on the "big four" – eczema and related disorders, psoriasis and other papulosquamous disorders, acne, and urticarial disorders – but many other skin conditions are also covered in detail.

Certain skin diseases have been excluded in order to keep the size of the book to manageable proportions. Connective tissue disorders will be discussed in another book to be published in the near future by Donica Publishing; sexually transmitted diseases and skin cancer are other major areas meriting separate consideration.

There are basically two ways of arranging dermatology books – by disease type or by body region. The latter approach has been popular with Chinese authors for some time, but in my opinion it is rather limiting since many skin disorders manifest in different parts of the body. Therefore, when the publishers suggested classification by disease type, I was happy to agree to their proposal. Although this classification implies acceptance of a more Western method of disease categorization, it is being increasingly adopted in teaching hospitals in China and has the additional advantage that it is more likely to be the classification initially used by patients (sometimes erroneously) at their first consultation.

Western medical terminology has also generally been adopted in this book for the description of lesions and clinical manifestations. Modern terminology is generally more precise and allows for more accurate recognition of the disease and pattern involved. Other than that, etiology and pathology, pattern identification, treatment principles, prescription formulae, and prescription explanations are all described using TCM terminology.

Before discussing individual conditions, the book starts with a detailed explanation of the physiology of the skin, the etiology of skin disorders, general methods of pattern identification (including a full description of various primary and secondary skin lesions), and the main treatment methods employed for skin disorders. It is recommended that practitioners read through these chapters first, since they form the basis for all subsequent sections.

The remainder of the main text of the book is divided into a number of chapters, each covering a particular category of skin disease. The approach adopted is the same for each section of each chapter. The section begins with a description of the clinical manifestations of the skin disorder in question, followed by differential diagnosis, where appropriate. The main part of each section relates to treatment.

Although herbal medicine (internal treatment, patent medicines and external treatment) usually takes on the major role, acupuncture, moxibustion, ear acupuncture, and seven-star needling also have a significant part to play in the treatment of a number of skin disorders. In China, a course of acupuncture treatment would normally be given on a daily basis. This may be possible in other countries in a hospital or hospice context; treatment at greater intervals is also perfectly feasible, although the effects may take longer to appear.

In terms of herbal treatment, the book attempts to offer clear identification of patterns, treatment principles and formulae used. The main symptoms and signs of each pattern are listed, and an explanation is given of the materia medica used in each prescription formula.

Since Chinese medicine is pattern-based, the skill of the practitioner lies in correct pattern identification and modification of the prescription to take account of the individual characteristics and clinical manifestations of each patient. It is impossible to cover all the possibilities in this book, but a few common modifications are presented.

Unless otherwise stated, a prescription is prepared by using one bag of ingredients per day and boiling twice in one liter of water to produce a decoction taken twice a day.

The ingredients of patent medicines and external treatment prescriptions are listed in appendices at the end of the book. A small number of these formulae may contain ingredients whose use may not be permitted in certain countries outside China. Where possible, alternatives for these preparations have been suggested in the text. However, in certain instances, notably in case histories and modern clinical experience reports, the original formulae have also been retained to give practitioners an insight into the way the particular condition involved would be treated in China (see also the note on names and legal status below).

The treatment description is followed by some brief clinical notes based on my own experiences. These frequently offer an alternative insight into the treatment

presented beforehand. Many diseases also include short excerpts from TCM classical literature, indicating how eminent doctors, ancient and modern, view the disease in question.

A major feature of the book is the inclusion of a number of case histories from other leading TCM dermatologists and a wide variety of clinical experience reports published in Chinese, mostly since the mid-1990s. As a result, practitioners can see the effect of different approaches and take them into consideration in their own practice.

These case histories and clinical experience reports are intended as a guide to practitioners and to stimulate their thought processes. In terms of clinical experience reports, I have generally preferred to focus on formulae or methods that can be employed on a daily basis in the clinic so as to provide practitioners with a more practical approach. However, it should be borne in mind that, even though these reports are better structured than in the past, they may not always be considered as meeting the criteria of Western medical research; they should therefore be viewed as useful pointers rather than as hard-and-fast rules. In particular, it is not always possible to give an accurate prognosis as to the length of treatment, but the likely time before results begin to be seen is stated where available.

The book therefore offers a balanced range of TCM treatment options for use in skin disorders. My own experience clearly indicates that Chinese medicine has a major role to play in dermatology and I would be very interested to hear readers' comments on the strategies adopted in this book and on their own experiences. These should be addressed in the first instance to the publishers at donica@donica.fsbusiness.co.uk.

A note on names and legal status

Acupuncture points are designated by the letter and number coding used in the National Acupuncture Points Standard of the People's Republic of China issued by the State Bureau of Technical Supervision.

Materia medica are referred to throughout the book by their Chinese name in pinyin and their pharmaceutical name in Latin. Different practitioners are used to different naming systems; however, by offering both pinyin and Latin, identification of the materia medica should be clear.

It is important at this point to draw readers' attention to the legal status of certain of the herbs included in this book. Although they are all available in China, a few herbs are subject to export restrictions and others are considered too toxic for use in some Western countries.

The situation regarding restrictions and bans tends to change over time and from country to country.

Materia medica that are included in Appendix I (all trade of wild species banned) and Appendix II (trade allowable with appropriate permits) of the Convention on International Trade in Endangered Species of Wild Fauna and Flora (CITES) are marked with an asterisk (*), as are other materia medica subject to restrictions or bans in certain countries as a result of their toxicity. Other animal and mineral materia medica are marked with the symbol ‡; in some countries, these substances cannot be sold in unlicensed medical preparations as herbs.

Readers should consult the appropriate authorities in their own countries for the latest developments. Inclusion of materia medica in this book does not imply that their use is permitted in all countries and in all circumstances. Practitioners should always check the contents of any patent medicines to ensure that they comply with the legal requirements of the country in which they practice.

Certain materia medica coming under these categories are used regularly in China to treat skin disorders, notably *Mu Tong* (Caulis Mutong) internally and *Zhu Sha* (Cinnabaris), *Qing Fen* (Calomelas) and *Xiong Huang* (Sulphur) externally. Where possible, alternative materia medica have been substituted in prescriptions or potential substitutes suggested. However, no alterations to formulae in clinical experience reports or case histories have been undertaken out of respect for the original authors' work.

Xu Yihou
Wuhan Hospital of Traditional Chinese Medicine, March 2004

Chapter 1

The skin and skin disorders in Traditional Chinese Medicine

Epidemiology of skin disorders
皮肤病的流行病学

It has been estimated that up to 25 percent of the population in Western countries may have a skin problem; however, the majority of these people do not seek professional medical advice. Of those who do, eczema, bacterial and viral infections, fungal infections, and acne account for almost two-thirds of cases.[i, ii]

The type, prevalence and incidence of skin diseases depend on a number of factors:

- Social and economic factors – most infectious diseases, including infectious diseases of the skin, are now more common in underdeveloped countries than in developed countries. On the other hand, industrialization has brought about an increase in the number of cases of occupation-related contact dermatitis. Changes in social habits can also have an effect; for example, the desire for a suntan has increased the number of cases of ultraviolet radiation-related skin disorders.

- Geographic factors – hot and humid climates predispose to bacterial and fungal infections and to sweating disorders such as miliaria rubra (prickly heat); exposure to ultraviolet radiation in sunny regions often results in skin damage in fairer-skinned individuals.

- Racial factors – skin tumors and photosensitive skin reactions occur more frequently in light-skinned than dark-skinned individuals; keloids are more common among black Africans; and vitiligo is more obvious on dark skin, even though incidence is roughly similar in all races.

- Age and gender – some skin conditions can occur at any age, but many others are age-related, occurring at a certain age or disappearing after a certain age is reached (see Table 1-1). In addition, certain skin disorders are more likely to affect a specific gender (see Table 1-2).

Table 1-1 Skin disorders and age

Age	Skin disorders
Infancy and childhood	Anaphylactoid purpura, atopic eczema, common warts (verruca vulgaris), diaper dermatitis (nappy rash), hemangioma, herpes simplex, ichthyosis, impetigo, keratosis pilaris, measles, nevus flammeus, pityriasis alba, tinea capitis (ringworm of the scalp), varicella (chickenpox)
Adolescence	Acne, melanocytic nevi, pityriasis rosea, psoriasis (plaque and guttate), seborrheic eczema, vitiligo
Early adulthood	Alopecia areata, dermatitis herpetiformis, erythema induratum (Bazin's disease), hidradenitis suppurativa, hyperhidrosis, perioral dermatitis, pityriasis versicolor, psoriasis, seborrhea, seborrheic eczema, tinea pedis (athlete's foot), vitiligo
Middle age	Alopecia areata, dermatitis herpetiformis, lichen planus, nodular prurigo, nummular eczema, palmoplantar pustulosis, pemphigus vulgaris, Raynaud's disease, rosacea, stasis eczema
Old age	Asteatotic eczema, bullous pemphigoid, chronic venous ulcer of the lower leg, erythema ab igne, herpes zoster (shingles), pemphigus vulgaris, pruritus, psoriasis, seborrheic eczema, stasis eczema

[i] H.C. Williams, *Dermatology*, in A. Stevens and J. Raftery (eds.), *Health Care Needs Assessment*, Series 2 (Oxford: Radcliffe Medical Press, 1997).
[ii] David J. Gawkrodger, *Dermatology*, 3rd ed. (Edinburgh: Churchill Livingstone, 2002).

Table 1-2 Skin disorders and gender

Gender	Skin disorders
Male	Dermatitis herpetiformis, keratosis pilaris, nummular eczema (discoid eczema), seborrheic eczema, sycosis barbae, tinea cruris (jock itch), tinea pedis (athlete's foot)
Female	Bromhidrosis, chronic venous ulcer of the lower leg, erythema induratum (Bazin's disease), hidradenitis suppurativa, melasma (chloasma), nodular prurigo, palmoplantar pustulosis, perioral dermatitis, pyoderma faciale, Raynaud's disease, rosacea, stasis eczema

Anatomy of the skin
皮肤结构

The skin is the largest organ of the body; it has a surface area of up to 2 square meters and an average weight of about 4kg. The skin is the barrier between the outside world and the internal constituents of the body, reacting to external changes such as external infection, trauma, friction, temperature changes, ultraviolet radiation, and irritants or allergens, and responding to internal stimuli such as genetic and psychological factors, internal diseases, internal infections, and administration of drugs.

Some of the most important functions of the skin are summarized in Table 1-3.

Table 1-3 Functions of the skin

Protects against chemicals, antigens and micro-organisms

Protects against mechanical injury

Reduces penetration of ultraviolet radiation

Prevents loss of body fluids

Regulates temperature

Acts as a sensory organ through specialized nerve endings

Assists in vitamin D synthesis

Subcutaneous fat acts as an insulator and calorie reserve

Appearance plays a role in body image

The skin is made up of three layers. The outer layer, the epidermis, is attached to and supported by connective tissue in the underlying dermis.

The dermis lies above the subcutis, consisting of connective tissue and subcutaneous fat, which can be up to 3cm thick on the abdomen.

The structure of the skin is illustrated in Figure 1-1.

Epidermis

The epidermis is a stratified squamous epithelium, consisting of four layers, with each layer made up in turn of several layers of tightly packed cells. The epidermis, which does not contain any blood vessels, is generally about 0.1mm thick, except on the palms and soles, where it may be up to 1mm thick.

The main cell in the epidermis, the keratinocyte, moves up from the basal layer to the horny layer; as dead surface cells are shed, they are replaced by cells moving up from below, thus keeping the thickness of the epidermis constant.

The deepest layer of the epidermis is the stratum basale (basal layer), which rests on a basement membrane attaching it to the dermis. The basal layer is composed essentially of keratinocytes, producing the protein keratin, with a much smaller number of melanocytes, which synthesize melanin and regulate pigmentation.

Cells in the basal layer are either dividing or non-dividing; those that divide move upward to the stratum spinosum (prickle cell layer), where keratin is synthesized.

The cells move upward to the stratum granulosum (granular layer), where they become flattened, lose their nuclei and become filled with keratin.

The dead cells then migrate upward to the outermost layer of the epidermis, the stratum corneum (horny layer), composed of sheets of flattened cells with no nucleus, known as corneocytes and held together by lipids, thus giving the epidermis its toughness. These corneocytes are eventually shed from the surface of the skin.

The structure of the epidermis is shown in Figure 1-2.

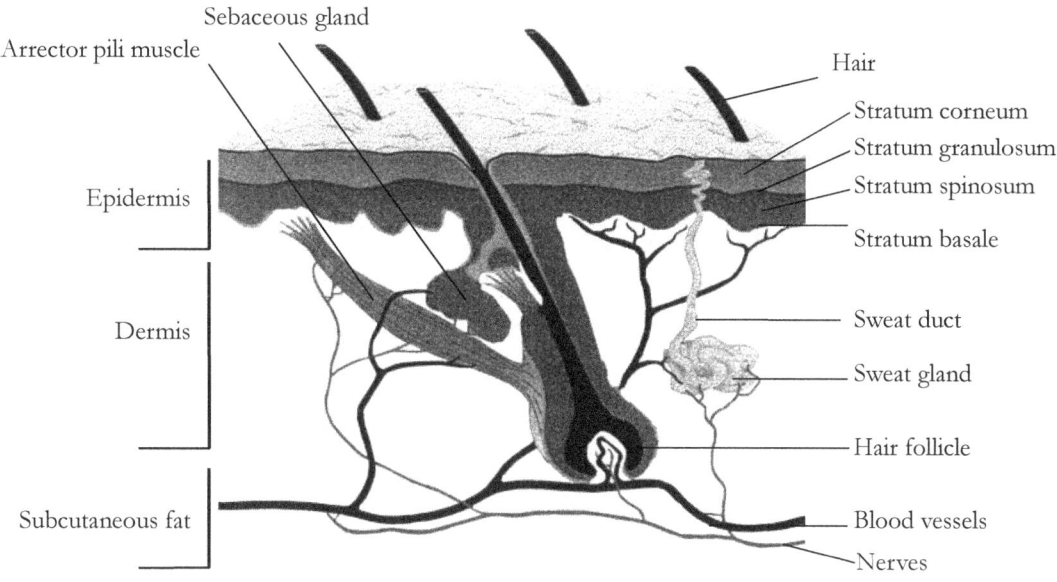

Figure 1-1 Structure of the skin

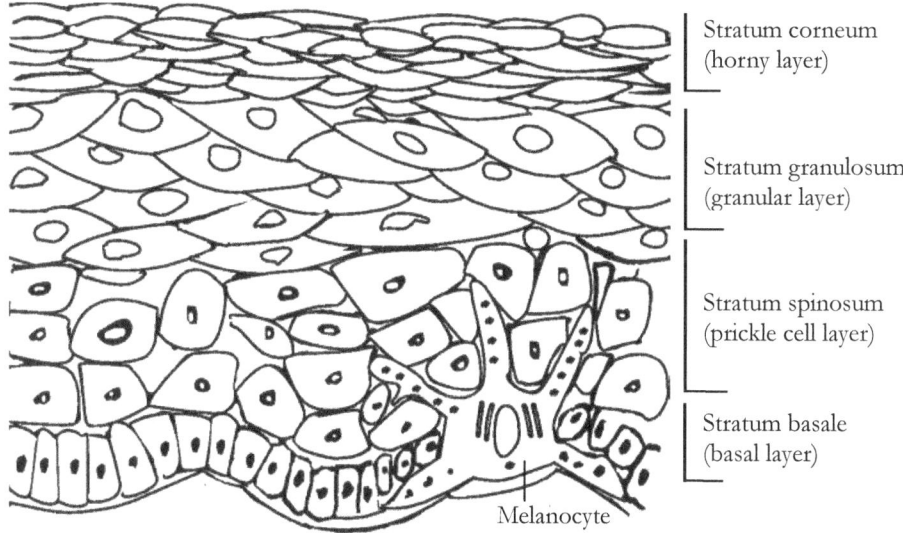

Figure 1-2 Structure of the epidermis

Dermis

The dermis is a tough layer of connective tissue supporting the epidermis structurally and nutritionally. Its thickness varies from 0.6mm on the eyelids to 3mm or more on the palms, soles and back. Upward projections of the dermis interlock with downward ridges of the epidermis in the papillary dermis, the upper layer of the dermis.

The deeper layer of the dermis, the reticular dermis, is made up principally of bundles of collagen, which provide toughness and strength; elasticity is provided by elastin fibers.

The dermis contains many of the structures that play a role in skin diseases; hair follicles and sebaceous and sweat glands have their roots deep in the dermis and pass through the epidermis to reach the skin surface.

The dermis also has a rich supply of blood vessels. Arteries in the deep plexus just above the subcutaneous fat branch upward to supply the sweat glands and the hair papillae. The superficial plexus is located in the papillary dermis and branches extend to the dermal papillae, where they form capillary loops. The cutaneous blood vessels play an important role in temperature regulation; under the influence of the sympathetic nervous system, the capillary loops can be bypassed to reduce surface heat loss when the body is too cold.

In addition, the skin has a plentiful supply of nerve fibers, most located near the dermo-epidermal junction; they function to detect pain, itching and temperature changes.

Physiology of the skin in Traditional Chinese Medicine
中医皮肤生理学

Function of the skin

The skin has several functions in TCM:
- The skin is the first line of defense of the body. In *Za Bing Yuan Liu Xi Zhu* [Enlightenment of the Origins of Miscellaneous Diseases], it says: "The skin covers the flesh to protect the sinews and bones."
- The skin governs the percolating and drainage of Body Fluids to allow the Essence and Qi to manifest externally. Maintaining an appropriate level of sweating through the pores allows the body's metabolism to function correctly.
- The skin maintains the normal activities of the body and safeguards the Zang-Fu organs by acting as a barrier to prevent external pathogenic factors from invading the body.

In *Su Wen: Pi Bu Lun* [Simple Questions: On Skin], it says: "Diseases start from the skin and hair. If they are attacked by external pathogenic factors, the interstices (*cou li*) may loosen and pathogenic factors can enter the interior and obstruct the Blood vessels, channels and network vessels; they may then be transmitted along the channels to the Zang-Fu organs and accumulate in the Stomach and Intestines." This highlights the importance of maintaining intact the defensive function of the skin.

Structure of the skin

Fu: The superficial layer of skin.
Ge: A thick layer of firm tissue beneath the superficial layer.
Cou li: Interstices, or the striae and connective tissue between the skin, flesh and muscles. The *cou li* are the gateway allowing the discharge of Body Fluids and the flow of Qi and Blood to the skin; they also function to resist invasion by external pathogenic factors.
Ji: The flesh and muscles under the skin, which control movement of the body.
Xuan fu: Literally, mysterious house or mysterious mansion, this is where the sweat gathers; it is also known as *han kong* (sweat pore), *qi men* (Qi gate), *yuan fu* (original house), or *gui men* (ghost gate). It corresponds to the apocrine and eccrine sweat glands and sebaceous glands, and their openings in the skin.
Mao fa: Fa refers to the hair on the head, *mao* refers to body hair, including the eyebrows, beard, axillary, and pubic hair.
Zhao jia: The nails, including both fingernails and toenails.

Relationship between the Zang-Fu organs and the skin

The skin has a close relationship with the Zang-Fu organs. In *Su Wen: Pi Bu Lun* [Simple Questions: On Skin], it says: "The skin is part of the vessels. If pathogenic factors settle in the skin and the interstices (*cou li*) are open, they will lodge in the network vessels; if the network vessels are full, they will enter the channels; if the channels are full, they will invade the Zang-Fu organs." In terms of the relationship between the color of the skin and the Zang-Fu organs, this chapter also says: "Predominantly bluish skin indicates pain; predominantly black skin indicates Bi syndrome; yellow and red skin indicates Heat; predominantly white skin indicates Cold." Therefore, observation of the skin color in different areas of the body will assist in making a diagnosis of diseases in the Zang-Fu organs.

THE HEART AND THE SKIN

The Heart governs the Blood vessels, opens into the tongue and its bloom is in the face. Blood depends on the pumping of the heart to circulate in the vessels throughout the body. The pumping of the heart depends on the flow of Heart Qi, which maintains the normal movement of the Blood in the vessels to supply the skin. If the function of the Heart in governing the Blood and Blood vessels is normal, the abundance of Blood vessels on the face means that the face is red and lustrous, the skin is moist and soft, and the tongue body is red with a moist coating. If Heart Qi is insufficient, the face is lusterless, dull or pale.

The Heart also governs the Spirit and this is closely related to the Heart governing the Blood and Blood vessels. When the Heart receives adequate nourishment from the Blood, it can function properly to govern the Spirit. In *Ling Shu: Ying Wei Sheng Hui* [The Miraculous Pivot: Generation of Nutritive and Defensive Qi], it says: "Blood is the Qi of the Spirit." Qi and Blood are the material source of the Spirit. Under normal circumstances, happiness will lead to harmony between Qi and Blood, but anxiety, worry and fear will damage the Heart. Heart-Fire generated by emotional problems can be transported through the Blood vessels and accumulate in the skin and flesh, thus causing skin diseases such as pemphigus vulgaris or urticaria.

The Heart opens into the tongue. Tongue diagnosis is important in the identification of patterns in the skin clinic. If the function of the Heart is normal, the tongue body is pink and moist, and the tongue is soft and moves flexibly. If Heart-Fire flames upward, the tongue body is red and mouth ulcers may occur.

THE LUNGS AND THE SKIN

The Lungs govern diffusion, open into the nose, and are connected with the skin and hair. They have the functions of transporting the Essence of Grain and Water from the Spleen and dissipating it throughout the body to reach the skin and hair, diffusing Wei Qi (Defensive Qi) to warm the flesh and nourish the skin, regulating the opening and closing of the interstices (*cou li*), and expelling sweat metabolized from the Body Fluids.

If the Lungs function normally, the skin and hair can be nourished so that the skin is dense and strong enough to repulse external pathogenic factors and the hair is shiny. If Lung Qi is Deficient and weak, the skin and hair will lack nourishment and moisture; the skin may turn rough and dry, and the hair will look withered. Pathogenic factors can easily invade the body, as the exterior is not consolidated, Wei Qi is too weak to maintain its defensive function and the interstices (*cou li*) are loose. This can result in diseases such as urticaria due to Wind-Heat, Wind-Cold or Wei Qi failing to consolidate the exterior.

If the diffusing function of the Lungs is normal, the sweat pores will be regulated correctly to meet the body's requirements. If Lung Qi is Deficient, Wei Qi will also be weak, impairing the regulation of sweating; spontaneous sweating or hyperhidrosis may develop. If the transmission of Wei Qi to the skin is obstructed, the interstices (*cou li*) will close, thus preventing sweating. If the Lungs' function of dispersing Body Fluids and the Essence of Grain and Water throughout the body is weakened, Body Fluids will collect in the Lungs to form Phlegm or may flood the skin and flesh to produce swelling as occurs in chronic eczema of the legs due to Lung Qi failing to diffuse Wei Qi and Damp-Heat pouring downward.

The Lungs open into the nose. If the Lungs are strong, breathing and the sense of smell will be normal. In *Ling Shu: Mai Du* [The Miraculous Pivot: Pulses], it says: "If the Lungs are harmonious, the nose can smell good or bad odors." If the Lungs are invaded by external pathogenic factors, this can result in impairment of the diffusing function, leading to skin diseases around the nose, such as rosacea caused by Wind-Heat attacking the Lungs due to Heat accumulating in the Lungs and Stomach.

THE SPLEEN AND THE SKIN

The Spleen governs the transportation and transformation of Grain and Water, opens into the mouth, and its bloom is in the lips. The transportation and transformation function depends on Spleen Qi. If Spleen Qi is exuberant, the transportation and transformation function is also exuberant and sufficient nutrients are supplied for the generation of Qi, Blood and Body Fluids so that the Zang-Fu organs and skin are nourished. If Spleen Qi is Deficient and weak, it cannot supply sufficient nutrients, thus resulting in Deficiency and depletion of Qi and Blood and insufficiency of Body Fluids, manifesting as lack of strength in the limbs and emaciation of the muscles.

The Spleen likes Dryness but hates Dampness. If the function of transporting and transforming water is weakened, water will collect internally resulting in Dampness being generated. Accumulation of internal Dampness obstructs the Spleen in bearing clear Qi upward and damages Spleen Yang, resulting in impairment of the Spleen's transportation and transformation function. Diseases due to Spleen Deficiency and obstruction of Dampness or Dampness causing impairment of the Spleen's transportation and transformation function include chronic eczema, pemphigus and keratosis follicularis (Darier's disease).

The Spleen also controls the Blood, which depends on the securing and containing function of Spleen Qi. If Spleen Qi is sufficient, the Spleen will be able to secure and contain the circulation of Blood within the Blood vessels. If Spleen Qi is Deficient, the Spleen cannot control the Blood properly and it may spill out from the vessels, resulting in such diseases as anaphylactoid purpura.

The Spleen opens into the mouth. If Spleen Qi is sufficient, the lips are red, moist and lustrous. If Spleen Qi is Deficient, the lips are pale and lusterless or possibly slightly yellow. If there is latent Heat and Fire in the Spleen, they can steam upward along the Spleen channel to the mouth and lips to cause mouth ulcers or perioral dermatitis.

THE LIVER AND THE SKIN

The Liver stores the Blood and governs the smooth flow of Qi; its bloom is in the nails. It has the function of regulating the activities of Qi by dredging and discharging; this is closely related to emotional stability. The Liver also works with Heart, Lung and Spleen Qi to promote Blood circulation throughout the body. If the Liver's functions are normal, Qi is regulated and can move freely, Qi and Blood are harmonious, the channels and network vessels are free, and the Zang-Fu organs can perform normally and in harmony. If these functions are impaired, the movement of Qi will be obstructed, resulting in depression and binding of Liver Qi and disturbance of the emotions, particularly anger; diseases such as melasma (chloasma) may result.

Healthy nails depend on nourishment by Liver-Blood. If Liver-Blood is sufficient, the nails are firm, red and shiny; if Liver-Blood is insufficient, the nails are soft, thin, dry, and dull, and may be deformed and cracked.

THE KIDNEYS AND THE SKIN

The Kidneys are very important organs as they are the root of Earlier Heaven and the root of Qi; they store the Essence, govern growth, control reproduction, and govern Water. Their bloom is in the hair (of the head), and they open into the ears and the anal and genital orifices.

The Essence is made up of Earlier Heaven Essence (*xian tian zhi jing*) inherited from the parents and Later Heaven Essence (*hou tian zhi jing*), extracted from food and used to promote the growth of the body. In *Su Wen: Shang Gu Tian Zhen Lun* [Simple Questions: On the Origins of Man], it says: "At the age of seven, girls have exuberant Kidney Qi; the permanent teeth appear and the hair grows. At the age of eight, boys have exuberant Kidney Qi; the hair and teeth grow. Essence can transform into Blood to nourish the hair." If Kidney Essence is sufficient, Blood is abundant, leading to black and shiny hair; if Kidney Essence is Deficient, the hair turns gray or dry or falls out.

In *Su Wen: Ni Tiao Lun* [Simple Questions: On Adverse Regulation], it says: "The Kidneys have the functions of storing Water and governing Body Fluids". Their function of Qi transformation transmits Water-Essence from food throughout the body to supplement the Blood and nourish the Zang-Fu organs and the skin and hair; the Kidneys also expel sweat and urination, metabolized from the Zang-Fu organs and the skin to maintain the balance of Water and Fluids. The moisture of the skin depends on the normal metabolism of the Body Fluids in the Kidneys. If the function of Qi transformation is impaired, the water that collects will spill to the skin to cause edema. If Kidney Qi is Deficient, Body Fluids are insufficient, leading to dry skin, as in ichthyosis vulgaris.

Relationship between Qi and Blood and the skin

Qi and Blood are the basic materials of construction of the body and the material foundation for maintaining the body's vital activities. In *Su Wen: Tiao Jing Lun* [Simple Questions: On Channel Regulation], it says: "Without Blood and Qi, there would be no life." Qi and Blood are very closely related; Qi generates Blood, whereas Blood nourishes Qi. Qi has a nourishing and warming function within the body; Blood has a nourishing and moistening function.

More specifically, Qi has the functions of promoting the production and movement of Blood, warming the Zang-Fu organs, the channels and network vessels, and the skin, sinews and bones, protecting the body from invasion by external pathogenic factors through the skin, hair, mouth, and nose, and securing and containing the Blood and sweat. Blood circulates with Qi all over the body and moistens the sinews, skin and flesh.

Ying Qi (Nutritive Qi) circulates with the Blood in the vessels and they function together to nourish the body and skin. Wei Qi (Defensive Qi) moves outside the vessels and under the skin to protect the flesh and exterior from invasion by external pathogenic factors, while warming and nourishing the flesh, skin and hair, and regulating sweating.

The movement of Blood in the vessels depends on the activities of Qi in moving and containing the Blood. If the moving function is too strong and the containing function not strong enough, the Blood will move quickly or spill from the vessels to cause bleeding. If the moving function is too weak and the containing function too strong, the Blood will move slowly or may stagnate, in which case Blood stasis will arise. Wu Jutong (1758-1836) said: "A physician who is good at treating Blood does not seek to treat Blood, which is substantial, but to treat Qi, which is insubstantial."

If Qi and Blood are in harmony, the body is healthy; if there is disharmony, diseases occur. Qi Deficiency will cause the skin and flesh to be undernourished and dry, and the hair to lack luster; Water and Dampness will collect and stagnate, resulting in swelling, vesicles and rough skin. Qi stagnation will inhibit the functional activities of Qi, resulting in black macules.

If the Blood is plentiful, the face will be red and moist, the skin moist, and the hair shiny; if the Blood is insufficient, the face will have a sallow yellow complexion, and the skin and hair will be dry; Blood Deficiency will cause scaly, dry and itchy skin; Blood stasis will cause rough and thickened skin, or hardened skin with scales such as in psoriasis.

Disharmony of Qi and Blood will cause upper body heat and lower body cold as well as upper body Excess and lower body Deficiency, resulting in such disorders as mouth ulcers, melasma (chloasma), nevus flammeus, and bromhidrosis.

Relationship between the channels and network vessels and the skin

The channels and network vessels are distributed throughout the body connecting the Zang-Fu organs to the exterior and functioning as a passageway for the movement of Qi and Blood. By circulating through the channels and vessels, Qi, Blood and Body Fluids can nourish the skin and flesh and the Zang-Fu organs.

Observation of the color of the skin at a certain location can help diagnose the disease in the channel. This can be taken as the starting point to identify which external pathogenic factors are invading the channel. The skin is closely associated with the channels and network vessels; in the treatment of skin disorders, consideration should therefore be given to the use of local points and channel conductor materia medica.

Etiology of skin disorders in Traditional Chinese Medicine
中医皮肤病病因

INVASION BY THE SIX PATHOGENIC FACTORS

There are six climatic factors in nature – Wind, Cold, Summerheat, Damp, Dryness, and Fire. Under normal conditions, they do not cause diseases; however, under abnormal circumstances, they can turn into pathogenic factors (also known as the Six Excesses), especially when the body resistance is weakened. These factors invade the body through the skin, body hair and flesh, or by being breathed in through the nose and mouth.

If Vital Qi (Zheng Qi) is insufficient to defeat the pathogenic factors and the function of the internal organs is damaged, internal Wind, Cold, Dampness, Dryness, and Fire (or Heat) can be generated and skin diseases may arise.

WIND

Huang Di Nei Jing [The Yellow Emperor's Classic of Internal Medicine] states: "Wind is the main cause of many diseases. It moves constantly and changes rapidly." Wind is Yang in nature, arises suddenly, moves swiftly, and blows upward; it tends to be more prevalent in spring, although it can occur in any season.

Predominance of Wind is likely to damage Yin, Blood and Body Fluids, resulting in such manifestations as dry skin, itching and desquamation. Skin lesions related to pathogenic Wind such wheals and scales usually have disseminated distribution with rapid onset and disappearance and are generally migratory.

Wind tends to combine with other pathogenic factors to invade the body, thus giving rise to the maxim that "Pathogenic Wind is the leading factor among the Six Excesses".

External Wind

External Wind can invade the body on its own, but more often combines with the other five pathogenic factors to attack as Wind-Cold, Summerheat-Wind, Wind-Damp, Wind-Dryness, or Wind-Fire. Symptoms caused by Wind appear suddenly and change rapidly with no fixed location.

Wind is in constant movement. It causes such skin conditions as urticaria, angioedema or pruritus. Since Wind moves upward, lesions involve the upper part of the body or the face and other areas of the head, as for example in seborrheic eczema of the scalp and face or pityriasis rosea on the chest and back.

The harsh and dry nature of Wind will lead to consumption of Yin and Blood. The skin is thus deprived of nourishment and bran-like scaling will appear such as in pityriasis alba.

Internal Wind

Internal Wind forms as a result of

- Blood Deficiency, in which case the Blood fails to nourish the Liver or emolliate the sinews;
- Heat Toxins damaging Yin;
- failure of Water (the Kidneys) to nourish Wood (the Liver).

Skin conditions caused by internal Wind include:

- seborrheic eczema due to Wind transforming into Dryness;
- diseases of the nails due to insufficiency of Liver-Blood;
- senile pruritus due to Qi and Blood Deficiency with rough and thick skin resulting from repeated scratching.

COLD

Cold is the main pathogenic factor in winter and is Yin in nature; it can be divided into external Cold and internal Cold. External Cold is mainly caused by cold weather; it invades the body to cause the Blood to congeal and Qi to stagnate. In skin diseases due to Cold, the skin is cold and lesions are white, dark red or bluish-purple in color. Internal Cold mostly develops as a result of Yang Deficiency of the Spleen and Kidneys, which then allows external Cold to invade. It is frequently difficult to distinguish between external and internal Cold as causative factors and they frequently combine to cause a disease. Accompanying symptoms and signs include thin and loose stools, long voidings of clear urine, and thin, clear phlegm.

External Cold

- External Cold invading the channels and network vessels impairs the normal circulation of Blood, leading for example to chilblains with purpura.
- If external Cold prevents Yang Qi from reaching the extremities of the limbs, the movement of Blood is inhibited, as for example in frostbite.
- The nature of pathogenic Cold is contracture and tautness. An invasion of pathogenic Cold may cause closure of the interstices (*cou li*) and reduce secretion of sweat. The skin feels cold and appears white due to contraction of the vessels, which prevents Qi and Blood from nourishing the skin properly, as for example in some patterns of Raynaud's disease.
- Cold congealing also results in Blood stasis and Blood congealing in the vessels, leading to subcutaneous swellings, which feel hard with a smooth surface. Manifestations include cold or bluish-purple limbs, hypertonicity of the sinews, nodules or masses, and severe pain, as for example in erythema induratum.

Internal Cold

- Internal Cold can also prevent Yang Qi from reaching the four limbs and the skin, leading to such symptoms as cold hands and feet or cyanosis of the extremities.
- If internal Cold congeals in the network vessels and obstructs the movement of Qi and Blood, the skin will become hard and swollen and ulceration may occur, as for example in morphea (localized scleroderma).

SUMMERHEAT

Summerheat is a Yang pathogenic factor and is hot in nature; it usually only occurs in summer. Although Summerheat can be included in the category of pathogenic Heat, it also has its own particular features; it bears upward and dissipates, consumes Yin and damages Body Fluids. Manifestations include profuse sweating, thirst, shortness of breath, and lassitude. Papules and vesicles are the characteristic skin lesions caused by invasion of Summerheat.

- Summerheat is caused by strong sunshine. In the hot summer, the sweat pores are open, which allows Summerheat to invade. It then steams upward, leading to redness and distension of the head, face and neck and causing such disorders as summer boils and miliaria rubra (prickly heat).
- Exposure to strong sunshine can cause injury to the skin. If the hot sun injures the skin, sunburn occurs.
- If Summerheat combines with Dampness and is retained in the flesh and interstices (*cou li*), it can lead to such disorders as impetigo and miliaria rubra. Accompanying symptoms and signs include a heavy head which feels bound up, generalized heaviness, a feeling of oppression in the chest, reduced appetite, thirst with no desire to drink, and diarrhea.

DAMPNESS

In *Shen She Zun Sheng Shu* [Master Shen's Book on the Importance of Respecting Life], Shen Jin'ao (1717-1776) said: "Dampness can be external or internal. Internal Dampness forms because of impairment of the Spleen's transportation and transformation function, exuberant Fire transforming into Damp-Heat or exuberant Water transforming into Dampness. External Dampness is caused by wet weather, living or working in damp conditions, dietary irregularities, or wearing clothes that are soaked in sweat." Thus it can be seen that external Dampness is related to climate and the environment, whereas internal Dampness is associated with exuberance or debilitation of Spleen Yin and Yang.

Dampness is a Yin pathogenic factor and is heavy, turbid and sticky in nature. Diseases due to Dampness often persist for long periods or recur frequently. Dizziness, poor appetite, distension and fullness of the abdomen, and heavy and tired limbs often appear as accompanying symptoms. Typical skin lesions include edema, vesicles or bullae, erosion, maceration, ulceration, exudation, and infiltration. Although Dampness usually affects the lower part of the body, it can cause diseases anywhere, as for example with retroauricular eczema, genital eczema and atopic eczema.

External Dampness

- People who live in a damp climate, work or live in a damp environment, or wear wet clothing as a result of sweating or being caught in the rain may be attacked by external pathogenic Dampness, manifesting as edema, vesicles and erosion (for example in eczema) or as maceration and erosion (for example in tinea pedis).
- The heavy and turbid nature of Dampness tends to cause skin diseases in the lower part of the body, as seen in disorders such as chronic eczema with thickening of the skin or nodular prurigo due to Damp-Heat pouring down. Although eczema may also involve the upper part of the body, in such cases Dampness will combine with Wind or Heat.
- Since Dampness is sticky and greasy, it is difficult to eliminate. Skin diseases caused by Dampness are difficult to treat and often recur; for example, acute eczema tends to develop into subacute and chronic eczema.

Internal Dampness

- Accumulation of Dampness transforms into Heat as seen in such disorders as eczema and erythema multiforme with vesicles and bullae mixed with erythema and red papules due to Damp-Heat accumulating in the Spleen and Stomach.
- When Damp-Heat steams upward to the head, it can cause such disorders as retroauricular eczema and perioral dermatitis.
- If Damp-Heat pouring down is obstructed, it can cause chronic leg ulcers.
- If Damp-Cold pours down, it can cause weeping chronic leg ulcers.

DRYNESS

Dryness is a Yang pathogenic factor and can be divided into external Dryness and internal Dryness. External Dryness is caused by dry weather (in China, traditionally occurring in late autumn) or in extremely dry, centrally-heated or air-conditioned environments; in addition, soap, detergents and chemicals can also cause dry skin. Internal Dryness results from consumption of Yin and Blood, often due to chronic diseases. In both cases, the skin is dry, rough and undernourished with patches of dry scale. The hair is dry, withered and lusterless. Consumption of Yin and Body Fluids accompanied by Cold will lead to cracking and fissuring of the skin.

External Dryness

Prevalence of Dryness results in dry skin with cracking and fissuring, or dry and itchy skin. External Dryness patterns are generally not very severe.

Internal Dryness

- If there is Dryness in the interior, Blood and Essence will dry up. Internal Dryness patterns are generally more severe than external Dryness patterns and are less easy to treat. Disorders caused by internal Dryness include ichthyosis vulgaris and the chronic phase of many types of eczema.
- Symptoms accompanying Dryness in the lower body include constipation and retention of urine.
- Wind-Dryness forms when Liver-Blood cannot nourish the sinews. It manifests as hypertonicity of the sinews and chapped and fissured hands and feet.
- Fire-Dryness forms as a result of latent Fire in the Spleen and manifests as constipation and chapped lips.
- Blood-Dryness forms when the Heart is impaired in its function of circulating the Blood, thus resulting in lack of nourishment of the skin and flesh; it manifests as itching, profuse dandruff, and loss of hair and beard.
- Deficiency-Dryness results from Yin Deficiency of the Stomach and Kidneys and manifests as scant urination and a dry, swollen throat.

FIRE

The pathogenic factors of Warmth, Heat and Fire belong to the same category but differ in degree. There is an ancient saying that "when pathogenic Warmth increases by a certain degree, it becomes pathogenic Heat; when pathogenic Heat reaches its maximum, it turns into pathogenic Fire." Heat and Fire Toxins are the main causes of suppurative skin diseases. In *Yi Zong Jin Jian: Wai Ke Xin Fa Yao Jue* [The Golden Mirror of Medicine: Essential Experiences in External Diseases], it says: "Abscesses are caused by Fire Toxins."

External Fire generally occurs in extremely hot conditions, whereas internal Fire is caused by disturbances of the Zang-Fu organs or Qi and Blood. Other external pathogenic factors or emotions that are intense, unexpressed or prolonged over time can give rise to pathogenic Fire. Fire tends to flame upward and skin lesions caused by Fire are usually distributed over the head, upper limbs and upper trunk, as is the case for example with furuncles and carbuncles, lichen simplex chronicus (neurodermatitis) and acne.

Diseases caused by Fire have a rapid onset, and change frequently and swiftly. The skin is bright red and feels hot; typical lesions, which tend to appear and disappear quickly, include erythema, red papules, purpura, and pustules. The extreme Heat of pathogenic Fire causes the tissues to putrefy, resulting in burning pain and various types of acute skin bleeding patterns due to Fire forcing the frenetic movement of Blood.

External Fire

- Wind-Heat may transform into Fire Toxins, as seen in such disorders as facial erysipelas.
- When Damp-Heat pours down, it can also transform into Fire Toxins as seen in such disorders as erysipelas of the lower limbs.
- Summerheat can also produce Fire and Toxins, as seen in such disorders as miliaria rubra (prickly heat) and furuncles.
- Fire Toxins may attack the body directly, for example in burns or erythema ab igne.

Internal Fire

- Heart-Fire flaming upward can result in such disorders as recurrent aphthous stomatitis (mouth ulcers).
- Fire in the Heart and Liver can result in such disorders as hyperhidrosis, herpes zoster (shingles) and folliculitis.
- Fire in the Liver and Gallbladder can result in such disorders as nipple eczema.
- Retention of Fire Toxins in the Heart and Spleen channels can lead to such disorders as dermatitis herpetiformis.
- Fire in the Lungs and Stomach can often result in such disorders as rosacea.
- If Fire is exuberant because of shortage of Water (with Water therefore failing to control Fire), disorders such as melanosis may develop on the face, exhibiting the color (black) of the organs involved, the Kidneys.

INVASION BY TOXIC PATHOGENIC FACTORS

Toxic pathogenic factors attack the body through the mouth and nose, or through the skin and mucous membranes. For example, viral, bacterial or fungal infections occur when a weak body is suddenly attacked by toxic pathogenic factors. Toxic pathogenic factors (both external and internal) can also frequently be taken to mean that a particular pathogenic factor is manifesting in an extreme way; for instance, the expression Heat Toxins implies that pathogenic Heat is very strong.

In TCM, this category also includes invasion by highly infectious pestilential epidemic pathogenic factors. Leprosy occurs when a Yin-natured pestilential toxic pathogenic factor attacks the body and is retained in the skin, vessels, flesh, sinews, and bones. Toxic pathogenic factors can also cause diseases through fetal infection, for instance, congenital syphilis. Fatal epidemic pathogenic factors in animals can be extremely toxic; cutaneous anthrax is a good example. Diseases caused by these pestilential epidemic pathogenic factors are beyond the scope of a non-specialized dermatology book.

DIETARY IRREGULARITIES

Rich, spicy, greasy, fried, and raw food can all lead to accumulation of Damp-Heat in the Spleen and Stomach and Fire Toxins in the interior. When these pathogenic factors move out to the skin and flesh, they can lead to a variety of skin conditions such as furuncles, eczema, herpes zoster (shingles), toxic erythema, and phytophotodermatitis.

Overindulgence in seafood, which is considered as stimulating food, can cause eczema and many other skin disorders, typically with erythema, papules and vesicles; excessive intake of spicy, greasy and sweet food can impair the Spleen's functions and generate internal Dampness and Heat, which is transported upward to the face to cause conditions such as acne, rosacea and seborrheic eczema.

EXCESSIVE SEXUAL ACTIVITY AND PHYSICAL LABOR

Giving birth to many children can damage the Chong and Ren vessels, resulting in Liver and Kidney Yin Deficiency and depletion of Body Fluids. Manifestations include dry mouth and eyes, aching and painful joints, and dry skin. Excessive physical exertion can damage the Spleen and lead to Deficiency of Original Qi (Yuan Qi), with the result that the Blood may not circulate properly. If this is accompanied by standing for long periods or carrying heavy loads, the veins may become varicose and chronic leg ulcers may result.

EMOTIONAL FACTORS

Psychological and emotional factors and sudden changes in the emotional state can lead to an imbalance between Yin and Yang, disharmony between Qi and Blood, and dysfunction of the Zang-Fu organs. Emotional strain can also cause skin diseases. Excessive anger damages the Liver, and excessive thought and preoccupation damage the Spleen. When emotional disturbances persist over a long period of time, Qi and

Blood may stagnate in the channels and network vessels, resulting in such diseases as alopecia areata, psoriasis and lichen simplex chronicus (neurodermatitis).

PARASITES

- Insect bites: Bites from mosquitoes, bedbugs, fleas, mites, and other insects can cause itching.
- The presence of parasites on or in the skin can also cause skin diseases, for instance scabies or lice infestation.
- Diseases caused by Worms include trichomoniasis,

manifesting as dampness and itching in the vagina, and tinea cruris.

ALLERGIES DUE TO CONSTITUTIONAL DEFICIENCY

- Allergies resulting from contact, for example, allergic contact dermatitis.
- Allergies resulting from food, for example, intake of *Hui Cai* (Chenopodium Album) or seafood.
- Allergies resulting from drugs, through oral administration, injection, inhalation, or infusion.

Pattern identification in the treatment of skin disorders
皮肤病的辩证治疗

Basic principles of pattern identification for skin disorders

Although the methods of diagnosis and pattern identification of skin disorders are generally similar to those used for internal diseases, there may be differences in emphasis in some instances.

PATTERN IDENTIFICATION ACCORDING TO THE EIGHT PRINCIPLES

The significance of pattern identification according to the Eight Principles (Yin-Yang, interior-exterior, Cold-Heat, Deficiency-Excess) is that the site of the disease can be located following the interior-exterior principle, the nature of the disease distinguished according to the Cold-Heat principle, and the relative strength between Vital Qi (Zheng Qi) and pathogenic factors assessed according to the Deficiency-Excess principle. Yin and Yang serve as a generalization of the other six principles, which is why the Eight Principles are also known as the Two Principles with Six Essential Items.

Pattern identification according to Yin and Yang

Yang Ke Gang Yao [A Summary of External Diseases] states that "The first and most important matter in external diseases is to differentiate between Yin and Yang."

- A Yang disease generally has an acute onset and short duration, and is located at a superficial site; the skin is inflamed or red, and feels hot or burning;

swellings are raised; pain is severe; the prognosis is good.
- A Yin disease has a gradual onset and long duration, and is located more deeply; the skin is dull red in color and does not feel hot; swellings are not raised; pain is dull; the prognosis is poor.

Pattern identification according to interior and exterior

Pattern identification according to the categories of interior and exterior serves to establish whether the site of the disease is deep or superficial, and whether the pathogenic factors are weak or strong. In general, a disease at a superficial site, such as furuncles, is easier to treat than a disease at a deep site, such as vasculitis.

Pattern identification according to Cold and Heat

- Cold-natured diseases such as Raynaud's disease may have systemic manifestations such as a cold body or limbs, a pallid complexion, a liking for warmth and an aversion to cold, a pale red tongue body with a white coating, and a slow pulse. Local manifestations include diffuse swelling, absence of any hot sensation of the skin, and no pain due to inflammation.
- Hot-natured diseases such as herpes zoster (shingles) and erysipelas may have systemic manifestations such as fever, red face, thirst with a desire for cold drinks, a liking for cold and an aversion to heat, a red tongue body with a dry yellow coating, and a rapid pulse. Local manifestations include obvious swelling, a high skin temperature, and severe pain due to inflammation.

Pattern identification according to Deficiency and Excess

Deficiency means Deficiency of Vital Qi (Zheng Qi), Excess means Excess of pathogenic factors. At the initial stage of skin diseases, pathogenic factors and Vital Qi are both strong and therefore fight against one another, resulting in an Excess pattern. In the later stages, there are two possibilities – either that the pathogenic factors have been eliminated, while Vital Qi has been damaged, or that there is a mixture of Deficiency and Excess because the constitution has been weakened and the pathogenic factors have become relatively stronger.

In *Wai Ke Shu Yao* [Essentials of External Diseases], it says: "Deficiency and Excess patterns vary considerably and a clear differentiation is essential. There is Deficiency or Excess of sores, of the Zang-Fu Organs, of Qi and Blood, of the upper and lower parts of the body, and of pathogenic factors and Vital Qi (Zheng Qi). They are all different from one another."

PATTERN IDENTIFICATION ACCORDING TO THE ZANG-FU ORGANS

The skin and Zang-Fu organs are closely related, giving rise to the statement in *Yang Ke Xin De Ji: Yang Zheng Zong Lun* [A Collection of Experiences in the Treatment of Sores: A Comprehensive Discussion on Sore Patterns] that "the Zang-Fu organs are situated in the interior and manifest on the exterior."

Heart patterns 心证

Characteristics: The Heart is situated in a deep location in the upper part of the body; the Ministerial Fire acts as its representative. Many diseases caused by Fire Toxins are related to the Heart channel. Mild Heat can result in itching, severe Heat in pain.

Clinical manifestations: Inflamed or red skin, a local burning sensation, erythema, erosion, bloody crusts, pus, nodules, and tongue ulcers; accompanying symptoms and signs include raging fever, delirium, psychological problems, and unconsciousness.

Disorders commonly involving the Heart: Acute eczema, bullous pemphigoid, erythroderma, hemangioma, herpes zoster (shingles), mouth ulcers, pemphigus vulgaris, pompholyx, urticaria.

Lung patterns 肺证

Characteristics: The Chinese character for the Lungs (*fei*) has a flesh radical and a phonetic component meaning "market". The Lungs control circulation in all the channels and vessels, and govern the skin and hair. Many deep wrinkles in the skin indicate weakness of the Lungs. This is a normal phenomenon in the elderly but abnormal in younger people. It can be regarded as an external sign to understand interior changes in the body.

Clinical manifestations: Wheals, papules, erythema, dry and scaling skin, and scratch marks; accompanying symptoms include dry nose and throat or dry cough.

Disorders commonly involving the Lungs: Acne, angioedema, atopic eczema, hyperhidrosis, pityriasis rubra pilaris, rosacea, urticaria.

Spleen patterns 脾证

Characteristics: The Chinese character for the Spleen (*pi*) has a flesh radical and a phonetic component meaning "assistance". The Spleen assists the Stomach to transform food. The Spleen likes Dryness and loathes Dampness. When Dampness is the main pathogenic factor causing disease, there is often an underlying factor of Spleen Yang Deficiency leading to impairment of the Spleen's normal transformation and transportation function.

Clinical manifestations: Papulovesicles, vesicles, exudation, erosion, keratoderma, atrophy, and subcutaneous nodules; these are frequently accompanied by indigestion, reduced appetite or anorexia, and loose stools or diarrhea.

Disorders commonly involving the Spleen: Anaphylactoid purpura, eczema, keratosis follicularis (Darier's disease), pemphigus, perioral dermatitis, recurrent aphthous stomatitis (mouth ulcers).

Liver patterns 肝证

Characteristics: The Chinese character for the Liver (*gan*) is made up of a flesh radical and a phonetic component meaning "interference". The Liver is an active organ that seldom calms down and is likely to interfere with the other organs. The Liver likes to be free of obstruction. Emotional disturbances and diseases affecting the hypochondrium, eyes and genitals are all related to the Liver channel. Other Liver patterns include Depression due to Qi stagnation, and hyperactive Fire generating Wind and causing convulsions.

Clinical manifestations: Papules, maculopapules, lichenification, pigmentation, and dry skin with scales; accompanying symptoms and signs include red eyes, intermittent pain in the epigastric and abdominal regions, itching, piercing pain in the hypochondrium, irascibility, and in more serious cases, spasms and convulsions of the arms and legs, and opisthotonos.

Disorders commonly involving the Liver: Disorders of the nails, herpes zoster (shingles), melanosis, melasma (chloasma), vitiligo.

Kidney patterns 肾证

Characteristics: The Chinese character for the Kidneys (*shen*) also has the meaning of "being responsible". The Kidneys govern the bones and have responsibility for the whole body. The weakness or strength of the Kidneys is of great importance for the body. The Kidneys are the root of Earlier Heaven (*xian tian*), and govern the urinary and reproductive functions; they store the essential substances without draining them. Most patterns involving the Kidneys are therefore Deficient in nature.

Clinical manifestations: Dark complexion, hair loss, cold and dark red skin, black macules, retarded development of the body, premature senility, forgetfulness, aching of the lower back, tinnitus, fear of cold, edema, and urinary and reproductive dysfunction.

Disorders commonly involving the Kidneys: Alopecia areata, chronic venous ulcer of the lower leg, ichthyosis vulgaris, melanosis, melasma (chloasma).

ZANG-FU ORGAN INTERRELATIONSHIP

The Zang-Fu organs do not function is isolation; they are related to and influence one another. In diagnosis, physiological and pathological changes in the main organ involved must be considered, as should its influence, negative or positive, on the other organs. A good understanding of the mutual influence of the Zang-Fu organs enhances diagnosis and treatment. The following relationships between Zang-Fu organs are commonly taken into consideration in the skin clinic.

Relationship between the Liver and the Spleen
Since these organs have a very close relationship, Liver disorders often affect the Spleen, resulting in a group of symptoms reflecting the disharmony between them such as distension in the stomach and abdomen and poor appetite. Treatment of these patterns usually starts with the Liver using ingredients such as *Chai Hu* (Radix Bupleuri), *Bai Shao* (Radix Paeoniae Lactiflorae), *Xiang Fu* (Rhizoma Cyperi Rotundi), *Jin Ju Ye* (Folium Fortunellae Margaritae), *Bo He* (Herba Menthae Haplocalycis), and *Fo Shou* (Fructus Citri Sarcodactylis). This treatment dredges the Liver and supports the Spleen.

Relationship between the Liver and the Kidneys
Kidney Yin controls Yin throughout the body. Insufficiency of Kidney Yin will always lead to insufficiency of Liver Yin and vice versa, thus giving rise to the adage that "the Liver and Kidneys share the same source". Simultaneous use of ingredients for nourishing Liver Yin and ingredients for nourishing Kidney Yin will achieve the most effective result.

Relationship between the Spleen and the Kidneys
Kidney Yang controls Yang throughout the body. Insufficiency of Kidney Yang will always lead to insufficiency of Spleen Yang and vice versa. Spleen and Kidney Yang Deficiency patterns reveal the mutual influence between the organs. Treating these patterns by adding ingredients for supplementing Kidney Yang to ingredients for supplementing Spleen Yang will achieve the most effective result.

Relationship between the Lungs and the Kidneys
The Lungs govern Qi and respiration and are also known as "the upper source of water". The Kidneys govern reception of Qi. Both the Kidneys and the Lungs are involved in diseases of the respiratory system and edema. If the disease is acute, the focus is put on the Lungs to treat the Manifestations (*biao*); if the disease is chronic, the focus is put on the Kidneys to treat the Root (*ben*).

PATTERN IDENTIFICATION ACCORDING TO THE WEI, QI, YING, AND XUE LEVELS

The terms Wei, Qi, Ying, and Xue first appeared in *Huang Di Nei Jing* [The Yellow Emperor's Classic of Internal Medicine] and were used essentially to summarize the body's physiological functions. Later, in his analysis of warm diseases, Ye Tianshi (1667-1746) developed the ideas into a pattern identification method to explain the progression of epidemic febrile diseases and provide a basis of reference for the use of ingredients based on this identification.

In practice, the theory of the Wei, Qi, Ying, and Xue levels allows many skin diseases to be classified and analyzed according to their clinical manifestations.

Systemic patterns
- Fever is a common pattern present in many acute skin diseases. In Excess patterns, it generally relates to exuberant Heat; the Qi level is involved. In Deficiency patterns, it indicates residual Heat lingering in the Ying level and both the Ying and Xue levels are involved.
- Mental confusion, delirious speech and fever as found in erythroderma indicate that Heat has entered the Pericardium channel; this condition is caused by the abnormal transmission or inward fall of pathogenic Heat.
- Convulsion of the limbs, lockjaw and opisthotonos are manifestations of tetany patterns, as may sometimes occur in certain severe drug eruptions in children, whereas counterflow cold of the limbs and coma are manifestations of reversal patterns as may occasionally occur in pemphigus. Both these types of pattern can result from exuberant Heat Toxins or from Deficiency-Wind stirring internally as a result of depletion of the Essence and Blood and failure of Water to nourish Wood.

Local patterns
- Macules whose color fades under pressure indicate Heat in the Qi level; if the color does not fade, this suggests Blood stasis in the Xue level.
- Skin which is bright red indicates exuberant Heat Toxins.

- Black macules represent severe Heat Toxins, with the patient in a very serious or critical state.
- Papules often form as a result of Heat in the Blood due to Wind-Heat, which involves the Stomach, or as a result of Damp obstruction, which involves the Lungs.

Tongue diagnosis
Tongue body
- A red tongue body is a sign of Heat pathogenic factors gradually entering the Ying level.
- A deep red tongue body indicates that Heat pathogenic factors have penetrated deep into the Ying level.

Tongue coating
The tongue coating mainly reflects the conditions of the Wei and Qi levels.
- A white tongue coating indicates a mild disease.
- A white, mold-like tongue coating marks a critical condition.
- A yellow tongue coating denotes interior Heat and indicates pathogenic factors in the Qi level in Excess-Heat patterns.
- A scorched-black dry tongue with prickles on the surface and a hard quality indicates severe Heat Toxins or Yang plundering true Yin.

Wei level patterns
Characteristics: Wei Qi (Defensive Qi) serves as the outermost defense of the body, protecting it from external invasion by pathogenic factors. If Wei Qi functions normally, the skin is moist and lustrous and the interstices (*cou li*) are dense so that external pathogenic factors cannot invade the body. If Wei Qi is weak, external pathogenic factors can easily invade. Pathogenic Wind attacking the Wei level leads to disharmony between Wei Qi and Ying Qi (Nutritive Qi).
Clinical manifestations: Wind-Heat patterns manifest as red wheals and itching, and in more severe cases, as swelling of the face and lips. Wind-Cold patterns manifest as pale red or whitish wheals with accompanying

symptoms such as slight fever, headache and discomfort in the throat.
Common skin disorders: Acute urticaria, cheilitis.

Qi level patterns
Characteristics: The transmission of Heat pathogenic factors from the exterior to the interior is manifested by two groups of symptoms – one resulting from Vital Qi (Zheng Qi) and pathogenic factors fighting one another, the other from Heat obstructing the functional activities of Qi. Patterns depend on the organ involved (see Table 1-4).
Clinical manifestations: Persistent raging fever and inflamed reddened skin covering the whole body or certain parts of it; accompanying symptoms include thirst with a desire for drinks and constipation.
Common skin disorders: See Table 1-4.

Ying level patterns
Characteristics: Ying level patterns are characterized by Vital Qi (Zheng Qi) Deficiency and depletion of Body Fluids. Pathogenic factors then seize the opportunity to invade the body.
Clinical manifestations: Large patches of erythema, and vesicles or bullae; accompanying symptoms and signs include high fever, irritability and restlessness, slight thirst, and delirious speech.
Common skin disorders: Acute eczema, bullous erythema multiforme, drug eruptions.

Xue level patterns
Characteristics: Heat pathogenic factors scorch the Xue level, leading to exuberant Heat in the Blood and the frenetic movement of Blood. As a result, blood spills out of the vessels to form macules (purpura). In addition, Heat can also disturb the Heart and Spirit, which may bring the disease process to a critical stage.
Clinical manifestations: Cutaneous purpura, or various bleeding patterns such as bleeding gums, blood in the stools and blood in the urine, possibly accompanied by mania or unconsciousness.

Table 1-4 Common diseases and Qi level pathology

Organ affected	Pathology	Common skin disorders
Lungs	Heat accumulating in the Lungs and obstructing Qi	Acne
Stomach	Exuberant Heat in the Stomach, Vital Qi (Zheng Qi) and pathogenic factors fighting one another	Toxic erythema
Liver	Retention of Heat in the Liver channel, Heat and Dampness fighting one another	Herpes zoster (shingles)
Kidneys	Non-transformation of Dampness in the Spleen, Dampness accumulating and generating Heat	Small vessel vasculitis

Table 1-5 Summary of the principles of pattern identification for skin disorders by phase

	Heat-transforming phase	Erythema phase	Entering the Ying level phase	Yin damage phase
Pattern identification according to the Eight Principles	Exterior Excess Heat	Interior Excess Heat	Interior Excess Heat	Interior Deficiency Heat
Pattern identification according to the Zang-Fu organs	Lungs	Lungs Stomach Intestines	Pericardium Stomach Liver	Liver Kidneys
Pattern identification according to the Wei, Qi, Ying, and Xue levels	Wei level, or moving from the Wei to the Qi level	Qi level or Qi and Xue levels	Moving from the Qi to the Ying level, or Ying level	Xue level
Main symptoms	Fever, large patches of erythema, papules, wheals	Erythema, ecchymoses	Low-grade fever, mental confusion, delirious speech, bleeding	Tetany, syncope, large amounts of scaling
Typical skin disorder	Acute urticaria	Scarlatiniform drug eruption	Inflammation due to insect bites	Erythroderma
Treatment	Diffuse the Lungs, clear Heat from the Qi level	Relieve Toxicity, reduce erythema	Clear Heat from the Ying level, protect Yin	Rescue Yin, calm the Liver and extinguish Wind
Typical prescription	*Yin Qiao San* (Honeysuckle and Forsythia Powder)	*Hua Ban Tang* (Decoction for Transforming Macules)	*Qing Ying Tang* (Decoction for Clearing Heat from the Ying Level)	*Ling Yang Gou Teng Tang* (Antelope Horn and Uncaria Decoction)

Common skin disorders: Purpura, secondary erythroderma.

Based on the discussion above, Table 1-5 summarizes the main points of pattern identification according to the Eight Principles, the Zang-Fu organs, and the Wei, Qi, Ying, and Xue levels.

PATTERN IDENTIFICATION ACCORDING TO QI AND BLOOD

Impairment of the functions of the Zang-Fu organs may affect the functions of Qi and Blood and vice versa. Pathological changes in Qi and Blood are closely associated with skin diseases.

Qi stagnation
Cause: Qi stagnation results from obstruction of Qi in the Zang-Fu organs and the channels and network vessels.
Clinical manifestations: Qi stagnation often manifests as local changes in pigmentation such as melasma (chloasma) due to Liver Depression and Qi stagnation and disharmony of Qi and Blood. Qi stagnation also manifests as pinpoint papules, nodules or cysts with painful or numb skin.

Accompanying symptoms and signs: Emotional depression, distension and fullness in the chest and abdomen, irregular periods, a pale tongue, and a wiry pulse.

Qi Deficiency
Cause: Qi Deficiency is often caused by a weak constitution (especially in the elderly), an irregular diet or chronic diseases.
Clinical manifestations: Qi Deficiency is characterized by flesh-colored or pink skin lesions, numb skin and thin nails.

- Deficiency of Spleen Qi, which fails to transport and transform accumulated Dampness, often underlies chronic eczema.
- Deficiency of Lung Qi, resulting in insecurity of Wei Qi and looseness of the interstices (*cou li*) allows pathogenic Wind to attack, and conditions such as chronic urticaria may arise.
- Qi Deficiency in the later stages of an illness may cause conditions such as pemphigus.

Accompanying symptoms and signs: A pale or sallow facial complexion, dizziness, palpitations, sleeplessness, spontaneous sweating, a pale tongue, and a thready and weak pulse.

Blood Deficiency

Cause: Blood Deficiency is caused by insufficient generation of Blood or profuse loss of Blood.

Clinical manifestations: Blood Deficiency is characterized by flesh-colored or pink skin lesions, dry, itchy and numb skin, and thin nails. It may cause skin disorders such as chronic eczema, folliculitis, pruritus, and alopecia areata.

Accompanying symptoms and signs: A somber white or sallow yellow facial complexion, pale and lusterless lips, nails and tongue, palpitations and sleeplessness, numbness of the hands and feet, scant menstruation, and a thready and weak pulse.

Blood stasis

Cause: Blood stasis is caused by blockage or stagnation of Qi in the channels and vessels, by prolonged Qi or Blood Deficiency, by Blood-Heat, or by Cold in the interior.

Clinical manifestations: Local fixed stabbing pain and numbness, thickened skin, dry and scaling skin, palpable masses, and purpura. Skin disorders that may be caused by Blood stasis include psoriasis, lichen planus, nodular prurigo, alopecia areata, and hemangioma.

Accompanying symptoms and signs: A dark complexion, purple lips and dry mouth with no desire for drinks, a dull purple tongue body, possibly with stasis marks, and a deep, moderate and rough pulse.

Blood-Dryness

Cause: Blood-Dryness is caused by Blood Deficiency transforming into Dryness or by an enduring illness damaging Yin and Blood.

Clinical manifestations: The skin is dry and rough with fissures and dry scaling. Blood-Dryness may cause skin disorders such as chronic eczema, atopic eczema, lichen simplex chronicus (neurodermatitis), and psoriasis.

Accompanying symptoms and signs: Dry mouth and tongue, dry eyes, dry stools, scant urine, and a thready and rough pulse.

Blood-Heat

Cause: Blood-Heat is caused by external contraction of pathogenic Heat, accumulation of Heat in the Zang-Fu organs, or pathogenic factors transforming into Heat and accumulating in the Xue level.

Clinical manifestations: Lesions are bright red and swollen, or hemorrhagic, or consist of large patches of flushing red skin with scaling. Skin disorders that may be caused by Blood-Heat include psoriasis, lichen simplex chronicus (neurodermatitis), anaphylactoid purpura, and drug eruptions.

Accompanying symptoms and signs: Dry mouth with no desire for drinks, constipation and reddish urine, or fever, irritability and restlessness, a red or dark red tongue body with a yellow coating, and a rapid pulse.

These six patterns identified according to Qi and Blood are common in the skin clinic. They can be considered individually or taken together, for example as Qi stagnation and Blood stasis, Blood Deficiency and Blood-Dryness, or Deficiency of Qi and Blood.

PATTERN IDENTIFICATION ACCORDING TO CHANNELS

The earliest records of the application of channel theory to identify skin disease patterns are found in documents on external diseases in the Ming Dynasty (1368-1644). In *Wai Ke Qi Xuan* [Revelations of the Mystery of External Diseases], it says: "The body structure consists of the skin, flesh, sinews, vessels, and bones (the Five Body Constituents). Different areas of the body surface are related to the internal organs by the channels and network vessels. ... In terms of the seven orifices, the eyes are associated with the Liver, the ears with the Kidneys, the nose with the Lungs, the mouth with the Spleen, and the tongue with the Heart (in other words, with the five Zang organs). External diseases reflect the channels and internal organs involved."

The channels and network vessels are passages for the movement of Qi and Blood. They have their source in the interior in the Zang-Fu organs, and they are distributed over the exterior body surface. They integrate the Zang-Fu organs, skin, blood vessels, sinews, bones, limbs, and the five sense organs into an organic entity. A balance is therefore achieved between the exterior and the interior, and the upper and lower parts of the body.

Pattern identification for skin diseases according to the theory of the channels and network vessels can be summarized as follows:

- **Pattern identification related to the occurrence and progression of skin diseases**

In *Dong Tian Ao Zhi (Wai Ke Mi Lu)* [Secret Records of External Diseases], it says: "If the Qi and Blood of the Zang-Fu organs fail to circulate properly, the channels and network vessels linking these organs will be obstructed and sores will be produced in the skin or flesh." This indicates that disorders of the Zang-Fu organs manifest in the exterior through the channels and network vessels. For example, the flaming of Fire in the Heart channel can lead to mouth and tongue ulcers; Phlegm congealing due to Spleen Deficiency can cause the growth of a fleshy goiter; and Lung-Heat steaming upward can result in rosacea.

- **Pattern identification related to the location of skin diseases**

In *Zheng Zhi Zhun Sheng: Yang Ke* [Standards of Diagnosis and Treatment: Skin Diseases], it says: "The human body has channels and network vessels just like a map has paths and boundaries. Treating diseases without a clear idea of the channels and network vessels is like drawing up a plan to arrest criminals without knowing the paths to follow to find them." It is clear that the purpose of pattern identification according to the channels and network vessels is also aimed at circumscribing the location of skin diseases. For example, facial acne often occurs in the area along the Stomach channel and can therefore be approached by treating the Stomach.

Generally speaking, lesions in sites rich in Qi and Blood are relatively easy to treat, whereas those in places rich in Qi but short of Blood are the most difficult to treat. Lesions in sites rich in Blood but short of Qi are treated first by supporting Vital Qi (Zheng Qi).

PATTERN IDENTIFICATION ACCORDING TO SYMPTOMS

Itching

Itching due to Wind

This pattern of itching usually involves the head, face, ears, and nose, but in severe cases the whole body may be affected.

- Itching due to Wind-Heat occurs suddenly and manifests as pinpoint to 2mm red papules. Scratching will cause slight bleeding, which dries up to form crusts; ulceration or erosion is rare. This type of itching is exacerbated by exposure to heat. The tongue body is red with a thin white coating; the pulse is floating and moderate, or floating and rapid.
- Itching due to Wind-Cold mainly involves exposed areas of the head, face, ears, hands, and feet. This type of itching occurs at certain times and in certain seasons, exacerbating in winter and improving in summer, and also aggravating in the morning and evening when the temperature is lower than in the middle of the day and the afternoon. Skin lesions manifest as an intricate crisscross network of white scratch marks with pale red papules and wheals. The tongue body is pale with a white coating; the pulse is tight.

Itching due to Dampness

Itching due to Dampness mainly involves the lower limbs, the scrotum, the vulva, and the webs between the toes. Skin lesions generally manifest as papulovesicles, vesicles or bullae, with erosion and yellow crusts. Pruritus results in the moist skin being scratched, causing profuse exudation. A vicious circle ensues, with itching resulting in excoriation, which in turn increases the severity of the itching and so on as the condition persists.

- Where Dampness is accompanied by Heat, the skin will be inflamed and slightly swollen, with pain more intense than itching.

- Where Dampness is accompanied by Cold, dull red or purplish-red skin will be thick and lichenified; itching will be more intense than pain.

Itching due to Heat

This pattern of itching has no fixed location. Skin lesions mostly manifest as widely disseminated red papules and erythema, which may become confluent. Other symptoms include sensations of burning heat and prickly itching, which lead to scratching. Excoriation produces oozing of blood, which dries up to form crusts. Pustular infection sometimes occurs, which can lead to the formation of boils.

Itching due to Dryness

Damage to or Deficiency of Yin and Blood after a warm-febrile disease generates Wind and Dryness, depriving the skin of nourishment. The dry skin results in paroxysmal itching. Exfoliation of bran-like scaling occurs after scratching.

Itching due to Blood stasis

This pattern of itching is only relieved by scratching until blood oozes from the excoriations. Skin lesions mainly manifest as dull red papules, which are either discretely distributed all over the body or coalesce into plaques. Lesions may also manifest as subcutaneous nodules.

Itching due to Deficiency

This condition manifests as generalized incessant itching accompanied by a sensation of formication.

- With Blood Deficiency, the skin is dry and itching is worse at night.
- With Qi Deficiency, itching is influenced by external pathogenic factors. For example, it can be provoked or exacerbated when there is a sudden change in the weather or as the seasons change.
- With Yang Deficiency, itching frequently occurs at the end of autumn and the beginning of winter. This type of itching is seen most often in middle-aged or elderly men.
- With Yin Deficiency, itching is constant. The skin is dry and lusterless. Exfoliation of bran-like scales occurs after scratching.

Itching due to Toxins

This type of itching mainly manifests as red papules or wheals with diffuse edema. Often caused by direct stimulation by Toxic substances, it usually occurs at fixed locations and gradually disappears after removal of the stimulating substance.

Itching due to insects or parasites

This type of itching chiefly involves the webs between the fingers and toes, the anus, the genitals, the lower abdomen, and the inframammary skin folds; in certain individuals, itching may be generalized. The condition tends to be worse during the night when many of these creatures become active. Itching caused by insects or parasites is often highly contagious.

Itching due to eating of certain foods

Food such as fish, prawns and crab may stir Wind to cause itching. Overeating of different kinds of meat such as beef, pork, lamb, and chicken makes it more difficult for the stomach to digest properly. With this type of itching, skin lesions manifest as red geographic wheals, edematous erythema, papules, vesicles and bullae, and bloody blisters. Accompanying symptoms include irritability and restlessness; itching is often intolerable. Without timely treatment, Toxic pathogenic factors may attack the interior to cause such systemic symptoms as vomiting, diarrhea and lassitude.

Itching due to consumption of alcohol

This type of itching is provoked immediately or a short time after drinking alcohol. Itching is accompanied by skin lesions manifesting as diffuse generalized erythema or pinpoint red morbilliform (measles-like) papules. As the alcohol Toxins are eliminated from the body by sweating or urination, the itching sensation and skin lesions will subside and subsequently disappear.

Pain

Heat-type pain

Exuberant Heat can cause stagnation of Qi and Blood in the channels and network vessels to produce pain. This type of pain is often accompanied by other symptoms such as a burning sensation and a preference for cold. The pain can be relieved with a cold compress of cool-natured materia medica. Heat-type pain is frequently seen in cases of erysipelas or furuncles.

Cold-type pain

This type of pain is usually accompanied by aversion to cold. Pain is aggravated by exposure to wind or cold. Application of dressings with warm or hot-natured materia medica helps to reduce the pain. Cold-type pain is often seen with chilblains and frostbite or at the initial and intermediate stages of Raynaud's disease.

Deficiency-type pain

This type of pain is mild and develops slowly. No distension is felt locally. Pain can be relieved by gentle local massage. Deficiency-type pain is seldom seen in skin diseases.

Excess-type pain

This type of pain is relatively intense and is accompanied by local distension. Touch or pressure is intolerable whatever the degree of pain. Excess-type pain occurs in conditions such as post-herpetic neuralgia.

Qi-type pain

This is a type of migratory pain which varies in response to emotional changes. It is seldom seen in skin diseases.

Blood-type pain

This type of pain has a fixed location; discomfort is exacerbated by touch or pressure. It can occur in conditions such as erythromelalgia.

Wind-type pain

This type of pain has no fixed location, and moves rapidly from one location to another. It is seen in conditions such as migratory arthralgia (moving Bi syndrome) or rheumatoid arthritis.

Suppuration-induced pain

This condition is characterized by throbbing pain or intense, distending pain. Pressure produces an undulating sensation. This type of pain often occurs during abscess formation in cases of furuncles or carbuncles.

Numbness

Numbness may result from

- Qi and Blood Deficiency depriving the channels and network vessels of nourishment
- Qi stagnation and Blood stasis
- retention of Cold, Damp or Phlegm in the channels and network vessels

PATTERN IDENTIFICATION ACCORDING TO SKIN LESIONS

PRIMARY LESIONS

Primary lesions are the initial or basic lesions of a skin eruption. Correct identification of primary lesions provides orientation for treatment and aids differential diagnosis.

Macules

Macules are circumscribed changes in skin color or texture up to 0.5 cm in size without elevation or depression; lesions of this type greater than 0.5 cm in size are known as **patches**.

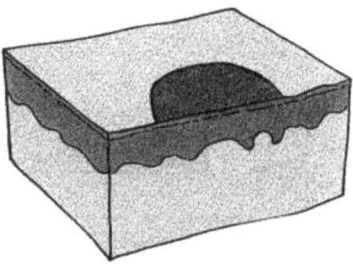

Red macules (erythema)

- Red is the color of Heat. A deep red color indicates predominance of Fire, a paler red indicates Heat.

Purplish-red macules are a sign of intense Heat or Blood stasis due to Heat.

- Red macules that blanch on pressure indicate Heat in the Qi level; if the color remains the same, this indicates Blood stasis in the Xue level.
- A few small macules indicate that Heat is not particularly strong; numerous larger macules (or patches) are a sign of more intense Heat.
- Recurrent crops of red macules indicate that Heat is intensifying.
- If the macules rapidly become confluent, Heat has entered the Ying level with consumption of Qi and Blood.
- Red macules appearing on the face and head indicate Wind-Heat, red macules on the lower limbs indicate Damp-Heat.
- If the red macules are itchy, Wind is involved.
- If the macules are scaly, Dryness is involved.
- If the macules are red and moist, the pathogenic factors are superficial and the disease can be treated more easily; if the macules are dark red, the pathogenic factors have already invaded deep into the body and the disease will be more difficult to treat.

Purple macules (purpura)

- Purple macules denote Heat retained in the Yang-ming channels.
- Purple macules due to the frenetic movement of hot Blood often occur in young adults; they have a sudden onset, no fixed location and do not fade under pressure.
- Pale purple macules due to Yang Deficiency of the Spleen and Kidneys generally appear on the legs and persist for long periods.
- Purple macules due to obstruction and stagnation of Blood first appear in childhood or adolescence. Some macules may be purplish-brown or bluish-purple.
- Purple macules due to Cold congealing and Blood stagnation appear on the face around the nose, on the ear lobe and on the dorsum of the hands and feet in young females. They are exacerbated in winter and alleviated in summer.
- Purple or purplish-red macules due to Damp-Heat pouring down occur most frequently in young females and involve the bilateral legs and thighs.

Black or dark brown macules

- Dark brown macules indicate Liver Depression.
- Black macules indicate extreme Heat Toxins.
- Brown macules due to Liver Depression and Qi stagnation appearing on the face, forehead and cheeks occur in melasma (chloasma) or melanosis.

The lesions have clearly-defined margins and do not fade under pressure.

- Small black macules due to insufficiency of Kidney Yin appear on the cheeks and forehead, behind the ears, on the forearms, and in the umbilical region in melanosis.

White macules

- Smooth white macules with clearly-defined margins but without scale are usually due to Qi stagnation or disharmony of Qi and Blood, for example in vitiligo. They are burning hot and red after exposure to the sun. The hairs inside the macules may turn white.
- White macules due to Summerheat-Damp often occur in the summer and appear as round white or grayish-white patches on the neck, axillae, chest, back, and extensor aspects of the limbs. The macules have a slightly shiny surface and are itchy. Fine scale is caused by scratching.

Papules

Papules are circumscribed palpable solid elevations of skin up to 0.5 cm in diameter; above this size they are known as **plaques**. Papules vary in appearance and may be pointed, rounded (domed), flat-topped, or umbilicated.

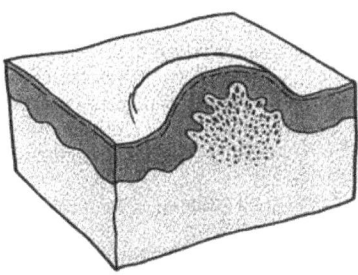

- Red papules are due to Heat; purplish-red papules are caused by exuberant Heat or Blood stasis due to Heat.
- If red papules are combined with red macules or bloody exudate is produced, this is a sign of Blood-Heat; if they are combined with vesicles or clear exudate is produced, Damp-Heat is indicated. Papules combined with pustules are caused by Heat Toxins.
- Hard papules and itchy lesions denote Wind-Heat.
- Flat-topped, hard purplish-red papules, as seen in lichen planus, are due to Blood stasis in the channels and vessels.
- In most cases, the Lungs, Spleen or Stomach are involved, as for example in acne, where papules on the face, usually in combination with open comedones (blackheads) or closed comedones (whiteheads) are due to accumulated Heat in the Lungs and Stomach.

Nodules

Nodules are round or oval circumscribed palpable solid lesions of varying color. They are larger than papules, measuring more than 0.5 cm in diameter in both width and depth. They are located below the skin surface and may involve any layer of the skin.

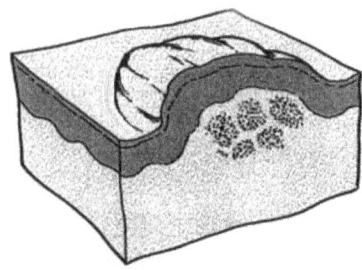

- Nodules may be caused by Phlegm congealing, Blood stasis or obstruction of the channels and network vessels.
- Palpable, slightly elevated nodules initially with overlying red skin, which gradually changes to dull red or purplish-red, indicate Qi stagnation and Blood stasis. Nodules appearing on the extensor aspects of the legs are numerous, small and superficial with overlying red or bright red skin. They tend to be acute, often appearing in spring, but generally do not rupture; this type of nodule is liable to recur. Nodules appearing on the flexor aspects of the legs are fewer, larger and deeper, with overlying purplish-red skin. They tend to be chronic, with exacerbation in winter and alleviation in summer; they often rupture and are difficult to cure.
- Nodules due to congealing and binding of Phlegm-Fire are firm and movable. They have a normal skin color and are painless. As they enlarge, the nodules become soft and can no longer be moved; the overlying skin turns deep red and there is a feeling of slight pain. Continual discharge of thin pus follows rupture as chronic ulceration results.
- Nodules due to Cold-Damp obstructing the network vessels commonly appear on the limbs in a linear distribution and gradually increase in number, becoming red and swollen. After rupture, thin yellow pus is discharged.
- Accumulation of Wind-Damp with prevalence of Wind will lead to nodular prurigo since exuberant Wind causes itching.

Pustules

Pustules are circumscribed elevations of skin of varying size containing a visible collection of pus. They may be round, spherical, conical, or umbilicated. Shallow pustules will not leave scars after healing, whereas deep-rooted pustules will. Pustules may be primary lesions, or may develop from papules or vesicles. They may indicate infection, but may also be sterile. Pustules are caused by internal and external factors.

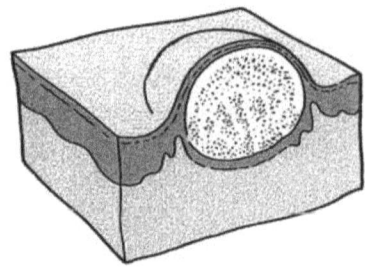

- Pustules with an internal origin are due to Heat transforming into Toxins after accumulating over a long period. Heat Toxins putrefy the flesh to form pus.
- Repeated crops of small pustules, which contain pale yellow fluid and occur in clusters, are due to the accumulation of Damp-Heat, as seen in palmoplantar pustulosis.
- Pustules due to accumulation of Heat in the Ying and Xue levels are superficial and appear on the top of erythema. The pinkish fluid in the pustules is a mixture of pus and blood. After rupture, the pustules dry up to form purulent bloody crusts.
- Toxic pathogenic factors may attack the exterior and cause pustules. Pustules due to Heat Toxins invading the skin and flesh are yellow with thin walls and clearly defined red margins. Rupture produces a discharge of sticky pus, which forms thick yellow crusts and may produce more pustules, as in impetigo.
- Pustules due to congealing of Damp Toxins initially manifest as vesicles, which turn into pustules. The thin-walled lesions often appear together on large erythematous patches, leaving an eroded surface following rupture as may occur in certain cases of herpes simplex. Exudation takes a long time to dry.

Vesicles and bullae

Vesicles are small circumscribed elevations of skin (up to 0.5 cm in diameter) containing fluid; bullae are similar to vesicles but are larger than 0.5 cm in diameter. Vesicles can develop into pustules or bullae. Vesicles and bullae may contain blood, serum or lymphatic fluid and their color changes according to the fluid contained.

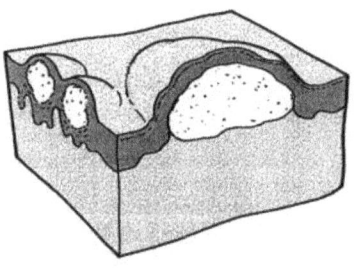

They may be semicircular, conical, flat-topped, umbilicated, or irregular in shape and may be subepidermal (as in bullous pemphigoid, see right lesion in illustration) or intraepidermal (as in pemphigus, see left lesions). The thin walls of vesicles and bullae break easily, leaving an eroded surface following rupture.

- Vesicles and bullae arise as a result of accumulation of Dampness in the skin and flesh.
- Vesicles due to accumulation of Wind-Damp in the skin are slightly red and are filled with a clear fluid. Generally very itchy, they do not occur at fixed locations, although distribution is denser in areas of profuse sweating. They commonly occur in spring, summer and autumn. When they rupture, exudation is slight.
- Vesicles due to accumulation of Damp-Heat are small and densely filled with fluid. The thin walls are taut and shiny. If the vesicles have no areola, Dampness is predominant, whereas a pale red areola indicates predominance of Heat. When the vesicles rupture, crusts form on the eroded surface, where new vesicles appear.
- Vesicles due to Water and Dampness flowing to the exterior are large with clear fluid which gradually becomes turbid. The walls of the vesicles are loose and thin and can break easily. After rupture, crusts slowly appear as the surface does not heal quickly. This type of vesicle is seen in herpes zoster (shingles), herpes simplex and varicella (chickenpox).
- Vesicles due to congealing and stagnation of Cold-Damp are white and usually appear on the hands and feet, the face and the lobe of the ear, as in chilblains. When they rupture, they are likely to erode and ulcerate and are difficult to treat.
- Bullae with loose walls and clear, thin fluid indicate Spleen Deficiency and exuberant Dampness, as in pemphigus. The lesions are pale red or yellowish white. Pain is mild.
- Bloody vesicles or bullae occur when Heat Toxins enter the Xue level and cause the frenetic movement of Blood, for example in herpes zoster (shingles).

Wheals
Wheals are circumscribed compressible elevated edematous lesions resulting from fluid infiltrating the dermis (dermal edema). Wheals are transient and generally disappear within a few hours; they are usually an indication of an urticarial disease. Lesions range in size from 3-4 mm to 10-12 cm in diameter, but some may be even larger. Wheals also vary in number and shape.

- Wheals due to Wind-Heat are red or pink and can spread rapidly throughout the body. They are exacerbated by heat and alleviated by cold.

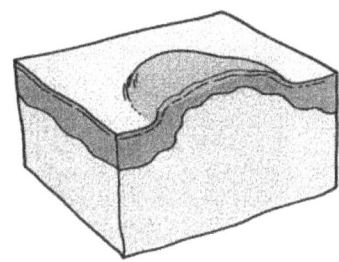

- Wheals due to Wind-Cold are pale white or porcelain white and are obvious on the exposed parts of the body. They are exacerbated by cold and alleviated by heat.
- Red or bright red linear wheals produced by scratching are due to Blood-Heat. They can appear on any part of the body. They are caused by the five emotions transforming into Fire, resulting in Blood-Heat generating Wind, which leads to damage to the Blood vessels.
- Dull red wheals appearing in areas under constant pressure are due to Blood stasis.
- Red wheals with acute onset and accompanying symptoms such as discomfort in the chest and stomach, abdominal distension and constipation are due to accumulated Heat in the Stomach and Intestines.
- Pale red or flesh-colored wheals that appear frequently and linger for months or years, increasing in severity with fatigue, are due to Deficiency of Qi and Blood.

Cysts
Cysts are spherical or elliptical lesions consisting of an epithelial-lined cavity containing fluid or semi-solid substances such as a mixture of fluid and cells or cellular products. They feel elastic on palpation. Cysts are generally caused by congealing of Phlegm and retention of Body Fluids, or by Blood stasis binding with Damp-Heat.

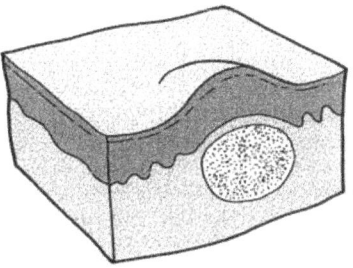

Tumors
Tumors are intradermal or subcutaneous masses more than 1 cm in diameter. They may be round, pedunculated or irregular in shape, soft or firm, elevated above the surface of the skin or merely palpable. Tumors may be benign or malignant. They may remain unchanged or expand gradually or finally rupture and ulcerate. Involution is rare. They generally result from Blood stasis,

Phlegm stagnation or turbid Qi being retained in the tissues. If these pathogenic factors break through into the interior and harm the Zang-Fu organs, Qi and Blood, they will become life-threatening.

SECONDARY LESIONS

Secondary lesions may develop from primary lesions during the evolution of skin disorders or during the treatment process, or result from scratching or infection.

Scales

Scales are accumulations of keratin from the thickened horny layer of the skin in the form of detached fragments or flakes. Normal epidermal cells renew themselves once every four weeks. Once they reach the horny layer (the stratum corneum), they are shed imperceptibly.

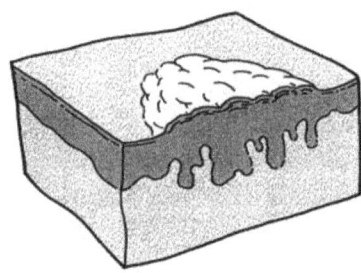

Scales can be furfuraceous (bran-like), exfoliative or ichthyotic, and either dry or greasy in nature.
- Dry, white scale is caused by Wind-Dryness due to Blood Deficiency, thus depriving the skin of nourishment.
- Fine, bran-like scale results from an invasion of Wind-Damp.
- Greasy, yellow scale is caused by Dampness accumulating in the skin.

The color of the skin under the scales also helps in pattern identification. Red skin under the scales indicates Blood-Heat, whereas a pinkish color is generally a sign of Blood-Dryness.

Erosion

Erosions develop following detachment of the epidermis in the case of vesicles, pustules or maceration, or rupture of the epidermis in the case of papules or small nodules, leaving a wet base exposed (for instance, after scratching or other injuries). Since erosions do not penetrate into the dermis, they heal without scarring.

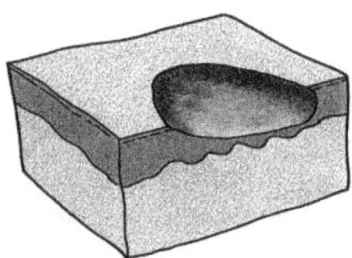

- Erosion with exudate indicates Spleen-Damp; if the exudate is yellow, this is a sign of exuberance of both Dampness and Heat.
- Erosion due to maceration of the skin between the fingers or toes or in the inguinal groove results from Damp-Heat transforming into Toxins.

Fissures

Fissures are linear clefts in the epidermis, often extending slightly into the dermis; they occur most frequently on the palms and heels, at the corners of the mouth, and in the perianal region.

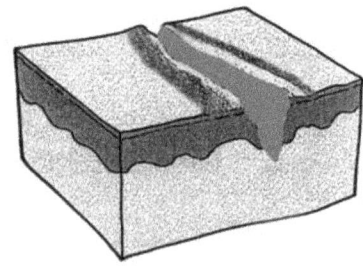

- Fissuring may be related to Cold and Dryness, since prevalence of Dryness leads to dry skin and prevalence of Cold results in fissures of the skin.
- Fissures can also occur as a result of prolonged consumption of Yin and damage to Body Fluids with consequent undernourishment of the skin.
- Fissures with bleeding are due to Blood-Heat and Wind-Dryness.

Lichenification

Lichenification manifests as an area of thickened epidermis with accentuated skin markings, giving the skin a leather or bark-like appearance. The plaque-like skin structure is due to the proliferation of keratin cells and hyperplasia of the horny layer as well as inflammatory cell infiltration of the dermis.

Lichenification develops due to the retention of Cold-Damp or stubborn Dampness in the skin and interstices (cou li), or can be caused by frequent scratching or rubbing.

Excoriations or scratch marks

Excoriations are erosions of the superficial layer of the skin caused by scratching; they are often linear. Exudation of serum or blood from the lesions will leave yellow or bloody crusts after drying.
- Bloody crusts following excoriation indicate Blood-Heat generating Wind.
- White linear lesions left by scratching are a sign of prevalence of Wind or internal Dryness.
- If the skin color is normal, but bleeding follows excoriation, this indicates Blood Deficiency generating Wind.

Crusts

Crusts are formed from dried exudate (serum, blood or pus) collecting on the skin surface. They can be thin or thick, soft or brittle.

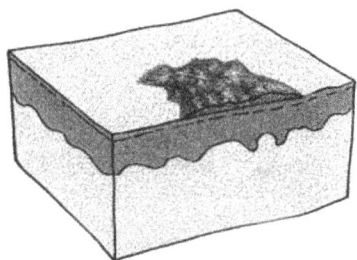

- Purulent crusts indicate that some Heat Toxins have not been cleared.
- Bloody crusts are a sign of residual Blood-Heat.
- Orange-yellow serous crusts indicate exuberance of both Dampness and Heat.

Ulcers

Ulcers are a circumscribed area of skin loss or destruction extending through the epidermis into the dermis and sometimes penetrating the subcutaneous fat. Ulcers heal with scarring. They generally occur as a result of the rupture of nodules or tumors, or due to trauma. The main causes of ulcers include exuberant Heat putrefying the flesh, or failure of the restorative function of Vital Qi (Zheng Qi).

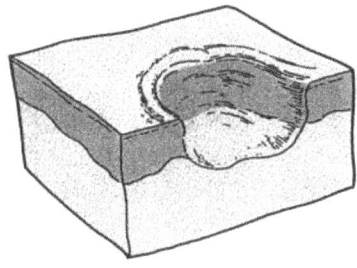

Scars

Scars result from the replacement of normal tissue by fibrous connective tissue at the site of an injury due to trauma, surgery, insect bites, or ulcers. They have a smooth appearance and lack normal skin markings. Scars are initially thick and red or rosy, but gradually become white and atrophic. Hyperplastic scars are elevated over the normal skin surface.

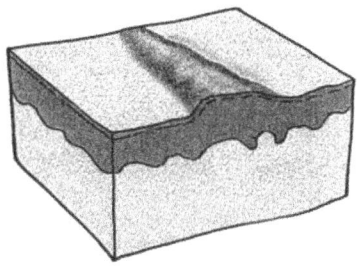

Maceration

Maceration occurs when the skin is soaked in water or remains moist for a long time, for example where a wet compress is maintained in place or the area between the fingers or toes remains damp for lengthy periods. As a result, the skin becomes soft and pale, and may fissure. Maceration is often an indication of Damp Toxins invading the skin or Damp-Heat pouring down.

Sclerosis

Sclerosis of the skin can be circumscribed or diffuse and is more perceptible on palpation than observation. It occurs as a result of Deficiency of Original Qi (Yuan Qi) and Cold, Damp, Phlegm, or Blood stasis obstructing the channels and network vessels.

Atrophy

Atrophy is thinning of the skin as a result of loss of the epidermis, dermis or subcutaneous fat. Atrophic skin is thin, translucent and wrinkled; blood vessels are normally easily visible in epidermal and dermal atrophy. Normal skin markings may be lost in epidermal atrophy, which is usually caused by Qi Deficiency. Elderly people with atrophic skin may retain skin markings; slight wrinkling may be present. This condition usually results from Lung Deficiency or insufficiency of Yin and Blood, leading to the skin being deprived of nourishment.

Abnormalities of pigmentation

These include secondary pigmentation and partial or complete secondary depigmentation. Secondary pigmentation is usually related to disharmony of Qi and Blood:

- A pale brown color indicates malnourishment of the skin due to Blood Deficiency
- A dark brown color is a sign of Kidney disorders or abdominal masses

Secondary depigmentation is generally an external manifestation of excessive or untimely Wind, Blood stasis or disorders of the Zang-Fu organs.

Definitions of other lesions

Abscess

An abscess is a localized collection of pus formed by necrosis of tissue in a cavity greater than 1cm in diameter.

Burrow

A burrow is a narrow, elevated, linear or tortuous tunnel in the skin produced by a parasite such as the scabies mite.

Comedo

A comedo is a plug of sebum and keratin lodged in the dilated orifice of a pilosebaceous gland. Open comedones are known as blackheads, closed comedones as whiteheads.

Table 1-6 Occurrence of skin disorders by body region

Scalp

Alopecia areata, atopic eczema (infantile), contact dermatitis, dermatitis herpetiformis, folliculitis, pediculosis, pemphigus, pityriasis rubra pilaris, plaque psoriasis, seborrhea, seborrheic eczema, tinea capitis (ringworm of the scalp), varicella (chickenpox)

Face

Acne, angioedema, chilblains, common warts (verruca vulgaris), contact dermatitis, erysipelas, folliculitis, hemangioma, herpes simplex, herpes zoster (shingles), measles, phytophotodermatitis, pityriasis rubra pilaris, polymorphic light eruption, pyoderma faciale, seborrhea, sunburn, varicella (chickenpox)

Forehead

Acne, atopic eczema (infantile), hyperhidrosis, keratosis follicularis (Darier's disease), melasma (chloasma), nevus flammeus, pityriasis alba, plane warts (verruca plana), rosacea

Eyelids

Contact dermatitis, eczema

Cheeks

Acne, atopic eczema (infantile), melasma (chloasma), pityriasis alba, rosacea

Chin

Acne, melasma (chloasma), perioral dermatitis, pityriasis alba, plane warts (verruca plana), rosacea, sycosis barbae

Ears

Chilblains, contact dermatitis, eczema, erysipelas, measles, seborrheic eczema

Nose (perinasal)

Impetigo, melasma (chloasma), rosacea, seborrheic eczema

Mouth (perioral)

Contact dermatitis, impetigo, melasma (chloasma), perioral dermatitis, pityriasis alba, plane warts (verruca plana)

Mouth (mucosa)

Herpetic stomatitis, lichen planus, oral candidiasis (thrush), pemphigus, recurrent aphthous stomatitis (mouth ulcers)

Lips

Angioedema, cheilitis

Neck

Atopic eczema (adult and childhood phase), contact dermatitis, furuncles, hemangioma, keratosis follicularis (Darier's disease), lichen simplex chronicus (neurodermatitis), measles, nevus flammeus, polymorphic light eruption, sunburn, tinea corporis (ringworm of the body), vitiligo

Trunk

Bullous pemphigoid, contact dermatitis, eczema, guttate psoriasis, herpes zoster (shingles), measles, nummular eczema (discoid eczema), papular urticaria, parapsoriasis (chronic superficial dermatitis), pediculosis, pemphigus, pityriasis lichenoides, pityriasis rosea, pityriasis rubra pilaris, sunburn, tinea corporis (ringworm of the body), urticaria, varicella (chickenpox)

Chest

Acne, eczema, keratosis follicularis (Darier's disease), pityriasis versicolor, polymorphic light eruption, seborrheic eczema

Back

Acne, eczema, keratosis follicularis (Darier's disease), nodular prurigo, pityriasis versicolor, plaque psoriasis, seborrheic eczema

Axillae

Bromhidrosis, bullous pemphigoid, chromhidrosis, erythrasma, flexural psoriasis, folliculitis, furuncles, hidradenitis suppurativa, hyperhidrosis, intertrigo, miliaria rubra, seborrheic eczema

Arms

Angioedema, bullous pemphigoid (flexor aspect), contact dermatitis, eczema, erythema multiforme (extensor aspect), guttate psoriasis, ichthyosis vulgaris (extensor aspect), impetigo, keratosis pilaris (upper arm), measles, nodular prurigo, nummular eczema (discoid eczema), papular urticaria, pityriasis lichenoides, pityriasis rubra pilaris, plaque psoriasis (extensor aspect), sunburn, tinea corporis (ringworm of the body), urticaria, varicella (chickenpox)

Forearms

Dermatitis herpetiformis, lichen planus (flexor aspect), lipoma, plane warts (verruca plana), polymorphic light eruption (extensor aspect)

Elbows

Atopic eczema (adult and childhood phase), lichen simplex chronicus (neurodermatitis), pemphigus, plaque psoriasis, scabies

Table 1-6 (*cont'd*) Occurrence of skin disorders by body region

Wrists
Atopic eczema (childhood phase), contact dermatitis, lichen planus (flexor aspect), lichen simplex chronicus (neurodermatitis), scabies, vitiligo

Hands
Callus, chilblains, contact dermatitis, erythema multiforme, scabies, tinea manuum (ringworm of the hands)

Dorsum of hands
Common warts (verruca vulgaris), nummular eczema (discoid eczema), phytophotodermatitis, plane warts (verruca plana), polymorphic light eruption, vitiligo

Palms
Eczema, hyperhidrosis, keratoderma, palmoplantar pustulosis, pompholyx, tinea manuum (ringworm of the hands)

Fingers
Common warts (verruca vulgaris), pompholyx, Raynaud's disease, scabies

Groin
Bullous pemphigoid, erythrasma, flexural psoriasis, folliculitis, furuncles, hidradenitis suppurativa, intertrigo, keratosis follicularis (Darier's disease), seborrheic eczema, tinea cruris (jock itch)

Genitals
Bromhidrosis, candidal balanitis, chromhidrosis, common warts (verruca vulgaris), contact dermatitis, diaper dermatitis (nappy rash), eczema, erythrasma, herpes simplex, hidradenitis suppurativa, hyperhidrosis, lichen simplex chronicus (neurodermatitis), pediculosis, pruritus, scabies

Perianal region
Diaper dermatitis (nappy rash), eczema, hidradenitis suppurativa, intertrigo, lichen simplex chronicus (neurodermatitis), pruritus

Buttocks
Anaphylactoid purpura, dermatitis herpetiformis, furuncles, keratosis pilaris, nummular eczema (discoid eczema), papular urticaria, parapsoriasis (chronic superficial dermatitis), scabies

Legs
Anaphylactoid purpura, angioedema, bullous pemphigoid (flexor aspect), erythema ab igne, erythema multiforme (extensor aspect), guttate psoriasis, ichthyosis vulgaris (extensor aspect), impetigo, measles, nodular prurigo, nummular eczema (discoid eczema), papular eczema, papular urticaria, parapsoriasis (chronic superficial dermatitis), pityriasis lichenoides, pityriasis rubra pilaris, plaque psoriasis (extensor aspect), sunburn, tinea corporis (ringworm of the body), urticaria, varicella (chickenpox)

Upper legs
Folliculitis, furuncles, keratosis pilaris, lipoma

Lower legs
Asteatotic eczema, chronic venous ulcer of the lower leg, ecthyma, erysipelas, erythema induratum, lichen planus, polymorphic light eruption, stasis eczema

Knees
Atopic eczema (adult and childhood phase), dermatitis herpetiformis, pemphigus, plaque psoriasis, vitiligo

Ankles
Atopic eczema (childhood phase), lichen planus, lichen simplex chronicus (neurodermatitis), scabies, stasis eczema

Feet
Chilblains, common warts (verruca vulgaris), contact dermatitis, erythema multiforme, scabies, tinea pedis (athlete's foot)

Soles
Callus, corns, eczema, hyperhidrosis, keratoderma, palmoplantar pustulosis, plantar warts (verruca plantaris), pompholyx, tinea pedis (athlete's foot)

Toes
Callus, corns, erythromelalgia, Raynaud's disease, tinea pedis (athlete's foot)

Nails
Alopecia areata, hangnail, lichen planus, psoriasis, pyogenic paronychia (whitlow), tinea unguium (ringworm of the nails)

Ecchymosis

An ecchymosis is a macular red or purple hemorrhage measuring more than 2mm in diameter in the skin or mucous membrane.

Keratosis

A keratosis is a horn-like thickening of the stratum corneum (horny layer).

Petechiae

Petechiae are pinhead circumscribed macules of blood in the skin.

Telangiectasia

This term is used to describe visible dilatation of small blood vessels in the skin.

LOCATION OF SKIN LESIONS

The location of skin lesions offers help for differential diagnosis and pattern identification. Certain disorders can occur at various body sites and distribution can be an important factor in diagnosis, pattern identification and subsequent treatment. For example, Damp-Heat can move upward to manifest as palpebral eczema or pour down to manifest as genital eczema. Some of the more common skin disorders and their distribution by body region are detailed in Table 1-6.

Examination of skin lesions

The following three points should be observed when examining skin lesions:

- First, conduct the observation in bright natural light whenever possible.
- Second, observe the skin carefully from different aspects and palpate with the fingers when required. Use a magnifying glass or microscope if necessary.
- Third, a thorough understanding of the characteristics of skin lesions is essential. Lesions should be noted in terms of the following aspects:
  - size, either in absolute measurements or in reference to the size of other suitable objects;
  - color, for example skin-colored, red, yellow, pale, or white;
  - consistency; palpate to test whether the lesions are soft or hard;
  - surface properties, for example smooth, rough, thorny, papillary, or cauliflower-like;
  - borders, for example sharply demarcated, irregular or indistinct;
  - morphology, for example round, oval, polygonal, umbilicated, or flat-topped;
  - configuration, for example discrete, confluent, grouped, linear, annular, or serpiginous;
  - distribution, for example unilateral, symmetrical, local, generalized, or along the course of nerves, blood vessels or channels.

Taking a history

Understanding the medical history and current condition through interrogation is a very important means of gaining first-hand information about the case, in particular for patients with a long medical history and a complicated condition. History-taking should cover the following points:

- General information: age, sex, date of birth, and the living and working environment.
- Chief presenting complaint: note the main features of the condition including the duration of the disease, the initial site of the disease and its subsequent spread, the appearance of the lesions and how this has evolved, accompanying sensations such as itching, pain or burning, and any factors alleviating or exacerbating the disease.
- Current condition: the main cause inducing the disorder in terms of exposure to climatic factors, improper diet (including alcohol intake), drug allergy, trauma or insect bites, or emotional factors must be established. It is essential to grasp the main symptoms and characteristics of the disease in order to make an analysis. In addition to the main symptoms, accompanying symptoms and signs need to be noted and previous prescriptions and their effect must be taken into account when arriving at a pattern identification.
- Previous medical history: understanding a patient's previous medical history will help to make a correct diagnosis in relation to the degree of severity of the current disorder. Patients should be asked about previous skin diseases and allergies. Any current or recent Western medication for internal or external use should also be noted.
- Family history: this is important for diagnosing diseases with a genetic component such as psoriasis or atopic eczema, or for infections or infestations such as scabies.
- Personal history: this includes the patient's occupation, dietary habits and lifestyle. Occupational factors or particular hobbies can result for example in contact dermatitis.
- Relationship history: a patient who has lost a partner tends to suffer from depression; women who have given birth to many children can suffer from insufficiency of the Kidneys.
- Menstrual history: generally speaking, lesions that increase in intensity or where itching becomes worse after menses are due to insufficiency of the Liver and Kidneys.

Chapter 2

Main treatment methods for skin disorders

Disease patterns and determination of treatment
病证结合论治

Treatment of skin disorders can be determined on the basis of pattern types, the stage of the disease, patterns indicated by formulae, or fixed prescriptions with modifications.

Determination of treatment on the basis of pattern types

Different patterns are identified for a disease and treatment is given on the basis of these patterns. In recent years, large numbers of clinical studies have been carried out and a great deal of experience accumulated, with the result that this method of determining treatment has been extended to a wide spectrum of diseases with good results.

This method is most suitable for complex diseases caused by multiple factors, with multiple organ involvement and multiple pathologies. The patterns present in such diseases are relatively easy to recognize in patients and treatment varies according to the patterns identified. For example, acne can be classified, based on the disease site and characteristic skin lesions, into different patterns such as Heat in the Lungs or Stomach, Blood-Heat, stagnation of Qi and Blood, and Blood stasis and binding of Phlegm. Each pattern has its own distinguishing features, which aid pattern identification and are helpful references for treatment.

Determination of treatment according to the disease stage

This method is used to determine treatment based on pattern identification according to the pathological changes occurring at different stages in the evolution of a particular disease. For example, measles passes through three phases – the pre-eruptive or initial fever phase, the eruptive phase, and the post-eruptive or recovery phase. Each phase lasts for three to five days, reflecting the different pathological changes in the natural course of measles; treatment principles therefore vary accordingly.

In the pre-eruptive phase, treatment follows the principle of venting papules with acrid and diffusing materia medica to help relieve Toxicity; in the eruptive phase, treatment focuses on relieving Toxicity and venting papules; and in the post-eruptive stage, the principle of nourishing Yin and clearing Heat is employed.

If the disease does not progress normally, for instance, where there is incomplete eruption of papules, disappearance of papules shortly after eruption, or the appearance of other symptoms such as a sudden drop in body temperature, rapid breathing and convulsions, this indicates exacerbation of the condition and appropriate measures should be taken as soon as possible (see Chapter 9).

Determination of treatment according to patterns indicated by formulae

In the early years of the Qing dynasty (1644-1911), Ke Yunbo concentrated on developing Zhang Zhongjing's method of treatment according to pattern identification as expounded in *Shang Han Za Bing Lun* [Treatise on Miscellaneous Cold Diseases]. He advocated the integration of diagnosis and treatment, associating prescriptions with patterns and naming patterns according to formulae. He held that Zhang Zhongjing must have taken formulae and patterns as the basis for pattern identification and treatment since he designated certain patterns as *Chai Hu Tang Zheng* (Bupleurum Decoction pattern) or *Gui Zhi Tang Zheng* (Cinnamon Twig Decoction pattern).

He also emphasized the use of a particular formula for the symptoms and signs of a particular pattern no matter which channel or disease might be involved. Examples include treatment with *Bai Hu Tang* (White Tiger Decoction) for *Bai Hu Tang Zheng* (White Tiger Decoction pattern), which presents with raging fever, profuse sweating, severe irritability and thirst, and a surging, large pulse; and treatment with *Xiao Chai Hu Tang* (Minor Bupleurum Decoction) for *Chai Hu Tang*

Zheng (Bupleurum Decoction pattern), which presents with a bitter taste in the mouth, dry throat, blurred vision, alternating fever and chills, bitter fullness in the chest and hypochondrium, irritability, and frequent retching.

Determination of treatment according to fixed prescriptions with modifications depending on pattern identification

This method, which is used frequently nowadays, takes a particular formula as the basic prescription for a particular disease and then modifies it depending on the clinical manifestations. It is suitable for diseases of short duration with a single etiology and pathology, and for diseases with a complicated etiology and long duration but whose pathology basically remains the same throughout its course.

For instance, *Liang Xue Xiao Feng San* (Powder for Cooling the Blood and Dispersing Wind) is used as one of the basic prescriptions for seborrheic eczema.

The basic formula is modified as follows:
- For large patches of erythema, add *Zi Cao* (Radix Arnebiae seu Lithospermi) and *Chi Shao* (Radix Paeoniae Rubra).
- For significant scaling, add *Cang Er Zi* (Fructus Xanthii Sibirici) and *He Shou Wu* (Radix Polygoni Multiflori).

Determination of treatment methods

Even though most skin diseases manifest primarily on the skin, both systemic and local factors need to be taken into consideration for pattern identification, and internal and external treatment are often combined. The internal treatment of skin diseases is similar in nature to that for internal diseases, but it also has its own specific characteristics. When combined with the principle of "putting particular emphasis on external treatment as one of the methods of treating external diseases," a unique diagnostic and treatment system for skin disorders comes into play.

Internal treatment
内治法

In *Lin Zheng Zhi Nan Yi An: Yang Ke* [Case Guide to Clinical Symptoms: Skin Diseases], it says: "Treatment of the external must be based on the internal; treatment of the internal is also treatment of the external." As a general principle, treatment should be given by seeking the cause from the patterns identified. Commonly used internal treatments for skin diseases include the methods of alleviating itching, regulating Dampness, relieving Toxicity, regulating the Blood, supplementing and nourishing, softening hardness, harmonizing and regulating, and consolidating and astringing.

Treatment principles

ALLEVIATING ITCHING

DISPELLING WIND TO ALLEVIATE ITCHING
One of the main treatment principles often referred to in books on TCM formulae is that "[various] skin disorders should be treated by diffusing and dissipating." The treatment principles and materia medica used depend on whether Wind combines with Heat or Cold.

- Itching due to disharmony between the Ying and Wei levels caused by Wind-Heat attacking the exterior

Treatment principle
Dredge Wind and clear Heat.

Commonly used prescription
Shu Feng Qing Re Tang (Decoction for Dredging Wind and Clearing Heat)

Commonly used materia medica
Bai Ji Li (Fructus Tribuli Terrestris)
Bo He (Herba Menthae Haplocalycis)
Chan Tui‡ (Periostracum Cicadae)
Fang Feng (Radix Ledebouriellae Divaricatae)
Fu Ping (Herba Spirodelae Polyrrhizae)
Jing Jie (Herba Schizonepetae Tenuifoliae)
Ju Hua (Flos Chrysanthemi Morifolii)
Niu Bang Zi (Fructus Arctii Lappae)

- Itching due to disharmony between the Ying and Wei levels caused by Wind-Cold invading the flesh

Treatment principle
Dissipate Cold to release the exterior.

Commonly used prescription
Ma Gui Ge Ban Tang (Ephedra and Cinnamon Twig Half-and-Half Decoction)

Commonly used materia medica

Bai Zhi (Radix Angelicae Dahuricae)
Du Huo (Radix Angelicae Pubescentis)
Gui Zhi (Ramulus Cinnamomi Cassiae)
*Ma Huang** (Herba Ephedrae)
Qiang Huo (Rhizoma et Radix Notopterygii)
Wei Ling Xian (Radix Clematidis)
*Xi Xin** (Herba cum Radice Asari)
Xin Yi Hua (Flos Magnoliae)

Modifications

1. For persistent itching complicated by Wind Toxins, add *Wu Shao She* ‡ (Zaocys Dhumnades), *Chan Tui* ‡ (Periostracum Cicadae) or other insect materia medica to restrain and eliminate the itching.
2. For severe itching complicated by Spleen Deficiency, add *Bai Zhu* (Rhizoma Atractylodis Macrocephalae), *Chen Pi* (Pericarpium Citri Reticulatae) and *Sha Ren* (Fructus Amomi) to fortify the Spleen.
3. For mild itching complicated by Qi Deficiency, add *Huang Qi* (Radix Astragali seu Hedysari), *Bai Zhu* (Rhizoma Atractylodis Macrocephalae) and *Da Zao* (Fructus Ziziphi Jujubae) to supplement Qi.

REGULATING DAMPNESS TO ALLEVIATE ITCHING

In *Yao Dui* [Compatibility of Medicines], Xu Zhicai (493-572) said, "Dryness can eliminate Dampness". Regulating Dampness to alleviate itching in skin diseases includes methods such as aromatically transforming Dampness, dispelling Dampness with warmth and acridity, and benefiting the movement of Dampness by bland percolation.

• Itching due to internal accumulation of Dampness in the Spleen plus external contraction of Wind

Treatment principle

Aromatically transform Dampness.

Commonly used prescription

Xie Huang San (Yellow-Draining Powder)

Commonly used materia medica

Huo Xiang (Herba Agastaches seu Pogostemi)
Pei Lan (Herba Eupatorii Fortunei)
Sha Ren (Fructus Amomi)
Yi Yi Ren (Semen Coicis Lachryma-jobi)

Modifications

1. For complications due to Damp-Heat, add ingredients such as *Yin Chen Hao* (Herba Artemisiae Scopariae), *Hua Shi*‡ (Talcum), *Bai Xian Pi* (Cortex Dictamni Dasycarpi Radicis), *Bian Xu* (Herba Polygoni Avicularis), *Jin Qian Cao* (Herba Lysimachiae), *Xi Xian Cao* (Herba Siegesbeckiae), and *Tu Fu Ling* (Rhizoma Smilacis Glabrae).

2. For complications due to Cold-Damp, add ingredients such as *Bi Xie* (Rhizoma Dioscoreae Hypoglaucae seu Septemlobae), *Bing Lang** (Semen Arecae Catechu), *Lu Lu Tong* (Fructus Liquidambaris), and *Hai Tong Pi* (Cortex Erythrinae).
3. For complications due to Blood-Heat, add ingredients such as *Jing Jie* (Herba Schizonepetae Tenuifoliae), *Yi Mu Cao* (Herba Leonuri Heterophylli), *Chi Shao* (Radix Paeoniae Rubra), *Hong Hua* (Flos Carthami Tinctorii), *Mu Dan Pi* (Cortex Moutan Radicis), and *Ling Xiao Hua* (Flos Campsitis).
4. For complications due to damage to Yin, add ingredients such as *He Shou Wu* (Radix Polygoni Multiflori), *Bai Shao* (Radix Paeoniae Lactiflorae), *Sheng Di Huang* (Radix Rehmanniae Glutinosae), *Shu Di Huang* (Radix Rehmanniae Glutinosae Conquita), and *Gou Teng* (Ramulus Uncariae cum Uncis).

CLEARING HEAT TO ALLEVIATE ITCHING

This method is recommended when pathogenic factors are between the Qi and Ying levels. Treatment aimed at thrusting the pathogenic factors outward will drive them toward the exterior, possibly aggravating itching; treatment aimed at cooling the interior will probably guide the pathogenic factors there or cause them to stagnate, again making it difficult to alleviate itching. Therefore the treatment principle of clearing Heat is an appropriate choice in such circumstances.

Treatment principle

Clear Heat.

Commonly used prescription

Xiao Feng San (Powder for Dispersing Wind)

Commonly used materia medica

Bai Xian Pi (Cortex Dictamni Dasycarpi Radicis)
Cang Er Zi (Fructus Xanthii Sibirici)
Han Shui Shi‡ (Calcitum)
Huang Qin (Radix Scutellariae Baicalensis)
Lian Qiao (Fructus Forsythiae Suspensae)
Lü Dou Yi (Testa Phaseoli Radiati)
Sheng Di Huang (Radix Rehmanniae Glutinosae)
Shi Gao‡ (Gypsum Fibrosum)
Xuan Shen (Radix Scrophulariae Ningpoensis)
Zhi Mu (Rhizoma Anemarrhenae Asphodeloidis)

Modifications

1. For severe Heat transforming into Toxins, add *Jiao Zhi Zi* (Fructus Gardeniae Jasminoidis, scorch-fried), *Ye Ju Hua* (Flos Chrysanthemi Indici), *Pu Gong Ying* (Herba Taraxaci cum Radice), *Jin Yin Hua* (Flos Lonicerae), and *Zi Hua Di Ding* (Herba Violae Yedoensitis).
2. For Heat combining with Damp Toxins, add *Huang Bai* (Cortex Phellodendri), *Che Qian Zi* (Semen Plantaginis), *Bi Xie* (Rhizoma Dioscoreae Hypoglaucae

seu Septemlobae), *Hai Jin Sha* (Spora Lygodii Japonici), *Jin Qian Cao* (Herba Lysimachiae), and *Can Sha*‡ (Excrementum Bombycis Mori).

3. For Heat combining with Wind, add *Qing Hao* (Herba Artemisiae Chinghao), *Chan Tui*‡ (Periostracum Cicadae), *Mu Zei* (Herba Equiseti Hiemalis), *Qing Xiang Zi* (Semen Celosiae Argenteae), *Sang Ye* (Folium Mori Albae), and *Niu Bang Zi* (Fructus Arctii Lappae).

MOISTENING DRYNESS TO ALLEVIATE ITCHING

Although itching due to Dryness can be caused internally through damage to the Essence and Blood, or externally by invasion of pathogenic Dryness, the basis of treatment for moistening Dryness to alleviate itching focuses on the Liver and Kidneys.

Treatment principle
Moisten Dryness, extinguish Wind and nourish the skin.

Commonly used prescription
Di Huang Yin Zi (Rehmannia Drink)

Commonly used materia medica
Bai He (Bulbus Lilii)
Bai Shao (Radix Paeoniae Lactiflorae)
E Jiao‡ (Gelatinum Corii Asini)
Gan Di Huang (Radix Rehmanniae Glutinosae Exsiccata)
Gou Qi Zi (Fructus Lycii)
Gou Teng (Ramulus Uncariae cum Uncis)
He Huan Pi (Cortex Albizziae Julibrissin)
He Shou Wu (Radix Polygoni Multiflori)
Hei Zhi Ma (Semen Sesami Indici)
Long Yan Rou (Arillus Euphoriae Longanae)
Mai Men Dong (Radix Ophiopogonis Japonici)
Sha Yuan Zi (Semen Astragali Complanati)
Shan Yao (Rhizoma Dioscoreae Oppositae)
Tian Men Dong (Radix Asparagi Cochinchinensis)
Ye Jiao Teng (Caulis Polygoni Multiflori)

Modifications
1. For concurrent Blood-Heat, add *Mu Dan Pi* (Cortex Moutan Radicis), *Zi Cao* (Radix Arnebiae seu Lithospermi) and *Bai Mao Gen* (Rhizoma Imperatae Cylindricae).
2. For concurrent Blood Deficiency, add *Sang Shen* (Fructus Mori Albae), *Xuan Shen* (Radix Scrophulariae Ningpoensis) and *Shu Di Huang* (Radix Rehmanniae Glutinosae Conquita).
3. For concurrent Blood stasis, add *Dan Shen* (Radix Salviae Miltiorrhizae), *Tao Ren* (Semen Persicae), *Hong Hua* (Flos Carthami Tinctorii), and *Su Mu* (Lignum Sappan).

TRANSFORMING BLOOD STASIS TO ALLEVIATE ITCHING

This method is used for itching resulting from inhibited movement of Qi in the channels and network vessels due to lumps caused by Qi stagnation and Blood stasis.

• If dark-colored blood oozes from stasis lumps after scratching, the treatment principle of invigorating the Blood and dissipating lumps should be employed.

Treatment principle
Invigorate the Blood and dissipate lumps.

Commonly used prescription
Tao Hong Si Wu Tang (Peach Kernel and Safflower Four Agents Decoction)

Commonly used materia medica

• For Blood stasis complicated by Heat

Bai Jiang Cao (Herba Patriniae cum Radice)
Chi Shao (Radix Paeoniae Rubra)
*Chuan Shan Jia** (Squama Manitis Pentadactylae)
Da Ji (Herba seu Radix Cirsii Japonici)
Dan Shen (Radix Salviae Miltiorrhizae)
Di Yu (Radix Sanguisorbae Officinalis)
Ling Xiao Hua (Flos Campsitis)
Mu Dan Pi (Cortex Moutan Radicis)
Pu Huang (Pollen Typhae)
Qian Cao Gen (Radix Rubiae Cordifoliae)
Shan Cha Hua (Flos Camelliae Japonicae)
Sheng Di Huang (Radix Rehmanniae Glutinosae)
Tao Ren (Semen Persicae)
Yi Mu Cao (Herba Leonuri Heterophylli)
Yu Jin (Radix Curcumae)

• For Blood stasis complicated by Dampness

Hua Rui Shi‡ (Ophicalcitum)
Lu Lu Tong (Fructus Liquidambaris)
Ma Bian Cao (Herba cum Radice Verbenae)

• For Blood stasis complicated by Cold

Chuan Xiong (Rhizoma Ligustici Chuanxiong)
Dang Gui (Radix Angelicae Sinensis)
Liu Ji Nu (Herba Artemisiae Anomalae)
Ru Xiang (Gummi Olibanum)
San Qi (Radix Notoginseng)
Shi Chang Pu (Rhizoma Acori Graminei)
Su Mu (Lignum Sappan)
Wang Bu Liu Xing (Semen Vaccariae Segetalis)
Xue Jie (Resina Draconis)
Zao Jiao Ci (Spina Gleditsiae Sinensis)
Ze Lan (Herba Lycopi Lucidi)

SUPPLEMENTING DEFICIENCY TO ALLEVIATE ITCHING

There is a common adage in TCM that "All pain is Excess in nature; all itching is Deficient in nature." It is very common to find itching due to Deficiency. In order to supplement Deficiency to alleviate itching, it is very important to determine whether it is Yin Deficiency, Yang Deficiency, Blood Deficiency, or Qi Deficiency that is involved.

- Itching due to Yin Deficiency

Treatment principle
Enrich Yin and extinguish Wind.

Commonly used prescription
Sha Shen Mai Dong Yin (Adenophora and Ophiopogon Beverage)

Commonly used materia medica
Gan Di Huang (Radix Rehmanniae Glutinosae Exsiccata)
Mai Men Dong (Radix Ophiopogonis Japonici)
Nan Sha Shen (Radix Adenophorae)
*Shi Hu** (Herba Dendrobii)
Tian Men Dong (Radix Asparagi Cochinchinensis)

- Itching due to Yang Deficiency

Treatment principle
Support Yang to alleviate itching

Commonly used prescription
Huang Qi Jian Zhong Tang (Astragalus Decoction for Fortifying the Middle)

Commonly used materia medica
Ba Ji Tian (Radix Morindae Officinalis)
Bu Gu Zhi (Fructus Psoraleae Corylifoliae)
Chen Xiang (Lignum Aquilariae Resinatum)
*Fu Zi** (Radix Lateralis Aconiti Carmichaeli Praeparata)
Rou Gui (Cortex Cinnamomi Cassiae)
Shan Zhu Yu (Fructus Corni Officinalis)
Xian Mao (Rhizoma Curculiginis Orchioidis)
Yin Yang Huo (Herba Epimedii)

- Itching due to Qi Deficiency

Treatment principle
Augment Qi to alleviate itching

Commonly used prescription
Si Jun Zi Tang (Four Gentlemen Decoction)

Commonly used materia medica
Bai Zhu (Rhizoma Atractylodis Macrocephalae)
Dang Shen (Radix Codonopsitis Pilosulae)
Dong Chong Xia Cao‡ (Cordyceps Sinensis)
Gan Cao (Radix Glycyrrhizae)
Huang Qi (Radix Astragali seu Hedysari)
Ren Shen (Radix Ginseng)
Shan Yao (Rhizoma Dioscoreae Oppositae)

- Itching due to Blood Deficiency

Treatment principle
Nourish the Blood to alleviate itching

Commonly used prescription
Si Wu Tang (Four Agents Decoction)

Commonly used materia medica
Bai Shao (Radix Paeoniae Lactiflorae)
Dang Gui (Radix Angelicae Sinensis)
E Jiao‡ (Gelatinum Corii Asini)
He Shou Wu (Radix Polygoni Multiflori)
Sang Shen (Fructus Mori Albae)
Shu Di Huang (Radix Rehmanniae Glutinosae Conquita)
Ye Jiao Teng (Caulis Polygoni Multiflori)

RELIEVING TOXICITY TO ALLEVIATE ITCHING

Mineral and metal ingredients have warm and harsh properties. Long-term internal administration will cause severe itching as a result of damage to Yin and consumption of Body Fluids.

Treatment principle
Protect Yin, relieve Toxicity, extinguish Wind, and alleviate itching.

Commonly used prescription
Jie Du Yang Yin Tang (Decoction for Relieving Toxicity and Nourishing Yin)

Commonly used materia medica
Bei Sha Shen (Radix Glehniae Littoralis)
Dan Shen (Radix Salviae Miltiorrhizae)
Di Gu Pi (Cortex Lycii Radicis)
Jin Yin Hua (Flos Lonicerae)
Mai Men Dong (Radix Ophiopogonis Japonici)
Nan Sha Shen (Radix Adenophorae)
Pu Gong Ying (Herba Taraxaci cum Radice)
Sheng Di Huang (Radix Rehmanniae Glutinosae)
*Shi Hu** (Herba Dendrobii)
Tian Men Dong (Radix Asparagi Cochinchinensis)
*Xi Yang Shen** (Radix Panacis Quinquefolii)
Xuan Shen (Radix Scrophulariae Ningpoensis)

KILLING WORMS TO ALLEVIATE ITCHING

Internal use of materia medica for expelling or killing Worms is only effective on intestinal parasites such as roundworm, pinworm and tapeworm.

Treatment principle
Killing Worms and alleviating itching

Commonly used prescription
Wu Mei Wan (Black Plum Pill)

Commonly used materia medica
*Bing Lang** (Semen Arecae Catechu)
Fei Zi (Semen Torreyae Grandis)
Lei Wan (Sclerotium Omphaliae Lapidescens)
Nan Gua Zi (Semen Cucurbitae Moschatae)
Shi Jun Zi (Fructus Quisqualis Indicae)

In addition, certain materia medica can be used externally to kill Worms and alleviate itching:

Ban Mao ‡ (Mylabris)
Chan Su ‡ (Venenum Bufonis)
Da Feng Zi (Semen Hydnocarpi)
Ku Fan ‡ (Alumen Praeparatum)
Li Lu (Radix et Rhizoma Veratri)
Liu Huang ‡ (Sulphur)
*Lu Hui** (Herba Aloes)
Mu Jin Pi (Cortex Hibisci Syriaci Radicis)
She Chuang Zi (Fructus Cnidii Monnieri)
Wu Gong ‡ (Scolopendra Subspinipes)

DISPERSING FOOD ACCUMULATION TO ALLEVIATE ITCHING

Itching can also be provoked by overindulgence in food such as fish, shellfish and other seafood, which are likely to stir Wind and impair the Stomach's digestive function.

Treatment principle
Disperse food accumulation and guide out stagnation.

Commonly used prescription
Bao He Wan (Preserving Harmony Pill)

Commonly used materia medica
Chen Pi (Pericarpium Citri Reticulatae)
Da Huang (Radix et Rhizoma Rhei)
Gu Ya (Fructus Setariae Italicae Germinatus)
Hu Huang Lian (Rhizoma Picrorhizae Scrophulariiflorae)
Ji Nei Jin ‡ (Endothelium Corneum Gigeriae Galli)
Mai Ya (Fructus Hordei Vulgaris Germinatus)
*Mu Xiang** (Radix Aucklandiae Lappae)
Pu Gong Ying (Herba Taraxaci cum Radice)
Shan Zha (Fructus Crataegi)
Shen Qu (Massa Fermentata)
Wu Yao (Radix Linderae Strychnifoliae)
Zi Su Ye (Folium Perillae Frutescentis)

DISPELLING THE EFFECTS OF ALCOHOL TO ALLEVIATE ITCHING

In *Pi Wei Lun* [A Treatise on the Spleen and Stomach], Li Gao said, "Alcohol is an invisible toxic substance that produces great heat." After drinking alcohol, especially after excess consumption of alcohol, Damp-Heat Toxins will accumulate in the Intestines and Stomach.

Treatment principle
Dispel the effects of alcohol by promoting urination.

Commonly used prescription
Ge Hua Jie Cheng Tang (Kudzu Flower Decoction for Resolving the Effects of Alcohol)

Commonly used materia medica
There are two means of relieving alcohol Toxicity by eliminating Dampness:

- Relief of alcohol Toxicity through the skin

Bai Bian Dou (Semen Dolichoris Lablab)
Bai Dou Kou (Fructus Amomi Kravanh)
Ding Xiang (Flos Caryophylli)
Gao Liang Jiang (Rhizoma Alpiniae Officinari)
Ge Hua (Flos Puerariae)
Rou Dou Kou (Semen Myristicae Fragrantis)
Sang Shen (Fructus Mori Albae)
Sha Ren (Fructus Amomi)
Shan Zha (Fructus Crataegi)
Wei Cao Guo (Fructus Tsaoko, roasted in fresh cinders)
Xi He Liu (Cacumen Tamaricis)

- Relief of alcohol Toxicity through urination

Bai Mao Gen (Rhizoma Imperatae Cylindricae)
Dan Zhu Ye (Herba Lophatheri Gracilis)
Fu Ling (Sclerotium Poriae Cocos)
Ze Xie (Rhizoma Alismatis Orientalis)
Zhu Ling (Sclerotium Polypori Umbellati)

OTHER MATERIA MEDICA FOR ALLEVIATING ITCHING

Books on Chinese materia medica down the ages indicate that materia medica derived from insects or from animals with scales or shells have the functions of clearing Heat and relieving Toxicity, extinguishing Wind and alleviating itching. Examples include *Ling Yang Jiao** (Cornu Antelopis), *Quan Xie* ‡ (Buthus Martensi), *Wu Gong* ‡ (Scolopendra Subspinipes), *Jiang Can* ‡ (Bombyx Batryticatus), *Feng Fang* ‡ (Nidus Vespae), *Wu Shao She* ‡ (Zaocys Dhumnades), *Qi She* ‡ (Agkistrodon), *Gui Ban** (Plastrum Testudinis), *Bie Jia** (Carapax Amydae Sinensis), and *Shui Zhi* ‡ (Hirudo seu Whitmania).

Clinical practice indicates that proper use of these materia medica can bring very good results, especially for chronic itching due to Wind Toxins. However, some patients may find that their itching is getting worse after internal use or external application of these ingredients. Therefore, prior to treatment, patients should be asked whether they have ever had a skin reaction after eating food such as fish, shellfish or chicken. Then ask whether in the past they have used materia medica derived from insects or from animals with scales or shells and whether there were any side-effects. Start the treatment with a small dose at the first visit and monitor results.

REGULATING DAMPNESS

When Dampness is severe, it should be dried or transformed, whereas mild manifestations of Dampness should be percolated or eliminated through urination. Persistent exudation may result in damage to Yin and consumption of Blood. It is also necessary to enrich Yin and eliminate Dampness.

FORTIFYING THE SPLEEN AND TRANSFORMING DAMPNESS

Clinical manifestations

Flooding of Dampness due to impairment of the functions of the Spleen manifests as papulovesicles, vesicles and exudation; the skin does not turn red and fever is not apparent.

Accompanying symptoms and signs

Poor appetite, oppression in the epigastric region, loose stools, and abdominal distension. The tongue body is pale with a thick and greasy coating; the pulse is soggy.

Treatment principle

Fortify the Spleen and transform Dampness.

Commonly used prescriptions

Chu Shi Wei Ling Tang (Poria Five Decoction for Eliminating Dampness and Calming the Stomach)

Xiang Ju Dan (Tangerine Peel and Cyperus Special Pill)

Commonly used materia medica

Bai Zhu (Rhizoma Atractylodis Macrocephalae)

Chao Bai Bian Dou (Semen Dolichoris Lablab, stir-fried)

Chen Pi (Pericarpium Citri Reticulatae)

Lian Zi (Semen Nelumbinis Nuciferae)

Qian Shi (Semen Euryales Ferocis)

Shan Yao (Rhizoma Dioscoreae Oppositae)

Ze Xie (Rhizoma Alismatis Orientalis)

CLEARING HEAT AND BENEFITING THE MOVEMENT OF DAMPNESS

Clinical manifestations

When Dampness and Heat are severe and spread all over the body, an acute condition will result, manifesting as erythema, vesicles, papulovesicles, exudation, severe erosion, and orange scabs. The main areas involved include the lower limbs, scrotum, vulva, anus, and the webs between the toes.

Accompanying symptoms and signs

Severe itching, constipation, and dry mouth and tongue. The tongue body is red with a yellow and greasy coating; the pulse is slippery.

Treatment principle

Clear Heat and benefit the elimination of Dampness.

Commonly used prescription

Long Dan Xie Gan Tang (Chinese Gentian Decoction for Draining the Liver)

This formula is usually modified by the addition of other ingredients such as *Bi Xie* (Rhizoma Dioscoreae Hypoglaucae seu Septemlobae), *Chi Fu Ling* (Sclerotium Poriae Cocos Rubrae), *Hua Shi* ‡ (Talcum), *Chi Xiao Dou* (Semen Phaseoli Calcarati), *Huang Bai* (Cortex Phellodendri), and *Bai Mao Gen* (Rhizoma Imperatae Cylindricae).

DISPELLING WIND AND DRYING DAMPNESS

Clinical manifestations

When Wind and Dampness combine to invade the skin and interstices (*cou li*), manifestations include thickened and lichenified skin, and intense itching; the disease tends to follow a protracted course. The tongue body is pale with a white coating; the pulse is wiry.

Treatment principle

Dispel Wind and dry Dampness.

Commonly used prescriptions

Cang Zhu Gao (Concentrated Atractylodes Syrup)

Chu Shi Wan (Pill for Eliminating Dampness)

Commonly used materia medica

Bai Xian Pi (Cortex Dictamni Dasycarpi Radicis)

Can Sha ‡ (Excrementum Bombycis Mori)

Cang Er Zi (Fructus Xanthii Sibirici)

Cang Zhu (Rhizoma Atractylodis)

Chen Pi (Pericarpium Citri Reticulatae)

Chi Shi Zhi ‡ (Halloysitum Rubrum)

Di Fu Zi (Fructus Kochiae Scopariae)

Hou Po (Cortex Magnoliae Officinalis)

Ku Shen (Radix Sophorae Flavescentis)

Wang Bu Liu Xing (Semen Vaccariae Segetalis)

Zhi Ke (Fructus Citri Aurantii)

ENRICHING YIN AND ELIMINATING DAMPNESS

Clinical manifestations

Persistent exudation damages Yin and consumes Body Fluids, eventually resulting in dry skin or desquamation. Yin and Body Fluids can also be depleted by long-term use of ingredients for benefiting the elimination of Dampness by bland percolation or bitter and cold materia medica for drying Dampness.

Accompanying symptoms and signs

A sensation of heat in the palms, soles and chest, dry mouth with a desire for drinks, and dry stools. The tongue body is red with a scant coating; the pulse is thready.

Treatment principle

Enrich Yin and eliminate Dampness.

Commonly used prescription

Zi Yin Chu Shi Tang (Decoction for Enriching Yin and Eliminating Dampness)

Commonly used materia medica

Bai Xian Pi (Cortex Dictamni Dasycarpi Radicis)

Dan Shen (Radix Salviae Miltiorrhizae)

Dang Gui (Radix Angelicae Sinensis)

Fu Ling (Sclerotium Poriae Cocos)

Mu Dan Pi (Cortex Moutan Radicis)
Nan Sha Shen (Radix Adenophorae)
She Chuang Zi (Fructus Cnidii Monnieri)
Sheng Di Huang (Radix Rehmanniae Glutinosae)
Xuan Shen (Radix Scrophulariae Ningpoensis)
Yi Yi Ren (Semen Coicis Lachryma-jobi)
Ze Xie (Rhizoma Alismatis Orientalis)

RELIEVING TOXICITY

Heat Toxins invading the body result in the four main symptoms of redness, swelling, heat, and pain. As the disease evolves, Heat destroys the flesh to form abscesses. Under normal circumstances, Blood-Heat should be treated by cooling the Blood and relieving Toxicity; Heat Toxins by clearing Heat and relieving Toxicity; Heat Toxins entering the Ying level by clearing Heat from the Ying level and relieving Toxicity; and Heat Toxins damaging Yin by increasing Body Fluids and relieving Toxicity.

COOLING THE BLOOD TO RELIEVE TOXICITY
Clinical manifestations
Intense Heat in the Blood is characterized by bright red, inflamed skin which feels as though it is burning; lesions manifest as papules and erythema.

Accompanying symptoms and signs
Delirious speech, irritability and restlessness, dry stools, and yellow or reddish urine. The tongue body is crimson with a scant coating; the pulse is slippery.

Treatment principle
Cool the Blood and relieve Toxicity.

Commonly used prescriptions
Xi Jiao Di Huang Tang (Rhinoceros Horn and Rehmannia Decoction)
Liang Xue Si Wu Tang (Four Agents Decoction for Cooling the Blood)

Commonly used materia medica
Bai Mao Gen (Rhizoma Imperatae Cylindricae)
Chi Shao (Radix Paeoniae Rubra)
Hong Hua (Flos Carthami Tinctorii)
Ling Xiao Hua (Flos Campsitis)
Mu Dan Pi (Cortex Moutan Radicis)
Sheng Di Huang (Radix Rehmanniae Glutinosae)
Zi Cao (Radix Arnebiae seu Lithospermi)

CLEARING HEAT TO RELIEVE TOXICITY
Clinical manifestations
Heat Toxins invading the skin manifest as reddening of the skin, swelling, a sensation of heat in the skin, pain, and protruding blisters with deep, solid roots. Patients usually have a robust constitution.

Accompanying symptoms and signs
Thirst with a desire for drinks, short voidings of reddish urine, and dry stools. The tongue body is red with a yellow coating; the pulse is surging and rapid.

Treatment principle
Clear Heat and relieve Toxicity.

Commonly used prescriptions
Wu Wei Xiao Du Yin (Five-Ingredient Beverage for Dispersing Toxicity)
Ye Ju Bai Du Tang (Wild Chrysanthemum Decoction for Vanquishing Toxicity)

Commonly used materia medica
Bai Hua She She Cao (Herba Hedyotidis Diffusae)
Bai Xian Pi (Cortex Dictamni Dasycarpi Radicis)
Ban Lan Gen (Radix Isatidis seu Baphicacanthi)
Chong Lou (Rhizoma Paridis)
Huang Bai (Cortex Phellodendri)
Huang Lian (Rhizoma Coptidis)
Huang Qin (Radix Scutellariae Baicalensis)
Jiao Zhi Zi (Fructus Gardeniae Jasminoidis, scorch-fried)
Jin Yin Hua (Flos Lonicerae)
Lian Qiao (Fructus Forsythiae Suspensae)
Lü Dou (Semen Phaseoli Radiati)
Niu Huang‡ (Calculus Bovis)
Pu Gong Ying (Herba Taraxaci cum Radice)
Qing Dai (Indigo Naturalis)
Sheng Ma (Rhizoma Cimicifugae)
Ye Ju Hua (Flos Chrysanthemi Indici)
Zhi Mu (Rhizoma Anemarrhenae Asphodeloidis)
Zi Hua Di Ding (Herba Violae Yedoensitis)

CLEARING HEAT FROM THE YING LEVEL AND RELIEVING TOXICITY
Clinical manifestations
Drug poisoning in the interior or Heat Toxins entering the Ying level manifest as large patches of erythema, inflammation and swelling.

Accompanying symptoms and signs
Persistent raging fever with convulsions, delirium and mania in severe cases. The tongue body is red with a scant coating; the pulse is thready and rapid.

Treatment principle
Clear Heat from the Ying level and relieve Toxicity.

Commonly used prescriptions
Qing Ying Tang (Decoction for Clearing Heat from the Ying Level)
Qing Gong Tang (Clearing the Palace Decoction)

Commonly used materia medica
Chi Shao (Radix Paeoniae Rubra)
Dan Zhu Ye (Herba Lophatheri Gracilis)

Han Shui Shi‡ (Calcitum)
Hu Po‡ (Succinum)
Jin Yin Hua (Flos Lonicerae)
Lian Qiao (Semen Forsythiae Suspensae)
Lian Zi Xin (Plumula Nelumbinis Nuciferae)
Lü Dou Yi (Testa Phaseoli Radiati)
Mai Men Dong (Radix Ophiopogonis Japonici)
Mu Dan Pi (Cortex Moutan Radicis)
Sheng Di Huang (Radix Rehmanniae Glutinosae)
Shi Gao‡ (Gypsum Fibrosum)
Xuan Shen (Radix Scrophulariae Ningpoensis)

INCREASING BODY FLUIDS AND RELIEVING TOXICITY
Clinical manifestations
When Heat Toxins enter the Ying level, they damage Yin and consume Body Fluids, leading to manifestations such as a sensation of burning heat on the skin and large patches of exfoliation, or bullae, severe erosion and fragile scabs.

Accompanying symptoms and signs
Fever, shortness of breath, fatigue, a faint and low voice, or unconsciousness in severe cases. The tongue body is red with a peeling coating; the pulse is thready and rapid.

Treatment principle
Increase Body Fluids and relieve Toxicity.

Commonly used prescription
Zeng Ye Jie Du Tang (Decoction for Increasing Body Fluids and Relieving Toxicity)

Commonly used materia medica
*Bie Jia** (Carapax Amydae Sinensis)
Chi Shao (Radix Paeoniae Rubra)
Gan Cao (Radix Glycyrrhizae)
Han Shui Shi‡ (Calcitum)
Hu Po‡ (Succinum)
Jin Yin Hua (Flos Lonicerae)
Lian Qiao (Fructus Forsythiae Suspensae)
*Ling Yang Jiao** (Cornu Antelopis)
Mai Men Dong (Radix Ophiopogonis Japonici)
Nan Sha Shen (Radix Adenophorae)
Sheng Di Huang (Radix Rehmanniae Glutinosae)
*Shi Hu** (Herba Dendrobii)
Shui Niu Jiao‡ (Cornu Bubali)
Tian Hua Fen (Radix Trichosanthis)
Xuan Shen (Radix Scrophulariae Ningpoensis)

REGULATING THE BLOOD
The Xue level is involved when there are manifestations such as erythema, nodules or blockage of the sweat pores. When regulating the Blood, a distinction must be made between materia medica for cooling the Blood,

invigorating the Blood and breaking up Blood stasis. It is nevertheless essential to remember the principle that "Qi is the commander of Blood; when Qi moves, Blood moves." The addition of materia medica for regulating Qi increases the effectiveness of materia medica for regulating the Blood.

COOLING THE BLOOD
Clinical manifestations
Erythema, which may coalesce into patches; in severe cases, erythroderma may develop.

Accompanying symptoms and signs
Fever and severe pruritus. The tongue body is red with a thin and white coating; the pulse is rapid.

Treatment principle
Cool the Blood and reduce erythema.

Commonly used prescription
Liang Xue Wu Gen Tang (Five Root Decoction for Cooling the Blood)

Commonly used materia medica
Bai Mao Gen (Rhizoma Imperatae Cylindricae)
Chi Shao (Radix Paeoniae Rubra)
Huai Hua (Flos Sophorae Japonicae)
Ling Xiao Hua (Flos Campsitis)
Mu Dan Pi (Cortex Moutan Radicis)
Qian Cao Gen (Radix Rubiae Cordifoliae)
Sheng Di Huang (Radix Rehmanniae Glutinosae)
Zi Cao (Radix Arnebiae seu Lithospermi)

INVIGORATING THE BLOOD
Clinical manifestations
Qi stagnation and Blood stasis obstruct the channels and network vessels, resulting in manifestations such as red or dark red skin, palpable nodules and lumps between the skin and membranes, and obvious tenderness.

Accompanying symptoms and signs
Pain in a fixed location or painful menstruation with large amounts of blood clots. The tongue body is dark with a white coating; the pulse is rough.

Treatment principle
Regulate Qi and invigorate the Blood.

Commonly used prescriptions
Xue Fu Zhu Yu Tang (Decoction for Expelling Stasis from the House of Blood)
Tong Jing Zhu Yu Tang (Decoction for Freeing the Channels and Expelling Blood Stasis)

Commonly used materia medica
Chi Shao (Radix Paeoniae Rubra)
Chuan Lian Zi (Fructus Meliae Toosendan)
Chuan Xiong (Rhizoma Ligustici Chuanxiong)

Dang Gui (Radix Angelicae Sinensis)
Hong Hua (Flos Carthami Tinctorii)
Ji Xue Teng (Caulis Spatholobi)
Jiu Zhi Da Huang (Radix et Rhizoma Rhei, processed with wine)
Mo Yao (Myrrha)
Qing Pi (Pericarpium Citri Reticulatae Viride)
Ru Xiang (Gummi Olibanum)
Wu Ling Zhi‡ (Excrementum Trogopteri)
Xiang Fu (Rhizoma Cyperi Rotundi)
Yan Hu Suo (Rhizoma Corydalis Yanhusuo)
Yu Jin (Radix Curcumae)

BREAKING UP BLOOD STASIS
Clinical manifestations
Blood stasis obstructing the channels and network vessels prevents the generation of new Blood, resulting in manifestations such as large, firm nodules that require a long time to disperse and dark red or normal-colored skin; other manifestations may include alopecia areata or stubborn urticaria.

Accompanying symptoms and signs
Pain in a fixed location or painful menstruation with large amounts of blood clots. The tongue body is dark with a white coating; the pulse is rough.

Treatment principle
Break up Blood stasis and free the network vessels.

Commonly used prescription
Da Huang Zhe Chong Wan (Rhubarb and Wingless Cockroach Pill)

Commonly used materia medica
Chuan Xiong (Rhizoma Ligustici Chuanxiong)
E Zhu (Rhizoma Curcumae)
Hong Hua (Flos Carthami Tinctorii)
Jiu Zhi Da Huang (Radix et Rhizoma Rhei, processed with wine)
San Leng (Rhizoma Sparganii Stoloniferi)
*She Xiang** (Secretio Moschi)
Shui Zhi‡ (Hirudo seu Whitmania)
Su Mu (Lignum Sappan)
Tao Ren (Semen Persicae)
Tu Bie Chong‡ (Eupolyphaga seu Steleophaga)

SUPPLEMENTING AND NOURISHING
This method aims to nourish and supplement Deficiency. It is often used in the later stages of diseases, when Deficiency is pronounced. Although Qi, Blood, Yin, or Yang Deficiency patterns may be involved, the general principle for supplementing Deficiency should always be borne in mind: "Employ sweet and warm materia medica for supplementation in Yang Deficiency patterns with Cold symptoms and signs; employ sweet and cool materia medica for supplementation in Yin Deficiency patterns with Heat symptoms and signs."

Supplementation methods include neutral supplementation, drastic supplementation, augmenting Qi, augmenting the Essence, nourishing the Blood vessels, strengthening the sinews and bones, nourishing the beard and hair, and keeping a healthy appearance. All types of debilitation, damage and Deficiency should be treated by supplementing methods, which function to supplement Qi and nourish the Blood, strengthen the body's energy, eliminate Deficiency and restore health.

When using supplementing materia medica, the relationship between Yin and Yang must always be borne in mind. In *Jing Yue Quan Shu* [The Complete Works of Zhang Jingyue], the author wrote: "When supplementing Yang, look for the Yin within Yang. Yang will then be assisted by Yin and can grow without limits. When supplementing Yin, look for the Yang within Yin. Yin will then increase with the assistance of Yang, and its source will never be exhausted."

SUPPORTING YANG
Clinical manifestations
Patterns of insufficiency of Yang Qi and a tendency towards prevalence of Yin-Cold are characterized by manifestations such as flat or sunken white sores, slowly evolving to form abscesses, which are difficult to heal after ulceration; further manifestations may include cold pale or bluish-purple extremities.

Accompanying symptoms and signs
Mental fatigue, aversion to cold, poor appetite, seminal emission, profuse vaginal discharge, loose stools, aching in the lower back, and limpness of the knees. The tongue body is pale with a white coating; the pulse is deep.

Treatment principle
Support Yang and dissipate Cold.

Commonly used prescriptions
- For predominance of Kidney Yang Deficiency, *Gui Fu Ba Wei Tang* (Cinnamon Bark and Aconite Eight-Ingredient Decoction)
- For predominance of Spleen Yang Deficiency, *Tuo Li Wen Zhong Tang* (Decoction for Drawing Toxins from the Interior and Warming the Middle)

Commonly used materia medica
Du Zhong (Cortex Eucommiae Ulmoidis)
*Fu Zi** (Radix Lateralis Aconiti Carmichaeli Praeparata)
Gan Jiang (Rhizoma Zingiberis Officinalis)
Ge Jie‡ (Gekko)
Gui Zhi (Ramulus Cinnamomi Cassiae)
Hu Tao Ren (Semen Juglandis Regiae)
Huang Qi (Radix Astragali seu Hedysari)
Lu Rong‡ (Cornu Cervi Parvum)

Rou Cong Rong (Herba Cistanches Deserticolae)
Rou Gui (Cortex Cinnamomi Cassiae)
Shan Zhu Yu (Fructus Corni Officinalis)
Tu Si Zi (Semen Cuscutae)
Wu Wei Zi (Fructus Schisandrae)
Wu Zhu Yu (Fructus Evodiae Rutaecarpae)
Yang Qi Shi‡ (Actinolitum)
Yin Yang Huo (Herba Epimedii)
Zi He Che‡ (Placenta Hominis)

ENRICHING (OR SUPPLEMENTING) YIN
Clinical manifestations
Yin Deficiency results in undernourishment of the skin leading to dry skin with scaling or desquamation accompanied by small amounts of exudation.

Accompanying symptoms and signs
Patterns of effulgent Yin Deficiency-Fire or constitutional insufficiency of Yin-Liquids are characterized by a dark and lusterless or haggard complexion, emaciation, low-grade fever, dry eyes, tidal fever, night sweating, dry cough, constipation due to lack of Body Fluids, blurred vision, tinnitus, dry mouth and throat, and limpness and aching of the lower back and knees. The tongue body is red with a scant coating; the pulse is thready.

Treatment principle
Enrich Yin and bear Fire downward.

Commonly used prescription
Liu Wei Di Huang Tang (Six-Ingredient Rehmannia Decoction)

Commonly used materia medica
Bai He (Bulbus Lilii)
Bie Jia* (Carapax Amydae Sinensis)
Dong Chong Xia Cao‡ (Cordyceps Sinensis)
Gou Qi Zi (Fructus Lycii)
Gui Ban* (Plastrum Testudinis)
Huang Jing (Rhizoma Polygonati)
Mai Men Dong (Radix Ophiopogonis Japonici)
Mu Dan Pi (Cortex Moutan Radicis)
Nan Sha Shen (Radix Adenophorae)
Nü Zhen Zi (Fructus Ligustri Lucidi)
Shi Hu* (Herba Dendrobii)
Shu Di Huang (Radix Rehmanniae Glutinosae Conquita)
Tian Men Dong (Radix Asparagi Cochinchinensis)
Xi Yang Shen* (Radix Panacis Quinquefolii)

Generally speaking, materia medica for enriching Yin are heavy and cloying. Where they are used, care should be taken to protect the Stomach and Spleen in order to avoid poor appetite and abdominal distension. To prevent further pathological changes, these materia medica should also be used with caution or not at all in cases of Yang Deficiency or predominance of Damp-Phlegm.

SUPPLEMENTING QI
Clinical manifestations
When Qi is Deficient, it is difficult to drive Toxins out through the exterior. The method of supplementing Qi is especially suitable for patients with chronic diseases with erosion of the skin or persistent, severe, non-healing ulcers.

Accompanying symptoms and signs
Pale complexion, lack of strength in the limbs, reduced appetite, loose stools, shortness of breath, reluctance to talk, lassitude, somnolence, dizziness and vertigo, blurred vision, thin clear exudate from abscesses, and non-healing sores. The tongue body is pale with a white coating; the pulse is weak.

Treatment principle
Supplement Qi.

Commonly used prescription
Si Jun Zi Tang (Four Gentlemen Decoction)

Commonly used materia medica
Bai Zhu (Rhizoma Atractylodis Macrocephalae)
Da Zao (Fructus Ziziphi Jujubae)
Dang Shen (Radix Codonopsitis Pilosulae)
Fu Ling (Sclerotium Poriae Cocos)
Huang Qi (Radix Astragali seu Hedysari)
Ren Shen (Radix Ginseng)
Shan Yao (Rhizoma Dioscoreae Oppositae)
Tai Zi Shen (Radix Pseudostellariae Heterophyllae)
Zhi Gan Cao (Radix Glycyrrhizae, mix-fried with honey)

SUPPLEMENTING THE BLOOD
Clinical manifestations
Blood Deficiency results externally in undernourishment of the skin, manifesting as dry skin and itching, and internally in disturbance of the Heart and Spirit, manifesting as palpitations, forgetfulness and insomnia.

Accompanying symptoms and signs
If Heat Toxins cause the frenetic movement of Blood, this can lead to symptoms such as spontaneous bleeding, blood in the urine and blood in the stool. The tongue body is pale with a thin white coating; the pulse is thready.

Treatment principle
Supplement the Blood.

Commonly used prescription
Si Wu Tang (Four Agents Decoction)

Commonly used materia medica
Bai Shao (Radix Paeoniae Lactiflorae)
Dang Gui (Radix Angelicae Sinensis)
E Jiao‡ (Gelatinum Corii Asini)
Gui Ban Jiao* (Gelatinum Plastri Testudinis)

He Shou Wu (Radix Polygoni Multiflori)
Ji Xue Teng (Caulis Spatholobi)
Long Yan Rou (Arillus Euphoriae Longanae)
Sang Shen (Fructus Mori Albae)
Shu Di Huang (Radix Rehmanniae Glutinosae Conquita)

As a general rule, supplementing preparations should not be used when pathogenic factors are exuberant but Vital Qi (Zheng Qi) has not yet become Deficient, otherwise they may strengthen the pathogenic factors. Nor should they be applied in cases of reduced appetite and poor digestion or Spleen and Stomach Deficiency. In such instances, the first step is to fortify the Spleen and harmonize the Stomach. Where Toxic pathogenic factors have not been completely eliminated, priority should be given to clearing these factors and relieving residual Toxicity while supplementing. This will prevent residual pathogenic factors from lingering or flaring up again.

SOFTENING HARDNESS
Clinical manifestations
Phlegm congealing into lumps causes obstruction of the channels and network vessels, leading to such manifestations as subcutaneous nodules or lumps with normal-colored or pale red skin, a sensation of mild heat in the lesion area and occasional stabbing pain.

Accompanying symptoms and signs
Distension in the stomach, oppression in the chest, shortness of breath, and poor appetite. The tongue body is dark with a white and greasy coating; the pulse is wiry and rough.

Treatment principle
Harmonize the Ying level and soften hardness.

Commonly used prescriptions
Xiang Bei Yang Rong Tang (Cyperus and Fritillaria Decoction for Nourishing Ying Qi)
Xiao Li Wan (Dispersing Scrofula Pill)

Commonly used materia medica
Bai Yao Zi (Tuber Stephaniae Cepharanthae)
Chen Pi (Pericarpium Citri Reticulatae)
Fu Ling (Sclerotium Poriae Cocos)
Hai Zao (Herba Sargassi)
Huang Yao Zi (Rhizoma Dioscoreae Bulbiferae)
Jiang Ban Xia (Rhizoma Pinelliae Ternatae, processed with ginger)
Kun Bu (Thallus Laminariae seu Eckloniae)
Mu Li‡ (Concha Ostreae)
Qing Pi (Pericarpium Citri Reticulatae Viride)
Shan Ci Gu (Pseudobulbus Shancigu)
Xia Ku Cao (Spica Prunellae Vulgaris)
Xiang Fu (Rhizoma Cyperi Rotundi)
Xuan Shen (Radix Scrophulariae Ningpoensis)

Zhe Bei Mu (Bulbus Fritillariae Thunbergii)

HARMONIZING AND REGULATING
This is a general term covering treatment methods for harmonizing Shaoyang, regulating and freeing the movement of Qi, regulating and harmonizing the Ying and Wei levels, and regulating the functions of the Zang-Fu organs. It includes methods for harmonizing Shaoyang, regulating and harmonizing the Ying and Wei levels, regulating and harmonizing the Liver and Spleen, and regulating and harmonizing the Intestines and Stomach.

HARMONIZING SHAOYANG
This method is mainly applied where Shaoyang functions are inhibited due to pathogenic factors invading the Gallbladder (Shaoyang) channel.

• Pathogenic factors transmitted from the exterior to the interior

Clinical manifestations
Itchy skin and intermittent wheals.

Accompanying symptoms and signs
Distension in the hypochondrium, dizziness, a bitter taste in the mouth, poor appetite, and dry throat. The tongue body is pale red with a thin white coating; the pulse is wiry.

Treatment principle
Harmonize Shaoyang.

Commonly used prescription
Xiao Chai Hu Tang (Minor Bupleurum Decoction)

Commonly used materia medica
Bai Mei Hua (Flos Mume Albus)
Chai Hu (Radix Bupleuri)
Chao Gu Ya (Fructus Setariae Italicae Germinatus, stir-fried)
Chao Mai Ya (Fructus Hordei Vulgaris Germinatus, stir-fried)
Huang Qin (Radix Scutellariae Baicalensis)
Jing Jie (Herba Schizonepetae Tenuifoliae)
Mei Gui Hua (Flos Rosae Rugosae)
Qing Hao (Herba Artemisiae Chinghao)
Yu Jin (Radix Curcumae)

• Retention of Summerheat in the Shaoyang channel accompanied by Phlegm-Damp

Clinical manifestations
Pale red papules or maculopapules appearing intermittently throughout the body, but more frequently in the antecubital and popliteal fossae, axillae and neck.

Accompanying symptoms and signs
Malaria-like alternating fever and chills with fever predominant, acid regurgitation and vomiting of bitter fluids, or vomiting of sticky, yellow phlegm. The tongue body is red with a yellow and greasy coating; the pulse is soggy.

Treatment principle
Harmonize Shaoyang, clear Summerheat and eliminate Dampness.

Commonly used prescription
Hao Qin Qing Dan Tang (Sweet Wormwood and Scutellaria Decoction for Clearing the Gallbladder)

Commonly used materia medica
Chen Pi (Pericarpium Citri Reticulatae)
Chi Fu Ling (Sclerotium Poriae Cocos Rubrae)
Fa Ban Xia (Rhizoma Pinelliae Ternatae Praeparata)
Gan Cao (Radix Glycyrrhizae)
Hua Shi‡ (Talcum)
Huang Qin (Radix Scutellariae Baicalensis)
Qing Dai (Indigo Naturalis)
Qing Hao (Herba Artemisiae Chinghao)
Zhi Ke (Fructus Citri Aurantii)
Zhu Ru (Caulis Bambusae in Taeniis)

REGULATING AND HARMONIZING THE YING AND WEI LEVELS

Clinical manifestations
Ying Qi moves inside the vessels, whereas Wei Qi moves outside the vessels. Manifestations of disharmony include itchy skin or obvious aggravation of wheals.

Accompanying symptoms and signs
Aversion to wind, occasional fever and profuse sweating. The tongue body is pale red with a thin white coating; the pulse is floating.

Treatment principle
Dispel Wind and dissipate Cold, regulate and harmonize the Ying and Wei levels.

Commonly used prescription
Gui Zhi Tang (Cinnamon Twig Decoction)

Commonly used materia medica
Bai Shao (Radix Paeoniae Lactiflorae)
Da Zao (Fructus Ziziphi Jujubae)
Gan Cao (Radix Glycyrrhizae)
Gui Zhi (Ramulus Cinnamomi Cassiae)
Sheng Jiang (Rhizoma Zingiberis Officinalis Recens)

REGULATING AND HARMONIZING THE LIVER AND SPLEEN

This method is suitable for patterns of binding Depression of Liver Qi leading to the Liver overwhelming the Spleen or patterns of Spleen Deficiency leading to impairment of the transportation function resulting in restrictions on the smooth flow of Liver Qi.

Clinical manifestations
Itching made worse by anxiety, with lichenification.

Accompanying symptoms and signs
Pain in the hypochondrium, depression, poor appetite, abdominal distension, irregular bowel movements, and cold limbs. The tongue body is pale red with a thin white coating; the pulse is wiry.

Treatment principle
Dredge the Liver and harmonize the Stomach, regulate Qi and dissipate lumps.

Commonly used prescription
Xiao Yao San (Free Wanderer Powder)

Commonly used materia medica
Bai Shao (Radix Paeoniae Lactiflorae)
Bai Zhu (Rhizoma Atractylodis Macrocephalae)
Chai Hu (Radix Bupleuri)
Chen Pi (Pericarpium Citri Reticulatae)
Dang Gui (Radix Angelicae Sinensis)
Fu Ling (Sclerotium Poriae Cocos)
Gan Cao (Radix Glycyrrhizae)
Xiang Fu (Rhizoma Cyperi Rotundi)
Zhi Ke (Fructus Citri Aurantii)

REGULATING AND HARMONIZING THE INTESTINES AND STOMACH

This method is suitable for patterns caused by pathogenic factors invading the Intestines and Stomach and presenting as Cold-Heat and Deficiency-Excess complexes and abnormality of both upward-bearing and downward-bearing functions.

Clinical manifestations
Urticaria may be an accompanying symptom for this pattern. If abdominal pain is severe, patches of red wheals may appear all over the body. These wheals usually disappear after the abdominal pain is alleviated.

Accompanying symptoms and signs
Pain or discomfort in the epigastric region or dry retching, nausea and vomiting, borborygmus, and diarrhea. The tongue body is pale red with a thin, yellow and greasy coating; the pulse is wiry and rapid.

Treatment principle
Open with acridity and bear downward with bitterness, regulate and harmonize the functional activities of Qi.

Commonly used prescription
Ban Xia Xie Xin Tang (Pinellia Decoction for Draining the Heart)

Commonly used materia medica
Da Zao (Fructus Ziziphi Jujubae)
Fa Ban Xia (Rhizoma Pinelliae Ternatae Praeparata)
Gan Jiang (Rhizoma Zingiberis Officinalis)
Huang Lian (Rhizoma Coptidis)
Huang Qin (Radix Scutellariae Baicalensis)

Ren Shen (Radix Ginseng)
Zhi Gan Cao (Radix Glycyrrhizae, mix-fried with honey)

CONSOLIDATING AND ASTRINGING

In skin disorders, this is an important treatment method for preventing loss of Blood by warming the Spleen to contain the Blood. This treatment is given for various bleeding patterns resulting from impairment of the Spleen's function in controlling the Blood due to insufficiency of Spleen Yang.

Clinical manifestations

Petechiae or ecchymoses with dark or pale-colored blood and cold limbs.

Accompanying symptoms and signs

A sallow complexion, fatigue, or poor appetite and loose stools. The tongue body is pale with a white coating; the pulse is deep, thready and forceless.

Treatment principle

Warm the Middle Burner and augment Qi, fortify the Spleen and stop bleeding.

Commonly used prescription

Huang Tu Tang (Yellow Earth Decoction)

Commonly used materia medica

Bai Zhu (Rhizoma Atractylodis Macrocephalae)
Dang Shen (Radix Codonopsitis Pilosulae)
E Jiao‡ (Gelatinum Corii Asini)
*Fu Zi** (Radix Lateralis Aconiti Carmichaeli Praeparata)
Gan Cao (Radix Glycyrrhizae)
Huang Qin (Radix Scutellariae Baicalensis)
Sheng Di Huang (Radix Rehmanniae Glutinosae)
Zao Xin Tu (Terra Flava Usta)

External treatment
外治法

Basic principles for the application of external medications

Evolution of diseases

The evolution of skin diseases and the factors that may influence this evolution must be taken into consideration. These factors include the etiology of the disease, the cold or hot nature of the disease, the patient's constitution, the area the patient originates from or lives in, diet, and personal hygiene.

Generally speaking, for acute diseases, for patients with a weak constitution, or for patients born or living in rainy, warm or hot climates where the interstices (*cou li*) are loose and diseases are more likely to be due to Damp-Heat, mild medications to clear Heat and transform Dampness should be used in order to avoid strongly irritating the skin.

For chronic diseases of a cold nature, for patients with a robust constitution, or for people born or living in cold or dry climates where the interstices (*cou li*) are dense and diseases are more likely to be due to Dryness and Cold, stronger medications can be used to shorten the course of diseases.

Tolerance of and reaction to external medications

Consideration should also be given to the age and gender of patients and the special characteristics of the skin condition in specific regions of the body. The skin on certain parts of the body such as the face, neck, genital region, and the flexor aspects of the limbs is more sensitive to external medications. The skin of infants and small children is much thinner and more delicate than adult skin and absorbs external medication more quickly.

Concentration of medications used

The concentration of external medications is very important in terms of absorption and the form of preparation.

- **Absorption:** Highly concentrated medications, especially those that are toxic, may be over-absorbed by the body through the skin, leading to drug poisoning. Traditionally the use of heavy metals in creams could cause drug poisoning when highly concentrated; however, these are generally no longer used outside China.
- **Form of preparation:** For materia medica used externally, a concentration appropriate to the form of preparation is needed to bring about the desired therapeutic effect. The experiences of both Chinese and Western TCM practitioners suggest that requirements for concentrations of wash preparations (aqueous lotions), wet compress preparations and preparations for steaming and washing are not particularly strict and concentrations can range from less than 40 percent to 100 percent. However, concentrations should be more strictly controlled for

other forms of preparation, ranging from 1 percent to 25 percent for ointments, from 25 percent to 35 percent for medicated pastes, and from 0.5 percent to 1 percent for medicated frost preparations.

As a general principle and for safety reasons, the concentration of external medications should start at a low level and then be increased gradually depending on patients' reactions and tolerance levels.

Types of preparation

External medications come in various forms. The most commonly used forms today include aqueous solutions (for washes, steam-washes, soaks, sitz baths, and wet compresses), powders, suspensions, steeps, tinctures, oils, emulsions, rubs, ointments, dressings, plasters, and fumigations. Each type of preparation has its own particular therapeutic effects, indications and precautions. The correct selection of the form of preparation of a medication will directly influence its therapeutic effectiveness.

Choice of preparation according to characteristics of skin lesions

The type of skin lesion is an important factor in the choice of the type of medication and its preparation. At the acute stage, powders or lotions are generally used for erythema and papules, whereas a wet compress is more effective for vesicles, erosion and exudation; at the subacute stage, oil pastes or ointments are often more effective; and at the chronic stage, ointments or plasters are recommended. Lotions and tinctures can be used for itching without obvious skin lesions. As the patient's condition evolves through a course of treatment, so the preparation used is likely to change.

Correct usage

Even if the preparation and form of medication is correct, the therapeutic result can still be affected if the medication is used wrongly. The practitioner must explain in detail to patients how to use the medication correctly, if necessary demonstrating the procedure to be followed. Practitioners should also make patients aware of possible reactions to the usage of medications. Medications should not be overprescribed, thus preventing waste if the medication is not used or loss of effectiveness if it is stored for too long.

Classification of materia medica for external application

Plant, animal and mineral ingredients can be used externally in the treatment of skin diseases, along with other substances employed as a vehicle (or base) for their application. These ingredients can be classified according to their functions and categories (see Table 2-1).

Substances commonly used as vehicles or bases are listed in Table 2-2.

Forms of medication for external application

AQUEOUS SOLUTION PREPARATIONS

These are liquid preparations with water as the solvent; they do not contain any undissolved powdered solids. These preparations can be divided into two categories – steeps and decoctions.

- Aqueous steeps are prepared by immersing and soaking the ingredients in water so that the ingredients themselves or the soluble elements they contain will dissolve. They can be used with or without filtration of the residues.
- Decoctions for washes are prepared by boiling the ingredients in water so that the ingredients themselves or the soluble elements they contain will dissolve in the liquid.

When preparing these solutions, the following aspects should be borne in mind:

- Materia medica should be cut into pieces or pounded to a coarse powder before decoction, especially those that are difficult to melt or dissolve such as resinous ingredients like *Ru Xiang* (Gummi Olibanum) and *Mo Yao* (Myrrha), or minerals and shells.
- Aromatic and volatile materia medica should only be decocted for a short time so that their active constituents are not lost. Minerals and shells need to be decocted for a long time.
- Materia medica that dissolve easily in water should be put in later than the others, or added to the decoction directly after removal of the residues. *Yang Yi Da Quan* [The Complete Book of External Diseases] records that *Ma Bian Cao* (Herba cum Radice Verbenae), *Li Zhi Cao* (Herba Salviae Plebeiae) and *Pu Gong Ying* (Herba Taraxaci cum Radice) were decocted initially, with *Duan Lü Fan*‡ (Melanteritum Rubrum) being added at the end to prepare an external wash for the treatment of hemorrhoids.
- Washes for the eyes or rinse preparations for the sinuses should be filtered before use in order to get rid of any particles.

Functions of aqueous solutions

Keeping the interstices (*cou li*) free of obstruction, freeing and regulating the Blood vessels, restraining exudation, cleansing lesions, flushing out pus, removing putridity and scales, eliminating bad smells, relieving Toxicity, and alleviating itching to aid healing of superficial lesions.

Table 2-1 Classification of materia medica according to function

---

Materia medica commonly used for alleviating itching

Ai Ye (Folium Artemisiae Argyi), *Bo He* (Herba Menthae Haplocalycis), *Bing Pian* (Borneolum), *Can Sha*‡ (Excrementum Bombycis Mori), *Cang Er Zi* (Fructus Xanthii Sibirici), *Di Fu Zi* (Fructus Kochiae Scopariae), *Ding Xiang* (Flos Caryophylli), *Feng Fang*‡ (Nidus Vespae), *Hua Jiao* (Pericarpium Zanthoxyli), *Jin Qian Cao* (Herba Lysimachiae), *Ku Shen* (Radix Sophorae Flavescentis), *Lu Lu Tong* (Fructus Liquidambaris), *Peng Sha*‡ (Borax), *She Chuang Zi* (Fructus Cnidii Monnieri), *Wei Ling Xian* (Radix Clematidis), *Wu Zhu Yu* (Fructus Evodiae Rutaecarpae), *Xiang Fu* (Rhizoma Cyperi Rotundi), *Yi Mu Cao* (Herba Leonuri Heterophylli), *Zao Jiao Ci* (Spina Gleditsiae Sinensis), and *Zhang Nao* (Camphora).

Materia medica commonly used for clearing Heat

Da Huang (Radix et Rhizoma Rhei), *Da Qing Ye* (Folium Isatidis seu Baphicacanthi), *Er Cha* (Pasta Acaciae seu Uncariae), *Fu Rong Ye* (Folium Hibisci Mutabilis), *Han Shui Shi*‡ (Calcitum), *Hu Zhang* (Radix et Rhizoma Polygoni Cuspidati), *Huang Bai* (Cortex Phellodendri), *Huang Lian* (Rhizoma Coptidis), *Huang Qin* (Radix Scutellariae Baicalensis), *Ma Chi Xian* (Herba Portulacae Oleraceae), *Pu Gong Ying* (Herba Taraxaci cum Radice), *Qing Dai* (Indigo Naturalis), *Zhi Zi* (Fructus Gardeniae Jasminoidis), and *Zi Hua Di Ding* (Herba Violae Yedoensitis).

Materia medica commonly used for absorbing Dampness

Bai Cao Shuang (Fuligo Herbarum Ustarum), *Can Sha*‡ (Excrementum Bombycis Mori), *Cang Zhu* (Rhizoma Atractylodis), *Chi Shi Zhi*‡ (Halloysitum Rubrum), *Duan Long Gu*‡ (Os Draconis Calcinatum), *Duan Mu Li*‡ (Concha Ostreae Calcinata), *Er Cha* (Pasta Acaciae seu Uncariae), *Ge Fen*‡ (Concha Meretricis seu Cyclinae Pulverata), *Hai Piao Xiao*‡ (Os Sepiae seu Sepiellae), *Hua Rui Shi*‡ (Ophicalcitum), *Hua Shi*‡ (Talcum), *Ku Fan*‡ (Alumen Praeparatum), *Lu Gan Shi*‡ (Calamina), *Wu Bei Zi*‡ (Galla Rhois Chinensis), and *Zao Xin Tu* (Terra Flava Usta).

Materia medica commonly used for dissipating Cold

Ai Ye (Folium Artemisiae Argyi), *Bai Fu Zi* (Rhizoma Typhonii Gigantei), *Bai Zhi* (Radix Angelicae Dahuricae), *Cang Er Zi* (Fructus Xanthii Sibirici), *Chan Su*‡ (Venenum Bufonis), *Chen Pi* (Pericarpium Citri Reticulatae), *Chuan Wu** (Radix Aconiti Carmichaeli), *Cong Bai* (Bulbus Allii Fistulosi), *Gan Jiang* (Rhizoma Zingiberis Officinalis), *Jiang Huang* (Rhizoma Curcumae Longae), *Ma Huang** (Herba Ephedrae), *Rou Gui* (Cortex Cinnamomi Cassiae), and *Wu Zhu Yu* (Fructus Evodiae Rutaecarpae).

Materia medica commonly used for moistening the skin

Bai Ji (Rhizoma Bletillae Striatae), *Bi Ma Zi* (Semen Ricini), *Da Feng Zi* (Semen Hydnocarpi), *Dang Gui* (Radix Angelicae Sinensis), *Feng Mi*‡ (Mel), *Gan Cao* (Radix Glycyrrhizae), *Hei Zhi Ma* (Semen Sesami Indici), *Hu Po*‡ (Succinum), *Hu Tao Ren* (Semen Juglandis Regiae), *Lu Hui** (Herba Aloes), *Mi La*‡ (Cera), *Sheng Di Huang* (Radix Rehmanniae Glutinosae), *Suan Zao Ren* (Semen Ziziphi Spinosae), *Tao Ren* (Semen Persicae), *Xing Ren* (Semen Pruni Armeniacae), *Zhen Zhu*‡ (Margarita), and pork lard‡ (*Zhu Zhi*, Adeps Suis).

Materia medica commonly used for generating flesh

Chi Shi Zhi‡ (Halloysitum Rubrum), *Dai Zhe Shi*‡ (Haematitum), *E Jiao*‡ (Gelatinum Corii Asini), *Hu Po*‡ (Succinum), *Hua Rui Shi*‡ (Ophicalcitum), *Mo Yao* (Myrrha), *Ru Xiang* (Gummi Olibanum), *Xue Jie* (Resina Draconis), *Xue Yu Tan*‡ (Crinis Carbonisatus Hominis), *Zhen Zhu*‡ (Margarita).

Materia medica commonly used for stopping bleeding

Bai Ji (Rhizoma Bletillae Striatae), *Ce Bai Ye* (Cacumen Biotae Orientalis), *Di Yu* (Radix Sanguisorbae Officinalis), *Liu Ji Nu* (Herba Artemisiae Anomalae), *Pu Huang* (Pollen Typhae), *San Qi* (Radix Notoginseng), *Shi Hui*‡ (Calx), *Si Gua Tan* (Fasciculus Vascularis Luffae Carbonisatus), *Wu Bei Zi*‡ (Galla Rhois Chinensis), *Xian He Cao* (Herba Agrimoniae Pilosae), *Xue Yu Tan*‡ (Crinis Carbonisatus Hominis), *Zi Cao* (Radix Arnebiae seu Lithospermi), and *Zong Lü Tan* (Fibra Carbonisata Trachycarpi Stipulae).

Materia medica commonly used for killing Worms

Bai Bu (Radix Stemonae), *Bing Lang** (Semen Arecae Catechu), *Chan Su*‡ (Venenum Bufonis), *Chuan Lian Zi* (Fructus Meliae Toosendan), *Da Feng Zi* (Semen Hydnocarpi), *He Shi* (Fructus Carpesii), *Ku Shen* (Radix Sophorae Flavescentis), *Li Lu* (Radix et Rhizoma Veratri), *Liu Huang*‡ (Sulphur), *Lu Lu Tong* (Fructus Liquidambaris), *Tu Jin Pi* (Cortex Pseudolaricis), *Wu Yi* (Fructus Praeparatio Ulmi), *Yang Ti Gen* (Radix Rumicis Crispi), and *Yuan Hua* (Flos Daphnes Genkwa).

Materia medica commonly used as corrosive agents

Duan Lü Fan‡ (Melanteritum Rubrum), *Mu Bie Zi* (Semen Momordicae Cochinchinensis), *Nao Sha*‡ (Sal Ammoniacum), *Shi Hui*‡ (Calx), *Wu Mei* (Fructus Pruni Mume), and *Ya Dan Zi* (Fructus Bruceae Javanicae).

Materia medica commonly used as blistering agents

Ba Dou (Semen Crotonis Tiglii) and *Ban Mao*‡ (Mylabris).

Materia medica commonly used as anesthetic agents

Ban Xia (Rhizoma Pinelliae Ternatae), *Cao Wu** (Radix Aconiti Kusnezoffii), *Chuan Wu** (Radix Aconiti Carmichaeli), *Ji Xing Zi* (Semen Impatientis Balsaminae), *Nao Yang Hua* (Flos Rhododendri Mollis), *Tian Nan Xing* (Rhizoma Arisaematis), and *Yang Jin Hua** (Flos Daturae).

Table 2-2 Substances commonly used as vehicles or bases

Animal substances ‡

Beef suet (*Niu Zhi*, Adeps Bovis), bovine marrow (*Niu Sui*, Medulla Bovis), egg white (*Ji Dan Qing*, Albumen Galli), Egg Yolk Oil (*Dan Huang You*), fish bile (*Yu Dan*, Bilis Pisci), fish oil (*Yu Zhi*, Oleum Pisci), honey (*Feng Mi*, Mel), pig's bile (*Zhu Dan Zhi*, Bilis Suis), pork lard (*Zhu Zhi*, Adeps Suis), sheep fat (*Yang Zhi*, Adeps Ovis), and yellow wax (*Huang La*, Cera Aurea).

Plant substances

Vegetables: Bitter gourd (*Ku Gua*, Fructus Momordicae Charantiae), Chinese chive (*Jiu Cai*, Folium Allii Tuberosi), Chinese leaf/pakchoi (*Da Bai Cai*, Fructus Brassicae Pekinensis), eggplant/aubergine (*Qie Zi*, Fructus Solani Melongenae), garlic (*Da Suan*, Bulbus Allii Sativi), luffa/dishcloth gourd (*Si Gua*, Fructus Luffae), luffa/dishcloth gourd leaf (*Si Gua Ye*, Folium Luffae), potato (*Ma Ling Shu*, Fructus Solani Tuberosi), radish (*Luo Bo*, Radix Raphani), shallot (*Qing Cong*, Herba Allii Fistulosi), tomato (*Xi Hong Shi*, Fructus Lycopersici Esculenti), and wax gourd (*Dong Gua*, Fructus Benincasae Hispidae).

Fruits: Apple (*Ping Guo*, Fructus Mali Pumilae), banana (*Xiang Jiao*, Fructus Musae), Chinese olive (*Gan Lan*, Fructus Canarii Albi), cucumber (*Huang Gua*, Fructus Cucumeris Sativi), strawberry (*Cao Mei*, Fructus Fragariae), water caltrop (*Ling Jiao*, Fructus et Radix Trapae), and water chestnut (*Bi Qi*, Cormus Heleocharitis).

Medicinal plants: Ban Zhi Lian (Herba Scutellariae Barbatae), *Lu Hui** (Herba Aloes), *Ma Chi Xian* (Herba Portulacae Oleraceae), *Pu Gong Ying* (Herba Taraxaci cum Radice), and *Qing Hao* (Herba Artemisiae Chinghao). Pound the fresh herbs to a pulp and press to obtain the juice.

Vegetable oils: Sesame oil, rapeseed oil (colza oil), sunflower oil, castor oil, olive oil, peppermint oil, and eucalyptus oil.

Distillates: Distillates of *Bo He* (Herba Menthae Haplocalycis), *Jin Yin Hua* (Flos Lonicerae), *Ju Hua* (Flos Chrysanthemi Morifolii), *Mo Li Hua* (Flos Jasmini), and *Qiang Wei Hua* (Flos Rosae Multiflorae).

Other substances

Alcohol, brown sugar dissolved in water, human milk ‡, rice water, tea, and vinegar.

Indications

Inflamed and swollen lesions, pronounced exudation (at the acute stage), suppurating lesions, profuse and thick scaling, itchy skin or itching in the genital and perianal areas, and as an antiseptic mouthwash.

Usage

Aqueous solution preparations are classified into various types according to their usage – washing and soaking preparations (including rinses, steam-washes, sitz baths, soaks, and wet compresses), lavage preparations (including douches and enemas), mouthwashes, preparations for direct topical application (also known as "sweeping" or "brushing" preparations in the classics) and eye-drops. Wet compresses and steam-washes are the most commonly used methods.

- The wet compress method was also known as the drenching method or wetting method in the past. There are detailed descriptions of the procedures and functions of wet compresses in *Wai Ke Da Cheng* [A Compendium of External Diseases], written by Qi Kun and published in 1655. These procedures and functions are still applicable in clinical practice today. Qi Kun explained the procedure as follows: "Fold a cotton or silk cloth seven or eight times. Moisten in a warm aqueous solution, then apply to the area of the lesions while it is still wet. Press it gently on the area with both hands for a short while. Change it when it cools down. Repeat the procedure four or five times. This method is useful for freeing the circulation of Qi and Blood, relieving Toxicity,

alleviating pain, dispelling Blood stasis, and removing putridity. This is an important manual skill and is essential for the treatment of large sores."

Nowadays, silk has been replaced by a bundle of six to eight layers of gauze, or a small towel folded in two. The material is first soaked in the medicated liquid before being pressed tightly against the lesions; the compress should be cold in spring, summer and autumn, and lukewarm in winter. Apply for 15-30 minutes three to five times a day.

- The steam-washing method starts by steaming the affected area with the hot liquid, while the peripheral areas are covered by a dry towel. When the liquid cools down, use it to soak and wash the affected area. The treatment lasts for 10-15 minutes each time and is performed once or twice a day.

General principles

- To soothe the skin and flesh and alleviate itching, use acrid and warm or acrid and hot materia medica, or materia medica with a dissipating function.
- To clear Heat, relieve Toxicity, and repress and kill bacteria, use bitter and cold materia medica which drain Fire.
- To control exudation and promote the healing of superficial erosions, use bitter and cold or sour and astringent materia medica.

Commonly used materia medica

- For weeping lesions present in the acute phase, materia medica such as *Bai Jiang Cao* (Herba Patriniae cum Radice), *Di Yu* (Radix Sanguisorbae Officinalis), *Huang Bai* (Cortex Phellodendri), *Huang Lian* (Rhizoma Coptidis), *Ma Chi Xian* (Herba Portulacae Oleraceae), *Shi Liu Pi** (Pericarpium Punicae Granati), and *Wu Bei Zi‡* (Galla Rhois Chinensis) can be used to prepare a decoction of a suitable concentration (as specified in the individual formulae) for a wet compress or a soak. This treatment relieves Toxicity, disperses swelling and controls exudation.

- For thickened lesions with skin like ox-hide or for severe and widespread itching, prepare a decoction for steam-washing with materia medica such as *Ai Ye* (Folium Artemisiae Argyi), *Cang Er Zi* (Fructus Xanthii Sibirici), *Chen Pi* (Pericarpium Citri Reticulatae), *Chu Tao Ye* (Folium Broussonetiae), *Ku Shen* (Radix Sophorae Flavescentis), *Lu Lu Tong* (Fructus Liquidambaris) *Wei Ling Xian* (Radix Clematidis), *Wu Jia Pi* (Cortex Acanthopanacis Gracilistyli Radicis), *Wu Zhu Yu* (Fructus Evodiae Rutaecarpae), *Xiang Fu* (Rhizoma Cyperi Rotundi), and *Xu Chang Qing* (Radix Cynanchi Paniculati). This treatment softens and moistens the skin, dissipates Wind, dispels Dampness, kills Worms, and alleviates itching.

Commonly used prescriptions

- For acute eczema, *Lu Lu Tong Shui Xi Ji* (Sweetgum Fruit Wash Preparation) or *Ma Chi Xian Shui Xi Ji* (Purslane Wash Preparation) can be used.
- For chronic eczema with severe itching, *Lu Hu Xi Ji* (Calamine and Giant Knotweed Wash Preparation) or *She Chuang Zi Xi Ji* (Cnidium Fruit Wash Preparation) can be used.
- For folliculitis, *Yuan Hua Shui Xi Ji* (Genkwa Wash Preparation) can be used.
- For hyperhidrosis of the hands and feet, *Ge Gen Shui Xi Ji* (Kudzu Vine Root Wash Preparation) can be used.
- For seborrheic alopecia, *Tou Gu Cao Shui Xi Ji* (Speranskia Wash Preparation) can be used.
- For the macerating type of tinea pedis, *Huang Ding Shui Xi Ji* (Siberian Solomonseal and Cloves Wash Preparation) can be used.
- For infectious skin diseases, *Cang Fu Shui Xi Ji* (Atractylodes and Broom Cypress Wash Preparation) can be used.
- For common warts (verruca vulgaris), *Xiang Mu Shui Xi Ji* (Cyperus and Scouring Rush Herb Wash Preparation) can be used.
- For psoriasis, *Cang Fu Shui Xi Ji* (Atractylodes and Broom Cypress Wash Preparation) or *Lu Lu Tong Shui Xi Ji* (Sweetgum Fruit Wash Preparation) can be used.

- For pruritus of the anus and vulva, *Zhi Yang Xi Fang Yi Hao* (No. 1 Wash Formula for Alleviating Itching) can be used.
- For seborrhea, *Shan Dou Gen Shui Xi Ji* (Subprostrate Sophora Root Wash Preparation) or *Zhi Yi Xi Fang* (Seborrhea Wash Formula) can be used.
- For herpetic stomatitis, *Qing Guo Shui Xi Ji* (Chinese Olive Wash Preparation) can be used.

Precautions

- Use the medicated lotions at an appropriate temperature. If they are too hot, they may scald the skin; if they are too cool, their action will not be strong enough. For areas with an uneven surface like the ears, nose, anus, and genitals, make sure there is tight contact between the wet compress and the skin, otherwise the treatment will fail in its objective.
- It is better to prepare the aqueous solutions as they are needed; they may deteriorate if they are stored for a lengthy period.
- In winter, patients should be kept warm to ensure that the condition does not worsen due to exposure to cold.

POWDER PREPARATIONS

Powder preparations are generally made by grinding one or more dried Chinese materia medica into a fine powder and filtering through a 100-120 mesh sieve, although there are also other specific processing methods.

Powder preparations made by grinding ingredients into a powder must be processed in one of the following ways to meet the requirements of clinical application:

- The ingredients must be ground until "no sound is heard while grinding". In other words, ground mineral or shell ingredients should not contain any coarse particles. The water-grinding method is normally used to grind insoluble minerals or shells into a fine powder. Crushed, coarse particles of a mineral are put into a container and ground with water. The suspension is then decanted. The procedure is repeated several times with water being added and the mineral ground again until no sediment of coarse particles is left. After the superfluous water is discarded, the precipitate is dried to obtain a very fine powder.

  No coarse residues should remain in ground animal ingredients, neither should visible plant fibers be contained in ground plant ingredients. Coarse particles in powdered preparations may irritate lesions and may also prevent the medication from functioning to its full extent.
- Certain ingredients can be ground together, others need to be ground separately. Precious ingredients or

highly toxic or corrosive ingredients should be ground separately first, and then added to the other ingredients and ground again in a mortar to mix them in completely.

- Ingredients that are difficult to grind into a fine powder should be processed by specific fine-mortar grinding methods.
  - Animal ingredients such as *Wu Gong*‡ (Scolopendra Subspinipes) and *Chuan Shan Jia** (Squama Manitis Pentadactylae) should be stir-fried until scorched and crisp, and then ground into a powder.
  - Resinous ingredients such as *Ru Xiang* (Gummi Olibanum) and *Mo Yao* (Myrrha) should be fried first to get rid of the oil they contain, and then ground into a powder.
  - Other ingredients like *Deng Xin Cao* (Medulla Junci Effusi) and *Tong Cao* (Medulla Tetrapanacis Papyriferi) should have their surface smeared with a layer of rice paste and left to dry in the sun before being ground into a powder.
  - Before grinding *Bing Pian* (Borneolum), wipe the mortar and pestle with a wet cloth.
- Follow the specific processing instructions for the ingredients as specified in the formulae. For example, *Ba Dou* (Semen Crotonis Tiglii) and *Bi Ma Zi* (Semen Ricini) can be used with or without the membrane; *Ban Mao*‡ (Mylabris) may be used with or without the feet and wings, and is sometimes used raw, sometimes stir-fried.
- Certain materia medica should be stored in an airtight container or kept away from light in order to preserve volatile components. This mostly concerns aromatic materia medica such as *Bing Pian* (Borneolum), *Bai Zhi* (Radix Angelicae Dahuricae) and *Chuan Xiong* (Rhizoma Ligustici Chuanxiong).

Other powder preparations are made by different processing methods:

- Some ingredients that are soluble in water can be made into powder through special filtration methods; for example, *Xi Gua Pi* (Exocarpium Citrulli Vulgaris) can be processed with *Mang Xiao*‡ (Mirabilitum) into watermelon frost, *Xi Gua Shuang* (Praeparatio Mirabiliti et Citrulli).[i]
- The juice of certain fresh materia medica can be dried and processed into a powder, for example *Cong Fen* (Chinese Green Onion Powder) or *Jiang Fen* (Ginger Powder).

- Some seeds are made into a powder by removing the oil and using the parts left over, such as *Ba Dou* (Semen Crotonis Tiglii), which can be processed into *Ba Dou Shuang* (Pulvis Crotonis Seminis).
- Some materia medica are made into powder through chemical changes. For example, the leaves and stems of *Qing Dai* (Indigo Naturalis) can be soaked in clean water in a porcelain container for 2-3 days until the leaves rot. The stems are the removed and 1kg of lime added for every 10kg of leaves. The ingredients are mixed thoroughly until the liquid turns purplish-red; the foam on the top is removed and dried in the sun.
- Other materia medica produce a powder by natural exudation, such as persimmon frost, *Shi Shuang* (Saccharum Kaki), which is processed from the fine white powder appearing on the surface of the fruit as it dries.

Functions of powder preparations

Clearing and cooling the body, soothing the skin and flesh, clearing Heat and relieving Toxicity, transforming putridity and generating flesh, alleviating pain, alleviating itching, and stopping bleeding.

Indications

Acute inflammatory skin diseases, erosion and ulceration of the skin and mucous membranes, abscesses before or after rupture, and bleeding.

Usage

Powder preparations can be applied in a number of different ways (see individual conditions for the most appropriate method of application).

- Sprinkle directly over the affected areas or the surface of the lesions.
- Spread directly over the affected areas with fresh *Sheng Jiang* (Rhizoma Zingiberis Officinalis Recens), *Lu Hui** (Herba Aloes), eggplant/aubergine (*Qie Di*, Pedicellus Solani Melongenae), cucumber (*Huang Gua*, Fructus Cucumeris Sativi), or other vegetables and squashes.
- Mix to a paste with the fresh juice of *Si Gua* (Fructus Luffae) or *Ma Chi Xian* (Herba Portulacae Oleraceae) or with the leaves of fresh Chinese cabbage/pakchoi (*Da Bai Cai*, Fructus Brassicae Pekinensis) and apply to the affected areas.
- Mix powder preparations with honey‡ (*Feng Mi*, Mel), vegetable oil (*Zhi Wu You*, Oleum Vegetale),[ii] egg white‡ (*Ji Dan Qing*, Albumen Galli), human milk‡ (*Ru Zhi*, Lac Hominis), vinegar (*Mi Cu*, Acetum

---

[i] The frost is prepared as follows: Place a watermelon in a clay container. Cut the top off the watermelon, fill it with *Mang Xiao*‡ (Mirabilitum) and replace it. Use a bamboo stick to hold the two parts of the watermelon together. Cover the container with a clay top and seal the join with brown paper strips and mud. Leave the container in a dark place for a few days. The watermelon frost will appear on the internal surface of the container and can be collected several times until no more frost appears.

[ii] Unless specified otherwise in the text, any readily available vegetable oil can be used in making this type of preparation.

Oryzae), alcohol (*Jiu*, Vinum seu Spiritus), the juice from selected materia medica, brown sugar dissolved in water, or cooled boiled water.

Commonly used materia medica

Bing Pian (Borneolum), *Duan Long Gu*‡ (Os Draconis Calcinatum), *Duan Mu Li*‡ (Concha Ostreae Calcinata), *Duan Shi Gao*‡ (Gypsum Fibrosum Calcinatum), *Er Cha* (Pasta Acaciae seu Uncariae), *Fu Hai Shi*‡ (Os Costaziae seu Pumex), *Hua Rui Shi*‡ (Ophicalcitum), *Hua Shi*‡ (Talcum), *Ku Fan*‡ (Alumen Praeparatum), *Lu Gan Shi*‡ (Calamina), *Qing Dai* (Indigo Naturalis), *Shi Hui*‡ (Calx), and *Zhen Zhu*‡ (Margarita).

Commonly used prescriptions

- For acute eczema, *Qing Dai San* (Indigo Powder) can be used.
- For atopic eczema, *Shi Zhen Fen* (Eczema Powder) can be used.
- For erysipelas, *Da Huang San* (Rhubarb Powder) can be used.
- For rosacea, *Dian Dao San* (Reversal Powder) can be used.
- For furuncles and carbuncles, *Yu Lu San* (Jade Dew Powder) or *Ru Yi Jin Huang San* (Agreeable Golden Yellow Powder) can be used.
- For diaper dermatitis (nappy rash), *Qing Liang Fen* (Cool Clearing Powder) can be used.
- For impetigo or folliculitis, *Er Bai San* (Two Whites Powder) can be used.
- For superficial ulcers, *Bing Shi San* (Borneol and Gypsum Powder) can be used.

Precautions

- Powder preparations for direct application to erosive or ulcerating lesions must be ground into a very fine powder or their effectiveness will be diminished.
- It is not advisable to apply powder preparations to areas of the head or body thickly covered by hair.
- Powder preparations should not be applied directly to vesicles or pustules, otherwise a pseudo-layer of crusts will form on the surface of lesions, making recovery difficult.

SUSPENSION PREPARATIONS

Also known as shake lotions, these preparations are made by mixing a certain amount of medicated powder insoluble in water with cold boiled water or distilled water. The powder will be deposited at the bottom of the bottle or other container after being stored for a certain period. Traditional suspension preparations are similar in some respects to modern preparations, but different in others. For instance, nowadays water, alcohol, vinegar, oil, the fresh juice from raw plants, and the body fluids of animals can be mixed to a paste with powdered materia medica for clinical application. The solid medicated powder is the main component of these preparations, which are applied directly to the lesions to form a thin layer on the surface.

Functions of suspension preparations

Clearing Heat and relieving Toxicity, absorbing Dampness and dissipating Wind, dispersing swelling and alleviating pain.

Indications

Acute inflammatory skin diseases with little or no exudation and erosion.

Usage

Usage of the preparations depends on the condition of the disease:

- For acute inflammatory skin diseases without exudation or erosion such as miliaria rubra, shake the medication before use, and brush it on the affected area two or three times a day.
- For lesions with slight erosion, mix the powdered materia medica to a paste with oil or the fresh juice of raw plant ingredients and apply immediately to the affected area directly once or twice a day.

Commonly used materia medica

*Bie Jia** (Carapax Amydae Sinensis), *Chi Shi Zhi*‡ (Halloysitum Rubrum), *Gui Ban** (Plastrum Testudinis), *Hua Shi*‡ (Talcum), *Huang Bai* (Cortex Phellodendri), *Huang Lian* (Rhizoma Coptidis), *Huang Qin* (Radix Scutellariae Baicalensis), *Liu Huang*‡ (Sulphur), *Lu Gan Shi*‡ (Calamina), and *Peng Sha*‡ (Borax).

Commonly used prescriptions

- For miliaria rubra, *Lu Hu Xi Ji* (Calamine and Giant Knotweed Wash Preparation) or *San Huang Xi Ji* (Three Yellows Wash Preparation) can be used.
- For acne, *Cuo Chuang Xi Ji* (Acne Wash Preparation) can be used.
- For pruritus or pityriasis rosea, *San Shi Shui* (Three Stones Lotion) can be used.

Precautions

- For elderly patients or patients with a weak constitution, do not cover more than one-third of the body surface in each treatment session, otherwise too much heat may be dispersed.
- Limit or avoid use of this kind of preparation in winter.
- When oil is used to prepare medications, staining of clothes or bed linen can occur.

INFUSION PREPARATIONS

These can be divided into wine-infusion preparations (tincture preparations) and vinegar-infusion preparations (soak preparations). In both instances, the materia medica are soaked in the liquid for at least seven days and used after the residue is removed.

- Tincture preparations are liquid medicinal preparations made with wine as the solvent; they do not contain any solids or powder. In China, *Huang Jiu* (Vinum Aureum), wine made from rice or millet, and *Bai Jiu* (Spiritus Incolor Granorum), spirits distilled from sorghum or maize, were traditionally used, but nowadays 50-75 percent ethyl alcohol is often employed instead of *Bai Jiu* (Spiritus Incolor Granorum).

- Soak preparations are liquid medicinal preparations made with vinegar as the solvent; they do not contain any solids or powder. Vinegar is made from various materials in different places, and so its name also varies. In the clinic, *Mi Cu* (Acetum Oryzae), rice vinegar, is generally used for this type of preparation.

Functions

Absorbing Dampness and dissipating Wind, killing Worms and alleviating itching, dissipating Blood stasis and dispersing swelling, stimulating pigmentation, invigorating the Blood and freeing the orifices.

Indications

Chronic skin diseases such as stubborn tinea, urticaria and pruritus; superficial fungal infections such as tinea corporis, tinea unguium and tinea manuum; hypopigmentation disorders such as vitiligo; and hair disorders such as alopecia areata.

Usage

- For tincture preparations, apply the medicated liquid directly to the affected area with a cotton swab or a fine brush once or twice a day.

- For soak preparations, steep the affected area with the medicated liquid for 15-30 minutes two or three times a day.

Commonly used materia medica

Bu Gu Zhi (Fructus Psoraleae Corylifoliae), *Fu Ping* (Herba Spirodelae Polyrrhizae), *Hua Jiao* (Pericarpium Zanthoxyli), *Huang Jing* (Rhizoma Polygonati), *Huo Xiang* (Herba Agastaches seu Pogostemi), *Ji Xing Zi* (Flos Impatientis Balsaminae), *Ku Shen* (Radix Sophorae Flavescentis), *Nao Yang Hua* (Flos Rhododendri Mollis), *Tu Jin Pi* (Cortex Pseudolaricis), *Wu Bei Zi*‡ (Galla Rhois Chinensis), *Yang Ti Gen* (Radix Rumicis Crispi), and *Zao Jiao* (Fructus Gleditsiae Sinensis).

Commonly used prescriptions

- For superficial fungal infections, *Tu Jin Pi Bai Bu Ding* (Golden Larch Bark and Stemona Root Tincture) can be used.

- For pruritus and urticaria, *Ku Shen Jiu* (Flavescent Sophora Root Wine) or *Bai Bu Ding* (Stemona Root Tincture) can be used.

- For pompholyx, *Tu Jin Pi Ding* (Golden Larch Bark Tincture) can be used.

- For alopecia areata, *Sheng Fa Ding* (Generating Hair Tincture) can be used.

- For tinea manuum, *Fu Ping Cu* (Duckweed Vinegar Preparation), *Cu Pao Fang* (Vinegar Soak Formula) or *Huo Xiang Jin Pao Ji* (Agastache/Patchouli Soak Preparation) can be used.

- For tinea unguium, *Cu Pao Fang* (Vinegar Soak Formula) or *E Zhang Feng Jin Pao Ji* (Soak Preparation for Goose-Foot Wind) can be used.

Precautions

- These preparations are contraindicated in cases of acute inflammatory skin diseases with broken skin and erosion.

- For chapped and fissured hands and feet, dilute the preparations before use to avoid causing stabbing pain or aggravating the condition.

OIL PREPARATIONS

Oil preparations are made by mixing medicated powders thoroughly into plant oils such as sesame oil or rapeseed oil, or by steeping materia medica in vegetable oil,[iii] frying until their surface is charred and then removing the residues before adding *Huang La* ‡ (Cera Aurea) or other types of wax.

Oil can also be extracted directly from animal or plant sources containing oil by the following methods:

- frying, for example *Dan Huang You* (Egg Yolk Oil)

- cold compression, for example *Song Mao You* (Pine Needle Oil)

- distillation of raw materia medica, for example oil distillate from *Hei Da Dou* (Semen Glycines Atrum) or rice bran.

Functions

Clearing Heat and relieving Toxicity, moistening the skin to prevent cracking, generating flesh and promoting hair growth, absorbing Dampness and closing sores.

Indications

Acute or subacute skin disorders with mild or moderate erosion and exudation; secondary infection, and abscesses due to infection by Toxins; and dry and chapped skin with desquamation.

Usage

- Apply the medicated oil preparation directly to the

[iii] Unless specified otherwise in the text, any readily available vegetable oil can be used in making this type of preparation.

affected area with a cotton swab or a fine brush two or three times a day.

- Alternatively, smear the oil on sterilized gauze, and apply the gauze to the affected area once a day.

Commonly used materia medica

Ce Bai Ye (Cacumen Biotae Orientalis), *Da Feng Zi* (Semen Hydnocarpi), *Duan Long Gu* ‡ (Os Draconis Calcinatum), *Duan Mu Li* ‡ (Concha Ostreae Calcinata), *Fu Rong Ye* (Folium Hibisci Mutabilis), *Gan Cao* (Radix Glycyrrhizae), *Hei Da Dou* (Semen Glycines Atrum), *Huang Lian* (Rhizoma Coptidis), *Qing Dai* (Indigo Naturalis), *Shan Dou Gen* (Radix Sophorae Tonkinensis), *Song Ye* (Folium Pini), *Xing Ren* (Semen Pruni Armeniacae), *Ya Dan Zi* (Fructus Bruceae Javanicae), egg yolk ‡ (*Ji Dan Huang*, Vitellus Galli), rice bran, and wheat bran.

Commonly used prescriptions

- For diaper dermatitis (nappy rash), *Zi Cao You* (Gromwell Root Oil) can be used.
- For erosive skin lesions or superficial, non-healing ulcers, *Dan Huang You* (Egg Yolk Oil) can be used.
- For acute eczema, *Huang Lian You* (Coptis Oil) can be used.
- For the infantile phase of atopic eczema, *Huang Ai You* (Coptis and Mugwort Leaf Oil) can be used.
- For profuse scaling on the head, *Shan Dou Gen You Ji* (Subprostrate Sophora Root Oil Preparation) can be used.
- To clean lesions and remove crusts, *Gan Cao You* (Licorice Oil) can be used.

Precautions

Keep clothes and bed linen away from oil preparations as much as possible to reduce the risk of staining.

EMULSION PREPARATIONS

Emulsion preparations are milky-white shake preparations containing a mixture of oil and water, which separate when left to stand.

Functions

Clearing Heat and relieving Toxicity, protecting the skin and alleviating itching, soothing the skin and flesh and dispersing swelling, reducing erythema and alleviating pain.

Indications

Acute inflammatory skin diseases; burns and scalds; specific injuries such as radiodermatitis and phototoxic dermatitis.

Usage

- Apply the medicated emulsion preparation directly to the affected area with a cotton swab or fine brush once or twice a day.

- Alternatively, smear the emulsion on sterilized gauze, and apply the gauze to the affected area once or twice a day.

Commonly used materia medica

Shi Hui ‡ (Calx), *Xian Lu Hui** (Herba Aloes Recens), *Xian Qing Hao* (Herba Artemisiae Chinghao Recens), *A La Bo Jiao* (Gum Arabic), *An Ye You* (Eucalyptus Oil), and certain plant oils such as olive oil, sesame oil and peanut oil.

Commonly used prescriptions

- For scalds and burns, use *Qing Liang Gao* (Cool Clearing Paste).
- For radiodermatitis, use *Lu Hui Ru Ji* (Aloe Cream).

Precautions

Emulsion preparations, especially those containing fresh plant juice, should be used as soon as possible once they are ready. These preparations tend to deteriorate rapidly.

RUB PREPARATIONS

Rub preparations are slices of plant tubers rubbed directly on the affected area or medicated powders applied with a slice of plant tuber.

Functions

Softening the skin and dissipating masses, moistening the skin and alleviating itching, and increasing pigmentation.

Indications

Skin diseases with extensive involvement, lichenification and itching such as stubborn tinea, chronic eczema, papular eczema, and psoriasis; and also for vitiligo.

Usage

Apply medicated powder to the affected area with a slice of plant tuber or pedicle; or mix medicated powder with oil to make a bolus, wrap it in a piece of cloth, and rub the affected area until it is slightly moist. Treat two or three times a day.

Commonly used materia medica

Cang Er Zi (Fructus Xanthii Sibirici), *Chen Pi* (Pericarpium Citri Reticulatae), *Liu Huang* ‡ (Sulphur), and *Wei Ling Xian* (Radix Clematidis); and application with fresh bitter gourd (*Ku Gua*, Fructus Momordicae Charantiae), cucumber (*Huang Gua*, Fructus Cucumeris Sativi), cucumber gourd (*Tu Gua*, Rhizoma Trichosanthis Cucumeroidis) eggplant/aubergine (*Qie Zi*, Fructus Solani Melongenae), and luffa/dishcloth gourd (*Si Gua*, Fructus Luffae).

Commonly used prescriptions

- For pityriasis versicolor, *Han Ban Ca Ji* (Sweat Macules Rub Preparation) is often used in China. *Bai Bu Ding* (Stemona Root Tincture) could be substituted in those countries where certain of the ingredients contained in *Han Ban Ca Ji* (Sweat Macules Rub Preparation) are not permitted.

- For localized pruritus, *San Shi Shui* (Three Stones Lotion) can be used as a rub preparation.
- For vitiligo, rub the affected area directly two or three times a day with fresh purple eggplant/aubergine or its pedicle.

Precautions

- The plant tubers or pedicles used must be fresh and moist.
- It is better to wrap the medicated powder in a piece of cloth made from natural fibers so that it will be hard enough to create friction, soften the skin and alleviate itching. Ordinary gauze is too soft when wet.

MASSAGE PREPARATIONS

A single ingredient or group of ingredients is ground into a very fine powder, mixed into a mud-like consistency with vegetable oil or animal fat and made into a bolus weighing 30-90 grams. Alternatively, the materia medica to be used can be boiled together to prepare a concentrated decoction used to massage the affected area.

Functions

Softening hardness and moistening the skin, killing Worms and alleviating itching, dispersing scales and softening the skin.

Indications

Disseminated lichen simplex chronicus (neurodermatitis) with thickened skin, nummular eczema of the hand, warts, and tinea manuum.

Usage

- Put the medicated bolus in the palms of the hands and use to rub the affected area backward and forward repeatedly.
- With decoctions, remove any materia medica with sharp points, and massage the affected area gently and evenly with the preparation two or three times a day.

Commonly used materia medica

Cang Er Zi (Fructus Xanthii Sibirici), *Cao Wu** (Radix Aconiti Kusnezoffii), *Chuan Wu** (Radix Aconiti Carmichaeli), *Gan Lan You* (Oleum Canarii Albi Fructi), *Gou Ji* (Rhizoma Cibotii Barometz), *Hai Piao Xiao‡* (Os Sepiae seu Sepiellae), *Man Jing Zi* (Fructus Viticis), *Mu Zei* (Herba Equiseti Hiemalis), *Wei Ling Xian* (Radix Clematidis), *Wu Zhu Yu* (Fructus Evodiae Rutaecarpae), *Xiang Fu* (Rhizoma Cyperi Rotundi), *Xiang You* (Oleum Sesami Seminis), pork lard ‡ (*Zhu Zhi*, Adeps Suis).

Commonly used prescriptions

- For warts, *Xiang Mu Shui Xi Ji* (Cyperus Rhizome and Scouring Rush Wash Preparation) can be used.

- For disseminated lichen simplex chronicus (neurodermatitis), *Cang Wu Cuo Yao* (Xanthium and Clamshell Massage Preparation) can be used.

Precautions

Massage the affected areas gently and evenly to prevent bleeding.

OINTMENTS

Ointments are prepared by grinding a single ingredient or group of ingredients to a fine powder, which is then mixed with a base substance to form a fine, smooth, evenly-dispersed semi-solid preparation.

The base used should meet the following requirements:

- It should be odorless and tasteless with stable properties that remain unaltered when stored for long periods.
- It should have an affinity to the skin without being oily or causing irritation.
- It should not change the properties of any added ingredients, but should preserve their homogeneity and benefit their penetrating and absorbing actions.

Traditionally, base substances included lard, vegetable oil, honey, wine, Vaseline®, vinegar, and lanolin; nowadays, Vaseline® and lanolin are usually used.

Ointments can be processed in different ways:

- **Mixing with different ingredients:** Powdered materia medica are mixed to a paste with oil of a low solidification threshold; for example, *San Miao San* (Mysterious Three Powder) mixed with *Su He Xiang* (Styrax Liquidus) as recorded in *Yi Zong Jin Jian* [The Golden Mirror of Medicine].

- **Grinding method:** Oil-rich seeds, animal fat or raw animal tissues are taken as the main ingredients; they are sometimes used as an excipient for other ingredients. The materia medica are then ground mechanically into a paste; for example, the corrosive medication *Wu Jin Gao* (Black-Gold Ointment), which is made by stir-frying *Ba Dou* (Semen Crotonis Tiglii) until black and then grinding it in a porcelain mortar until it becomes a paste, as recorded in *Zheng Zhi Zhun Sheng* [Standards of Diagnosis and Treatment].

- **Frying method:** The ingredients are fried in vegetable oil or animal fat to extract their non-solid constituents. The residues are removed from the medicated oil and *Mi La‡* (Cera) is added; once it has melted, the paste is ready for use. *Lü La Gao* (Green Wax Ointment), recorded in *Yang Yi Da Quan* [The Complete Book of External Diseases], is made by this process.

Functions

Clearing Heat and relieving Toxicity, moistening the skin to prevent cracking, dispersing swelling and alleviating pain, softening hardness and dissipating lumps, and generating skin and flesh.

Indications

Local limitation and absorption of deep inflammatory conditions; dry, chapped and fissured skin; thickened skin and lichenification; and suppurative or post-suppurative lesions.

Usage

- **Direct application:** Gently apply a thin layer of ointment directly to the affected area. If the skin is thick, first tap with a plum-blossom needle and then apply the ointment. This treatment will be more effective if the area is covered after application.
- **Indirect application (dressing):** Spread a layer of ointment on a piece of sterilized gauze, and then apply the dressing to the affected area; alternatively, sprinkle medicated powder on sterilized gauze, and then apply the dressing. Renew the dressing once or twice a day.

Commonly used materia medica

Bing Pian (Borneolum), *Bo He* (Herba Menthae Haplocalycis), *Dang Gui* (Radix Angelicae Sinensis), *Duan Long Gu* ‡ (Os Draconis Calcinatum), *Ge Fen* ‡ (Concha Meretricis seu Cyclinae Pulverata), *Huang La* ‡ (Cera Aurea), *Huang Lian* (Rhizoma Coptidis), *Jiang Huang* (Rhizoma Curcumae Longae), *Ku Lian Pi* (Cortex Meliae Radicis), *Ku Fan* ‡ (Alumen Praeparatum), *Lang Du* (Radix Euphorbiae Fischerianae), *She Chuang Zi* (Fructus Cnidii Monnieri), *Wu Bei Zi* ‡ (Galla Rhois Chinensis), *Wu Mei* (Fructus Pruni Mume), and *Zi Cao* (Radix Arnebiae seu Lithospermi).

Commonly used prescriptions

- For tinea capitis, *Tu Chuang Gao* (Bald Scalp Sore Paste) can be used.
- For eczema, *Qing Dai Gao* (Indigo Paste), *Shi Du Gao* (Damp Toxin Paste) or *Lang Du Gao* (Chinese Wolfsbane Paste) can be used.
- For the infantile phase of atopic eczema, characterized by large erythematous patches with profuse bran-like scaling and severe itching, *Run Ji Gao* (Flesh-Moistening Paste) or *Wu Yun Gao* (Black Cloud Paste) can be used.
- For seborrheic eczema, *Wu Shi Gao* (Five-Stone Paste) or *Dang Gui Gao* (Chinese Angelica Root Paste) can be used.
- For lichen simplex chronicus (neurodermatitis) with thickened lesions, *Hei Dou Liu You Ruan Gao* (Black Soybean and Vaseline® Ointment) can be used.
- For eczema of the scrotum, *Ku Shen Gao* (Flavescent Sophora Root Paste) or *Lang Du Gao* (Chinese Wolfsbane Paste) can be used.

- For ichthyosis vulgaris with severe keratinization or fissuring, *Run Ji Gao* (Flesh-Moistening Paste) can be used.
- For superficial ulcers on the skin, *Huang Lian Ruan Gao* (Coptis Ointment) can be used.
- For the early stage of pyogenic infections with red, hot, swollen, and painful lesions, *Ru Yi Jin Huang San* (Agreeable Golden Yellow Powder) can be used mixed into a paste with vegetable oil.

Precautions

Direct or indirect application of ointments is contra-indicated for lesions with profuse exudation or severe erosion.

PLASTER PREPARATIONS

Plaster preparations are produced by soaking the ingredients in vegetable oil (preferably sesame oil, as it has a low boiling point) and then frying them in the oil until the surface of the ingredients is charred. The residues are then removed from the medicated oil, which is boiled again to reach 400°C. The heat is turned off and *Qian Dan* ‡ (Minium) added. The mixture is stirred vigorously until it reaches a medicated plaster consistency. Plaster preparations are extremely viscous; they feel hard at normal temperatures, but become as soft as ointment when heated. Plasters normally come in two shapes, either flat or in stick form (medicated stick), which can be cut into small pieces and used for small, widely disseminated lesions. Plaster preparations are effective and very easy to use.

Medicated plasters can be used to treat the exterior or the interior depending on the thickness of the paste layer:

- Plasters for treating the exterior have a thin layer of medicated plaster and have the functions of dispersing swelling, draining pus, dispelling putridity, alleviating pain, generating flesh, keeping out Wind, and protecting tissues. They should be changed once a day.
- Plasters for treating the interior have a thick layer of medicated plaster and have the functions of expelling Wind-Cold, harmonizing Qi and Blood, dispersing focal distension caused by Phlegm, strengthening the sinews and bones, and dissipating Blood stasis. They are usually changed once a week or once a month.

Functions

Softening hardness and dissipating lumps, arresting Wind and alleviating itching, protecting the skin and preventing cracking, draining pus and dispelling putridity, generating flesh and alleviating pain, expelling Cold and alleviating Bi syndrome.

Indications
Chronic, circumscribed skin diseases with thickening of the skin such as nodular prurigo and circumscribed lichen simplex chronicus (neurodermatitis); superficial ulcers; and skin diseases with isolated, highly proliferative, keratotic lesions such as tinea unguium, warts and keloids.

Usage
- Cut a piece of hard plaster to fit the lesion. Heat the plaster preparation to soften it, and then apply tightly over the lesion. Change the plaster once every one or two days.
- If a medicated stick is to be used, heat it up to soften it, cut a piece off and press into a flat layer the size of the lesion. Apply it tightly over the lesion. Change the medicated stick plaster once every three to five days.

Commonly used materia medica
Bai Fu Zi (Rhizoma Typhonii Gigantei), *Bai Guo* (Semen Ginkgo Bilobae), *Ban Mao* ‡ (Mylabris), *Cao Wu** (Radix Aconiti Kusnezoffii), *Chan Su*‡ (Venenum Bufonis), *Chuan Wu** (Radix Aconiti Carmichaeli), *Ji Xing Zi* (Semen Impatientis Balsaminae), *Ku Xing Ren* (Semen Pruni Armeniacae Amarum), *Mo Yao* (Myrrha), *Nao Sha* ‡ (Sal Ammoniacum), *Quan Xie* ‡ (Buthus Martensi), *Ru Xiang* (Gummi Olibanum), *Su Mu* (Lignum Sappan), *Teng Huang* (Resina Garciniae), *Tian Nan Xing* (Rhizoma Arisaematis), *Tou Gu Cao* (Herba Speranskiae seu Impatientis), *Wu Gong*‡ (Scolopendra Subspinipes), and *Zao Jiao* (Fructus Gleditsiae Sinensis).

Commonly used prescriptions
- For keloids, *Hei Se Ba Gao Gun* (Black Medicated Plaster Stick) can be used. iv
- For tinea unguium, ingrown nail and pyogenic paronychia (whitlow), *Ba Jia Gao* (Nail-Removing Plaster) can be used.
- For erythema induratum, *Yang He Jie Ning Gao* (Harmonious Yang Decongealing Plaster) can be used. v
- For nodular prurigo, *Kang Fu Ying Gao* (Healthy Skin Plaster) can be used. vi
- For chronic venous ulcers of the lower limb, *Dong Fang Yi Hao Yao Gao* (Oriental Medicated Plaster No. 1) can be used.

Precautions
Spread the medicated plaster evenly so that it fits over the lesion. If after application of the plaster, erythema, papules, papulovesicles, or vesicles appear, possibly accompanied by exudation and erosion, these are manifestations of *gao yao feng* (plaster Wind). Stop using the preparations immediately and treat as irritant contact dermatitis.

FUMING AND STEAMING PREPARATIONS
Fuming preparations include fumigation preparations; steaming preparations include steam treatments and hot compresses.

Fuming preparations were first recorded in *Huang Di Nei Jing* [The Yellow Emperor's Classic of Internal Medicine]: "If Yang Qi is retained in the exterior, treat it by steaming." *Gu Jin Tu Shu Ji Cheng Yi Bu Quan Lu: Yong Ju Ding Du Men* [Complete Medical Works of the Library Collection, Ancient and Modern: Toxicity of Yong and Ju Abscesses and Clove Sores] gave a more detailed explanation: "Mix powdered *Jiang Xiang* (Lignum Dalbergiae Odoriferae) and powdered *Feng Xiang Zhi* (Resina Liquidambaris) thoroughly in a pan to make pills the size of marbles. Put the pills in an incense burner; use paper to make the opening of the burner into a tube. Burn the pills slowly like ambergris. Keep the opening of the burner over the lesion so that it can be fumigated by the smoke. Stop for a moment if the patient feels tired, and then continue." More recently, Professor Zhao Bingnan has used *Xuan Zheng Xun Yao* (Fumigation Preparation for Tinea) to treat lichen simplex chronicus (neurodermatitis) with good results.

Steaming preparations work by decocting the materia medica and allowing the steam to rise to the lesions. The heated decoction can also be used as a hot compress on the affected area.

Functions
Freeing the movement of Qi and Blood, warming the channels and freeing the network vessels, killing Worms and alleviating itching, flushing out putridity and generating flesh.

Indications
Thickened and lichenified skin, chronic non-healing ulcers, and pruritus.

Usage
- When using fumigation preparations, either hermetically seal off the thick smoke and fumigate the lesions alone, or protect the mouth, nose, ears, and

iv In those countries where the use of certain ingredients employed in the preparation of *Hei Se Ba Gao Gun* (Black Medicated Plaster Stick) is not permitted, *Hei Bu Yao Gao* (Black Cloth Medicated Paste) can be applied instead.
v In those countries where the use of certain ingredients employed in the preparation of *Yang He Jie Ning Gao* (Harmonious Yang Decongealing Plaster) is not permitted, *Zi Se Xiao Zhong Gao* (Purple Paste for Dispersing Swelling) can be applied instead.
vi In those countries where the use of certain ingredients employed in the preparation of *Kang Fu Ying Gao* (Healthy Skin Plaster) is not permitted, *Hei Bu Yao Gao* (Black Cloth Medicated Paste) can be applied instead.

eyes and let the smoke fumigate all the other parts of the body.

- When using steaming preparations, cover the area around the lesions with a towel, then steam the affected area with the boiling liquid. Once the liquid has cooled down, it can be used to wash the lesions.

Commonly used materia medica

Ai Ye (Folium Artemisiae Argyi), *Bai Jie Zi* (Semen Sinapis Albae), *Bai Lian* (Radix Ampelopsis Japonicae), *Cang Zhu* (Rhizoma Atractylodis), *Chuan Xiong* (Rhizoma Ligustici Chuanxiong), *He Shi* (Fructus Carpesii), *Da Feng Zi* (Semen Hydnocarpi), *Huang Qi* (Radix Astragali seu Hedysari), *Ku Shen* (Radix Sophorae Flavescentis), *Liu Huang*‡ (Sulphur), *Nao Yang Hua* (Flos Rhododendri Mollis), *Pao Jiang* (Rhizoma Zingiberis Officinalis Praeparata), *Rou Gui Fen* (Cortex Cinnamomi Cassiae, powdered), *Song Xiang* (Resina Pini), *Wu Bei Zi*‡ (Galla Rhois Chinensis), and *Xi Xin** (Herba cum Radice Asari).

Commonly used prescriptions

- For lichen simplex chronicus (neurodermatitis), Zhao Bingnan's fumigation technique can be used (see Chapter 3).
- Prescriptions for steaming and soaking the affected area can help in the treatment of chilblains (see Chapter 17) and Raynaud's disease (see Chapter 7).
- For chronic non-healing ulcers, *Hui Yang Xun Yao* (Yang-Returning Fuming Preparation) can be used.

Precautions

- Fuming and steaming preparations are contra-indicated or are to be used with caution in cases of acute inflammatory diseases, asthma, bronchitis or other respiratory problems, or primary hypertension, and where patients are extremely weak.
- The smoke produced by medicated fumigation preparations may irritate the mucous membranes; the mouth, nose and eyes should therefore be covered.

Acupuncture and moxibustion
针灸疗法

ACUPUNCTURE

Information on those acupuncture points most commonly used in the treatment of skin disorders can be found in Appendix 3.

Principles of combination of points

The general principles of combination of points are also applicable to acupuncture points used for skin disorders. Certain of these principles are discussed in greater detail below. Details of other principles – such as combining *yuan* (source) and *luo* (network) points, combining front-*mu* and back-*shu* points, selection of exterior-interior related channel points, and selection of left and right points, points on the front or back, upper or lower points, lateral points for disorders of the center, and central points for disorders of the limbs – can be found in standard acupuncture textbooks.

SELECTION OF POINTS ACCORDING TO PATTERN IDENTIFICATION

Patterns can be identified on the basis of the Zang-Fu organ involved and the etiology and pathology of the disease; the points are then selected accordingly. For example, LR-3 Taichong is selected to drain Fire in the Liver and Gallbladder to dredge the Liver and regulate Qi with the reducing method and to enrich and supplement Liver-Blood with the reinforcing method in order to treat diseases such as vulval pruritus and melasma; and SP-9 Yinlingquan is selected to benefit the movement of Dampness and disperse swelling with the reducing method and to warm and supplement Spleen Yang, augment Qi and support the Spleen with the reinforcing method in order to treat diseases such as pruritus and eczema.

SELECTION OF POINTS ON THE AFFECTED CHANNELS

When a disorder occurs in a channel or vessel related to a particular Zang-Fu organ, acupuncture points on that channel or vessel can be selected for treatment. For example, TB-4 Yangchi is selected to warm Yang and dissipate Cold to treat Raynaud's disease, BL-20 Pishu is selected to transform Dampness and fortify the Spleen to treat urticaria due to Dampness invading the Spleen channel, and ST-5 Daying is selected to treat herpes zoster of the lower jaw.

SELECTION OF POINTS ON THE SAME CHANNEL

With this method, also known as the method of combining points on the same channel, two or three acupuncture points on the same channel are selected for the treatment. For example, LI-11 Quchi and LI-4 Hegu are selected for diseases of the scalp or face such as acne and psoriasis, and SP-6 Sanyinjiao and SP-9 Yinlingquan for problems in the genital region or lower limbs such as vulval pruritus or chronic venous ulcer of the lower leg.

COMBINATION OF LOCAL AND DISTAL POINTS

This method uses local points in the diseased area in combination with distal points situated far away from the affected area. This treatment regulates both systemic and local functions. For example, LI-20 Yingxiang is used with LI-4 Hegu for acne; and CV-4 Guanyuan can be used with GV-26 Shuigou for mouth ulcers. In acute diseases, use distal points first, then local points; for chronic diseases, use local points before distal points.

SELECTION OF TENDER SPOTS AS POINTS

This method locates tender points and uses them for acupuncture treatment. The "Ashi points" first described in the Tang dynasty (618-907) are a good example. Nowadays, acupuncture treatment of skin disorders often refers to Ashi points, which are used for example in the treatment of herpes zoster, warts, eczema, and lichen simplex chronicus (neurodermatitis).

SELECTION OF EMPIRICAL POINTS

Some points have a specific effect on certain diseases. A good example is described in the *Song of the Four Command Points*, which summarizes the experiences of acupuncturists prior to the Ming dynasty (1368-1644). According to the song, ST-36 Zusanli is used to treat diseases in the abdomen, BL-40 Weizhong to treat disorders of the back and lower back, LU-7 Lieque to treat diseases of the head and neck, and LI-4 Hegu to treat diseases of the face and mouth.

Empirical points are also frequently used in treating skin disorders; examples include LI-11 Quchi and SP-10 Xuehai for localized lichen simplex chronicus (neurodermatitis), GV-14 Dazhui or BL-25 Dachangshu for urticaria, TB-13 Naohui, SI-16 Tianchuang and BL-21 Weishu for pityriasis rosea, and KI-1 Yongquan for small vessel vasculitis.

SELECTION OF POINTS ACCORDING TO LESIONS

• Skin diseases with an acute onset are often due to pathogenic Wind settling in the skin and flesh, and manifesting as erythema, papules and wheals, accompanied by itching.

Treatment principle

Dispel Wind to alleviate itching.

Point selection

Acupuncture point selection is mainly based on the Bladder, Gallbladder and Large Intestine channels and can include points such as GB-20 Fengchi, BL-12 Fengmen, LI-11 Quchi, and GB-31 Fengshi. The reducing method is applied.

Modifications

1. Moxibustion can be combined with acupuncture for Wind-Cold patterns.
2. Where Damp combines with Wind to invade and vesicles appear, add SP-9 Yinlingquan.
3. For restless sleep, add HT-7 Shenmen.

• Bright red or purple lesions with a sensation of burning heat and pain due to accumulation of pathogenic Fire and Heat in the skin and flesh.

Treatment principle

Clear Heat and cool the Blood.

Point selection

Acupuncture point selection is mainly based on the Large Intestine and Spleen channels and can include points such as LI-11 Quchi, LI-4 Hegu, SP-10 Xuehai, SP-6 Sanyinjiao, and BL-15 Xinshu. The reducing method is applied.

Modification

For erosions with exudation, add BL-20 Pishu and SP-9 Yinlingquan.

• Lesions characterized by tidal reddening and swelling with a sensation of burning heat and pain (possibly with suppuration) due to exuberant Heat Toxins causing Qi stagnation and Blood stasis and disharmony of the Ying and Wei levels.

Treatment principle

Clear Heat and relieve Toxicity, cool the Blood and dissipate Blood stasis.

Point selection

Acupuncture point selection is mainly based on the Governor Vessel and the Large Intestine and Stomach channels and can include points such as GV-14 Dazhui, GV-10 Lingtai, LI-11 Quchi, ST-36 Zusanli, SP-10 Xuehai, and local points in the affected area. The reducing method is applied. Bleeding therapy may be combined to cause slight bleeding and expel Toxins.

Modifications

1. For red, swollen and painful lesions on the head and face, add LI-4 Hegu.

2. For lesions on the upper limbs with severe swelling, add LU-5 Chize.

3. For lesions on the lower limbs, add BL-40 Weizhong.

• Erythema, papules, vesicles, exudation, and erosion due to accumulation of Damp-Heat in the skin and flesh.

Treatment principle
Clear Heat and eliminate Dampness.

Point selection
Acupuncture point selection is mainly based on the Large Intestine, Stomach and Spleen channels and can include points such as LI-11 Quchi, ST-44 Neiting, SP-9 Yinlingquan, SP-6 Sanyinjiao, SP-10 Xuehai, and local points in the affected area. The reducing method is applied.

Modifications
1. For lesions on the face and neck, add GB-20 Fengchi, LI-4 Hegu and SJ-5 Waiguan.
2. For constipation, add SJ-6 Zhigou.
3. Where Dampness is stronger than Heat, moxibustion can be applied.

• Ecchymosis, white patches, pigmentation, warts, nodules, lichenification, or chronic ulceration due to obstruction of the channels and network vessels, thus resulting in congealing and stagnation of Qi and Blood.

Treatment principle
Invigorate the Blood and transform Blood stasis, soften hardness and dissipate lumps.

Point selection
Local lesion areas and acupuncture points related to the lesions are selected in addition to BL-17 Geshu and SP-10 Xuehai, which are key acupuncture points for regulating the Blood. The reducing method is applied in combination with moxibustion.

• Dry and lichenified skin with desquamation and itching accompanied by dry hair or hair loss due to Blood Deficiency and Wind-Dryness or Yin deficiency and Blood-Dryness.

Treatment principle
Nourish the Blood and moisten the skin.

Point selection
Acupuncture points are mainly selected on the back (principally the Bladder channel) and along the Large Intestine and Stomach channels and can include points such as BL-17 Geshu, BL-20 Pishu, BL-23 Shenshu, GB-20 Fengchi, LI-11 Quchi, ST-36 Zusanli, and SP-6 Sanyinjiao. The reinforcing method is applied.

• Ulcerating sores with dull and pale flesh, or open sores, or recurrent urticaria, or plaques of dull pale papules, or dry skin with itching due to insufficiency of Qi and Blood.

Treatment principle
Supplement Qi and augment the Blood.

Point selection
Acupuncture points are mainly selected on the back and along the Conception Vessel and Stomach channel and can include points such as BL-17 Geshu, CV-6 Qihai, BL-20 Pishu, SP-10 Xuehai, and ST-36 Zusanli. The reinforcing method is applied. Moxibustion can be added.

• Alopecia areata and melasma (chloasma) due to depletion of the Liver and Kidneys resulting in insufficiency of Essence and Blood.

Treatment principle
Supplement and boost the Liver and Kidneys.

Point selection
Acupuncture points are mainly selected on the back, along the Kidney channel and in the affected areas and can include points such as BL-18 Ganshu, BL-23 Shenshu, KI-3 Taixi, and SP-6 Sanyinjiao. The reinforcing method is applied.

• Dull white or bluish-purple lesions with a lower skin temperature and numbness and pain due to debilitation of Yang Qi, Cold congealing and Qi stagnation.

Treatment principle
Warm Yang and dispel Cold.

Point selection
Acupuncture points are mainly selected on the back, the Governor and Conception Vessels and the Large Intestine and Stomach channels and can include points such as BL-20 Pishu, BL-23 Shenshu, GV-14 Dazhui, GV-4 Mingmen, and CV-4 Guanyuan. The reinforcing method is applied. Moxibustion can be added.

• Itchy skin, lichenification and scrofula due to Depression and binding of Liver Qi and impairment of the functional activities of Qi.

Treatment principle
Soothe the Liver and regulate Qi.

Point selection
Acupuncture points are mainly selected on the back, along the Liver channel and in the affected areas and can include points such as BL-18 Ganshu, LR-14 Qimen, GB-20 Fengchi, LR-2 Xingjian, and SP-10 Xuehai. The reducing method is applied. Suspended moxibustion can be added for local lesions.

Technique

For skin disorders, needling direction and depth and insertion techniques are assumed to be standard unless otherwise indicated in the disorder concerned.

The reinforcing, reducing and even methods are all used for skin disorders. The regulatory functions of acupuncture in terms of supplementing Deficiency (reinforcing method) and draining Excess (reducing method) vary according to the speed of needle insertion, whether the needle is inserted directly or gradually by levels, the strength and speed with which the needle is lifted and thrust, the direction and angle of needle rotation, needling depth and direction, the number of needle rotations, retention time, and whether the needling direction follows or runs counter to the course of the channel. The even method is applicable for conditions with both Deficiency and Excess, or for patients with a Deficient constitution but an Excess pattern. Other techniques are described in footnotes to specific skin disorders, as appropriate.

When Qi is obtained, the needling sensation can manifest as soreness, distension or numbness in or radiating from the points, or with a sensation like an electric shock.

The strength of the conduction of the needling sensation influences the effectiveness of the treatment:

- Points on the head will often produce a heavy or tight sensation, which spreads around the points.
- Points on the face usually produce a sensation of localized distending pain.
- Points on the neck produce sore or numb sensations or a sensation like an electric shock; these sensations often radiate to the head, shoulder and chest.
- Points on the chest and back produce sensations of heaviness, numbness or distension, which radiate along the ribs to the hypochondrium or upper abdomen.
- Points on the lower back produce sensations of numbness, distension or heaviness, which generally spread to the lower abdomen and legs.
- Points on the lower abdomen usually produce sensations of heaviness, soreness and numbness, which spread downward.
- Points on the limbs produce sore or numb sensations or a sensation like an electric shock. The sensation at points located above the knee or elbow usually spreads to the distal part of the limbs; the sensation at points located below the knee or elbow either also spreads to the distal part of the limbs, or spreads to both the proximal and distal parts of the limbs.

Needle retention time, needle manipulation, the length of a treatment session, and the number of treatment sessions required vary among disorders and are detailed in the relevant section.

MOXIBUSTION

MOXIBUSTION WITH MOXA

This method of moxibustion uses moxa floss made from mugwort leaves, *Ai Ye* (Folium Artemisiae Argyi).

Direct cone moxibustion

Moxa cones made of moxa floss are burnt during moxibustion. In direct cone moxibustion, the moxa cones are placed directly on the skin and burnt. This type of moxibustion aims to achieve a warming effect. Small or medium-sized moxa cones are generally used; they are burnt until the skin becomes red but not scorched, giving patients a pleasant warm feeling. This method is suitable for diseases such as warts (verrucae), lichen simplex chronicus (neurodermatitis), tinea unguium (ringworm of the nail), and Raynaud's disease.

Indirect cone moxibustion on a medium

With this method, a layer of animal, plant or mineral material is placed between the skin and the moxa cone. The most common media used for indirect moxibustion include ginger, garlic, scallion, or salt. This method can be used for urticaria, erysipelas, folliculitis, lichen simplex chronicus (neurodermatitis), and chilblains.

Suspended moxibustion with a moxa roll (or moxa stick)

Moxa rolls (or sticks) are made by using paper to wrap moxa floss into a cylindrical shape. Treatment is performed by burning one end of the moxa roll and applying it close to acupuncture points or affected areas.

With suspended moxibustion (also known as gentle moxibustion, circling moxibustion or sparrow-pecking moxibustion), the moxa roll is held near the end that is burning and moved close to the acupuncture point or affected area. The burning moxa roll is kept suspended over the point or area, or moved backward and forward or in circles, or moved up and down like a sparrow pecking its food. This method is suitable for such conditions as chronic eczema, furuncles, chronic venous ulcer of the lower leg, chilblains, and melanosis.

Warm-needling moxibustion

A 2 cm piece of moxa roll is cut off and fixed to the top of the needle handle about 2-3 cm above the skin surface. It is then burnt from the bottom and the ash removed after the moxa has finished burning. After a short pause, the needle is withdrawn. This method can be used for conditions such as Raynaud's disease.

MOXIBUSTION WITH NON-MOXA MATERIALS

This method of moxibustion uses materials other than moxa.

Natural moxibustion

This method involves the application to certain acupuncture points of medicinal materials that are strongly irritating to the skin, thus causing blistering. Materials commonly used include mashed *Da Suan* (Bulbus Allii Sativi), *Bai Jie Zi* (Semen Sinapis Albae), *Ban Mao‡* (Mylabris), *Bai Hu Jiao* (Fructus Piperis Albicatus), and *Wei Ling Xian* (Radix Clematidis). Natural moxibustion is used in China to treat conditions such as localized psoriasis and lichen simplex chronicus (neurodermatitis).

Moxibustion with *Deng Xin Cao* (Medulla Junci Effusi)

This method involves burning *Deng Xin Cao* (Medulla Junci Effusi) after soaking it in sesame oil or other types of vegetable oil, and then pressing it quickly against certain acupuncture points. In China, it is used to treat pruritus and furuncles.

Other treatment methods
其他疗法

EAR ACUPUNCTURE

Needles

Three types of needles are commonly used in ear acupuncture treatment:

- Filiform needles – usually gauge nos. 26, 28 and 30, 1-3 cm in length.
- Thumbtack needles – usually made of 30-gauge stainless steel wire; the needle body is 2-3 mm long and is connected to an annular head.
- Intradermal needles – made of 35-gauge stainless steel wire, these needles are 1.0-1.5 cm long with a cap on top.

Techniques

- Filiform needles are inserted into specific ear points on the auricle. Successful ear acupuncture requires accurate location of ear points and sterilization of the points. The ear is held steady with one hand, with the index finger supporting locations at the back of the ear corresponding to the points in front. Rotate the needle during insertion and make sure that the cartilage is not penetrated. Retention time varies according to the disease. Withdraw the needles slowly to reduce bleeding to a minimum. Press the needling hole with a dry sterilized cotton ball after the needle is withdrawn. This treatment can be used for urticaria, furuncles, warts (verrucae), hyperhidrosis, alopecia areata, recurrent aphthous stomatitis (mouth ulcers), lichen planus, or pruritus.
- With the seed-embedding technique, seeds such as *Wang Bu Liu Xing* (Semen Vaccariae Segetalis), *Lai Fu Zi* (Semen Raphani Sativi), *Jie Zi* (Semen Brassicae Junceae), *Su Mi* (Semen Setariae Italicae), or *Lü Dou* (Semen Phaseoli Radiati) are embedded at ear points and held in place with adhesive plaster or tape. Patients should be reminded to press the embedded seeds for one minute three to five times a day. This treatment can be used for urticaria, acne, miliaria rubra, hyperhidrosis, or small vessel vasculitis.
- With the needle-embedding technique, sterilized thumbtack needles or intradermal needles are inserted with hemostatic forceps at the points selected and held in place with adhesive plaster or tape. The needles are usually retained for one to five days, but never for more than seven. Needle embedding at ear points is not recommended in summer when sweating is likely. Immediate management should be given in cases of infection with redness and swelling. This treatment can be used for hyperhidrosis, keratosis follicularis, vitiligo, or urticaria.
- The pricking to bleed technique can also be employed at ear points. After routine sterilization of the points, prick with a three-edged needle to produce one to two drops of blood. Bleeding is performed once every five to seven days. This treatment can be used for melasma (chloasma).

Commonly used points

Spleen, Stomach, Liver, Heart, Lungs, Kidneys, Ear-Shenmen, Endocrine, Subcortex, Adrenal Gland, and Sympathetic Nerve.

Precautions

- Strict sterilization of instruments and points is essential. If local infection is not treated correctly, the whole ear may become infected, resulting in suppuration, or perichondritis in severe cases.

- In rare cases, patients may experience very severe pain after needles are inserted into the ear points. Withdrawal of the needles often helps to alleviate the pain. If it remains, massage the ear gently until the pain stops.
- Ear acupuncture should not be given to patients with lesions on the ear.

SEVEN-STAR NEEDLING

Types of needle

- **Lotus receptacle:** The shape of the needle resembles the head of a lotus seed. The head of the needle is circular, 1.5-2.0 cm in diameter, and divided into two planes. Seven stainless steel needles are distributed evenly over the surface of one side of the head; another five needles are attached to the other side of the head in a bunch. A fine flexible handle, 20 cm long, is attached between the two planes of the head.
- **Cylindrical:** This instrument consists of a metal tube 5-6 cm long and 3-4 cm in diameter. Several rows of short needles are fixed to the surface of the tube, to which a 15-20 cm handle is attached.
- **Motor-driven:** This instrument consists of a rectangular box containing a tiny electric motor; a number of needles and a handle are attached to the box. The motor drives a crankshaft to cause the handle to move with a tapping motion. The tapping frequency can be adjusted by a frequency regulator button.

Techniques

- Hold the needle handle with the right hand. The index finger presses directly against the top of the handle, while the thumb and the middle finger hold the handle and the ring finger and little finger secure the end of the handle at the minor thenar eminence. The instrument is tapped by flexing and extending the wrist evenly and rhythmically at a frequency of 90-120 times per minute. The lesions are tapped along a straight line from left to right and then from right to left, or from top to bottom, or from the center to the periphery.
- **Mild stimulation:** Tap quickly but gently and rhythmically by not allowing the handle to rise too far when it springs back after hitting the skin. Flexion and extension of the wrist are limited, generating a relatively weak force for tapping. The skin tapped will become slightly flushed and red. This is a reinforcing method and is recommended for treating the head and face and for the elderly, children and people with a weak constitution. For skin disorders, it can also be used to treat tinea cruris, furuncles and keloids.
- **Strong stimulation:** Tap slowly and rhythmically by allowing the handle to rise quite high when it springs back after hitting the skin. Flexion and extension of the wrist are ample, generating a relatively strong force for tapping. The skin tapped will have a pronounced red color and there may be slight bleeding. This is a reducing method and is recommended for treating the back and limbs and for young and middle-aged people. For skin disorders, it can also be used to treat vitiligo and eczema.

Precautions

- The needling instrument must be properly sterilized prior to treatment. Single-use disposable needles should be used if available, otherwise cutaneous needling instruments must be sterilized before re-use to prevent cross-infection.
- After treatment, the lesions should be covered by sterilized gauze and held in place with adhesive plaster to prevent secondary infection.

Note on plum-blossom needling

Plum-blossom needling is similar to seven-star needling, except that the head of the instrument contains five short, fine stainless steel needles grouped in a pattern resembling the petals of a plum blossom. The technique is the same as that for seven-star needling. Plum-blossom needling is used to treat skin disorders such as tinea corporis, herpes zoster, plane warts, and alopecia areata.

ACUPUNCTURE POINT LASER THERAPY

The helium-neon laser apparatus is the apparatus used most frequently for laser therapy at acupuncture points, although a carbon dioxide, argon-ion or helium-cadmium apparatus is sometimes used. The helium-neon laser can stimulate the activity of various enzymes, increase the level of phagocytes, red blood cells and hemoglobin in the blood, accelerate vascular development, and promote the healing of wounds and ulcers. It can penetrate the skin to stimulate the nerve ends, thus helping to speed up the regeneration of diseased tissue.

For skin disorders, point laser therapy can be used to treat urticaria, rosacea, alopecia areata, papular urticaria (insect bites), annular erythema, and chronic venous ulcer of the lower leg.

PRICKING TO BLEED THERAPY

Instruments

- Large, medium or small stainless steel three-edged needles are generally used for pricking the blood vessels and network vessels to cause significant amounts of bleeding.
- Short, thick filiform needles (gauge no. 26-28, length 0.5-1.0 cun) are generally used to prick acupuncture points such as the twelve *jing* (well) points and EX-UE-11 Shixuan [vii] to cause slight bleeding.

Points used

- Peripheral bleeding, the most commonly used method, is performed at points such as the twelve *jing* (well) points, EX-UE-11 Shixuan,[vii] GV-26 Shuigou, GB-14 Yangbai, and Ear Apex.
- Superficial veins can also be bled at points such as PC-3 Quze, LU-5 Chize, BL-40 Weizhong, EX-HN-5 Taiyang,[viii] and the posterior auricular vein.

Techniques

- Point pricking is applied most often in peripheral bleeding. After routine local sterilization, the point is pricked by a three-edged or thick needle to release a little blood and is then withdrawn immediately.
- Moderate pricking is used for bleeding of the small veins.
- Pricking and cupping are often combined for bleeding therapy on the trunk and proximal limbs, for example to treat insect bites or pityriasis rosea.

Frequency

- Acute diseases should be treated once a day for two or three days.
- Chronic conditions may have an interval of two to three days or even one to two weeks between treatment sessions.
- The frequency of bleeding therapy should be adjusted in accordance with the nature of the disease, the age and constitution of patients, the amount of bleeding, and the results achieved.

Functions

- Abating fever, mainly for fever in Excess-Heat patterns resulting from external invasion or Yang exuberance.
- Alleviating pain, for example for headache or sore throat.
- Dispersing swelling, for example for angioedema.
- Relieving Toxicity, for example from insect bites and stings.
- Stopping bleeding, for example with nosebleeds or bleeding gums.
- Invigorating the Blood, for example in treating alopecia areata or Raynaud's disease.
- Dissipating Blood stasis obstructing the network vessels, for example in vitiligo.
- Clearing Heat and cooling the Blood, for example in treating pityriasis rosea, psoriasis or folliculitis.

- Alleviating itching, for example in pruritus or eczema.
- Clearing Heat from the Lungs, for example in treating acne and rosacea.

Precautions

- A full explanation of the procedures should be given to patients prior to treatment to obtain their consent.
- Bleeding treatment is contraindicated for patients with severe anemia, low blood pressure, hemorrhagic diseases, varicose veins, and hemangioma.
- Deep pricking must be avoided.
- Strict sterilization is required to avoid infection.

CUPPING THERAPY
Methods

- With fire-cupping, burning a flame inside the cup drives the air out. Negative pressure is produced inside cups so that when inverted they will suck up the skin when placed on the body. In skin disorders, fire-cupping can be used to treat pityriasis rosea or folliculitis.
- Flash-cupping is a variant of the fire-cupping method. Once the skin has been sucked up, remove the cup and then replace repeatedly so that the skin is again sucked up each time. This will cause tidal reddening of the skin. In skin disorders, this method is mostly used for psoriasis.
- With medicated cupping, the prescribed materia medica are put in a cloth bag, which is placed in water and boiled until the required concentration is achieved. Bamboo cups are put into the medicated liquid and boiled for another 5-10 minutes. The cups are taken out of the water with tongs or tweezers, shaken to remove surplus liquid and pressed quickly onto the skin. In skin disorders, this method can be used for urticaria.
- Cupping can be combined with the pricking-to-bleed method. First, bleed the area with a three-edged needle; then employ fire-cupping. This combination can be used in the treatment of acne, folliculitis, insect bites, psoriasis, pityriasis rosea, and vitiligo.
- Cupping is also often used in combination with acupuncture. Insert the needles at the points. Carry out reinforcing or reducing techniques as required and retain the needles. Then, use fire-cupping to place cups on the skin centered on the needles. Acupuncture and cupping therapy can be combined in the treatment of psoriasis.

[vii] M-UE-1 according to the system employed by the Shanghai College of Traditional Chinese Medicine.
[viii] M-HN-9 according to the system employed by the Shanghai College of Traditional Chinese Medicine.

Diet therapy
饮食疗法

In addition to application of Chinese materia medica and acupuncture in the treatment of skin diseases, Traditional Chinese Medicine also emphasizes the importance of diet therapy in order to supplement treatment or to prevent occurrence in the first place.

In TCM, inappropriate diet is one of the major causes of skin diseases. Therefore, a thorough understanding of the nature of diet therapy and its impact on skin diseases is essential for all dermatologists so that it can be applied in their own practice and guidance provided for patients.

NATURE AND FLAVOR OF FOOD
As with Chinese materia medica, food can be classified according to its nature and flavor. Diet therapy can therefore be integrated with the patient's condition and underlying disease pattern and the treatment prescribed.

In TCM, food can be classified into one of the four natures or can be considered as neutral (see Table 2-3).

Food can also be classified into one or more of the five flavors (see Table 2-4).

TCM also considers that excessive intake of spicy, stimulating and greasy food impairs the functions of the Spleen and leads to many skin diseases. Examples of these foods are listed below.

Spicy food
Chilli, garlic, ginger (fresh), mustard, pepper, and spring onion.

Stimulating food
Bamboo shoots, Chinese chives (*Xie Bai*, Bulbus Allii Macrostemi), coriander, mushroom, mustard leaf; lamb; fish, crab and shrimp; and alcohol.

Greasy food
Butter, cream, cheese, deep-fried food, lamb, and pork.

Table 2-3 Classification of food according to nature

Cold
Foods with a cold nature include bamboo root, bitter gourd, cucumber, kelp, lotus root, purslane (*Ma Chi Xian*, Herba Portulacae Oleraceae), seaweed, sugarcane, tomato, water chestnut, wax gourd, and wild rice stem; banana, grapefruit, mulberry, muskmelon, persimmon, and water melon; crab; pig's intestines; prepared soybeans and soy sauce.

Cool
Foods with a cool nature include celery, colza, eggplant/aubergine, luffa/dishcloth gourd (*Si Gua*, Fructus Luffae), mushroom, spinach, water caltrop, white radish (mooli), and winter gourd; barley, bean curd, buckwheat, coix seed (*Yi Yi Ren*, Semen Coicis Lachryma-jobi), millet, mung bean, wax gourd seed (*Dong Gua Ren*, Semen Benincasae Hispidae), and wheat; apple, Buddha's hand (*Fo Shou*, Fructus Citri Sarcodactylis), loquat, mango, orange, pear, and tangerine; tea; pork rind; duck's eggs; all raw and cold vegetables and fruit; and cold drinks.

Hot
Foods with a hot nature include chilli, Chinese prickly ash (*Hua Jiao*, Pericarpium Zanthoxyli), cinnamon bark, and pepper.

Warm
Foods with a warm nature include Chinese chives, fennel seed, garlic, ginger (fresh), leaf mustard, pumpkin, rapeseed, scallion, and spring onion; polished glutinous rice; almond, apricot, black plum, cherry, chestnut, Chinese date (*Da Zao*, Fructus Ziziphi Jujubae), litchee, longan pulp (dried), peach, pomegranate, and walnut kernel; chicken, ham, lamb, and pig's liver; goat's milk, goose eggs; crucian carp, trout, eel, prawns, sea cucumber, and shrimps; alcohol and vinegar.

Neutral
Foods with a neutral nature include black jelly fungus (wood ears), cabbage, carrot, celery, Chinese leaf (pakchoi), day-lily buds, lotus leaf (*He Ye*, Folium Nelumbinis Nuciferae), onion, peas, potato, rutabaga, shiitake mushrooms, sweet potato, and yellow jelly fungus; aduki bean, black sesame seed, black soybean, rice, and sweet corn; Chinese olive (*Gan Lan*, Fructus Canarii Albi), fig, ginkgo nut, grapes, hazelnut, lotus seed (*Lian Zi*, Semen Nelumbinis Nuciferae), peanuts, plum, pumpkin seed (*Nan Gua Zi*, Semen Cucurbitae Moschatae), and torreya nut (*Fei Zi*, Semen Torreyae Grandis); beef, duck, goose, pig's kidney, pork, quail; chicken's eggs and quail's eggs; cow's milk; jellyfish, loach and yellow croaker; royal jelly, honey and granulated sugar.

Table 2-4 Classification of food according to flavor

Acrid

Foods with an acrid flavor include celery, chilli, Chinese chives (*Xie Bai*, Bulbus Allii Macrostemi), cinnamon bark, day-lily buds, garlic, ginger (fresh), leaf mustard, onion, pepper, rapeseed, scallion, spring onion, and white radish (mooli). Acrid foods have a dissipating function and can expel external pathogenic factors; they can be used for instance in the treatment of urticaria due to Wind or Cold.

Sour

Foods with a sour flavor include purslane (*Ma Chi Xian*, Herba Portulacae Oleraceae) and tomato; apricot, black plum (*Wu Mei*, Fructus Pruni Mume), coconut, grapefruit, hawthorn fruit, litchee, loquat, orange, peach, pear, pomegranate, and tangerine; trout; vinegar; and royal jelly. Sour foods have an astringent function and can be used for instance in the treatment of profuse sweating.

Bitter

Foods with a bitter flavor include bitter gourd, lotus leaf (*He Ye*, Folium Nelumbinis Nuciferae) and seaweed; almond, ginkgo nut and peach kernel (*Tao Ren*, Semen Persicae); pig's liver; prepared soybean; tea; alcohol and vinegar. Bitter foods can clear Heat and dispel Dampness and can be used for instance in the treatment of various types of eczema due to Damp-Heat.

Sweet

Foods with a sweet flavor include bamboo root, broad bean, carrot, celery, Chinese leaf (pakchoi), cucumber, day-lily buds, eggplant/aubergine, jelly fungus, lotus root, luffa/dishcloth gourd (*Si Gua*, Fructus Luffae), peas, potato, shiitake mushrooms, spinach, sweet potato, tomato, wax gourd, wild rice stem; aduki bean, bean curd, black bean, black sesame seed, coix seed (*Yi Yi Ren*, Semen Coicis Lachryma-jobi), glutinous rice, millet, mung bean, rice, soybean, and sweet corn; apple, apricot, banana, cherry, chestnut, Chinese date (*Da Zao*, Fructus Ziziphi Jujubae), Chinese olive (*Gan Lan*, Fructus Canarii Albi), coconut, fig, gingko nut, hawthorn fruit, hazelnut, litchee, longan pulp (dried), lotus seed (*Lian Zi*, Semen Nelumbinis Nuciferae), mulberry fruit, muskmelon, orange, peach, peanuts, pear, plum, pomegranate, pumpkin seed (*Nan Gua Zi*, Semen Cucurbitae Moschatae), torreya nut (*Fei Zi*, Semen Torreyae Grandis), walnut, water chestnut, and water melon; beef, chicken, duck, goose, ham, lamb, pig's kidney, pig's liver, pork, and quail; chicken, duck and quail eggs; jellyfish, loach, trout, and yellow croaker; royal jelly, honey and granulated white sugar. Sweet foods have a supplementing and harmonizing function and can be used in the treatment of skin disorders due to Spleen Deficiency such as pruritus, lichen planus, chronic eczema, asteatotic eczema, perianal eczema, and dermatitis herpetiformis.

Salty

Foods with a salty flavor include cucumber, kelp and seaweed; barley and millet; duck, ham, pig's kidney, and pork; crab, loach and jellyfish; soy sauce; and salt. Salty foods soften hardness and dissipate lumps and can be used in the treatment of skin disorders manifesting with nodules or cysts such as cystic acne, erythema induratum and lipoma.

RELATIONSHIP OF FOOD TO SKIN DISORDERS

As the lists above indicate, food can be cold, cool, hot, warm or neutral in nature and acrid, sour, bitter, sweet, or salty in taste. Diseases are normally identified according to the Eight Principles as Interior-Exterior, Excess-Deficiency, Heat-Cold, and Yin-Yang. The nature and taste of food should match the pattern of the disease; otherwise, if the food contradicts the pattern of the disease, the condition will worsen.

In *Jin Kui Yao Lue* [Synopsis of Prescriptions from the Golden Cabinet], Zhang Zhongjing said: "The flavor of food taken may fit the pattern of the disease or endanger the body. If it fits the pattern of the disease, the body can be supplemented; if it endangers the body, disease will result." Therefore, the application of diet therapy for skin diseases should be based on the patient's constitution and the pattern of the disease in order to help

cure the disease; in other words, use supplementation in cases of Deficiency, drainage in cases of Excess, Heat in cases of Cold, and Cold in cases of Heat.

- For skin disorders characterized by Cold patterns such as Raynaud's disease and cold urticaria, food and drink of a cold or cool nature (including raw and cold vegetables and fruit, and cold drinks) should be avoided and preference given to food and drink of a hot, warm or neutral nature with a supplementing function and high in nutrition.

- For skin disorders such as folliculitis, herpes zoster, herpes simplex, ecthyma, measles, varicella (chickenpox), and miliaria rubra, characterized by Heat patterns with lesions manifesting as erythema and vesicles accompanied by exudation, erosion and itching, food of a warm or hot nature with an acrid and spicy taste or stimulating food such as chilli, spring onion, lamb, seafood, cheese, butter, and strong tea should be avoided, as should alcohol and cigarettes. Intake of food of a cool or cold nature should be increased.

- For Yang Deficiency skin disorders such as chilblains or Raynaud's disease with lesions manifesting as pale and cold limbs, food and drink of a warm or hot nature with a supplementing function is recommended. Food and drink of a cold or cool nature should be avoided.

- For skin disorders caused by exuberant Fire due to Yin Deficiency such as recurrent aphthous stomatitis (mouth ulcers) or drug eruptions with lesions manifesting as swelling, pain, itching, erythema, pustules, scaling, or erosion, food of a warm or hot nature or stimulating food such as deep-fried, greasy and sweet food, seafood, strong tea, coffee, and alcohol should be avoided. Light and cool food and drink with a moistening function is recommended such as water melon juice, chestnut juice, fresh vegetables and fruit, and congee.

- For lesions manifesting as itching in diseases such as urticaria, lichen simplex chronicus (neurodermatitis), scabies, and papular urticaria, acrid and spicy foods should be avoided.

- For lesions manifesting as vesicles, exudation or erosion due to accumulation of Dampness in the Spleen and Stomach, as seen for example in atopic eczema, perianal eczema or erythema multiforme, sweet and greasy food should be avoided. Light food such as fresh vegetables and fruit or congee made with *Yi Yi Ren* (Semen Coicis Lachryma-jobi) and *Chen Pi* (Pericarpium Citri Reticulatae) is recommended.

- The above principles may need to be adapted for skin diseases of a more complicated etiology and for patients of different constitutions. For example, patients with eczema should generally avoid acrid, spicy, raw, cold, and stimulating food such as seafood and cheese; patients with psoriasis should avoid acrid, spicy and stimulating food such as seafood and alcohol; and patients with acne, rosacea, seborrheic alopecia, or seborrheic eczema should avoid acrid, spicy, greasy, and sweet food (in particular, chocolate).

- Different people have different constitutions. In general, people with oily or greasy skin should eat more cool or neutral foods and cut down on intake of foods of a warm or hot nature, whereas neutral foods combined with small amounts of foods of a warm or hot nature may be beneficial to people with dry skin.

FOOD FUNCTIONS

Foods with the function of dispersing inflammation

Colza (rape), garlic, lotus leaf (*He Ye*, Folium Nelumbinis Nuciferae), reed rhizome (*Lu Gen*, Rhizoma Phragmitis Communis), purslane (*Ma Chi Xian*, Herba Portulacae Oleraceae), spinach root, and wax gourd seed (*Dong Gua Ren*, Semen Benincasae Hispidae) can be used for inflammatory skin disorders characterized by swollen, hot and painful skin.

Foods with the function of relieving Toxicity

- Bitter gourd, cucumber, green plum, mung bean (*Lü Dou*, Semen Phaseoli Radiati), pineapple, tomato, water melon, and wax gourd clear Heat and relieve Toxicity.

- Fresh ginger (*Sheng Jiang*, Rhizoma Zingiberis Officinalis Recens) and rice vinegar (*Mi Cu*, Acetum Oryzae) relieve fish and crab Toxins (food poisoning).

- Tea, white hyacinth bean (*Bai Bian Dou*, Semen Dolichoris Lablab) and mung bean (*Lü Dou*, Semen Phaseoli Radiati) relieve Toxicity induced by drugs.

- Garlic inhibits and kills bacteria to relieve Toxicity.

- Honey (*Feng Mi*, Mel) relieves all kinds of Toxicity.

These foods can be used in the treatment of skin disorders characterized by erythema and vesicles.

Foods with the function of dispelling Dampness and benefiting the movement of water

Foods such as aduki bean (*Chi Xiao Dou*, Semen Phaseoli Calcarati), corn silk (*Yu Mi Xu*, Stylus Zeae Mays), mung bean (*Lü Dou*, Semen Phaseoli Radiati), trichosanthes fruit (*Gua Lou*, Fructus Tricosanthis), water melon, and carp can be used for skin disorders characterized by vesicles and lichenoid changes.

Foods with the function of fortifying the Spleen and increasing the appetite

Barley sprouts (*Mai Ya*, Fructus Hordei Vulgaris Germinatus), black plum (*Wu Mei*, Fructus Pruni Mume), Chinese prickly ash (*Hua Jiao*, Pericarpium Zanthoxyli), fennel seed (*Xiao Hui Xiang*, Fructus Foeniculi Vulgaris), fresh ginger (*Sheng Jiang*, Rhizoma Zingiberis Officinalis Recens), garlic, hawthorn fruit (*Shan Zha*, Fructus Crataegi), spring onion, tangerine peel (*Chen Pi*, Pericarpium Citri Reticulatae), and vinegar can be used for skin disorders such as eczema.

Foods with supplementing and augmenting functions

- Chinese dates (*Da Zao*, Fructus Ziziphi Jujubae), Chinese yam (*Shan Yao*, Rhizoma Dioscoreae Oppositae), malt sugar (*Yi Tang*, Saccharon Granorum), lotus seeds (*Lian Zi*, Semen Nelumbinis Nuciferae), and peanuts have the function of supplementing the Spleen and Stomach and can be used for skin disorders such as eczema.

- Chinese leek seeds, lamb, prawns, sea cucumber, and walnuts supplement Kidney Yang and can be used for skin disorders such as melasma (chloasma).

- Chinese dates (*Da Zao*, Fructus Ziziphi Jujubae), litchees, mulberry fruit (*Sang Shen*, Fructus Mori Albae), and longan fruit (*Long Yan Rou*, Arillus Euphoriae Longanae) supplement the Blood and can be used for skin disorders such as alopecia.
- Black jelly fungus supplements Yin and can be used for skin disorders such as mouth ulcers.

Foods with the function of venting papules

Carrots, chestnuts, crucian carp, prawns (fresh), shiitake mushrooms, and yellow croaker have the function of venting papules. For instance, carrots and chestnuts can be used in the treatment of skin disorders such as measles in the pre-eruptive phase and varicella (chicken-pox).

Foods with the function of expelling Worms

Black plum (*Wu Mei*, Fructus Pruni Mume), carrots, garlic, and pumpkin seed (*Nan Gua Zi*, Semen Cucurbitae Moschatae) can be used in the treatment of skin disorders caused by parasites.

Chapter 3

Eczema and dermatitis

Eczema is a common non-infective skin disease characterized by an inflammatory skin reaction to various internal and external stimuli with such typical manifestations as erythema and vesiculation, which may lead to exudation and crusting. Lesions tend to be circumscribed in the chronic phase with infiltration, lichenification and severe itching; recurrence is frequent.

The term eczema has a long history, originating from the Greek word "ekzein" meaning "to boil", a reference to the vesiculation that occurs in acute conditions. In recent years, there has been much discussion over the use of the terms "eczema" and "dermatitis". Strictly speaking, as dermatitis refers more generally to inflammation of the skin, it is a broader term than eczema, which is just one type of inflammation.

One reason for this discussion is that eczema and dermatitis, as strictly defined, are very similar in terms of pathological changes and are not easy to distinguish from one another according to the clinical manifestations. For example, the condition may initially present as contact dermatitis, but skin lesions may appear eczematous over the long term with repeated onset. A number of types of occupational contact dermatitis may have chronic eczematous manifestations. Primary contact dermatitis due to long-term contact with mild irritants may also manifest as eczema, for example, hand eczema in women due to frequent contact with soap or washing-up liquids.

Although eczema and contact dermatitis have many common features, they also differ in a number of aspects. For example, contact dermatitis generally presents initially as an acute condition, while eczema is more often a chronic process characterized by infiltration and lichenification. Contact dermatitis is self-limited and will heal soon after the causative factors are removed, whereas the origin of eczema is often unclear and the condition tends to recur. The causes of contact dermatitis are relatively straightforward once the trigger factor has been identified, while eczema tends to be more complicated and more closely related to the body's constitution.

This blurring of distinctions among causes and manifestations tends these days to mean that the majority of practitioners use the terms eczema and dermatitis more or less interchangeably, possibly with a preference for eczema when talking to patients. In this chapter, therefore, atopic eczema is the same as atopic dermatitis, seborrheic eczema is the same as seborrheic dermatitis, and so on.

The etiology of eczema is very complex, often involving an interaction of external and internal factors:

- External factors such as climate and the environment can play a role in the occurrence of eczema, which can be triggered by external stimuli such as sunlight, ultraviolet light, cold, heat, dryness, profuse sweating, scratching, friction, exposure to various kinds of animal fur, plants and chemicals, and contact with products used on a daily basis such as facial creams, soaps, cosmetics, and artificial fibers. Some foods may also aggravate the condition.

- Internal factors leading to eczema include chronic gastrointestinal disorders, stress, insomnia, overexertion, and emotional disturbances. Infection, metabolic disturbance and endocrine dysfunction can all trigger or aggravate eczema.

In terms of pathology, eczema is a delayed allergic reaction provoked by a complex of internal and external factors. Patients with a particular body constitution may have an inherited susceptibility to eczema. The disease may also be affected by the individual's general health condition and environmental factors. For example, patients sometimes have an adverse reaction to many non-harmful stimuli at work or elsewhere in their daily lives; for instance, some foods can make eczema worse.

Patients may be hypersensitive with a positive reaction to a number of substances in patch tests. Even after removal of the sensitizing agents, the eczema will take a long time to disappear. However, some patients are able to change the body's degree of reactivity through exercise or a change in their immediate environment and may avoid eczema when exposed to stimuli that used to cause the disease in the past. This is an indication of the complex nature of the pathology of eczema.

Since eczema is a reaction pattern, different stimuli can cause the skin to react in similar ways, often at the same time. This means that classification of the type of eczema seen in the clinic is often difficult. Classification of eczema according to the morphology or phase of the eruption provides a useful description of the type of lesion involved and offers clues to their TCM treatment. This book adopts a classification that combines those categorizations generally listed in modern Western medical textbooks with modifications or additions to take account of a TCM pattern identification-based approach.

Thus, this chapter begins with the description and treatment of general features of eczema according to whether the condition is acute, subacute or chronic. Many of the common patterns of eczema described later in the chapter also share these general features. The TCM treatment recommended for these patterns can then be taken into consideration when deciding on a treatment strategy for a particular type of eczema.

The chapter then discusses two particular forms of eczema that are difficult to classify – papular eczema, which TCM considers as a separate eczema pattern, and infectious eczematoid dermatitis, which can result from infection of the lesions of eczema.

Following this, the chapter focuses on a number of common eczematous conditions arranged according to a classification that currently appears to have achieved a broad consensus in the West. Some particular types of eczema are classified by body site at the end of the chapter as an aid to TCM analysis of eczematous conditions.

In TCM, the causative factors of eczema are generally divided into three main categories:

- External pathogenic factors (especially Wind, Dampness or Heat) settling in the skin.
  - Prevalence of Wind manifests as multiple lesions and pronounced itching.
  - Prevalence of Dampness manifests as lingering non-healing lesions mainly located in the lower part of the body.
  - Prevalence of Heat manifests as red and swollen skin, possibly leading to infection by Toxins.
- Internal factors involving the Heart, Spleen and Kidneys – dysfunction of these three organs leads to impairment of the metabolic function. As a result, pathogenic factors such as Damp-Heat move out to the skin and interstices (*cou li*).
  - Where there is hyperactivity of Heart-Fire, lesions are red, inflamed and extremely itchy.
  - Where there is severe Dampness resulting from Spleen dysfunction, maceration and erosion occur.
  - Persistence of the disease will result in Kidney Deficiency (Kidney Yin or Kidney Yang Deficiency).
- Dietary irregularities – overintake of spicy, greasy or rich food can lead to depletion of Yin-Liquids and binding of Damp-Heat.

In TCM, eczema is also known as *shi zhen* (Damp eruption), *feng shi chuang* (Wind-Damp sore) or *jin yin chuang* (wet spreading sore). Particular categories of eczema have different names (see the relevant sections below).

Basic patterns of eczema
湿疹

Most of the types of eczema described below share certain general features and these features or basic patterns (acute, subacute and chronic) are described in the first part of this chapter.

Clinical manifestations

Acute eczema

- Various skin lesions – erythema, papules, papulovesicles, and vesicles – can be present at the same time; one of these types of lesion may predominate.
- Vesicles may rupture spontaneously to cause pinpoint erosion with thick sticky discharge. Yellowish punctate transparent crusts form as the erosion and weeping dry up.

- Repeated occurrence of the disease will gradually lead to the involvement of a larger area. Erosion develops as a result of scratching, with weeping and maceration occurring locally as the condition worsens.
- In cases of secondary infection, vesicles will change into pustules filled with turbid fluid; these pustules will dry up to form purulent yellow crusts. Nearby lymph nodes are swollen and painful.
- Acute eczema can be further subdivided according to the predominant lesion.
  - *Erythematous eczema:* Mostly present at the initial stage with lesions characterized by localized reddening with ill-defined borders, sometimes accompanied by slight swelling.

- *Papular eczema*: Clusters of red papules a few millimeters in diameter mixed with tiny vesicles are present on an erythematous base. Bloody crusts form after scratching.
- *Vesicular eczema*: Clusters of small domed or pointed vesicles with underlying edema are present on an erythematous base. Pinpoint erosion occurs after vesicles rupture.
- *Pustular eczema*: After secondary infection, the clear fluid in the vesicles turns turbid and purulent. Thick greenish-yellow purulent crusts form after the lesions dry up.
- *Erosive eczema*: Excoriation of vesicles or pustules results in serous, bloody or pustular exudate with erosion of varying area.
- *Crusting eczema*: White, gray, yellow, or greenish-yellow crusts form after vesicular, pustular and erosive lesions dry up.
- *Desquamative eczema*: Bran-like or fine scaling may occur when the conditions described above heal.

Subacute eczema

- This condition often evolves from persistent acute eczema. Compared with acute eczema, it is characterized by less erythema and swelling, fewer vesicles, generally smaller papules, and more scaling.
- Other manifestations include some small areas of erosion due to excoriation, some exudation of clear fluid, crusts, and severe itching.
- Subacute eczema tends to develop into chronic eczema, but may also develop features of acute eczema due to external stimuli.

Chronic eczema

- This condition often evolves from recurring acute or subacute eczema.
- Characteristic lesions manifest as dry, rough, thickened, and scaling skin, deepening and widening of the cleavage lines of the skin, and hyperpigmentation or hypopigmentation.
- Itching may be moderate or intense; repeated scratching or rubbing of the skin often results in obvious lichenification, which in itself is itchy, resulting in self-perpetuation of the condition.

Differential diagnosis

Psoriasis

Psoriasis usually involves the extensor aspect of the limbs, especially the extensor aspect of the elbows and knees, but sometimes spreads to affect the whole body. The nails and scalp may also be involved. At the initial stage, bright red or dark red macules, maculopapules or papules appear with a shiny, wax-like surface, coalescing to form well demarcated round or oval plaques ranging from a few millimeters to several centimeters in size. These plaques are subsequently covered by large dry silvery-white laminated scales. If the scales are removed, bleeding points appear (Auspitz's sign). The lesions of psoriasis are likely to be more clearly defined than those of eczema.

Lichen planus

Eruptions usually involve the flexor surfaces of the wrists and forearms, and the lower legs around and above the ankles. Lesions manifest as intensely pruritic 2-10 mm flat-topped dull red shiny papules with an irregular, sharply defined angulated border. The surface of the lesions exhibits a lacy white pattern of lines (Wickham's striae). Mucous membranes are involved in 40-60 percent of individuals, commonly manifesting as grayish-white papules or Wickham's striae on the buccal mucosa, lips and tongue.

Lichen simplex chronicus (neurodermatitis)

Chronic eczema needs to be differentiated from lichen simplex chronicus, which tends to occur in easily reached areas of the body such as the nape of the neck, wrists and ankles. Lesions generally manifest as a single irregular or polygonal-shaped plaque with intermingled red flat papules. The skin in the affected area is rough with deepened skin creases (lichenification). In chronic cases, the lichenified areas become brown and are covered by dry fine scales.

Scabies

Scabies is characterized by the development of vesicles and burrows in the skin at any site, characteristically at the wrist, the web of the fingers and the lower abdomen, with intense itching at night. Eczema lacks the grayish linear, curved or serpiginous burrows characteristic of scabies.

Fungal infections

The differential diagnosis varies depending on the location of the lesions (see Chapter 11 for individual conditions). The classic tinea pattern presents as single or multiple sharply circumscribed circular, semicircular or concentric lesions which gradually heal in the center but are elevated at the borders with clusters of red papules or papulovesicles. Tinea manuum and tinea pedis are usually asymmetrical.

Drug eruptions

Drug eruptions have a sudden onset and extensive skin lesions. The causative factor can usually be clearly related to an allergic reaction to certain drugs.

Table 3-1 Differential diagnosis of acute eczema and contact dermatitis

	Acute eczema	Contact dermatitis
Etiology	Complex, may involve both internal and external factors	Identification of irritant or allergy-inducing agents aids diagnosis
Location	Involvement may be extensive, especially in children	Generally localized initially to direct contact areas (most frequently, the hands and face), but may spread elsewhere in cases of allergic contact dermatitis
Skin lesions	Polymorphic with diffuse, ill-defined borders	Lesions similar to those of acute or chronic eczema, but usually more localized
Duration of disease	Relatively long, frequently becomes chronic	May be acute or chronic; removal of contact with causative factor aids recovery
Recurrence	Common	Can be triggered by further contact with causative factor

Contact dermatitis

Table 3-1 compares acute eczema and contact dermatitis. Differentiation is often difficult, but is helpful from a TCM treatment viewpoint.

Etiology and pathology

Eczema can be caused by both internal and external factors, but internal factors are usually more important and include Heart-Fire, Spleen-Damp, Liver-Wind, and other imbalances in the Zang-Fu organs. Wind and Dampness are the main external factors.

Heat in the Heart channel

The Heart governs the Blood vessels. Emotional disturbances may generate Heat, which, when retained for a long period, transforms into Fire. Fire lies latent in the Ying and Xue levels, generating internal Blood-Heat. Exuberant Heat generates Wind, which then attacks the skin to cause eczema.

Dietary irregularities

- An improper diet with excessive intake of tea, alcohol, fish, seafood, or spicy food may stir Wind and impair the Spleen's transportation and transformation function, resulting in the generation of internal Dampness, which then transforms into Heat.
- Overeating of cold and raw food (including fruit) damages Spleen Yang and generates Water and Dampness internally. Spleen Deficiency and Heart-Fire then bind together to cause the disease.

Wind

Blood-Dryness generating Wind may arise as a result of:

- Damp-Heat accumulating internally complicated by an invasion by external Wind
- persistent exudation leading to damage to Yin and consumption of Blood
- excessive intake of spicy, aromatic or dry food

Persistent damage to Yin and consumption of Blood lead to lack of nourishment of Liver-Blood; Wind is generated internally and prevalence of Wind gives rise to Dryness.

Acute phase

In the acute phase, Wind, Heat and Dampness are the main causative factors:

- Wind patterns are characterized by rapid changes and manifest as itching of varying intensity
- Heat patterns are characterized by movement toward the exterior and manifest as erythema and papules
- Damp patterns are characterized by heaviness and turbidity, with Dampness gathering in the skin and manifesting as vesicles; as Dampness tends to be sticky and greasy, it is difficult to eliminate

Chronic phase

When the disease reaches the chronic phase, Damp-Heat has accumulated internally over a long period. Heat damages the Ying level, exudation of water damages Yin, and damage to Yin and consumption of Blood lead to Dryness, manifesting as gradual lichenification, dry skin, desquamation, or fissuring. Therefore in order to treat Blood-Dryness, accumulated Dampness must be eliminated first, thus allowing the skin to be properly nourished.

Pattern identification and treatment

INTERNAL TREATMENT

WIND PREDOMINATING OVER DAMPNESS (ACUTE PHASE)

Symptoms are usually worse on the upper body, manifesting as red papules and a small number of vesicles, mild exudation, and incessant itching. The tongue body is red with a thin white coating; the pulse is wiry and slippery.

Treatment principle

Dispel Wind and eliminate Dampness.

Prescription

XIAO FENG SAN JIA JIAN
Powder for Dispersing Wind, with modifications

Jing Jie (Herba Schizonepetae Tenuifoliae) 6g
Ku Shen (Radix Sophorae Flavescentis) 6g
Chan Tui ‡ (Periostracum Cicadae) 6g
Zhi Mu (Rhizoma Anemarrhenae Asphodeloidis) 6g
Gan Cao (Radix Glycyrrhizae) 6g
Fang Feng (Radix Ledebouriellae Divaricatae) 10g
Dang Gui (Radix Angelicae Sinensis) 10g
Cang Zhu (Rhizoma Atractylodis) 10g
Chao Niu Bang Zi (Fructus Arctii Lappae, stir-fried) 10g
Sheng Di Huang (Radix Rehmanniae Glutinosae) 12g
Shi Gao ‡ (Gypsum Fibrosum) 12g, decocted for 30 minutes before adding the other ingredients
Bai Xian Pi (Cortex Dictamni Dasycarpi Radicis) 12g
Tong Cao (Medulla Tetrapanacis Papyriferi) 3g

Explanation

- *Jing Jie* (Herba Schizonepetae Tenuifoliae), *Chan Tui* ‡ (Periostracum Cicadae), *Fang Feng* (Radix Ledebouriellae Divaricatae), and *Chao Niu Bang Zi* (Fructus Arctii Lappae, stir-fried) dredge Wind and alleviate itching.
- *Ku Shen* (Radix Sophorae Flavescentis), *Cang Zhu* (Rhizoma Atractylodis) and *Shi Gao* ‡ (Gypsum Fibrosum) clear Heat and dry Dampness.
- *Zhi Mu* (Rhizoma Anemarrhenae Asphodeloidis), *Sheng Di Huang* (Radix Rehmanniae Glutinosae), *Tong Cao* (Medulla Tetrapanacis Papyriferi), and *Gan Cao* (Radix Glycyrrhizae) clear Heart-Heat and cool the Blood.
- *Dang Gui* (Radix Angelicae Sinensis) and *Bai Xian Pi* (Cortex Dictamni Dasycarpi Radicis) eliminate Dampness and alleviate itching.
- Itching will disappear once Wind is dissipated, Heat is cleared and Dampness is transformed.

HEAT PREDOMINATING OVER DAMPNESS (ACUTE PHASE)

This pattern is characterized by acute onset, inflammation, numerous red 1-2 mm papules and a few vesicles, with a sensation of scorching heat. Accompanying symptoms and signs include irritability, thirst, itching, short voidings of reddish urine, and constipation. The tongue body is red with a thin yellow coating; the pulse is slippery and rapid.

Treatment principle

Clear Heat and eliminate Dampness.

Prescription

LIANG XUE CHU SHI TANG JIA JIAN
Decoction for Cooling the Blood and Eliminating Dampness, with modifications

Sheng Di Huang (Radix Rehmanniae Glutinosae) 15g
Ren Dong Teng (Caulis Lonicerae Japonicae) 15g
Bai Xian Pi (Cortex Dictamni Dasycarpi Radicis) 15g
Liu Yi San (Six-To-One Powder) 15g, wrapped
Mu Dan Pi (Cortex Moutan Radicis) 10g
Chi Shao (Radix Paeoniae Rubra) 10g
Hai Tong Pi (Cortex Erythrinae) 10g
Di Fu Zi (Fructus Kochiae Scopariae) 10g
Xi Xian Cao (Herba Siegesbeckiae) 12g
Chi Xiao Dou (Semen Phaseoli Calcarati) 12g
Lian Zi Xin (Plumula Nelumbinis Nuciferae) 6g

Explanation

- *Sheng Di Huang* (Radix Rehmanniae Glutinosae), *Mu Dan Pi* (Cortex Moutan Radicis), *Chi Shao* (Radix Paeoniae Rubra), and *Chi Xiao Dou* (Semen Phaseoli Calcarati) cool the Blood and clear Heat, transform Dampness and alleviate itching.
- *Ren Dong Teng* (Caulis Lonicerae Japonicae), *Bai Xian Pi* (Cortex Dictamni Dasycarpi Radicis), *Xi Xian Cao* (Herba Siegesbeckiae), *Hai Tong Pi* (Cortex Erythrinae), and *Di Fu Zi* (Fructus Kochiae Scopariae) relieve Toxicity and eliminate Dampness, dissipate Wind and alleviate itching.
- *Liu Yi San* (Six-To-One Powder) and *Lian Zi Xin* (Plumula Nelumbinis Nuciferae) clear Heat from the Heart and guide out reddish urine.
- The skin will stop feeling itchy once Heat Toxins have been expelled through the urine.

DAMP-HEAT (ACUTE PHASE)

This pattern is characterized by acute onset and short duration. Various types of lesion – erythema, papules, vesicles, erosion, and exudation – may appear simultaneously or in succession at any body site; borders are indistinct. Accompanying symptoms and signs include severe itching, dry throat with no desire for drinks or irritability with thirst, constipation, and yellow urine. The tongue body is red with a thin yellow coating, slightly greasy at the root; the pulse is slippery and rapid, or wiry and slippery.

Treatment principle

Clear Heat and benefit the movement of Dampness, dissipate Wind and alleviate itching.

Prescription

LONG DAN XIE GAN TANG JIA JIAN

Chinese Gentian Decoction for Draining the Liver, with modifications

Chao Long Dan Cao (Radix Gentianae Scabrae, stir-fried) 6g
Huang Qin (Radix Scutellariae Baicalensis) 6g
Chai Hu (Radix Bupleuri) 6g
Jing Jie (Herba Schizonepetae Tenuifoliae) 6g
Chan Tui ‡ (Periostracum Cicadae) 6g
Sheng Di Huang (Radix Rehmanniae Glutinosae) 15g
Ze Xie (Rhizoma Alismatis Orientalis) 15g
Bai Xian Pi (Cortex Dictamni Dasycarpi Radicis) 15g
Che Qian Zi (Semen Plantaginis) 10g, wrapped
Jiao Zhi Zi (Fructus Gardeniae Jasminoidis, scorch-fried) 10g
Chi Shao (Radix Paeoniae Rubra) 10g
Fang Feng (Radix Ledebouriellae Divaricatae) 10g

Explanation

- *Huang Qin* (Radix Scutellariae Baicalensis), *Chao Long Dan Cao* (Radix Gentianae Scabrae, stir-fried), *Jiao Zhi Zi* (Fructus Gardeniae Jasminoidis, scorch-fried), *Sheng Di Huang* (Radix Rehmanniae Glutinosae), and *Chi Shao* (Radix Paeoniae Rubra) clear Heat and cool the Blood.

- *Ze Xie* (Rhizoma Alismatis Orientalis), *Che Qian Zi* (Semen Plantaginis) and *Bai Xian Pi* (Cortex Dictamni Dasycarpi Radicis) transform Dampness and relieve Toxicity.

- *Chai Hu* (Radix Bupleuri), *Jing Jie* (Herba Schizonepetae Tenuifoliae), *Fang Feng* (Radix Ledebouriellae Divaricatae), and *Chan Tui* ‡ (Periostracum Cicadae) dredge Wind and alleviate itching.

DAMPNESS PREDOMINATING OVER HEAT (SUBACUTE/CHRONIC PHASE)

This pattern usually manifests in the lower body with a dull, pale skin and numerous vesicles with exudation on rupture after scratching. Accompanying symptoms and signs include itching, poor appetite, thin and loose stools, and lassitude. The tongue body is pale with a thin white coating; the pulse is thready and moderate.

Treatment principle

Fortify the Spleen and regulate Dampness.

Prescription

CHU SHI WEI LING TANG JIA JIAN

Poria Five Decoction for Eliminating Dampness and Calming the Stomach, with modifications

Cang Zhu (Rhizoma Atractylodis) 10g
Chen Pi (Pericarpium Citri Reticulatae) 10g
Hou Po (Cortex Magnoliae Officinalis) 10g
Chao Zhi Ke (Fructus Citri Aurantii, stir-fried) 10g
Sheng Di Huang (Radix Rehmanniae Glutinosae) 12g
Fu Ling Pi (Cortex Poriae Cocos) 12g
Che Qian Zi (Semen Plantaginis) 12g, wrapped
Zhu Ling (Sclerotium Polypori Umbellati) 12g
Chi Xiao Dou (Semen Phaseoli Calcarati) 15g
Yi Yi Ren (Semen Coicis Lachryma-jobi) 15g
Ze Xie (Rhizoma Alismatis Orientalis) 15g
Sha Ren (Fructus Amomi) 8g, added 10 minutes before the end of the decoction process

Explanation

- *Cang Zhu* (Rhizoma Atractylodis), *Chen Pi* (Pericarpium Citri Reticulatae), *Hou Po* (Cortex Magnoliae Officinalis), *Chao Zhi Ke* (Fructus Citri Aurantii, stir-fried), and *Sha Ren* (Fructus Amomi) fortify the Spleen and regulate Dampness.

- *Fu Ling Pi* (Cortex Poriae Cocos), *Che Qian Zi* (Semen Plantaginis), *Zhu Ling* (Sclerotium Polypori Umbellati), *Yi Yi Ren* (Semen Coicis Lachryma-jobi), and *Ze Xie* (Rhizoma Alismatis Orientalis) clear Heat and benefit the movement of Dampness.

- *Chi Xiao Dou* (Semen Phaseoli Calcarati) and *Sheng Di Huang* (Radix Rehmanniae Glutinosae) cool the Blood and eliminate Dampness.

DAMP OBSTRUCTION DUE TO SPLEEN DEFICIENCY (CHRONIC PHASE)

The disease is of long duration, with lesions presenting as discrete pale red or dull red macules or papules, with a few vesicles or papulovesicles and occasional exudation of fluid. Scaling and crusting occur as the lesions dry. Accompanying symptoms and signs include intense itching, epigastric discomfort, poor appetite, a sallow facial complexion, loose stools, and scant urine. The tongue body is pale red with a greasy white or greasy yellow coating; the pulse is deep, soggy, wiry, and slippery.

Treatment principle

Fortify the Spleen and eliminate Dampness.

Prescription

JIAN PI CHU SHI TANG JIA JIAN

Decoction for Fortifying the Spleen and Eliminating Dampness, with modifications

Fu Ling Pi (Cortex Poriae Cocos) 15g
Yin Chen Hao (Herba Artemisiae Scopariae) 15g
Sheng Di Huang (Radix Rehmanniae Glutinosae) 15g
Bai Zhu (Rhizoma Atractylodis Macrocephalae) 12g
Huang Qin (Radix Scutellariae Baicalensis) 12g
Jiao Zhi Zi (Fructus Gardeniae Jasminoidis, scorch-fried) 12g
Chao Zhi Ke (Fructus Citri Aurantii, stir-fried) 12g
Bai Xian Pi (Cortex Dictamni Dasycarpi Radicis) 12g

BASIC PATTERNS OF ECZEMA 75

Chi Xiao Dou (Semen Phaseoli Calcarati) 30g
Yi Yi Ren (Semen Coicis Lachryma-jobi) 10g
Chao Mai Ya (Fructus Hordei Vulgaris Germinatus, stir-fried) 10g
Chao Gu Ya (Fructus Setariae Italicae Germinatus, stir-fried) 10g

Explanation

- *Fu Ling Pi* (Cortex Poriae Cocos), *Bai Zhu* (Rhizoma Atractylodis Macrocephalae), *Yi Yi Ren* (Semen Coicis Lachryma-jobi), *Chao Mai Ya* (Fructus Hordei Vulgaris Germinatus, stir-fried), and *Chao Gu Ya* (Fructus Setariae Italicae Germinatus, stir-fried) support the Spleen and transform Dampness.
- *Huang Qin* (Radix Scutellariae Baicalensis), *Jiao Zhi Zi* (Fructus Gardeniae Jasminoidis, scorch-fried) and *Sheng Di Huang* (Radix Rehmanniae Glutinosae) clear Heat and relieve Damp-Heat.
- *Yin Chen Hao* (Herba Artemisiae Scopariae), *Bai Xian Pi* (Cortex Dictamni Dasycarpi Radicis), *Chi Xiao Dou* (Semen Phaseoli Calcarati), and *Chao Zhi Ke* (Fructus Citri Aurantii, stir-fried) transform Dampness and clear Heat.

BLOOD-DRYNESS DUE TO DAMAGE TO YIN WITH ACCUMULATION OF DAMPNESS (CHRONIC PHASE)

This condition is lingering and recurrent. Lesions are dull red or dirty gray, and the skin is rough, infiltrated or lichenified with scratch marks, crusting or scaling, or small amounts of exudation. Accompanying symptoms and signs include difficulty in falling asleep because of the intense itching, mental exhaustion, dry throat, and thirst. The tongue body is dry and red with a thin coating or no coating; the pulse is thready and slippery, or wiry and thready.

Treatment principle

Enrich Yin and nourish the Blood, eliminate Dampness and alleviate itching.

Prescription
ZI YIN CHU SHI TANG JIA JIAN
Decoction for Enriching Yin and Eliminating Dampness, with modifications

Sheng Di Huang (Radix Rehmanniae Glutinosae) 30g
Xuan Shen (Radix Scrophulariae Ningpoensis) 10g
Dang Gui (Radix Angelicae Sinensis) 10g
Dan Shen (Radix Salviae Miltiorrhizae) 10g
She Chuang Zi (Fructus Cnidii Monnieri) 10g
Fu Ling (Sclerotium Poriae Cocos) 12g
Ze Xie (Rhizoma Alismatis Orientalis) 12g
Bai Xian Pi (Cortex Dictamni Dasycarpi Radicis) 12g
Chao Bai Bian Dou (Semen Dolichoris Lablab, stir-fried) 15g

Shan Yao (Rhizoma Dioscoreae Oppositae) 15g
Yi Yi Ren (Semen Coicis Lachryma-jobi) 15g
Yi Mu Cao (Herba Leonuri Heterophylli) 9g
Xu Chang Qing (Radix Cynanchi Paniculati) 9g

Explanation

- *Sheng Di Huang* (Radix Rehmanniae Glutinosae), *Xuan Shen* (Radix Scrophulariae Ningpoensis) and *Shan Yao* (Rhizoma Dioscoreae Oppositae) enrich Yin and protect Body Fluids.
- *Fu Ling* (Sclerotium Poriae Cocos), *Yi Yi Ren* (Semen Coicis Lachryma-jobi) and *Chao Bai Bian Dou* (Semen Dolichoris Lablab, stir-fried) transform Dampness and moisten Dryness.
- *Dang Gui* (Radix Angelicae Sinensis), *Yi Mu Cao* (Herba Leonuri Heterophylli), *Xu Chang Qing* (Radix Cynanchi Paniculati), and *Dan Shen* (Radix Salviae Miltiorrhizae) invigorate the Blood to alleviate itching.
- *Bai Xian Pi* (Cortex Dictamni Dasycarpi Radicis), *Ze Xie* (Rhizoma Alismatis Orientalis) and *She Chuang Zi* (Fructus Cnidii Monnieri) transform Dampness to alleviate itching.
- This prescription can be applied to all chronic cases.

General modifications

1. For abdominal fullness, add *Hou Po* (Cortex Magnoliae Officinalis), *Da Fu Pi* (Pericarpium Arecae Catechu) and *Mei Gui Hua* (Flos Rosae Rugosae).
2. For poor appetite, add *Pei Lan* (Herba Eupatorii Fortunei), *Chao Mai Ya* (Fructus Hordei Vulgaris Germinatus, stir-fried), *Chao Gu Ya* (Fructus Setariae Italicae Germinatus, stir-fried), and *Ji Nei Jin*‡ (Endothelium Corneum Gigeriae Galli).
3. For dry throat and thirst, add *Mai Men Dong* (Radix Ophiopogonis Japonici), *Yu Zhu* (Rhizoma Polygonati Odorati) and *Shi Hu** (Herba Dendrobii).
4. For severe, incessant itching, add *Wu Shao She*‡ (Zaocys Dhumnades) and *Xu Chang Qing* (Radix Cynanchi Paniculati).
5. For insomnia due to itching, add *Suan Zao Ren* (Semen Ziziphi Spinosae), *Ye Jiao Teng* (Caulis Polygoni Multiflori), *Long Gu*‡ (Os Draconis), and *Mu Li*‡ (Concha Ostreae).
6. For loose stools, add *Bai Bian Dou* (Semen Dolichoris Lablab), *Shan Yao* (Rhizoma Dioscoreae Oppositae) and *Yin Yang Huo* (Herba Epimedii).
7. For lichenified lesions, add *Chi Shao* (Radix Paeoniae Rubra), *Tao Ren* (Semen Persicae), *Dan Shen* (Radix Salviae Miltiorrhizae), *Ze Lan* (Herba Lycopi Lucidi), *Di Long*‡ (Lumbricus), *Zao Jiao Ci* (Spina Gleditsiae Sinensis), and *Chuan Shan Jia** (Squama Manitis Pentadactylae).

8. For erythema and a burning sensation accompanying an acute recurrence, add *Di Gu Pi* (Cortex Lycii Radicis), *Chi Shao* (Radix Paeoniae Rubra), *Dan Shen* (Radix Salviae Miltiorrhizae), and *Zi Cao* (Radix Arnebiae seu Lithospermi).

9. For lesions on the face and head, add *Chuan Xiong* (Rhizoma Ligustici Chuanxiong), *Qiang Huo* (Rhizoma et Radix Notopterygii) and *Bai Zhi* (Radix Angelicae Dahuricae).

10. For lesions on the breasts and around the umbilicus, add *Yin Chen Hao* (Herba Artemisiae Scopariae), *Tu Da Huang* (Radix Rumicis Madaio) and *Che Qian Zi* (Semen Plantaginis).

11. For lesions on the arms and legs, add *Sang Zhi* (Ramulus Mori Albae), *Chuan Niu Xi* (Radix Cyathulae Officinalis) and *Ren Dong Teng* (Caulis Lonicerae Japonicae).

12. For lesions on the lower leg with varicose veins and black skin, add *Ze Lan* (Herba Lycopi Lucidi), *E Zhu* (Rhizoma Curcumae) and *Chuan Niu Xi* (Radix Cyathulae Officinalis).

PATENT HERBAL MEDICINES

Acute stage

- Take five tablets of *Qing Jie Pian* (Clearing and Relieving Tablet) twice a day with lukewarm boiled water.

- Select one or two of the following – *Er Miao Wan* (Mysterious Two Pill), *San Miao Wan* (Mysterious Three Pill), *Long Dan Xie Gan Wan* (Chinese Gentian Pill for Draining the Liver) and *Fang Feng Tong Sheng San* (Ledebouriella Powder that Sagely Unblocks) – and take 4.5g orally with lukewarm boiled water twice a day.

Chronic stage

- Take five tablets of *Dang Gui Pian* (Chinese Angelica Root Tablet) twice a day with lukewarm boiled water.

- Take 3g of *Wu She Zhi Yang Wan* (Black-Tail Snake Pill for Alleviating Itching) twice a day with lukewarm boiled water.

EXTERNAL TREATMENT

Acute stage

- Before rupture of papules and vesicles, use *Lu Lu Tong Shui Xi Ji* (Sweetgum Fruit Wash Preparation) to prepare a decoction for use as a wet compress for 15 minutes; then apply *Shi Zhen Yi Hao Gao* (No. 1 Eczema Paste). Treat twice a day.

- For lesions with erosion and large amounts of exudate, prepare a 10 percent aqueous solution with *Huang Bai* (Cortex Phellodendri); or prepare a decoction with equal amounts of *Ma Chi Xian* (Herba Portulacae Oleraceae) and *Di Yu* (Radix Sanguisorbae Officinalis), or with *Pu Gong Ying* (Herba Taraxaci cum Radice) 60g and *Ye Ju Hua* (Flos Chrysanthemi Indici) 15g. When cooled, apply these preparations as a wet compress on the lesions for 15 minutes, two to five times a day.

- For erythema, papules and vesicles with a little exudation, apply *San Huang Xi Ji* (Three Yellows Wash Preparation) five or six times a day, or apply *Qing Dai San* (Indigo Powder) four or five times a day.

- For erosion, pustules and crusting, mix *Qing Dai San* (Indigo Powder) with *Xiang You* (Oleum Sesami Seminis) and apply to the affected area three times a day; alternatively, *Huang Lian You* (Coptis Oil) may be applied.

Subacute stage

- Mix *San Huang Xi Ji* (Three Yellows Wash Preparation) or *Qing Dai San* (Indigo Powder) with *Xiang You* (Oleum Sesami Seminis) and apply to the affected area three times a day.

Chronic stage

- Apply *Qing Dai Gao* (Indigo Paste) or *Pi Zhi Gao* (Skin Grease) to the lesions. For patients with varicose veins in the lower leg, wrap the leg in a bandage.

- Apply *Qing Dai Gao* (Indigo Paste) to the affected area once a day and heat with a hair dryer for 10 minutes.

- Mix *Mao Yan Cao Gao* (Crescent Euphorbia Paste) with *Qing Dai Gao* (Indigo Paste) in a 1:4 ratio and apply to the lesions twice a day.

- If itching is severe, use *Lu Hu Xi Ji* (Calamine and Giant Knotweed Wash Preparation) or *She Chuang Zi Xi Ji* (Cnidium Fruit Wash Preparation) as an external wash three to five times a day.

- If the condition is of long duration with lichenification and severe itching, apply *Zhi Yang Fen* (Powder for Alleviating Itching) directly on the affected area, or mix the powder into a paste with vegetable oil before application. Treat once or twice a day.

- For lesions with lichenification and scaling, apply *Shi Du Gao* (Damp Toxin Paste) or *Hei Dou Liu You Ruan Gao* (Black Soybean and Vaseline® Ointment) to the affected area once or twice a day.

- For dry lesions with fissuring, apply *Lang Du Gao* (Chinese Wolfsbane Paste) once or twice a day.

ACUPUNCTURE

Selection of points on the affected channels

Main points: LI-11 Quchi, SP-10 Xuehai and BL-40 Weizhong.

Auxiliary points: PC-7 Daling, LI-15 Jianyu and PC-3 Quze.

Combined local and distal points
Points: CV-3 Zhongji, SP-10 Xuehai, SP-6 Sanyinjiao, LR-5 Ligou, and LR-1 Dadun.

Selection of points according to pattern identification
Damp-Heat: GV-13 Taodao, BL-13 Feishu, LI-11 Quchi, HT-7 Shenmen, and SP-9 Yinlingquan.
Damp obstruction: ST-36 Zusanli, SP-6 Sanyinjiao, CV-12 Zhongwan, and SP-8 Diji.
Blood-Dryness: PC-4 Ximen, ST-36 Zusanli, SP-6 Sanyinjiao, and SP-2 Dadu.

Selection of points according to disease stage
Chronic stage: ST-36 Zusanli, SP-9 Yinlingquan, LI-11 Quchi, and SP-10 Xuehai.
Acute stage: Add GV-14 Dazhui, BL-13 Feishu, BL-40 Weizhong, and SP-6 Sanyinjiao to the points selected for the chronic stage.

Explanation
The points in the four groups fall into three categories:
- ST-36 Zusanli, PC-3 Quze, SP-9 Yinlingquan, GV-14 Dazhui, CV-12 Zhongwan, and SP-8 Diji clear Heat and transform Dampness.
- LI-11 Quchi, BL-13 Feishu, PC-7 Daling, LI-15 Jianyu, LR-1 Dadun, LR-5 Ligou, and GV-13 Taodao dredge Wind and disperse swelling.
- SP-10 Xuehai, BL-40 Weizhong, SP-6 Sanyinjiao, CV-3 Zhongji, PC-4 Ximen, HT-7 Shenmen, and SP-2 Dadu cool the Blood and reduce erythema.

MOXIBUSTION
Main points: LI-11 Quchi and SP-10 Xuehai.
Auxiliary points: LI-15 Jianyu, GB-30 Huantiao, LI-4 Hegu, GV-20 Baihui, GV-14 Dazhui, and Ashi points (sites of intense itching).
Technique: Give gentle moxibustion with a moxa stick at each point for 10-15 minutes once a day. However, keep moxibustion at points on the head and face to a minimum.

EAR ACUPUNCTURE
Points: Lung, Adrenal Gland, Endocrine, Spleen, Ear-Shenmen, and ear points corresponding to the sites of lesions on the body.
Technique: Needle three or four of the points. Retain the needles for 30 minutes. Treat once a day.

ELECTRO-ACUPUNCTURE
Point: Ashi points (the site of the lesions).
Technique: Insert four 1.5 cun no. 32 filiform needles obliquely around the Ashi points toward the center of the lesion to a depth of 1.0 cun. Connect to an electro-acupuncture apparatus and increase the current gradually according to the tolerance level of individual patients. Treat for 20 minutes once a day or every other day.

ENCIRCLEMENT NEEDLING
Point: Ashi points (the site of the lesions).
Technique: Insert several filiform needles obliquely from the border of the lesions toward the center, with one needle inserted perpendicularly in the center. Retain the needles for 30 minutes after obtaining Qi. Treat once every two days. This method is recommended for chronic eczema.

PLUM-BLOSSOM NEEDLING
Prescription 1
Points: LI-11 Quchi, EX-B-2 Jiaji 1st-17th,[i] the sites of lesions, the medial aspect of the lower leg, LI-4 Hegu, and ST-36 Zusanli.
Technique: Produce strong stimulation on both sides of the spine between T_1 and L_5, but only moderate stimulation at the other areas and points. Treat once every other day.

Prescription 2
Points: Ashi points (the site of the lesions).
Technique: Tap gently from the edge to the center of the lesions until there is slight exudation or bleeding. Treat once every two or three days. This treatment is recommended for chronic eczema.

Clinical notes

- Acute eczema usually appears at a time of confrontation between Vital Qi (Zheng Qi) and pathogenic factors. Materia medica selected for internal usage should be those that drain Fire with cold and bitterness and those that benefit the movement of Dampness and alleviate itching.

- Subacute eczema appears at a time when Vital Qi (Zheng Qi) and pathogenic factors are intermingling. The primary treatment principle is to clear Heat and drain Fire, and support the Spleen and transform Dampness, with the secondary considerations of dissipating Wind and alleviating itching, enriching Yin and eliminating Dampness, or invigorating the Blood and alleviating itching. The condition is often complicated at this stage:
  - If itching is worse, herbs for dissipating Wind to alleviate itching should predominate.

---

[i] M-BW-35 according to the system employed by the Shanghai College of Traditional Chinese Medicine.

- If exudation is worse, herbs for enriching Yin should predominate in order to inhibit exudation of Body Fluids.
- If lesions are thick, herbs for invigorating the Blood should predominate in order to transform Blood stasis to soften the skin.

Materia medica for primary and secondary treatment should be used in approximately equal proportions.

- Chronic eczema usually appears at a time of Deficiency of Vital Qi (Zheng Qi) and debilitation of pathogenic factors. Treatment should focus on supporting the Spleen to transform Dampness or enriching Yin to eliminate Dampness with the secondary consideration of dissipating or extinguishing Wind to alleviate itching.
- When treating this condition, careful differentiation must be made among Wind, Dampness, Heat, and Deficiency patterns.
  - Severe itching denotes that Wind is predominant, with the treatment principle being to dredge Wind.
  - Erosion and exudation indicate that Dampness is predominant, with the treatment principle being to clear and transform Dampness.
  - Redness, swelling, pain, and itching imply that Heat is predominant, with the treatment principle being to clear Heat Toxins
  - Yin Deficiency patterns manifest as dryness and itching, with the treatment principle being to nourish Yin and moisten Dryness.
- External treatment should be based on two major principles:
  - Medications should start from lower concentrations, gradually increasing to higher concentrations, especially for infants and weak patients and in areas where the skin is delicate.
  - Apply a wet compress or wash for symptoms of a wet nature such as exudation and erosion; and use relatively drier medications such as ointments for symptoms of a dry nature including thickening or lichenification of the skin or fissuring.
- Acupuncture and moxibustion are effective in dispersing swelling and alleviating itching while helping the lesions to heal and can therefore be used as supporting treatment.
- Eczema is likely to recur. It leaves no scar after the lesions have disappeared.

Advice for the patient

- Avoid washing with hot water. Do not wash with soap and avoid contact with washing powder.
- Remove intake of fish, shellfish, seafood, spicy food, or alcohol from the diet.
- Avoid scratching the lesions to prevent the possibility of secondary infection.

Case histories

Case 1

Patient
Male, aged 30.

Clinical manifestations
Two weeks previously, red papules had appeared on the patient's abdomen. The lesions were itchy, especially at night. Scratching led to spreading of the lesions and exudation of yellow fluid. In some areas of the skin, the papules became confluent, forming large patches, with the lesions gradually extending to the lower back and trunk. Accompanying symptoms and signs included dry stools, yellow urine and dry mouth with no desire for drinks.

Examination revealed small red papules distributed over pale red erythematous patches on the chest and back. Clusters of 1-2 mm papules were found on the lower abdomen and lower back interspersed with small vesicles. The tops of some of the papules had been broken by scratching; small amounts of exudate had oozed out and dried up to form crusts. Similar lesions were also noted on the buttocks. The tongue body was normal with a thin white coating; the pulse was deep, thready and slightly rapid.

Diagnosis
Acute eczema (*shi zhen*).

Pattern identification
Damp-Heat accumulating over a long period and transforming into Heat, with Heat predominating over Dampness.

Treatment principle
Clear Heat, cool the Blood and benefit the movement of Dampness.

Prescription ingredients
Long Dan Cao (Radix Gentianae Scabrae) 15g
Huang Qin (Radix Scutellariae Baicalensis) 15g
Zhi Zi (Fructus Gardeniae Jasminoidis) 15g
Sheng Di Huang (Radix Rehmanniae Glutinosae) 30g
Chi Shao (Radix Paeoniae Rubra) 25g
Yin Chen Hao (Herba Artemisiae Scopariae) 25g
Zi Cao (Radix Arnebiae seu Lithospermi) 15g
Di Fu Zi (Fructus Kochiae Scopariae) 15g
Bai Mao Gen (Rhizoma Imperatae Cylindricae) 25g
Gan Cao (Radix Glycyrrhizae) 10g

One bag a day was used to prepare a decoction, taken twice a day.

Second visit
After 21 bags of the decoction, lesions were gradually beginning to subside and the color of the papules was becoming

paler. A few small red papules had appeared on the abdomen and groin; wheal-like lesions were also occasionally evident.

Treatment principle
Clear Heat, cool the Blood and benefit the movement of Dampness, nourish the Blood and cool the Liver.

Prescription ingredients
Long Dan Cao (Radix Gentianae Scabrae) 15g
Huang Qin (Radix Scutellariae Baicalensis) 15g
Sheng Di Huang (Radix Rehmanniae Glutinosae) 30g
Chi Shao (Radix Paeoniae Rubra) 25g
Dang Gui (Radix Angelicae Sinensis) 20g
Yin Chen Hao (Herba Artemisiae Scopariae) 25g
Nü Zhen Zi (Fructus Ligustri Lucidi) 25g
Han Lian Cao (Herba Ecliptae Prostratae) 20g
Bai Ji Li (Fructus Tribuli Terrestris) 15g
Gan Cao (Radix Glycyrrhizae) 10g

Outcome
After another 15 bags of the decoction, the lesions had disappeared.

Discussion
See Case 2 below. [1]

Case 2
Patient
Male, aged 28.

Clinical manifestations
Ten days previously, papules and vesicles had appeared suddenly all over the patient's body. Scratching led to exudation, which had worsened in the last two or three days. Rupture of the vesicles resulted in yellow exudate and an erosive surface. Accompanying symptoms and signs included thirst, dry stools and short voidings of reddish urine.

Examination revealed pinpoint to 2mm red papules and vesicles distributed over the face, neck, trunk, and limbs. Some of the lesions had become confluent with erosion and marked exudation. The patient had a temperature of 37.7°C. The tongue body was red at the tip with a white coating; the right pulse was surging and large, the left pulse was wiry and slippery.

Diagnosis
Acute eczema (*jin yin chuang*).

Pattern identification
Accumulated Dampness retained over a long period had transformed into Heat, with neither Dampness nor Heat predominating.

Treatment principle
Clear Heat and benefit the movement of Dampness.

Prescription ingredients
Long Dan Cao (Radix Gentianae Scabrae) 15g
Huang Qin (Radix Scutellariae Baicalensis) 15g
Huang Bai (Cortex Phellodendri) 20g
Ze Xie (Rhizoma Alismatis Orientalis) 15g
Yin Chen Hao (Herba Artemisiae Scopariae) 15g

Che Qian Zi (Semen Plantaginis) 20g
Zhi Zi (Fructus Gardeniae Jasminoidis) 15g
Gan Di Huang (Radix Rehmanniae Glutinosae Exsiccata) 30g
Zi Hua Di Ding (Herba Violae Yedoensitis) 20g
Dan Zhu Ye (Herba Lophatheri Gracilis) 20g
Da Qing Ye (Folium Isatidis seu Baphicacanthi) 20g

External treatment
After using a decoction of *Ma Chi Xian* (Herba Portulacae Oleraceae) 30g as a wet compress, *Qu Shi San* (Powder for Dispelling Dampness) was mixed with *Gan Cao You* (Licorice Oil) for application to the affected areas.

Outcome
After six bags of the decoction, the lesions were beginning to improve and after another 26 bags, they had disappeared.

Discussion
In both these cases, Damp-Heat patterns were involved. Internal accumulation of Dampness should be considered as the Root and its retention and transformation into Heat as the Manifestation. In line with the principle of treating the Manifestations in acute cases, large doses of materia medica for clearing Heat and cooling the Blood were used such as *Long Dan Cao* (Radix Gentianae Scabrae), *Huang Qin* (Radix Scutellariae Baicalensis), *Zhi Zi* (Fructus Gardeniae Jasminoidis), *Huang Bai* (Cortex Phellodendri), *Sheng Di Huang* (Radix Rehmanniae Glutinosae), *Da Qing Ye* (Folium Isatidis seu Baphicacanthi), and *Chi Shao* (Radix Paeoniae Rubra). Other materia medica for clearing Heat and benefiting the movement of Dampness such as *Yin Chen Hao* (Herba Artemisiae Scopariae), *Ze Xie* (Rhizoma Alismatis Orientalis), *Di Fu Zi* (Fructus Kochiae Scopariae), and *Bai Mao Gen* (Rhizoma Imperatae Cylindricae) were included so that the Root and Manifestations were treated at the same time. [2]

Case 3
Patient
Female, aged 52.

Clinical manifestations
Ten days before the first consultation, the patient had been caught in the rain. The following day, her legs felt heavy and the medial aspects were itchy. Red papules and vesicles 2-3 mm in diameter appeared locally after scratching, and the itching became worse. Exudation occurred in the areas where the skin had been broken by scratching. Gradually, the whole body was involved. The patient, who was overweight, could not sleep because of the itching. Accompanying symptoms and signs included a bitter taste in the mouth, irritability, short voidings of reddish urine, and difficult bowel movements.

Examination revealed erythema with surface exudate and crusting present in two locations on the medial aspect of the legs, the largest patches being 3-5 cm in diameter. Discrete 2-3 mm papules and vesicles were also found on the legs, scalp, face, and trunk. The exudate was yellowish-white in color. The tongue body was red with a yellow and greasy coating; the pulse was slippery and rapid.

Diagnosis
Acute eczema (*feng shi chuang*).

Pattern identification

Exuberant Damp-Heat.

Treatment principle

Dredge Wind, clear Heat and benefit the movement of Dampness.

Acupuncture points

LI-11 Quchi, SP-10 Xuehai and SP-9 Yinlingquan.

Technique

The needles were inserted perpendicularly to a depth of 1.0-1.5 cun at LI-11 Quchi and SP-10 Xuehai and to a depth of 0.5-1.2 cun at SP-9 Yinlingquan, with manipulation by the lifting and thrusting reducing method for one minute after insertion. The needles were retained for 30 minutes. Treatment took place daily.

Outcome

After two days of treatment, itching was reduced; after three further treatments, some of the papules and vesicles had been dispersed; after another four treatments, crusts fell off; and after nine more treatments, the itching had stopped, the papules and vesicles had disappeared, and the skin had recovered its normal appearance.

Discussion

The patient's obesity was due to accumulation of Damp-Heat. After being caught in the rain and wading through water, an external invasion of Wind-Damp took place. External and internal pathogenic factors combined and interacted with each other to cause exuberant Damp-Heat. When this Damp-Heat flooded to the skin and flesh, papular and vesicular eruptions occurred with itching and exudation. Internally, the Damp-Heat was encumbering Spleen Yang. Accompanying symptoms and signs of a bitter taste in the mouth, irritability, short voidings of reddish urine, difficult bowel movements, a red tongue body with a yellow and greasy coating, and a slippery and rapid pulse were all signs of exuberant Damp-Heat. [3]

Case 4
Patient

Male, aged 34.

Clinical manifestations

Two weeks previously after drinking alcohol, itchy papules and vesicles with watery exudate appeared all over the patient's body, causing him considerable discomfort day and night. Accompanying symptoms and signs included a bitter taste in the mouth, nausea, abdominal distension, loss of appetite, lassitude, dizziness, and loose stools. As the condition persisted, erosion and exudation worsened, with the patient using one roll of toilet paper a day to try to dry up the lesions.

Examination revealed papules and vesicles distributed over large patches of edematous erythema on the trunk and limbs with significant erosion and exudation. Crusting and scaling could be seen in a few areas. The tongue body was pale with a white and greasy coating; the pulse was wiry and slippery.

Diagnosis

Subacute eczema (*jin yin chuang*).

Pattern identification

Damp-Heat accumulating internally with Dampness predominating over Heat.

Treatment principle

Clear the Spleen, eliminate Dampness and clear Heat.

Prescription ingredients

Bai Zhu (Rhizoma Atractylodis Macrocephalae) 10g
Zhi Ke (Fructus Citri Aurantii) 10g
Yi Yi Ren (Semen Coicis Lachryma-jobi) 30g
Chi Fu Ling (Sclerotium Poriae Cocos Rubrae) 15g
Dong Gua Pi (Epicarpium Benincasae Hispidae) 15g
Bai Xian Pi (Cortex Dictamni Dasycarpi Radicis) 30g
Ku Shen (Radix Sophorae Flavescentis) 15g
Che Qian Zi (Semen Plantaginis) 15g
Ze Xie (Rhizoma Alismatis Orientalis) 15g
Yin Chen Hao (Herba Artemisiae Scopariae) 30g
Huang Qin (Radix Scutellariae Baicalensis) 10g
Zhi Zi (Fructus Gardeniae Jasminoidis) 10g
Liu Yi San (Six-To-One Powder) 30g, wrapped

One bag a day was used to prepare a decoction, taken twice a day.

External treatment

A decoction was prepared with *Ma Chi Xian* (Herba Portulacae Oleraceae) 30g and *Huang Bai* (Cortex Phellodendri) 30g and applied warm to the affected areas as a damp compress.

Outcome

After three bags of the decoction, edema had been reduced and there was less exudation. Since itching had improved, the patient was able to sleep for a few hours. After another four bags, itching disappeared, erosion gradually diminished and exudation stopped. The patient was told to drink another seven bags, after which the symptoms had disappeared, leaving a small amount of scaling over the lesions.

Discussion

This was essentially a case of exuberant Dampness due to Spleen Deficiency. The patient had a normal constitution, but after drinking alcohol, Damp-Heat accumulated internally, subsequently encumbering the Spleen and impairing its transformation and transportation function with the result that Water and Dampness accumulated to obstruct the skin and flesh. The key treatment principle therefore was to clear Heat from the Spleen and eliminate Dampness.

In the prescription, *Bai Zhu* (Rhizoma Atractylodis Macrocephalae), *Zhi Ke* (Fructus Citri Aurantii), *Yi Yi Ren* (Semen Coicis Lachryma-jobi), *Chi Fu Ling* (Sclerotium Poriae Cocos Rubrae), *Dong Gua Pi* (Epicarpium Benincasae Hispidae), *Bai Xian Pi* (Cortex Dictamni Dasycarpi Radicis), *Ku Shen* (Radix Sophorae Flavescentis), *Ze Xie* (Rhizoma Alismatis Orientalis), *Che Qian Zi* (Semen Plantaginis), and large a dosage of *Yin Chen Hao* (Herba Artemisiae Scopariae) were used to benefit the movement of Dampness and clear Heat. They were assisted by *Huang Qin* (Radix Scutellariae Baicalensis) and *Zhi Zi* (Fructus Gardeniae Jasminoidis), which clear Heat from the Lungs and Middle Burner. [4]

Case 5
Patient
Male, aged 38.

Clinical manifestations
One month before the consultation, the patient abraded the skin on the left elbow in a bicycle accident. He immediately felt local itching, which became more severe day by day and spread to the whole arm with exudation. After another five or six days, the disease spread throughout the body, with papules evident on the ears, trunk and other areas. The patient was often away from home on business trips and had an excessive consumption of certain food such as lamb, fish and seafood. He had suffered from chronic eczema on the left lower leg for 18 years. Accompanying symptoms included poor digestion, dry stools and yellow urine.

Except for the palm and the dorsum of the hand, the skin on the upper limb was dull red with moist ulceration and profuse exudation. Vesicles and papulovesicles with crusts were densely distributed on the borders of the ulcers. Discrete, small red papules and papulovesicles were found on the ears and trunk. A patch of chronic infiltrating 1.0-1.5 cm coin-shaped lesions was evident on the left lower leg. The tongue body was red with a thin white coating; the pulse was wiry and slippery.

Diagnosis
Acute flare-up of chronic eczema (*jin yin chuang*).

Pattern identification
Spreading of Damp-Heat due to Spleen Deficiency and Heart-Fire.

Treatment principle
Benefit the movement of Dampness and clear Heat.

Prescription ingredients
Sheng Di Huang (Radix Rehmanniae Glutinosae) 30g
Pu Gong Ying (Herba Taraxaci cum Radice) 15g
Long Dan Cao (Radix Gentianae Scabrae) 9g
Huang Qin (Radix Scutellariae Baicalensis) 9g
Fu Ling Pi (Cortex Poriae Cocos) 9g
Liu Yi San (Six-To-One Powder) 9g, wrapped
Tong Cao (Medulla Tetrapanacis Papyriferi) 6g
Da Huang (Radix et Rhizoma Rhei) 6g, added 10 minutes
   before the end of the decoction process
Jin Yin Hua (Flos Lonicerae) 12g

One bag a day was used to prepare a decoction, taken twice a day. In addition, a cool wet compress was prepared with a decoction of *Di Yu* (Radix Sanguisorbae Officinalis) 30g and *Ma Chi Xian* (Herba Portulacae Oleraceae) 30g.

Second visit
After three days, exudation had diminished, but there was still inflammation and swelling. *Mu Dan Pi* (Cortex Moutan Radicis) 9g, *Chi Shao* (Radix Paeoniae Rubra) 9g and *Ze Xie* (Rhizoma Alismatis Orientalis) 9g were added to the original prescription to cool the Blood and eliminate Dampness. Four bags were prescribed. The compress remained the same.

Third visit
The day before the third consultation, the patient ate a bowl of shrimp and egg soup. Exudation increased, lesions spread to the shoulder, and small, discrete groups of papulovesicles were observed in the popliteal fossae. *Long Dan Cao* (Radix Gentianae Scabrae) was removed from the original prescription and *Cang Zhu* (Rhizoma Atractylodis) 9g, *Chen Pi* (Pericarpium Citri Reticulatae) 6g, *Huang Bai* (Cortex Phellodendri) 6g, and *Hou Po* (Cortex Magnoliae Officinalis) 6g were added for the purpose of fortifying the Spleen and draining Dampness. The external application remained the same.

Fourth visit
After another five days, the lesions on the left arm were localized and exudation had decreased markedly. Erosions were bright red, and most were re-epithelializing. Lesions in other areas had almost disappeared. The appetite had improved, but the patient still complained of poor sleep and constipation. The prescription was then amended.

Prescription ingredients
Sheng Di Huang (Radix Rehmanniae Glutinosae) 30g
Mu Dan Pi (Cortex Moutan Radicis) 9g
Chi Shao (Radix Paeoniae Rubra) 9g
Chi Fu Ling (Sclerotium Poriae Cocos Rubrae) 9g
Ze Xie (Rhizoma Alismatis Orientalis) 9g
Cang Zhu (Rhizoma Atractylodis) 9g
Che Qian Zi (Semen Plantaginis) 9g, wrapped
Liu Yi San (Six-To-One Powder) 9g, wrapped
Huang Bai (Cortex Phellodendri) 6g
Da Huang (Radix et Rhizoma Rhei) 6g, added 10 minutes
   before the end of the decoction process
Pu Gong Ying (Herba Taraxaci cum Radice) 15g
Jin Yin Hua (Flos Lonicerae) 12g

Fifth visit
After a further five days of drinking the decoction, the lesions on the left arm had virtually disappeared, but exudation had manifested due to rupture after scratching while the patient was asleep. The prescription was therefore modified by removing *Jin Yin Hua* (Flos Lonicerae) and adding *Bai Xian Pi* (Cortex Dictamni Dasycarpi Radicis) 9g and *Di Fu Zi* (Fructus Kochiae Scopariae) 9g.

Sixth visit
Five days later, the patient only felt itching on the central part of the left forearm. The skin of the lesions in the other areas had returned to normal. *Dang Gui* (Radix Angelicae Sinensis) 9g, *Feng Fang* (Nidus Vespae) 9g and *Chan Tui* ‡ (Periostracum Cicadae) 6g were added to the previous prescription to nourish the Blood and dissipate Wind.

Outcome
After another five days, the skin was clear. [5]

Case 6
Patient
Male, aged 47.

Clinical manifestations

Six years ago, itchy dark red papules began to appear all over the patient's body with occasional exudation. The condition had recurred on numerous occasions since then. One year ago, the patient had been hospitalized for treatment with steroids, but his condition did not improve. Itching had become more intense, preventing him from sleeping properly. Other symptoms included generalized pain, fatigue and poor appetite.

Examination revealed dark red papules distributed all over the body except the face. The skin was rough with deepening of the cleavage lines of the skin and lichenification; some dark brown pigmentation was evident. Excoriations and bloody crusts were also noted in some places. The tongue body was red with a white and greasy coating; the pulse was wiry and slippery.

Diagnosis

Chronic eczema (*jin yin chuang*).

Pattern identification

Internal accumulation of Damp Toxins spreading to the skin and flesh.

Treatment principle

Eliminate Dampness and moisten the skin, relieve Toxicity and alleviate itching.

Prescription ingredients

Quan Xie ‡ (Buthus Martensi) 3g
Bai Xian Pi (Cortex Dictamni Dasycarpi Radicis) 15g
Di Fu Zi (Fructus Kochiae Scopariae) 12g
Mu Jin Pi (Cortex Hibisci Syriaci Radicis) 9g
Gan Di Huang (Radix Rehmanniae Glutinosae Exsiccata) 18g
Wei Ling Xian (Radix Clematidis) 9g
Huai Hua (Flos Sophorae Japonicae) 12g
Cang Er Zi (Fructus Xanthii Sibirici) 6g
Ku Shen (Radix Sophorae Flavescentis) 12g
Chen Pi (Pericarpium Citri Reticulatae) 6g

One bag a day was used to prepare a decoction, taken twice a day.

External treatment

A decoction of *Long Dan Cao* (Radix Gentianae Scabrae) 75g, *Xi Xian Cao* (Herba Siegesbeckiae) 25g and *Hua Jiao* (Pericarpium Zanthoxyli) 10g was used as an external wash.

Second visit

After ten bags of the decoction, itching was somewhat moderated, but the other symptoms were unchanged. The treatment principle and prescription were changed.

Treatment principle

Clear Heat and eliminate Dampness.

Prescription

LONG DAN XIE GAN TANG JIA JIAN

Chinese Gentian Decoction for Draining the Liver, with modifications

Long Dan Cao (Radix Gentianae Scabrae) 9g
Da Huang (Radix et Rhizoma Rhei) 9g
Huang Bai (Cortex Phellodendri) 9g
Huang Qin (Radix Scutellariae Baicalensis) 9g
Mu Jin Pi (Cortex Hibisci Syriaci Radicis) 12g
Bai Zhu (Rhizoma Atractylodis Macrocephalae) 12g
Chi Fu Ling (Sclerotium Poriae Cocos Rubrae) 12g
Bai Xian Pi (Cortex Dictamni Dasycarpi Radicis) 30g
Gan Di Huang (Radix Rehmanniae Glutinosae Exsiccata) 18g
Huai Hua (Flos Sophorae Japonicae) 12g
Cang Er Zi (Fructus Xanthii Sibirici) 6g

External treatment

Gan Cao You (Licorice Oil) and *Ru Yi Jin Huang San* (Agreeable Golden Yellow Powder) were applied externally to the affected areas.

Third visit

After fifteen bags of the decoction, the condition had still not improved significantly and so the prescription was changed again.

Treatment principle

Dissipate Wind and alleviate itching, clear Heat in the Blood and relieve Toxicity.

Prescription

QIN JIAO WAN FANG JIA JIAN

Large-Leaf Gentian Pill Formula, with modifications

Wu She ‡ (Zaocys Dhumnades) 9g
Qin Jiao (Radix Gentianae Macrophyllae) 15g
Fang Feng (Radix Ledebouriellae Divaricatae) 9g
Huang Qi (Radix Astragali seu Hedysari) 15g
Ku Shen (Radix Sophorae Flavescentis) 15g
Lou Lu (Radix Rhapontici seu Echinopsis) 9g
Huang Lian (Rhizoma Coptidis) 6g
Bai Xian Pi (Cortex Dictamni Dasycarpi Radicis) 18g
Wei Ling Xian (Radix Clematidis) 18g

Outcome

After twenty bags of the decoction, the condition showed obvious improvement with the surface of the lesions becoming thinner and softer and itching having practically disappeared. The patient was then prescribed *Qin Jiao Wan* (Large-Leaf Gentian Pill) for another two weeks, after which itching had disappeared completely and the skin had returned to normal.

Discussion

In this case of chronic eczema, the original prescription had to be changed twice before treatment was successful. Wind-Damp Toxins had accumulated and entered the Xue level and Vital Qi (Zheng Qi) had become debilitated. However, the treatment principle of eliminating Dampness and moistening the skin, relieving Toxicity and alleviating itching only had a moderate effect on the condition. The rough and thick skin with obvious excoriations and bloody crusts indicated retention of Damp-Heat with accumulated Toxins entering the Xue level. The treatment principle was finally amended to dissipating Wind and alleviating itching, clearing Heat in the Blood and relieving Toxicity, for which *Qin Jiao Wan Fang Jia Jian* (Large-Leaf Gentian Pill Formula, with modifications) was used. [6]

Case 7
Patient
Male, aged 62.

Clinical manifestations
For 20 years, the patient had suffered from itchy eruptions on the hands and lower legs. The condition was exacerbated in winter and when severe, scratching would break the lesions and result in watery exudate. In the past few days, itching had intensified and the lesions multiplied after excessive intake of alcohol. Accompanying symptoms and signs included irritability, a sensation of heat in the palms, soles and center of the chest, thirst with no desire for drinks, constipation, and insomnia.

Examination revealed patches of dark red, rough, lichenified skin on the wrists, the dorsum of the hands and the medial aspect of the lower legs with excoriations, bloody crusts, and slight erosion and exudation. Lichenification, fissuring, pigmentation, and some scaling was evident on the palms and soles. Patches of scaling erythema were distributed on the trunk and limbs. The tongue body was dark red with a white coating; the pulse was deep, thready and slightly rapid.

Diagnosis
Chronic eczema (*shi zhen*).

Pattern identification
Damp-Heat transforming into Fire and consuming Yin-Blood, resulting in Wind-Dryness due to Blood Deficiency, thus depriving the skin of nourishment.

Treatment principle
Nourish the Blood and dispel Wind, foster Yin and moisten Dryness, eliminate Dampness and alleviate itching.

Prescription ingredients
Dang Gui (Radix Angelicae Sinensis) 10g
Ye Jiao Teng (Caulis Polygoni Multiflori) 30g
Bai Shao (Radix Paeoniae Lactiflorae) 15g
Chi Shao (Radix Paeoniae Rubra) 15g
Bai Xian Pi (Cortex Dictamni Dasycarpi Radicis) 30g
Sheng Di Huang (Radix Rehmanniae Glutinosae) 30g
Gua Lou (Fructus Trichosanthis) 30g
Xuan Shen (Radix Scrophulariae Ningpoensis) 15g
Mu Dan Pi (Cortex Moutan Radicis) 15g
Nü Zhen Zi (Fructus Ligustri Lucidi) 15g
Han Lian Cao (Herba Ecliptae Prostratae) 15g
Ku Shen (Radix Sophorae Flavescentis) 15g
Jiang Huang (Rhizoma Curcumae Longae) 10g
Mu Gua (Fructus Chaenomelis) 10g

One bag a day was used to prepare a decoction, taken twice a day.

External treatment
Cang Er Zi (Fructus Xanthii Sibirici) 15g
Di Fu Zi (Fructus Kochiae Scopariae) 15g
She Chuang Zi (Fructus Cnidii Monnieri) 15g
Ma Chi Xian (Herba Portulacae Oleraceae) 30g
Ku Shen (Radix Sophorae Flavescentis) 15g
Bai Bu (Radix Stemonae) 10g

Ku Fan‡ (Alumen Praeparatum) 10g
Zao Jiao (Fructus Gleditsiae Sinensis) 10g
Huang Bai (Cortex Phellodendri) 10g
Ce Bai Ye (Cacumen Biotae Orientalis) 15g

A decoction prepared with these ingredients was allowed to cool to lukewarm and then used to soak the feet and hands. *Huang Lian Ruan Gao* (Coptis Ointment), *5% Hei Dou Liu You Ruan Gao* (Black Soybean and Vaseline® Ointment) and *5% Shui Yang Suan Ruan Gao* (Salicylic Acid Ointment) were applied alternately to the areas of dry skin.

Second visit
After seven bags of the decoction, itching had lessened and the lesions had begun to disappear. The patient was able to sleep and bowel movement was normal. The prescription was modified by removing *Gua Lou* (Fructus Trichosanthis) and adding *Yi Yi Ren* (Semen Coicis Lachryma-jobi) 30g. External treatment was not modified.

Outcome
After 14 bags of the decoction, most of the lesions had disappeared apart from some lichenified areas on the lower legs. The patient was told to take *Chu Shi Wan* (Pill for Eliminating Dampness) 6g and *Qin Jiao Wan* (Large-Leaf Gentian Pill) 6g twice a day until all the lesions disappeared.[7]

Literature excerpt

According to Ma Lianxiang in *Dang Dai Ming Yi Lin Zheng Jing Hua: Pi Fu Bing Zhuan Ji* [A Selection of Clinical Experiences of Famous Contemporary Practitioners: Skin Disease Specialists]: "The main pathology of eczema relates to Dampness, Toxins and Wind. However, the key pathological factor for stubborn eczema is Heat Toxins lying latent in the Xue level. Over time, this gradually results in the consumption of Yin and Blood, eventually leading to Blood Deficiency generating Wind. In the treatment, *He Shou Wu* (Radix Polygoni Multiflori) is used as the sovereign ingredient to nourish the Blood and dispel Wind; *Chan Pi*‡ (Corium Bufonis) and *Xu Chang Qing* (Radix Cynanchi Paniculati) are used as minister ingredients to clear Heat from the Xue level and relieve Toxicity; *Ye Ju Hua* (Flos Chrysanthemi Indici), *Di Fu Zi* (Fructus Kochiae Scopariae), *Bai Xian Pi* (Cortex Dictamni Dasycarpi Radicis), *Yi Yi Ren* (Semen Coicis Lachryma-jobi), *Fu Ling Pi* (Cortex Poriae Cocos), *Cang Zhu* (Rhizoma Atractylodis), *Xi Xian Cao* (Herba Siegesbeckiae), and *Huang Bai* (Cortex Phellodendri) are used as assistant ingredients to benefit the movement of Dampness and alleviate itching; and *Gan Cao* (Radix Glycyrrhizae) is used as the envoy to regulate the other ingredients and harmonize the Middle Burner. The ingredients in this combination will function together to nourish the Blood, dispel Wind, clear Heat, and relieve Toxicity."

Modern clinical experience

TREATMENT METHODS APPLICABLE TO ALL STAGES OF ECZEMA

INTERNAL ADMINISTRATION OF SOLUBLE GRANULES

Dai prescribed *Pi Yan Er Hao Chong Ji* (No. 2 Soluble Granules for Dermatitis) for 90 eczema patients. [8]

Prescription ingredients

Sheng Di Huang (Radix Rehmanniae Glutinosae) 10g
Xuan Shen (Radix Scrophulariae Ningpoensis) 10g
Shi Gao‡ (Gypsum Fibrosum) 10g
Zhi Mu (Rhizoma Anemarrhenae Asphodeloidis) 10g
Bai Mao Gen (Rhizoma Imperatae Cylindricae) 15g
Jing Jie (Herba Schizonepetae Tenuifoliae) 6g
Fang Feng (Radix Ledebouriellae Divaricatae) 6g
Jin Yin Hua (Flos Lonicerae) 15g
Niu Bang Zi (Fructus Arctii Lappae) 6g
Ju Hua (Flos Chrysanthemi Morifolii) 10g
Gan Cao (Radix Glycyrrhizae) 6g
Shui Niu Jiao‡ (Cornu Bubali) 30g
Sheng Ma (Rhizoma Cimicifugae) 6g

Five grams of the granules were taken twice a day. Treatment was effective for 71 of the 90 patients (78.9 percent).

COMBINED INTERNAL AND EXTERNAL TREATMENT

1. **Mo** combined internal and external decoctions to treat eczema. [9]

Internal prescription ingredients

Bai Xian Pi (Cortex Dictamni Dasycarpi Radicis) 30g
Di Fu Zi (Fructus Kochiae Scopariae) 30g
Chi Xiao Dou (Semen Phaseoli Calcarati) 30g
Jin Yin Hua (Flos Lonicerae) 20g
Da Qing Ye (Folium Isatidis seu Baphicacanthi) 20g
Chi Shao (Radix Paeoniae Rubra) 10g
Hua Shi‡ (Talcum) 10g
Jing Jie (Herba Schizonepetae Tenuifoliae) 10g
Fang Feng (Radix Ledebouriellae Divaricatae) 10g
Chan Tui‡ (Periostracum Cicadae) 6g

One bag a day was used to prepare a decoction, taken twice a day.

External prescription ingredients

Ku Shen (Radix Sophorae Flavescentis) 60g
Ju Hua (Flos Chrysanthemi Morifolii) 60g
She Chuang Zi (Fructus Cnidii Monnieri) 30g
Jin Yin Hua (Flos Lonicerae) 30g
Di Fu Zi (Fructus Kochiae Scopariae) 20g
Bai Zhi (Radix Angelicae Dahuricae) 15g
Huang Bai (Cortex Phellodendri) 15g
Shi Chang Pu (Rhizoma Acori Graminei) 10g

The ingredients were wrapped in gauze and decocted in 500ml of water for 20 minutes. The decoction was then strained and used to steam and wash the affected areas for 20 minutes, twice a day. Dosages were halved for children under 10. Results were seen after three weeks.

2. **Wang** also combined internal and external prescriptions. [10]

Internal prescription ingredients

Fang Feng (Radix Ledebouriellae Divaricatae) 12g
Chuan Xiong (Rhizoma Ligustici Chuanxiong) 12g
Tong Cao (Medulla Tetrapanacis Papyriferi) 12g
Chan Tui‡ (Periostracum Cicadae) 12g
Dang Gui (Radix Angelicae Sinensis) 9g
Sheng Di Huang (Radix Rehmanniae Glutinosae) 9g
Da Huang (Radix et Rhizoma Rhei) 30g
Ku Shen (Radix Sophorae Flavescentis) 30g
Gan Cao (Radix Glycyrrhizae) 6g

One bag a day was used to prepare a decoction, taken twice a day.

External prescription ingredients

Ku Shen (Radix Sophorae Flavescentis) 60g
Da Huang (Radix et Rhizoma Rhei) 50g
Hei Zhi Ma (Semen Sesami Indici) 50g
Di Fu Zi (Fructus Kochiae Scopariae) 40g
Chan Tui‡ (Periostracum Cicadae) 30g
Sheng Di Huang (Radix Rehmanniae Glutinosae) 30g
Dang Gui (Radix Angelicae Sinensis) 30g
Dan Shen (Radix Salviae Miltiorrhizae) 30g
Chuan Xiong (Rhizoma Ligustici Chuanxiong) 30g
Fu Ling (Sclerotium Poriae Cocos) 30g
Fang Feng (Radix Ledebouriellae Divaricatae) 30g
Shi Chang Pu (Rhizoma Acori Graminei) 20g
Tong Cao (Medulla Tetrapanacis Papyriferi) 20g

The ingredients were decocted in 2000ml of water to obtain 1000ml of liquid, which was then diluted in water in a ratio of 1:10 and used to bathe the affected areas for 30 minutes once or twice a day. Results were seen between three days and one month.

ACUPUNCTURE

Cui treated 28 cases of eczema with acupuncture. [11]
Main points: LI-11 Quchi, SP-10 Xuehai and GV-14 Dazhui.

Auxiliary points

- For Wind, Dampness and Heat patterns, add GB-31 Fengshi and ST-25 Tianshu.

- For encumbrance of Dampness due to Spleen Deficiency, add ST-36 Zusanli.
- For internal Heat due to Yin Deficiency, add SP-6 Sanyinjiao and KI-3 Taixi.
- For obstruction due to Wind-Damp, add BL-40 Weizhong.

Technique: The reducing method was applied for Wind, Dampness and Heat patterns, and the even method for all other conditions. Plum-blossom needling was also administered locally. Treatment was given twice daily for six days, after which only three patients had not shown any effect.

ACUTE ECZEMA

CLASSICAL FORMULA USED IN A NEW WAY

Li treated 116 cases of acute eczema with *Xie Xin Tang Jia Wei* (Draining the Heart Decoction, with additions). [12]

Prescription ingredients

Da Huang (Radix et Rhizoma Rhei) 10g, added 10 minutes before the end of the decoction process
Zi Cao (Radix Arnebiae seu Lithospermi) 10g
Mu Dan Pi (Cortex Moutan Radicis) 10g
Huang Qin (Radix Scutellariae Baicalensis) 10g
Huang Lian (Rhizoma Coptidis) 6g
Yin Chen Hao (Herba Artemisiae Scopariae) 15g
Hua Shi‡ (Talcum) 15g
Bai Xian Pi (Cortex Dictamni Dasycarpi Radicis) 15g
Di Fu Zi (Fructus Kochiae Scopariae) 15g
Gan Cao (Radix Glycyrrhizae) 6g

One bag a day was used to prepare a decoction, taken twice a day.

External prescription ingredients

Huang Lian (Rhizoma Coptidis)
Ku Fan‡ (Alumen Praeparatum)
Liu Huang‡ (Sulphur)

Gan Cao (Radix Glycyrrhizae)
The ingredients were mixed together in the proportions of 5:1:1:1 and ground into a very fine powder for direct external application to the lesions twice a day.

A course of treatment (internal and external prescriptions) lasted for one week and results were evaluated after one to three weeks; 80 patients were cured (69.0 percent), 30 experienced some improvement (25.9 percent) and 6 showed no improvement (5.1 percent).

EXTERNAL APPLICATION OF A SINGLE INGREDIENT

Fu prepared *Lai Fu Zi Gao* (Radish Seed Paste) by stir-frying 60g of *Lai Fu Zi* (Semen Raphani Sativi) with sand for 30 minutes, allowing it to cool and grinding it into a fine powder before mixing to a paste with an appropriate amount of cottonseed oil (*Mian Zi You,* Oleum Gossypii Seminis). The medicated paste was applied to the lesions once a day for one week. [13]

CHRONIC ECZEMA

INTERNAL TREATMENT

Luo prescribed *Ku Shen Wu She Tang Jia Jian* (Flavescent Sophora Root and Black-Tail Snake Decoction, with modifications). [14]

Prescription ingredients

Ku Shen (Radix Sophorae Flavescentis) 9g
Wu She‡ (Zaocys Dhumnades) 22g, reduced by 2/3 for children
Dang Gui (Radix Angelicae Sinensis) 9g
Sheng Di Huang (Radix Rehmanniae Glutinosae) 15g
Mu Dan Pi (Cortex Moutan Radicis) 9g
Chi Shao (Radix Paeoniae Rubra) 9g

One bag a day was used to prepare a decoction, taken twice a day. Results were seen after eight weeks.

Papular eczema
丘疹性湿疹

TCM usually considers papular eczema as a separate eczematous condition with Wind playing a major role in each of the patterns involved.

This condition is also known as *xue feng chuang* (Blood-Wind sore).

Clinical manifestations

- Papular eczema mainly occurs on the legs, but in severe cases the entire body is likely to be involved.

- At the initial stage, lesions present as 1-2 mm papules or papulovesicles. Excoriation produces exudation of blood or clear fluid.
- Itching is intense, being worst at night.

Differential diagnosis

See Basic patterns of eczema above.

Etiology and pathology

- Chronic emotional problems can lead to Qi stagnation, which can then generate Heart-Fire. The Heart governs Fire and the Blood. Exuberant Heart-Fire will result in Heat in the Blood and the generation of Wind. When this Wind moves to the exterior, it will provoke severe itching.
- If Damp-Heat in the Liver and Spleen channels is complicated by an invasion of external Wind, it will move to the skin and be retained in the Lung channel.
- Prolonged retention of Wind-Heat in the Lung channel leads to Blood-Dryness and damages the Blood. This in turn results in Blood Deficiency and lack of Body Fluids, with the skin therefore being deprived of normal nourishment.

Pattern identification and treatment

INTERNAL TREATMENT

EXUBERANT WIND DUE TO HEAT IN THE BLOOD

The initial stage is characterized by 1-2 mm red papules with intense itching. Excoriation produces oozing of blood. Symptoms are worse at night. Accompanying symptoms and signs include sleeplessness, irritability and thirst. The tongue body is red with a thin coating; the pulse is wiry and rapid.

Treatment principle
Cool the Blood and clear Heat, dissipate Wind and alleviate itching.

Prescription
XIAO FENG SAN JIA JIAN
Powder for Dispersing Wind, with modifications

Dang Gui (Radix Angelicae Sinensis) 6g
Fang Feng (Radix Ledebouriellae Divaricatae) 6g
Chan Tui ‡ (Periostracum Cicadae) 6g
Ku Shen (Radix Sophorae Flavescentis) 6g
Jing Jie (Herba Schizonepetae Tenuifoliae) 6g
Sheng Di Huang (Radix Rehmanniae Glutinosae) 12g

Shi Gao ‡ (Gypsum Fibrosum) 12g, decocted for 30 minutes before adding the other ingredients
Niu Bang Zi (Fructus Arctii Lappae) 12g
Cang Zhu (Rhizoma Atractylodis) 10g
Hei Zhi Ma (Semen Sesami Indici) 10g
Gou Teng (Ramulus Uncariae cum Uncis) 10g
Xu Chang Qing (Radix Cynanchi Paniculati) 10g
Gan Cao (Radix Glycyrrhizae) 3g
Tong Cao (Medulla Tetrapanacis Papyriferi) 3g

Explanation
- *Jing Jie* (Herba Schizonepetae Tenuifoliae), *Fang Feng* (Radix Ledebouriellae Divaricatae), *Chan Tui* ‡ (Periostracum Cicadae), and *Niu Bang Zi* (Fructus Arctii Lappae) dredge Wind and clear Heat, and dissipate Wind-Heat through the skin.
- *Gou Teng* (Ramulus Uncariae cum Uncis), *Xu Chang Qing* (Radix Cynanchi Paniculati) and *Hei Zhi Ma* (Semen Sesami Indici) extinguish interior Wind due to Deficiency and alleviate itching.
- *Sheng Di Huang* (Radix Rehmanniae Glutinosae) and *Dang Gui* (Radix Angelicae Sinensis) nourish the Blood and moisten Dryness.
- *Shi Gao* ‡ (Gypsum Fibrosum) clears Heat from the Qi level.
- *Ku Shen* (Radix Sophorae Flavescentis) and *Cang Zhu* (Rhizoma Atractylodis) dry Dampness and alleviate itching.
- *Gan Cao* (Radix Glycyrrhizae) and *Tong Cao* (Medulla Tetrapanacis Papyriferi) clear Heat from the Heart and promote urination.

DAMP-HEAT ACCOMPANIED BY INVASION OF EXTERNAL WIND

In contrast to the first pattern, this pattern has prevalence of Dampness rather than Wind. It is characterized by 1-2 mm red papules; scratching produces exudation of clear fluid or blood. Itching is comparatively severe. Accompanying symptoms and signs include irritability and restlessness, thirst, dry stools, and yellow urine. The tongue body is red with a thin yellow coating; the pulse is wiry and slippery.

Treatment principle
Cool the Blood and dispel Wind, percolate Dampness and alleviate itching.

Prescription
LIANG XUE CHU SHI TANG JIA JIAN
Decoction for Cooling the Blood and Eliminating Dampness, with modifications

Sheng Di Huang (Radix Rehmanniae Glutinosae) 15g
Ren Dong Teng (Caulis Lonicerae Japonicae) 15g
Bai Xian Pi (Cortex Dictamni Dasycarpi Radicis) 15g

Mu Dan Pi (Cortex Moutan Radicis) 10g
Chi Shao (Radix Paeoniae Rubra) 10g
Xi Xian Cao (Herba Siegesbeckiae) 10g
Di Fu Zi (Fructus Kochiae Scopariae) 10g
Fu Ling Pi (Cortex Poriae Cocos) 10g
Chi Xiao Dou (Semen Phaseoli Calcarati) 30g
Lian Qiao (Fructus Forsythiae Suspensae) 12g
Hai Tong Pi (Cortex Erythrinae) 12g
Yi Yi Ren (Semen Coicis Lachryma-jobi) 12g

Explanation

- *Sheng Di Huang* (Radix Rehmanniae Glutinosae), *Mu Dan Pi* (Cortex Moutan Radicis), *Chi Shao* (Radix Paeoniae Rubra), *Lian Qiao* (Fructus Forsythiae Suspensae), and *Chi Xiao Dou* (Semen Phaseoli Calcarati) clear Heat from the Heart and cool the Blood, relieve Toxicity and reduce eruptions.
- *Ren Dong Teng* (Caulis Lonicerae Japonicae), *Bai Xian Pi* (Cortex Dictamni Dasycarpi Radicis), *Hai Tong Pi* (Cortex Erythrinae), *Di Fu Zi* (Fructus Kochiae Scopariae), and *Xi Xian Cao* (Herba Siegesbeckiae) free the network vessels and dissipate Wind, transform Dampness and alleviate itching.
- *Yi Yi Ren* (Semen Coicis Lachryma-jobi) and *Fu Ling Pi* (Cortex Poriae Cocos) support the Spleen and percolate Dampness.

BLOOD DEFICIENCY AND WIND-DRYNESS

The skin is dry with bran-like scale. Ecchymosis due to scratching occurs in some areas. Patients experience itching that worsens at night. The tongue body is pale, or purple with stasis macules; the tongue has a scant coating. The pulse is deficient and thready.

Treatment principle

Nourish the Blood and dispel Wind, moisten Dryness and alleviate itching.

Prescription

DANG GUI YIN ZI JIA JIAN

Chinese Angelica Root Drink, with modifications

Dang Gui (Radix Angelicae Sinensis) 12g
Shu Di Huang (Radix Rehmanniae Glutinosae Conquita) 12g
Bai Shao (Radix Paeoniae Lactiflorae) 12g
Bai Ji Li (Fructus Tribuli Terrestris) 12g
He Shou Wu (Radix Polygoni Multiflori) 15g
Huang Qi (Radix Astragali seu Hedysari) 15g
Lian Zi Xin (Plumula Nelumbinis Nuciferae) 4.5g
Jing Jie (Herba Schizonepetae Tenuifoliae) 6g
Fang Feng (Radix Ledebouriellae Divaricatae) 6g
Chuan Xiong (Rhizoma Ligustici Chuanxiong) 6g
Chan Tui‡ (Periostracum Cicadae) 6g

Long Gu‡ (Os Draconis) 30g
Mu Li‡ (Concha Ostreae) 30g
Shan Yao (Rhizoma Dioscoreae Oppositae) 30g
Hei Zhi Ma (Semen Sesami Indici) 30g

Explanation

- *Dang Gui* (Radix Angelicae Sinensis), *Shu Di Huang* (Radix Rehmanniae Glutinosae Conquita), *Bai Shao* (Radix Paeoniae Lactiflorae), *Chuan Xiong* (Rhizoma Ligustici Chuanxiong), *Shan Yao* (Rhizoma Dioscoreae Oppositae), *Hei Zhi Ma* (Semen Sesami Indici), *He Shou Wu* (Radix Polygoni Multiflori), and *Huang Qi* (Radix Astragali seu Hedysari) nourish the Blood and moisten Dryness.
- *Fang Feng* (Radix Ledebouriellae Divaricatae), *Jing Jie* (Herba Schizonepetae Tenuifoliae), *Bai Ji Li* (Fructus Tribuli Terrestris), and *Chan Tui*‡ (Periostracum Cicadae) dissipate Wind and alleviate itching.
- *Long Gu*‡ (Os Draconis) and *Mu Li*‡ (Concha Ostreae) calm the Liver with their heavy, settling properties to extinguish interior Wind.
- *Lian Zi Xin* (Plumula Nelumbinis Nuciferae) clears Heart-Fire and guides out reddish urine.

EXTERNAL TREATMENT

- For red papules, apply *Ku Shen Jiu* (Flavescent Sophora Root Wine) or *Lu Hu Xi Ji* (Calamine and Giant Knotweed Wash Preparation) to the affected area twice a day.
- For lesions with dry skin and itching, apply *Huang Lian Ruan Gao* (Coptis Ointment) or *Run Ji Gao* (Flesh-Moistening Paste) twice a day.
- For lesions with slight exudation of clear fluid, prepare a decoction with *Ma Chi Xian* (Herba Portulacae Oleraceae) and *Huang Bai* (Cortex Phellodendri) and apply as a cold compress once a day.

Clinical notes

- Papular eczema can be caused by the interaction of Wind-Heat, Damp-Heat and Heat in the Blood. For pattern identification purposes, it is important to recognize which is the predominant factor.
  - If Wind-Heat predominates, the Lung is the main organ involved, and treatment should focus on diffusing and dissipating pathogenic factors.
  - If Damp-Heat predominates, the Spleen is the main organ involved, and treatment should focus on transforming Dampness.
  - If Heat in the Blood predominates, the Heart is the main organ involved, and treatment should focus on cooling the Blood.

When treating all three patterns, it is important to keep the following maxim in mind: "Treat the Blood first to treat Wind. When the Blood is moving, Wind will automatically disappear."

- External medications for papular eczema vary according to the lesions involved:
  - use medicated wine preparations or wash preparations for papules
  - use ointments for dry, itchy lesions
  - use powder preparations mixed with oil to treat lesions with exudation and severe itching, such as *Qu Shi San* (Powder for Dispelling Dampness) mixed with *Gan Cao You* (Licorice Oil). In the author's experience, mixing powder with oil is particularly effective when severe itching accompanies exudation since the mixture can achieve the effects of promoting contraction and moistening the skin to alleviate itching.

Advice for the patient

- Avoid greasy, spicy and fried food and alcohol.

- Avoid scratching the lesions to prevent secondary infection.
- Wear cotton clothing next to the skin.
- Avoid washing with soap and hot water.

Literature excerpt

In *Yi Zong Jin Jian: Wai Ke Xin Fa Yao Jue* [The Golden Mirror of Medicine: Essential Methods for the Treatment of External Diseases], it says: "*Xue feng chuang* (Blood-Wind sore) occurs because Damp-Heat in the Liver and Spleen channels, when attacked by invading external Wind, moves to the skin and is retained in the Lung channel. Manifestations include millet-sized, intensely itchy sores all over the body. Scratching the lesions causes exudation with thick discharge, leading to maceration in patches. Accompanying symptoms and signs include irritability and restlessness, thirst, and itching, which is worse at night."

Infectious eczematoid dermatitis
传染性湿疹样皮炎

This condition presents as a scaling or oozing eruption due to bacterial infection (usually staphylococcal), in which the process is continued by sensitization as well as by infection. Significant bacterial colonization of lesions is common in all types of eczema although infection is most common in seborrheic, nummular and atopic eczema.

In TCM, infectious eczematoid dermatitis is considered as a type of *shi du yang* (Damp Toxin sore).

Clinical manifestations

- The eczematoid lesion is usually induced by a primary suppurative focus such as otitis media, skin ulcers or pressure sores.
- Purulent discharge from the primary focus may give rise to eczematoid lesions such as papules, papulovesicles, vesicles, pustules, erosion, and purulent crusts around the focus.
- Lesions may spread following excoriation.

- Severe cases may present with fever, dilatation of local lymph glands and leucocytosis.
- Itching varies from moderate to severe.

Differential diagnosis

Infectious eczematoid dermatitis is difficult to differentiate from contact dermatitis, especially at the acute stage or where sensitization causes an allergic reaction. Identification of possible causes is usually the best guide to differentiation and treatment.

Etiology and pathology

- Dietary irregularities, including a predilection for tea and alcohol, seafood and spicy food, cause failure of the Spleen's transportation function resulting in Damp-Heat accumulating internally. When this condition is complicated by concurrent external contraction of Wind Toxins, the disease may occur.

- Infectious eczematoid dermatitis is often related to congenital factors, especially in those people with a constitutional tendency toward internal exuberance of Heat Toxins. Emotional stress, a rash and impatient nature, or irritability and restlessness cause Qi Depression that subsequently transforms into Fire. Since the Heart governs Fire and the Blood vessels, intense internal Heart-Fire causes Heat in the Xue level, thus giving rise to the disease.

- When the disease reaches the chronic phase, Damp-Heat has accumulated internally over a long period, causing damage to Yin and consumption of Blood that leads to Dryness, manifesting as gradual lichenification and desquamation.

Pattern identification and treatment

INTERNAL TREATMENT

BINDING OF DAMP-HEAT
Inflammatory papules and papulovesicles spread throughout the body; some lesions may have exudation and erosion. Itching is likely to be severe. Accompanying symptoms and signs include a bitter taste in the mouth, irritability, a sensation of burning heat all over the body, and yellow urine. The tongue body is red with a thin yellow coating; the pulse is thready and rapid.

Treatment principle
Clear Heat and benefit the movement of Dampness.

Prescription
LONG DAN XIE GAN TANG JIA JIAN
Chinese Gentian Decoction for Draining the Liver, with modifications

Long Dan Cao (Radix Gentianae Scabrae) 6g
Zhi Zi (Fructus Gardeniae Jasminoidis) 6g
Huang Qin (Radix Scutellariae Baicalensis) 6g
Huang Bai (Cortex Phellodendri) 6g
Chai Hu (Radix Bupleuri) 6g
Sheng Di Huang (Radix Rehmanniae Glutinosae) 15g
Mu Dan Pi (Cortex Moutan Radicis) 10g
Che Qian Zi (Semen Plantaginis) 10g
Chi Fu Ling (Sclerotium Poriae Cocos Rubrae) 10g
Gou Teng (Ramulus Uncariae cum Uncis) 10g
Chi Xiao Dou (Semen Phaseoli Calcarati) 30g

Explanation
- *Long Dan Cao* (Radix Gentianae Scabrae), *Zhi Zi* (Fructus Gardeniae Jasminoidis), *Sheng Di Huang* (Radix Rehmanniae Glutinosae), *Mu Dan Pi* (Cortex Moutan Radicis), and *Huang Bai* (Cortex Phellodendri) clear Heat from the Liver and drain Fire.

- *Che Qian Zi* (Semen Plantaginis), *Chi Fu Ling* (Sclerotium Poriae Cocos Rubrae) and *Chi Xiao Dou* (Semen Phaseoli Calcarati) benefit the movement of Dampness and clear Heat.

- *Gou Teng* (Ramulus Uncariae cum Uncis) extinguishes Wind and alleviates itching.

- *Huang Qin* (Radix Scutellariae Baicalensis) and *Chai Hu* (Radix Bupleuri) free the exterior and interior to clear internal Heat and thrust external pathogenic factors outward.

BLOOD-DRYNESS DUE TO YIN DEFICIENCY
The disease is protracted or recurrent. The skin is dry with desquamation and some lichenification; in some places, scratch marks are clearly visible with bloody scaling. Itching is present, worse at night, thus making sleep difficult. The tongue body is red with a scant coating; the pulse is thready and rapid.

Treatment principle
Enrich Yin and moisten Dryness, extinguish Wind and alleviate itching.

Prescription
ZI YIN CHU SHI TANG JIA JIAN
Decoction for Enriching Yin and Eliminating Dampness, with modifications

Sheng Di Huang (Radix Rehmanniae Glutinosae) 12g
He Shou Wu (Radix Polygoni Multiflori) 12g
Bai Shao (Radix Paeoniae Lactiflorae) 12g
Gou Teng (Ramulus Uncariae cum Uncis) 12g
Zhen Zhu Mu ‡ (Concha Margaritifera) 30g, decocted for 30 minutes before adding the other ingredients
Ye Jiao Teng (Caulis Polygoni Multiflori) 10g
Fu Shen (Sclerotium Poriae Cocos cum Ligno Hospite) 10g
Nü Zhen Zi (Fructus Ligustri Lucidi) 10g
Gou Qi Zi (Fructus Lycii) 10g
Suan Zao Ren (Semen Ziziphi Spinosae) 10g
Huang Lian (Rhizoma Coptidis) 3g
Lian Zi Xin (Plumula Nelumbinis Nuciferae) 3g

Explanation
- *He Shou Wu* (Radix Polygoni Multiflori), *Bai Shao* (Radix Paeoniae Lactiflorae), *Nü Zhen Zi* (Fructus Ligustri Lucidi), *Gou Qi Zi* (Fructus Lycii), and *Sheng Di Huang* (Radix Rehmanniae Glutinosae) enrich Yin and moisten Dryness, nourish the Blood and emolliate the Liver.

- *Zhen Zhu Mu* ‡ (Concha Margaritifera) and *Gou Teng* (Ramulus Uncariae cum Uncis) act in combination as heavy settlers to extinguish Wind and alleviate itching.

- *Ye Jiao Teng* (Caulis Polygoni Multiflori), *Fu Shen* (Sclerotium Poriae Cocos cum Ligno Hospite),

Huang Lian (Rhizoma Coptidis), *Lian Zi Xin* (Plumula Nelumbinis Nuciferae), and *Suan Zao Ren* (Semen Ziziphi Spinosae) clear the Heart and drain Fire to quiet the Spirit.

EXTERNAL TREATMENT

- For lesions with exudation and erosion or infected abscesses, apply *Ma Chi Xian Shui Xi Ji* (Purslane Wash Preparation) as a wet compress two or three times a day.
- For dry and itchy skin, apply a thin coating of *Huang Lian Ruan Gao* (Coptis Ointment) once or twice a day.

Clinical notes

- At the initial stage of the disease when Damp-Heat is predominant, treatment should focus on clearing Heat and transforming Dampness, relieving Toxicity and alleviating itching. It is important to bring erosive lesions with exudation under control as soon as possible.
- At the later stage, the disease is characterized by recurrent attacks and treatment should focus on enriching Yin and eliminating Dampness, supporting the Spleen and consolidating the Root. At this stage, it is better to use heavy settlers for alleviating itching while reducing the amount of materia medica with the function of arresting Wind.
- The ancient physicians concluded that extreme Dryness is like Dampness, in that Dryness and Dampness may cause the same disease with similar signs. Many patients have eczema or dermatitis for years and prolonged treatment does not result in a cure. The more materia medica for benefiting the movement of Dampness that are applied, the worse erosion and exudation become. Therefore, the most effective treatment principle is to eliminate Dampness by enriching Yin with *Zi Yin Chu Shi Tang* (Decoction for Enriching Yin and Eliminating Dampness).
- Action should be taken to prevent and treat the primary infection.

Advice for the patient

- During treatment, avoid eating fish, shellfish, seafood, and spicy food and do not drink alcohol, coffee or strong tea.

- Do not wash with hot water and avoid scratching the lesion in order to prevent secondary infection.

Case history

Patient
Female, aged 67.

Clinical manifestations
The patient had suffered from eczema on the left leg with itching and exudation for eight years. Two weeks before the consultation, a lesion had appeared on the left leg after rupture of the skin due to scratching after itching. The patient had begun to feel uncomfortable after a bath, and the lesion on the leg started to become red and swollen. She found it difficult to sleep because of the severe itching and pain. Three days later, an itchy skin eruption had spread throughout the body; scratching produced exudate. The swelling on the left leg was so bad that the patient could no longer walk. By the time of the consultation, some of the lesions were cracked with exudation of yellow fluid. Accompanying symptoms and signs included no desire for food and drink, a dry mouth with a bitter taste, occasional nausea, constipation with bowel movements once every two or three days, and scanty yellow or reddish urine.

Examination revealed erythematous patches of varying shapes and sizes distributed on the trunk and limbs. Pink 2-3 mm papules and 3-4 mm vesicles were distributed individually and in clusters in the spaces between the patches. Some of the lesions had been broken by scratching, resulting in fresh red erosions and crusting. Yellow exudate was visible in some fissures. The skin was red, shiny and taut. The lower left leg was very red and swollen and movement of the leg was limited by the swelling. The tongue body was pale red with a white coating that turned yellow and greasy in the center; the pulse was slippery and rapid.

Pattern identification
Damp-Heat accumulating internally and external contraction of Toxic pathogenic factors.

Treatment principle
Clear Heat and benefit the movement of Dampness, cool the Blood and relieve Toxicity.

Prescription ingredients
Jin Yin Hua (Flos Lonicerae) 15g
*Han Fang Ji** (Radix Stephaniae Tetrandrae) 15g [ii]
Bai Zhu (Rhizoma Atractylodis Macrocephalae) 15g
Ze Xie (Rhizoma Alismatis Orientalis) 15g
Che Qian Cao (Herba Plantaginis) 15g
Long Dan Cao (Radix Gentianae Scabrae) 6g
Gan Di Huang (Radix Rehmanniae Glutinosae Exsiccata) 30g
Bai Mao Gen (Rhizoma Imperatae Cylindricae) 30g
Yi Yi Ren (Semen Coicis Lachryma-jobi) 30g
Liu Yi San (Six-To-One Powder) 30g

[ii] In those countries where the supply, importation or use of *Han Fang Ji** (Radix Stephaniae Tetrandrae) is not permitted, it can be replaced in this prescription by *Tong Cao* (Medulla Tetrapanacis Papyriferi).

One bag a day was used to prepare a decoction, taken twice a day.

External treatment

- A decoction was prepared with *Long Dan Cao* (Radix Gentianae Scabrae) 60g, *Huang Bai* (Cortex Phellodendri) 30g, *Hua Jiao* (Pericarpium Zanthoxyli) 9g, and *Zi Hua Di Ding* (Herba Violae Yedoensitis) 30g for use as a wet compress.
- *Gui Ban San* (Tortoise Plastron Powder) 12g and *Qu Shi San* (Powder for Dispelling Dampness) 60g were mixed with *Gan Cao You* (Licorice Oil) for local application. [iii]
- *Qin Bai Gao* (Scutellaria and Phellodendron Paste) was applied to locations with erythema.

Second visit

After three days, the patient's appetite was better, bowel movement had returned to normal and the urine was slightly yellow. Since itching had been reduced, sleep had improved. Generalized erythema had clearly decreased and the swelling of the left leg was diminishing. Most of the erosive area had been covered by new pink skin and exudation had stopped. However, new eruptions had occurred in some areas. The yellow, greasy tongue coating had been reduced; the pulse was slippery and slightly rapid.

Modifications to prescription

Long Dan Cao (Radix Gentianae Scabrae), *Gan Di Huang* (Radix Rehmanniae Glutinosae Exsiccata), *Liu Yi San* (Six-To-One Powder), and *Bai Mao Gen* (Rhizoma Imperatae Cylindricae) were removed, and *Yin Chen Hao* (Herba Artemisiae Scopariae) 30g, *Bai Xian Pi* (Cortex Dictamni Dasycarpi Radicis) 15g, *Gan Cao* (Radix Glycyrrhizae) 9g, and *Hou Po* (Cortex Magnoliae Officinalis) 9g were added. The external application was the same as before.

Third visit

After another three days, the appetite was normal and the urine was clear. The lesions on the trunk and limbs had basically disappeared with desquamation in many areas. No new rashes were observed. The swelling on the left lower leg had disappeared and the diameter was the same as the right leg.

Treatment principle

Dissipate Wind and alleviate itching.

Prescription
QUAN CHONG FANG JIA JIAN

Scorpion Formula, with modifications

Quan Xie ‡ (Buthus Martensi, crushed) 6g
Bai Ji Li (Fructus Tribuli Terrestris) 30g
Bai Xian Pi (Cortex Dictamni Dasycarpi Radicis) 30g
Dang Gui (Radix Angelicae Sinensis) 9g
Hou Po (Cortex Magnoliae Officinalis) 9g
Ze Xie (Rhizoma Alismatis Orientalis) 9g
Ku Shen (Radix Sophorae Flavescentis) 9g

Fang Feng (Radix Ledebouriellae Divaricatae) 9g
Yi Yi Ren (Semen Coicis Lachryma-jobi) 15g
Cang Zhu (Rhizoma Atractylodis) 15g
Bai Zhu (Rhizoma Atractylodis Macrocephalae) 15g
Huang Bai (Cortex Phellodendri) 15g
Zhi Ke (Fructus Citri Aurantii) 6g

External treatment

Qin Bai Gao (Scutellaria and Phellodendron Paste) was applied externally to alleviate itching.

Outcome

After three bags of this prescription, all the symptoms had disappeared except for a little desquamation. The lesion on the lower left leg was basically cured; all that remained was two fingernail-sized slightly lichenified areas with desquamation and occasional itching. The patient was given *Chu Shi Wan* (Pill for Eliminating Dampness) 6g and *Qin Jiao Wan* (Large-Leaf Gentian Pill) 6g twice a day for oral administration to consolidate the cure. [15]

Modern clinical experience

TREATMENT ACCORDING TO PATTERN IDENTIFICATION

1. Guan adopted the treatment principle of clearing Heat and benefiting the movement of Dampness, dispelling Wind and relieving Toxicity to treat this condition. Materia medica commonly used in his prescriptions included:

Long Dan Cao (Radix Gentianae Scabrae)
Zhi Zi (Fructus Gardeniae Jasminoidis)
Huang Qin (Radix Scutellariae Baicalensis)
Huang Bai (Cortex Phellodendri)
Dang Gui (Radix Angelicae Sinensis)
Da Qing Ye (Folium Isatidis seu Baphicacanthi)
Sheng Di Huang (Radix Rehmanniae Glutinosae)
Tong Cao (Medulla Tetrapanacis Papyriferi)
Ze Xie (Rhizoma Alismatis Orientalis)
Che Qian Zi (Semen Plantaginis)
Gan Cao (Radix Glycyrrhizae)

For suppurative infections, *Zi Hua Di Ding* (Herba Violae Yedoensitis), *Pu Gong Ying* (Herba Taraxaci cum Radice), *Jin Yin Hua* (Flos Lonicerae), *Chong Lou* (Rhizoma Paridis), and *Ban Zhi Lian* (Herba Scutellariae Barbatae) were added. [16]

2. According to the theory that "all painful and itching sores are ascribed to the Heart" (one of the Nineteen Pathogenic Principles), **Zhu Renkang** used *Sheng Di Huang* (Radix Rehmanniae Glutinosae), *Mu Dan Pi*

[iii] In those countries where certain ingredients contained in *Gui Ban San* (Tortoise Plastron Powder) mean that its use is not permitted, *Xin San Miao San* (New Mysterious Three Powder) can be substituted.

(Cortex Moutan Radicis) and *Chi Shao* (Radix Paeoniae Rubra) to cool the Blood; *Shi Gao*‡ (Gypsum Fibrosum), *Zhi Mu* (Rhizoma Anemarrhenae Asphodeloidis) and *Lian Qiao* (Fructus Forsythiae Suspensae) to clear Heat from the flesh; and *Huang Lian* (Rhizoma Coptidis) and *Dan Zhu Ye* (Herba Lophatheri Gracilis) to clear Heart-Fire. *Ku Shen* (Radix Sophorae Flavescentis), *Chi Fu Ling* (Sclerotium Poriae Cocos Rubrae), *Tong Cao* (Medulla Tetrapanacis Papyriferi), *Bai Xian Pi* (Cortex Dictamni Dasycarpi Radicis), and *Di Fu Zi* (Fructus Kochiae Scopariae) were used as assistants to eliminate Dampness and alleviate itching. For dry and itchy skin, he added materia medica for nourishing the Blood and moistening Dryness. The prescription contains no materia medica for treating Wind in order to avoid mutual exacerbation of Wind and Fire. [17]

COMBINED TCM AND WESTERN MEDICINE TREATMENT

The **Dermatology Department of Guangdong TCM Hospital** treated 21 cases of infectious eczematoid dermatitis (19 male and 2 female) by combining TCM and Western medicine methods. The duration of the disease up to the date of treatment varied from 3 days to 28 days. Most of the patients had infectious foci on the lower limbs. Five cases had accompanying symptoms of fever, ten had a high white blood cell count, and three had proteinuria. Most patients had a red tongue with a yellow coating, and a rapid or slippery and rapid pulse. Internal and external treatments were used in parallel. [18]

Treatment principle

Clear Heat and benefit the movement of Dampness, cool the Blood and relieve Toxicity.

Internal prescription ingredients

Jin Yin Hua (Flos Lonicerae) 15g
Sheng Di Huang (Radix Rehmanniae Glutinosae) 15g
Bi Xie (Rhizoma Dioscoreae Hypoglaucae seu Septemlobae) 15g

Tu Fu Ling (Rhizoma Smilacis Glabrae) 15g
Ye Ju Hua (Flos Chrysanthemi Indici) 15g
Pu Gong Ying (Herba Taraxaci cum Radice) 15g
Tong Cao (Medulla Tetrapanacis Papyriferi) 12g
Chi Shao (Radix Paeoniae Rubra) 12g
Hua Shi‡ (Talcum) 25g
Yu Zhu (Rhizoma Polygonati Odorati) 8g

One bag a day was used to prepare a decoction, taken twice a day.

External prescription ingredients

Da Huang (Radix et Rhizoma Rhei) 30g
Di Yu (Radix Sanguisorbae Officinalis) 30g
Ku Shen (Radix Sophorae Flavescentis) 30g
Hei Mian Shen (Radix Breyniae Fruticosae) 30g
Wu Bei Zi‡ (Galla Rhois Chinensis) 30g

These ingredients were decocted in 1500-2000ml of water for use lukewarm as an external wash.

Western medicine

Western drugs used in the treatment included chlorpheniramine maleate, cyproheptadine, berberine, and erythromycin.

Most patients started to show an improvement in their condition after three days and all had begun to improve after seven days. The overall length of treatment ranged from 7 days to 54 days, averaging 19 days.

The authors of the report consider that although infectious eczematoid dermatitis is not recognized as such in TCM, it has elements of *jin yin chuang* (wet spreading sore), *feng shi chuang* (Wind-Damp sore) or *huang shui chuang* (yellow water sore). All of these sores are caused by Damp-Heat accumulating internally followed by an invasion of external Heat Toxins. Damp-Heat combines with the Heat Toxins to attack the skin and flesh. The treatment principle should focus therefore on giving equal weight to clearing Damp-Heat and eliminating Heat Toxins.

Contact dermatitis
接触性皮炎

Contact dermatitis arises as a result of an allergic reaction to certain substances (allergic contact dermatitis) or exposure to or contact with an irritant (irritant contact dermatitis). The condition is generally a delayed and cumulative response to a trigger factor through development of type IV hypersensitivity (cell-mediated immune reactions). Contact dermatitis is common in both industrial and domestic environments; irritants account for many more cases than allergens.

Common causes of irritant or allergic contact dermatitis are listed in Table 3-2.

Table 3-2 Common causes of irritant or allergic contact dermatitis

Irritant contact dermatitis

Water

Frictional abrasives or abrasive dusts

Chemicals (alkalis more than acids)

Solvents

Oils

Detergents

Soaps

Coarse fibers or sawdust

Extremes of temperature

Low environmental humidity

Allergic contact dermatitis

Nickel in jewelry, zips, jean studs, coins or watch straps

Chromate in cement, paint, anticorrosives, some leathers, or tattoo pigments

Rubber additives in tires, footwear, gloves, or condoms

Fragrances in cosmetics, soaps or detergents

Preservatives in water-based products such as cosmetics, toiletries and cooling fluids

Paraphenylene diamine in dyes for hair or clothing

Epoxy resin in adhesives and plastics

Colophony in sticking plaster, glue or polishes

Plants such as poison ivy, poison oak or primula (see also Phytophotodermatitis in Chapter 17)

Topical medication, particularly antibiotics (e.g. neomycin)

In terms of TCM etiology and pathology, contact dermatitis is caused by internal accumulation of Damp-Heat complicated by an invasion of external Heat Toxins at a time when the constitution is weakened by reduction of tolerance of toxic or allergic substances. Internal Damp-Heat and external Heat Toxins combine and accumulate in the skin and flesh to produce a variety of lesions.

Clinical manifestations and lesions vary depending on the relative weakness of the constitution, the strength of the accumulated Damp-Heat, the intensity of the Heat Toxins, and the specific contact location. Where Heat Toxins settle in the skin, the main lesion will be erythema; where the condition is caused by accumulation of Damp-Heat, lesions will include erythema, vesicles and edema.

The appearance of dermatitis at various body sites is an indication of possible contact with the factor triggering the reaction, as detailed in Table 3-3.

Table 3-3 Body sites with possible causes of contact dermatitis

Body site	Allergens or irritants responsible
Head	Shampoos, hair dyes
Face and eyes	Cosmetics
Ears	Earrings, topical medication
Mouth	Lipstick, toothpaste
Neck	Necklace
Trunk	Clothing dyes, deodorant, bra fastenings, jean studs
Arms	Plants, water
Wrists	Bracelets, watch straps
Hands	Water, cleaning materials, rubber gloves, rings, nail varnish
Genitals	Condoms, toiletries
Feet	Footwear

Although the original site of the eruption provides an idea of the likely cause, subsequent spread to other sites may confuse the picture.

In classical TCM texts, contact dermatitis was related to the type of substance then likely to cause the disease. In terms of allergic contact dermatitis, this was lacquer or lead-based cosmetic powders, whereas for irritant contact dermatitis, it was more likely to be friction-induced. These days, contact dermatitis is much more likely to be caused by the various chemical substances used in industrial processes, dyes, toiletries, and cosmetics, or by certain medications; irritant contact dermatitis develops from the use of agents such as alkalis, detergents, oils, or organic solvents. Notwith- standing the differences in etiological agents, the TCM treatment methods remain similar.

Irritant contact dermatitis
刺激性接触性皮炎

Irritant contact dermatitis is generally caused by expo- sure to strong irritants such as solvents, coarse fibers and resins, which cause a rapid and acute reaction, or by repeated exposure to mild irritants such as water, soaps, detergents, heat, and abrasives, which may require sev- eral months or years to elicit a reactive response (often on the hands, particularly on the dorsum). The intensity of the dermatitis is usually related to the strength of the irritant and the length of exposure. Unlike in allergic contact dermatitis, prior sensitization is not necessary, although patients with a history of atopic eczema are more likely to develop irritant contact dermatitis.

In the home, women with young children are most likely to be affected as a result of frequent contact with water and detergents; in the workplace, irritant contact dermatitis occurs most frequently among hairdressers, catering staff, nurses, chemical plant workers, and metal workers. In many instances, those affected are unable to give up their work or abandon their household chores, with the result that the skin is unable to regain its nor- mal barrier function.

This section deals with one example of irritant contact dermatitis known in TCM as *gao yao feng* (plaster Wind).

Clinical manifestations

- Lesions occur in areas formerly in contact with medicated plasters. The borders of the lesions are clearly defined, corresponding to the shape of the dressing.
- Local reddening and swelling occurs, accompanied by vesicles, erosion and exudation in severe cases.
- Pruritus is likely to be severe, possibly with a burning sensation.

Differential diagnosis

Irritant contact dermatitis is difficult to differentiate from allergic contact dermatitis and atopic eczema. Identification of possible causes is usually the best guide to differentiation and treatment.

Etiology and pathology

Internal accumulation of Dampness combined with contact with external Toxins causes damage to the skin.

Pattern identification and treatment

INTERNAL TREATMENT

HEAT TOXINS AND DAMPNESS ACCUMULATING IN THE SKIN
Lesions are inflamed and swollen with papulovesicles, exudation and erosion, and local itching. Tongue and pulse are normal.

Treatment principle
Transform Dampness and relieve Toxicity.

Prescription
LIANG XUE JIE DU TANG JIA JIAN
Decoction for Cooling the Blood and Relieving Toxicity, with modifications

Sheng Di Huang (Radix Rehmanniae Glutinosae) 12g
Fu Ling Pi (Cortex Poriae Cocos) 12g
Lian Qiao (Fructus Forsythiae Suspensae) 12g
Chi Xiao Dou (Semen Phaseoli Calcarati) 12g
Mu Dan Pi (Cortex Moutan Radicis) 6g
Chi Shao (Radix Paeoniae Rubra) 6g
Zi Cao (Radix Arnebiae seu Lithospermi) 6g
Lian Zi Xin (Plumula Nelumbinis Nuciferae) 6g
Chan Tui‡ (Periostracum Cicadae) 3g
Fu Ping (Herba Spirodelae Polyrrhizae) 3g
Gan Cao (Radix Glycyrrhizae) 3g
Bai Mao Gen (Rhizoma Imperatae Cylindricae) 15g
Bai Xian Pi (Cortex Dictamni Dasycarpi Radicis) 15g
Che Qian Cao (Herba Plantaginis) 15g

Explanation
- *Fu Ling Pi* (Cortex Poriae Cocos), *Chi Xiao Dou* (Semen Phaseoli Calcarati), *Bai Mao Gen* (Rhizoma Imperatae Cylindricae), and *Che Qian Cao* (Herba Plantaginis) clear Heat and benefit the movement of Dampness.

- *Sheng Di Huang* (Radix Rehmanniae Glutinosae), *Mu Dan Pi* (Cortex Moutan Radicis), *Chi Shao* (Radix Paeoniae Rubra), *Zi Cao* (Radix Arnebiae seu Lithospermi), and *Bai Mao Gen* (Rhizoma Imperatae Cylindricae) cool the Blood and reduce erythema.
- *Lian Qiao* (Fructus Forsythiae Suspensae), *Gan Cao* (Radix Glycyrrhizae), *Lian Zi Xin* (Plumula Nelumbinis Nuciferae), *Chan Tui*‡ (Periostracum Cicadae), *Fu Ping* (Herba Spirodelae Polyrrhizae), and *Bai Xian Pi* (Cortex Dictamni Dasycarpi Radicis) dredge Wind and alleviate itching, relieve Toxicity and disperse swelling.

EXTERNAL TREATMENT

- For severe erosion and exudation, prepare a decoction with *Shi Liu Pi** (Pericarpium Punicae Granati) 12g, *Ma Chi Xian* (Herba Portulacae Oleraceae) 12g and *Xuan Ming Fen* ‡ (Mirabilitum Depuratum) 15g for use as a wet compress for 15-20 minutes two or three times a day.
- For local dryness and severe itching, apply *Huang Lian Ruan Gao* (Coptis Ointment) externally once or twice a day.

Clinical notes

- Mild conditions can be cured if the affected area is treated first with a wet compress and then by external application of *Huang Lian Ruan Gao* (Coptis Ointment).
- Internal treatment should be added for severe cases.

Advice for the patient

- Avoid contact with sensitizing substances including medications used externally.
- In other types of irritant contact dermatitis, suitable protective clothing or gloves should be worn.
- After contact with irritant substances or substances of unknown chemical composition, wash the local area immediately with a suitable cleansing agent.
- Individuals with a history of contact dermatitis should be advised to bear this in mind when choosing a career.

Allergic contact dermatitis
变态反应性接触性皮炎

Allergic contact dermatitis is a delayed hypersensitivity reaction (type IV hypersensitivity, or cell-mediated immune reaction). This type of hypersensitive reaction is caused by sensitized lymphocytes. When the body is exposed to an antigen, T-lymphocytes become sensitized and divide and multiply to form effector lymphocytes. The antigen is recognized by the sensitized lymphocytes on subsequent exposure. Interaction between the antigen and these lymphocytes leads to the release of cytokines (soluble molecules that mediate action between cells). Cytokine release results in inflammatory cells (mainly T-lymphocytes) accumulating in the dermis and epidermis. Tissue damage is usually at its greatest two or three days afterward.

Once previous contact has been established with the allergen, any area of the skin can react to further contact and elicit the allergy. Common causes of this type of allergy include dyes, metals (such as nickel and chromium), plants (such as primula or ragweed), chemicals (such as formaldehyde), rubber additives, latex, fragrances, preservatives in cosmetics and toiletries, and topical medications (for example, antibiotics and steroids).

It may be possible to gain an idea of the likely allergen responsible for this type of contact dermatitis at the initial stage by noting the site of the lesion, but this may be more difficult as the condition evolves and lesions spread elsewhere. Questioning the patient about his or her profession and possible contact with typical allergens can help to establish a diagnosis before proceeding to pattern identification.

In TCM, since this condition was originally caused by contact with or exposure to lacquer, it is still often referred to as *qi chuang* (lacquer sore).

This section gives three examples of the TCM treatment of allergic contact dermatitis – lacquer sore, cosmetic dermatitis and hair dye dermatitis. The treatment principles detailed are also applicable to other types of allergic contact dermatitis.

Lacquer sore
漆疮

Clinical manifestations

Contact dermatitis

- Previous contact with lacquer is required to induce the allergy. Once it has developed, re-exposure to the substance will result in the appearance of symptoms a few hours to several days later. Typical manifestations include a burning sensation and a prickly itching feeling in the area exposed. Lesions then develop as erythema, edema, and small papules and papulovesicles, rapidly evolving into vesicles full of fluid.
- Rupture of the vesicles results in erosion and yellow crusts. In some cases, lesions may spread throughout the body.
- Swelling is especially obvious in areas where the skin is loose such as the eyelids and scrotum.
- In severe cases, accompanying symptoms and signs include dizziness, headache, lassitude, thirst, poor appetite, palpitations, and fever.
- Once sensitization has occurred, desensitization is rarely possible.

Dermatitis urticans (urticaria-like skin eruptions)

- This condition usually appears several days after the onset of acute contact dermatitis and may occur on the original lesion.
- Scratching produces wheals or dermographism. Lesions disappear slowly.

Differential diagnosis

Tinea manuum

Contact dermatitis of the hands should be differentiated from tinea manuum, where lesions mainly involve the center of the palm and the palmar aspect of the fingers. At the initial stage, small transparent pinpoint vesicles appear, which quickly rupture with a small amount of exudate. They soon dry up and are covered with layers of white scale. Later, the affected skin becomes dry, rough and thick, and may crack or fissure. Tinea manuum is usually asymmetrical and is frequently seen in association with tinea pedis.

Phytophotodermatitis

This condition occurs on exposure to sunlight after ingesting or coming into contact with plants (such as giant hogweed, carrot, parsnip, celery, fennel, or common rue) containing light-sensitizing substances known as psoralens (furanocoumarins). It is most common in spring and summer when furanocoumarins are highest and UV exposure is the greatest. Bizarre inflammatory patterns and linear streaks of hyperpigmentation are key clues to diagnosing phytophotodermatitis, with eruptions mostly manifesting in exposed areas.

Facial erysipelas

Acute contact dermatitis of the face should be differentiated from facial erysipelas, where there is no history of contact with allergens. The appearance of skin lesions is preceded by a prodromal phase of fever, chills and malaise, usually lasting between 4 and 48 hours. Lesions initially manifest as localized bright red or purplish-red edematous erythema with irregular, sharply demarcated and rapidly expanding borders. The surface of the lesions is tense, shiny and hot. The eruption reaches a peak in 5-7 days and then subsides gradually over the following one to two weeks.

Etiology and pathology

Contact with Toxins

Lacquer, acrid in flavor and hot in nature, is a Toxic substance. People with congenital insufficiency, looseness of the skin and interstices (*cou li*) and instability of the sweat pores will suffer from lacquer poisoning if they touch a lacquer tree or come into contact with lacquer.

Exuberant Wind-Heat

Acrid, hot and toxic substances such as lacquer can stir Wind and generate Fire. Lacquer can attack the skin and interstices (*cou li*) and its Toxins can constrain the Liver channel and spread to the skin and flesh, manifesting as inflammation, vesicular eruptions, edema, and pruritus. In *Dong Tian Ao Zhi (Wai Ke Mi Lu)* [Secret Records of External Diseases], it says: "Patients with lacquer sores usually contract the disease after smelling lacquer ... Lung Qi will be constrained after attack by inhalation of the smell ... This will result in itchy skin."

Heat Toxins mixed with Dampness

Invasion of lacquer Toxins due to constitutional Deficiency and looseness of the skin and interstices (*cou li*) leads to binding of Dampness and Heat, which cannot be drained internally or thrust outward through the exterior. As a result, Damp-Heat is retained in the skin, flesh, channels, and network vessels, thus causing the disease.

Pattern identification and treatment

INTERNAL TREATMENT

EXUBERANT WIND-HEAT

Inflamed and swollen skin, papules, edema and wheals, with severe itching, appear on the wrists, the sides of the fingers, the dorsum of the hands, and the forearm. The condition worsens after scratching. The tongue body is red with a thin yellow coating; the pulse is floating and rapid.

Treatment principle
Clear Heat and disperse Wind.

Prescription
XIAO FENG SAN JIA JIAN
Powder for Dispersing Wind, with modifications

Jing Jie (Herba Schizonepetae Tenuifoliae) 6g
Ku Shen (Radix Sophorae Flavescentis) 6g
Chan Tui‡ (Periostracum Cicadae) 6g
Zhi Mu (Rhizoma Anemarrhenae Asphodeloidis) 6g
Tong Cao (Medulla Tetrapanacis Papyriferi) 6g
Sheng Di Huang (Radix Rehmanniae Glutinosae) 10g
Fang Feng (Radix Ledebouriellae Divaricatae) 10g
Chao Niu Bang Zi (Fructus Arctii Lappae, stir-fried) 10g
Chi Fu Ling (Sclerotium Poriae Cocos Rubrae) 10g
Shi Gao‡ (Gypsum Fibrosum) 15g, decocted for 30 minutes before adding the other ingredients
Da Qing Ye (Folium Isatidis seu Baphicacanthi) 12g

Explanation
- Jing Jie (Herba Schizonepetae Tenuifoliae), Chan Tui‡ (Periostracum Cicadae), Fang Feng (Radix Ledebouriellae Divaricatae), and Chao Niu Bang Zi (Fructus Arctii Lappae, stir-fried) dredge Wind and disperse swelling to alleviate itching.
- Zhi Mu (Rhizoma Anemarrhenae Asphodeloidis), Da Qing Ye (Folium Isatidis seu Baphicacanthi), Shi Gao‡ (Gypsum Fibrosum), and Sheng Di Huang (Radix Rehmanniae Glutinosae) clear Heat from the Qi level and cool the Blood to reduce erythema.
- Tong Cao (Medulla Tetrapanacis Papyriferi), Ku Shen (Radix Sophorae Flavescentis) and Chi Fu Ling (Sclerotium Poriae Cocos Rubrae) benefit the movement of Dampness and transform Toxicity to clear Heat.

HEAT TOXINS MIXED WITH DAMPNESS

This pattern manifests as sudden onset of redness, swelling, a burning sensation, and prickly itching in the area in contact with lacquer. Lesions develop into papules, papulovesicles and clusters of vesicles. In severe cases, bullae or hemorrhagic blisters may appear; if they rupture, exudation, erosion or superficial ulceration may ensue. The tongue body is red with a yellow coating; the pulse is slippery and rapid.

Treatment principle
Clear Heat and relieve Toxicity, transform Dampness and disperse swelling.

Prescription
HUA BAN JIE DU TANG JIA JIAN
Decoction for Transforming Erythema and Relieving Toxicity, with modifications

Xuan Shen (Radix Scrophulariae Ningpoensis) 6g
Chao Zhi Mu (Rhizoma Anemarrhenae Asphodeloidis, stir-fried) 6g
Chao Huang Lian (Rhizoma Coptidis, stir-fried) 6g
Sheng Ma (Rhizoma Cimicifugae) 6g
Shi Gao‡ (Gypsum Fibrosum) 15g, decocted for 30 minutes before adding the other ingredients
Chao Niu Bang Zi (Fructus Arctii Lappae, stir-fried) 10g
Fang Feng (Radix Ledebouriellae Divaricatae) 10g
Fu Ping (Herba Spirodelae Polyrrhizae) 10g
Bai Mao Gen (Rhizoma Imperatae Cylindricae) 30g
Lian Zi Xin (Plumula Nelumbinis Nuciferae) 4.5g

Explanation
- Shi Gao‡ (Gypsum Fibrosum), Chao Zhi Mu (Rhizoma Anemarrhenae Asphodeloidis, stir-fried), Xuan Shen (Radix Scrophulariae Ningpoensis), Chao Huang Lian (Rhizoma Coptidis, stir-fried), and Lian Zi Xin (Plumula Nelumbinis Nuciferae) clear Heat from the Qi level and relieve Toxicity, enrich Yin and protect Body Fluids.
- Sheng Ma (Rhizoma Cimicifugae), Chao Niu Bang Zi (Fructus Arctii Lappae, stir-fried), Fang Feng (Radix Ledebouriellae Divaricatae), Fu Ping (Herba Spirodelae Polyrrhizae), and Bai Mao Gen (Rhizoma Imperatae Cylindricae) dissipate Wind and disperse swelling, eliminate Dampness and alleviate itching.

General modifications
1. For severe edema, add Fu Ling Pi (Cortex Poriae Cocos), Hua Shi‡ (Talcum) and Dong Gua Pi (Epicarpium Benincasae Hispidae).
2. For relatively severe Heat Toxins, add Lü Dou Yi (Testa Phaseoli Radiati) and Chao Huang Bai (Cortex Phellodendri, stir-fried).
3. For intense itching, add Bai Zhi (Radix Angelicae Dahuricae), Qiang Huo (Rhizoma et Radix Notopterygii), Bai Xian Pi (Cortex Dictamni Dasycarpi Radicis), and Gou Teng (Ramulus Uncariae cum Uncis).
4. For lesions on the upper body, add Sang Ye (Folium Mori Albae) and Ju Hua (Flos Chrysanthemi Morifolii).

5. For lesions on the lower body, add *Long Dan Cao* (Radix Gentianae Scabrae) and *Qing Pi* (Pericarpium Citri Reticulatae Viride).

EXTERNAL TREATMENT

- For lesions manifesting mainly as erythema and papules, wash the affected area with *Lu Hu Xi Ji* (Calamine and Giant Knotweed Wash Preparation) or *San Huang Xi Ji* (Three Yellows Wash Preparation) twice a day.
- For lesions manifesting as papulovesicles or vesicles with exudation and erosion, prepare a decoction with *Di Yu* (Radix Sanguisorbae Officinalis) 15g and *Huang Bai* (Cortex Phellodendri) 15g and use as a cold compress for 15 minutes twice a day. Then, mix *Qing Dai San* (Indigo Powder) or *Yu Lu San* (Jade Dew Powder) into a paste with vegetable oil for external application twice a day. Treat until the lesions heal.

ACUPUNCTURE

Points: LU-5 Chize, LI-11 Quchi, PC-3 Quze, and BL-40 Weizhong.

Technique: Apply the reducing method and retain the needles for 30 minutes after obtaining Qi. Manipulate the needles three to five times during this period. Treat once a day. A course consists of five treatment sessions. The therapeutic result is better if BL-40 Weizhong is pricked to cause a small amount of bleeding.

Explanation

These points are selected to clear Heat and transform Dampness, disperse Wind and alleviate itching. Pricking BL-40 Weizhong to cause bleeding works very well for draining Fire and relieving Toxicity, invigorating the Blood and reducing erythema.

Clinical notes

- In the acute phase (as described in the patterns above), the treatment principle should focus on dredging Wind and dispersing swelling, cooling the Blood and alleviating itching. If there is obvious exudation, add materia medica for clearing Heat and transforming Dampness to assist in relieving Toxicity.
- Once contact with allergy-inducing substances is avoided, contact dermatitis can be treated by applying materia medica for clearing and transforming Damp-Heat, cooling the Blood and relieving Toxicity in prescriptions such as *Long Dan Xie Gan Tang* (Chinese Gentian Decoction for Draining the Liver) and *Liang Xue Si Wu Tang* (Four Agents Decoction for Cooling the Blood).
- Appropriate acupuncture treatment is effective for dispersing swelling and alleviating itching.
- External treatment is important to enhance the therapeutic effect.

Advice for the patient

- Avoid contact with known allergens.
- Individuals with a history of contact dermatitis should be advised to bear this in mind when choosing a career.
- If there is local redness, swelling and exudation, do not wash the lesion with hot water, avoid scratching, and do not eat spicy or irritating food.

Literature excerpt

According to *Wai Ke Zheng Zong* [An Orthodox Manual of External Diseases]: "Lacquer sore can be caused by a variety of factors. Some people are affected by contact with lacquer and some are not. Lacquer is an acrid, hot, toxic substance. If the exterior of the body is weak, the Toxins can invade to cause the disease. Itching appears first; after scratching, the disease gradually comes to resemble *yin zhen* (dormant papules, or urticaria). Lesions spread quickly throughout the body, manifesting as erosive patches with exudation and pain. In severe cases, alternating chills and fever may be accompanying symptoms. Hot baths and spicy food must be avoided, otherwise the disease may become stubborn."

Cosmetic dermatitis
化妆品皮炎

This type of allergic contact dermatitis is caused by exposure to or contact with fragrances and preservatives in toiletries or cosmetics.

In TCM, this condition is also known as *hua fen chuang* (pollen sore).

Clinical manifestations

- This disease is most common in women who use cosmetics.

- At the initial stage, a dense distribution of tiny red or pale red papules appears in the region of the face where make-up is habitually applied. Patches with ill-defined margins may form.
- Itching of varying intensity usually accompanies the eruption.
- Pigmentation and rough skin are likely if the disease persists.

Etiology and pathology

The condition is caused by constitutional insufficiency and looseness of the interstices (*cou li*) complicated by external contraction of Wind Toxins or contact with Toxic substances.

Pattern identification and treatment

INTERNAL TREATMENT

DAMP TOXINS ACCUMULATING IN THE SKIN

Tiny pinpoint papules appear on the face, which becomes inflamed and slightly itchy.

Treatment principle
Relieve Toxicity and improve the countenance.

Prescription
LÜ DOU JIE DU TANG JIA JIAN
Mung Bean Decoction for Relieving Toxicity, with modifications

Lü Dou Yi (Testa Phaseoli Radiati) 30g

Dong Gua Ren (Semen Benincasae Hispidae) 30g
Shan Yao (Rhizoma Dioscoreae Oppositae) 30g
Fu Ling (Sclerotium Poriae Cocos) 10g
Chao Bai Bian Dou (Semen Dolichoris Lablab, stir-fried) 10g
Chai Hu (Radix Bupleuri) 10g
Sheng Ma (Rhizoma Cimicifugae) 10g
Dang Gui Wei (Extremitas Radicis Angelicae Sinensis) 6g
Chao Bai Shao (Radix Paeoniae Lactiflorae, stir-fried) 6g
Gan Cao (Radix Glycyrrhizae) 6g
Hong Hua (Flos Carthami Tinctorii) 6g
Ling Xiao Hua (Flos Campsitis) 6g

Explanation
- *Lü Dou Yi* (Testa Phaseoli Radiati), *Chai Hu* (Radix Bupleuri), *Sheng Ma* (Rhizoma Cimicifugae), and *Gan Cao* (Radix Glycyrrhizae) clear Heat and relieve Toxicity.
- *Dong Gua Ren* (Semen Benincasae Hispidae), *Fu Ling* (Sclerotium Poriae Cocos), *Shan Yao* (Rhizoma Dioscoreae Oppositae), and *Chao Bai Bian Dou* (Semen Dolichoris Lablab, stir-fried) fortify the Spleen and eliminate Dampness.
- *Dang Gui Wei* (Extremitas Radicis Angelicae Sinensis), *Chao Bai Shao* (Radix Paeoniae Lactiflorae, stir-fried), *Hong Hua* (Flos Carthami Tinctorii), and *Ling Xiao Hua* (Flos Campsitis) cool the Blood and relieve Toxicity.

EXTERNAL TREATMENT
Apply *Bing Pian Lu Gan Shi Xi Ji* (Borneol and Calamine Wash Preparation) to the face every night before going to bed. Wash off the following morning.

Hair dye dermatitis
染发皮炎

Hair dye dermatitis is another example of allergic contact dermatitis that has been treated down the ages by TCM. Nowadays, this type of contact dermatitis is caused by allergy to paraphenylene diamine contained in hair dye products.

Clinical manifestations

- The patient has a history of dyeing the hair before onset of the disease.
- Onset is acute. Mild cases are characterized by erythema, papules or vesicles, severe cases by redness, swelling, pustules, erosion, and exudation.
- Lesions mainly involve the scalp, hair line, face, ear lobe, and neck.
- Severe itching and a burning sensation are common.
- Accompanying symptoms and signs include red and swollen eyes with conjunctival congestion, fever, aversion to cold, and nausea.
- Once the remaining hair dye is removed from the affected area, the condition will improve after one to two weeks.

Etiology and pathology

When the skin and interstices (*cou li*) are loose, pathogenic Wind-Damp-Heat can invade to bring about the condition.

Pattern identification and treatment

INTERNAL TREATMENT

DAMP-HEAT

The scalp is bright red and swollen with exudation and erosion. Pain and itching are common. The tongue body is red with a thin yellow coating; the pulse is moderate and rapid.

Treatment principle
Clear Heat and eliminate Dampness.

Prescription
CHU SHI WEI LING TANG JIA JIAN
Poria Five Decoction for Eliminating Dampness and Calming the Stomach, with modifications

Fu Ling (Sclerotium Poriae Cocos) 10g
Chen Pi (Pericarpium Citri Reticulatae) 10g
Cang Zhu (Rhizoma Atractylodis) 10g
Fang Feng (Radix Ledebouriellae Divaricatae) 10g
Sheng Di Huang (Radix Rehmanniae Glutinosae) 15g
Huang Qin (Radix Scutellariae) 6g
Zhi Zi (Fructus Gardeniae Jasminoidis) 6g
Chan Tui‡ (Periostracum Cicadae) 6g
Ku Shen (Radix Sophorae Flavescentis) 6g
Chao Huai Hua (Flos Sophorae Japonicae, stir-fried)12g
Bai Mao Gen (Rhizoma Imperatae Cylindricae) 12g

Explanation
- Fu Ling (Sclerotium Poriae Cocos), Chen Pi (Pericarpium Citri Reticulatae) and Cang Zhu (Rhizoma Atractylodis) fortify the Spleen and eliminate Dampness.
- Sheng Di Huang (Radix Rehmanniae Glutinosae), Zhi Zi (Fructus Gardeniae Jasminoidis), Huang Qin (Radix Scutellariae), Chao Huai Hua (Flos Sophorae Japonicae, stir-fried), and Bai Mao Gen (Rhizoma Imperatae Cylindricae) cool the Blood and relieve Toxicity.
- Fang Feng (Radix Ledebouriellae Divaricatae), Chan Tui‡ (Periostracum Cicadae) and Ku Shen (Radix Sophorae Flavescentis) eliminate Wind and alleviate itching.

WIND-HEAT

The scalp is itchy with dry and scaling skin and dry hair. The tongue body is red with a scant coating; the pulse is floating and rapid.

Treatment principle
Dredge Wind and clear Heat.

Prescription
XIAO FENG SAN JIA JIAN
Powder for Dispersing Wind, with modifications

Fang Feng (Radix Ledebouriellae Divaricatae) 6g
Jing Jie (Herba Schizonepetae Tenuifoliae) 6g
Ku Shen (Radix Sophorae Flavescentis) 6g
Sheng Di Huang (Radix Rehmanniae Glutinosae) 10g
Huang Qin (Radix Scutellariae) 10g
Qiang Huo (Rhizoma et Radix Notopterygii) 10g
Bai Fu Zi (Rhizoma Typhonii Gigantei) 10g
Tian Ma* (Rhizoma Gastrodiae Elatae) 12g
Ju Hua (Flos Chrysanthemi Morifolii) 12g
Sang Ye (Folium Mori Albae) 12g
Bai Mao Gen (Rhizoma Imperatae Cylindricae) 12g
Sheng Ma (Rhizoma Cimicifugae) 3g
Shi Chang Pu (Rhizoma Acori Graminei) 3g

Explanation
- Fang Feng (Radix Ledebouriellae Divaricatae), Jing Jie (Herba Schizonepetae Tenuifoliae), Qiang Huo (Rhizoma et Radix Notopterygii), Bai Fu Zi (Rhizoma Typhonii Gigantei), Tian Ma* (Rhizoma Gastrodiae Elatae), Ju Hua (Flos Chrysanthemi Morifolii), Sang Ye (Folium Mori Albae), and Sheng Ma (Rhizoma Cimicifugae) dredge Wind and clear Heat.
- Sheng Di Huang (Radix Rehmanniae Glutinosae), Huang Qin (Radix Scutellariae) and Bai Mao Gen (Rhizoma Imperatae Cylindricae) clear Heat and cool the Blood.
- Ku Shen (Radix Sophorae Flavescentis) and Shi Chang Pu (Rhizoma Acori Graminei) dredge Wind and alleviate itching

EXTERNAL TREATMENT

- For pronounced redness and swelling with exudation, apply a wet compress of Sang Bai Pi Shui Xi Ji (White Mulberry Root Bark Wash Preparation) for 24 hours and then rinse off.
- For dry and scaly lesions with severe itching, apply Huang Lian Ruan Gao (Coptis Ointment) twice a day.

Case histories

Case 1

Patient
Female, aged 56.

Clinical manifestations
Four days previously, a few hours after dyeing her hair, the patient's scalp and facial skin became red and itchy. By the next day, the affected area had become swollen and was covered with small vesicles; it was difficult to open the eyes, which were unbearably itchy. The patient took prednisone and applied a medicinal lotion, but the condition showed little improvement. The swelling and redness became worse and there was obvious exudation. Accompanying symptoms and signs included insomnia, poor appetite, dry stools, and short voidings of reddish urine.

Examination revealed that the patient's scalp, face, ears, and hands were red and swollen and were covered by clusters of vesicles and bullae with exudation. The eyelids were obviously swollen; conjunctival hyperemia was noted. Touching the face produced a burning sensation. The tongue body was red with a slightly yellow coating; the pulse was wiry, slippery and rapid.

Diagnosis
Allergic contact dermatitis caused by hair dye (*ran fa pi yan*).

Pattern identification
Internal accumulation of Damp-Heat with infection by Toxins.

Treatment principle
Clear Heat and cool the Blood, relieve Toxicity and benefit the movement of Dampness.

Prescription ingredients
Long Dan Cao (Radix Gentianae Scabrae) 10g
Huang Qin (Radix Scutellariae Baicalensis) 15g
Sheng Di Huang (Radix Rehmanniae Glutinosae) 30g
Mu Dan Pi (Cortex Moutan Radicis) 15g
Bai Mao Gen (Rhizoma Imperatae Cylindricae) 30g
Ye Ju Hua (Flos Chrysanthemi Indici) 10g
Ma Chi Xian (Herba Portulacae Oleraceae) 30g
Bai Jiang Cao (Herba Patriniae cum Radice) 30g
Yi Yi Ren (Semen Coicis Lachryma-jobi) 30g
Che Qian Zi (Semen Plantaginis) 15g
Ze Xie (Rhizoma Alismatis Orientalis) 15g
Dong Gua Pi (Epicarpium Benincasae Hispidae) 15g
Che Qian Cao (Herba Plantaginis) 30g
Bai Xian Pi (Cortex Dictamni Dasycarpi Radicis) 30g
Ku Shen (Radix Sophorae Flavescentis) 15g
Shi Gao ‡ (Gypsum Fibrosum) 30g, decocted for 30 minutes before adding the other ingredients

One bag a day was used to prepare a decoction, taken twice a day.

External treatment
A decoction was prepared with *Ma Chi Xian* (Herba Portulacae Oleraceae) 30g and *Huang Bai* (Cortex Phellodendri) 10g and allowed to cool. The hair was moved away from the affected area as much as possible and the decoction then applied as a cold compress for 30 minutes two to four times a day. Tetracycline ointment was applied to the eyes.

Second visit
After two bags of the internal decoction, the redness and swelling of the face was showing an obvious improvement, the blisters had dried, and the eyes could open slightly. The appetite became better and bowel movement returned to normal. The tongue body was red with a white coating; the pulse was wiry, slippery and rapid. The patient was told to continue with the prescription.

Further visits
Three days later, the swelling on the face had completely disappeared. The skin was still slightly red with bran-like scaling and slight itching. After taking seven bags of the decoction, all the symptoms disappeared, including the blisters on the hands. [19]

Case 2
Patient
Female, aged 28.

Clinical manifestations
Four days previously, the patient's arms touched a newly painted desk. A few hours later, a red eruption appeared on those areas of the arms which had touched the desk; the skin became itchy and swollen and the patient experienced a burning pain. By the following day, the eruption had affected all of the arms with the appearance of erythematous patches and vesicles. Itching had worsened and the face and eyelids had become swollen. Accompanying symptoms included thirst with no desire for drinks. Stool and urine were both normal.

Examination revealed 1-2 mm vesicles and a small amount of pale yellow exudate on the sides of the arms with a less dense distribution on the face, chest and abdomen. The tongue body was pale red with a white coating; the pulse was wiry and rapid.

Diagnosis
Allergic contact dermatitis (*qi chuang*).

Pattern identification
Internal accumulation of Damp-Heat with infection by Toxins.

Treatment principle
Clear Heat and cool the Blood, relieve Toxicity and eliminate Dampness.

Prescription ingredients
Long Dan Cao (Radix Gentianae Scabrae) 10g
Huang Qin (Radix Scutellariae Baicalensis) 10g
Sheng Di Huang (Radix Rehmanniae Glutinosae) 15g
Mu Dan Pi (Cortex Moutan Radicis) 15g
Ma Chi Xian (Herba Portulacae Oleraceae) 30g
Ban Lan Gen (Radix Isatidis seu Baphicacanthi) 30g
Sang Bai Pi (Cortex Mori Albae Radicis) 15g
Tong Cao (Medulla Tetrapanacis Papyriferi) 10g
Ze Xie (Rhizoma Alismatis Orientalis) 15g
Dong Gua Pi (Epicarpium Benincasae Hispidae) 15g
Liu Yi San (Six-To-One Powder) 30g, wrapped
Jiang Huang (Rhizoma Curcumae Longae) 10g

One bag a day was used to prepare a decoction, taken twice a day.

External treatment
A decoction was prepared with *Ma Chi Xian* (Herba Portulacae Oleraceae) 30g, allowed to cool and applied to the affected area as a cold compress for 30 minutes four times a day. *Gan Cao You* (Licorice Oil) was then applied to dispel Dampness.

Second visit
After taking three bags of the decoction, the erythema on the face, chest and abdomen had clearly improved, and the redness and swelling were much less. The burning sensation had disappeared. The patient was told to continue with the prescription.

Outcome

After taking another three bags of the decoction, the lesions had virtually disappeared apart from a small amount of desquamation.

Discussion

Contact dermatitis is an acute inflammation that occurs after the skin comes into contact with certain substances. It can be classified into two types: original stimulation (irritant contact dermatitis) and abnormal reaction (allergic contact dermatitis). The former occurs because substances such as strong acids or alkalis are so stimulating that anybody coming into contact with them can be affected over time; the latter is basically slight stimulation causing an allergic reaction in a limited number of people who are physically allergic to the substance.

In TCM, contact dermatitis is named differently according to the different substances that are touched. For instance, those cases caused by touching medicated plaster are called *gao yao feng* (plaster Wind), those caused by touching paint or lacquer are known as *qi chuang* (lacquer sore). According to TCM theory, this type of disease occurs mainly because the human body is frail by nature; when the interstices (*cou li*) are loose, the skin may be invaded by external Heat Toxins that accumulate in the skin.

The first case is an allergic inflammation of the skin caused by contact with a substance that induces a rapid response in the area of the skin that has touched the substance, the affected area then becoming inflamed, swollen and itchy. It is clearly distinguished from the unaffected area in which there is no inflammation or only slight inflammation. Clinical manifestations include redness and swelling with a sensation of burning heat, dry stools and short voidings of reddish urine. The pulse is rapid, wiry and slippery, and the tongue body is red with a yellow coating.

There are obvious signs of Dampness, Heat and Toxins. The treatment principle therefore focuses on clearing Heat, relieving Toxicity and cooling the Blood with the secondary consideration of benefiting the movement of Dampness and dispersing swelling. In the prescription, *Long Dan Cao* (Radix Gentianae Scabrae), *Huang Qin* (Radix Scutellariae Baicalensis) and *Shi Gao* ‡ (Gypsum Fibrosum) are used to clear Heat and relieve Toxicity; *Sheng Di Huang* (Radix Rehmanniae Glutinosae), *Mu Dan Pi* (Cortex Moutan Radicis) and *Bai Mao Gen* (Rhizoma Imperatae Cylindricae) cool the Blood and clear Heat; and *Bai Xian* Pi (Cortex Dictamni Dasycarpi Radicis), *Ze Xie* (Rhizoma Alismatis Orientalis), *Ku Shen* (Radix Sophorae Flavescentis), *Che Qian Zi* (Semen Plantaginis), and *Dong Gua Pi* (Epicarpium Benincasae Hispidae) benefit the movement of Dampness and clear Heat.

To treat skin diseases caused by allergy to certain substances, the patient must avoid the substance causing the allergy. It is very important to treat the affected area. The substance causing the allergy should first be cleared from the location, followed by external application of a soothing medication (cream or ointment). Mild materia medica of a cool nature can then be applied in a cold compress to relieve the inflammation. Any medication that may cause allergy or stimulation should be avoided because improper use will only exacerbate the disease. [20]

Modern clinical experience

INTERNAL TREATMENT

Fang formulated a prescription to treat 30 cases of contact dermatitis – fourteen caused by cosmetics, nine by paint, three by anti-pruritus drugs and four by other substances. [21]

Prescription

QU FENG ZHI YANG TANG

Decoction for Dispelling Wind and Alleviating Itching

Di Gu Pi (Cortex Lycii Radicis) 30g
Sang Bai Pi (Cortex Mori Albae Radicis) 12g
Ze Xie (Rhizoma Alismatis Orientalis) 12g
Bai Mao Gen (Rhizoma Imperatae Cylindricae) 12g
Lü Dou Yi (Testa Phaseoli Radiati) 12g
Sang Ye (Folium Mori Albae) 9g
Huang Qin (Radix Scutellariae Baicalensis) 9g

One bag a day was used to prepare a decoction, taken twice a day. Results were seen after two weeks.

TREATMENT OF CONTACT DERMATITIS DUE TO DYES

1. **Wang** treated contact dermatitis due to dyes with an internal prescription. [22]

Prescription

QING RE JIE DU TANG JIA JIAN

Decoction for Clearing Heat and Relieving Toxicity, with modifications

Jing Jie (Herba Schizonepetae Tenuifoliae) 10g
Fang Feng (Radix Ledebouriellae Divaricatae) 10g
Bai Xian Pi (Cortex Dictamni Dasycarpi Radicis) 12g
Sheng Di Huang (Radix Rehmanniae Glutinosae) 20g
Ye Jiao Teng (Caulis Polygoni Multiflori) 20g
Jin Yin Hua (Flos Lonicerae) 30g
Pu Gong Ying (Herba Taraxaci cum Radice) 30g
Lian Qiao (Fructus Forsythiae Suspensae) 15g
Chan Tui ‡ (Periostracum Cicadae) 9g
Gan Cao (Radix Glycyrrhizae) 6g

Modifications

1. For obvious Heat patterns, *Mu Dan Pi* (Cortex Moutan Radicis) 10g and *Chi Shao* (Radix Paeoniae Rubra) 10g were added.
2. For severe Damp-Heat, *Ze Xie* (Rhizoma Alismatis Orientalis) 10g, *Huang Qin* (Radix Scutellariae Baicalensis) 10g and *Fu Ling Pi* (Cortex Poriae Cocos) 20g were added.

One bag a day was used to prepare a decoction, taken twice a day. Results were seen after two to nine bags (six bags on average).

2. Liu treated contact dermatitis due to dyes with a combination of TCM and Western medicine. [23]

Western medicine
10% calcium gluconate 10ml, vitamin C 2g and dexamethasone 5mg were mixed with 50% glucose solution 40ml for an intravenous drip, which was given once a day.

TCM prescription for internal use
QU FENG CHU SHI TANG
Decoction for Dispelling Wind and Eliminating Dampness

Jin Yin Hua (Flos Lonicerae) 20g
Lian Qiao (Fructus Forsythiae Suspensae) 12g
Pu Gong Ying (Herba Taraxaci cum Radice) 12g
Mu Dan Pi (Cortex Moutan Radicis) 12g
Tu Fu Ling (Rhizoma Smilacis Glabrae) 12g
Jing Jie (Herba Schizonepetae Tenuifoliae) 10g
Fang Feng (Radix Ledebouriellae Divaricatae) 10g
Ku Shen (Radix Sophorae Flavescentis) 10g

Bai Xian Pi (Cortex Dictamni Dasycarpi Radicis) 12g
She Chuang Zi (Fructus Cnidii Monnieri) 12g
Chan Tui ‡ (Periostracum Cicadae) 9g

One bag a day was used to prepare a decoction, taken twice a day.

TCM prescription for external application as a local wash

Ku Shen (Radix Sophorae Flavescentis) 30g
Di Fu Zi (Fructus Kochiae Scopariae) 30g
Bai Xian Pi (Cortex Dictamni Dasycarpi Radicis) 30g
She Chuang Zi (Fructus Cnidii Monnieri) 30g
Pu Gong Ying (Herba Taraxaci cum Radice) 30g
Huang Bai (Cortex Phellodendri) 15g
Ku Fan ‡ (Alumen Praeparatum) 15g
He Shi (Fructus Carpesii) 20g

Results were seen after ten days.

Atopic eczema
异位性湿疹

This is a chronic, recurrent, pruritic, and inflammatory skin disease associated with genetic factors and is also known as hereditary allergic dermatitis. Characteristics of the disease include:
- family history of susceptibility to asthma, hay fever, urticaria, and eczema
- allergy to heterologous protein
- high serum immunoglobulin (IgE) levels
- an increase in the number of eosinophil leucocytes in the blood.
  In TCM, this disease is also known as *si wan feng* (four bends Wind), where the bends refer to the antecubital and popliteal fossae.

Clinical manifestations

- Atopic eczema affects at least 3 percent of infants in Western countries, but onset may be delayed until later. Females outnumber males by up to 2:1. Some 60-70 percent of those likely to develop the condition will have done so before the age of 12 months. Two-thirds of patients have a family history of atopy. Remission occurs by the age of 15 in around three-quarters of patients, but some relapse later. This condition is rare in the elderly.

- Exposure to extreme cold and heat, sweating, emotional disturbance, and contact with woolen articles can trigger pruritus.
- Some patients are more prone to develop bacterial or viral infections.
- The disease occurs in different age groups, each with their own particular characteristics:

Infantile phase (from one month to two years)
- The main sites of involvement include the cheeks, forehead and scalp. In a few cases, involvement may spread to the trunk and limbs. Severe itching from lesions induces crying and disturbs sleep.
- Fat babies who tend to sweat are more likely to suffer from an exudative-type condition. Lesions manifest as erythema and a dense distribution of pinpoint papules, papulovesicles and vesicles with exudation. Thick or thin yellow crusts form when the exudate dries up. A moist, bright red erosive base will often show once crusts fall off due to rubbing or scratching provoked by itching.
- Thin, weak babies are more likely to suffer from a dry-type condition. Lesions are characterized by pale red or dark red erythematous patches, a dense distribution of small papules without vesicles, dryness without obvious exudation, and grayish-white bran-like scales

on the surface of the lesions. Slight infiltration, licheni-fication, fissuring, scratch marks, or bloody crusting will be present in a persistent condition.

Childhood phase (from 3 to 12 years)

- The antecubital and popliteal fossae, neck, wrists, and ankles are the main sites involved.
- Lichenification, excoriations and dry skin are frequent.
- Sleep may be affected.
- In some cases, small, firm papules are found on the back and the extensor aspects of the limbs; exco-riation may lead to bloody crusting and pigmentation.

Adolescent and adult phase (from 12 years to early 20's)

- The condition occurs mostly in the antecubital and popliteal fossae, and the anterior and lateral aspects of the neck.
- Circumscribed dry lesions appear with infiltration, thickening and lichenification, and pigmentation as a sequel.
- The hands may also be involved after contact with irritants.

Differential diagnosis

Infantile seborrheic eczema

This condition often occurs in babies shortly after birth. Lesions manifest as grayish-yellow or brownish-yellow oily scales partially or completely covering the scalp (known as cradle cap). Itching is present, but not pronounced.

Contact dermatitis

Atopic eczema is difficult to differentiate from irritant or allergic contact dermatitis, especially at the chronic stage. Identification of possible causes is usually the best guide to differentiation and treatment. Individuals with a history of atopic eczema are often more suscep-tible to irritants causing dermatitis.

Etiology and pathology

- This condition is due to constitutional insufficiency and Deficiency of the Lungs and Spleen complicated by external contraction of Wind, Dampness and Heat, which are obstructed in the skin and flesh. An enduring condition will cause damage to Yin and Body Fluids resulting in Yin Deficiency and Blood-Dryness.
- The mother's preference for fatty, sweet, spicy, or fried food or overindulgence in fish and seafood during pregnancy or lactation will result in impair-ment of the Spleen's transportation function and the generation of Damp-Heat in the interior. The

mother will pass on the Heat Toxins and turbid sub-stances in the blood to the baby through breast-feeding. If this is complicated by improper feeding and nursing after birth, Damp-Heat may move to the skin and flesh to cause the disease. Dampness tends to predominate in plump babies, Heat in thin and weak babies.

- Constitutional weakness plus the child's preference for an inappropriate diet of fish, seafood and spicy food will damage the Spleen and Stomach and result in the generation of internal Damp-Heat. Where this Damp-Heat moves outward to accumulate in the skin and flesh and is complicated by invasion of pathogenic Wind, Dampness or Heat, or Toxic sub-stances such as dust mites or pollen, red papules and vesicles may appear suddenly. Where impairment of the Spleen's transportation and transformation func-tion results in Damp-Heat accumulating in the interior, this Damp-Heat may be retained over a long period, resulting in a chronic disease with repeated recurrence.
- Congenital (Earlier Heaven) insufficiency leads to Liver and Kidney Deficiency. Lack of proper care after birth (Later Heaven) results in damage to the Spleen and Lungs. Damage to the Spleen leads to deficiency of the source for generating transfor-mation of Qi and Blood; damage to the Lungs causes weakness of Wei Qi (Defensive Qi). As a result, it is easy for external pathogenic factors to invade. At the initial stage, these factors are obstructed in the skin and interstices (*cou li*), causing dryness and itching; at the later stage, Yin is dam-aged and Blood is consumed, making the skin rough and leathery.

Pattern identification and treatment

INTERNAL TREATMENT

DAMP-HEAT IN INFANTS (PREDOMINANCE OF DAMPNESS)

Fat babies are particularly likely to be affected. The main sites of involvement include the face, head and neck, but the condition may spread to other areas. Lesions are marked by erythema, papules and vesicles with thick exudation. As the disease develops, crusts appear and itching becomes increasingly pronounced, leading to disturbance of sleep patterns. Accompanying symptoms and signs include constipation and short voidings of yellow urine. The tongue body is pale red with a thin yellow coating; the pulse is slippery and rapid.

Treatment principle

Clear Heat, transform Dampness and alleviate itching.

Prescription
XIE HUANG SAN JIA JIAN
Yellow-Draining Powder, with modifications

Huo Xiang (Herba Agastaches seu Pogostemi) 6g
Chao Huang Bai (Cortex Phellodendri, stir-fried) 6g
Fu Ling Pi (Cortex Poriae Cocos) 6g
Chao Huang Qin (Radix Scutellariae Baicalensis, stir-fried) 6g
Shi Gao ‡ (Gypsum Fibrosum) 10g, decocted for 30 minutes before adding the other ingredients
Shan Yao (Rhizoma Dioscoreae Oppositae) 4.5g
Fang Feng (Radix Ledebouriellae Divaricatae) 4.5g
Jiao Zhi Zi (Fructus Gardeniae Jasminoidis, scorch-fried) 4.5g
Gan Cao (Radix Glycyrrhizae) 3g

Explanation
- *Huo Xiang* (Herba Agastaches seu Pogostemi), *Fu Ling Pi* (Cortex Poriae Cocos) and *Shan Yao* (Rhizoma Dioscoreae Oppositae) transform Dampness.
- *Shi Gao* ‡ (Gypsum Fibrosum), *Chao Huang Bai* (Cortex Phellodendri, stir-fried), *Chao Huang Qin* (Radix Scutellariae Baicalensis, stir-fried), and *Jiao Zhi Zi* (Fructus Gardeniae Jasminoidis, scorch-fried) clear Heat from the Heart and drain Fire.
- *Fang Feng* (Radix Ledebouriellae Divaricatae) and *Gan Cao* (Radix Glycyrrhizae) dredge Wind and alleviate itching.

FETAL HEAT
This pattern is more common in thin, weak, undernourished babies with a yellow complexion. Lesions, which are usually located on the scalp, face or neck, but may occasionally spread to the trunk and limbs, are characterized by papules and large pale red or dark red erythematous patches covered by oily scales or crusts. The skin is rough and itchy, disturbing sleep. Scratching provoked by itching will cause slight bleeding or result in the formation of bloody crusts. Some babies have accompanying symptoms of indigestion, manifesting as vomiting of milk shortly after feeding, and loose stools, possibly with undigested food. The tongue body is pale red with a scant coating; the pulse is moderate.

Treatment principle
Clear Heat from the Heart and guide out reddish urine, support the Spleen and foster Yin.

Prescription
SAN XIN DAO CHI SAN JIA JIAN
Three Plumules Powder for Guiding Out Reddish Urine

Lian Qiao Xin (Plumula Forsythiae Suspensae) 3g
Zhi Zi Xin (Plumula Gardeniae Jasminoidis) 3g
Lian Zi Xin (Plumula Nelumbinis Nuciferae) 6g
Sheng Di Huang (Radix Rehmanniae Glutinosae) 6g
Xuan Shen (Radix Scrophulariae Ningpoensis) 6g

Chan Tui ‡ (Periostracum Cicadae) 6g
Shan Yao (Rhizoma Dioscoreae Oppositae) 10g
Bai Zhu (Rhizoma Atractylodis Macrocephalae) 10g
Chao Bai Shao (Radix Paeoniae Lactiflorae, stir-fried) 10g
Chao Gu Ya (Fructus Setariae Italicae Germinatus, stir-fried) 10g
Chao Mai Ya (Fructus Hordei Vulgaris Germinatus, stir-fried) 10g
Gan Cao (Radix Glycyrrhizae) 4.5g
Deng Xin Cao (Medulla Junci Effusi) 5g

Explanation
- *Lian Qiao Xin* (Plumula Forsythiae Suspensae), *Zhi Zi Xin* (Plumula Gardeniae Jasminoidis), *Lian Zi Xin* (Plumula Nelumbinis Nuciferae), and *Deng Xin Cao* (Medulla Junci Effusi) clear Heart-Heat and guide out reddish urine, relieve Toxicity and reduce fever.
- *Chan Tui* ‡ (Periostracum Cicadae) dissipates Wind and alleviates itching.
- *Sheng Di Huang* (Radix Rehmanniae Glutinosae), *Xuan Shen* (Radix Scrophulariae Ningpoensis), *Shan Yao* (Rhizoma Dioscoreae Oppositae), and *Chao Bai Shao* (Radix Paeoniae Lactiflorae, stir-fried) enrich Yin and protect Body Fluids.
- *Bai Zhu* (Rhizoma Atractylodis Macrocephalae), *Chao Gu Ya* (Fructus Setariae Italicae Germinatus, stir-fried), *Chao Mai Ya* (Fructus Hordei Vulgaris Germinatus, stir-fried), and *Gan Cao* (Radix Glycyrrhizae) fortify the Spleen and support the Stomach.

DAMP-HEAT IN CHILDREN
Lesions mainly involve the antecubital and popliteal fossae and are characterized by pinpoint papules, papulovesicles and vesicles, some of which coalesce; slight infiltration and severe itching are likely. Bleeding or exudation follows rupture of the skin after scratching. The tongue body is red with a thin yellow coating; the pulse is soggy and rapid.

Treatment principle
Clear Heat and dispel Dampness, support Vital Qi (Zheng Qi) and alleviate itching.

Prescription
CHU SHI WEI LING TANG JIA JIAN
Poria Five Decoction for Eliminating Dampness and Calming the Stomach, with modifications

Fu Ling Pi (Cortex Poriae Cocos) 10g
Chao Huang Bai (Cortex Phellodendri, stir-fried) 10g
Chen Pi (Pericarpium Citri Reticulatae) 10g
Ku Shen (Radix Sophorae Flavescentis) 10g
Zhu Ling (Sclerotium Polypori Umbellati) 12g
Di Fu Zi (Fructus Kochiae Scopariae) 12g
Bai Xian Pi (Cortex Dictamni Dasycarpi Radicis) 12g

Huang Qi (Radix Astragali seu Hedysari) 12g
Yi Yi Ren (Semen Coicis Lachryma-jobi) 15g
Chi Xiao Dou (Semen Phaseoli Calcarati) 15g
Cang Er Zi (Fructus Xanthii Sibirici) 6g
Chan Tui ‡ (Periostracum Cicadae) 6g

Explanation

- *Chen Pi* (Pericarpium Citri Reticulatae), *Ku Shen* (Radix Sophorae Flavescentis), *Chao Huang Bai* (Cortex Phellodendri, stir-fried), *Chi Xiao Dou* (Semen Phaseoli Calcarati), *Fu Ling Pi* (Cortex Poriae Cocos), and *Zhu Ling* (Sclerotium Polypori Umbellati) dry Dampness and clear Heat.
- *Yi Yi Ren* (Semen Coicis Lachryma-jobi) and *Huang Qi* (Radix Astragali seu Hedysari) augment Qi and support the Spleen.
- *Di Fu Zi* (Fructus Kochiae Scopariae), *Bai Xian Pi* (Cortex Dictamni Dasycarpi Radicis), *Cang Er Zi* (Fructus Xanthii Sibirici), and *Chan Tui* ‡ (Periostracum Cicadae) eliminate Dampness and relieve Toxicity, dissipate Wind and alleviate itching.

SPLEEN AND STOMACH DEFICIENCY

This pattern is seen more frequently in children and adults with a weak constitution and is liable to recur. Lesions present as papules and vesicles with erosion and exudation; the skin is dry and rough with some scaling and localized itching. Accompanying symptoms and signs include a pale complexion, lassitude, poor appetite, abdominal distension, and diarrhea. The tongue body is pale with a greasy coating; the pulse is thready and weak or deep and slippery.

Treatment principle

Fortify the Spleen and eliminate Dampness.

Prescription

JIAN PI CHU SHI TANG HE CHU SHI WEI LING TANG JIA JIAN
Decoction for Fortifying the Spleen and Eliminating Dampness Combined With Poria Five Decoction for Eliminating Dampness and Calming the Stomach, with modifications

Chao Bai Zhu (Rhizoma Atractylodis Macrocephalae, stir-fried) 10g
Cang Zhu (Rhizoma Atractylodis) 10g
Hou Po (Cortex Magnoliae Officinalis) 10g
Chen Pi (Pericarpium Citri Reticulatae) 10g
Fu Ling (Sclerotium Poriae Cocos) 12g
Ze Xie (Rhizoma Alismatis Orientalis) 12g
Zhu Ling (Sclerotium Polypori Umbellati) 10g
Liu Yi San (Six-To-One Powder) 10g, wrapped
Di Fu Zi (Fructus Kochiae Scopariae) 15g
Bai Xian Pi (Cortex Dictamni Dasycarpi Radicis) 15g

Explanation

- *Cang Zhu* (Rhizoma Atractylodis), *Hou Po* (Cortex Magnoliae Officinalis), *Chen Pi* (Pericarpium Citri Reticulatae), and *Chao Bai Zhu* (Rhizoma Atractylodis Macrocephalae, stir-fried) fortify the Spleen and eliminate Dampness.
- *Zhu Ling* (Sclerotium Polypori Umbellati), *Ze Xie* (Rhizoma Alismatis Orientalis), *Fu Ling* (Sclerotium Poriae Cocos), and *Liu Yi San* (Six-To-One Powder) benefit the movement of Dampness.
- *Di Fu Zi* (Fructus Kochiae Scopariae) and *Bai Xian Pi* (Cortex Dictamni Dasycarpi Radicis) dissipate Wind to alleviate itching.

BLOOD-DRYNESS

This pattern generally occurs in the adult phase. The elbow, knee and neck are the main areas involved. Lesions manifest as thickening and lichenification with ill-defined borders. Dry and cracked skin is likely. Slight bleeding or exudation occurs after scratching or rubbing. Itching is severe, especially at night. The tongue body is pale red with a scant coating; the pulse is thready and rapid.

Treatment principle

Enrich Yin and eliminate Dampness, moisten Dryness and alleviate itching.

Prescription

ZI YIN CHU SHI TANG JIA JIAN
Decoction for Enriching Yin and Eliminating Dampness, with modifications

Dang Gui (Radix Angelicae Sinensis) 6g
Chao Bai Shao (Radix Paeoniae Lactiflorae, stir-fried) 6g
Chai Hu (Radix Bupleuri) 6g
Huang Qin (Radix Scutellariae Baicalensis) 6g
Shu Di Huang (Radix Rehmanniae Glutinosae Conquita) 15g
Di Gu Pi (Cortex Lycii Radicis) 15g
Yi Mu Cao (Herba Leonuri Heterophylli) 15g
Chao Zhi Mu (Rhizoma Anemarrhenae Asphodeloidis, stir-fried) 10g
Ze Xie (Rhizoma Alismatis Orientalis) 10g
Fang Feng (Radix Ledebouriellae Divaricatae) 10g
He Shou Wu (Radix Polygoni Multiflori) 10g
Gan Cao (Radix Glycyrrhizae) 10g

Explanation

- *Dang Gui* (Radix Angelicae Sinensis), *Chao Bai Shao* (Radix Paeoniae Lactiflorae, stir-fried), *Shu Di Huang* (Radix Rehmanniae Glutinosae Conquita), *Gan Cao* (Radix Glycyrrhizae), and *He Shou Wu* (Radix Polygoni Multiflori) nourish the Blood and moisten Dryness.
- *Chao Zhi Mu* (Rhizoma Anemarrhenae Asphodeloidis, stir-fried), *Di Gu Pi* (Cortex Lycii Radicis),

Huang Qin (Radix Scutellariae Baicalensis), and *Chai Hu* (Radix Bupleuri) clear retained Heat from the skin and interstices (*cou li*).

- *Yi Mu Cao* (Herba Leonuri Heterophylli) and *Fang Feng* (Radix Ledebouriellae Divaricatae) invigorate the Blood, dissipate Wind and alleviate itching.
- *Ze Xie* (Rhizoma Alismatis Orientalis) benefits the movement of water but does not damage Yin.

General modifications

1. For profuse exudate, add *Tong Cao* (Medulla Tetrapanacis Papyriferi), *Dong Gua Pi* (Epicarpium Benincasae Hispidae) and *Bai Mao Gen* (Rhizoma Imperatae Cylindricae).
2. For severe itching, add *Qiang Huo* (Rhizoma et Radix Notopterygii), *Wu Shao She* ‡ (Zaocys Dhumnades) and *Chan Tui* ‡ (Periostracum Cicadae).
3. For thickening and lichenification of the skin, add *Chi Shi Zhi* ‡ (Halloysitum Rubrum), *Dan Shen* (Radix Salviae Miltiorrhizae), *Ji Xue Teng* (Caulis Spatholobi), and *Ye Jiao Teng* (Caulis Polygoni Multiflori).
4. For asthma, add *Wu Wei Zi* (Fructus Schisandrae), *Kuan Dong Hua* (Flos Tussilaginis Farfarae), *Chao Zhi Ke* (Fructus Citri Aurantii, stir-fried), and *Shan Zhu Yu* (Fructus Corni Officinalis).
5. For hay fever (allergic rhinitis), add *Xin Yi Hua* (Flos Magnoliae), *Man Jing Zi* (Fructus Viticis) and *Bai Zhi* (Radix Angelicae Dahuricae).

PATENT HERBAL MEDICINES

- For fetal Heat or Damp-Heat patterns in infants, take *Wang Shi Bao Chi Wan* (Master Wang's Red Pill for Protecting Infants) one pill per month of age from six months upward (for example, nine pills for infants aged nine months), twice a day.
- For Damp-Heat patterns in children, take *Long Dan Xie Gang Wan* (Chinese Gentian Pill for Draining the Liver) 3g, twice a day, using the version excluding *Mu Tong*** (Caulis Mutong).
- Where conditions are complicated by hay fever, take five tablets of *Bi Yan Pian* (Nasal Inflammation Tablet) two or three times a day.

EXTERNAL TREATMENT

- For lesions in the infantile phase characterized by erythema, papules, vesicles, exudation, and erosion, prepare a decoction with equal amounts of *Di Yu* (Radix Sanguisorbae Officinalis) and *Guan Zhong*** (Rhizoma Dryopteris Crassirhizomae) for use as a wet compress on the affected area for 15 minutes two to four times a day. Then apply *Qing Dai Gao* (Indigo Paste), *Di Hu Hu* (Sanguisorba and Giant Knotweed Paste), *Huang Ai You* (Coptis and Mug-

wort Leaf Oil), or *Qu Shi San* (Powder for Dispelling Dampness) mixed with vegetable oil.
- For lesions in the infantile phase characterized by large erythematous patches with profuse bran-like scaling and severe itching, apply *Run Ji Gao* (Flesh-Moistening Paste), *Huang Lian Ruan Gao* (Coptis Ointment) or *Wu Yun Gao* (Black Cloud Paste) to the affected area once or twice a day.
- For the childhood phase, apply *Hei Dou Liu You Ruan Gao* (Black Soybean and Vaseline® Ointment), *Huang Lian Ruan Gao* (Coptis Ointment) or *Wu Shi Gao* (Five-Stone Paste) to the affected area once or twice a day.
- For the adult phase, use *Hu Po Er Wu Hu Gao* (Two Blacks Paste with Amber) for slight exudation, *Run Ji Gao* (Flesh-Moistening Paste) in combination with *Shi Zhen Fen* (Eczema Powder) for dryness and fissuring, and *Lu Hu Xi Ji* (Calamine and Giant Knotweed Wash Preparation) for relatively severe itching but no exudation. Apply these medications to the affected area once or twice a day.

Clinical notes

- Treatment for atopic eczema depends on whether the condition occurs in the infantile, childhood or adult phase.
  - In the infantile phase, treatment is based on the principle of clearing fetal Heat and relieving Toxicity with the focus on the Heart.
  - In the childhood phase, treatment is based on the principle of clearing and regulating Damp-Heat with the focus on the Spleen.
  - In the adult phase, treatment is based on the principle of emolliating the Liver and extinguishing Wind with the focus on the Liver and Kidneys.
- Pruritus is the most significant and distressing symptom of this disease. No matter which phase the disease occurs in, the treatment should also include materia medica to extinguish Wind and alleviate itching such as *Gou Teng* (Ramulus Uncariae cum Uncis) or *Bai Ji Li* (Fructus Tribuli Terrestris), or materia medica to quiet the Spirit and alleviate itching such as *Ye Jiao Teng* (Caulis Polygoni Multiflori), *He Huan Pi* (Cortex Albizziae Julibrissin) or *Suan Zao Ren* (Semen Ziziphi Spinosae). Great care should be exercised when using ingredients with the sole function of dissipating Wind and alleviating itching such as *Wei Ling Xian* (Radix Clematidis) and *Xu Chang Qing* (Radix Cynanchi Paniculati) because these herbs can damage Yin and consume Blood.
- It is difficult to give medications to babies. One option is for the mother to take the medication

instead so that it will work on the baby through the milk after breast-feeding. Alternatively, feed the decoction spoonful by spoonful throughout the day.

- Combining external treatment with internal treatment is helpful in controlling the development of the disease and healing lesions.
- When applying medications to the face, avoid coming into contact with the eyes or mouth in order to prevent possible irritation.

Advice for the patient

- During the infantile stage, monitor the infant's digestive function. Avoid intake of food that may cause an allergic reaction.
- Avoid washing the infant with hot water. Put gloves on the infant while sleeping to prevent scratching.
- At all stages, try to avoid irritation by external stimuli, for example due to tight clothing, washing with hot water or scratching.
- Keep the room temperature comfortable, but not too hot.
- Avoid stress or overexerting the body and maintain an optimistic mood.

Case history

Patient
Female, aged 15.

Clinical manifestations
The patient had suffered for more than ten years from generalized itchy pimples with exudation. Physical examination revealed densely distributed red papules on the limbs and trunk, with erosion in some places. Discharge of sticky exudate, blood and pus with the formation of yellow crusts was also evident. The area around the lesions was red with scratch marks. Erosion was more pronounced on the legs and was affecting leg movement. The tongue body was pale with a thin white coating; the pulse was deep and wiry.

Pattern identification
Internal accumulation of Damp Toxins, external invasion of Wind and disharmony of Qi and Blood in the chronic phase of atopic eczema.

Treatment principle
Relieve Toxicity and eliminate Dampness, dissipate Wind and alleviate itching while supporting Vital Qi (Zheng Qi), dispelling pathogenic factors and harmonizing Qi and Blood.

Prescription ingredients
Wu Shao She‡ (Zaocys Dhumnades) 3g

Qin Jiao (Radix Gentianae Macrophyllae) 6g
Huang Lian (Rhizoma Coptidis) 6g
Da Huang (Radix et Rhizoma Rhei) 6g
Bai Xian Pi (Cortex Dictamni Dasycarpi Radicis) 6g
Fang Feng (Radix Ledebouriellae Divaricatae) 6g
Ku Shen (Radix Sophorae Flavescentis) 10g
Lou Lu (Radix Rhapontici seu Echinopsis) 10g
Huang Qi (Radix Astragali seu Hedysari) 10g
Cang Zhu (Rhizoma Atractylodis) 12g
Bai Zhu (Rhizoma Atractylodis Macrocephalae) 12g

One bag a day was used to prepare a decoction, taken twice a day.

External treatment
Xi Shi Xin Ba Gao (Dilute Plaster Preparation) was prescribed for external application. iv

Follow-up treatment
After 12 bags, the patient had less itching and most skin eruptions had subsided. Hypopigmentation had occurred in some places. However, there were still densely-distributed papules on both legs. The treatment was changed to oral administration of *Qin Jiao Wan* (Large-Leaf Gentian Pill), *Chu Shi Wan* (Pill for Eliminating Dampness) and *Xiang Ju Dan* (Tangerine Peel and Cyperus Special Pill) combined with external application of *Tuo Se Ba Gao Gun* (Decolorizing Medicated Plaster Stick). iv

Outcome
After another month of treatment, the skin was almost back to normal and the itching had disappeared. The patient continued with the same treatment for three months to consolidate the cure. [24]

Literature excerpt

In *Yi Zong Jin Jian: Wai Ke Xin Fa Yao Jue* [The Golden Mirror of Medicine: Essential Methods for the Treatment of External Diseases], it says: "*Si wan feng* (four bends Wind) often occurs in the popliteal fossae and around the ankles with one attack each month. In appearance, it is similar to *feng xuan* (Wind tinea [tinea corporis]). The disease occurs because of Wind invading the interstices (*cou li*). It is characterized by severe itching, which provokes scratching. Exudation follows if the skin is ruptured by scratching, which gives the disease an appearance similar to *shi xuan* (Damp tinea [acute eczema]). For treatment, prepare a one-liter decoction of barley (*Da Mai*, Fructus Hordei) for steaming and then washing the affected areas. Follow this with external application of *San Miao San* (Mysterious Three Powder) to percolate Dampness and kill Worms. This type of treatment helps to alleviate itching and the disease will gradually be cured."

---

iv Alternatively, *Hei Se Ba Gao Gun* (Black Medicated Plaster Stick) or *Huang Lian Ruan Gao* (Coptis Ointment) could be used.

Modern clinical experience

TREATMENT ACCORDING TO PATTERN IDENTIFICATION

1. **Zhang Zhili** differentiated among three patterns in the treatment of atopic eczema: [25]

- **Internal accumulation of Damp-Heat due to Spleen Deficiency and Stomach-Heat**

This pattern is seen more often in the infantile phase of atopic eczema. Materia medica he commonly used to treat this pattern included:

Huang Lian (Rhizoma Coptidis) 6g
Huang Qin (Radix Scutellariae Baicalensis) 10g
Ma Chi Xian (Herba Portulacae Oleraceae) 15g
Bai Xian Pi (Cortex Dictamni Dasycarpi Radicis) 15g
Bai Zhu (Rhizoma Atractylodis Macrocephalae) 10g
Zhi Ke (Fructus Citri Aurantii) 10g
Yi Yi Ren (Semen Coicis Lachryma-jobi) 15g
Jiao Zhi Zi (Fructus Gardeniae Jasminoidis, scorch-fried) 6g
Jiao Bing Lang* (Semen Arecae Catechu, scorch-fried) 6g
Ji Nei Jin‡ (Endothelium Corneum Gigeriae Galli) 10g

For local management, *Ma Chi Xian* (Herba Portulacae Oleraceae) 30g was decocted for use as a wet compress. This was followed by external application of *Qu Shi San* (Powder for Dispelling Dampness) and *Huang Lian Ruan Gao* (Coptis Ointment).

- **Food stagnation due to Spleen Deficiency with accumulation of Dampness**

This pattern is seen more often seen in the childhood phase of atopic eczema. Materia medica he commonly used to treat this pattern included:

Bai Zhu (Rhizoma Atractylodis Macrocephalae) 6g
Fu Ling (Sclerotium Poriae Cocos) 6g
Yi Yi Ren (Semen Coicis Lachryma-jobi) 6g
Zhi Ke (Fructus Citri Aurantii) 10g
Bai Xian Pi (Cortex Dictamni Dasycarpi Radicis) 6g
Ku Shen (Radix Sophorae Flavescentis) 6g
Che Qian Zi (Semen Plantaginis) 10g
Ze Xie (Rhizoma Alismatis Orientalis) 10g
Jiao Bing Lang* (Semen Arecae Catechu, scorch-fried) 6g
Jiao Shan Zha (Fructus Crataegi, scorch-fried) 6g
Jiao Shen Qu (Massa Fermentata, scorch-fried) 6g
Jiao Mai Ya (Fructus Hordei Vulgaris Germinatus, scorch-fried) 6g
Ji Nei Jin‡ (Endothelium Corneum Gigeriae Galli) 6g
Chao Lai Fu Zi (Semen Raphani Sativi, stir-fried) 6g

Local management was essentially the same as for the infantile phase. For rough skin, 5% *Hei Dou Liu You Ruan Gao* (Black Soybean and Vaseline® Ointment) can be used with *Huang Lian Ruan Gao* (Coptis Ointment); for lichenification, 5% salicylic acid ointment was used with *Huang Lian Ruan Gao* (Coptis Ointment).

- **Spleen Deficiency and Blood-Dryness leading to obstruction of Wind-Damp and depriving the skin and flesh of nourishment**

This pattern is more often seen in the adolescent and adult phase of atopic eczema. Materia medica he commonly used to treat this pattern included:

Bai Zhu (Rhizoma Atractylodis Macrocephalae) 10g
Fu Ling (Sclerotium Poriae Cocos) 10g
Yi Yi Ren (Semen Coicis Lachryma-jobi) 15g
Zhi Ke (Fructus Citri Aurantii) 10g
Hou Po (Cortex Magnoliae Officinalis) 6g
Dang Gui (Radix Angelicae Sinensis) 15g
Ye Jiao Teng (Caulis Polygoni Multiflori) 15g
Chi Shao (Radix Paeoniae Rubra) 10g
Bai Shao (Radix Paeoniae Lactiflorae) 10g
Bai Ji Li (Fructus Tribuli Terrestris) 15g
Bai Xian Pi (Cortex Dictamni Dasycarpi Radicis) 30g
Ku Shen (Radix Sophorae Flavescentis) 15g
Fang Feng (Radix Ledebouriellae Divaricatae) 6g

Huang Lian Ruan Gao (Coptis Ointment) was recommended for local management.

2. **Wang** also differentiated among three patterns when giving treatment. [26]

- **Damp-Heat**

Treatment principle

Clear and transform Damp-Heat while fortifying the Spleen, dispersing food stagnation and guiding out accumulation.

Prescription ingredients

Jin Yin Hua (Flos Lonicerae) 6g
Ye Ju Hua (Flos Chrysanthemi Indici) 6g
Ban Lan Gen (Radix Isatidis seu Baphicacanthi) 6g
Ma Chi Xian (Herba Portulacae Oleraceae) 6g
Bai Xian Pi (Cortex Dictamni Dasycarpi Radicis) 6g
Dan Zhu Ye (Herba Lophatheri Gracilis) 2g
Deng Xin Cao (Medulla Junci Effusi) 2g
Jiao Shan Zha (Fructus Crataegi, scorch-fried) 8g
Jiao Shen Qu (Massa Fermentata, scorch-fried) 8g
Jiao Mai Ya (Fructus Hordei Vulgaris Germinatus, scorch-fried) 8g
Jiao Bing Lang* (Semen Arecae Catechu, scorch-fried) 8g

- **Spleen Deficiency**

Treatment principle

Fortify the Spleen, disperse food stagnation and guide out accumulation.

Prescription ingredients

Fu Ling (Sclerotium Poriae Cocos) 6g
Bai Zhu (Rhizoma Atractylodis Macrocephalae) 6g
Bai Bian Dou (Semen Dolichoris Lablab) 6g
Yi Yi Ren (Semen Coicis Lachryma-jobi) 6g
Chen Pi (Pericarpium Citri Reticulatae) 6g
Ma Chi Xian (Herba Portulacae Oleraceae) 4g
Bai Mao Gen (Rhizoma Imperatae Cylindricae) 4g
Mu Dan Pi (Cortex Moutan Radicis) 4g
Bai Xian Pi (Cortex Dictamni Dasycarpi Radicis) 8g
Jiao Shan Zha (Fructus Crataegi, scorch-fried) 8g
Jiao Shen Qu (Massa Fermentata, scorch-fried) 8g
Jiao Mai Ya (Fructus Hordei Vulgaris Germinatus, scorch-fried) 8g

- **Blood-Dryness**

Treatment principle

Cool and nourish the Blood and moisten Dryness, clear Heat and relieve Toxicity, fortify the Spleen, disperse food stagnation and guide out accumulation.

Prescription ingredients

Sheng Di Huang (Radix Rehmanniae Glutinosae) 10g
Bai Shao (Radix Paeoniae Lactiflorae) 6g
Mai Men Dong (Radix Ophiopogonis Japonici) 6g
Mu Dan Pi (Cortex Moutan Radicis) 6g
Bai Mao Gen (Rhizoma Imperatae Cylindricae) 6g
Ban Lan Gen (Radix Isatidis seu Baphicacanthi) 6g
Huang Bai (Cortex Phellodendri) 6g
Jiao Shan Zha (Fructus Crataegi, scorch-fried) 8g
Jiao Shen Qu (Massa Fermentata, scorch-fried) 8g
Jiao Mai Ya (Fructus Hordei Vulgaris Germinatus, scorch-fried) 8g
Bai Zhu (Rhizoma Atractylodis Macrocephalae) 6g

EMPIRICAL FORMULAE

1. **Liu** treated atopic eczema with an empirical formula accompanied by an external wash.[27]

Internal treatment prescription
YANG XUE QU FENG TANG
Decoction for Nourishing the Blood and Dispelling Wind

Zhi He Shou Wu (Radix Polygoni Multiflori Praeparata) 30g
Dang Gui (Radix Angelicae Sinensis) 15g
Ji Xue Teng (Caulis Spatholobi) 15g
Bai Xian Pi (Cortex Dictamni Dasycarpi Radicis) 15g
Di Fu Zi (Fructus Kochiae Scopariae) 15g
Bai Ji Li (Fructus Tribuli Terrestris) 15g
Xu Chang Qing (Radix Cynanchi Paniculati) 10g
Jing Jie (Herba Schizonepetae Tenuifoliae) 10g
Quan Xie‡ (Buthus Martensi) 10g
Wu Shao She‡ (Zaocys Dhumnades) 10g

One bag a day was used to prepare a decoction, taken twice a day. A course of treatment consisted of 20 consecutive days, with a five-day break between courses. The treatment was continued for two to three courses.

External prescription ingredients

Ku Shen (Radix Sophorae Flavescentis) 30g
Bai Xian Pi (Cortex Dictamni Dasycarpi Radicis) 15g
Di Fu Zi (Fructus Kochiae Scopariae) 15g
Hua Jiao (Pericarpium Zanthoxyli) 15g
Ku Fan‡ (Alumen Praeparatum) 15g
Bai Bu (Radix Stemonae) 15g

The ingredients were soaked in 1000ml of 75 percent alcohol for one week. After removing the residues, the medicated liquid was applied to wash the affected area two or three times a day.

2. **Dong** reported on his treatment of infantile atopic eczema.[28]

Prescription
QI MIAO YIN
Marvelous Beverage

Huang Qi (Radix Astragali seu Hedysari) 3g
Bai Zhu (Rhizoma Atractylodis Macrocephalae) 3g
Fang Feng (Radix Ledebouriellae Divaricatae) 3g
Gan Cao (Radix Glycyrrhizae) 3g
Mu Dan Pi (Cortex Moutan Radicis) 3g
Zhi Zi (Fructus Gardeniae Jasminoidis) 3g
Di Fu Zi (Fructus Kochiae Scopariae) 3g
Hong Hua (Flos Carthami Tinctorii) 2g

Modifications

1. *Jin Yin Hua* (Flos Lonicerae) 6g and *Huang Lian* (Rhizoma Coptidis) 3g were added for accumulation of Damp-Heat.
2. *Yu Li Ren* (Semen Pruni) 3g and *E Jiao*‡ (Gelatinum Corii Asini) 3g were added for Blood-Dryness due to Yin Deficiency.

The ingredients were decocted twice in 500ml of water to obtain a 200ml decoction, with 100ml taken morning and evening. The ingredients were decocted again in 2000ml of water to obtain a preparation for an external wash once a day.

Of 41 Damp-Heat pattern cases, 21 recovered completely, 16 experienced some improvement and 4 had no improvement; of the 35 cases with a pattern of Blood-Dryness due to Yin Deficiency, 15 recovered completely, 15 experienced some improvement and 5 had no improvement.

3. **Yu** prepared *Pi Yan Xiao Jing Yin Er Hao* (No. 2 Dermatitis Dispersing Beverage) to treat atopic eczema.[29]

Prescription ingredients

Cang Zhu (Rhizoma Atractylodis) 2g
Dang Gui (Radix Angelicae Sinensis) 2g
Che Qian Zi (Semen Plantaginis) 2g
Huang Qin (Radix Scutellariae Baicalensis) 2g
Chai Hu (Radix Bupleuri) 2g

Each bag therefore contained 10 grams. One bag each time was prescribed for patients in the 5-9 year age group, one and half bags each time for patients in the 10-14 age group, and two bags each time for patients older than 14. The bags were used to prepare a decoction taken three times a day for three months.

Observations that a decrease in CD₃, CD₈ and IgE occurred with *Pi Yan Xiao Jing Yin Er Hao* (No. 2 Dermatitis Dispersing Beverage) indicated that it may be effective against inflammation and delayed allergic reaction.

4. **Zhan** reported on his treatment of atopic eczema at the infantile stage. [30]

Prescription
SHU FENG QU SHI TANG
Decoction for Dredging Wind and Dispelling Dampness

Ren Dong Teng (Caulis Lonicerae Japonicae) 9g
Chao Huang Qin (Radix Scutellariae Baicalensis, stir-fried) 2g
Chan Tui‡ (Periostracum Cicadae) 2g
Chao Zhi Ke (Fructus Citri Aurantii, stir-fried) 2g
Chen Pi (Pericarpium Citri Reticulatae) 2g
Chao Jiang Can‡ (Bombyx Batryticatus, stir-fried) 6g
Bai Xian Pi (Cortex Dictamni Dasycarpi Radicis) 6g
Chao Bai Zhu (Rhizoma Atractylodis Macrocephalae, stir-fried) 5g
Chao Cang Zhu (Rhizoma Atractylodis, stir-fried) 5g
Huo Xiang (Herba Agastaches seu Pogostemi) 5g

Modifications
1. For severe Heat, *Zhi Zi Pi* (Cortex Gardeniae Jasminoidis) and *Bai Mao Gen* (Rhizoma Imperatae Cylindricae) were added.
2. For severe Wind, *Fang Feng* (Radix Ledebouriellae Divaricatae) and *Sang Ye* (Folium Mori Albae) were added.
3. For severe Dampness, *Yi Yi Ren* (Semen Coicis Lachryma-jobi) was added.
4. For smelly stools, *Shan Zha Tan* (Fructus Crataegi Carbonisatus) was added.

One bag a day was used to prepare a decoction, taken twice a day. Initial results were seen after two weeks.

5. **Zhang** combined *Ge Gen Qin Lian Tang* (Kudzu, Scutellaria and Coptis Decoction) and *Ping Wei San Jia Wei* (Calming the Stomach Powder, with additions) to treat the infantile phase of atopic eczema. [31]

Prescription ingredients

Ge Gen (Radix Puerariae) 10g
Huang Qin (Radix Scutellariae Baicalensis) 6g
Chen Pi (Pericarpium Citri Reticulatae) 5g
Cang Zhu (Rhizoma Atractylodis) 5g
Huang Lian (Rhizoma Coptidis) 3g
Hou Po (Cortex Magnoliae Officinalis) 3g
Gan Cao (Radix Glycyrrhizae) 3g

Modifications
1. *Ren Dong Teng* (Caulis Lonicerae Japonicae) was added to clear Heat and relieve Toxicity.
2. *Chan Tui*‡ (Periostracum Cicadae) was added to clear Heat and dredge Wind.
3. *Hong Hua* (Flos Carthami Tinctorii) was added to invigorate and nourish the Blood.

One bag a day was used to prepare a decoction for oral administration at four different times during the day.

Ge Gen Qin Lian Tang (Kudzu, Scutellaria and Coptis Decoction) has the functions of releasing the flesh and clearing Heat, and *Ping Wei San Jia Wei* (Calming the Stomach Powder, with additions) arouses the Spleen and dispels Dampness. This is an example of combining ingredients of a hot and cold nature to treat this disease.

EXTERNAL TREATMENT (INFANTILE PHASE)

1. **Peng** prepared an external wash to treat atopic eczema in infants. [32]

Prescription ingredients

Ku Shen (Radix Sophorae Flavescentis) 15g
Huang Lian (Rhizoma Coptidis) 15g
Huang Bai (Cortex Phellodendri) 15g
She Chuang Zi (Fructus Cnidii Monnieri) 12g
Di Fu Zi (Fructus Kochiae Scopariae) 12g
Bai Xian Pi (Cortex Dictamni Dasycarpi Radicis) 12g
Wu Bei Zi‡ (Galla Rhois Chinensis) 10g
Ming Fan‡ (Alumen) 6g
Bing Pian (Borneolum) 2g

The ingredients were decocted in 1500ml of water for 30 minutes to obtain 1000ml of decoction. When it had cooled to around 40°C, it was used to wash the affected areas twice daily for five days.

Modifications
1. *Fang Feng* (Radix Ledebouriellae Divaricatae) 15g was added for severe itching.
2. *Hua Shi*‡ (Talcum) 15g was added for profuse exudation.

2. **Qian** formulated a decoction for use as an external wash and wet compress. [33]

Prescription ingredients

Jin Yin Hua (Flos Lonicerae) 20g
Wu Mei (Fructus Pruni Mume) 20g
Lian Qiao (Fructus Forsythiae Suspensae) 15g
Bai Xian Pi (Cortex Dictamni Dasycarpi Radicis) 15g
Pu Gong Ying (Herba Taraxaci cum Radice) 30g
*Ma Huang** (Herba Ephedrae) 10g

One bag a day was used to prepare a decoction for application to the affected areas twice a day.

COMBINED INTERNAL AND EXTERNAL TREATMENT

Fu treated atopic eczema with a combination of internal and external medications. [34]

- **Internal treatment for acute conditions characterized by erythema, papules, erosion, and exudation**

Treatment principle
Clear Heat and relieve Toxicity, fortify the Spleen and eliminate Dampness.

Prescription
PI YAN YI HAO
Dermatitis Formula No. 1

Jin Yin Hua (Flos Lonicerae) 30g
Fu Ling (Sclerotium Poriae Cocos) 30g
Yi Yi Ren (Semen Coicis Lachryma-jobi) 30g
Lian Qiao (Fructus Forsythiae Suspensae) 15g
Ze Xie (Rhizoma Alismatis Orientalis) 15g
Dan Zhu Ye (Herba Lophatheri Gracilis) 10g
Huang Lian (Rhizoma Coptidis) 10g
Bai Zhu (Rhizoma Atractylodis Macrocephalae) 10g
Gan Cao (Radix Glycyrrhizae) 10g

The ingredients were ground into a very fine powder. Six grams of the powdered mixture were infused in hot boiled water for 30 minutes three times a day; after the tea had cooled, the residues were removed and the tea was drunk.

- **Internal treatment for conditions at the remission stage or for conditions marked by dry skin and fine, thin scales**

Treatment principle
Fortify the Spleen and augment Qi, enrich Yin and nourish the Blood

Prescription
PI YAN ER HAO
Dermatitis Formula No. 2

Bai Zhu (Rhizoma Atractylodis Macrocephalae) 10g
Gan Cao (Radix Glycyrrhizae) 10g

Tai Zi Shen (Radix Pseudostellariae Heterophyllae) 15g
Xuan Shen (Radix Scrophulariae Ningpoensis) 15g
Dang Gui (Radix Angelicae Sinensis) 15g
Sheng Di Huang (Radix Rehmanniae Glutinosae) 30g
Fu Ling (Sclerotium Poriae Cocos) 30g
Duan Long Gu‡ (Os Draconis Calcinatum) 30g
Duan Mu Li‡ (Concha Ostreae Calcinata) 30g

The ingredients were ground into a very fine powder. Three times a day, six grams of the powdered mixture were wrapped in a cloth and decocted for five minutes. The decoction was then filtered and drunk.

- **External treatment of erosive and exudative lesions**

Prescription
SHI FU FANG
Wet Compress Formula

Ye Ju Hua (Flos Chrysanthemi Indici) 15g
Gan Cao (Radix Glycyrrhizae) 15g
Bai Zhi (Radix Angelicae Dahuricae) 15g
Ku Shen (Radix Sophorae Flavescentis) 30g
Huang Bai (Cortex Phellodendri) 30g

These ingredients were decocted and the resulting liquid was used as a cold wet compress.

- **External treatment of erythematous, papular and scaly lesions**

Prescription
HUANG FU SHUANG
Yellow Skin Frost

Huang Lian (Rhizoma Coptidis) 15g
Bo He (Herba Menthae Haplocalycis) 15g
Huang Bai (Cortex Phellodendri) 30g
Gan Cao (Radix Glycyrrhizae) 30g

A cold cream was prepared from a filtered decoction of the ingredients.

COMBINED TREATMENT WITH TCM AND WESTERN MEDICINE

Zheng treated atopic eczema with TCM on a pattern identification basis combined with Western medicine. [35]

- **Damp-Heat**

Treatment principle
Clear Heat, benefit the movement of Dampness and dispel Wind.

Prescription ingredients

Long Dan Cao (Radix Gentianae Scabrae) 20g
Ma Chi Xian (Herba Portulacae Oleraceae) 20g
Di Yu (Radix Sanguisorbae Officinalis) 14g
Ku Shen (Radix Sophorae Flavescentis) 14g

Fang Feng (Radix Ledebouriellae Divaricatae) 14g
Tong Cao (Medulla Tetrapanacis Papyriferi) 14g
Di Fu Zi (Fructus Kochiae Scopariae) 16g
Jing Jie (Herba Schizonepetae Tenuifoliae) 16g
Sha Yuan Zi (Semen Astragali Complanati) 16g
Bai Zhu (Rhizoma Atractylodis Macrocephalae) 12g
Zi Cao (Radix Arnebiae seu Lithospermi) 18g
Hua Shi ‡ (Talcum) 18g

- **Exuberant Wind due to Spleen Deficiency**

Treatment principle
Fortify the Spleen, eliminate Dampness and dispel Wind.

Prescription ingredients
Huang Qi (Radix Astragali seu Hedysari) 20g
Bai Zhu (Rhizoma Atractylodis Macrocephalae) 14g
Cang Zhu (Rhizoma Atractylodis) 14g
Hou Po (Cortex Magnoliae Officinalis) 14g
Fang Feng (Radix Ledebouriellae Divaricatae) 14g
Chai Hu (Radix Bupleuri) 14g
Bi Xie (Rhizoma Dioscoreae Hypoglaucae seu Septemlobae) 18g
Bai Xian Pi (Cortex Dictamni Dasycarpi Radicis) 18g
Tong Cao (Medulla Tetrapanacis Papyriferi) 16g
Jing Jie (Herba Schizonepetae Tenuifoliae) 16g
Di Fu Zi (Fructus Kochiae Scopariae) 16g

Chan Tui ‡ (Periostracum Cicadae) 10g

- **Blood-Dryness due to Spleen Deficiency**

Treatment principle
Nourish the Blood, dispel Wind and fortify the Spleen.

Prescription ingredients
Huang Qi (Radix Astragali seu Hedysari) 20g
Sheng Di Huang (Radix Rehmanniae Glutinosae) 20g
Shu Di Huang (Radix Rehmanniae Glutinosae Conquita) 20g
Dang Gui (Radix Angelicae Sinensis) 16g
Fu Ling (Sclerotium Poriae Cocos) 16g
Bo He (Herba Menthae Haplocalycis) 16g
Hong Hua (Flos Carthami Tinctorii) 12g
Fang Feng (Radix Ledebouriellae Divaricatae) 12g
Chuan Xiong (Rhizoma Ligustici Chuanxiong) 14g
Zhi Mu (Rhizoma Anemarrhenae Asphodeloidis) 14g
Chan Tui ‡ (Periostracum Cicadae) 10g
Di Fu Zi (Fructus Kochiae Scopariae) 18g

For all patterns, one bag a day of the ingredients was used to prepare a decoction for internal administration twice a day. The residues were decocted again with the addition of *Guan Zhong** (Rhizoma Dryopteris Crassirhizomae) 18g for use as an external wash.

Western medicines used included antihistamines, hormones, tranquilizers, calcium preparations, and vitamin C.

Seborrheic eczema
脂溢性湿疹

Seborrheic eczema (also known as seborrheic dermatitis) is a chronic inflammatory condition mainly affecting hair-bearing areas of the head and body, where sebaceous glands are most numerous, and often manifesting with greasy yellowish scales. It should be noted that seborrheic eczema is unrelated to seborrhea. Overgrowth of pityrosporum yeast organisms may be important in the development of the condition.

In TCM, seborrheic eczema of the scalp is also known as *zou pi qu chuang* (wandering skin sore), seborrheic eczema of the face as *mian you feng* (wandering Wind of the face) and seborrheic eczema of the chest as *niu kou feng* (buttonhole Wind).

Clinical manifestations

- Seborrheic eczema mostly occurs in young and

middle-aged people or obese individuals, but flexural involvement is more common in the elderly.
- The main sites of involvement are areas of the skin with abundant sebaceous activity such as the scalp and retroauricular region.
- There are three common patterns, which may merge together:

Scalp and facial involvement
- The disease often starts on the scalp and may spread gradually to the eyebrows and nasolabial folds, with an itchy red or yellowish-red scaly or exudative erythematous eruption affecting the scalp and scalp margins, the sides of the nose, the eyebrows, and the ears.
- This condition, which may be associated with blepharitis or otitis externa, is most common in young adult males. It may be accompanied by marked dandruff.

Petaloid

- A dry, scaly, often yellowish eczema appears over the presternal and interscapular areas.
- This may be accompanied by extensive follicular papules or pustules on the trunk (also known as seborrheic folliculitis).

Flexural

- In this pattern, there is involvement of the axillae, groins, umbilical region, and submammary areas with a moist intertrigo, often colonized by *Candida albicans*.
- This condition is seen most often in the elderly.

- In severe cases, there is intense itching, damp ulceration and the formation of opaque, greasy crusts.
- In young infants, seborrheic eczema manifests as grayish-yellow or brownish-yellow oily scales partially or completely covering the scalp (known as cradle cap). Flexural lesions of moist scaly erythema may also be present.
- Seborrheic eczema is difficult to cure and may persist for years with frequent recurrences.

Differential diagnosis

Psoriasis

It is often very difficult to distinguish between scalp psoriasis and seborrheic eczema of the scalp, although the latter tends to affect the anterior margin of the scalp and is likely to spread to the ears and face. Psoriasis is characterized by well-defined erythematous lesions with mica-like silvery-white scales and punctate bleeding when scales are removed. It is most common on the extensor surfaces of the elbows and knees and in the hair-bearing scalp.

Tinea capitis (ringworm of the scalp)

Most cases of tinea capitis begin with one or several patches of scaling or alopecia. In "gray patch ringworm", the lesions are characterized by round or irregular scaly lesions of grayish-white patches. Hairs usually break off 3-4 mm above the skin surface with white sheaths left at the root of the affected hairs. The scalp is not inflamed and healing occurs without scarring.

Pityriasis versicolor

Pityriasis versicolor is more common in young adults and mainly occurs on the chest and back, but may also spread to the upper arms, neck and abdomen. Involvement of the scalp and face is rare. Lesions, which may be pale white, pale red, yellowish-brown or dark brown, start with multiple small macules, which soon enlarge to round or oval macular nail-sized patches covered by a layer of fine scaling.

Rosacea

Lesions in rosacea normally involve the nose, chin, cheeks, and forehead. At the initial stage, temporary flushing and erythema interspersed with discrete inflamed pinhead papules and pustules appear. As the condition develops, the erythema does not fade and telangiectasia occurs. Rosacea lacks the scaling that is usually characteristic of seborrheic eczema.

Etiology and pathology

Overindulgence in greasy, sweet or spicy food or emotional disturbances impair the transformation function of the Spleen and Stomach, resulting in the generation of internal Dampness, which then transforms into Heat. Damp-Heat moves upward along the channels to the head and face or outward to other areas of the body, where it accumulates and obstructs the skin and interstices (*cou li*). Where this is accompanied by an external invasion of Wind-Heat, internal and external pathogenic factors combine and interact on each other to cause the disease.

Exuberant Heat and Wind-Dryness

Where exuberant Heat predominates over external Wind, the disease manifests as exuberant Heat and Wind-Dryness, with lesions characterized by erythema, papules and grayish scaling.

Accumulation of Damp-Heat

Where accumulation of internal Damp-Heat predominates over external Wind-Heat, the disease manifests as a Damp-Heat pattern and lesions are characterized by erythema, papules and greasy scaling.

Pattern identification and treatment

INTERNAL TREATMENT

EXUBERANT HEAT AND WIND-DRYNESS

Discrete red papules appearing on pale red or yellowish-red erythematous patches are covered by grayish-white bran-like scaling. Mild to moderate local itching may be present. The tongue body is red with a thin coating; the pulse is rapid.

Treatment principle

Clear Heat and cool the Blood, dispel Wind and alleviate itching.

Prescription

LIANG XUE XIAO FENG SAN JIA JIAN

Powder for Cooling the Blood and Dispersing Wind, with modifications

Sheng Di Huang (Radix Rehmanniae Glutinosae) 30g
Mu Dan Pi (Cortex Moutan Radicis) 10g
Ku Shen (Radix Sophorae Flavescentis) 10g
Huang Qin (Radix Scutellariae Baicalensis) 10g
Jin Yin Hua (Flos Lonicerae) 10g
Zhi Mu (Rhizoma Anemarrhenae Asphodeloidis) 10g
Shi Gao ‡ (Gypsum Fibrosum) 30g, decocted for 30 minutes before adding the other ingredients
Jing Jie (Herba Schizonepetae Tenuifoliae) 10g
Chan Tui ‡ (Periostracum Cicadae) 6g
Bai Ji Li (Fructus Tribuli Terrestris) 12g

Explanation

- *Sheng Di Huang* (Radix Rehmanniae Glutinosae), *Mu Dan Pi* (Cortex Moutan Radicis), *Huang Qin* (Radix Scutellariae Baicalensis), *Jin Yin Hua* (Flos Lonicerae), *Zhi Mu* (Rhizoma Anemarrhenae Asphodeloidis), and *Shi Gao* ‡ (Gypsum Fibrosum) clear Heat and cool the Blood.
- *Ku Shen* (Radix Sophorae Flavescentis), *Jing Jie* (Herba Schizonepetae Tenuifoliae), *Chan Tui* ‡ (Periostracum Cicadae), and *Bai Ji Li* (Fructus Tribuli Terrestris) dispel Wind and alleviate itching.

Modifications

1. For large patches of erythema, add *Zi Cao* (Radix Arnebiae seu Lithospermi) and *Chi Shao* (Radix Paeoniae Rubra).
2. For significant scaling, add *Cang Er Zi* (Fructus Xanthii Sibirici) and *He Shou Wu* (Radix Polygoni Multiflori).

DAMP-HEAT ACCUMULATING IN THE EXTERIOR

Lesions manifest as large red or yellowish-red erythema on the scalp, face, chest, and back, behind the ears, and in the axillae and inguinal grooves. A few discrete papules may be present. The erythema is covered by greasy scale and some exudate may be seen. Patients experience severe itching. Accompanying symptoms and signs include irritability, poor appetite, dry throat with no desire for drinks, a bitter taste in the mouth, and short voidings of reddish urine. The tongue body is red with a yellow and slightly greasy coating; the pulse is wiry and slippery.

Treatment principle

Clear Heat and transform Dampness, dredge Wind and alleviate itching.

Prescription

XIE HUANG SAN JIA JIAN

Yellow-Draining Powder, with modifications

Shi Gao ‡ (Gypsum Fibrosum) 15g, decocted for 30 minutes before adding the other ingredients

Huo Xiang (Herba Agastaches seu Pogostemi) 15g
Sheng Di Huang (Radix Rehmanniae Glutinosae) 15g
Yin Chen Hao (Herba Artemisiae Scopariae) 15g
Fang Feng (Radix Ledebouriellae Divaricatae) 10g
Jing Jie (Herba Schizonepetae Tenuifoliae) 10g
Jiao Zhi Zi (Fructus Gardeniae Jasminoidis, scorch-fried) 10g
Huang Qin (Radix Scutellariae Baicalensis) 10g
Chi Fu Ling (Sclerotium Poriae Cocos Rubrae) 10g
Chan Tui ‡ (Periostracum Cicadae) 4.5g
Deng Xin Cao (Medulla Junci Effusi) 4.5g
Dan Zhu Ye (Herba Lophatheri Gracilis) 4.5g
Bai Mao Gen (Rhizoma Imperatae Cylindricae) 30g

Explanation

- *Huo Xiang* (Herba Agastaches seu Pogostemi), *Yin Chen Hao* (Herba Artemisiae Scopariae) and *Huang Qin* (Radix Scutellariae Baicalensis) clear Heat and transform Dampness.
- *Shi Gao* ‡ (Gypsum Fibrosum), *Jiao Zhi Zi* (Fructus Gardeniae Jasminoidis, scorch-fried), *Deng Xin Cao* (Medulla Junci Effusi), and *Dan Zhu Ye* (Herba Lophatheri Gracilis) clear Heat from the Qi level.
- *Jing Jie* (Herba Schizonepetae Tenuifoliae), *Fang Feng* (Radix Ledebouriellae Divaricatae) and *Chan Tui* ‡ (Periostracum Cicadae) dissipate Wind and alleviate itching.
- *Sheng Di Huang* (Radix Rehmanniae Glutinosae), *Bai Mao Gen* (Rhizoma Imperatae Cylindricae) and *Chi Fu Ling* (Sclerotium Poriae Cocos Rubrae) cool the Blood and reduce erythema.

Modifications

1. For large patches of erythema, add *Mu Dan Pi* (Cortex Moutan Radicis) or *Zhi Mu* (Rhizoma Anemarrhenae Asphodeloidis).
2. For erosion and exudation, add *Di Yu* (Radix Sanguisorbae Officinalis) and *Cang Zhu* (Rhizoma Atractylodis).

EXTERNAL TREATMENT

- For erythema with profuse scaling, apply *Wu Shi Gao* (Five-Stone Paste) to the affected area once or twice a day or use an aqueous suspension of *Yu Ji San* (Jade Flesh Powder) to wash the face in the morning and evening.
- For profuse white or greasy scales on the scalp, wash the affected area with *Tou Gu Cao Shui Xi Ji* (Speranskia Wash Preparation) once a day or every other day.
- For lesions with mild erosion and exudation, prepare a decoction with *Di Yu Shi Fu Tang* (Sanguisorba Wet Compress Decoction) and apply as a cold compress to the affected area for 30 minutes once or twice a day until the lesions heal.

- For dry skin with profuse white scales, apply *Run Ji Gao* (Flesh-Moistening Paste) or *Dang Gui Gao* (Chinese Angelica Root Paste) to the lesions once or twice a day.

Clinical notes

- For internal treatment, it is important for pattern differentiation to determine whether Damp-Heat or pathogenic Wind is predominant:
  - If Damp-Heat predominates, there will be some thick, foul-smelling exudate and the formation of greasy yellow scale. Treatment should therefore focus on eliminating Dampness and clearing Heat.
  - If pathogenic Wind predominates, there will be a relatively large amount of scaling, which is replaced after being shed following scratching. Treatment in this case should concentrate on enriching Yin, moistening Dryness, extinguishing Wind, and alleviating itching.
- External treatment helps to inhibit exudation, alleviate itching and heal lesions.

Advice for the patient

- In the acute phase, avoid washing with hot water or using strong, irritant external medications.
- Reduce intake of greasy and sweet food, or fish, shellfish and other seafood. Increase the intake of vegetables. It is important to keep bowel movements regular.
- Although this disease tends to linger, it can be cured after one or two months of continuous treatment.

Case history

Patient
Female, aged 33.

Clinical manifestations
The patient had been suffering from generalized skin lesions with intermittent remission and relapse for more than ten years. Examination revealed yellowish-red erythema on the head and face including the area around the nose. Lesions in this area exhibited slight infiltration, covered by a small amount of bran-like scaling; there was also excoriation with bloody crusts. Infiltrated erythema with a slightly moist surface was also present in the right axilla, below the breasts and in the popliteal fossae. The tongue body was enlarged with a thin white coating; the pulse was slippery and thready.

Pattern identification
Retention of Damp-Heat in the skin and Blood-Dryness.

Treatment principle
Benefit the movement of Dampness and clear Heat, cool and nourish the Blood.

Prescription ingredients
Chao Long Dan Cao (Radix Gentianae Scabrae, stir-fried) 10g
Huang Qin (Radix Scutellariae Baicalensis) 10g
Chai Hu (Radix Bupleuri) 10g
Chi Shao (Radix Paeoniae Rubra) 10g
Bai Shao (Radix Paeoniae Lactiflorae) 10g
Yin Chen Hao (Herba Artemisiae Scopariae) 15g
Di Fu Zi (Fructus Kochiae Scopariae) 15g
He Shou Wu (Radix Polygoni Multiflori) 15g
Zi Cao (Radix Arnebiae seu Lithospermi) 15g
Ze Xie (Rhizoma Alismatis Orientalis) 12g
Dang Gui (Radix Angelicae Sinensis) 12g
Gan Cao (Radix Glycyrrhizae) 6g
Sheng Di Huang (Radix Rehmanniae Glutinosae) 50g

One bag a day was used to prepare a decoction, taken twice a day.

Follow-up treatment
After 20 bags of the prescription, the lesions under the axilla and below the breasts were receding, but the itching remained. The hair was dry. There was still some exudate where the skin in the affected area was broken due to scratching.

Treatment principle
Nourish the Blood and eliminate Damp-Heat.

Prescription ingredients
Ci Shi‡ (Magnetitum) 30g
Sheng Di Huang (Radix Rehmanniae Glutinosae) 30g
Long Gu‡ (Os Draconis) 30g
Mu Li‡ (Concha Ostreae) 30g
Dang Gui (Radix Angelicae Sinensis) 30g
Suan Zao Ren (Semen Ziziphi Spinosae) 30g
Yin Chen Hao (Herba Artemisiae Scopariae) 30g
Di Fu Zi (Fructus Kochiae Scopariae) 30g
Chi Shao (Radix Paeoniae Rubra) 18g
Bai Shao (Radix Paeoniae Lactiflorae) 18g
Chuan Xiong (Rhizoma Ligustici Chuanxiong) 10g
Chai Hu (Radix Bupleuri) 10g
Chao Long Dan Cao (Radix Gentianae Scabrae, stir-fried) 10g
Gan Cao (Radix Glycyrrhizae) 6g

Outcome
After 30 bags of the new prescription, the condition was relieved.

Discussion
This condition, which had recurred persistently for more than ten years with moist erythema, infiltration, scaling, and itching, is an example of Dampness accumulating in the body over a long period and transforming into Heat. Damp-Heat had moved out to the skin to cause the problem. The long case history and the pulse and tongue conditions indicated an enduring illness damaging Yin and consuming Blood, resulting in Blood-Heat due to Deficiency with Blood Deficiency

depriving the skin of nourishment. After the first prescription achieved a good effect in relieving most of the symptoms, pathogenic factors were weakened but Vital Qi (Zheng Qi) was still Deficient and so the treatment principle was changed to nourishing the Blood and eliminating Damp-Heat. [36]

Literature excerpt

According to *Zhu Ren Kang Lin Chuang Jing Yan Ji* [A Collection of Zhu Renkang's Clinical Experiences]: "The initial stage of the disease is marked by reddened and slightly swollen skin, itching and desquamation. The tongue body is red with a thin white or thin yellow coating; the pulse is wiry and slippery. Pattern identification indicates Heat in the Blood and Dryness due to Wind. Treatment should follow the principle of cooling the Blood and clearing Heat, dispersing Wind and moistening Dryness. *Sheng Di Huang* (Radix Rehmanniae Glutinosae), *Dan Shen* (Radix Salviae Miltiorrhizae) and *Chi Shao* (Radix Paeoniae Rubra) are used to cool the Blood; *Shi Gao* ‡ (Gypsum Fibrosum) and *Zhi Mu* (Rhizoma Anemarrhenae Asphodeloidis) to clear Heat from the skin and flesh; *Jing Jie* (Herba Schizonepetae Tenuifoliae), *Chan Tui* ‡ (Periostracum Cicadae) and *Bai Ji Li* (Fructus Tribuli Terrestris) to disperse Wind; *Dang Gui* (Radix Angelicae Sinensis), *Huo Ma Ren* (Semen Cannabis Sativae) and *Gan Cao* (Radix Glycyrrhizae) to moisten Dryness; and *Ku Shen* (Radix Sophorae Flavescentis) and *Bai Xian Pi* (Cortex Dictamni Dasycarpi Radicis) to alleviate itching.

"If the disease has persisted for a number of years and is characterized by dry, dark, lichenified skin, layers of scales, itching, broken skin due to scratching, constipation, a pale tongue body with a clean coating, and a wiry and thready pulse, this indicates a pattern of Blood Deficiency and Dryness due to Wind. Treatment should follow the principle of nourishing the Blood and moistening Dryness, dispersing Wind and alleviating itching. *Shu Di Huang* (Radix Rehmanniae Glutinosae Conquita), *Dang Gui* (Radix Angelicae Sinensis), *Dan Shen* (Radix Salviae Miltiorrhizae), *Bai Shao* (Radix Paeoniae Lactiflorae), *He Shou Wu* (Radix Polygoni Multiflori), and *Mai Men Dong* (Radix Ophiopogonis Japonici) are used to nourish the Blood and enrich Yin; *Zhi Ke* (Fructus Citri Aurantii), *Huo Ma Ren* (Semen Cannabis Sativae) and *Gan Cao* (Radix Glycyrrhizae) to moisten Dryness; and *Bai Ji Li* (Fructus Tribuli Terrestris) and *Bai Xian Pi* (Cortex Dictamni Dasycarpi Radicis) to disperse Wind and alleviate itching."

Modern clinical experience

INTERNAL TREATMENT

Wang Yiqian identified three different patterns and treatment principles for seborrheic eczema. [37]

- **Blood Deficiency and Wind-Dryness**

Treatment principle

Invigorate the Blood and free the network vessels, nourish the Blood and dispel Wind.

Prescription ingredients

Dang Gui (Radix Angelicae Sinensis) 9g
Chuan Xiong (Rhizoma Ligustici Chuanxiong) 9g
Chi Shao (Radix Paeoniae Rubra) 9g
Bai Shao (Radix Paeoniae Lactiflorae) 9g
Shu Di Huang (Radix Rehmanniae Glutinosae Conquita) 9g
Tao Ren (Semen Persicae) 9g
Hong Hua (Flos Carthami Tinctorii) 6g
Chai Hu (Radix Bupleuri) 6g
Hei Zhi Ma (Semen Sesami Indici) 12g

- **Damp-Heat in the Heart channel**

Treatment principle

Clear Heat from the Heart, enrich Body Fluids, transform Dampness and alleviate itching.

Prescription ingredients

Huang Lian (Rhizoma Coptidis) 4.5g
Sheng Di Huang (Radix Rehmanniae Glutinosae) 15g
Di Fu Zi (Fructus Kochiae Scopariae) 12g
Gan Cao (Radix Glycyrrhizae) 9g
Jiang Can ‡ (Bombyx Batryticatus) 9g
Bai Xian Pi (Cortex Dictamni Dasycarpi Radicis) 9g
Ye Ju Hua (Flos Chrysanthemi Indici) 9g

- **Qi fall in the Middle Burner, insufficiency of the Spleen and Stomach**

Treatment principle

Bear Yang upward, dissipate Fire, consolidate the exterior, and moisten Dryness.

Prescription ingredients

Dang Shen (Radix Codonopsitis Pilosulae) 30g
Bai Zhu (Rhizoma Atractylodis Macrocephalae) 9g
Bai Shao (Radix Paeoniae Lactiflorae) 9g
Fang Feng (Radix Ledebouriellae Divaricatae) 9g
Zhi Gan Cao (Radix Glycyrrhizae, mix-fried with honey) 6g
Sheng Ma (Rhizoma Cimicifugae) 6g
Chai Hu (Radix Bupleuri) 6g
Ge Gen (Radix Puerariae) 12g

One bag a day was used to prepare a decoction, taken twice a day. A course of treatment consisted of seven bags. Results were usually seen after one to three courses.

COMBINED INTERNAL AND EXTERNAL TREATMENT

Wu treated 34 cases of seborrheic eczema by combining internal and external treatment. [38]

Internal treatment prescription
JIA WEI YU NÜ JIAN
Augmented Jade Lady Brew

Sheng Di Huang (Radix Rehmanniae Glutinosae) 30g
Shu Di Huang (Radix Rehmanniae Glutinosae Conquita) 30g
Shi Gao‡ (Gypsum Fibrosum) 30g, decocted for 30 minutes before adding the other ingredients
Niu Xi (Radix Achyranthis Bidentatae) 15g
Mai Men Dong (Radix Ophiopogonis Japonici) 15g
Di Gu Pi (Cortex Lycii Radicis) 15g
Mu Dan Pi (Cortex Moutan Radicis) 15g
Shan Zhu Yu (Fructus Corni Officinalis) 10g
Gou Qi Zi (Fructus Lycii) 10g
Zhi Mu (Rhizoma Anemarrhenae Asphodeloidis) 10g
Ze Xie (Rhizoma Alismatis Orientalis) 6g
Bai Ji Li (Fructus Tribuli Terrestris) 18g
Gan Cao (Radix Glycyrrhizae) 4g

One bag a day was used to prepare a decoction, taken twice a day.

External treatment prescription ingredients

Huang Jing (Rhizoma Polygonati) 30g
Ku Shen (Radix Sophorae Flavescentis) 30g
Wu Bei Zi‡ (Galla Rhois Chinensis) 15g
Xu Chang Qing (Radix Cynanchi Paniculati) 20g

The decoction was used to wash the affected areas once or twice a day. Where this was effective, improvements were seen within two weeks.

EXTERNAL TREATMENT

1. **Yuan** treated seborrheic eczema with an external wash and soak. [39]

Prescription
JIA WEI HUANG LIAN JIE DU TANG
Augmented Coptis Decoction for Relieving Toxicity

Huang Lian (Rhizoma Coptidis) 10g
Huang Qin (Radix Scutellariae Baicalensis) 10g
Huang Bai (Cortex Phellodendri) 10g
Jin Yin Hua (Flos Lonicerae) 10g
Zhi Zi (Fructus Gardeniae Jasminoidis) 12g
Mo Yao (Myrrha) 12g
Ru Xiang (Olibanum) 12g
Ku Shen (Radix Sophorae Flavescentis) 20g
*Chuan Shan Jia** (Squama Manitis Pentadactylae) 6g
Gui Zhi (Ramulus Cinnamomi Cassiae) 6g

One bag a day was decocted to obtain 500ml of liquid, which was divided into three portions. In the morning and at noon, 150ml of the decoction was added to 200ml of boiled water and used to wash the affected area for 15-20 minutes. The remaining 200ml was mixed with 300ml of boiled water and used as a soak for 15 minutes each evening, after which a towel soaked in the decoction was applied as a wet compress for 30 minutes. Results began to be seen after seven days.

2. **Song** prepared a medicated bath that can be used for infants and children. [40]

Prescription ingredients

Ku Shen (Radix Sophorae Flavescentis) 20-30g
Huang Bai (Cortex Phellodendri) 15-20g
Huang Qin (Radix Scutellariae Baicalensis) 20g
Jing Jie (Herba Schizonepetae Tenuifoliae) 20g
Jin Yin Hua (Flos Lonicerae) 30g
Sang Bai Pi (Cortex Mori Albae Radicis) 30g
Di Fu Zi (Fructus Kochiae Scopariae) 30g
Cang Zhu (Rhizoma Atractylodis) 15g
Bai Zhi (Radix Angelicae Dahuricae) 15g
Fang Feng (Radix Ledebouriellae Divaricatae) 15g
Shi Chang Pu (Rhizoma Acori Graminei) 15g
Bo He (Herba Menthae Haplocalycis) 15g

Each day, one bag of the ingredients was decocted in one liter of water over a mild heat for 20 minutes and then left to cool. For patients with thick crusts and scales, *Gan Lan You* (Oleum Canarii Albi Seminis) was applied to the lesions for one hour before they were washed with the medicated liquid to remove the crusts, dead skin and oil. The liquid was then filtered to remove the residue before being poured into bathwater whose temperature had been regulated to 38°C. The child was put in the bath for 30-50 minutes, or a thick gauze cloth soaked in the medicated liquid was used as a wet compress, or the liquid was applied directly to the lesions. Five days made up a course of treatment. Results were seen after four courses.

3. **Zhang** treated 50 cases of seborrheic eczema with a steam-wash. [41]

Prescription
QU XIE TANG
Decoction for Removing Scales

Ku Shen (Radix Sophorae Flavescentis) 20g
Bai Xian Pi (Cortex Dictamni Dasycarpi Radicis) 20g
Di Fu Zi (Fructus Kochiae Scopariae) 20g
Bai Zhi (Radix Angelicae Dahuricae) 20g
Da Huang (Radix et Rhizoma Rhei) 15g
Tu Jin Pi (Cortex Pseudolaricis) 15g
Hua Jiao (Pericarpium Zanthoxyli) 15g
Huang Bai (Cortex Phellodendri) 15g
Ce Bai Ye (Cacumen Biotae Orientalis) 30g
Lian Qiao (Fructus Forsythiae Suspensae) 25g

A decoction of the ingredients was used to steam and wash the affected area for 30 minutes a day. Three days made up a course of treatment. Results were seen after one or two courses.

Nummular eczema (discoid eczema)
钱币状湿疹

This type of eczema is characterized by multiple, extremely itchy coin-shaped inflammatory lesions. Onset is usually gradual with no obvious precipitating factor.

In TCM, this condition is also known as *qian bi shi zhen* (coin-sized Damp eruption).

Clinical manifestations

- Nummular eczema affects adults of all ages, but most particularly middle-aged males. It is often exacerbated in winter and alleviated in summer.
- It mainly involves the limbs, but may also occur on the dorsum of the hands, the buttocks and the trunk.
- At the initial stage, a few isolated lesions appear on the legs, followed by multiple lesions with haphazard distribution.
- Lesions manifest as sharply demarcated, coin-shaped plaques 1-5 cm in diameter formed from the confluence of densely distributed red papules or vesicles.
- Lesions may be acute with clear or bloody exudate and crusting, or chronic with erythema and scaling.
- Itching is usually severe.
- The condition persists for months or years and often recurs at the site of previous plaques.

Differential diagnosis

Psoriasis
In psoriasis, lesions usually involve the scalp and the extensor aspect of the limbs, especially the extensor aspect of the elbows and knees. At the initial stage, bright red or dark red macules, maculopapules or papules appear with a shiny, wax-like surface, which is subsequently covered by silvery-white scales. Nummular eczema does not involve the scalp nor does it have the silvery scales characteristic of psoriasis.

Tinea corporis
Lesions usually involve the trunk, face or neck. They start with grouped red papules or papulovesicles, which increase gradually in number and size and spread outward to form single or multiple sharply circumscribed circular, semicircular or concentric erythema. Lesions gradually heal in the center but are elevated at the borders (the "active edge") with clusters of red papules or papulovesicles. Thin, fine scaling may be noted sometimes. This condition tends to be more severe in summer.

Etiology and pathology

Cold-Damp obstruction
Cold-Damp pathogenic factors invade the skin and obstruct the channels and network vessels to cause local Qi stagnation and accumulation of Cold-Damp, resulting in exudation and severe itching.

Dampness restricting Spleen Yang
Devitalized Spleen Yang is easily restricted by Dampness to cause Damp obstruction in the Middle Burner, resulting in red papules on the trunk, or to cause Dampness to pour down, resulting in red papules on the buttocks. Since the Spleen governs the four limbs, Dampness also moves outward to the lower limbs and the dorsum of the hands.

Pattern identification and treatment

INTERNAL TREATMENT

COLD-DAMP OBSTRUCTION
Lesions mainly involve the lower limbs and are characterized by coin-like, slightly raised, dull red plaques. Excoriation results in slight watery exudate. The tongue body is pale red with a thin white coating; the pulse is moderate and thready.

Treatment principle
Dissipate Cold and dry Dampness.

Prescription
SHENG YANG CHU SHI FANG FENG TANG JIA JIAN
Ledebouriella Decoction for Bearing Yang Upward and Eliminating Dampness, with modifications

Cang Zhu (Rhizoma Atractylodis) 12g
Wu Yao (Radix Linderae Strychnifoliae) 12g

Fang Feng (Radix Ledebouriellae Divaricatae) 12g
Fu Ling (Sclerotium Poriae Cocos) 10g
Chao Bai Zhu (Rhizoma Atractylodis Macrocephalae, stir-fried) 10g
Chuan Niu Xi (Radix Cyathulae Officinalis) 10g
Bi Xie (Rhizoma Dioscoreae Hypoglaucae seu Septemlobae) 10g
Dang Gui (Radix Angelicae Sinensis) 10g
Chao Bai Shao (Radix Paeoniae Lactiflorae, stir-fried) 10g
Jiang Ban Xia (Rhizoma Pinelliae Ternatae, processed with ginger) 10g
Xiao Hui Xiang (Fructus Foeniculi Vulgaris) 10g
Wu Zhu Yu (Fructus Evodiae Rutaecarpae) 6g
Chuan Xiong (Rhizoma Ligustici Chuanxiong) 6g
Qing Pi (Pericarpium Citri Reticulatae Viride) 6g

Explanation

- *Chao Bai Zhu* (Rhizoma Atractylodis Macrocephalae, stir-fried), *Cang Zhu* (Rhizoma Atractylodis), *Jiang Ban Xia* (Rhizoma Pinelliae Ternatae, processed with ginger), *Wu Zhu Yu* (Fructus Evodiae Rutaecarpae), *Wu Yao* (Radix Linderae Strychnifoliae), and *Xiao Hui Xiang* (Fructus Foeniculi Vulgaris) warm Spleen Yang to dissipate Cold externally and transform Dampness internally to treat the Root.
- *Dang Gui* (Radix Angelicae Sinensis) and *Chao Bai Shao* (Radix Paeoniae Lactiflorae, stir-fried) nourish the Blood and moisten the skin.
- *Chuan Niu Xi* (Radix Cyathulae Officinalis) guides the effect of the other materia medica downward and also strengthens the Dampness-percolating function of *Bi Xie* (Rhizoma Dioscoreae Hypoglaucae seu Septemlobae), *Fu Ling* (Sclerotium Poriae Cocos) and *Fang Feng* (Radix Ledebouriellae Divaricatae).
- *Qing Pi* (Pericarpium Citri Reticulatae Viride) and *Chuan Xiong* (Rhizoma Ligustici Chuanxiong) soothe the Liver and regulate Qi. If Qi can move freely, it is difficult for pathogenic factors to collect and the disease can be treated.

DAMPNESS RESTRICTING SPLEEN YANG

Lesions mainly involve the dorsum of the hand, the trunk, the buttocks, and the lower limbs and are characterized by round, slightly raised, rough plaques with a dry, scaly surface. Itching varies in intensity from moderate to severe and the condition is difficult to treat. The tongue body is pale red with a scant coating; the pulse is deep and thready.

Treatment principle

Warm Yang and benefit the movement of Dampness.

Prescription

SHI WEI REN SHEN SAN JIA JIAN

Ten-Ingredient Ginseng Powder, with modifications

Dang Shen (Radix Codonopsitis Pilosulae) 10g

Chao Bai Zhu (Rhizoma Atractylodis Macrocephalae, stir-fried) 10g
Fu Ling (Sclerotium Poriae Cocos) 10g
Jiang Ban Xia (Rhizoma Pinelliae Ternatae, processed with ginger) 10g
Chao Bai Shao (Radix Paeoniae Lactiflorae, stir-fried) 10g
Chai Hu (Radix Bupleuri) 6g
Gan Cao (Radix Glycyrrhizae) 6g
Hou Po (Cortex Magnoliae Officinalis) 4g
Chen Pi (Pericarpium Citri Reticulatae) 5g
Gui Zhi (Ramulus Cinnamomi Cassiae) 5g
Gan Jiang (Rhizoma Zingiberis Officinalis) 3g
Da Zao (Fructus Ziziphi Jujubae) 15g

Explanation

- *Dang Shen* (Radix Codonopsitis Pilosulae), *Fu Ling* (Sclerotium Poriae Cocos), *Chao Bai Zhu* (Rhizoma Atractylodis Macrocephalae, stir-fried), and *Gan Cao* (Radix Glycyrrhizae) supplement Qi and boost the Spleen and Stomach.
- *Hou Po* (Cortex Magnoliae Officinalis), *Chen Pi* (Pericarpium Citri Reticulatae) and *Jiang Ban Xia* (Rhizoma Pinelliae Ternatae, processed with ginger) dry Dampness and regulate Qi, thus depriving Dampness of a place to collect.
- *Gan Jiang* (Rhizoma Zingiberis Officinalis), *Da Zao* (Fructus Ziziphi Jujubae), *Gui Zhi* (Ramulus Cinnamomi Cassiae), *Chao Bai Shao* (Radix Paeoniae Lactiflorae, stir-fried), and *Chai Hu* (Radix Bupleuri) harmonize the Ying and Wei levels, support the Spleen and reinforce Yang. A supplementing effect can be achieved in Deficiency patterns and a draining effect in Excess patterns. This is in accordance with the principle that a healthy Spleen dries Dampness.

EXTERNAL TREATMENT

- At the acute stage, use *Ma Chi Xian Shui Xi Ji* (Purslane Wash Preparation) as a cold wash for 15 minutes once a day.
- For slight exudation, use *Hu Po Er Wu Hu Gao* (Two Blacks Paste with Amber); for dryness and fissuring, use *Run Ji Gao* (Flesh-Moistening Paste) in combination with *Shi Zhen Fen* (Eczema Powder). Apply these medications to the affected area once or twice a day.

Clinical notes

- Internal treatment for nummular eczema mainly emphasizes supporting the Spleen. Materia medica with sweet and warm properties should be prescribed alongside herbs for percolating Dampness such as *Bi Xie* (Rhizoma Dioscoreae Hypoglaucae seu Septemlobae).

- This condition tends to recur frequently. Treatment should be based on the principle of repeating the prescription if it achieved a satisfactory effect in previous occurrences.

Advice for the patient

- Do not use hot water to wash the affected areas, otherwise the condition will worsen.

- Avoid eating stimulating food such as fish, cheese and butter.
- Strengthen the body by doing more physical exercise.
- Avoid using creams containing steroids.

Hand and foot eczema
手足湿疹

This section provides a general description of various commonly seen patterns of eczema on the hand or foot and the TCM treatment applicable to such conditions. Reference should also be made to other sections dealing with eczematous manifestations on the hands or feet – acute or chronic eczema, contact dermatitis (irritant or allergic), atopic eczema, pompholyx, and recurrent focal palmar peeling (keratolysis exfoliativa).

Clinical manifestations

- This condition mainly occurs on the palm, the sole, and the area between the fingers and toes.
- Skin lesions can be classified into four types:
  - damp type – papules and papulovesicles, exudation, and maceration on rupture after scratching.
  - dry type – the skin is dry, cracked and lichenified with obvious keratosis.
  - enduring type – the disease is of long duration and repeated recurrence with intermittent remission and aggravation; it may be seen with the other types.
  - infection by microorganisms – lesions of this type progress rapidly from papulovesicles to yellow or white pustules; pain and itching are present.

Differential diagnosis

Tinea manuum
This condition often occurs on one hand initially, later involving both hands in severe cases. Lesions may have well-defined borders. Microscopic examination for fungi is positive. The condition is aggravated in summer and alleviated in winter.

Etiology and pathology

Accumulation of Damp-Heat
Dietary irregularities such as excessive intake of fish, seafood, and fried or greasy food will lead to impairment of the transportation and transformation function of the Spleen, especially when there is constitutional weakness and Spleen and Stomach Deficiency. As a result, Damp-Heat will accumulate inside the body and may spread to the hands and feet to cause eczema.

Wind and Dampness fighting each other
Looseness of the skin and interstices (*cou li*) allows external pathogenic Wind-Damp to invade. Wind and Dampness fight each other in the fleshy exterior to cause the disease. In *Zhu Bing Yuan Hou Lun* [A General Treatise on the Causes and Symptoms of Diseases], it says: "When the exterior is Deficient, external Wind-Damp seizes the opportunity to invade. These pathogenic factors are then confronted by Qi and Blood, and bind and accumulate inside the body to cause sores. This condition usually involves the hands and feet and resembles the fruits of *Wu Zhu Yu* (Fructus Evodiae Rutaecarpae). It is characterized by pain, itching, formation of sores after scratching, yellow exudate, maceration and erosion, and intermittent remission and aggravation of the symptoms."

Wind-Dryness due to Blood Deficiency
Heat in the Spleen and Stomach with Wind predominating over Dampness may lead to consumption of Blood and damage to Yin. The skin will therefore be deprived of nourishment as a result of generation of Wind and transformation into Dryness. In *Wai Ke Zhen Quan* [True Notes on External Diseases], it says:

"The condition characterized by dryness, itching and desquamation in the center of the palm, sometimes accompanied by cracks due to dryness and slight pain, is known as *zhang xin feng* (palm Heart Wind). It occurs because of Heat in the Spleen and Stomach and generation of Wind due to Blood Deficiency, thus depriving the skin of nourishment."

Damp-Heat Toxins

External contact with water, and living or working in a humid or wet environment can result in pathogenic Dampness predominating over Wind. Dampness and Heat bind and accumulate to transform into Toxins. When the skin is affected by Damp-Heat Toxins, clusters of yellow or white pustules appear accompanied by pain and itching. This condition is persistent with intermittent remission and aggravation.

Pattern identification and treatment

INTERNAL TREATMENT

DAMP-HEAT ACCUMULATING INTERNALLY

Lesions mainly manifest as papules, papulovesicles and vesicles. Exudation occurs on rupture of the lesions after scratching; in severe cases, maceration and crust formation may result. Accompanying symptoms and signs include dry stools, short voidings of yellow urine and severe itching. The tongue body is red with a thin yellow or yellow and greasy coating; the pulse is soggy and rapid.

Treatment principle

Clear Heat and percolate Dampness.

Prescription
HUANG LIAN JIE DU TANG JIA JIAN

Coptis Decoction for Relieving Toxicity, with modifications

Chao Huang Lian (Rhizoma Coptidis, stir-fried) 6g
Jiao Zhi Zi (Fructus Gardeniae Jasminoidis, scorch-fried) 6g
Sang Zhi (Ramulus Mori Albae) 6g
Chao Huang Qin (Radix Scutellariae Baicalensis, stir-fried) 10g
Chao Huang Bai (Cortex Phellodendri, stir-fried) 10g
Bai Mao Gen (Rhizoma Imperatae Cylindricae) 10g
Yi Yi Ren (Semen Coicis Lachryma-jobi) 15g
Shan Yao (Rhizoma Dioscoreae Oppositae) 15g
Chi Xiao Dou (Semen Phaseoli Calcarati) 15g

Explanation

- *Chao Huang Lian* (Rhizoma Coptidis, stir-fried), *Chao Huang Qin* (Radix Scutellariae Baicalensis, stir-fried), *Jiao Zhi Zi* (Fructus Gardeniae Jasminoidis, scorch-fried), and *Chao Huang Bai* (Cortex Phellodendri, stir-fried) clear Heat and drain Fire.

- *Bai Mao Gen* (Rhizoma Imperatae Cylindricae), *Shan Yao* (Rhizoma Dioscoreae Oppositae), *Yi Yi Ren* (Semen Coicis Lachryma-jobi), and *Chi Xiao Dou* (Semen Phaseoli Calcarati) cool the Blood and transform Dampness.

- *Sang Zhi* (Ramulus Mori Albae) dissipates Wind and alleviates itching and guides the other ingredients to the site of the disease.

WIND AND DAMPNESS FIGHTING EACH OTHER

The skin is dry, cracked, thickened, and lichenified with desquamation or occasional eruption of new papules and vesicles. Accompanying symptoms include itching or general malaise. The tongue body is pale red with a scant coating; the pulse is thready and rapid.

Treatment principle

Dispel Wind and overcome Dampness with the secondary consideration of moistening Dryness and alleviating itching.

Prescription
QU FENG DI HUANG WAN JIA JIAN

Rehmannia Pill for Dispelling Wind, with modifications

Sheng Di Huang (Radix Rehmanniae Glutinosae) 15g
Shu Di Huang (Radix Rehmanniae Glutinosae Conquita) 15g
Bai Ji Li (Fructus Tribuli Terrestris) 12g
Jiao Zhi Mu (Rhizoma Anemarrhenae Asphodeloidis, scorch-fried) 10g
Gou Qi Zi (Fructus Lycii) 10g
Sang Shen (Fructus Mori Albae) 10g
Gou Teng (Ramulus Uncariae cum Uncis) 10g
He Shou Wu (Radix Polygoni Multiflori) 10g
Fang Feng (Radix Ledebouriellae Divaricatae) 10g
Xu Chang Qing (Radix Cynanchi Paniculati) 10g
Wei Ling Xian (Radix Clematidis) 10g
Tu Si Zi (Semen Cuscutae) 6g
Du Huo (Radix Angelicae Pubescentis) 6g
Jiang Huang (Rhizoma Curcumae Longae) 6g
Sang Zhi (Ramulus Mori Albae) 6g
Chuan Niu Xi (Radix Cyathulae Officinalis) 6g

Explanation

- *Sheng Di Huang* (Radix Rehmanniae Glutinosae), *Shu Di Huang* (Radix Rehmanniae Glutinosae Conquita), *Jiao Zhi Mu* (Rhizoma Anemarrhenae Asphodeloidis, scorch-fried), *He Shou Wu* (Radix Polygoni Multiflori), *Tu Si Zi* (Semen Cuscutae), *Sang Shen* (Fructus Mori Albae), and *Gou Qi Zi* (Fructus Lycii) enrich Yin and moisten Dryness.

- *Bai Ji Li* (Fructus Tribuli Terrestris), *Fang Feng* (Radix Ledebouriellae Divaricatae), *Xu Chang Qing* (Radix Cynanchi Paniculati), *Gou Teng* (Ramulus Uncariae cum Uncis), *Wei Ling Xian* (Radix Clematidis), and *Du Huo* (Radix Angelicae Pubescentis) expel Wind and alleviate itching.

- *Xu Chang Qing* (Radix Cynanchi Paniculati), *Wei Ling Xian* (Radix Clematidis) and *Du Huo* (Radix Angelicae Pubescentis) dispel Wind and overcome Dampness.
- *Sang Zhi* (Ramulus Mori Albae), *Jiang Huang* (Rhizoma Curcumae Longae) and *Chuan Niu Xi* (Radix Cyathulae Officinalis) guide all the ingredients to the hands and feet to increase the effectiveness of the treatment.

WIND-DRYNESS DUE TO BLOOD DEFICIENCY

This condition is persistent and recurrent with intermittent remission and aggravation. The skin is rough with occasional desquamation and scaling, or may be dry, cracked and painful. The tongue body is red with a scant coating or no coating; the pulse is deficient, thready and rapid.

Treatment principle
Nourish the Blood and moisten Dryness, enrich Yin and eliminate Dampness.

Prescription
ZI YIN CHU SHI TANG JIA JIAN
Decoction for Enriching Yin and Eliminating Dampness, with modifications

Sheng Di Huang (Radix Rehmanniae Glutinosae) 15g
Dang Gui (Radix Angelicae Sinensis) 10g
Nan Sha Shen (Radix Adenophorae) 10g
Hei Da Dou (Semen Glycines Atrum) 10g
He Shou Wu (Radix Polygoni Multiflori) 10g
Gou Teng (Ramulus Uncariae cum Uncis) 10g
Shan Yao (Rhizoma Dioscoreae Oppositae) 10g
Dan Shen (Radix Salviae Miltiorrhizae) 12g
Bai Xian Pi (Cortex Dictamni Dasycarpi Radicis) 12g
She Chuang Zi (Fructus Cnidii Monnieri) 12g
Fu Ling Pi (Cortex Poriae Cocos) 9g
Ze Xie (Rhizoma Alismatis Orientalis) 9g
Sang Zhi (Ramulus Mori Albae) 9g
Chi Xiao Dou (Semen Phaseoli Calcarati) 30g

Explanation
- *Sheng Di Huang* (Radix Rehmanniae Glutinosae), *Dang Gui* (Radix Angelicae Sinensis) and *Dan Shen* (Radix Salviae Miltiorrhizae) nourish and invigorate the Blood.
- *Nan Sha Shen* (Radix Adenophorae), *He Shou Wu* (Radix Polygoni Multiflori), *Hei Da Dou* (Semen Glycines Atrum), and *Shan Yao* (Rhizoma Dioscoreae Oppositae) enrich Yin and moisten Dryness.
- *Gou Teng* (Ramulus Uncariae cum Uncis), *Bai Xian Pi* (Cortex Dictamni Dasycarpi Radicis), *She Chuang Zi*

(Fructus Cnidii Monnieri), and *Sang Zhi* (Ramulus Mori Albae) dissipate Wind and alleviate itching.
- *Fu Ling Pi* (Cortex Poriae Cocos), *Chi Xiao Dou* (Semen Phaseoli Calcarati) and *Ze Xie* (Rhizoma Alismatis Orientalis) transform Dampness and clear Heat.

DAMP-HEAT TRANSFORMING INTO TOXINS

This pattern manifests as clusters of recurrent vesicles and pustules on the palms and soles, with yellow exudate on rupture after scratching. Local itching and pain are likely. Lesions have intermittent remission and aggravation. The tongue body is red with a thin yellow coating; the pulse is soggy and rapid.

Treatment principle
Clear Heat and relieve Toxicity, transform Dampness and alleviate itching.

Prescription
YE JU BAI DU TANG JIA JIAN
Wild Chrysanthemum Decoction for Vanquishing Toxicity, with modifications

Ye Ju Hua (Flos Chrysanthemi Indici) 12g
Ban Zhi Lian (Herba Scutellariae Barbatae) 12g
Lian Zi Xin (Plumula Nelumbinis Nuciferae) 12g
Zi Hua Di Ding (Herba Violae Yedoensitis) 12g
Xi Xian Cao (Herba Siegesbeckiae) 15g
Fu Ling Pi (Cortex Poriae Cocos) 15g
Jin Yin Hua (Flos Lonicerae) 15g
Bai Hua She She Cao (Herba Hedyotidis Diffusae) 15g
Chi Xiao Dou (Semen Phaseoli Calcarati) 30g
Jiao Zhi Zi (Fructus Gardeniae Jasminoidis, scorch-fried) 6g

Explanation
- *Ye Ju Hua* (Flos Chrysanthemi Indici), *Ban Zhi Lian* (Herba Scutellariae Barbatae), *Zi Hua Di Ding* (Herba Violae Yedoensitis), *Bai Hua She She Cao* (Herba Hedyotidis Diffusae), and *Jin Yin Hua* (Flos Lonicerae) clear Heat and relieve Toxicity.
- *Lian Zi Xin* (Plumula Nelumbinis Nuciferae), *Zhi Zi* (Fructus Gardeniae Jasminoidis) and *Chi Xiao Dou* (Semen Phaseoli Calcarati) clear Heat from the Heart and relieve Toxicity.
- *Fu Ling Pi* (Cortex Poriae Cocos) and *Xi Xian Cao* (Herba Siegesbeckiae) transform Dampness, dissipate Wind and alleviate itching.

EXTERNAL TREATMENT
- For lesions characterized by papulovesicles and pustules, prepare a decoction of *Lu Lu Tong Shui Xi Ji* (Sweetgum Fruit Wash Preparation) or *Cang Fu Shui Xi Ji* (Atractylodes and Broom Cypress Wash Preparation) for use as a soak or wet compress.

- For damp-type lesions, mix *Qu Shi San* (Powder for Dispelling Dampness) with vegetable oil for external application, or use *Wu Shi Gao* (Five-Stone Paste).
- For dry-type lesions, apply *Huang Lian Ruan Gao* (Coptis Ointment) or *Run Ji Gao* (Flesh-Moistening Paste); see also the clinical notes below.
- For lichenified skin, apply *Hei Dou Liu You Ruan Gao* (Black Soybean and Vaseline® Ointment).
- For enduring lesions, apply *Li Lu Gao* (Veratrum Root Paste) to the affected area.

Clinical notes

- In external treatment of this condition, it is important to differentiate between dry and damp types:
  - Dry-type lesions are characterized by local lichenification with hyperkeratosis and painful fissuring. Treatment should start with medicated soaks before using pastes or ointments, which is the main recommendation for this type.
  - Damp-type lesions are characterized by exudation and erosion with severe itching. Treatment is based on medicated wash preparations used as soaks or wet compresses several times a day. However, if exudation and erosion are not severe, medicated pastes or ointments can be used instead.
- Internal treatment should focus on the Heart and Spleen. Where itching is severe, put the emphasis on clearing Heat from the Heart and draining Fire. Where Dampness predominates, put the emphasis on supporting the Spleen and drying Dampness. In both cases, adding channel conductors will enable the treatment to function more rapidly.
- The prognosis is good if the condition is managed properly, but recurrence is likely.

Advice for the patient

- Cut down or eliminate intake of fish, seafood, and greasy and fried food.
- Avoid washing affected areas with strongly alkaline soap or hot water.
- Avoid contact with down, wool or nylon products.

Case history

Patient
Female, aged 26.

Clinical manifestations
The patient had been suffering from repeated attacks of eczema on both hands for many years. More recently, she had been in contact at work with a chemical that caused extensive erythema, papules, vesicles, itching, erosion, and crusting with involvement extending to the forearms. Treatment with lotions for tinea made her condition worse. She also received outpatient treatment at the hospital with calcium gluconate plus the external application of steroid ointments, but there was no effect.

At the time of the consultation, the patient had a dense distribution of vesicles, some of which were red, swollen and eroded. She had been constipated for two days and had a dry mouth and thirst. The tongue body was red with a thin coating; the pulse was wiry and thready.

Pattern identification
Damp-Heat accumulating internally and moving outward to the skin and flesh.

Treatment principle
Clear Heat and benefit the movement of Dampness.

Prescription ingredients
Sheng Di Huang (Radix Rehmanniae Glutinosae) 12g
Yin Chen Hao (Herba Artemisiae Scopariae) 12g
Ku Shen (Radix Sophorae Flavescentis) 12g
Chi Shao (Radix Paeoniae Rubra) 10g
Mu Dan Pi (Cortex Moutan Radicis) 10g
Da Huang (Radix et Rhizoma Rhei) 10g, added 10 minutes before the end of the decoction process
Pu Gong Ying (Herba Taraxaci cum Radice) 30g
Bai Mao Gen (Rhizoma Imperatae Cylindricae) 30g
Gan Cao (Radix Glycyrrhizae) 3g

One bag a day was decocted three times with the first two decoctions being drunk and the third used as a wet compress.

Second visit
After five days, there was less exudation and skin lesions were alleviated in most areas. Crusts had formed in some places, but itching was still present and some small vesicles remained. The prescription was modified with the addition of *Bai Xian Pi* (Cortex Dictamni Dasycarpi Radicis) 12g. *Qing Dai San* (Indigo Powder) mixed with *Xiang You* (Oleum Sesami Seminis) was applied externally.

Third visit
Seven days later, the skin was dry with desquamation; itching had been alleviated and the lesions were almost cleared. The prescription was changed to *Long Dan Xie Gan Wan* (Chinese Gentian Pill for Draining the Liver) 5g twice a day, and *Di Long Pian* (Earthworm Tablet), five 0.3g tablets three times a day for three weeks. External treatment was changed to *Huang Lian Ruan Gao* (Coptis Ointment). [42]

Modern clinical experience

SOAKS

1. **Lu** ground 200g of the bark of *Lei Gong Teng* (Radix Tripterygii Wilfordii) into a coarse powder and decocted it in 1000 ml of water for 30 minutes. After allowing the

decoction to cool, it was used to soak the affected hand and foot for 15-30 minutes, two or three times a day. The same decoction and its residue were used for one week. Four weeks of treatment made up a course.

The decoction was used to treat 56 patients with hand and foot eczema – 25 with subacute eczema involving the dorsal aspects of the fingers and toes and the peri-ungual areas and characterized by papules and vesicles, and 31 with eczema fissum on the palms and soles. After one month of treatment, significant improvement or complete healing of the lesions occurred. [43]

2. Alternative prescriptions for external application as soaks have also been recommended. [44]

Prescription 1

Ku Shen (Radix Sophorae Flavescentis) 15g
Huang Bai (Cortex Phellodendri) 15g
Jing Jie (Herba Schizonepetae Tenuifoliae) 12g
Fang Feng (Radix Ledebouriellae Divaricatae) 12g

Prescription 2

Fang Feng (Radix Ledebouriellae Divaricatae) 6g

Fu Ping (Herba Spirodelae Polyrrhizae) 6g
Ku Shen (Radix Sophorae Flavescentis) 12g
Huang Bai (Cortex Phellodendri) 10g
Cang Zhu (Rhizoma Atractylodis) 10g
Di Fu Zi (Fructus Kochiae Scopariae) 15g

Where Damp-Heat predominated and lesions had yellow exudate, the prescription was modified by adding *Yi Yi Ren* (Semen Coicis Lachryma-jobi) 30g, *Ma Chi Xian* (Herba Portulacae Oleraceae) 20-30g and *Ku Fan*‡ (Alumen Praeparatum) 6g.

Prescription 3
KU SHEN TANG
Flavescent Sophora Root Decoction

Cang Zhu (Rhizoma Atractylodis) 30g
Ku Shen (Radix Sophorae Flavescentis) 30g
Chang Shan (Radix Dichroae Febrifugae) 30g
Shang Lu (Radix Phytolaccae) 30g
Qian Niu Zi (Semen Pharbitidis) 20g

All these decoctions were used to soak the affected hand or foot for 20 minutes, once or twice a day.

Pompholyx
汗疱疹

Pompholyx is an acute vesicular type of eczema, which attacks the palms, the sides of the fingers and the soles of the feet, particularly in warm weather or in individuals who sweat profusely. Affected individuals frequently have an atopic background. Lesions manifest as clusters of deep-seated vesicles on non-erythematous skin, accompanied by a sensation of burning heat and intense itching. Scaling and desquamation follow after the blisters dry up. Recurrence is frequent.

In TCM, pompholyx is also known as *ma yi wo* (ant's nest).

Clinical manifestations

- The disease tends to occur most frequently toward the end of spring and the beginning of summer with exacerbation during the summer. It sometimes heals spontaneously in winter. It attacks at a similar time each year.
- There is usually symmetrical involvement of the palms, the lateral fingers, the tips of the fingers, and less frequently the soles of the feet.
- At the initial stage, lesions manifest as a sudden eruption of deep-seated domed vesicles, 1-5 mm in diameter, raised slightly above the skin surface; inflammation is absent.
- Vesicles are filled with a clear and glistening fluid, which may occasionally turn turbid.
- Scaling and peeling follow drying of the vesicles; new skin is thin, tender and painful.
- Itching varies from moderate to severe; a sensation of burning heat is normally present.
- This condition recurs frequently over long periods.

Differential diagnosis

Recurrent focal palmar peeling (keratolysis exfoliativa)
Lesions mainly manifest as exfoliation of the palms and soles, and are therefore quite similar to the healing phase of pompholyx. However, vesicles are never seen.

Palmoplantar pustulosis (pustular psoriasis)
This disease tends to involve the soles, particularly the plantar arch, more than the palms. Lesions manifest as symmetrical erythema covered by small vesicles, which rapidly evolve into numerous deep, sterile 3-10 mm pustules of varying colors. Brown crusts will form in about ten days as the pustules dry up spontaneously. After crusts fall off, new pustules form underneath scales.

Trichophytid reaction
This is an eruption representing an allergic reaction to dermatophyte infection elsewhere in the body. Vesicles are relatively shallow with comparatively thin walls. There will be some active foci of infection with *Trychophyton* species at a distant site (for example, in tinea pedis). Once they are eliminated, the trichophytid reaction will disappear.

Etiology and pathology

Excessive thought and preoccupation predisposes to damage to the Heart and Spleen. When Spleen Qi is Deficient, the Spleen is impaired in its transformation and transportation function, allowing Damp-Heat to accumulate internally. Where this is complicated by external contraction of Summerheat-Damp, the internal and external pathogenic factors will combine. Since they cannot be expelled or drained, they steam to block the skin and interstices (*cou li*) and flow along the channels and network vessels to the palms and soles.

Pattern identification and treatment

INTERNAL TREATMENT

ACCUMULATION OF DAMP-HEAT
The disease is of relatively short duration and is characterized by groups of vesicles containing a clear fluid, which occasionally turns turbid. Pruritus and a sensation of burning heat are experienced. Accompanying symptoms and signs include abdominal distension, poor appetite, irregular bowel movements, and short voidings of yellow urine. The tongue body is red with a thin, yellow and slightly greasy coating; the pulse is slippery and rapid.

Treatment principle
Clear Heat and transform Dampness, support the Spleen and relieve Toxicity.

Prescription
XIE HUANG SAN JIA JIAN
Yellow-Draining Powder, with modifications

Huo Xiang (Herba Agastaches seu Pogostemi) 15g
Pei Lan (Herba Eupatorii Fortunei) 15g

Yi Yi Ren (Semen Coicis Lachryma-jobi) 15g
Chao Huang Lian (Rhizoma Coptidis, stir-fried) 6g
Jiao Zhi Zi (Fructus Gardeniae Jasminoidis, scorch-fried) 6g
Tong Cao (Medulla Tetrapanacis Papyriferi) 6g
Ze Xie (Rhizoma Alismatis Orientalis) 12g
Lian Qiao (Fructus Forsythiae Suspensae) 12g
Che Qian Zi (Semen Plantaginis) 12g, wrapped
Liu Yi San (Six-To-One Powder) 12g, wrapped
Shan Yao (Radix Dioscoreae Oppositae) 30g
Bai Xian Pi (Cortex Dictamni Dasycarpi Radicis) 10g
Jin Yin Hua (Flos Lonicerae) 10g
Huang Qin (Radix Scutellariae Baicalensis) 10g
Sang Zhi (Ramulus Mori Albae) 4.5g

Explanation
- *Huo Xiang* (Herba Agastaches seu Pogostemi), *Pei Lan* (Herba Eupatorii Fortunei), *Yi Yi Ren* (Semen Coicis Lachryma-jobi), *Jiao Zhi Zi* (Fructus Gardeniae Jasminoidis, scorch-fried), *Huang Qin* (Radix Scutellariae Baicalensis), and *Shan Yao* (Radix Dioscoreae Oppositae) clear Heat and transform Dampness, support the Spleen and transform turbidity.
- *Chao Huang Lian* (Rhizoma Coptidis, stir-fried), *Tong Cao* (Medulla Tetrapanacis Papyriferi), *Ze Xie* (Rhizoma Alismatis Orientalis), *Che Qian Zi* (Semen Plantaginis), and *Liu Yi San* (Six-To-One Powder) benefit the movement of Dampness and relieve Toxicity.
- *Bai Xian Pi* (Cortex Dictamni Dasycarpi Radicis) eliminates Dampness and alleviates itching.
- *Lian Qiao* (Fructus Forsythiae Suspensae) and *Jin Yin Hua* (Flos Lonicerae) clear Heat and relieve Toxicity.
- *Sang Zhi* (Ramulus Mori Albae) guides the other ingredients to the extremities.

HEART AND SPLEEN DEFICIENCY
With this pattern, the disease lasts for a long time or recurs every year, manifesting as dry blisters with layers of desquamation and exposure of tender skin, sometimes with a sensation of burning pain. Accompanying symptoms and signs include lassitude, listlessness, reduced appetite, shortness of breath, and occasional sweating on exertion. The tongue body is pale red with a scant coating; the pulse is deficient and thready.

Treatment principle
Supplement the Heart and boost the Spleen, constrain sweating and alleviate itching.

Prescription
GUI PI TANG JIA JIAN
Decoction for Restoring the Spleen, with modifications

Huang Qi (Radix Astragali seu Hedysari) 12g
Dang Shen (Radix Codonopsitis Pilosulae) 12g

Fu Ling (Sclerotium Poriae Cocos) 12g
Suan Zao Ren (Semen Ziziphi Spinosae) 12g
Bai Zi Ren (Semen Biotae Orientalis) 12g
Fang Feng (Radix Ledebouriellae Divaricatae) 10g
Bai Zhu (Rhizoma Atractylodis Macrocephalae) 10g
Mai Men Dong (Radix Ophiopogonis Japonici) 10g
Wu Wei Zi (Fructus Schisandrae) 10g
Duan Long Gu ‡ (Os Draconis Calcinatum) 30g
Duan Mu Li ‡ (Concha Ostreae Calcinata) 30g
Lian Zi Xin (Plumula Nelumbinis Nuciferae) 6g
Yuan Zhi (Radix Polygalae Tenuifoliae) 6g

Explanation

- *Huang Qi* (Radix Astragali seu Hedysari), *Dang Shen* (Radix Codonopsitis Pilosulae), *Fu Ling* (Sclerotium Poriae Cocos), *Bai Zhu* (Rhizoma Atractylodis Macrocephalae), *Suan Zao Ren* (Semen Ziziphi Spinosae), and *Bai Zi Ren* (Semen Biotae Orientalis) supplement the Heart and boost the Spleen, quiet the Spirit and sharpen the wits.

- *Fang Feng* (Radix Ledebouriellae Divaricatae), *Bai Zhu* (Rhizoma Atractylodis Macrocephalae), *Wu Wei Zi* (Fructus Schisandrae), *Duan Long Gu* ‡ (Os Draconis Calcinatum), and *Duan Mu Li* ‡ (Concha Ostreae Calcinata) constrain sweating and alleviate itching.

- *Lian Zi Xin* (Plumula Nelumbinis Nuciferae), *Mai Men Dong* (Radix Ophiopogonis Japonici) and *Yuan Zhi* (Radix Polygalae Tenuifoliae) clear Heat from the Heart.

EXTERNAL TREATMENT

- At the initial stage with vesicles, itching and pain, soak the affected area in a warm decoction of *Ge Gen Shui Xi Ji* (Kudzu Vine Root Wash Preparation), then apply *Bai Bu Ding* (Stemona Root Tincture) or 10% *Tu Jin Pi Ding* (Golden Larch Bark Tincture) to the area two or three times a day.

- If tender skin is exposed with a sensation of burning heat and pain, apply *Huang Lian Ruan Gao* (Coptis Ointment) once or twice a day.

- For groups of deep-seated vesicles with scaling following drying of the vesicles, accompanied by itching and a sensation of burning heat, prepare a decoction of *Wang Bu Liu Xing* (Semen Vaccariae Segetalis) 30g and *Ming Fan* ‡ (Alumen) 9g and use it to soak the hand for 15 minutes twice a day for one week.

ACUPUNCTURE

Main points: LI-4 Hegu, PC-8 Laogong, SI-3 Houxi, EX-UE-9 Baxie,ᵛ EX-LE-10 Bafeng,ᵛⁱ and KI-1 Yongquan.

Auxiliary points: LI-11 Quchi, TB-5 Waiguan, ST-36 Zusanli, and ST-41 Jiexi.

Technique: Apply the reducing method. Retain the needles for 30 minutes. Treat once a day. A course consists of seven treatment sessions.

Explanation

- LI-4 Hegu, PC-8 Laogong and KI-1 Yongquan clear Heat and eliminate Dampness.

- LI-11 Quchi, TB-5 Waiguan, SI-3 Houxi, and ST-41 Jiexi benefit the movement of Dampness and relieve Toxicity.

- ST-36 Zusanli augments Qi and eliminates Dampness.

- EX-UE-9 Baxie and EX-LE-10 Bafeng disperse swelling and alleviate itching.

Clinical notes

Both internal and external treatments are indicated for this disease. Internal treatment focuses on the Heart and Spleen with the treatment principle of clearing Heat and transforming Dampness, relieving Toxicity and draining Fire. External treatment aims to eliminate and dry Dampness, soften the skin and alleviate itching.

Advice for the patient

- Change the diet to include more milk products and meat soups to increase nutrition.

- Try to avoid mood swings, excessive brooding and stress.

- Avoid alcohol, spicy foods, fish, and other stimulating food.

- Do not use strongly alkaline soap and do not wash with hot water.

- Do not break the vesicles or tear away the peeling skin, as infection may occur.

Case history

Patient
Male, aged 32.

Clinical manifestations
Vesicles appeared on the palm of both hands two months previously. After the vesicles broke, scaling and peeling followed. The condition had recurred for a number of years. The patient's hands were always sweating. He had been given TCM treatment elsewhere at different times with separate prescriptions, one based on the treatment principle of clearing

---

ᵛ M-UE-22 according to the system employed by the Shanghai College of Traditional Chinese Medicine.
ᵛⁱ M-LE-8 according to the system employed by the Shanghai College of Traditional Chinese Medicine.

Heat and relieving Toxicity, the other based on promoting the movement of Dampness and dissipating Wind. With these prescriptions, the condition sometimes improved initially, but would then worsen.

Pattern identification
Accumulation of Damp-Heat.

Treatment principle
Benefit the movement of Dampness, clear Heat and relieve Toxicity.

Prescription
LONG DAN XIE GAN TANG JIA JIAN
Chinese Gentian Decoction for Draining the Liver, with modifications

Long Dan Cao (Radix Gentianae Scabrae) 9g
Zhi Zi (Fructus Gardeniae Jasminoidis) 9g
Fu Ling (Sclerotium Poriae Cocos) 9g

Ze Xie (Rhizoma Alismatis Orientalis) 9g
Lian Qiao (Fructus Forsythiae Suspensae) 9g
Che Qian Zi (Semen Plantaginis) 9g, wrapped
Huang Qin (Radix Scutellariae Baicalensis) 9g
Liu Yi San (Six-To-One Powder) 9g, wrapped
Bi Xie (Rhizoma Dioscoreae Hypoglaucae seu Septemlobae) 9g
Bai Xian Pi (Cortex Dictamni Dasycarpi Radicis) 9g
Jin Yin Hua (Flos Lonicerae) 9g
Tong Cao (Medulla Tetrapanacis Papyriferi) 4.5g
Sheng Di Huang (Radix Rehmanniae Glutinosae) 15g
Pu Gong Ying (Herba Taraxaci cum Radice) 15g

One bag a day was used to prepare a decoction, taken twice a day.

Outcome
After seven bags, no new vesicles had appeared, and existing vesicles had begun to disappear. The patient was told to continue with the same prescription for another 14 days to consolidate the improvement. [45]

Recurrent focal palmar peeling (keratolysis exfoliativa)
剥脱性角质松解症

Recurrent focal palmar peeling is a commonly seen chronic skin disease and is considered by most authorities to be a mild form of pompholyx. The horny layer of the palms and soles separates from the layer beneath, resulting in peeling and exfoliation.

Clinical manifestations

- This condition occurs most often in adults and is associated with hyperhidrosis of the hands and feet and pompholyx.
- It tends to occur at the end of spring and the beginning of summer or at the end of autumn and the beginning of winter.
- The condition mainly involves the palms bilaterally, less often the soles of the feet.
- At the initial stage, lesions appear as pinpoint white spots containing no fluid. The lesions gradually extend and eventually produce scaling and peeling. The center of the scaly area may turn red and tender.
- After desquamation of the horny layer, the skin underneath returns to normal. The cycle lasts 3-6 weeks. The condition resolves spontaneously, but may recur once or more a year.

Differential diagnosis

Pompholyx
There is usually symmetrical involvement of the palms, the lateral fingers, the tips of the fingers, and less frequently the soles of the feet. At the initial stage, lesions manifest as a sudden eruption of deep-seated domed vesicles. Vesicles are filled with a clear and glistening fluid. Scaling and peeling follow drying of the vesicles. Itching varies from moderate to severe.

Tinea manuum
Lesions mainly involve the center of the palm and the palmar aspect of the fingers. Small transparent pinpoint vesicles appear, which quickly rupture with a small amount of exudate. They soon dry up and are covered with layers of white scale. Later, local skin becomes dry, rough and thick, and may crack or fissure. It is often difficult to differentiate from extensive, recurrent focal palmar peeling without mycological examination.

Etiology and pathology

When the Spleen is Deficient, internal pathogenic Damp-Heat is generated. This obstructs the palms and soles and accumulates to cause Damp stagnation, resulting in lack of nourishment for the skin and subsequent dry skin and recurrent desquamation.

Pattern identification and treatment

INTERNAL TREATMENT

DAMP-HEAT ACCUMULATING IN THE SKIN

This pattern is characterized by a chronic condition recurring several times a year. Lesions tend to coalesce to form large areas of white scale. Accompanying symptoms and signs include profuse sweating, irritability and restlessness, and heat in the center of the palms. The tongue body is red with a scant coating; the pulse is thready and rapid.

Treatment principle
Moisten Dryness with cold and sweetness, blandly percolate stagnated Dampness.

Prescription
YE SHI YANG WEI TANG JIA JIAN
Ye's Decoction for Nourishing the Stomach, with modifications

Nan Sha Shen (Radix Adenophorae) 15g
Shi Hu* (Herba Dendrobii) 15g
Tian Men Dong (Radix Asparagi Cochinchinensis) 15g
Bai Shao (Radix Paeoniae Lactiflorae) 10g
Yu Zhu (Rhizoma Polygonati Odorati) 10g
Sheng Di Huang (Radix Rehmanniae Glutinosae) 10g
Yi Yi Ren (Semen Coicis Lachryma-jobi) 30g
Dong Gua Pi (Epicarpium Benincasae Hispidae) 30g
Chi Xiao Dou (Semen Phaseoli Calcarati) 30g
Sang Zhi (Ramulus Mori Albae) 6g
Si Gua Luo (Fasciculus Vascularis Luffae) 6g
Lian Zi Xin (Plumula Nelumbinis Nuciferae) 6g

Explanation
- *Nan Sha Shen* (Radix Adenophorae) and *Shi Hu** (Herba Dendrobii) nourish the Stomach and generate Body Fluids.

- *Tian Men Dong* (Radix Asparagi Cochinchinensis) and *Yu Zhu* (Rhizoma Polygonati Odorati) moisten Dryness and generate Body Fluids.
- *Sheng Di Huang* (Radix Rehmanniae Glutinosae) and *Bai Shao* (Radix Paeoniae Lactiflorae) enrich Yin and nourish the Blood.
- *Yi Yi Ren* (Semen Coicis Lachryma-jobi), *Chi Xiao Dou* (Semen Phaseoli Calcarati) and *Dong Gua Pi* (Epicarpium Benincasae Hispidae) benefit the movement of water and percolate Dampness.
- *Sang Zhi* (Ramulus Mori Albae) and *Si Gua Luo* (Fasciculus Vascularis Luffae) transform Dampness and free the network vessels.
- *Lian Zi Xin* (Plumula Nelumbinis Nuciferae) nourishes the Heart and quiets the Spirit to eliminate irritability.

EXTERNAL TREATMENT
To treat dry and scaling palms, prepare the decoction below, which has the effect of eliminating Dampness and dissipating Wind, moistening Dryness and softening the skin.

Prescription ingredients

Chen Pi (Pericarpium Citri Reticulatae) 30g
Gou Ji (Rhizoma Cibotii Barometz) 30g
Wu Bei Zi‡ (Galla Rhois Chinensis) 15g
Cang Er Zi (Fructus Xanthii Sibirici) 15g
Jin Qian Cao (Herba Lysimachiae) 15g

Use warm to soak the affected area for 10-15 minutes once or twice a day. After soaking, apply *Huang Lian Ruan Gao* (Coptis Ointment).

EAR ACUPUNCTURE WITH SEEDS
Points: Ear-Shenmen, Sympathetic Nerve, Heart, and Hand.
Technique: Attach *Wang Bu Liu Xing* (Semen Vaccariae Segetalis) seeds to the points with adhesive tape and ask the patient to press the seeds for one minute three to five times a day. This can help to reduce the extent of scaling.

Asteatotic eczema
皮脂缺乏湿疹

Asteatotic eczema is a type of chronic eczema that occurs predominantly in elderly patients, mostly those with a history of dry skin and chapping. Other contributory factors include excessive washing of the affected area and dry environments in winter, especially those related to central heating. The condition often coexists with varicose vein of the lower legs.

Clinical manifestations

- Asteatotic eczema is most common in winter and improves in summer.
- Although any skin site may be affected, the condition occurs most frequently on the lower legs.
- Dry skin is the first sign, followed by faint erythema that progresses to inflamed eczematous papules coalescing to form large plaques. A network of thin red superficial cracks and fissures appears in a "crazy paving" pattern (eczema craquelé). The skin may be painful and itchy.
- Severe, persistent inflammation may produce exudation and crusting with stinging or burning pain.

Differential diagnosis

Stasis eczema
Most patients are middle-aged or elderly with varicose veins in the leg. The condition manifests initially as mild edema in the lower third of the lower leg, and erythema or brown pigmentation on the anterior aspect of the tibia and around the ankle. Eczematoid lesions (papules, vesicles, erosion, exudation, and crusts) appear subsequently. At the chronic stage, the skin becomes dry, thick and lichenified with desquamation and fissuring. Ulceration may eventually appear on the distal part of the lower leg.

Etiology and pathology

Dietary irregularities damage the Spleen and Stomach, resulting in generation of Dampness and retention of Fluids. Water and Dampness collect to encumber the Spleen, thus impairing its transportation and transformation function and causing the internal accumulation of Damp-Heat. Long-term accumulation of Damp-Heat consumes Yin and damages the Blood to cause Blood Deficiency and Wind-Dryness as well as Spleen

Deficiency and Blood stasis. Lack of nourishment leads to the skin becoming persistently thick and fissured.

Pattern identification and treatment

INTERNAL TREATMENT

SPLEEN DEFICIENCY AND BLOOD-DRYNESS
This pattern is characteristic of a prolonged illness. Lesions manifest as thick red plaques with rough and fissured skin and obvious excoriations. There may be exudation and crusting; itching may be intense. Accompanying symptoms and signs include fatigue and lack of strength, poor appetite, insomnia, and profuse dreaming. The tongue is pale with an enlarged body and a white coating; the pulse is deep and moderate.

Treatment principle
Fortify the Spleen and dry Dampness, nourish and invigorate the Blood, and transform Blood stasis.

Prescription
JIAN PI RUN FU TANG JIA JIAN
Decoction for Fortifying the Spleen and Moistening the Skin, with modifications

Dang Shen (Radix Codonopsitis Pilosulae) 10g
Fu Ling (Sclerotium Poriae Cocos) 10g
Bai Zhu (Rhizoma Atractylodis Macrocephalae) 10g
Dang Gui (Radix Angelicae Sinensis) 10g
Chi Shao (Radix Paeoniae Rubra) 10g
Bai Shao (Radix Paeoniae Lactiflorae) 10g
Shu Di Huang (Radix Rehmanniae Glutinosae Conquita) 10g
Dan Shen (Radix Salviae Miltiorrhizae) 15g
Ji Xue Teng (Caulis Spatholobi) 15g
Bai Xian Pi (Cortex Dictamni Dasycarpi Radicis) 30g
Ku Shen (Radix Sophorae Flavescentis) 15g
Ye Jiao Teng (Caulis Polygoni Multiflori) 30g
Bai Ji Li (Fructus Tribuli Terrestris) 30g
Di Fu Zi (Fructus Kochiae Scopariae) 15g
Chen Pi (Pericarpium Citri Reticulatae) 10g
Zhi Shi (Fructus Citri Aurantii) 10g

Explanation
- *Dang Shen* (Radix Codonopsitis Pilosulae), *Fu Ling* (Sclerotium Poriae Cocos) and *Bai Zhu* (Rhizoma Atractylodis Macrocephalae) fortify the Spleen, augment Qi and dry Dampness.

- *Dang Gui* (Radix Angelicae Sinensis), *Shu Di Huang* (Radix Rehmanniae Glutinosae Conquita), *Chi Shao* (Radix Paeoniae Rubra), *Bai Shao* (Radix Paeoniae Lactiflorae), *Dan Shen* (Radix Salviae Miltiorrhizae), and *Ji Xue Teng* (Caulis Spatholobi) nourish and invigorate the Blood and transform Blood stasis.
- *Di Fu Zi* (Fructus Kochiae Scopariae), *Bai Xian Pi* (Cortex Dictamni Dasycarpi Radicis) and *Ku Shen* (Radix Sophorae Flavescentis) are key herbs in the treatment of itchy skin; they clear Heat and relieve Toxicity, dispel Wind and eliminate Dampness.
- *Ye Jiao Teng* (Caulis Polygoni Multiflori) and *Bai Ji Li* (Fructus Tribuli Terrestris) nourish the Blood and quiet the Spirit, and dredge Wind to alleviate itching.
- *Chen Pi* (Pericarpium Citri Reticulatae) and *Zhi Shi* (Fructus Citri Aurantii) regulate Qi and fortify the Spleen.

EXTERNAL TREATMENT
- To dry Dampness and moisten the skin, wash the affected area with the following decoction for 15 minutes once a day.

Prescription
CANG FU SHUI XI JI
Atractylodes and Broom Cypress Wash Preparation

Cang Er Zi (Fructus Xanthii Sibirici) 15g
Di Fu Zi (Fructus Kochiae Scopariae) 15g
Tu Jin Pi (Cortex Pseudolaricis) 15g
She Chuang Zi (Fructus Cnidii Monnieri) 15g
Ku Shen (Radix Sophorae Flavescentis) 15g
Bai Bu (Radix Stemonae) 15g
Ku Fan‡ (Alumen Praeparatum) 6g

- Apply *Huang Lian Ruan Gao* (Coptis Ointment) to the affected areas twice a day to clear Heat and relieve Toxicity.

Advice for the patient

- Strengthen the body by doing physical exercises such as *tai ji quan* or walking.
- Massage the skin to promote the circulation of blood and improve the supply of blood to the skin.
- Elderly people should take steps to prevent or have treatment for underlying chronic conditions such as nephritis, diabetes, indigestion, or insomnia.
- Eat less stimulating food such as fish, prawn and crab, and increase the intake of fresh vegetables and fruit.
- Do not use alkaline soap. Shower or bath in warm rather than hot water. Do not soak the body in the bath for too long. Apply moisturizing cream after baths or showers.
- Keep warm.

Stasis eczema
瘀滞性湿疹

Stasis eczema is also known as gravitational eczema, varicose eczema or venous eczema; where it is accompanied by chronic ulceration of the lower leg, the condition is sometimes referred to as varicose syndrome.

This condition is caused by varicosities of the leg, which lead to venous congestion and increased capillary permeability, resulting in edema, local hypoxia, malnutrition of local tissues, and local pruritus. External irritation such as scratching or trauma may trigger the disease. Lesions can easily develop into ulcers, which often remain unhealed for a long time or occasionally become malignant.

In TCM, stasis dermatitis is also known as *xia zhu chuang* (pouring downward sore) or *shi du chuang* (Damp Toxin sore).

Clinical manifestations

- Most patients are middle-aged or elderly with a long history of varicose veins of the leg. Women are more usually affected than men.
- The condition is often preceded by heaviness or aching in the leg aggravated by prolonged standing or walking.
- At the initial stage, the main manifestations are mild edema in the lower third of the lower leg, and erythema or brown pigmentation on the anterior aspect of the tibia and around the ankle. Eczematoid lesions (papules, vesicles, erosion, exudation, and crusts) appear subsequently.

- At the chronic stage, the skin becomes dry, thick and lichenified with desquamation and fissuring.
- Ulceration may eventually appear on the distal part of the lower leg. This condition is very difficult to cure and may occasionally develop into squamous carcinoma in some patients.
- Pruritus of varying intensity is present.
- The disease is of long duration and is difficult to cure; relapse is frequent.

Etiology and pathology

Damp-Heat pouring down
Damp-Heat from the Spleen and Stomach pour downward along the channels to the legs, inhibiting the movement of Qi and Blood and obstructing the channels and network vessels in the skin and interstices (*cou li*).

Externally-contracted Toxic pathogenic factors
Pathogenic Wind-Damp Toxins stream between the tibia and the knee joints, gradually binding with internal Damp-Heat and transforming into Heat Toxins to cause the disease.

Blood Deficiency and Wind-Dryness
If the disease endures, it may damage Yin and consume Blood to deprive the skin and interstices (*cou li*) of nourishment.

Pattern identification and treatment

INTERNAL TREATMENT

ACUTE STAGE (DAMP-HEAT POURING DOWN)
Edematous erythema, papulovesicles and small vesicles with slight exudation and erosion can be found on the leg. Severe cases present with redness, swelling, a burning sensation, and discharge of pus and fluid. Accompanying symptoms include slight fever and general malaise. The tongue body is red with a yellow and greasy coating; the pulse is wiry and rapid.

Treatment principle
Clear Heat and transform Dampness, harmonize the Blood and relieve Toxicity.

Prescription
SAN MIAO WAN HE WU WEI XIAO DU YIN JIA JIAN
Mysterious Three Pill Combined With Five-Ingredient Beverage for Dispersing Toxicity, with modifications

Cang Zhu (Rhizoma Atractylodis) 10g
Huang Bai (Cortex Phellodendri) 10g
Da Fu Pi (Pericarpium Arecae Catechu) 10g
Dang Gui (Radix Angelicae Sinensis) 10g
Dan Shen (Radix Salviae Miltiorrhizae) 12g
Ze Lan (Herba Lycopi Lucidi) 12g
Bai Xian Pi (Cortex Dictamni Dasycarpi Radicis) 12g
Ren Dong Teng (Caulis Lonicerae Japonicae) 15g
Pu Gong Ying (Herba Taraxaci cum Radice) 15g
Zi Hua Di Ding (Herba Violae Yedoensitis) 15g
Chuan Niu Xi (Radix Cyathulae Officinalis) 6g
Qing Pi (Pericarpium Citri Reticulatae Viride) 6g
Chi Xiao Dou (Semen Phaseoli Calcarati) 30g

Explanation
- *Cang Zhu* (Rhizoma Atractylodis), *Huang Bai* (Cortex Phellodendri) and *Da Fu Pi* (Pericarpium Arecae Catechu) clear Heat and dry Dampness.
- *Dan Shen* (Radix Salviae Miltiorrhizae), *Ze Lan* (Herba Lycopi Lucidi), *Chuan Niu Xi* (Radix Cyathulae Officinalis), *Qing Pi* (Pericarpium Citri Reticulatae Viride), *Dang Gui* (Radix Angelicae Sinensis), and *Chi Xiao Dou* (Semen Phaseoli Calcarati) regulate Qi and harmonize the Blood, transform Blood stasis and free the network vessels.
- *Ren Dong Teng* (Caulis Lonicerae Japonicae), *Pu Gong Ying* (Herba Taraxaci cum Radice) and *Zi Hua Di Ding* (Herba Violae Yedoensitis) clear Heat and relieve Toxicity.
- *Bai Xian Pi* (Cortex Dictamni Dasycarpi Radicis) transforms Dampness and alleviates itching.

CHRONIC STAGE (WIND-DRYNESS DUE TO BLOOD DEFICIENCY)
The disease is of long duration. The skin is dry, rough and lichenified with desquamation and marked pigmentation. Itching of varying intensity occurs. The tongue body is pale red with a scant coating; the pulse is deficient and thready.

Treatment principle
Enrich the Liver and supplement the Kidneys, free the network vessels and alleviate itching.

Prescription
GUI FU BA WEI TANG JIA JIAN
Cinnamon Bark and Aconite Eight-Ingredient Decoction, with modifications

Rou Gui (Cortex Cinnamomi Cassiae) 3g
Gan Jiang (Rhizoma Zingiberis Officinalis) 6g
Shu Di Huang (Radix Rehmanniae Glutinosae Conquita) 10g
Shan Zhu Yu (Fructus Corni Officinalis) 10g
Ze Xie (Rhizoma Alismatis Orientalis) 10g
Fu Ling (Sclerotium Poriae Cocos) 10g
Chuan Xiong (Rhizoma Ligustici Chuanxiong) 4.5g
Yi Yi Ren (Semen Coicis Lachryma-jobi) 30g

Ren Dong Teng (Caulis Lonicerae Japonicae) 30g
Chi Xiao Dou (Semen Phaseoli Calcarati) 30g

Explanation

- *Rou Gui* (Cortex Cinnamomi Cassiae) and *Gan Jiang* (Rhizoma Zingiberis Officinalis) warm Yang and dissipate Cold.
- *Shu Di Huang* (Radix Rehmanniae Glutinosae Conquita) and *Shan Zhu Yu* (Fructus Corni Officinalis) enrich the Kidneys and emolliate the Liver.
- *Ze Xie* (Rhizoma Alismatis Orientalis), *Fu Ling* (Sclerotium Poriae Cocos) and *Yi Yi Ren* (Semen Coicis Lachryma-jobi) clear Heat and benefit the movement of Dampness.
- *Ren Dong Teng* (Caulis Lonicerae Japonicae), *Chi Xiao Dou* (Semen Phaseoli Calcarati) and *Chuan Xiong* (Rhizoma Ligustici Chuanxiong) relieve Toxicity and transform Blood stasis.
- The prescription includes more herbs with the function of enriching Yin and moistening Dryness than with the function of warming Yang and dissipating Cold with the result that Deficient Blood can be supplemented and Wind-Dryness moistened. The disease can then be eliminated.

EXTERNAL TREATMENT

- If there are signs of infection, such as exudation and erosion, apply *Ma Chi Xian Shui Xi Ji* (Purslane Wash Preparation) as a wet compress two or three times a day. After exudation has been controlled, mix *Shi Zhen Fen* (Eczema Powder) into a paste with vegetable oil and apply to the lesions once or twice a day.
- For pruritus with slightly dry skin or desquamation, apply *Shi Zhen Yi Hao Gao* (No. 1 Eczema Paste) or *Qing Dai Gao* (Indigo Paste) once or twice a day.

Clinical notes

- For cases due to infection, try to control the development of the disease as soon as possible and prevent ulceration, otherwise the condition will persist for some time.
- For enduring cases that are difficult to cure, treatment to invigorate the Blood should be supplemented by external treatment of the affected area in order to shorten the duration of the disease.

Advice for the patient

- Most patients with this condition are middle-aged or elderly or have to stand for long periods during the day. While undergoing treatment they should therefore wear compression hosiery or elevate the legs above the level of the rest of the body when recumbent.
- Patients with varicose veins may benefit from vein surgery when the lesions are in the recovery phase.
- Avoid scratching and trauma to prevent recurrence or aggravation of the condition.

Literature excerpt

In *Sheng Ji Zong Lu* [General Collection for Holy Relief], it says: "Where pathogenic Wind-Damp Toxins prevail, they congeal in the Ying and Wei levels, where they are retained. Toxins pour down in the channels and network vessels to the legs between the knees and the feet, resulting in swelling and hardening of the skin, and nodes forming and developing into sores with incessant discharge of pus and fluid. The condition is persistent and recurrent. Since Toxins pour down like water, this gives rise to the name *xia zhu chuang* (pouring downward sore)."

Modern clinical experience

TREATMENT ACCORDING TO PATTERN IDENTIFICATION

Gu proposed internal treatment according to the principle of harmonizing the Ying level, clearing Heat and benefiting the movement of Dampness. [46]

Prescription ingredients

Dan Shen (Radix Salviae Miltiorrhizae) 15g
Ze Lan (Herba Lycopi Lucidi) 10g
Dang Gui (Radix Angelicae Sinensis) 10g
Bai Xian Pi (Cortex Dictamni Dasycarpi Radicis) 15g
Ku Shen (Radix Sophorae Flavescentis) 10g
Cang Zhu (Rhizoma Atractylodis) 10g
Yi Yi Ren (Semen Coicis Lachryma-jobi) 15g
Chi Xiao Dou (Semen Phaseoli Calcarati) 20g
Liu Yi San (Six-To-One Powder) 15g

Modifications

1. For acute cases, he added *Sheng Di Huang* (Radix Rehmanniae Glutinosae), *Chi Shao* (Radix Paeoniae Rubra) and *Di Gu Pi* (Cortex Lycii Radicis).
2. For subacute cases, he added *Tu Fu Ling* (Rhizoma Smilacis Glabrae), *Jiao Bai Zhu* (Rhizoma Atractylodis Macrocephalae, scorch-fried) and *Che Qian Cao* (Herba Plantaginis).
3. For chronic cases, he added *Yi Mu Cao* (Herba Leonuri Heterophylli), *Yu Zhu* (Rhizoma Polygonati Odorati), *Sheng Di Huang* (Radix Rehmanniae Glutinosae), and *Shu Di Huang* (Radix Rehmanniae Glutinosae Conquita).

Lichen simplex chronicus (neurodermatitis)
神经性皮炎

Lichen simplex chronicus (neurodermatitis) is a chronic inflammatory skin disease characterized by paroxysms of pruritus and the development of lichenoid changes of the skin. The disease occurs from repeated scratching or rubbing, either as a habit or in response to stress. There is no underlying dermatological disorder.

In TCM, lichen simplex chronicus is also known as *niu pi xuan* (oxhide tinea) or *she ling chuang* (collar sore).

Clinical manifestations

- This condition tends to occur on the nape of the neck, the wrists, the elbows, the ankles, and the anogenital region. It may also spread to the limbs, the areas around the eyes and the sacrococcygeal region.
- It is more common in adults and is unrelated to season.
- Lesions generally manifest as single or multiple irregular or polygonal-shaped plaques with intermingled slightly elevated red papules. The skin in the affected area is rough with deepened skin creases (lichenification).
- In chronic cases, the lichenified areas become brown (due to hemosiderin deposition) and are covered by fine dry scales.
- There is severe pruritus, which is worse during the night.
- The disease tends be chronic with repeated attacks.

Differential diagnosis

Psoriasis
Psoriasis is usually more widespread than lichen simplex chronicus, involving the extensor aspect of the limbs, especially the extensor aspect of the elbows and knees, and sometimes spreading to affect the whole body. The nails and scalp may also be involved. At the initial stage, bright red or dark red macules, maculopapules or papules appear with a shiny, wax-like surface, coalescing to form well demarcated round or oval plaques ranging from a few millimeters to several centimeters in size. These plaques are subsequently covered by large dry silvery-white laminated scales. If the scales are removed, bleeding points appear (Auspitz's sign). The lesions of psoriasis are usually much less itchy than those of lichen simplex chronicus.

Chronic eczema
This condition often evolves from recurring acute or subacute eczema. Characteristic lesions manifest as dry, rough, thickened, and scaling skin, deepening and widening of the cleavage lines of the skin, and hyperpigmentation or hypopigmentation. Itching may be moderate or intense; repeated scratching or rubbing of the skin often results in obvious lichenification. Although more usual in easily reached areas, chronic eczema tends to be more widespread than lichen simplex chronicus.

Lichen planus
Eruptions usually involve the flexor surfaces of the wrists and forearms, and the lower legs around and above the ankles. Lesions manifest as intensely pruritic 2-10 mm flat-topped dull red shiny papules. The surface of the lesions exhibits a lacy white pattern of lines (Wickham's striae). Lesions that persist, most frequently on the shins, may develop into confluent hypertrophic plaques that can resemble the lesions of lichen simplex chronicus, with a coarse surface covered by scales. Mucous membranes are involved in 40-60% of lichen planus cases.

Etiology and pathology

- Emotional factors such as emotional depression, nervous tension, irritability, and stress can lead to stagnation of Qi, which transforms into Heat and generates Fire. Fire and Heat accumulate and lie latent in the Ying and Xue levels, leading to exuberant Heat in the Blood, which then generates Wind. Exuberant Wind causes Dryness, which manifests as severe itching with dryness and desquamation.
- Enduring Blood-Heat gradually damages Yin and Blood, resulting in insufficiency of Ying Qi (Nutritive Qi) and Blood and impairing movement in the channels and vessels. As a result, the skin and flesh are deprived of normal nourishment so that lesions manifest as thickened and rough plaques. Blood Deficiency may also generate Wind, which causes Dryness, leading to itching and scales.
- If Pathogenic Wind-Damp-Heat invades the exterior and is retained in the flesh and interstices (*cou li*) rather than being dispersed, it can transform into Heat, resulting in exuberant Heat in the Ying and Xue levels. When pathogenic Wind is retained for a

long period in the interstices (*cou li*), it causes disharmony in the channels and vessels. When movement in the channels and vessels is impaired, the disease will become chronic.

- Friction caused by clothing and scratching may also aggravate the disease, causing lichenification.

Pattern identification and treatment

INTERNAL TREATMENT

EXUBERANT WIND DUE TO BLOOD-HEAT

At the initial stage, lesions manifest as slightly elevated flat-topped red papules, which quickly become confluent to form red plaques with well-defined borders. The skin becomes rough, deepened skin creases appear and a thin layer of fine dry scales covers the plaques. Severe itching and excoriation lead to bloody crusts. Accompanying symptoms and signs include restlessness, dry mouth, thirst, and poor sleep. The tongue body is red with a thin yellow coating; the pulse is wiry and slippery or slippery and rapid.

Treatment principle
Clear Heat and cool the Blood, disperse Wind and alleviate itching.

Prescription
XIAO FENG SAN JIA JIAN
Powder for Dispersing Wind, with modifications

Jing Jie (Herba Schizonepetae Tenuifoliae) 6g
Fang Feng (Radix Ledebouriellae Divaricatae) 6g
Ku Shen (Radix Sophorae Flavescentis) 6g
Chao Niu Bang Zi (Fructus Arctii Lappae, stir-fried) 10g
Sheng Di Huang (Radix Rehmanniae Glutinosae) 10g
Dan Shen (Radix Salviae Miltiorrhizae) 10g
Chao Mu Dan Pi (Cortex Moutan Radicis, stir-fried) 10g
Shi Gao‡ (Gypsum Fibrosum) 12g, decocted for 30 minutes before adding the other ingredients
Fu Ling Pi (Cortex Poriae Cocos) 12g
Di Fu Zi (Fructus Kochiae Scopariae) 12g
Bai Xian Pi (Cortex Dictamni Dasycarpi Radicis) 12g

Explanation
- *Jing Jie* (Herba Schizonepetae Tenuifoliae), *Fang Feng* (Radix Ledebouriellae Divaricatae) and *Chao Niu Bang Zi* (Fructus Arctii Lappae, stir-fried) dissipate Wind and alleviate itching.
- *Sheng Di Huang* (Radix Rehmanniae Glutinosae), *Dan Shen* (Radix Salviae Miltiorrhizae) and *Chao Mu Dan Pi* (Cortex Moutan Radicis, stir-fried) cool and invigorate the Blood, moisten the skin and reduce erythema.

- *Shi Gao*‡ (Gypsum Fibrosum) and *Fu Ling Pi* (Cortex Poriae Cocos) clear Heat from the Qi level and reduce fever.
- *Di Fu Zi* (Fructus Kochiae Scopariae), *Bai Xian Pi* (Cortex Dictamni Dasycarpi Radicis) and *Ku Shen* (Radix Sophorae Flavescentis) alleviate itching, relieve Toxicity and dissipate Wind.

BLOOD-DRYNESS DUE TO YIN DEFICIENCY

Lesions, which may be multiple, manifest as pale red or grayish-white thick dry plaques with a rough surface covered by dry scales. The skin is lichenified. There is severe itching, which is worse during the night and disturbs sleep. This is a chronic condition with lesions that resist treatment or recur after remission. The tongue body is red with a scant coating; the pulse is deficient and thready.

Treatment principle
Nourish Yin, moisten the skin, extinguish Wind, and alleviate itching.

Prescription
SI WU RUN FU TANG JIA JIAN
Four Agents Decoction for Moistening the Skin, with modifications

Dang Gui (Radix Angelicae Sinensis) 10g
Hei Zhi Ma (Semen Sesami Indici) 10g
Qin Jiao (Radix Gentianae Macrophyllae) 10g
Chao Bai Shao (Radix Paeoniae Lactiflorae, stir-fried) 12g
Gan Di Huang (Radix Rehmanniae Glutinosae Exsiccata) 12g
He Shou Wu (Radix Polygoni Multiflori) 12g
Gou Teng (Ramulus Uncariae cum Uncis) 12g
Dai Zhe Shi‡ (Haematitum) 15g, decocted for 30 minutes before adding the other ingredients
Zhen Zhu Mu‡ (Concha Margaritifera) 15g
Nan Sha Shen (Radix Adenophorae) 15g
Suan Zao Ren (Semen Ziziphi Spinosae) 6g
Shan Yao (Radix Dioscoreae Oppositae) 30g

Explanation
- *Dang Gui* (Radix Angelicae Sinensis), *Chao Bai Shao* (Radix Paeoniae Lactiflorae, stir-fried), *Gan Di Huang* (Radix Rehmanniae Glutinosae Exsiccata), and *He Shou Wu* (Radix Polygoni Multiflori) nourish the Blood and moisten Dryness.
- *Hei Zhi Ma* (Semen Sesami Indici), *Nan Sha Shen* (Radix Adenophorae) and *Shan Yao* (Radix Dioscoreae Oppositae) enrich Yin and moisten Dryness.
- *Gou Teng* (Ramulus Uncariae cum Uncis) and *Qin Jiao* (Radix Gentianae Macrophyllae) extinguish Wind and alleviate itching.
- *Dai Zhe Shi*‡ (Haematitum), *Zhen Zhu Mu*‡ (Concha Margaritifera) and *Suan Zao Ren* (Semen Ziziphi

Spinosae) calm the Liver, extinguish Wind and quiet the Spirit to strengthen the effect in alleviating itching.

ACCUMULATION OF WIND-DAMP

In this chronic pattern which responds poorly to treatment, lesions manifest as thickened, infiltrative, lichenified plaques resembling the skin on the neck of an ox (hence one of the names for this condition in Chinese – *niu pi xuan*, or oxhide tinea). Local itching is intense. The tongue body is red or crimson with a scant coating. The pulse is deep and rough.

Treatment principle

Arrest Wind, transform Dampness, clear Heat, and alleviate itching.

Prescription

WU SHE QU FENG TANG JIA JIAN

Black-Tail Snake Decoction for Expelling Wind, with modifications

Wu Shao She ‡ (Zaocys Dhumnades) 10g
Jing Jie (Herba Schizonepetae Tenuifoliae) 10g
Huang Qin (Radix Scutellariae Baicalensis) 10g
Qiang Huo (Rhizoma et Radix Notopterygii) 10g
Fang Feng (Radix Ledebouriellae Divaricatae) 12g
Lian Qiao (Fructus Forsythiae Suspensae) 12g
Jin Yin Hua (Flos Lonicerae) 12g
Chan Tui ‡ (Periostracum Cicadae) 6g
Gan Cao (Radix Glycyrrhizae) 6g
Ku Shen (Radix Sophorae Flavescentis) 4.5g
Xu Chang Qing (Radix Cynanchi Paniculati) 30g
Chi Xiao Dou (Semen Phaseoli Calcarati) 30g

Explanation

- *Wu Shao She* ‡ (Zaocys Dhumnades), *Jing Jie* (Herba Schizonepetae Tenuifoliae), *Qiang Huo* (Rhizoma et Radix Notopterygii), *Fang Feng* (Radix Ledebouriellae Divaricatae), *Chan Tui* ‡ (Periostracum Cicadae), *Ku Shen* (Radix Sophorae Flavescentis), and *Xu Chang Qing* (Radix Cynanchi Paniculati) dissipate Wind and dispel Dampness, and arrest Wind to alleviate itching.

- *Huang Qin* (Radix Scutellariae Baicalensis), *Lian Qiao* (Fructus Forsythiae Suspensae), *Jin Yin Hua* (Flos Lonicerae), *Gan Cao* (Radix Glycyrrhizae), and *Chi Xiao Dou* (Semen Phaseoli Calcarati) clear Heat and relieve Toxicity, invigorate the Blood and reduce eruptions.

General modifications

1. For tension, irritability or sudden outbursts of anger, add *Mu Li* ‡ (Concha Ostreae), *Long Gu* ‡ (Os Draconis), *He Huan Pi* (Cortex Albizziae Julibrissin), *Wu Wei Zi* (Fructus Schisandrae Chinensis), and *Ye Jiao Teng* (Caulis Polygoni Multiflori).

2. For gastrointestinal dysfunction, add *Chao Zhi Ke* (Fructus Citri Aurantii, stir-fried), *Bai Zhu* (Rhizoma Atractylodis Macrocephalae) and *Chen Pi* (Pericarpium Citri Reticulatae).

3. For menstrual irregularities, add *Yi Mu Cao* (Herba Leonuri Heterophylli), *Wu Yao* (Radix Linderae Strychnifoliae), *Zhi Xiang Fu* (Rhizoma Cyperi Rotundi, processed), and *Yue Ji Hua* (Flos et Fructus Rosae Chinensis).

4. For thickened skin with deep crease lines, add *Chi Shi Zhi* ‡ (Halloysitum Rubrum), *Jiu Zhi Da Huang* (Radix et Rhizoma Rhei, processed with alcohol), *Tao Ren* (Semen Persicae), *Cang Zhu* (Rhizoma Atractylodis), and *Chuan Shan Jia** (Squama Manitis Pentadactylae).

5. For predominance of Wind-Heat, add *Fu Ping* (Herba Lemnae seu Spirodelae) and *Chan Tui* ‡ (Periostracum Cicadae).

6. For predominance of Cold-Damp, add *Yi Yi Ren* (Semen Coicis Lachryma-jobi), *Wei Ling Xian* (Radix Clematidis) and *Ma Huang** (Herba Ephedrae).

7. For predominance of Wind Toxins, add *Cang Er Zi* (Fructus Xanthii Sibirici), *Quan Xie* ‡ (Buthus Martensi) or *Gou Teng* (Ramulus Uncariae cum Uncis), and *Wu Shao She* ‡ (Zaocys Dhumnades).

8. For insomnia, add *Bai Zi Ren* (Semen Biotae Orientalis), *Yuan Zhi* (Radix Polygalae Tenuifoliae) and *Hu Po* ‡ (Succinum).

EXTERNAL TREATMENT

- For circumscribed lesions with severe itching, apply *Bai Bu Ding* (Stemona Root Tincture), *Ban Mao Cu Jin Ji* (Mylabris Vinegar Steep Preparation) or *Qing Liang Gao* (Cool Clearing Paste) twice a day.

- For thin lesions, apply *Huang Lian Ruan Gao* (Coptis Ointment) twice a day.

- For thickened lesions, apply *Hei Dou Liu You Ruan Gao* (Black Soybean and Vaseline® Ointment) twice a day.

- For disseminated lesions, apply *Cang Wu Cuo Yao* (Xanthium and Clamshell Massage Preparation); see Appendix 5 for details.

- Zhao Bingnan suggested the following fumigation method:

Prescription ingredients

Cang Zhu (Rhizoma Atractylodis) 9g
Ku Shen (Radix Sophorae Flavescentis) 9g
Huang Bai (Cortex Phellodendri) 9g
Fang Feng (Radix Ledebouriellae Divaricatae) 9g
Da Feng Zi (Semen Hydnocarpi) 30g
Bai Xian Pi (Cortex Dictamni Dasycarpi Radicis) 30g
Song Xiang (Resina Pini) 12g
He Shi (Fructus Carpesii) 12g
Wu Bei Zi ‡ (Galla Rhois Chinensis) 15g

Grind the ingredients into a powder and roll up in a piece of thick paper. Light the roll and fume the affected areas for 15-30 minutes, once or twice a day. The heat produced by the burning roll should be adjusted according to the patient's tolerance level.

ACUPUNCTURE

Empirical points

Main points: LI-11 Quchi and SP-10 Xuehai.

Auxiliary points: LI-4 Hegu, SP-6 Sanyinjiao and Ashi points (lesion sites).

Technique: Apply the even method. Retain the needles for 30 minutes after obtaining Qi. Treat once a day. A course consists of ten treatment sessions.

Indications: This method is used for localized lichen simplex chronicus (neurodermatitis).

Selection of points on the affected channels

Points: GB-20 Fengchi, BL-10 Tianzhu, GV-16 Fengfu, GV-15 Yamen, GV-14 Dazhui, LI-11 Quchi, PC-6 Neiguan, LI-4 Hegu, BL-40 Weizhong, ST-36 Zusanli, and SP-10 Xuehai.

Technique: Select five or six of the points and apply the reducing method. Retain the needles for 30 minutes after obtaining Qi. Treat once a day. A course consists of ten treatment sessions.

Indications: This method is used for disseminated lichen simplex chronicus (neurodermatitis).

Explanation

- LI-11 Quchi, LI-4 Hegu, GV-14 Dazhui, GV-16 Fengfu, GB-20 Fengchi, and BL-10 Tianzhu dissipate Wind and alleviate itching.
- SP-10 Xuehai, SP-6 Sanyinjiao and ST-36 Zusanli nourish the Blood and moisten Dryness.
- GV-15 Yamen, PC-6 Neiguan and BL-10 Xuehai quiet the Spirit and settle the Mind.
- BL-40 Weizhong drains Heat and relieves Toxicity.

MOXIBUSTION

Direct moxibustion

Points: Ashi points (the site of the lesions).

Technique

- *Moxa cones:* Place five to seven moxa cones around the Ashi points relatively equidistant from each other and burn.
- *Moxa sticks:* Hold an ignited moxa stick over the area of the lesions, adjusting the temperature according to the patient's tolerance level.

Indirect moxibustion with moxa cones

Points: Ashi points (the site of the lesions).

Technique: Position a slice of fresh ginger or garlic over each of the Ashi points. Place the moxa cones on top of the slices and burn three to five cones at each point. Treat once a day. A course consists of ten treatment sessions.

ENCIRCLEMENT NEEDLING

Points: Ashi points (the site of the lesions).

Technique: Insert 1 cun filiform needles obliquely above, below and to the left and right of the Ashi points (four needles in total). Retain for 30 minutes after obtaining Qi. Treat once every other day. A course consists of five treatment sessions.

Indications: This method is used for localized lichen simplex chronicus (neurodermatitis).

ENCIRCLEMENT NEEDLING WITH ELECTRO-ACUPUNCTURE

Points: Ashi points (the site of the lesions).

Technique: Insert 1 cun filiform needles obliquely above, below and to the left and right of the Ashi points with their tips all directed toward the center of the lesions (four needles in total). Adjust the frequency according to the patient's tolerance level. Retain the needles for 15-30 minutes. Treat once a day or every other day. A course consists of ten treatment sessions.

Clinical notes

- Combining internal and external treatments is recommended for best results. Internal medications should be prescribed according to syndrome differentiation. External medications should differ according to whether the lesions are localized or disseminated. Acupuncture and moxibustion have a good effect in quieting the Spirit and alleviating itching.

- Where the condition is caused by emotional factors, treatment should focus more on nourishing the Blood and quieting the Spirit, or on settling fright and quieting the Spirit. For recurrent dry and scaly skin, the treatment principle should focus more on invigorating the Blood and transforming Blood stasis.

- To consolidate the improvement, continue with internal treatment for one or two months even when the lesions are resolving and itching has subsided, otherwise relapse is possible.

Advice for the patient

- Emotional factors play an important part in the etiology of this disease, and so avoiding mental stress is essential; patients may have to be prepared to alter their lifestyle to achieve this.

- Physical abrasions can trigger the condition, and so avoiding mechanical and physical irritants is important.
- Dietary factors can aggravate any skin condition, hence spicy food and overindulgence in coffee, strong tea or alcohol should be avoided.

Case histories

Case 1

Patient
Female, aged 42.

Clinical manifestations
The patient had experienced itchiness on the nape of the neck for six months. The itching, which was severe at night, had gradually spread to the bilateral antecubital and popliteal fossae and the leg. The skin had become rough and thickened. Accompanying symptoms and signs included irritability and irascibility, restless sleep, a bitter taste in the mouth, dry throat, and menstrual irregularities.

Examination revealed thickened, scaly, dark red, hyperpigmented plaques on the nape of the neck, the antecubital and popliteal fossae and the extensor aspect of the leg with obvious ridges and without clear margins. Rubbing and scratch marks were evident. The tongue body was red at the margins and tip with a slightly yellow coating; the pulse was wiry and slippery.

Pattern identification
Constrained Liver Qi combined with external contraction of pathogenic Wind leading to enduring Depression transforming into Fire.

Treatment principle
Soothe the Liver and regulate Qi, clear Heat and dissipate Wind.

Prescription ingredients
Chai Hu (Radix Bupleuri) 10g
Zhi Ke (Fructus Citri Aurantii) 10g
Long Dan Cao (Radix Gentianae Scabrae) 10g
Zhi Zi (Fructus Gardeniae Jasminoidis) 10g
Sheng Di Huang (Radix Rehmanniae Glutinosae) 15g
Mu Dan Pi (Cortex Moutan Radicis) 10g
Chi Shao (Radix Paeoniae Rubra) 10g
Bai Shao (Radix Paeoniae Lactiflorae) 10g
Dang Gui (Radix Angelicae Sinensis) 10g
Ye Jiao Teng (Caulis Polygoni Multiflori) 30g
Gou Teng (Ramulus Uncariae cum Uncis) 10g
Fang Feng (Radix Ledebouriellae Divaricatae) 10g

One bag a day was used to prepare a decoction, taken twice a day.

External treatment
Xiong Huang Jie Du San Ding Ji (Realgar Powder Tincture Preparation for Relieving Toxicity)[vii] was applied to the affected areas twice a day.

Second visit
After seven bags of the decoction, itching was reduced and the patient was less irritable. The prescription was modified by removing *Long Dan Cao* (Radix Gentianae Scabrae), *Zhi Zi* (Fructus Gardeniae Jasminoidis) and *Gou Teng* (Ramulus Uncariae cum Uncis) and adding *Quan Xie*‡ (Buthus Martensi) 6g, *Zao Jiao Ci* (Spina Gleditsiae Sinensis) 6g, *Xu Chang Qing* (Radix Cynanchi Paniculati) 15g, and *Bai Ji Li* (Fructus Tribuli Terrestris) 30g.

External treatment
Tao Ye Xi Ji (Paper Mulberry Leaf Wash Preparation) was prescribed to wash the affected areas for 15 minutes once a day.

Outcome
After 14 bags of the modified decoction, itching had stopped and the lesions had resolved.

Discussion
Zhang Zhili considers that emotional and mental factors are a major cause of this disease among women in modern society. Generalized itching and dark red skin lesions arise because of emotional problems and Depression binding Liver Qi. If these factors are complicated by external contraction of pathogenic Wind, enduring Depression transforms into Fire, which attacks the skin and flesh to cause the condition.

Irritability, irascibility, a bitter taste in the mouth, and a dry throat are caused by Liver-Fire flaming upward and menstrual irregularities result from impairment of the Liver's dredging and drainage function and inhibition of the functional activities of Qi.

Chai Hu (Radix Bupleuri) and *Zhi Ke* (Fructus Citri Aurantii) soothe the Liver and regulate Qi; *Long Dan Cao* (Radix Gentianae Scabrae) and *Zhi Zi* (Fructus Gardeniae Jasminoidis) clear and drain Liver-Fire; *Sheng Di Huang* (Radix Rehmanniae Glutinosae) and *Mu Dan Pi* (Cortex Moutan Radicis) cool the Blood and clear Heat; *Dang Gui* (Radix Angelicae Sinensis), *Chi Shao* (Radix Paeoniae Rubra), *Bai Shao* (Radix Paeoniae Lactiflorae), *Ye Jiao Teng* (Caulis Polygoni Multiflori), and *Gou Teng* (Ramulus Uncariae cum Uncis) nourish and invigorate the Blood and extinguish Wind to alleviate itching; and *Fang Feng* (Radix Ledebouriellae Divaricatae) dissipates Wind to alleviate itching.

After repressing Liver-Fire, *Dang Gui* (Radix Angelicae Sinensis), *Sheng Di Huang* (Radix Rehmanniae Glutinosae), *Chi Shao* (Radix Paeoniae Rubra), *Bai Shao* (Radix Paeoniae Lactiflorae), and *Mu Dan Pi* (Cortex Moutan Radicis) nourish the Blood and emolliate the Liver to treat the Root. The combination of *Quan Xie*‡ (Buthus Martensi), *Xu Chang Qing* (Radix Cynanchi Paniculati), *Bai Ji Li* (Fructus Tribuli Terrestris), and *Zao Jiao Ci* (Spina Gleditsiae Sinensis) nourishes the Blood and expels Wind to alleviate itching while dispelling any residual Wind in the Blood. [47]

---

vii In those countries where the use of *Xiong Huang* (Realgar) is not permitted, *Bai Bu Ding* (Stemona Tincture) can be substituted.

Case 2
Patient
Male, aged 45.

Clinical manifestations
The patient had been suffering from intermittent recurrent itching in the nape of the neck for three years. Itching was worse at night and made it difficult for him to fall asleep. The patient had been given injections of calcium gluconate and steroid creams for external use before coming to the TCM hospital. His condition was still not under control.

Examination revealed an elliptical lesion 4 x 6 cm on the nape of the neck with obvious ridges, lichenification, excoriations, and crusting. The tongue body was pale with a thin white coating; the pulse was soggy and moderate.

Pattern identification
Accumulation and obstruction of Wind-Damp causing lack of nourishment of the skin and flesh.

Treatment principle
Dispel Wind and benefit the movement of Dampness, nourish the Blood and moisten the skin.

Prescription ingredients
*Tian Ma** (Rhizoma Gastrodiae Elatae) 6g
Gou Teng (Ramulus Uncariae cum Uncis) 6g
Fang Feng (Radix Ledebouriellae Divaricatae) 10g
Fu Ping (Herba Spirodelae Polyrrhizae) 6g
Bai Ji Li (Fructus Tribuli Terrestris) 15g
Ku Shen (Radix Sophorae Flavescentis) 15g
Bai Xian Pi (Cortex Dictamni Dasycarpi Radicis) 15g
Qin Jiao (Radix Gentianae Macrophyllae) 15g
Di Fu Zi (Fructus Kochiae Scopariae) 15g
Dang Gui (Radix Angelicae Sinensis) 10g
Ye Jiao Teng (Caulis Polygoni Multiflori) 30g
Sheng Di Huang (Radix Rehmanniae Glutinosae) 15g

One bag a day was used to prepare a decoction, taken twice a day.

External treatment
Zhi Yang Gao (Paste for Alleviating Itching) was applied to the affected area in the morning, 5% *Hei Dou Liu You Ruan Gao* (Black Soybean and Vaseline® Ointment) in the evening.

Second visit
After seven bags of the decoction, itching was significantly alleviated and the lesion had become thinner. The prescription was modified by replacing *Sheng Di Huang* (Radix Rehmanniae Glutinosae) by *Shu Di Huang* (Radix Rehmanniae Glutinosae Conquita) 10g. External treatment continued as before.

Outcome
After another 14 bags of the decoction, the lesion disappeared completely.

Discussion
Lichen simplex chronicus in this patient was caused by accumulation and obstruction of Wind-Damp and lack of nourishment of the skin and flesh due to pathogenic Wind settling in the skin and flesh. Retention of pathogenic Wind in the skin and flesh over time consumes and damages Yin and Blood, leading to lack of nourishment of the skin and flesh and resulting in a condition that is generally slow to respond to treatment.

This case was based on the principle of treating Wind to treat the Blood. By nourishing the Blood and moistening the skin, Wind is eliminated automatically by moving the Blood. *Quan Chong Fang* (Scorpion Formula), modified here and consisting of *Tian Ma** (Rhizoma Gastrodiae Elatae), *Gou Teng* (Ramulus Uncariae cum Uncis), *Bai Ji Li* (Fructus Tribuli Terrestris), *Ku Shen* (Radix Sophorae Flavescentis), and *Bai Xian Pi* (Cortex Dictamni Dasycarpi Radicis), is the core of the treatment; when combined with *Dang Gui* (Radix Angelicae Sinensis), *Ye Jiao Teng* (Caulis Polygoni Multiflori) and *Sheng Di Huang* (Radix Rehmanniae Glutinosae), it nourishes the Blood and moistens the skin. *Fang Feng* (Radix Ledebouriellae Divaricatae), *Qin Jiao* (Radix Gentianae Macrophyllae) and *Di Fu Zi* (Fructus Kochiae Scopariae) dissipate Wind to alleviate itching, and *Fu Ping* (Herba Spirodelae Polyrrhizae) expels Wind and eliminates Dampness to alleviate itching. After achieving a satisfactory effect on the first visit, *Sheng Di Huang* (Radix Rehmanniae Glutinosae) was replaced by *Shu Di Huang* (Radix Rehmanniae Glutinosae Conquita) to strengthen the effect in nourishing the Blood. [48]

Case 3
Patient
Male, aged 64.

Clinical manifestations
The patient was suffering from itching that had gradually worsened over the previous four years and had spread from the nape of the neck to the back of the shoulders. Itching was severe and unrelenting. The conditioned had intensified in the past month due to overwork and insomnia. Unbearable generalized itching had made it difficult to sleep at all during the night.

Examination revealed a thickened and lichenified lesion 8 x 4 cm on the nape of the neck and smaller lesions on the trunk and the extensor aspects of the limbs; lesions had a rough surface with obvious ridges. The local skin was pigmented with excoriations and crusting. The tongue body was pale red with a white coating; the pulse was thready and moderate.

Pattern identification
Wind-Dryness due to Blood Deficiency, leading to lack of nourishment of the skin and flesh.

Treatment principle
Nourish the Blood and dredge Wind, moisten the skin and alleviate itching.

Prescription ingredients
Dang Gui (Radix Angelicae Sinensis) 10g
Chuan Xiong (Rhizoma Ligustici Chuanxiong) 10g
Chi Shao (Radix Paeoniae Rubra) 10g
Bai Shao (Radix Paeoniae Lactiflorae) 10g
Ye Jiao Teng (Caulis Polygoni Multiflori) 30g
Ji Xue Teng (Caulis Spatholobi) 15g

Bai Ji Li (Fructus Tribuli Terrestris) 30g
Hong Hua (Flos Carthami Tinctorii) 10g
Ku Shen (Radix Sophorae Flavescentis) 15g
Bai Xian Pi (Cortex Dictamni Dasycarpi Radicis) 30g
Fang Feng (Radix Ledebouriellae Divaricatae) 10g
Fu Ping (Herba Spirodelae Polyrrhizae) 10g
Quan Xie ‡ (Buthus Martensi) 6g

One bag a day was used to prepare a decoction, taken twice a day.

External treatment
Bai Bu Ding (Stemona Root Tincture) 60ml was applied to the affected areas twice a day.

Second visit
After seven bags of the decoction, itching and excoriations were significantly reduced but sleep was still poor. The prescription was modified by removing *Fang Feng* (Radix Ledebouriellae Divaricatae) and *Fu Ping* (Herba Spirodelae Polyrrhizae) and adding *Zhen Zhu Mu* ‡ (Concha Margaritifera) 30g and *Chao Suan Zao Ren* (Semen Ziziphi Spinosae, stir-fried) 15g.

Third visit
After another 14 bags of the decoction, the itching was alleviated and sleep significantly improved; excoriations continued to decrease. The patient was told to continue with the prescription for another 14 bags. External treatment was changed to 5% *Hei Dou Liu You Ruan Gao* (Black Soybean and Vaseline® Ointment) and 10% urea ointment applied alternately to the affected areas.

Outcome
After two weeks, the lesions had disappeared leaving slight pigmentation.

Discussion
Older patients often have a weak constitution and insufficiency of the Heart and Spleen. Insufficiency of Heart-Blood causes Blood Deficiency and Wind-Dryness, resulting in lack of nourishment of the skin and flesh. *Dang Gui* (Radix Angelicae Sinensis), *Chuan Xiong* (Rhizoma Ligustici Chuanxiong), *Bai Ji Li* (Semen Sinapis Albae), *Chi Shao* (Radix Paeoniae Rubra), and *Bai Shao* (Radix Paeoniae Lactiflorae) nourish the Blood and moisten the skin; *Ye Jiao Teng* (Caulis Polygoni Multiflori), *Zhen Zhu Mu* ‡ (Concha Margaritifera) and *Chao Suan Zao Ren* (Semen Ziziphi Spinosae, stir-fried) nourish the Blood, boost the Heart and quiet the Spirit to alleviate itching; *Ji Xue Teng* (Caulis Spatholobi) and *Hong Hua* (Flos Carthami Tinctorii) nourish and invigorate the Blood and moisten Dryness; *Fang Feng* (Radix Ledebouriellae Divaricatae), *Bai Xian Pi* (Cortex Dictamni Dasycarpi Radicis), *Fu Ping* (Herba Spirodelae Polyrrhizae), *Ku Shen* (Radix Sophorae Flavescentis), and *Quan Xie* ‡ (Buthus Martensi) expel Wind and eliminate Dampness to alleviate itching. The overall prescription was formulated to nourish the Blood and moisten the skin, expel Wind and eliminate Dampness to alleviate itching and achieved a satisfactory effect in the treatment of this obstinate disease. [49]

Literature excerpt

In *Wai Ke Zheng Zong* [An Orthodox Manual of External Diseases], it says: "Persistent tinea is often due to Wind, Heat, Dampness, and Worms… *Niu pi xuan* (oxhide tinea) resembles hard thick oxhide, and feels like a rotten log. This disease occurs because of Blood-Dryness and Wind Toxins and involves the Spleen and Lung Channels. Treat initially with *Xiao Feng San* (Powder for Dispersing Wind) with the addition of *Fu Ping* (Herba Spirodelae Polyrrhizae) 30g. Meanwhile, the juice extracted from *Cong Bai* (Bulbus Allii Fistulosi) and *Dan Dou Chi* (Semen Sojae Praeparatum) is used to guide the ingredients to the exterior through their dispersing function. For chronic conditions, treat with *Shou Wu Wan* (Fleeceflower Root Pill) and *La Fan Wan* (Wax and Alum Pill) and external application of *Tu Da Huang Gao* (Madaio Dock Root Paste) and *Tu Jin Pi San* (Golden Larch Bark Powder). The condition resolves slowly."

Modern clinical experience

Internal treatment is the main treatment for the disseminated type of lichen simplex chronicus, whereas external treatment is suggested for the localized type.

INTERNAL TREATMENT
Chen treated lichen simplex chronicus patterns of exuberant Wind due to Blood Deficiency. [50]

Prescription
YANG XUE QU FENG TANG
Decoction for Nourishing the Blood and Dispelling Wind

Sheng Di Huang (Radix Rehmanniae Glutinosae) 20g
Dan Shen (Radix Salviae Miltiorrhizae) 20g
Mu Dan Pi (Cortex Moutan Radicis) 10g
Bai Xian Pi (Cortex Dictamni Dasycarpi Radicis) 10g
Xi Xian Cao (Herba Siegesbeckiae) 10g
Dang Gui (Radix Angelicae Sinensis) 10g
Wei Ling Xian (Radix Clematidis) 10g
Gou Teng (Ramulus Uncariae cum Uncis) 10g
Ji Xue Teng (Caulis Spatholobi) 15g
Ye Jiao Teng (Caulis Polygoni Multiflori) 15g
He Shou Wu (Radix Polygoni Multiflori) 15g
Di Fu Zi (Fructus Kochiae Scopariae) 12g

One bag a day was used to prepare a decoction, taken twice a day. Results were obtained within two weeks where this prescription proved effective.

COMBINED INTERNAL AND EXTERNAL TREATMENT
Lu treated the condition internally and externally. [51]

Internal treatment prescription

Dang Gui (Radix Angelicae Sinensis) 10g

Chi Shao (Radix Paeoniae Rubra) 10g

Chuan Xiong (Rhizoma Ligustici Chuanxiong) 10g

Niu Xi (Radix Achyranthis Bidentatae) 10g

Sheng Di Huang (Radix Rehmanniae Glutinosae) 30g

Shu Di Huang (Radix Rehmanniae Glutinosae Conquita) 30g

Dan Shen (Radix Salviae Miltiorrhizae) 30g

Yi Yi Ren (Semen Coicis Lachryma-jobi) 30g

Bai Xian Pi (Cortex Dictamni Dasycarpi Radicis) 15g

One bag a day was used to prepare a decoction, taken twice a day. A course of treatment lasted ten days.

External treatment prescription

Lu Lu Tong (Fructus Liquidambaris) 30g

Xiang Fu (Rhizoma Cyperi Rotundi) 30g

Wu Zhu Yu (Fructus Evodiae Rutaecarpae) 15g

Mu Zei (Herba Equiseti Hiemalis) 10g

A decoction of these ingredients was used to steam and wash the affected area. Results were seen after two courses.

EXTERNAL TREATMENT

1. **Zhang** prescribed external application of *Di Tai Cha Ji* (Anti-Lichen Rub Preparation). [52]

Prescription ingredients

*Ma Qian Zi** (Semen Nux-Vomicae) 3g

*Sheng Cao Wu** (Radix Aconiti Kusnezoffii Cruda) 3g

Wu Bei Zi‡ (Galla Rhois Chinensis) 3g

*Xi Xin** (Herba cum Radice Asari) 3g

Huang Bai (Cortex Phellodendri) 6g

Ban Xia (Rhizoma Pinelliae Ternatae) 6g

Tian Nan Xing (Rhizoma Arisaematis) 6g

The ingredients were ground into a fine powder and soaked in 30 percent Cresol and Soap Solution 150ml, 95 percent alcohol 50ml and castor oil 20ml for five days. The medication was then applied externally directly on the lesions with gauze or cotton buds, three to four times a day for seven days.

2. **Wang** steeped *Zi Cao* (Radix Arnebiae seu Lithospermi) in *Xiang You* (Oleum Sesami Seminis) in a ratio of 1:2 for 15 days. The oil was then filtered and used externally on lesions three to six times a day. After one month of treatment, paroxysmal itching was relieved and plaques and lichenification were reduced. After two to two and half months of treatment, the skin in the affected area returned to normal and itching disappeared. The medication proved effective for lesions in the nape of the neck and the anogenital region. No recurrence was reported in follow-up visits between six months and four years. [53]

COMBINED TCM AND WESTERN MEDICINE TREATMENT

Chen combined TCM and Western medicine in the treatment of lichen simplex chronicus. [54]

TCM prescription ingredients

Jing Jie (Herba Schizonepetae Tenuifoliae) 9g

Fang Feng (Radix Ledebouriellae Divaricatae) 9g

Zhi Zi (Fructus Gardeniae Jasminoidis) 6g

Ku Shen (Radix Sophorae Flavescentis) 6g

Dang Gui (Radix Angelicae Sinensis) 9g

Mu Dan Pi (Cortex Moutan Radicis) 9g

Ci Shi‡ (Magnetitum) 15g

Mu Li‡ (Concha Ostreae) 15g

Gan Cao (Radix Glycyrrhizae) 3g

One bag a day was used to prepare a decoction, taken twice a day.

Western medicine

Beclometasone dipropionate ointment was applied externally.[viii] Results were seen between 10 and 20 days. Recurrence affected 10 percent of patients after treatment was ended.

SEVEN-STAR NEEDLING COMBINED WITH MOXIBUSTION

Ma reported on treatment of the condition with a seven-star needle, preferring it to the encirclement needling method. After routine disinfection of the affected area, he tapped heavily but slowly from the peripheral area of the lesions to the center until the skin reddened and there was slight bleeding. He removed the blood with a cotton ball, ignited a pure moxa stick and circled the area about 2cm above the lesions for 10-15 minutes. Treatment was given once every other day. Results were seen after 10 sessions. [55]

---

viii This medicine is a prescription drug and can only be prescribed by registered doctors.

Diaper dermatitis (nappy rash)
尿布皮炎

Diaper dermatitis is a cutaneous inflammation within the diaper (nappy) area, usually due to chemical irritation (ammoniacal dermatitis), often complicated by candidal infection. Ammoniacal dermatitis is caused by the skin being in prolonged contact with wet, soiled diapers, with bacteria in the stool reacting with the urine to form irritant ammonia. The use of disposable super-absorbent diapers has helped to reduce the incidence of this condition in recent years.

In TCM, diaper dermatitis is also known as *yan kao chuang* (buttock-submerging sore).

Clinical manifestations

- Skin lesions occur in the diaper area, mainly the genital region, the buttocks, the perineum, and the medial aspect of the thigh. The skin folds are spared.
- Lesions, which coincide with the diaper area, initially manifest as moist glazed erythema with clearly-defined borders. Papules, vesicles and erosion occur subsequently; in severe cases, superficial ulceration may be present.
- Secondary infection with *Candida albicans* is common, manifesting as erythematous papules or pustules.
- Some babies may be restless and cry a great deal due to pain and general discomfort; other symptoms can include fever and lack of appetite.

Differential diagnosis

Intertrigo
This disease is common in babies. Skin lesions, usually located in the skin folds, manifest as erythema with distinct margins, erosion and exudation. Satellite candidal lesions are often present outside the main distribution of lesions.

Infantile seborrheic eczema
This condition occurs in babies shortly after birth and affects the skin folds including the groin as well as the scalp and neck. Flexural lesions manifest as moist, clearly demarcated erythema. Itching is present, but not pronounced.

Etiology and pathology

- A baby's skin is delicate and tender. If the diaper is not changed promptly after defecation or urination, the feces and urine will produce foul, turbid Damp-Heat, which will attack the skin and cause diaper dermatitis.
- The disease may also result from wearing diapers that have not been dried properly after washing. As a result, Fire pathogenic factors may not have been completely eliminated and Wind and Heat may combine to irritate the skin.

Pattern identification and treatment

INTERNAL TREATMENT

ACCUMULATION OF DAMP-HEAT
The affected area is red and swollen with 1-2 mm papules and vesicles, and some erosion and exudation. Accompanying symptoms and signs include persistent crying, restlessness, constipation, reddish urine, and mouth and tongue ulcers. The tongue body is red with a yellow coating; the pulse is soggy and rapid.

Treatment principle
Clear Heat and benefit the movement of Dampness, cool the Blood and relieve Toxicity.

Prescription
DAO CHI SAN JIA JIAN
Powder for Guiding Out Reddish Urine, with modifications

Sheng Di Huang (Radix Rehmanniae Glutinosae) 10g
Tong Cao (Medulla Tetrapanacis Papyriferi) 2g
Zhi Zi (Fructus Gardeniae Jasminoidis) 6g
Chuan Niu Xi (Radix Cyathulae Officinalis) 6g
Jin Yin Hua (Flos Lonicerae) 6g
Lian Qiao (Fructus Forsythiae Suspensae) 6g
Chi Shao (Radix Paeoniae Rubra) 3g
Huang Bai (Cortex Phellodendri) 3g
Deng Xin Cao (Medulla Junci Effusi) 5g
Bai Mao Gen (Rhizoma Imperatae Cylindricae) 12g

Explanation
- *Sheng Di Huang* (Radix Rehmanniae Glutinosae), *Tong Cao* (Medulla Tetrapanacis Papyriferi), *Zhi Zi* (Fructus Gardeniae Jasminoidis), *Deng Xin Cao* (Medulla Junci Effusi), and *Bai Mao Gen* (Rhizoma Imperatae Cylindricae) clear Heat from the Heart and guide out reddish urine, cool the Blood and reduce erythema.
- *Chuan Niu Xi* (Radix Cyathulae Officinalis), *Jin Yin Hua* (Flos Lonicerae), *Lian Qiao* (Fructus Forsythiae Suspensae), *Chi Shao* (Radix Paeoniae Rubra), and

Huang Bai (Cortex Phellodendri) transform Dampness and relieve Toxicity, disperse swelling and alleviate pain.

INFECTION BY TOXINS

Maceration occurs when the wet diaper is left in place for a long time. This gradually results in papulovesicles, pustules and erosion appearing in the affected area, possibly with superficial ulceration in severe cases. There is a sensation of burning heat and stabbing pain. Accompanying symptoms include fever and constipation. The tongue body is red with a scant coating; the pulse is rapid.

Treatment principle

Clear Heat and benefit the movement of Dampness, relieve Toxicity and alleviate pain.

Prescription
YIN HUA GAN CAO TANG JIA JIAN
Honeysuckle and Licorice Decoction, with modifications

Jin Yin Hua (Flos Lonicerae) 12g
Ye Ju Hua (Flos Chrysanthemi Indici) 12g
Yi Yi Ren (Semen Coicis Lachryma-jobi) 12g
Gan Cao (Radix Glycyrrhizae) 6g
Chao Long Dan Cao (Radix Gentianae Scabrae, stir-fried) 6g
Chi Fu Ling (Sclerotium Poriae Cocos Rubrae) 6g
Che Qian Zi (Semen Plantaginis) 6g, wrapped
Lü Dou Yi (Testa Phaseoli Radiati) 15g
Huang Qi (Radix Astragali seu Hedysari) 10g
Chi Xiao Dou (Semen Phaseoli Calcarati) 10g

Explanation
* *Jin Yin Hua* (Flos Lonicerae), *Ye Ju Hua* (Flos Chrysanthemi Indici), *Gan Cao* (Radix Glycyrrhizae), and *Chi Xiao Dou* (Semen Phaseoli Calcarati) clear Heat and relieve Toxicity.
* *Yi Yi Ren* (Semen Coicis Lachryma-jobi), *Chi Fu Ling* (Sclerotium Poriae Cocos Rubrae) and *Che Qian Zi* (Semen Plantaginis) benefit the movement of Dampness and transform Toxicity.
* *Chao Long Dan Cao* (Radix Gentianae Scabrae, stir-fried) and *Che Qian Zi* (Semen Plantaginis) clear and drain Damp-Heat from the Liver and Gallbladder.
* *Lü Dou Yi* (Testa Phaseoli Radiati) clears Damp-Heat from the Heart channel.
* *Huang Qi* (Radix Astragali seu Hedysari) supports Vital Qi (Zheng Qi) to reinforce the effect of ingredients for clearing Heat and relieving Toxicity.

General modifications
1. For fever, add *Shi Gao* ‡ (Gypsum Fibrosum) and *Zhi Mu* (Rhizoma Anemarrhenae Asphodeloidis).
2. For constipation, add *Da Huang* (Radix et Rhizoma Rhei) and *Xuan Shen* (Radix Scrophulariae Ningpoensis).
3. For crying and restlessness, add *Chan Tui* ‡ (Periostracum Cicadae) and *Mu Li* ‡ (Concha Ostreae).
4. For reddish urine, add *Liu Yi San* (Six-To-One Powder).
5. For severe local redness and swelling, add *Zi Cao* (Radix Arnebiae seu Lithospermi).

EXTERNAL TREATMENT
* If lesions manifest as erosion, exudation and superficial ulceration, select two or three materia medica from the following – *Ye Ju Hua* (Flos Chrysanthemi Indici), *Pu Gong Ying* (Herba Taraxaci cum Radice), *Huang Lian* (Rhizoma Coptidis), *Shi Liu Pi** (Pericarpium Punicae Granati), *Wu Bei Zi* ‡ (Galla Rhois Chinensis), *Huang Bai* (Cortex Phellodendri), and *Gan Cao* (Radix Glycyrrhizae) – and prepare a decoction for use as a wash or wet compress on the affected area for 15-30 minutes two or three times a day. Then apply *Zi Cao You* (Gromwell Root Oil) and *Qing Dai Gao* (Indigo Paste) to the lesions.
* If the affected area is red, swollen and painful, apply *Huang Lian Ruan Gao* (Coptis Ointment), *Zi Lian Gao* (Gromwell Root and Coptis Paste) or *Qing Liang Gao* (Cool Clearing Paste) externally. Then spread *Qing Liang Fen* (Cool Clearing Powder), *Ku Fan Fen* (Prepared Alum Powder), *Yan Kao San* (Buttock-Submerging Sore Powder), or *Fu Long Gan San* (Oven Earth Powder) over the lesions.

Clinical notes
* In treating diaper dermatitis, TCM emphasizes clearing Heat and cooling the Blood, transforming Dampness and relieving Toxicity since it is essential to bring the symptoms under control as soon as possible and avoid erosion and exudation.
* It is difficult to give medications to babies and infants. For infants less than 1 year old, give 5-10ml of the decoction three to five times a day; for infants aged 1-2, give 10-15ml three to five times a day.

Advice for the carer
* Keep the affected area dry and clean.
* Use superabsorbent disposable diapers if possible and change them frequently. If cloth diapers are used, they should be washed and dried thoroughly and changed frequently.
* Avoid the application of irritating medications.

Literature excerpt

In *Dong Tian Ao Zhi (Wai Ke Mi Lu)* [Secret Records of External Diseases], it says: "How can a newborn child have much internal Damp-Heat? However, since it has to urinate and defecate in a diaper, it is difficult to keep the lower body dry and Dampness and Heat will collect there. Diaper dermatitis occurs because the mother does not look after the baby properly, tightly enveloping it in quilts so that the baby cannot move about after urination and defecation; this is a particular problem in the heat of summer. Instead of clearing Damp-Heat from the interior, external treatment will be more effective. Mix some very finely-powdered *Zao Xin Tu* (Terra Flava Usta) with a little *Hua Shi* ‡ (Talcum), spread over the lesions and cover with a piece of tissue."

Modern clinical experience

EXTERNAL APPLICATION OF OILS

1. **Zheng** used *Dan Huang You* (Egg Yolk Oil) to treat erosive diaper dermatitis. The oil was obtained by placing an egg yolk in an iron spoon and cooking it over a mild heat until it turned dark brown and produced a sticky, dark brown oil. The erosion was washed with 3 percent hydrogen peroxide solution and physiological saline before sterile gauze dipped in the yolk oil was applied to the lesions. The gauze was replaced each time the diaper was changed. Results were seen in mild rashes after one day; and in severe rashes after three days. [56]

2. **He** reported on the use of his version of *Zi Cao You* (Gromwell Root Oil) in the treatment of diaper dermatitis. The oil was prepared with one portion of *Zi Cao* (Radix Arnebiae seu Lithospermi) to two portions of rapeseed oil (colza oil). After soaking the herb in the oil for one hour, the mixture was steamed for another hour. The oil was allowed to cool before the residue was removed. The oil was applied to the diaper area three or four times a day. A course of treatment lasted for seven days. During the treatment, diapers were changed frequently and the diaper area kept dry. Results were usually seen within one course of treatment. [57]

3. **Li** treated diaper dermatitis with an infusion prepared according to his own formula, followed by application of his version of *Zi Cao You* (Gromwell Root Oil). The infusion was made with *Jin Yin Hua* (Flos Lonicerae) 6g, *Bai Ji** (Rhizoma Bletillae Striatae) 6g and *Ye Ju Hua* (Flos Chrysanthemi Indici) 6g, which were soaked in boiled water for ten minutes before the liquid was drained off for use.

Zi Cao You (Gromwell Root Oil) was prepared with *Zi Cao* (Radix Arnebiae seu Lithospermi) 50g, Vaseline® 50g and *Xiang You* (Oleum Sesami Seminis) 450ml. *Zi Cao* (Radix Arnebiae seu Lithospermi) was steeped in *Xiang You* (Oleum Sesami Seminis) overnight and then cooked over a low heat until scorched; the herb was removed and the oil mixed with Vaseline®.

The infusion was used to wash the affected area. After the area was dried, *Zi Cao You* (Gromwell Root Oil) was applied, and the area then exposed to an incandescent lamp or far-infrared lamp for 10 minutes. When the skin dried, *Zi Cao You* (Gromwell Root Oil) was again applied. This treatment was given twice a day for a week. [58]

EXTERNAL TREATMENT WITH MEDICATED POWDER

Cai treated diaper dermatitis with finely-ground *Hua Shi* ‡ (Talcum) 100g and *Qing Dai* (Indigo Naturalis) 50g. After the affected area was washed with warm water, the powder mix was applied two or three times a day for three days. [59]

Palpebral eczema
眼睑湿疹

Palpebral eczema may occur in conjunction with seborrheic eczema and may be associated with blepharitis. It may also be a manifestation of contact dermatitis, for example due to an allergic reaction to cosmetics applied to the eyelid.

In TCM, palpebral eczema is also known as *feng chi chuang yi* (red Wind sore).

Clinical manifestations

- Sites of involvement are circumscribed to the eyelid area.
- The condition manifests initially as local reddening of the skin, with pinpoint papules, papulovesicles

and vesicles subsequently appearing. Erosion occurs on rupture of the vesicles, resulting in a bright red color around the ruptured lesions. Patients also experience pain and itching.

- The disease tends to persist with intermittent remission and aggravation. Delayed or inappropriate treatment may result in conjunctivitis.

Etiology and pathology

Wind-Heat in the Spleen channel

Excessive intake of pungent or spicy food leads to accumulation of Heat in the Spleen and Stomach. Where this is complicated by an invasion of external Wind, internal Heat is stirred up and attacks upward into the eyes. Wind and Heat fight and settle in the eyelids to cause the disease.

Wind-Heat attacking upward

If external Wind, Dampness and Heat invade when Damp-Heat is steaming in the Spleen and Stomach, the three pathogenic factors will be retained in the Xue level and accumulate in the skin of the eyelids to cause the disease.

Damp-Heat

If stimulating food such as fish, prawns, cheese, or butter is eaten when internal Heat is relatively strong, internal and external factors will combine to spread to the skin and flesh.

Infection by Toxins

The disease may also occur after infection by Toxins as a result of frequent rubbing of the skin after contact with Toxic substances.

Pattern identification and treatment

INTERNAL TREATMENT

WIND-HEAT IN THE SPLEEN CHANNEL

This pattern manifests as redness, a burning sensation, itching, and painful and swollen eyelids with vesicles and sticky exudate. The tongue body is red with a thin, white and greasy coating; the pulse is rapid.

Treatment principle

Clear Heat from the Spleen and eliminate Wind.

Prescription

CHU FENG QING PI YIN JIA JIAN

Beverage for Eliminating Wind and Clearing Heat from the Spleen, with modifications

Lian Qiao (Fructus Forsythiae Suspensae) 12g
Fang Feng (Radix Ledebouriellae Divaricatae) 12g
Xuan Shen (Radix Scrophulariae Ningpoensis) 12g

Sheng Di Huang (Radix Rehmanniae Glutinosae) 12g
Huang Qin (Radix Scutellariae Baicalensis) 10g
Jie Geng (Radix Platycodi Grandiflori) 10g
Jing Jie (Herba Schizonepetae Tenuifoliae) 10g
Zhi Mu (Rhizoma Anemarrhenae Asphodeloidis) 10g
Chi Shao (Radix Paeoniae Rubra) 10g
Jiao Zhi Zi (Fructus Gardeniae Jasminoidis, scorch-fried) 6g
Chong Wei Zi (Semen Leonuri Heterophylli) 6g

Explanation

- *Lian Qiao* (Fructus Forsythiae Suspensae), *Xuan Shen* (Radix Scrophulariae Ningpoensis), *Sheng Di Huang* (Radix Rehmanniae Glutinosae), *Zhi Mu* (Rhizoma Anemarrhenae Asphodeloidis), and *Huang Qin* (Radix Scutellariae Baicalensis) nourish Yin, clear Heat and relieve Toxicity.
- *Jing Jie* (Herba Schizonepetae Tenuifoliae), *Fang Feng* (Radix Ledebouriellae Divaricatae), *Jie Geng* (Radix Platycodi Grandiflori), and *Chong Wei Zi* (Semen Leonuri Heterophylli), dredge Wind and alleviate itching.
- *Chi Shao* (Radix Paeoniae Rubra) and *Jiao Zhi Zi* (Fructus Gardeniae Jasminoidis, scorch-fried) clear Heat and cool the Blood.

WIND-HEAT ATTACKING UPWARD

Lesions on the eyelids are characterized by redness, dryness and itching, or painful inflammation and local ulceration. The tongue body is red with a thin, white and greasy coating; the pulse is floating and rapid.

Treatment principle

Clear Heat and relieve Toxicity, dredge Wind and dissipate pathogenic factors.

Prescription

PU JI XIAO DU YIN JIA JIAN

Universal Salvation Beverage for Dispersing Toxicity, with modifications

Huang Qin (Radix Scutellariae Baicalensis) 12g
Xuan Shen (Radix Scrophulariae Ningpoensis) 12g
Ban Lan Gen (Radix Isatidis seu Baphicacanthi) 12g
Sheng Di Huang (Radix Rehmanniae Glutinosae) 12g
Lian Qiao (Fructus Forsythiae Suspensae) 12g
Huang Lian (Rhizoma Coptidis) 6g
Sheng Ma (Rhizoma Cimicifugae) 6g
Chen Pi (Pericarpium Citri Reticulatae) 6g
Ma Bo (Sclerotium Lasiosphaerae seu Calvatiae) 6g
Chao Niu Bang Zi (Fructus Arctii Lappae, stir-fried) 10g
Chai Hu (Radix Bupleuri) 10g
Chi Shao (Radix Paeoniae Rubra) 10g

Explanation

- *Huang Qin* (Radix Scutellariae Baicalensis), *Ban Lan Gen* (Radix Isatidis seu Baphicacanthi), *Ma Bo* (Sclerotium Lasiosphaerae seu Calvatiae), *Huang Lian*

(Rhizoma Coptidis), and *Xuan Shen* (Radix Scrophulariae Ningpoensis) clear Heat and relieve Toxicity.

- *Sheng Di Huang* (Radix Rehmanniae Glutinosae), *Chi Shao* (Radix Paeoniae Rubra) and *Lian Qiao* (Fructus Forsythiae Suspensae) clear Heat from the Heart and cool the Blood.

- *Chen Pi* (Pericarpium Citri Reticulatae), *Chao Niu Bang Zi* (Fructus Arctii Lappae, stir-fried), *Chai Hu* (Radix Bupleuri), and *Sheng Ma* (Rhizoma Cimicifugae) dredge Wind and dissipate pathogenic factors.

DAMP-HEAT

Lesions are erosive with purple, bloody, purulent, and foul-smelling exudate and the formation of moist crusts. Eyelids tend to be swollen rather than itchy. The tongue body is red with a yellow and greasy coating; the pulse is rapid and soggy.

Treatment principle

Clear Heat and eliminate Dampness.

Prescription
CHU SHI TANG JIA JIAN

Decoction for Eliminating Dampness, with modifications

Lian Qiao (Fructus Forsythiae Suspensae) 10g
Fu Ling (Sclerotium Poriae Cocos) 10g
Fang Feng (Radix Ledebouriellae Divaricatae) 10g
Chao Zhi Ke (Fructus Citri Aurantii, stir-fried) 10g
Hua Shi ‡ (Talcum) 15g, wrapped
Che Qian Zi (Semen Plantaginis) 12g, wrapped
Huang Lian (Rhizoma Coptidis) 6g
Tong Cao (Medulla Tetrapanacis Papyriferi) 6g
Jing Jie (Herba Schizonepetae Tenuifoliae) 6g
Gan Cao (Radix Glycyrrhizae) 6g

Explanation

- *Lian Qiao* (Fructus Forsythiae Suspensae), *Huang Lian* (Rhizoma Coptidis) and *Gan Cao* (Radix Glycyrrhizae) clear Heat from the Heart and relieve Toxicity.

- *Jing Jie* (Herba Schizonepetae Tenuifoliae), *Fang Feng* (Radix Ledebouriellae Divaricatae) and *Chao Zhi Ke* (Fructus Citri Aurantii, stir-fried) dredge Wind and clear Heat.

- *Fu Ling* (Sclerotium Poriae Cocos), *Tong Cao* (Medulla Tetrapanacis Papyriferi), *Hua Shi* ‡ (Talcum), and *Che Qian Zi* (Semen Plantaginis) benefit the movement of Dampness and promote urination.

General modifications

1. For severe itching, add *Cang Er Zi* (Fructus Xanthii Sibirici), *Chan Tui* ‡ (Periostracum Cicadae), *She Tui* ‡ (Exuviae Serpentis), and *Di Fu Zi* (Fructus Kochiae Scopariae).

2. For lesions with redness and severe pain, add *Chi Shao* (Radix Paeoniae Rubra) and *Mu Dan Pi* (Cortex Moutan Radicis).

3. For ulcerating lesions with bloody or purulent exudate, add *Tu Fu Ling* (Rhizoma Smilacis Glabrae), *Jin Yin Hua* (Flos Lonicerae), *Pu Gong Ying* (Herba Taraxaci cum Radice), and *Zi Hua Di Ding* (Herba Violae Yedoensitis).

EXTERNAL TREATMENT

- For red and dry lesions or erosive lesions with small amounts of sticky exudate, apply *Qing Dai* (Indigo Naturalis) mixed to a paste with *Xiang You* (Oleum Sesami Seminis).

- For lesions with profuse sticky exudate, apply powdered *Hua Shi* ‡ (Talcum) or refined *Lu Gan Shi* ‡ (Calamina) to eliminate Dampness and clear Heat.

Clinical notes

- When prescribing ingredients for internal administration, consideration should be given to differentiating among Wind, Heat and Dampness patterns:
  - Conditions presenting with puffiness and severe itching of the eyelids should generally be treated with materia medica for dredging Wind and alleviating itching.
  - Conditions presenting with red and painful eyelids should generally be treated with materia medica for clearing Heat and relieving Toxicity.
  - Conditions presenting with erosion and exudation on the eyelids should generally be treated with materia medica for transforming Dampness and clearing Heat.
  In practice, ingredients are chosen according to the relative severity of the various manifestations.

- Ingredients used externally should be pure in quality and processed into a very fine powder, preferably by the traditional water-grinding method (see the section on powder preparations on page 48). Avoid local irritation that may aggravate the condition.

- Palpebral eczema is one of the more common diseases of the eyelid. It frequently occurs after local skin contact with irritant substances such as perfumed cosmetics, hair dyes and adhesive plasters or due to long-term application of certain types of ointment or solutions for treating eye diseases.

Advice for the patient

- Keep the local area clean.
- Make sure that exudate does not seep into the eyes.

Literature excerpt

In *Yi Zong Jin Jian: Yan Ke Xin Fa Yao Jue* [The Golden Mirror of Medicine: Essential Methods for the Treatment of Eye Diseases], it says: "*Feng chi chuang yi* (red Wind sore) occurs in the eyelid with redness and erosion but does not initially involve the pupil. It is caused by Wind-Heat in the Spleen channel. *Si Wu Tang Jia Jian* (Four Agents Decoction, with modifications) is the recom- mended treatment, consisting of *Sheng Di Huang* (Radix Rehmanniae Glutinosae), *Ku Shen* (Radix Sophorae Flavescentis), *Niu Bang Zi* (Fructus Arctii Lappae), *Bo He* (Herba Menthae Haplocalycis), *Fang Feng* (Radix Lede- bouriellae Divaricatae), *Dang Gui* (Radix Angelicae Sinen- sis), *Chi Shao* (Radix Paeoniae Rubra), *Tian Hua Fen* (Radix Trichosanthis), *Lian Qiao* (Fructus Forsythiae Sus- pensae), *Jing Jie Sui* (Spica Schizonepetae Tenuifoliae), and *Chuan Xiong* (Rhizoma Ligustici Chuanxiong)."

Retroauricular eczema
耳后湿疹

Eczema in the skin folds behind the ear may be a mani- festation of atopic eczema or seborrheic eczema. It needs to be distinguished from psoriasis affecting the retroauricular fold; psoriasis in this area may not exhibit the same degree of scaling as the psoriatic lesions which are almost invariably present at other locations.

In TCM, this condition is also known as *yue shi chuang* (periodic corroding sore).

Clinical manifestations

- This condition usually occurs in the folds at the back of the ear, but may also spread to involve the rest of the ear.
- Children are particularly likely to be affected.
- The initial stage is characterized by erythema and papulovesicles.
- The condition usually becomes chronic with scaling.
- Itching is severe.

Differential diagnosis

Contact dermatitis
There is an obvious history of contact with external stimuli, such as hair dyes. This condition manifests as red and swollen skin, vesicles and exudation.

Infectious eczematoid dermatitis
Purulent discharge from a primary focus (for example, otitis media) may give rise to eczematoid lesions such as papules, papulovesicles, vesicles, pustules, crusting, and profuse exudate. Lesions may spread following excoria- tion.

Etiology and pathology

- The Gallbladder and Stomach channels pass through the area around the ear. The Liver and Gallbladder stand in interior-exterior relationship, as do the Spleen and Stomach.
- Dietary irregularities such as excessive intake of fish, seafood and greasy food will lead to impairment of the Spleen's transportation and transformation func- tion. As a result, Damp-Heat will accumulate and move upward along the channels to the area around the ear to produce the lesions.
- Prolonged accumulation of Damp-Heat in the Liver and Gallbladder transforms into Dryness. This results in damage to Yin and Blood, which leads to Blood-Dryness due to Yin Deficiency.

Pattern identification and treatment

INTERNAL TREATMENT

DAMP-HEAT ACCUMULATING IN THE SKIN
This pattern has a sudden onset, manifesting as small patches of erythema with infiltration. Lesions in the folds of the ear may fissure with small amounts of exu- date and moist crusts, causing maceration and severe local pain and itching. Accompanying symptoms and signs include a bitter taste in the mouth, dry mouth, constipation, and short voidings of yellow urine. The tongue body is red with a thin, yellow and slightly greasy coating; the pulse is slippery and rapid.

Treatment principle

Clear Heat, dispel Dampness and alleviate itching.

Prescription

LONG DAN XIE GAN TANG JIA JIAN

Chinese Gentian Decoction for Draining the Liver, with modifications

Chao Long Dan Cao (Radix Gentianae Scabrae, stir-fried) 10g
Huang Qin (Radix Scutellariae Baicalensis) 10g
Che Qian Zi (Semen Plantaginis) 10g, wrapped
Chao Mu Dan Pi (Cortex Moutan Radicis, stir-fried) 10g
Jiao Zhi Zi (Fructus Gardeniae Jasminoidis, scorch-fried) 10g
Sheng Di Huang (Radix Rehmanniae Glutinosae) 30g
Bai Mao Gen (Rhizoma Imperatae Cylindricae) 15g
Liu Yi San (Six-To-One Powder) 12g, wrapped in *He Ye* (Folium Nelumbinis Nuciferae) ix
Chai Hu (Radix Bupleuri) 6g
Tong Cao (Medulla Tetrapanacis Papyriferi) 6g

Explanation

• *Chao Long Dan Cao* (Radix Gentianae Scabrae, stir-fried), *Jiao Zhi Zi* (Fructus Gardeniae Jasminoidis, scorch-fried), *Chai Hu* (Radix Bupleuri), *Huang Qin* (Radix Scutellariae Baicalensis), and *Tong Cao* (Medulla Tetrapanacis Papyriferi) clear and drain Damp-Heat from the Liver and Gallbladder.

• *Sheng Di Huang* (Radix Rehmanniae Glutinosae), *Chao Mu Dan Pi* (Cortex Moutan Radicis, stir-fried) and *Bai Mao Gen* (Rhizoma Imperatae Cylindricae) clear Heat and cool the Blood.

• *Che Qian Zi* (Semen Plantaginis) and *Liu Yi San* (Six-To-One Powder) guide Heat downward to clear Heat from the Fu organs.

BLOOD-DRYNESS DUE TO YIN DEFICIENCY

This condition is lingering and recurrent, with thickened skin, fissuring of the ear folds, recurrent scaling, and lancinating pain. Accompanying symptoms and signs include dry rough skin with itching and a dry mouth. The tongue body is red and dry with a scant coating; the pulse is thready and rapid.

Treatment principle

Enrich Yin and nourish the Blood, moisten Dryness and eliminate Dampness.

Prescription

ZI YIN CHU SHI TANG JIA JIAN

Decoction for Enriching Yin and Eliminating Dampness, with modifications

Sheng Di Huang (Radix Rehmanniae Glutinosae) 30g
Xuan Shen (Radix Scrophulariae Ningpoensis) 15g
Dang Gui (Radix Angelicae Sinensis) 15g
Dan Shen (Radix Salviae Miltiorrhizae) 12g
Fu Ling (Sclerotium Poriae Cocos) 12g
Ze Xie (Rhizoma Alismatis Orientalis) 12g
Bai Xian Pi (Cortex Dictamni Dasycarpi Radicis) 10g
Di Fu Zi (Fructus Kochiae Scopariae) 10g
Gou Teng (Ramulus Uncariae cum Uncis) 10g
Chai Hu (Radix Bupleuri) 6g
Chao Bai Shao (Radix Paeoniae Lactiflorae, stir-fried) 6g

Explanation

• *Sheng Di Huang* (Radix Rehmanniae Glutinosae), *Xuan Shen* (Radix Scrophulariae Ningpoensis), *Dang Gui* (Radix Angelicae Sinensis), *Chao Bai Shao* (Radix Paeoniae Lactiflorae, stir-fried), and *Dan Shen* (Radix Salviae Miltiorrhizae) nourish the Blood and moisten the skin, enrich Yin and moisten Dryness.

• *Fu Ling* (Sclerotium Poriae Cocos) and *Ze Xie* (Rhizoma Alismatis Orientalis) support the Spleen and transform Dampness.

• *Bai Xian Pi* (Cortex Dictamni Dasycarpi Radicis), *Gou Teng* (Ramulus Uncariae cum Uncis), *Di Fu Zi* (Fructus Kochiae Scopariae), and *Chai Hu* (Radix Bupleuri) transform Dampness and relieve Toxicity, dissipate Wind and alleviate itching.

EXTERNAL TREATMENT

• In the acute phase with exudation, use *Lu Lu Tong Shui Xi Ji* (Sweetgum Fruit Wash Preparation) or prepare a decoction with *Di Yu* (Radix Sanguisorbae Officinalis) 15g, *Huang Bai* (Cortex Phellodendri) 10g and *Pu Gong Ying* (Herba Taraxaci cum Radice) 10g for use a wet compress on the affected area two or three times a day.

• Once exudation from the lesions has begun to diminish, but there is still slight erosion, mix *Qu Shi San* (Powder for Dispelling Dampness) or *Jie Du Dan* (Special Powder for Relieving Toxicity) to a paste with *Xiang You* (Oleum Sesami Seminis) for application to the lesions.

• When exudation and erosion have improved, but there is still slight erosion, apply *Di Hu Hu* (Sanguisorba and Giant Knotweed Paste) to the affected area.

Clinical notes

Treatment for lesions around the ear depends on whether a Deficiency or an Excess pattern is involved.

• Excess patterns are generally of short duration and are characterized by erythema, obvious exudation and relatively severe itching. Treatment should focus

---

ix If fresh leaves are not available, soak dried *He Ye* (Folium Nelumbinis Nuciferae) overnight before use.

on the Liver and Gallbladder with formulae such as *Long Dan Xie Gan Tang* (Chinese Gentian Decoction for Draining the Liver) or *Chai Hu Qing Gan Yin* (Bupleurum Beverage for Clearing the Liver).

- Deficiency patterns are generally of long duration and are characterized by dry, lichenified lesions with desquamation and itching with intermittent remission and exacerbation. Treatment should concentrate on the Spleen and Kidneys with formulae such as *Zhi Bai Di Huang Tang* (Anemarrhena, Phellodendron and Rehmannia Decoction) or *Zi Yin Chu Shi Tang* (Decoction for Enriching Yin and Eliminating Dampness).

Advice for the patient

- Keep the affected areas clean. Avoid washing with hot water.
- Avoid greasy and spicy foods and alcohol.
- If the disease is associated with a certain trigger, such as wearing glasses, early treatment results in a better prognosis.

Case history

Patient
Male, aged 52.

Clinical manifestations
The patient had been suffering from exudation, redness and itching in both retroauricular areas for about a month. Treatment with Western medicine had not proved effective. At the time of the first consultation, the lesions had begun to spread to the face and arms. Accompanying symptoms included thirst and constipation. Physical examination revealed diffuse erythema with ill-defined borders in both retroauricular areas; the erythema was covered by dense groupings of pinpoint papules and vesicles. Erosion, exudation and crusting were also present in the affected areas. Small discrete patches of vesicular lesions had appeared on the neck, nose, forearms, and dorsum of the hand. The tongue coating was yellow and greasy.

Diagnosis
Acute eczema beginning as retroauricular eczema (*yue shi chuang* developing into *jin yin chuang*).

Pattern identification
Retention of Damp-Heat in the Liver and Gallbladder.

Treatment principle
Clear Heat and benefit the movement of Dampness.

Prescription
LONG DAN XIE GAN TANG JIA JIAN
Chinese Gentian Decoction for Draining the Liver, with modifications

Long Dan Cao (Radix Gentianae Scabrae) 6g

Huang Qin (Radix Scutellariae Baicalensis) 9g
Sheng Di Huang (Radix Rehmanniae Glutinosae) 9g
Mu Dan Pi (Cortex Moutan Radicis) 9g
Chi Shao (Radix Paeoniae Rubra) 9g
Bi Xie (Rhizoma Dioscoreae Hypoglaucae seu Septemlobae) 9g
Yi Yi Ren (Semen Coicis Lachryma-jobi) 9g
Che Qian Zi (Semen Plantaginis) 9g
Chai Hu (Radix Bupleuri) 6g

One bag a day was used to prepare a decoction, taken twice a day.

External treatment
Pi Yan Xi Ji (Dermatitis Wash Preparation) for use as a wash and *Huang Ling Dan* (Yellow Spirit Special Pill) crushed and mixed to a paste with *Xiang You* (Oleum Sesami Seminis) for application to the affected areas.

Outcome
The patient's condition showed some improvement after following this treatment, but new eruptions were still occurring. The tongue body was red. The patient was given another five bags of the same prescription, after which his condition began to show considerable improvement; the lesions were drying up with crusting and desquamation, and there was less itching and burning sensation. The patient was given ten more bags of the prescription. By this time, his skin was almost clear. He was then given the patent herbal medicine *Chu Shi Wan* (Pill for Eliminating Dampness) to consolidate the treatment. [60]

Modern clinical experience

EXTERNAL TREATMENT WITH POWDERS

1. **Chen** prescribed *Shan Jia San* (Pangolin Powder) to treat retroauricular eczema. The powder was prepared from equal proportions of *Chuan Shan Jia** (Squama Manitis Pentadactylae), *Hu Huang Lian* (Rhizoma Picrorhizae Scrophulariiflorae), *Xue Jie* (Resina Draconis), and *Da Huang* (Radix et Rhizoma Rhei). These ingredients were ground into a powder and made into a paste with *Xiang You* (Oleum Sesami Seminis) for external application to the affected area once a day. [61]

2. **Hao** prescribed *Ku Qing Song San* (Prepared Alum, Indigo and Rosin Powder) to treat retroauricular eczema. The powder was prepared with *Ku Fan*‡ (Alumen Praeparatum) 15g, *Qing Dai* (Indigo Naturalis) 6g and *Song Xiang* (Resina Pini) 9g. These ingredients were ground into a very fine powder and mixed into a paste with vegetable oil for external application once a day. Results were seen within five days. A few patients with secondary infection required treatment with antibiotics. [62]

EXTERNAL TREATMENT WITH PATENT MEDICINE

Yang reported on treatment with *Xi Gua Shuang* (Watermelon Frost), produced by the Guilin TCM

Pharmaceutical Factory, which was applied to the affected area twice a day. The frost was made from *Xi Gua Shuang* (Praeparatio Mirabiliti et Citrulli), *Huang Lian* (Rhizoma Coptidis), *Huang Qin* (Radix Scutellariae Baicalensis), *Shan Dou Gen* (Radix Sophorae Tonkinensis), and *Bing Pian* (Borneolum). Results were seen within seven days. [63]

EXTERNAL TREATMENT WITH MEDICATED PASTE

Zhen treated retroauricular eczema with *Lian Bing Gao* (Coptis and Borneol Paste). [64]

Prescription ingredients

Huang Lian (Rhizoma Coptidis) 50g
Da Huang (Radix et Rhizoma Rhei) 25g
Huang Bai (Cortex Phellodendri) 30g
Gan Cao (Radix Glycyrrhizae) 20g

The ingredients were ground into a very fine powder and mixed into a paste with *Bing Pian* (Borneolum) 10g and vegetable oil. The paste was applied externally to the affected area once a day for three to five days.

EXTERNAL TREATMENT WITH WASH PREPARATIONS

1. **Ren** prepared a decoction for use as a wash. [65]

Prescription ingredients

Huang Bai (Cortex Phellodendri) 10g
Che Qian Zi (Semen Plantaginis) 10g, wrapped
Chi Shao (Radix Paeoniae Rubra) 10g
Ku Shen (Radix Sophorae Flavescentis) 10g
Di Fu Zi (Fructus Kochiae Scopariae) 10g

Gan Cao (Radix Glycyrrhizae) 5g

The decoction was used as a wash once a day to treat damp erosive lesions in the retroauricular region. The treatment was more effective if two teaspoons of the decoction were also taken orally while the wash was being applied. Treatment was given at the same time with a TDP electromagnetic wave treatment apparatus produced by Ba Shan Apparatus Factory, Chongqing. The apparatus was placed 30cm away from the affected ear and used for 30 minutes per session. The skin temperature was controlled within the 30-40°C range. Treatment was given once a day. Ten treatments made up a course.

2. **Wang** treated retroauricular eczema with a wet compress. [66]

Prescription
XIAO SHI TANG
Decoction for Dispersing Dampness

Di Fu Zi (Fructus Kochiae Scopariae) 20g
She Chuang Zi (Fructus Cnidii Monnieri) 20g
Ku Shen (Radix Sophorae Flavescentis) 20g
Huang Bai (Cortex Phellodendri) 20g

The ingredients were decocted initially for 30 minutes and the liquid drained off; they were then decocted a second time for 20 minutes and the liquid was again drained off. The two liquids were mixed together and boiled down to 50ml to be used as a wet compress on the affected area once or twice a day. A course of treatment lasted for three days. Patients were advised to give up smoking, alcohol, spring onions, garlic, and spicy food during treatment.

Nipple eczema
乳头湿疹

Nipple eczema is usually bilateral, and mainly affects women up to the age of 30. It is more common in atopic subjects.

Breast feeding is a common precipitant, but the condition can also be caused by topical agents including medicaments, perfumes and nail varnish.

It is important to exclude the differential diagnoses of scabies infection and Paget's disease of the nipple (see below).

In TCM, this condition is also known as *ru tou feng* (nipple Wind).

Clinical manifestations

- Dark red maculopapules appear on the nipples and areolae with slight exudation and erosion or dryness and desquamation.

- Lesions present with pain and itching. Where this condition occurs in nursing mothers, stabbing or lancinating pain occurs when the baby sucks milk.

- Nipple eczema may also develop due to neglect of personal hygiene by nursing mothers and the irritant effect of milk and infant saliva. As the nipples are often immersed in milk, erosion and fissuring can occur. Candidal infection is also common in this situation.

Differential diagnosis

Scabies
Although scabies usually involves the sides of the fingers, the webs between the fingers and the sides of the hands, it may spread to other areas including the nipples within one to two weeks. Severe itching develops after four to six weeks; itching is worse on exposure to heat or at night. Nipple eczema lacks the grayish linear, curved or serpiginous burrows characteristic of scabies.

Paget's disease of the nipple
This condition occurs in breast cancer. Incidence increases with age, mostly affecting women in their forties or older. The lesion presents as a sharply demarcated red plaque that spreads slowly around the nipple and areola. It is generally unilateral, whereas eczema usually affects both nipples. Differentiation is important as the underlying cancer must be treated without delay.

Etiology and pathology

- The congenital constitution of some women is exuberant Heat. If they suffer damage to the seven emotions, Liver Yang will become hyperactive and transform into Fire, or Heat will accumulate in the Liver channel. Since Fire in the Liver and Gallbladder cannot be drained, nipple eczema will result.
- Nursing mothers are particularly prone to nipple eczema. The inverted nipples of nursing mothers make it difficult for babies to suck milk. Poor positioning of the baby on the breast and hard sucking may cause the nipples to crack, resulting in infection by Heat Toxins.

Pattern identification and treatment

INTERNAL TREATMENT

DAMP-HEAT IN THE LIVER AND GALLBLADDER
This pattern is characterized by reddening of the skin of the nipple, papulovesicles, exudation and erosion, and intolerable stabbing pain in the nipple area. Accompanying symptoms and signs include a bitter taste in the mouth, constipation or short voidings of yellow urine.

The tongue body is red with a thin yellow coating; the pulse is wiry and rapid.

Treatment principle
Clear Heat from the Liver and transform Dampness.

Prescription
LONG DAN XIE GAN TANG JIA JIAN
Chinese Gentian Decoction for Draining the Liver, with modifications

Chao Long Dan Cao (Radix Gentianae Scabrae, stir-fried) 6g
Jiao Zhi Zi (Fructus Gardeniae Jasminoidis, scorch-fried) 6g
Chai Hu (Radix Bupleuri) 6g
Tong Cao (Medulla Tetrapanacis Papyriferi) 6g
Sheng Di Huang (Radix Rehmanniae Glutinosae) 10g
Fu Ling Pi (Cortex Poriae Cocos) 10g
Chi Shao (Radix Paeoniae Rubra) 10g
Che Qian Zi (Semen Plantaginis) 10g
Fang Feng (Radix Ledebouriellae Divaricatae) 10g
Bai Xian Pi (Cortex Dictamni Dasycarpi Radicis) 12g
Gou Teng (Ramulus Uncariae cum Uncis) 12g
Yi Yi Ren (Semen Coicis Lachryma-jobi) 12g
Gan Cao (Radix Glycyrrhizae) 3g

Explanation
- *Jiao Zhi Zi* (Fructus Gardeniae Jasminoidis, scorch-fried), *Chao Long Dan Cao* (Radix Gentianae Scabrae, stir-fried) and *Chai Hu* (Radix Bupleuri) clear and drain Damp-Heat from the Liver and Gallbladder.
- *Sheng Di Huang* (Radix Rehmanniae Glutinosae) and *Chi Shao* (Radix Paeoniae Rubra) cool the Blood and reduce erythema.
- *Che Qian Zi* (Semen Plantaginis), *Tong Cao* (Medulla Tetrapanacis Papyriferi), *Fu Ling Pi* (Cortex Poriae Cocos), and *Yi Yi Ren* (Semen Coicis Lachryma-jobi) clear Heat and benefit the movement of Dampness.
- *Fang Feng* (Radix Ledebouriellae Divaricatae), *Gou Teng* (Ramulus Uncariae cum Uncis) and *Bai Xian Pi* (Cortex Dictamni Dasycarpi Radicis) dredge Wind and alleviate itching, eliminate Dampness and relieve Toxicity.
- *Gan Cao* (Radix Glycyrrhizae) regulates and harmonizes the actions of the other materia medica to reduce their cold and bitter nature.

HEAT AND DRYNESS DUE TO SPLEEN DEFICIENCY
Symptoms include dryness and desquamation of the areolae and surrounding areas, sometimes with cracking or fissuring of the nipple with intolerable stabbing pain. Accompanying symptoms and signs include a bitter taste in the mouth, constipation or short voidings of yellow urine. The tongue body is pale red; the pulse is soggy and thready.

Treatment principle

Support the Spleen and moisten Dryness.

Prescription

YI WEI TANG JIA JIAN

Decoction for Boosting the Stomach, with modifications

Bei Sha Shen (Radix Glehniae Littoralis) 12g
Tian Men Dong (Radix Asparagi Cochinchinensis) 12g
Mai Men Dong (Radix Ophiopogonis Japonici) 12g
*Shi Hu** (Herba Dendrobii) 12g
Yu Zhu (Rhizoma Polygonati Odorati) 12g
Sheng Di Huang (Radix Rehmanniae Glutinosae) 12g
Fang Feng (Radix Ledebouriellae Divaricatae) 6g
Chan Tui‡ (Periostracum Cicadae) 6g
Lian Zi Xin (Plumula Nelumbinis Nuciferae) 6g
Shan Yao (Rhizoma Dioscoreae Oppositae) 15g
Chi Xiao Dou (Semen Phaseoli Calcarati) 15g
Chao Bai Bian Dou (Semen Dolichoris Lablab, stir-fried) 15g

Explanation

- *Bei Sha Shen* (Radix Glehniae Littoralis), *Tian Men Dong* (Radix Asparagi Cochinchinensis), *Mai Men Dong* (Radix Ophiopogonis Japonici), *Shi Hu** (Herba Dendrobii), *Yu Zhu* (Rhizoma Polygonati Odorati), and *Sheng Di Huang* (Radix Rehmanniae Glutinosae) nourish the Stomach with cold and sweetness and moisten the skin.

- *Shan Yao* (Rhizoma Dioscoreae Oppositae), *Chao Bai Bian Dou* (Semen Dolichoris Lablab, stir-fried) and *Chi Xiao Dou* (Semen Phaseoli Calcarati) support the Spleen and moisten Dryness.

- *Fang Feng* (Radix Ledebouriellae Divaricatae) and *Chan Tui*‡ (Periostracum Cicadae) dredge Wind and alleviate itching.

- *Lian Zi Xin* (Plumula Nelumbinis Nuciferae) clears Heat from the Heart and relieves Toxicity.

EXTERNAL TREATMENT

- For lesions with severe exudation and erosion, first prepare a decoction with *Wu Bei Zi*‡ (Galla Rhois Chinensis) 10g, *Wu Zhu Yu* (Fructus Evodiae Rutaecarpae) 10g and *Can Sha*‡ (Excrementum Bombycis Mori) 6g and use as a wet compress. When exudation has lessened, apply *Dan Huang You* (Egg Yolk Oil) until the lesions heal.

- For dry lesions with desquamation and stabbing pain, apply *Huang Lian Ruan Gao* (Coptis Ointment) two or three times a day.

Clinical notes

- The nipple and areolae are governed by the Liver and Gallbladder channels. At the initial stage, the emphasis in internal treatment should be put on clearing Heat from the Liver and draining Fire; treatment should subsequently focus on nourishing Yin and emolliating the Liver.

- External medications should be mild and moist in nature and effective in alleviating itching. Avoid using strong ingredients with an acrid flavor and hot nature, otherwise the skin will be irritated.

Advice for the patient

Use mild external medications to avoid irritating the skin.

Literature excerpt

In *Yang Ke Xin De Ji: Bian Ru Yong Ru Ju Lun* [A Collection of Experiences in the Treatment of Sores: Discussions on Differentiation between Breast Abscesses and Deep-Rooted Breast Abscesses], it says: "*Ru tou feng* (nipple Wind) is characterized by dryness and cracking of the nipple with severe lancinating pain, or with bleeding or thick exudate, or with the formation of yellow crusts. It is caused by emotional disturbances such as anger or depression leading to retention of Fire in the Liver channel. The disease may occur before or after delivery. *Xiao Yao San* (Free Wanderer Powder) is recommended for internal treatment and powdered *Bai Zhi* (Radix Angelicae Dahuricae) cooked in milk for external treatment."

Modern clinical experience

EXTERNAL TREATMENT

1. **Li** treated 35 patients with *Ru Feng San* (Nipple Wind Powder). [67]

Prescription ingredients

Ru Xiang (Gummi Olibanum) 15g
Wei Wu Mei (Fructus Pruni Mume, roasted) 15g
Ma Bo (Sclerotium Lasiosphaerae seu Calvatiae) 15g
San Qi (Radix Notoginseng) 6g
Zhe Bei Mu (Bulbus Fritillariae Thunbergii) 12g
Wu Gong‡ (Scolopendra Subspinipes) 3 pieces

To prepare the medication, *Ma Bo* (Sclerotium Lasiosphaerae seu Calvatiae) was oven-dried at a low heat, *Wu Mei* (Fructus Pruni Mume) charred into ash and *Ru Xiang* (Gummi Olibanum) ground into a very fine powder. They were then mixed with the other ingredients; the mixture was ground again into a fine powder and stored in a bottle ready for use.

Modifications

1. For lesions with severe itching, he added charred, ground *Qie Zi* (Fructus Solani Melongenae) 2g.
2. For lesions with profuse purulent exudate, he added powdered *Lu Gan Shi* ‡ (Calamina) 5g.

Before treatment, physiological saline was used to clean the lesions; approximately 1g of the powder was then applied to the surface of lesions with a piece of sterilized cotton once or twice a day. Nursing mothers were treated up to three times a day; however, they were reminded to clean the nipples with saline and then rinse with water before breast-feeding in order to avoid the baby swallowing any of the medicated powder.

2. **Wang** used *San Shi San* (Three Stones Powder) prepared with equal proportions of *Lu Gan Shi* ‡ (Calamina), *Hua Rui Shi* ‡ (Ophicalcitum) and *Han Shui Shi* ‡ (Calcitum), to which *Bing Pian* (Borneolum) was added in a proportion of 1:3. The ingredients were ground into a fine powder and mixed into a paste with vegetable oil for direct external application to the affected area two or three times a day until the condition cleared. [68]

3. **Shan Canggui** treated nipple eczema with *Zhu Hong San* (Vermilion Powder). [69]

Prescription ingredients

Hua Shi ‡ (Talcum) 30g, ground with water
Ru Xiang (Gummi Olibanum) 30g
Ge Fen ‡ (Concha Meretricis seu Cyclinae Pulverata) 30g
Huang Lian (Rhizoma Coptidis) 30g
Duan Shi Gao ‡ (Gypsum Fibrosum Calcinatum) 30g
Bing Pian (Borneolum) 3g

The powder was mixed with vegetable oil for external application to the lesions once or twice a day.

Genital eczema
生殖器湿疹

There are varying causes of genital eczema. In the infant, seborrheic eczema and diaper dermatitis (nappy rash) are both common conditions. In older children, other forms of "endogenous" eczema can occur, particularly in atopic individuals. Adults are affected by seborrheic eczema, irritant contact dermatitis (for example, from soaps and detergents), and allergic contact dermatitis (commonly due to medicaments, perfumes and clothing constituents). The genital area is also a common site for lichen simplex chronicus (neurodermatitis).

In TCM, vulvar eczema is also known as *yin shi chuang* (genital Damp sore) and eczema of the scrotum as *shen nang feng* (Kidney sac Wind, or scrotal Wind).

Clinical manifestations

- This condition originates in the genital region (the scrotum in men and the vulva in women) and may sometimes spread from there to the perianal area.

Vulvar eczema

- Lesions mainly involve the labia majora or the crural folds between the top of the thigh and the labia majora.
- Typical manifestations include redness, swelling, erosion and exudation, lichenification, infiltration, and hyperpigmentation or hypopigmentation due to scratching and rubbing.
- Infection is common, resulting in vulvitis, urethritis and cystitis.
- This condition tends to become chronic due to irritation from menstruation and vaginal secretions.

Eczema of the scrotum

- In acute cases, lesions are generally dark red, glistening, moist, and weeping (often soaking the underwear), with swelling and crusting.
- In chronic cases, lesions dry up and lichenify with deepening and widening of the skin creases, resembling a walnut shell. Thin crusts or scales may appear with inflammatory hyperpigmentation; scratching may also result in hypopigmentation.
- Sleep may be disturbed due to severe itching in the affected area.

Differential diagnosis

Lichen planus

Lesions manifest as purplish-red lichenoid changes to the skin with involvement of the labia majora and minora. Wickham's striae (lace-like white surface markings) are distinguishing features of lichen planus.

Tinea cruris (jock itch)

This disease occurs almost exclusively in males. The lesion appears as a red scaly patch that spreads gradually from the crural fold to the thigh and the buttocks, but rarely involves the scrotum. Small vesicles or pustules may form at the border of the lesion, while the center heals, sometimes with temporary pigmentation. There is often intolerable local itching.

Candidiasis

Candidiasis in the genital region occurs more often in women. The lesion has no well-defined border. It often involves the mucous membranes and skin folds with a sticky, white secretion. Where men are affected, the infection is more likely to spread to the scrotum than is the case with tinea cruris.

Etiology and pathology

- The Liver and Kidney channels pass through the genital region. When turbid Dampness forms due to Spleen Deficiency and accumulates to transform into Heat, Damp-Heat can flow along the Liver channel to the genitals, spreading moisture and itching. In addition, Kidney Yang Deficiency will impair transportation of Spleen Yang, leading to Dampness pouring down to the genital region; again, accumulation of Dampness will result in Heat.

- Depletion and Deficiency in the Kidney channel may allow external Wind-Heat to invade, leading to dryness, itching and possibly fissuring in the genital region.

Pattern identification and treatment

INTERNAL TREATMENT

DAMP-HEAT IN THE LIVER AND SPLEEN

Lesions are dark red, moist, swollen, and deeply infiltrated. Rupture of the lesions after scratching leads to exudation of fluid and possibly erosion. Itching is severe, and the itching and erosion aggravate one another. The tongue body is pale red with a thin yellow coating; the pulse is soggy, thready and rapid.

Treatment principle

Clear Heat from the Liver and support the Spleen, dispel Dampness and alleviate itching.

Prescription
ZHI BAI DI HUANG TANG JIA JIAN
Anemarrhena, Phellodendron and Rehmannia Decoction, with modifications

Yan Shui Chao Huang Bai (Cortex Phellodendri, stir-fried with brine) 6g

Chao Cang Zhu (Rhizoma Atractylodis, stir-fried) 6g
Xiao Hui Xiang (Fructus Foeniculi Vulgaris) 6g
Chao Mu Dan Pi (Cortex Moutan Radicis, stir-fried) 6g
Sheng Di Huang (Radix Rehmanniae Glutinosae) 12g
Shan Zhu Yu (Fructus Corni Officinalis) 12g
Chi Fu Ling (Sclerotium Poriae Cocos Rubrae) 12g
Shan Yao (Rhizoma Dioscoreae Oppositae) 30g
Chao Du Zhong (Cortex Eucommiae Ulmoidis, stir-fried) 10g
Xu Duan (Radix Dipsaci) 10g
She Chuang Zi (Fructus Cnidii Monnieri) 10g

Explanation

- *Yan Shui Chao Huang Bai* (Cortex Phellodendri, stir-fried with brine), *Sheng Di Huang* (Radix Rehmanniae Glutinosae) and *Chao Mu Dan Pi* (Cortex Moutan Radicis, stir-fried) nourish Yin and clear Heat.

- *Chao Cang Zhu* (Rhizoma Atractylodis, stir-fried), *Chi Fu Ling* (Sclerotium Poriae Cocos Rubrae) and *Shan Yao* (Rhizoma Dioscoreae Oppositae) support the Spleen and transform Dampness.

- *Shan Zhu Yu* (Fructus Corni Officinalis), *Xiao Hui Xiang* (Fructus Foeniculi Vulgaris), *She Chuang Zi* (Fructus Cnidii Monnieri), *Xu Duan* (Radix Dipsaci), and *Chao Du Zhong* (Cortex Eucommiae Ulmoidis, stir-fried) warm Yang and supplement the Kidneys, dissipate Cold and alleviate itching.

INVASION OF WIND DUE TO KIDNEY YIN DEFICIENCY

The disease is of long duration. Skin lesions are dry, lichenified, rough, and fissured. Patients experience itching, which worsens at night. Some female patients develop atrophy or hypopigmentation of the labia majora and minora, and some male patients may suffer from impotence. The tongue body is pale red with a scant coating; the pulse is deficient and thready.

Treatment principle

Supplement Deficiency and boost the Kidneys, extinguish Wind and alleviate itching.

Prescription
SAN CAI FENG SUI DAN JIA JIAN
Heaven, Human and Earth Pill for Sealing the Marrow, with modifications

Tian Men Dong (Radix Asparagi Cochinchinensis) 12g
Shu Di Huang (Radix Rehmanniae Glutinosae Conquita) 12g
Xuan Shen (Radix Scrophulariae Ningpoensis) 10g
Huang Bai (Cortex Phellodendri) 10g
Dang Shen (Radix Codonopsitis Pilosulae) 10g
Fu Shen (Sclerotium Poriae Cocos cum Ligno Hospite) 10g
Chao Cang Zhu (Rhizoma Atractylodis, stir-fried) 10g
Sha Ren (Fructus Amomi) 6g, added 5 minutes before the end of the decoction process

Chao Du Zhong (Cortex Eucommiae Ulmoidis, stir-fried) 10g
Wu Wei Zi (Fructus Schisandrae) 6g
Shan Zhu Yu (Fructus Corni Officinalis) 6g
Shan Yao (Rhizoma Dioscoreae Oppositae) 30g
Long Gu‡ (Os Draconis) 30g
Mu Li‡ (Concha Ostreae) 30g

Explanation

- *Tian Men Dong* (Radix Asparagi Cochinchinensis), *Shu Di Huang* (Radix Rehmanniae Glutinosae Conquita), *Xuan Shen* (Radix Scrophulariae Ningpoensis), *Wu Wei Zi* (Fructus Schisandrae), *Dang Shen* (Radix Codonopsitis Pilosulae), *Fu Shen* (Sclerotium Poriae Cocos cum Ligno Hospite), and *Shan Yao* (Rhizoma Dioscoreae Oppositae) supplement the Spleen and boost the Kidneys.

- *Chao Du Zhong* (Cortex Eucommiae Ulmoidis, stir-fried), *Wu Wei Zi* (Fructus Schisandrae), *Shan Zhu Yu* (Fructus Corni Officinalis), and *Huang Bai* (Cortex Phellodendri) enrich and supplement the Liver and Kidneys.

- *Sha Ren* (Fructus Amomi) and *Chao Cang Zhu* (Rhizoma Atractylodis, stir-fried) support Yang with warmth and acridity, dissipate Cold and alleviate itching.

- With their heavy, settling properties, *Long Gu* ‡ (Os Draconis) and *Mu Li* ‡ (Concha Ostreae) promote contraction of sores in the genital region.

General modifications

1. For severe itching making sleep difficult, add *Chao Huang Lian* (Rhizoma Coptidis, stir-fried), *Suan Zao Ren* (Semen Ziziphi Spinosae), *He Huan Pi* (Cortex Albizziae Julibrissin), and *Gou Teng* (Ramulus Uncariae cum Uncis).
2. For turbid vaginal discharge, add *Chun Pi* (Cortex Ailanthi Altissimae), *Jin Ying Zi* (Fructus Rosae Laevigatae) and *Qian Shi* (Semen Euryales Ferocis).
3. For dry and cracked skin, add *Di Gu Pi* (Cortex Lycii Radicis), *Gou Qi Zi* (Fructus Lycii), *Sang Shen* (Fructus Mori Albae), *He Shou Wu* (Radix Polygoni Multiflori), and *Tu Si Zi* (Semen Cuscutae).

EXTERNAL TREATMENT

For lichenified lesions with severe itching, apply *Lang Du Gao* (Chinese Wolfsbane Paste), *Ku Shen Gao* (Flavescent Sophora Root Paste) or *Li Lu Gao* (Veratrum Root Paste) to the affected area.

Clinical notes

- TCM emphasizes the Liver and Kidneys in the treatment of genital eczema.

- At the initial stage of the disease, Damp-Heat in the Liver channel is likely to be the predominant pattern. *Long Dan Xie Gan Tang* (Chinese Gentian Decoction for Draining the Liver) can be used as an alternative to the recommended prescription.

- At the later stage, the predominant pattern is more likely to be depletion and Deficiency in the Kidney channel. For Kidney Yin Deficiency, *Mai Wei Di Huang Tang* (Ophiopogon and Rehmannia Decoction) can be used as an alternative to the recommended prescription.

In both cases, the addition of ingredients to extinguish Wind and alleviate itching will increase the effectiveness of the treatment.

- Oozing, erosive and itchy lesions are usually attributed to Damp-Heat in the Liver channel and the treatment principle is therefore based on clearing Heat from the Liver and draining Fire. For persistent conditions, with lichenification and itching that worsens at night, treatment should be based on boosting the Kidneys and extinguishing Wind.

- Factors inducing the occurrence or aggravation of the disease should be investigated. These factors can include personal habits (such as wearing tight underwear that prevents the evaporation of sweat), the working environment (such as working in very hot or damp conditions), emotional disturbances, or relevant previous medical history.

Advice for the patient

- Avoid external stimuli triggering the condition such as washing with hot water, excessive scratching, contact with underwear made of synthetic fibers, and spicy food and alcohol.

- Patients need to be made aware of the need to restrain sexual activity, otherwise a condition which is at the recovery stage may become aggravated or recurrent.

Case history

Patient
Male, aged 34.

Clinical manifestations
The patient had suffered from moisture, erosion, exudation, and itching in the scrotum for seven years. When the condition was severe, he felt discomfort when sitting or lying; work and rest were disturbed. The condition had worsened in the last three weeks, his underwear was soaked by exudate and walking was difficult. Accompanying symptoms and signs included dizziness, fatigue, poor appetite, oppression in the

chest and epigastrium, and defecation with a sensation of incomplete evacuation.

Examination revealed rough, swollen and lichenified skin on both sides of the scrotum with widespread erosion and exudation. Excoriations and bloody crusts were noted, as was an unpleasant smell. The skin on the medial aspects of the thighs was thick, rough and pigmented with lichenoid eruptions. The tongue body was pale and enlarged with tooth marks and a greasy white coating that was slightly yellow in the center; the pulse was wiry and slippery.

Diagnosis
Eczema of the scrotum (*shen nang feng*).

Pattern identification
Accumulation of Dampness due to Spleen Deficiency with Dampness then transforming into Heat and Damp-Heat pouring down.

Treatment principle
Fortify the Spleen and eliminate Dampness, clear Heat, relieve Toxicity and cool the Blood.

Prescription ingredients
Huo Xiang (Herba Agastaches seu Pogostemi) 10g
Yin Chen Hao (Herba Artemisiae Scopariae) 30g
Bai Zhu (Rhizoma Atractylodis Macrocephalae) 10g
Zhi Ke (Fructus Citri Aurantii) 10g
Yi Yi Ren (Semen Coicis Lachryma-jobi) 30g
Che Qian Cao (Herba Plantaginis) 30g
Ze Xie (Rhizoma Alismatis Orientalis) 15g
*Fang Ji** (Radix Stephaniae Tetrandrae) 10g [x]
Ku Shen (Radix Sophorae Flavescentis) 15g
Tong Cao (Medulla Tetrapanacis Papyriferi) 6g
Huang Bai (Cortex Phellodendri) 10g
Long Dan Cao (Radix Gentianae Scabrae) 6g
Sheng Di Huang (Radix Rehmanniae Glutinosae) 15g
Mu Dan Pi (Cortex Moutan Radicis) 15g
Liu Yi San (Six-To-One Powder) 30g, wrapped
Di Fu Zi (Fructus Kochiae Scopariae) 15g

One bag a day was used to prepare a decoction, taken twice a day.

External treatment
Ma Chi Xian (Herba Portulacae Oleraceae) 30g
Huang Bai (Cortex Phellodendri) 30g
Ku Shen (Radix Sophorae Flavescentis) 15g
She Chuang Zi (Fructus Cnidii Monnieri) 15g
Bai Bu (Radix Stemonae) 10g

A decoction prepared with these ingredients was used to wash the affected areas. This was followed by application of *Qu Shi San* (Powder for Dispelling Dampness) mixed to a paste with *Gan Cao You* (Licorice Oil).

Second visit
After three bags of the decoction, there was a pronounced reduction in erosion and exudation; itching was subsiding, allowing the patient to sleep better. After another seven bags, lesions had improved, swelling was reduced, urine and stool were normal, the tongue body was pale with a white coating, and the pulse was moderate.

The prescription was modified by removing *Tong Cao* (Medulla Tetrapanacis Papyriferi), *Yin Chen Hao* (Herba Artemisiae Scopariae), *Long Dan Cao* (Radix Gentianae Scabrae), and *Fang Ji** (Radix Stephaniae Tetrandrae), and adding *Dang Gui* (Radix Angelicae Sinensis) 10g, *Ye Jiao Teng* (Caulis Polygoni Multiflori) 30g and *Dan Shen* (Radix Salviae Miltiorrhizae) 15g.

External treatment was changed to *Huang Lian Ruan Gao* (Coptis Ointment) and 5% *Hei Dou Liu You Ruan Gao* (Black Soybean and Vaseline® Ointment), which were mixed together for application to the affected area.

Outcome
After 14 bags of the second decoction, itching had stopped, the skin had dried up, crusts had been shed, and the swelling had disappeared. The patient took *Chu Shi Wan* (Pill for Eliminating Dampness) 6g and *Qin Jiao Wan* (Large-Leaf Gentian Pill) 6g twice a day for three weeks until all the lesions disappeared. [70]

Modern clinical experience

COMBINED INTERNAL AND EXTERNAL TREATMENT

1. **Zeng** treated eczema of the scrotum with classical formulae. [71]

Internal treatment prescription
JIA WEI SI MIAO TANG
Augmented Mysterious Four Decoction

Huang Bai (Cortex Phellodendri) 12g
Cang Zhu (Rhizoma Atractylodis) 12g
Niu Xi (Radix Achyranthis Bidentatae) 10g
Zhi Zi (Fructus Gardeniae Jasminoidis) 10g
Dang Gui (Radix Angelicae Sinensis) 10g
Fang Feng (Radix Ledebouriellae Divaricatae) 10g
Yi Yi Ren (Semen Coicis Lachryma-jobi) 20g
Fu Ling (Sclerotium Poriae Cocos) 20g
Sheng Di Huang (Radix Rehmanniae Glutinosae) 20g
Bai Xian Pi (Cortex Dictamni Dasycarpi Radicis) 15g

One bag a day was used to prepare a decoction, taken twice a day.

Modifications
1. For dryness and desquamation, *Di Gu Pi* (Cortex Lycii Radicis) 12g, *He Shou Wu* (Radix Polygoni Multiflori) 15g and *Gou Qi Zi* (Fructus Lycii) 12g were added.

---

[x] In those countries where it is illegal to use *Fang Ji** (Radix Stephaniae Tetrandrae), it can be substituted in this prescription by *Che Qian Zi* (Semen Plantaginis) 15g.

2. For severe itching making sleep difficult, *Suan Zao Ren* (Semen Ziziphi Spinosae) 10g and *He Huan Pi* (Cortex Albizziae Julibrissin) 10g were added.

3. For excessive exudate, *Che Qian Zi* (Semen Plantaginis) 15g, *Tong Cao* (Medulla Tetrapanacis Papyriferi) 10g and *Ze Xie* (Rhizoma Alismatis Orientalis) 10g were added.

4. For constipation, *Da Huang* (Radix et Rhizoma Rhei) 6g was added 10 minutes before the end of the decoction process.

External treatment prescription
DI FU ZI XI FANG
Broom Cypress Fruit Wash Preparation

Di Fu Zi (Fructus Kochiae Scopariae) 20g
Wu Bei Zi‡ (Galla Rhois Chinensis) 20g
Hai Tong Pi (Cortex Erythrinae) 10g
Bo He (Herba Menthae Haplocalycis) 6g
Bai Zhi (Radix Angelicae Dahuricae) 4g

The prepared decoction was allowed to cool until luke-warm and then used as an external wash for five minutes twice a day.

Seven days of the combined internal and external treatment constituted a course. The combined approach produced results within three weeks.

2. **Lü** also used a classical formula to treat eczema of the scrotum. [72]

Prescription
LONG DAN XIE GAN TANG JIA WEI
Chinese Gentian Decoction for Draining the Liver, with additions

Long Dan Cao (Radix Gentianae Scabrae) 10g
Ze Xie (Rhizoma Alismatis Orientalis) 10g
Tong Cao (Medulla Tetrapanacis Papyriferi) 10g
Dang Gui (Radix Angelicae Sinensis) 10g
Chai Hu (Radix Bupleuri) 10g
Huang Qin (Radix Scutellariae Baicalensis) 10g
Zhi Zi (Fructus Gardeniae Jasminoidis) 10g
Che Qian Zi (Semen Plantaginis) 10g, wrapped
Ku Shen (Radix Sophorae Flavescentis) 15g
Cang Zhu (Rhizoma Atractylodis) 15g
Bai Xian Pi (Cortex Dictamni Dasycarpi Radicis) 15g
Di Fu Zi (Fructus Kochiae Scopariae) 15g
Da Huang (Radix et Rhizoma Rhei) 6g, added 10 minutes before the end of the decoction process
Gan Cao (Radix Glycyrrhizae) 6g
Sheng Di Huang (Radix Rehmanniae Glutinosae) 20g

One bag a day was used to prepare a decoction, taken twice a day. The residues were decocted again for use as a wash for the affected area. Between nine and twenty bags were needed to see results.

EXTERNAL TREATMENT
Forms of medication for local treatment include wet compress preparations, steam-wash preparations and pastes.

1. **Huang** treated eczema of the scrotum with *Liu Pi Tang* (Six Bark Decoction). [73]

Prescription ingredients

Di Gu Pi (Cortex Lycii Radicis) 30g
Bai Xian Pi (Cortex Dictamni Dasycarpi Radicis) 30g
Huang Bai (Cortex Phellodendri) 30g
Tu Jin Pi (Cortex Pseudolaricis) 15g
Mu Dan Pi (Cortex Moutan Radicis) 15g
*Shi Liu Pi** (Pericarpium Punicae Granati) 50g

Modifications
1. For the acute phase, *Ku Shen* (Radix Sophorae Flavescentis) was added.
2. For the chronic phase, *She Chuang Zi* (Fructus Cnidii Monnieri) and *Mang Xiao*‡ (Mirabilitum) were added.
3. For infection, *Pu Gong Ying* (Herba Taraxaci cum Radice) was added.

The ingredients were used to prepare a decoction for steam-washing the affected area for 30 minutes, once in the morning and once in the evening. Results were seen in the majority of patients after twenty days of treatment.

2. **Zeng** prepared a decoction for use as a wet compress or soak to treat eczema of the scrotum. [74]

Prescription ingredients

Ku Shen (Radix Sophorae Flavescentis) 30g
Di Fu Zi (Fructus Kochiae Scopariae) 30g
Bai Xian Pi (Cortex Dictamni Dasycarpi Radicis) 30g
Wu Bei Zi‡ (Galla Rhois Chinensis) 30g
Huang Bai (Cortex Phellodendri) 30g
Ku Fan‡ (Alumen Praeparatum) 30g
Tu Fu Ling (Rhizoma Smilacis Glabrae) 30g
Fang Feng (Radix Ledebouriellae Divaricatae) 30g

Two bags a day were used to prepare a decoction for use as a wet compress or soak seven or eight times a day. Results were seen within five days.

3. **Yang** prepared a decoction for external use to treat genital eczema. [75]

Prescription ingredients

Huang Bai (Cortex Phellodendri) 30g
Ye Ju Hua (Flos Chrysanthemi Indici) 30g
She Chuang Zi (Fructus Cnidii Monnieri) 30g
Cang Er Zi (Fructus Xanthii Sibirici) 30g

Dan Shen (Radix Salviae Miltiorrhizae) 30g
Hu Zhang (Radix et Rhizoma Polygoni Cuspidati) 20g
Ku Shen (Radix Sophorae Flavescentis) 20g
Bo He (Herba Menthae Haplocalycis) 20g
Chai Hu (Radix Bupleuri) 20g
Fu Ling (Sclerotium Poriae Cocos) 20g
Dang Gui (Radix Angelicae Sinensis) 20g
Huang Lian (Rhizoma Coptidis) 15g

One bag a day was used and decocted three times; the liquids collected were mixed together and used first for steaming and then for washing the affected area for 20-30 minutes twice a day. For lesions with exudation, the decoction was cooled before use as a wet compress. Results were seen within 10 days.

4. **Yu** combined an external wash with a powder preparation to treat genital eczema. [76]

External wash ingredients

Jing Jie (Herba Schizonepetae Tenuifoliae) 15g
Fang Feng (Radix Ledebouriellae Divaricatae) 15g
Tou Gu Cao (Herba Speranskiae seu Impatientis) 15g
Mang Xiao ‡ (Mirabilitum) 15g
Bai Zhi (Radix Angelicae Dahuricae) 15g
Dang Gui (Radix Angelicae Sinensis) 15g
Hua Jiao (Pericarpium Zanthoxyli) 15g
Ai Ye (Folium Artemisiae Argyi) 30g
Ku Shen (Radix Sophorae Flavescentis) 30g
She Chuang Zi (Fructus Cnidii Monnieri) 30g

After decocting for 20 minutes, the preparation was used as a wash for 20-30 minutes twice a day. In the acute phase, the decoction was used as a cold wet compress; in the chronic phase, it was used first to steam and then to wash the affected area.

Powder preparation ingredients

Long Gu ‡ (Os Draconis) 30g
Da Huang (Radix et Rhizoma Rhei) 15g
Bing Pian (Borneolum) 3g
Zhen Zhu Fen ‡ (Pearl Powder) 3g

These ingredients were ground into a very fine powder and applied twice a day to the affected area when it was still warm after washing with the medicated decoction prepared with the first prescription. Where this treatment was effective, results were seen within 10 days.

COMBINED USE OF TCM AND WESTERN MEDICINE

Han treated eczema of the scrotum by combining TCM and Western medicine. [77]

TCM prescription ingredients

Ku Shen (Radix Sophorae Flavescentis) 30g
She Chuang Zi (Fructus Cnidii Monnieri) 30g
Di Fu Zi (Fructus Kochiae Scopariae) 30g
Jing Jie (Herba Schizonepetae Tenuifoliae) 20g
Fang Feng (Radix Ledebouriellae Divaricatae) 20g
Bai Xian Pi (Cortex Dictamni Dasycarpi Radicis) 20g
Chan Tui ‡ (Periostracum Cicadae) 15g

If there was secondary infection resulting in abscesses, *Jin Yin Hua* (Flos Lonicerae) 30g, *Ju Hua* (Flos Chrysanthemi Morifolii) 30g and *Lian Qiao* (Fructus Forsythiae Suspensae) 20g were added.

The ingredients were used to prepare a decoction for steam-washing the affected areas for 30 minutes every evening.

A medium-potency steroid cream, fluocinolone acetonide, was applied to the lesions after the skin had dried. Results were seen after 15 days.

Perianal eczema
肛周湿疹

Perianal eczema is an eczematoid change around the anus usually due to poor anal hygiene, irritation from repeated washing (especially with soap or detergent), worm infection, or hemorrhoids

Topical medicaments (especially those containing local anesthetic agents or antibiotics) and perfumed toiletries are commonly responsible for contact hypersensitivity reactions at this site.

In TCM, this condition is also known as *han huo chuang* (Cold-Fire sore).

Clinical manifestations

- This condition mostly occurs in middle-aged or older men.
- Acute conditions are characterized by moisture, erosion and exudation, whereas lichenification, infiltration and radial fissuring accompanied by depigmentation or pain are typical manifestations in the chronic phase.

- Severe itching makes sleep difficult.

Differential diagnosis

Tinea cruris (jock itch)
This disease occurs almost exclusively in males. The lesion appears as a red scaly patch that spreads gradually to the thigh and the buttocks from the crural fold. There is often intolerable local itching.

Flexural psoriasis
This type of psoriasis usually affects older people, women more than men. Lesions can involve the ano-genital region and other body flexures and manifest as well-demarcated, red, glistening plaques without scaling.

Lichen simplex chronicus (neurodermatitis)
This condition, which should be differentiated from the chronic stage of perianal eczema, occurs as a result of constant scratching to alleviate pruritus, the anogenital region being one of the sites of predilection. Lesions generally manifest as a single irregular or polygonal-shaped plaque. The skin in the affected area is rough with deepened skin creases and very little exudation.

Etiology and pathology

Damp-Heat
A preference for spicy, greasy and rich food, or excessive intake of greasy food and alcohol will lead to Dampness and Heat binding and gradually transforming into Fire and Heat Toxins. Damp-Heat pours down to the Large Intestine and gradually generates Worms, eventually resulting in redness, exudation and erosion of the skin and mucous membranes around the anus.

Spleen Deficiency
Spleen Deficiency impairs the transportation and transformation function leading to internal generation of Dampness, which pours down to cause perianal eczema.

Wind-Dryness
Long-term accumulation of Damp-Heat consumes Yin and damages the Blood to cause Blood Deficiency and Wind-Dryness. Lack of nourishment leads to the skin becoming dry and fissured.

Pattern identification and treatment

INTERNAL TREATMENT

DAMP-HEAT
Pruritus occurs around the anus. Excoriation leads to maceration in the perianal area. The tongue body is red with a greasy, turbid coating; the pulse is slippery.

Treatment principle
Kill Worms and alleviate itching, clear and transform Damp-Heat.

Prescription
ZHUI CHONG WAN JIA JIAN
Pill for Expelling Worms, with modifications

Da Fu Pi (Pericarpium Arecae Catechu) 6g
Lei Wan (Sclerotium Omphaliae Lapidescens) 6g
Ku Lian Pi (Cortex Meliae Radicis) 6g
Shi Jun Zi (Fructus Quisqualis Indicae) 10g
Chen Pi (Pericarpium Citri Reticulatae) 10g
Chao Huang Bai (Cortex Phellodendri, stir-fried) 10g
Chao Long Dan Cao (Radix Gentianae Scabrae, stir-fried) 10g
Fu Ling (Sclerotium Poriae Cocos) 10g
Chao Zhi Ke (Fructus Citri Aurantii, stir-fried) 12g
Shu Da Huang (Radix et Rhizoma Rhei Conquitae) 4.5g, added 10 minutes before the end of the decoction process

Explanation
- *Chao Long Dan Cao* (Radix Gentianae Scabrae, stir-fried), *Chao Huang Bai* (Cortex Phellodendri, stir-fried) and *Fu Ling* (Sclerotium Poriae Cocos) clear Heat and transform Dampness.
- *Da Fu Pi* (Pericarpium Arecae Catechu), *Lei Wan* (Sclerotium Omphaliae Lapidescens), *Ku Lian Pi* (Cortex Meliae Radicis), and *Shi Jun Zi* (Fructus Quisqualis Indicae) kill Worms and alleviate itching.
- *Chen Pi* (Pericarpium Citri Reticulatae), *Chao Zhi Ke* (Fructus Citri Aurantii, stir-fried) and *Shu Da Huang* (Radix et Rhizoma Rhei Conquitae) regulate Qi and free the Fu organs.
- Once Damp-Heat Toxins have been removed, the itching will disappear spontaneously.

SPLEEN DEFICIENCY
This pattern manifests as prickly itching around the anus, which worsens at night, or as macerated and blanched skin, or as dry, painful and cracked skin around the anus. Accompanying symptoms and signs include a lusterless white facial complexion, emaciation, irritability and restlessness, anxiety, abnormal appetite, and loose stools. The tongue body is pale red with a scant coating; the pulse is wiry and thready.

Treatment principle
Augment Qi and fortify the Spleen, support Vital Qi (Zheng Qi) and alleviate itching.

Prescription
SI JUN ZI TANG JIA WEI
Four Gentlemen Decoction, with additions

Sha Ren (Fructus Amomi) 6g, added 5 minutes before the end of the decoction process

Huang Lian (Rhizoma Coptidis) 6g
Chen Pi (Pericarpium Citri Reticulatae) 12g
Dang Shen (Radix Codonopsitis Pilosulae) 12g
Bai Zhu (Rhizoma Atractylodis Macrocephalae) 12g
Shan Yao (Rhizoma Dioscoreae Oppositae) 12g
Fu Ling (Sclerotium Poriae Cocos) 10g
Shen Qu (Massa Fermentata) 10g
Lian Zi Xin (Plumula Nelumbinis Nuciferae) 10g
Gan Cao (Radix Glycyrrhizae) 10g

Explanation

- *Dang Shen* (Radix Codonopsitis Pilosulae), *Fu Ling* (Sclerotium Poriae Cocos), *Bai Zhu* (Rhizoma Atractylodis Macrocephalae), *Gan Cao* (Radix Glycyrrhizae), and *Shan Yao* (Rhizoma Dioscoreae Oppositae) augment Qi and support the Spleen.
- *Sha Ren* (Fructus Amomi) and *Chen Pi* (Pericarpium Citri Reticulatae) regulate Qi and transform Dampness.
- *Huang Lian* (Rhizoma Coptidis) and *Lian Zi Xin* (Plumula Nelumbinis Nuciferae) drain Fire and relieve Toxicity.
- *Shen Qu* (Massa Fermentata) expels pathogenic factors and disperses food accumulation.
- If Spleen Qi is strong enough to perform its normal transportation function, Damp-Heat can be eliminated.

WIND-DRYNESS

The skin and mucous membranes around the anus are red, dry, cracked, lichenified, and itchy. Excoriations with bloody crusts are evident. Accompanying symptoms and signs include dry mouth with a desire for drinks and stools that are sometimes dry and sometimes loose. The tongue body is red with a scant coating; the pulse is floating and rapid.

Treatment principle

Dredge Wind and moisten Dryness, extinguish Wind and alleviate itching.

Prescription

YANG XUE RUN FU TANG JIA JIAN

Decoction for Nourishing the Blood and Moistening the Skin, with modifications

Dang Gui (Radix Angelicae Sinensis) 10g
Bai Shao (Radix Paeoniae Lactiflorae) 10g
He Shou Wu (Radix Polygoni Multiflori) 10g
Hei Zhi Ma (Semen Sesami Indici) 10g
Shu Di Huang (Radix Rehmanniae Glutinosae Conquita) 10g
Gou Teng (Ramulus Uncariae cum Uncis) 12g
Bai Ji Li (Fructus Tribuli Terrestris) 12g
Huang Qin (Radix Scutellariae Baicalensis) 6g
Ku Shen (Radix Sophorae Flavescentis) 6g

Explanation

- *Dang Gui* (Radix Angelicae Sinensis), *Bai Shao* (Radix Paeoniae Lactiflorae), *He Shou Wu* (Radix Polygoni Multiflori), and *Shu Di Huang* (Radix Rehmanniae Glutinosae Conquita) enrich Yin and moisten Dryness.
- *Gou Teng* (Ramulus Uncariae cum Uncis) and *Bai Ji Li* (Fructus Tribuli Terrestris) extinguish Wind and alleviate itching.
- *Hei Zhi Ma* (Semen Sesami Indici) moistens Dryness and frees the bowels.
- *Huang Qin* (Radix Scutellariae Baicalensis) and *Ku Shen* (Radix Sophorae Flavescentis) clear Heat and relieve Toxicity, dry Dampness and alleviate itching.

General modifications

1. For poor appetite and food accumulation, add *Shan Zha* (Fructus Crataegi) and *Mai Ya* (Fructus Hordei Vulgaris Germinatus).
2. For nausea and abdominal pain, add *Ji Nei Jin*‡ (Endothelium Corneum Gigeriae Galli) and *Lai Fu Zi* (Semen Raphani Sativi).
3. For persistent non-healing lesions, add *Chao Du Zhong* (Cortex Eucommiae Ulmoidis, stir-fried), *Xiao Hui Xiang* (Fructus Foeniculi Vulgaris) and *Chen Xiang* (Lignum Aquilariae Resinatum).
4. For irritability and mental confusion, add *Ye Jiao Teng* (Caulis Polygoni Multiflori) and *He Huan Pi* (Cortex Albizziae Julibrissin).

EXTERNAL TREATMENT

- For damp ulceration in the perianal area, select two or three herbs from *Jiu Cai* (Folium Allii Tuberosi), *Chuan Lian Zi* (Fructus Meliae Toosendan), *Bian Xu* (Herba Polygoni Avicularis), *Tao Ye* (Folium Persicae), *She Chuang Zi* (Fructus Cnidii Monnieri), and *Ma Chi Xian* (Herba Portulacae Oleraceae) and prepare a decoction for use as a wet compress on the affected area.
- For dryness, desquamation and itching in the perianal area, select one of the following materia medica – powdered *Bing Lang** (Semen Arecae Catechu), powdered *Shi Jun Zi* (Fructus Quisqualis Indicae), powdered *Bai Bu* (Radix Stemonae), and powdered *He Shi* (Fructus Carpesii) – and mix into a paste with vegetable oil. Apply the medicated paste directly to the perianal area.

ACUPUNCTURE

Main point: EX-LE-3 Baichongwo.[xi]
Auxiliary point: BL-25 Dachangshu.

[xi] M-LE-34 according to the system employed by the Shanghai College of Traditional Chinese Medicine.

Technique: Apply the reducing method to the points. Retain the needles for 30 minutes after obtaining Qi, stimulating them three to five times during this period. Treat once a day. A course consists of ten treatment sessions.

Explanation

EX-LE-3 Baichongwo and BL-25 Dachangshu expel Wind and eliminate Dampness, disperse swelling and alleviate itching.

MOXIBUSTION

Point: Ashi point (the perianal area).
Technique: Apply an ignited moxa stick to the affected area, adjusting the temperature according to the patient's tolerance level. Treat for five to ten minutes once a day. This treatment is suitable for the stage of chronic eczematoid changes around the anus.

Clinical notes

- When treating this condition, the main focus is placed on external treatment. Best results are generally achieved by combining decoctions for use as a wet compress and external application of ointments. Medications selected for external application should not be stimulating in the form in which they are used.

- Internal treatment can play a certain supporting role and is especially necessary for conditions complicated by disharmony of the Zang-Fu organs.

- Acupuncture and moxibustion are effective in alleviating itching and appropriate use will help to achieve a good result.

- Give prior treatment to primary diseases such as hemorrhoids, anal fistulae and perianal boils.

Advice for the patient

- Pay close attention to personal hygiene. Take baths or showers regularly, cut the fingernails frequently and change underwear daily. Wash hands before meals and after using the toilet.

- Avoid spicy food and alcohol during the treatment.

Modern clinical experience

COMBINED INTERNAL AND EXTERNAL TREATMENT

1. **Dong** combined internal treatment according to pattern identification with steam-washing of the affected area. [78]

- For **Damp-Heat** patterns, he recommended the following materia medica:

Chao Huang Bai (Cortex Phellodendri, stir-fried) 10g
Cang Zhu (Rhizoma Atractylodis) 6g
Ku Shen (Radix Sophorae Flavescentis) 15g
Qin Jiao (Radix Gentianae Macrophyllae) 10g
Jing Jie (Herba Schizonepetae Tenuifoliae) 10g
Di Fu Zi (Fructus Kochiae Scopariae) 10g
Fang Feng (Radix Ledebouriellae Divaricatae) 6g
Bai Xian Pi (Cortex Dictamni Dasycarpi Radicis) 30g

Other materia medica such as *Jin Yin Hua* (Flos Lonicerae) 10g, *Bai Mao Gen* (Rhizoma Imperatae Cylindricae) 30g, *Fu Ling* (Sclerotium Poriae Cocos) 10g, and *Yi Yi Ren* (Semen Coicis Lachryma-jobi) 30g could be added depending on the strength of the Damp-Heat.

- For **Blood Deficiency and Wind-Dryness** patterns, he recommended the following materia medica:

Dang Shen (Radix Codonopsitis Pilosulae) 10g
Cang Zhu (Rhizoma Atractylodis) 6g
Fu Ling (Sclerotium Poriae Cocos) 10g
Dang Gui (Radix Angelicae Sinensis) 15g
Sheng Di Huang (Radix Rehmanniae Glutinosae) 15g
Fang Feng (Radix Ledebouriellae Divaricatae) 10g
Hong Hua (Flos Carthami Tinctorii) 10g
Ku Shen (Radix Sophorae Flavescentis) 15g

Prescriptions for localized steam-washing depended on the stage of the disease:

- **Acute stage**

Ku Shen (Radix Sophorae Flavescentis) 15g
Hua Jiao (Pericarpium Zanthoxyli) 6g
Huang Bai (Cortex Phellodendri) 15g
Tu Fu Ling (Rhizoma Smilacis Glabrae) 30g
Cang Zhu (Rhizoma Atractylodis) 6g
Di Fu Zi (Fructus Kochiae Scopariae) 15g
She Chuang Zi (Fructus Cnidii Monnieri) 6g
Bai Xian Pi (Cortex Dictamni Dasycarpi Radicis) 30g
Bing Pian (Borneolum) 10g, added 5 minutes before the end of the decoction process

- **Chronic stage**

Dang Gui (Radix Angelicae Sinensis) 15g
Bai Shao (Radix Paeoniae Lactiflorae) 15g
Sheng Di Huang (Radix Rehmanniae Glutinosae) 15g
Cang Zhu (Rhizoma Atractylodis) 10g
Tu Fu Ling (Rhizoma Smilacis Glabrae) 30g
Huang Qin (Radix Scutellariae Baicalensis) 10g
Fang Feng (Radix Ledebouriellae Divaricatae) 10g
Chan Tui‡ (Periostracum Cicadae) 10g
She Chuang Zi (Fructus Cnidii Monnieri) 15g

Bing Pian (Borneolum) 10g, added 5 minutes before the end of the decoction process

Results were seen after 20 days on average (in a range from 10 to 60 days).

2. **Ye** combined internal treatment with a sitz bath. [79]

Internal prescription ingredients

Dang Gui (Radix Angelicae Sinensis) 10g
Chuan Xiong (Rhizoma Ligustici Chuanxiong) 10g
Bai Shao (Radix Paeoniae Lactiflorae) 10g
Chi Shao (Radix Paeoniae Rubra) 10g
Shu Di Huang (Radix Rehmanniae Glutinosae Conquita) 15g
Tao Ren (Semen Persicae) 10g
Hong Hua (Flos Carthami Tinctorii) 10g
He Shou Wu (Radix Polygoni Multiflori) 15g
Bai Xian Pi (Cortex Dictamni Dasycarpi Radicis) 30g
Fang Feng (Radix Ledebouriellae Divaricatae) 10g
Chan Tui ‡ (Periostracum Cicadae) 10g
Jiang Can ‡ (Bombyx Batryticatus) 10g

One bag a day was used to prepare a decoction, taken three times a day.

Sitz bath prescription ingredients

Ku Shen (Radix Sophorae Flavescentis) 50g
Huang Bai (Cortex Phellodendri) 50g
Bai Xian Pi (Cortex Dictamni Dasycarpi Radicis) 200g
Di Fu Zi (Fructus Kochiae Scopariae) 100g
She Chuang Zi (Fructus Cnidii Monnieri) 50g
Wu Bei Zi ‡ (Galla Rhois Chinensis) 20g
Da Huang (Radix et Rhizoma Rhei) 20g
Ku Fan ‡ (Alumen Praeparatum) 50g

The ingredients were decocted in 10 liters of water to prepare a sitz bath taken twice a day, 10-20 minutes each time. The course of treatment ranged from one to three weeks.

EXTERNAL TREATMENT

1. **Xie** treated perianal eczema with a sitz bath and a powder for external application. [80]

Bath prescription
SHI ZHEN TANG ZUO YU
Eczema Decoction Sitz Bath

Tu Fu Ling (Rhizoma Smilacis Glabrae) 30g
Bai Jiang Cao (Herba Patriniae cum Radice) 30g
Bai Xian Pi (Cortex Dictamni Dasycarpi Radicis) 30g
Di Fu Zi (Fructus Kochiae Scopariae) 30g
Ma Chi Xian (Herba Portulacae Oleraceae) 30g
Bian Xu (Herba Polygoni Avicularis) 30g
Ye Ju Hua (Flos Chrysanthemi Indici) 30g
Hua Shi ‡ (Talcum) 30g

Ku Shen (Radix Sophorae Flavescentis) 60g
Jin Yin Hua (Flos Lonicerae) 40g
She Chuang Zi (Fructus Cnidii Monnieri) 20g
Chan Tui ‡ (Periostracum Cicadae) 20g
Cang Er Zi (Fructus Xanthii Sibirici) 20g
Hua Jiao (Pericarpium Zanthoxyli) 20g
Ku Fan ‡ (Alumen Praeparatum) 15g
Bing Pian (Borneolum) 9g, added to the prepared decoction

All the ingredients except *Bing Pian* (Borneolum) were decocted in water for 20 minutes. After *Bing Pian* (Borneolum) was added, the liquid was divided into two portions. The decoction was first used to steam the affected area, then as a 20-30 minute sitz bath, two or three times a day.

Powder prescription
SHI ZHEN SAN
Eczema Powder

Ku Fan ‡ (Alumen Praeparatum) 10g
Hua Shi ‡ (Talcum) 20g
Da Huang (Radix et Rhizoma Rhei) 20g
Huang Bai (Cortex Phellodendri) 20g
Duan Shi Gao ‡ (Gypsum Fibrosum Calcinatum) 40g
Bing Pian (Borneolum) 2g

The ingredients were ground together into a very fine powder, and used for lesions with exudation; for lesions without exudation, the powder was mixed with vegetable oil before application. The period of treatment required ranged from five to eight days. Recurrence was rare.

2. **Li** combined application of *Huang Bai Ku Shen Cha Ji* (Phellodendron and Flavescent Sophora Root Rub Preparation) and *Huang Bai Zhi Yang Gao* (Phellodendron Paste for Alleviating Itching). [81]

Rub prescription
HUANG BAI KU SHEN CHA JI
Phellodendron and Flavescent Sophora Root Rub Preparation

Huang Bai (Cortex Phellodendri) 20g
Ku Shen (Radix Sophorae Flavescentis) 20g
Da Huang (Radix et Rhizoma Rhei) 20g
Hua Jiao (Pericarpium Zanthoxyli) 15g
Cang Zhu (Rhizoma Atractylodis) 15g
She Chuang Zi (Fructus Cnidii Monnieri) 15g
Bai Zhi (Radix Angelicae Dahuricae) 15g

These ingredients were ground into a very fine powder, wrapped in a cloth and soaked in a tightly-sealed container with 5kg of *Chen Cu* (Acetum Vetum) for three months. The residues were then removed and the medicated liquid was stored in a bottle ready for use.

Paste prescription
HUANG BAI ZHI YANG GAO
Phellodendron Paste for Alleviating Itching

Huang Bai (Cortex Phellodendri)
Ku Fan‡ (Alumen Praeparatum)
Bing Pian (Borneolum)
Duan Shi Gao‡ (Gypsum Fibrosum Calcinatum)

The paste was prepared by grinding equal amounts of the ingredients into a powder and mixing into a paste with Vaseline® in a ratio of 1:4.

The medications were used to treat erosive and exudative lesions. After washing the affected area with lukewarm water, *Huang Bai Ku Shen Cha Ji* (Phellodendron and Flavescent Sophora Root Rub Preparation) was applied first. Once this had dried, *Huang Bai Zhi Yang Gao* (Phellodendron Paste for Alleviating Itching) was used. Treatment was given once in the morning and once in the evening. The treatment period required ranged from ten days to two months.

3. **Tian** treated pruritic perianal eczema with *Er Huang San* (Two Yellows Powder). The powder was prepared by grinding *Pu Huang* (Pollen Typhae) 100g and *Liu Huang*‡ (Sulphur) 25g into a fine powder. After washing the eczematous or itchy perianal area with lukewarm water, the powder was applied with a piece of dry gauze. The gauze was also used to massage the affected area gently for one or two minutes after application of the medication, after which the area was covered by fresh gauze. Treatment was given once in the morning and once in the evening. Where this method was effective, significant improvement was seen within 10 days. [82]

References

1. Beijing Hospital of Traditional Chinese Medicine, *Zhao Bing Nan Lin Chuang Jing Yan Ji* [A Collection of Zhao Bingnan's Clinical Experiences] (Beijing: People's Medical Publishing House, 1975), 130.
2. Ibid., 132.
3. Tianjin College of Traditional Chinese Medicine First Affiliated Hospital, *Shi Xue Min Zhen Jiu Lin Zheng Ji Yan* [A Collection of Shi Xuemin's Clinical Experiences in Acupuncture and Moxibustion] (Tianjin: Tianjin Science and Technology Publishing House, 1990), 466.
4. An Jiafeng and Zhang Peng, *Zhang Zhi Li Pi Fu Bing Yi An Xuan Cui* [A Collection of Zhang Zhili's Skin Disease Cases] (Beijing: People's Medical Publishing House, 1994), 108.
5. Traditional Chinese Medicine Research Academy: Beijing Guang'anmen Hospital, *Zhu Ren Kang Lin Chuang Jing Yan Ji* [A Collection of Zhu Renkang's Clinical Experiences] (Beijing: People's Medical Publishing House, 1979), 97.
6. Beijing Hospital of Traditional Chinese Medicine, *Zhao Bing Nan Lin Chuang Jing Yan Ji*, 138.
7. An Jiafeng and Zhang Peng, *Zhang Zhi Li Pi Fu Bing Yi An Xuan Cui*, 110.
8. Dai Qin, *Zhong Yao Zhi Liao Fan Fa Xing Shi Zhen 126 Li Liao Xiao Fen Xi* [Analysis of the Therapeutic Results of 126 Cases of Extensive Eczema Treated with Chinese Materia Medica], *Tian Jin Zhong Yi* [Tianjin Journal of Traditional Chinese Medicine] 16, 1 (1999): 17.
9. Mo Zhigang, *Zhong Yao Nei Fu Wai Xi Zhi Liao Shi Zhen 110 Li* [Internal Treatment and External Washes with Chinese Materia Medica in the Treatment of 110 Cases of Eczema], *Guang Xi Zhong Yi Yao* [Guangxi Journal of Traditional Chinese Medicine and Materia Medica] 20, 2 (1997): 6.
10. Wang Yanxu, *Nei Wai He Zhi Shi Zhen 30 Li* [Treatment of 30 Cases of Eczema with Combined Internal and External Treatment], *He Nan Zhong Yi* [Henan Journal of Traditional Chinese Medicine] 16, 6 (1996): 372.
11. Cui Yongqiang, *Zhen Ci Zhi Liao Shi Zhen 28 Li Lin Chuang Guan Cha* [Clinical Observation of 28 Cases of Eczema Treated by Acupuncture], *Zhong Guo Zhen Jiu* [Chinese Journal of Acupuncture and Moxibustion] 16, 7 (1996): 17-18.
12. Li Ming, *Xie Xin Tang Jia Wei Zhi Liao Ji Xing Shi Zhen 116 Li Lin Chuang Liao Xiao Guan Cha* [Clinical Observation of the Therapeutic Effect in 116 Cases of Acute Eczema Treated with Augmented *Xie Xin Tang* (Draining the Heart Decoction)], *Yun Nan Zhong Yi Zhong Yao Za Zhi* [Yunnan Journal of Traditional Chinese Medicine and Materia Medica] 17, 6 (1996): 22.
13. Fu Yushan, *Ji Xing Shi Zhen Wai Yong Lai Fu Zi* [External Use of *Lai Fu Zi* (Semen Raphani Sativi) for Acute Eczema], *Zhong Yi Za Zhi* [Journal of Traditional Chinese Medicine] 39, 8 (1998): 475.
14. Luo Yuming, *Ku Shen Wu She Tang Jia Jian Zhi Liao 110 Li Lin Chuang Guan Cha* [Clinical Observation of the Treatment of 110 Cases of Eczema with Modified *Ku Shen Wu She Tang* (Flavescent Sophora Root and Black-Tail Snake Decoction)], *Jiang Xi Zhong Yi Yao* [Jiangxi Journal of Traditional Chinese Medicine] 2 (1985): 23.
15. Beijing Hospital of Traditional Chinese Medicine, *Zhao Bing Nan Lin Chuang Jing Yan Ji*, 118.
16. Guan Fen, *Shi Yong Zhong Yi Pi Fu Bing Xue* [Practical Dermatology in Traditional Chinese Medicine] (Lanzhou: Gansu People's Publishing House, 1986), 147.
17. Traditional Chinese Medicine Research Academy: Beijing Guang'anmen Hospital, *Zhu Ren Kang Lin Chuang Jing Yan Ji*, 97.
18. Dermatology Department of Guangdong TCM Hospital, *Chuan Ran Xing Shi Zhen Yang Pi Yan 21 Li Zhi Liao Xiao Jie* [Summary of Treatment of 21 Cases of Infectious

Eczematoid Dermatitis], *Shi Yong Yi Xue Za Zhi* [Journal of Practical Medicine] 2, 2 (1986): 34.

19. An Jiafeng and Zhang Peng, *Zhang Zhi Li Pi Fu Bing Yi An Xuan Cui*, 135.

20. Ibid., 137.

21. Fang Peiying, *Zi Ni Qu Feng Zhi Yang Tang Zhi Liao Jie Chu Xing Pi Yan 30 Li* [Treatment of 30 Cases of Contact Dermatitis with the Empirical Prescription *Qu Feng Zhi Yang Tang* (Decoction for Dispelling Wind and Alleviating Itching)], *Shang Hai Zhong Yi Yao Za Zhi* [Shanghai Journal of Traditional Chinese Medicine and Materia Medica] 2 (1996): 35.

22. Wang Yuzhen, *Qing Re Jie Du Tang Zhi Liao Ran Fa Ji Zhi Jie Chu Xing Pi Yan 30 Li* [Treatment of 30 Cases of Contact Dermatitis due to Dyes with *Qing Re Jie Du Tang* (Decoction for Clearing Heat and Relieving Toxicity)], *Zhong Guo Zhong Xi Yi Jie He Za Zhi* [Journal of Integrated TCM and Western Medicine] 18, 1 (1994): 62.

23. Liu Wei, *Zhong Xi Yi Jie He Zhi Liao Ran Fa Suo Zhi Jie Chu Xing Pi Yan 32 Li* [Treatment of 32 Cases of Contact Dermatitis due to Dyes with a Combination of TCM and Western Medicine], *Liao Ning Zhong Yi Za Zhi* [Liaoning Journal of Traditional Chinese Medicine] 25, 2 (1998): 76.

24. Beijing Hospital of Traditional Chinese Medicine, *Zhao Bing Nan Lin Chuang Jing Yan Ji*, 149.

25. Zhang Peng, *Zhang Zhi Li Zhi Liao Yi Wei Xing Pi Yan Jing Yan* [Zhang Zhili's Experiences in Treating Atopic Eczema], *Zhong Yi Za Zhi* [Journal of Traditional Chinese Medicine] 39, 8 (1998): 402-4.

26. Wang Ping, *Xiao Er Shi Zhen Ji Yi Wei Xing Pi Yan Zhi Liao Ti Hui* [Experiences in Treating Infantile Eczema and Atopic Eczema], *Shi Yong Zhong Xi Yi Jie He Za Zhi* [Practical Journal of Integrated TCM and Western Medicine] 11, 7 (1998): 620.

27. Liu Tianji, *Yang Xue Qu Feng Tang Zhi Liao Yi Wei Xing Pi Yan 60 Li* [Treatment of 60 Cases of Atopic Eczema with *Yang Xue Qu Feng Tang* (Decoction for Nourishing the Blood and Dispelling Wind)], *Si Chuan Zhong Yi* [Sichuan Journal of Traditional Chinese Medicine] 16, 9 (1998): 29.

28. Dong Ziliang, *Qi Miao Yin Zhi Liao Yi Chuan Guo Min Xing Pi Yan Lin Chuang Guan Cha* [Clinical Observation of the Treatment of Atopic Eczema with *Qi Miao Yin* (Marvelous Beverage)], *Zhong Guo Zhong Yi Yao Xin Xi Za Zhi* [Traditional Chinese Medicine and Materia Medica News] 4, 12 (1997): 36-37.

29. Yu Shigen, *Pi Yan Xiao Jing Yin Er Hao Zhi Liao Yi Wei Xing Pi Yan De Lin Chuang He Shi Yan Yan Jiu* [Clinical and Experimental Study on the Treatment of Atopic Eczema with *Pi Yan Xiao Jing Yin Er Hao* (No. 2 Dermatitis Dispersing Beverage)], *Zhong Yi Za Zhi* [Journal of Traditional Chinese Medicine] 40, 3 (1999): 165-7.

30. Zhan Naijun, *Shu Feng Qu Shi Zhi Liao Ying You Er Shi Zhen 36 Li* [Treatment of 36 Cases of Eczema in Infants and Young Children with the Principles of Dredging Wind and Dispelling Dampness], *Zhe Jiang Zhong Yi Za Zhi* [Zhejiang Journal of Traditional Chinese Medicine] 29, 6 (1994): 262.

31. Zhang Xiangxin, *Ge Gen Qin Lian Tang He Ping Wei San Jia Wei Zhi Liao Ying Er Shi Zhen* [Treatment of Infantile Eczema by Combining *Ge Gen Qin Lian Tang* (Kudzu, Scutellaria and Coptis Decoction) and Augmented *Ping Wei San* (Calming the Stomach Powder)], *Si Chuan Zhong Yi* [Sichuan Journal of Traditional Chinese Medicine] 7 (1987): 12.

32. Peng Jinfang, *Qu Feng Zhi Yang Tang Zhi Liao Ying Er Shi Zhen 139 Li* [Treatment of 139 Cases of Infantile Eczema with *Qu Feng Zhi Yang Tang* (Decoction for Dispelling Wind and Alleviating Itching)], *Guang Xi Zhong Yi Yao* [Guangxi Journal of Traditional Chinese Medicine and Materia Medica] 22, 4 (1999): 27.

33. Qian Chunmei, *Zhong Yao Wai Xi Zhi Liao Ying Er Shi Zhen* [Treatment of Infantile Eczema with Chinese Materia Medica External Wash Preparations], *Jiang Su Zhong Yi* [Jiangsu Journal of Traditional Chinese Medicine] 20, 9 (1999): 46.

34. Fu Hongwei, *Zhong Yao Nei Wai He Zhi Ying You Er Yi Wei Xing Pi Yan 160 Li – Fu Xi Yao Zhi Liao 100 Li Dui Zhao* [Chinese Materia Medica Used in Combined Internal and External Treatment of 160 Cases of Infantile Atopic Eczema – Attachment of Comparative Treatment of 100 Cases with Western Medications], *Zhe Jiang Zhong Yi Za Zhi* [Zhejiang Journal of Traditional Chinese Medicine] 34, 8 (1999): 334.

35. Zheng Jida, *Zhong Xi Yi Jie He Zhi Liao Yi Wei Xing Pi Yan 36 Li* [Treatment of 36 Cases of Atopic Eczema with a Combination of TCM and Western Medicine], *Guang Xi Zhong Yi Yao* [Guangxi Journal of Traditional Chinese Medicine and Materia Medica] 19, 2 (1996): 15-16.

36. Beijing Hospital of Traditional Chinese Medicine, *Zhao Bing Nan Lin Chuang Jing Yan Ji Yao*, 137.

37. Cao Yan, *Wang Yi Qian Zhi Liao Zhi Yi Xing Pi Yan San Fa* [Wang Yiqian's Three Methods for Treating Seborrheic Eczema], *Jiang Su Zhong Yi* [Jiangsu Journal of Traditional Chinese Medicine] 18, 1 (1997): 7-8.

38. Wu Yin, *Yu Nü Jian Jia Wei Zhi Liao Zhi Yi Xing Pi Yan 34 Li* [Treatment of 34 Cases of Seborrheic Eczema with Augmented *Yu Nü Jian* (Jade Lady Brew)], *Si Chuan Zhong Yi* [Sichuan Journal of Traditional Chinese Medicine] 15, 12 (1997): 43.

39. Yuan Mingze, *Jia Wei Huang Lian Jie Du Tang Zhi Liao Zhi Yi Xing Pi Yan* [Treatment of Seborrheic Eczema with *Jia Wei Huang Lian Jie Du Tang* (Augmented Coptis Decoction for Relieving Toxicity)], *Hu Bei Zhong Yi Za Zhi* [Hubei Journal of Traditional Chinese Medicine] 20, 3 (1998): 35.

40. Song Guoxu, *Yao Yu Zhi Liao Ying Er Zhi Yi Xing Pi Yan 42 Li* [Treatment of 42 Cases of Infantile Seborrheic Eczema with a Medicated Bath], *Zhong Hua Shi Yong Zhong Xi Yi Za Zhi* [Practical Journal of Traditional Chinese Medicine and Western Medicine] 12, 5 (1999): 866.

41. Zhang Jianxin, *Zhong Yao Qu Xie Tang Zhi Liao Zhi Yi Xing Pi Yan 50 Li* [Treatment of 50 Cases of Seborrheic Eczema with *Qu Xie Tang* (Decoction for Removing Scales)], *Zhong Yi Wai Zhi Za Zhi* [Journal of Traditional Chinese Medicine External Treatments] 6, 2 (1997): 47.

42. Gu Bohua, *Wai Ke Jing Yan Xuan* [A Selection of Experiences in the Treatment of External Diseases] (Shanghai: Shanghai People's Publishing House, 1977), 2.

43. Lu Shubo, *Lei Gong Teng Wai Pi Jian Ye Jin Pao Zhi Liao Shou Zu Shi Zhen 56 Li* [Treatment of 56 Cases of Hand and Foot Eczema with a Soak Prepared from a Decoction of Thunder God Vine Bark], *Zhong Guo Pi Fu Xing Bing Xue Za Zhi* [Chinese Journal of Dermatology and Venereology] 10, 5 (1996): 304.

44. Cheng Qiusheng et al., *Pi Fu Bing Zhong Yi Xi Zi Liao Fa* [Soak Therapies for Traditional Chinese Medicine Treatment of Skin Diseases] (Xi'an: Northwest University Publishing House, 1993), 123-4.

45. Traditional Chinese Medicine Research Academy: Beijing Guang'anmen Hospital, *Zhu Ren Kang Lin Chuang Jing Yan Ji*, 222.

46. Gu Bohua, *Shi Yong Zhong Yi Wai Ke Xue* [Practical Treatment of External Diseases with Traditional Chinese Medicine] (Shanghai: Shanghai Science and Technology Publishing House, 1985), 460.

47. An Jiafeng and Zhang Peng, *Zhang Zhi Li Pi Fu Bing Yi An Xuan Cui*, 152.

48. Zhang Zhili, *Zhang Zhi Li Pi Fu Bing Lin Chuang Jing Yan Ji Yao* [A Collection of Zhang Zhili's Clinical Experiences in the Treatment of Skin Diseases] (Beijing: People's Medical Publishing House, 2001), 276.

49. An Jiafeng and Zhang Peng, *Zhang Zhi Li Pi Fu Bing Yi An Xuan Cui*, 153.

50. Chen Sufei, *Zi Ni Yang Yue Qu Feng Tang Zhi Liao Shen Jing Xing Pi Yan 60 Li* [Treatment of 60 Cases of Neurodermatitis with the Empirical Prescription *Yang Yue Qu Feng Tang* (Decoction for Nourishing the Blood and Dispelling Wind)], *Guang Xi Zhong Yi Za Zhi* [Guangxi Journal of Traditional Chinese Medicine] 21, 2 (1998): 29.

51. Lu Jianxiu, *Shen Jing Xing Pi Yan 68 Li Liao Xiao Fen Xi* [Analysis of the Therapeutic Effect in 68 Cases of Neurodermatitis], *He Nan Zhong Yi* [Henan Journal of Traditional Chinese Medicine] 14, 4 (1994): 254.

52. Zhang Li, *Di Tai Cha Ji Zhi Liao Shen Jing Xing Pi Yan 60 Li* [Treatment of 60 Cases of Neurodermatitis with *Di Tai Ca Ji* (Anti-Lichen Rub Preparation)], *Zhong Yi Wai Zhi Za Zhi* [Journal of Traditional Chinese Medicine External Treatments] 7, 1 (1998): 21.

53. Wang Wenli, *Zi Cao Zhi Liao Shen Jing Xing Pi Yan You Te Xiao* [Specific Effect of *Zi Cao* (Radix Arnebiae seu Lithospermi) in the Treatment of Neurodermatitis], *Zhong Yi Za Zhi* [Journal of Traditional Chinese Medicine] 37, 9 (1996): 519.

54. Chen Sitai, *Zhong Xi Yi Jie He Zhi Liao Shen Jing Xing Pi Yan 73 Li* [Treatment of 73 Cases of Neurodermatitis with a Combination of Traditional Chinese Medicine and Western Medicine], *Zhong Ji Yi Kan* [Intermediate Grade Medical Journal] 31, 11 (1996): 51-52.

55. Ma Tianwei, *Qi Xing Zhen Jia Ai Tiao Jiu Zhi Liao Ju Xian Xing Shen Jing Xing Pi Yan 63 Li* [Treatment of 63 Cases of Circumscribed Neurodermatitis with Seven-Star Needling and Moxibustion with a Moxa Stick], *Zhong Guo Zhen Jiu* [Chinese Journal of Acupuncture and Moxibustion] 11, 9 (1996): 19-20.

56. Zheng Huasheng, *Dan Huang You Wai Zhi Niao Bu Pi Yan Mi Lan* [External Treatment of Erosive Diaper Dermatitis with *Dan Huang You* (Egg Yolk Oil)], *Yun Nan Zhong Yi Za Zhi* [Yunnan Journal of Traditional Chinese Medicine] 15, 3 (1994): 29.

57. He Yan, *Zi Cao You Zhi Liao Ying Er Niao Bu Xing Pi Yan 78 Li* [Treatment of 78 Cases of Infantile Diaper Dermatitis with *Zi Cao You* (Gromwell Root Oil)], *Xin Jiang Zhong Yi Yao* [Xinjiang Journal of Traditional Chinese Medicine and Materia Medica] 18, 6 (1998): 341.

58. Li Ya, *Zhong Yao Zong He Zhi Liao Xin Sheng Er Niao Bu Pi Yan* [Summary of Treatment of Diaper Dermatitis in Newborns with Chinese Materia Medica], *Shan Dong Zhong Yi Za Zhi* [Shandong Journal of Traditional Chinese Medicine] 17, 4 (1998): 186.

59. Cai Xiaohua, *Zhong Yao Wai Fu Zhi Liao Niao Bu Pi Yan 78 Li* [Treatment of 78 Cases of Diaper Dermatitis with External Application of Chinese Materia Medica], *Guang Dong Yi Xue* [Guangdong Journal of Medicine] 19, 10 (1998): 736.

60. Guan Fen, *Shi Yong Zhong Yi Pi Fu Bing Xue* [Practical Dermatology in Traditional Chinese Medicine] (Lanzhou: Gansu People's Publishing House, 1981), 140.

61. Chen Bingqiang, *Shan Jia San Zhi Liao Wai Er Shi Zhen Lin Chuang Guan Cha* [Clinical Observation of the Treatment of Ear Eczema with *Shan Jia San* (Pangolin Powder)], *He Nan Zhong Yi* [Henan Journal of Traditional Chinese Medicine] 18, 6 (1998): 394-5.

62. Hao Xingdun, *Ku Qing Song San Zhi Liao Wai Er Shi Zhen* [Treatment of Ear Eczema with *Ku Qing Song San* (Prepared Alum, Indigo and Rosin Powder)], *Shan Dong Zhong Yi Za Zhi* [Shandong Journal of Traditional Chinese Medicine] 17, 12 (1998): 571.

63. Yang Liping, *Xi Gua Shuang Zhi Liao Er Bi Bu Shi Zhen Bing Gan Ran 32 Li* [*Xi Gua Shuang* (Watermelon Frost) in the Treatment of 32 Cases of Ear and Nose Eczema Complicated by Infection], *Zhong Guo Zhong Xi Yi Jie He Za Zhi* [Journal of Integrated TCM and Western Medicine] 16, 3 (1996): 181.

64. Zhen Xianfu, *Lian Bing Gao Zhi Liao Wai Er Shi Zhen 20 Li* [Treatment of 20 Cases of Ear Eczema with *Lian Bing Gao* (Coptis and Borneol Paste)], *Si Chuan Zhong Yi* [Sichuan Journal of Traditional Chinese Medicine] 9 (1996): 50.

65. Ren Sixiu, *Zhong Yao Jia Li Liao Zhi Liao Xiao Er Er Bu Shi Zhen* [Treatment of Ear Eczema in Children with a Combination of Chinese Materia Medica and Physiotherapy], *Hei Long Jiang Zhong Yi Yao* [Heilongjiang Journal of Traditional Chinese Medicine and Materia Medica] 3 (1999): 20.

66. Wang Yueru, *Zi Ni Xiao Shi Tang Zhi Liao Er Bu Shi Zhen 67 Li Lin Chuang Guan Cha* [Clinical Observation of 67 Cases of Ear Eczema Treated with *Xiao Shi Tang* (Decoction for Dispersing Dampness)], *He Bei Zhong Yi* [Hebei Journal of Traditional Chinese Medicine] 17, 4 (1995): 31-32.

67. Li Sheng'an, *Ru Feng San Zhi Liao Ru Tou Jun Lie Zheng 35 Li* [Treatment of 35 Cases of Cracked Nipples with *Ru Feng San* (Nipple Wind Powder)], *Zhong Yi Za Zhi* [Journal of Traditional Chinese Medicine] 11 (1980): 78.

68. Wang Honghai, *San Shi San Zhi Liao Ru Tou Jun Lie* [Treatment of Cracked Nipples with *San Shi San* (Three Stones Powder)], *Xin Zhong Yi* [New Journal of Traditional Chinese Medicine] 6 (1974): 253.

69. Xu Yihou, *Shan Cang Gui Wai Ke Jing Yan Ji* [A Collection of Shan Canggui's Experiences in Treating External Diseases] (Wuhan: Hubei Science and Technology Publishing House, 1984), 119.

70. Zhang Zhili, *Zhang Zhi Li Pi Fu Bing Lin Chuang Jing Yan Ji Yao*, 244.

71. Zeng Yi, *Jia Wei Si Miao Tang Zhi Liao Yin Nang Shi Zhen 50 Li* [Treatment of 50 Cases of Eczema of the Scrotum with *Jia Wei Si Miao Tang* (Augmented Mysterious Four Decoction)], *Zhong Guo Pi Fu Xing Bing Xue Za Zhi* [Chinese Journal of Dermatology and Venereology] 11, 1 (1997): 47.

72. Lü Yipei, *Long Dan Xie Gan Tang Jia Wei Zhi Liao Ji Xing Yin Nang Shi Zhen 29 Li* [Treatment of 29 Cases of Acute Eczema of the Scrotum with Augmented *Long Dan Xie Gan Tang* (Chinese Gentian Decoction for Draining the Liver)], *Guang Xi Zhong Yi Yao* [Guangxi Journal of Traditional Chinese Medicine and Materia Medica], 21, 1 (1998): 37.

73. Huang Xianxun, *Liu Pi Tang Xun Xi Zhi Liao Yin Nang Shi Zhen 47 Li* [Steam-Wash Treatment of 47 Cases of Eczema of the Scrotum with *Liu Pi Tang* (Six Bark Decoction)], *Zhong Yi Wai Zhi Za Zhi* [Journal of Traditional Chinese Medicine External Treatments] 5, 1 (1996): 9.

74. Zeng Xiaoyue, *Qing Re Shou Lian Qu Shi Wei Zhu Zhi Liao Ji Xing Yin Nang Shi Zhen 72 Li* [Treatment of 72 Cases of Acute Eczema of the Scrotum by Focusing on Clearing Heat, Promoting Contraction and Dispelling Dampness], *Zhong Yi Wai Zhi Za Zhi* [Journal of Traditional Chinese Medicine External Treatments] 8, 2 (1999): 23.

75. Yang Fang'e, *Zhong Yao Ta Zi Fa Zhi Liao Wai Yin Shi Zhen 30 Li* [Treatment of 30 Cases of Genital Eczema with a Soak Prepared with Chinese Materia Medica], *Shan Xi Zhong Yi Xue Yuan Xue Bao* [Journal of Shanxi College of Traditional Chinese Medicine] 19, 4 (1996): 4.

76. Yu Qingyun, *Zhong Yao Wai Yong Zhi Liao Wai Yin Shi Zhen 60 Li* [Chinese Materia Medica in the External Treatment of 60 Cases of Genital Eczema], *Zhong Guo Zhong Xi Yi Jie He Za Zhi* [Journal of Integrated TCM and Western Medicine] 18, 4 (1998): 250.

77. Han Jingshui, *Zhong Xi Yi Jie He Zhi Liao Wan Gu Xing Yin Nang Shi Zhen 34 Li* [Combination of TCM and Western Medicine in the Treatment of 34 Cases of Stubborn Eczema of the Scrotum], *Shan Dong Yi Yao* [Shandong Journal of Medicine] 39, 12 (1999): 10.

78. Dong Xiaochun, *Bian Zheng Zhi Liao Gang Men Shi Zhen 80 Li* [Treatment of 80 Cases of Perianal Eczema Based on Pattern Identification], *Yun Nan Zhong Yi Zhong Yao Za Zhi* [Yunnan Journal of Traditional Chinese Medicine and Materia Medica] 20, 4 (1999): 21-22.

79. Ye Zhadong, *Zhong Yi Yao Zhi Liao Gang Men Man Xing Shi Zhen 55 Li* [Treatment of 55 Cases of Chronic Perianal Eczema with Traditional Chinese Medicine and Materia Medica], *Zhong Yi Wai Zhi Za Zhi* [Journal of Traditional Chinese Medicine External Treatments] 7, 1 (1998): 13.

80. Xie Deying, *Zi Ni Shi Zhen Tang Zuo Yu Zhi Liao Ji Xing Gang Men Shi Zhen 52 Li* [Treatment of 52 Cases of Acute Perianal Eczema with the Empirical Prescription *Shi Zhen Tang Zuo Yu* (Eczema Decoction Sitz Bath)], *Gui Yang Zhong Yi Xue Yuan Xue Bao* [Journal of Guiyang College of Traditional Chinese Medicine] 20, 3 (1998): 33-34.

81. Li Xiaoya, *Huang Bai Ku Shen Cha Ji Zhi Liao Gang Men Shi Zhen 36 Li* [Treatment of 36 Cases of Perianal Eczema with *Huang Bai Ku Shen Cha Ji* (Phellodendron and Flavescent Sophora Root Rub Preparation)], *Tian Jin Zhong Yi* [Tianjin Journal of Traditional Chinese Medicine] 16, 4 (1999): 38-39.

82. Tian Zhenguo, *Er Huang San Zhi Liao Gang Men Shi Zhen Sao Yang 20 Li* [Treatment of 20 Cases of Pruritic Anal Eczema with *Er Huang San* (Two Yellows Powder)], *Liao Ning Zhong Yi Za Zhi* [Liaoning Journal of Traditional Chinese Medicine] 23, 1 (1996): 25.

Chapter 4

Psoriasis and other papulosquamous disorders

Papulosquamous diseases are characterized by scaling, papules and plaques. Papulosquamous eruptions are raised, scaly and sharply marginated. Some diseases such as psoriasis present with large silvery-white scales; others such as the pityriasis conditions have much finer, bran-like scaling.

According to Traditional Chinese Medicine, there are several main causes of the type of skin disorder characterized by the presence of papular lesions and scaling:

- External pathogenic factors (principally Wind-Heat or Wind-Cold), which settle in the skin and flesh, disturb the normal diffusion of Qi by the Lungs and Spleen. These pathogenic factors then obstruct the channels and network vessels and stagnate in the skin and interstices (*cou li*), depriving the skin and flesh of nourishment.
- Dietary irregularities or internal damage due to the emotions can lead to Blood-Heat accumulating internally. Where this occurs over a period of time, Blood-Heat becomes exuberant, leading to generation of Wind. Prevalence of Wind gives rise to Dryness, preventing adequate nourishment of the skin and flesh.

- Qi stagnation and Blood stasis caused by Wind, Damp and Heat pathogenic factors being retained over a long period or by internal damage due to the emotions deprive the skin and flesh of nourishment.
- An improper diet can impair the normal functions of the Spleen and Stomach and generate internal Damp-Heat. If the body is attacked by external Wind, then Damp, Heat and Wind will combine to obstruct the skin and flesh and stagnate in the channels and network vessels to deprive the skin and flesh of nourishment.
- Exuberant Heart-Fire complicated by an invasion of Wind-Heat leads to transformation into Toxins. Heat Toxins gradually enter the Ying and Xue levels to consume Body Fluids, thus impeding correct nourishment of the skin and flesh. Insufficiency of Lung Yin and impairment of the transformation of Qi also results in Body Fluids not being disseminated correctly to nourish the skin and flesh.
- Yin Deficiency of the Liver and Kidneys leads to insufficiency of the Essence and Blood with the skin being deprived of moisture and nourishment and consequently becoming dry with desquamation.

Psoriasis
银屑病

Psoriasis is a chronic, recurrent inflammatory skin disease characterized by well-defined erythematous plaques topped by large, adherent silvery scales. It has a prevalence worldwide of 1 to 3 percent, although it is commoner in Europe and North America than in Africa and Asia.

The disease arises when the cells in the epidermis proliferate at many times their usual rate. Keratinocytes normally take 14 days to progress from differentiation in the basal layer of the epidermis to the stratum cor-

neum (the horny layer), where after another 14 days they die and are shed. In psoriasis, the turnover period is reduced to four days. Although the cycle time of individual cells does not change much, the number of cells is vastly expanded, resulting in the scaly appearance of psoriatic plaques.

The cause of these changes is still not completely clear, but research has indicated that they are related to hereditary, immunologic, metabolic, and endocrine factors.

There is a genetic component – when one parent has psoriasis, there is a 15-25 percent probability of the child developing the disease; this probability rises to 50-60 percent when both parents are affected. Incidence is unrelated to gender.

Infection may also play a role, although psoriasis itself is neither infectious nor contagious. An acute attack or aggravation of the disease is often triggered by inflammation of the upper respiratory tract or tonsillitis, most frequently in association with group A beta-hemolytic streptococcal infection.

Stress, trauma such as a scratch or surgical scar (the Koebner phenomenon), environmental influences, drugs such as lithium and antimalarials, and infection by the HIV virus affect the course and severity of the disease.

In TCM, this disease is also known as *bai bi* (white crust).

Clinical manifestations

- Psoriasis can start at any age, although it is rare in children under 10. Onset usually peaks between 15 and 30, but a second peak occurs between 55 and 60.
- Psoriasis can present in a variety of patterns:

Plaque psoriasis

- The most common type of psoriasis usually involves the extensor aspect of the limbs (especially the extensor aspect of the elbows and knees), the lower back and the scalp.
- Lesions are well demarcated and vary greatly in number, size and shape. Sometimes only a small area is affected without any obvious changes over a long period, sometimes the whole body is affected.
- At the initial stage, bright red or dark red macules, maculopapules or papules appear with a shiny, wax-like surface, coalescing to form round or oval plaques from a few millimeters to several centimeters in size. These plaques are subsequently covered by large dry silvery-white laminated mica-like scales.
- If the waxy scale is removed, a thin red translucent moist layer is revealed; removal of this layer will produce pinpoint bleeding points (Auspitz's sign).
- On the scalp, areas of scaling are interspersed with normal skin. The scaly area often extends beyond the scalp margin.
- In up to 50 percent of cases, pathological changes to the finger and toe nails occur (pitting, distal separation from the nail bed, discoloration, and subungual hyperkeratosis).

Guttate psoriasis

- This form of psoriasis is associated with group A streptococcal infection and occurs most frequently in adolescents and young adults.
- The disease is characterized by the sudden onset of numerous uniform, small, round, symmetrically distributed plaques, which resemble drops of wax on the skin.
- Lesions are usually found on the trunk or limbs.
- Lesions become larger after the acute phase and the disease may develop into chronic plaque psoriasis.

Flexural psoriasis

- This type of psoriasis usually affects older people, women more than men.
- Lesions involve the axillae, submammary folds and anogenital region and manifest as well-demarcated, red, glistening plaques without scaling.

Pustular psoriasis

This disease, which is not commonly encountered in the TCM clinic, has two forms:

- Generalized pustular psoriasis is a rare condition usually only seen in late middle age or old age. It manifests as widespread scaly patches covered by numerous densely distributed yellowish sterile pustules ranging in size from pinpoint to over 10mm. Patches sometimes become confluent. Accompanying features include high fever and painful and swollen joints. Generalized pustular psoriasis is a life-threatening medical condition with abrupt onset and requires hospital admission.
- Localized pustular psoriasis (palmoplantar pustulosis) is limited to the palms and soles, with symmetrically distributed erythema covered by numerous pustules ranging in size from 3 to 10mm. Brown crusts form after five to seven days as the sterile pustules dry up and desquamation follows. After the crusts fall off, new pustules form underneath scales. This disease is discussed in more detail later in this chapter.

Erythrodermic psoriasis

- This type of psoriasis (also known as psoriatic exfoliative dermatitis) occurs in up to about 2 percent of cases of chronic psoriasis.
- Precipitating factors include inappropriate treatment of psoriasis with systemic corticosteroids, strongly irritant topical medications, or the abuse of diaphoretics.
- There is generalized intense inflammation with red or dark red skin. Scales peel off from the lesions. Hyperkeratosis results in broken scales on the palms and soles. The disease tends to persist for months and is difficult to heal.

- Some patients have a fever and metabolic upsets, sometimes with damage to the liver and kidneys or cardiac failure.
- Erythrodermic psoriasis is a serious disease usually requiring hospital admission.

Psoriatic arthritis
- This complication of psoriasis occurs in up to 5 percent of cases, with a higher incidence occurring in colder climates.
- It generally occurs as a consequence of chronic psoriasis or in a period of aggravation of the disease after repeated attacks.
- Various patterns of joint involvement may be seen. It affects both large and small joints, especially the small joints of the fingers. Symptoms include pain, swelling, and rigidity or deformity of the joints. Specific changes may be seen on X-ray.

Differential diagnosis

PLAQUE PSORIASIS

Hypertrophic lichen planus
Eruptions in lichen planus usually involve the flexor surfaces of the wrists and forearms, and the lower legs around and above the ankles. Lesions manifest as intensely pruritic dull red flat-topped shiny papules with an irregular, sharply defined angulated border. Lesions that persist, most frequently on the shins, may develop into confluent hypertrophic plaques. These lesions can become hyperkeratotic with a coarse surface covered by dull scales.

Lichen simplex chronicus (neurodermatitis)
Plaque psoriasis on the elbows and knees should be differentiated from lichen simplex chronicus, where lesions generally manifest as a single irregular or polygonal-shaped plaque with intermingled red papules. The skin in the affected area is rough with deepened skin creases. In chronic cases, the lichenified areas become brown and are covered by dry fine scales.

Nummular eczema
Nummular eczema mainly involves the limbs, but may also occur on the dorsum of the hands, the buttocks and the trunk; the scalp and the extensor aspects of the elbows and knees are generally spared. Lesions manifest as very itchy, sharply demarcated, coin-shaped plaques 1-5 cm in diameter formed from the confluence of densely distributed red papules or vesicles. Lesions may be acute with clear or bloody exudate and crusting, or chronic with erythema and scaling, which is less waxy than that found in psoriasis.

Pityriasis rubra pilaris
This disorder begins with redness and bran-like scaling of the scalp and face and subsequently develops to involve the trunk and limbs, especially the extensor aspects. Lesions manifest as pink or red pinpoint to 0.5mm follicular, keratotic papules. As the papules increase in number, they merge into large red plaques covered by grayish-white scale. Some areas of skin may be spared by the plaques, but red plugged follicles are likely to be evident in these areas. The skin on the palms and soles becomes thick, yellow and keratinized with fissuring. Follicular plugging and thickening of the palms and soles are absent in psoriasis.

Parapsoriasis (chronic superficial dermatitis)
The scaling in chronic superficial dermatitis is much less marked than in psoriasis. The lesions, which manifest as pale red, yellowish-red or purplish-brown patches or plaques with clearly-defined margins, are typically more asymmetrical than those of psoriasis and, once established, tend not to change in size.

OTHER TYPES OF PSORIASIS
Pityriasis rosea
Guttate psoriasis should be differentiated from pityriasis rosea. In pityriasis rosea, a herald patch generally precedes the rash. Lesions are usually confined to the trunk and proximal extremities; they are oval rather than round and tend to be oriented along skin lines. Lesions are covered by a thin layer of bran-like scales. A "collarette" ring of fine scale often remains within the border of the lesions.

Seborrheic eczema
Scalp and flexural psoriasis should be differentiated from seborrheic eczema, where the main condition is an itchy red or yellowish-red scaly or exudative erythematous eruption affecting the scalp and scalp margins, the sides of the nose, the eyebrows, and the ears. It may be accompanied by dry scaly eczema over the presternal and interscapular areas or involvement of the axillae, groins and submammary areas with a moist intertrigo, often colonized by *Candida albicans*. Psoriasis does not usually involve the face and plaques on the scalp are not as extensive as in seborrheic eczema.

Intertrigo
Flexural psoriasis should be differentiated from intertrigo, which also involves the axillae, the submammary folds and the genital region and mainly affects the elderly. Lesions manifest as pink, moist, glistening plaques with distinct margins, erosion and exudation, often accompanied by painful fissuring in the skin creases. Satellite candidal lesions are often present outside the main distribution of lesions.

Tinea unguium

Nail psoriasis needs to be differentiated from tinea unguium. At the initial stage, the distal part of the fingernail or toenail becomes lusterless with gradual thickening and atrophy, finally separating from the nail bed. In severe cases, fungal infection leads to the nail becoming decayed, fragmented or deformed. The nail plate becomes brittle and easily broken with an uneven surface. Toenails, especially the nail of the big toe, are usually more affected than fingernails. It is rare for all nails to be affected and pitting is absent. Tinea unguium is often accompanied by tinea manuum or tinea pedis.

Etiology and pathology

At the initial stage, the disease manifests as pathological changes involving the Xue level, including Blood-Heat, Blood-Dryness and Blood stasis. Once the disease becomes persistent, it is characterized by debilitation or hyperactivity of the Zang-Fu organs, especially the Liver and Kidneys.

External pathogenic factors settling in the flesh

External pathogenic Wind, Cold, Damp, Heat or Dryness may settle in the skin and flesh to influence the normal diffusion of Qi by the Lungs and Spleen. These pathogenic factors can also obstruct the channels and network vessels and stagnate in the skin and interstices (*cou li*), depriving the skin and flesh of nourishment.

Blood-Heat

Where Blood-Heat has accumulated in the body over a period of time, exuberant Blood-Heat generates Wind and prevalence of Wind gives rise to Dryness, depriving the skin and flesh of nourishment. The same effect occurs where accumulation of Blood-Heat or Heat Toxins leads to depletion of Body Fluids, resulting in Yin Deficiency and Blood-Dryness; this is seen more often where psoriasis has become chronic.

Internal damage due to the seven emotions

Enduring repression of the seven emotions results in transformation into Fire. Fire or Heat Toxins can then disturb the Ying and Xue levels, and move outward to the exterior to block the sweat pores. This will eventually result in Qi stagnation and Blood stasis and give rise to the disease.

Dietary irregularities

Overindulgence in spicy foods, fish, seafood, and chicken and goose or other foods which tend to stir Wind leads to disharmony between the Spleen and Stomach, resulting in Qi stagnation and binding of Damp and Heat. When these are thrust outward to reach the skin, the disease will occur.

Disharmony of the Chong and Ren vessels

Since the Chong and Ren vessels pertain to the Liver and Kidneys, disharmony may arise between them as a result of menstruation or childbirth leading to an imbalance between Yin and Yang of the Liver and Kidneys. This will manifest as internal Heat due to Yin Deficiency or external Cold due to Yang Deficiency. If the condition persists, complex patterns of dual Deficiency of Yin and Yang, true Cold and false Heat or true Heat and false Cold can develop.

Pattern identification and treatment

INTERNAL TREATMENT[i]

WIND-HEAT

This pattern occurs in the early stages of an initial attack or subsequent episode of plaque psoriasis. Red or dark red maculopapules, papules or small erythematous patches develop quickly on the trunk and limbs, sometimes also spreading to the scalp or scalp margin. The surface of the lesions is covered by silvery-white scales that can be peeled off easily to reveal small bleeding points (Auspitz's sign). Accompanying symptoms and signs include itching, fever, thirst, and a sore and dry throat. The tongue body is red with a thin yellow coating; the pulse is floating and rapid.

Treatment principle

Dredge Wind and release the exterior, clear Heat and cool the Blood.

Prescription
XIAO FENG SAN JIA JIAN
Powder for Dispersing Wind, with modifications

Ku Shen (Radix Sophorae Flavescentis) 6g
Zhi Mu (Rhizoma Anemarrhenae Asphodeloidis) 6g
Jing Jie (Herba Schizonepetae Tenuifoliae) 6g
Fang Feng (Radix Ledebouriellae Divaricatae) 6g
Chan Tui ‡ (Periostracum Cicadae) 6g
Sheng Di Huang (Radix Rehmanniae Glutinosae) 10g
Mu Dan Pi (Cortex Moutan Radicis) 10g
Chao Niu Bang Zi (Fructus Arctii Lappae, stir-fried) 10g
Huang Qin (Radix Scutellariae Baicalensis) 10g
Hong Hua (Flos Carthami Tinctorii) 4.5g
Ling Xiao Hua (Flos Campsitis) 4.5g

---

i Generalized pustular psoriasis and erythrodermic psoriasis are serious conditions normally requiring hospitalization; TCM treatment is therefore likely to be carried out in conjunction with Western medicine.

Explanation

- *Jing Jie* (Herba Schizonepetae Tenuifoliae), *Chan Tui* ‡ (Periostracum Cicadae), *Fang Feng* (Radix Ledebouriellae Divaricatae), and *Chao Niu Bang Zi* (Fructus Arctii Lappae, stir-fried) dissipate Wind and alleviate itching.
- *Zhi Mu* (Rhizoma Anemarrhenae Asphodeloidis) and *Huang Qin* (Radix Scutellariae Baicalensis) clear and drain Heat from the Lungs.
- *Sheng Di Huang* (Radix Rehmanniae Glutinosae), *Mu Dan Pi* (Cortex Moutan Radicis), *Hong Hua* (Flos Carthami Tinctorii), and *Ling Xiao Hua* (Flos Campsitis) cool the Blood and reduce erythema.
- *Ku Shen* (Radix Sophorae Flavescentis) expels Wind and alleviates itching, dispels Dampness and relieves Toxicity.

WIND-COLD

This pattern occurs in an initial episode of plaque or guttate psoriasis. Lesions appear as dots or coin-shaped discs or coalesce into red patches covered by scales that are easy to peel off. The pattern may occur in any season but is relatively severe in winter, usually moderating or subsiding in summer. The tongue body is pale red with a thin white coating; the pulse is floating and tight.

Treatment principle
Dredge Wind and dissipate Cold, invigorate the Blood and regulate the Ying level.

Prescription
SI WU MA HUANG TANG JIA JIAN
Four Agents Ephedra Decoction, with modifications

Ma Huang* (Herba Ephedrae) 6g
Gui Zhi (Ramulus Cinnamomi Cassiae) 6g
Xing Ren (Semen Pruni Armeniacae) 6g
Chuan Xiong (Rhizoma Ligustici Chuanxiong) 6g
Dang Gui (Radix Angelicae Sinensis) 12g
Bai Shao (Radix Paeoniae Lactiflorae) 12g
Sheng Di Huang (Radix Rehmanniae Glutinosae) 12g
Bei Sha Shen (Radix Glehniae Littoralis) 12g
Sheng Jiang (Rhizoma Zingiberis Officinalis Recens) 10g
Da Zao (Fructus Ziziphi Jujubae) 15g

Explanation

- *Ma Huang** (Herba Ephedrae), *Gui Zhi* (Ramulus Cinnamomi Cassiae), *Xing Ren* (Semen Pruni Armeniacae), *Da Zao* (Fructus Ziziphi Jujubae), and *Sheng Jiang* (Rhizoma Zingiberis Officinalis Recens) warm Yang and dissipate Cold, and harmonize the Ying and Wei levels.
- *Chuan Xiong* (Rhizoma Ligustici Chuanxiong) invigorates the Blood and dispels Wind.

- *Dang Gui* (Radix Angelicae Sinensis), *Bai Shao* (Radix Paeoniae Lactiflorae) and *Sheng Di Huang* (Radix Rehmanniae Glutinosae) nourish and invigorate the Blood, free the network vessels and reduce lesions.
- *Bei Sha Shen* (Radix Glehniae Littoralis) clears Heat from the Lungs and nourishes Lung Yin, and prevents pathogenic factors from entering the interior.

BLOOD-HEAT

This pattern occurs in the early stages of an initial attack or subsequent episode of guttate or plaque psoriasis. Lesions manifests as bright red or dark red papules, maculopapules or macular patches of varying sizes scattered throughout the body or distributed mostly on the trunk and limbs. Sometimes lesions start on the scalp before spreading gradually to other parts of the body. New lesions appear continuously, covered by silvery-white scales that shed easily when dry and elicit the characteristic Auspitz's sign on removal of the underlying moist layer. Accompanying symptoms and signs include itching, irritability, thirst, constipation, and short voidings of yellow urine. The tongue body is red with a thin yellow coating; the pulse is wiry and rapid, or slippery and rapid.

Treatment principle
Cool the Blood and relieve Toxicity, invigorate the Blood and reduce erythema.

Prescription
YIN HUA HU ZHANG TANG JIA JIAN
Honeysuckle and Giant Knotweed Decoction, with modifications

Jin Yin Hua (Flos Lonicerae) 15g
Hu Zhang (Radix et Rhizoma Polygoni Cuspidati) 15g
Dan Shen (Radix Salviae Miltiorrhizae) 15g
Ji Xue Teng (Caulis Spatholobi) 15g
Sheng Di Huang (Radix Rehmanniae Glutinosae) 12g
Dang Gui Wei (Extremitas Radicis Angelicae Sinensis) 12g
Chi Shao (Radix Paeoniae Rubra) 12g
Huai Hua (Flos Sophorae Japonicae) 12g
Da Qing Ye (Folium Isatidis seu Baphicacanthi) 10g
Mu Dan Pi (Cortex Moutan Radicis) 10g
Zi Cao (Radix Arnebiae seu Lithospermi) 10g
Bei Dou Gen (Rhizoma Menispermi) 10g
Nan Sha Shen (Radix Adenophorae) 10g

Explanation

- *Sheng Di Huang* (Radix Rehmanniae Glutinosae), *Chi Shao* (Radix Paeoniae Rubra), *Dang Gui Wei* (Extremitas Radicis Angelicae Sinensis), *Mu Dan Pi* (Cortex Moutan Radicis), and *Zi Cao* (Radix Arnebiae seu Lithospermi) cool the Blood and reduce erythema.

- *Jin Yin Hua* (Flos Lonicerae), *Da Qing Ye* (Folium Isatidis seu Baphicacanthi) and *Bei Dou Gen* (Rhizoma Menispermi) clear Heat and relieve Toxicity.
- *Ji Xue Teng* (Caulis Spatholobi), *Hu Zhang* (Radix et Rhizoma Polygoni Cuspidati) and *Dan Shen* (Radix Salviae Miltiorrhizae) transform Blood stasis and free the network vessels.
- *Huai Hua* (Flos Sophorae Japonicae) and *Nan Sha Shen* (Radix Adenophorae) relieve Toxicity and protect Yin.

BLOOD STASIS

In this plaque psoriasis pattern, the disease is of relatively long duration. Lesions are dull red, hard and thick, mostly forming coin-shaped plaques, but with some resembling oyster shells. They are covered by thick, dry, relatively adherent silvery-white scales. Old lesions tend to remain fixed in size and position and new lesions seldom appear. Accompanying symptoms and signs include itching of varying intensity or absence of itching, and a dry mouth with no desire for drinks. The tongue body is dull purple or dark red with stasis marks and a thin white or thin yellow coating; the pulse is wiry and choppy, or deep and choppy.

Treatment principle

Invigorate the Blood and transform Blood stasis, free the network vessels and dissipate lumps.

Prescription
HUANG QI DAN SHEN TANG JIA JIAN
Astragalus and Red Sage Decoction, with modifications

Dan Shen (Radix Salviae Miltiorrhizae) 15g
Ze Lan (Herba Lycopi Lucidi) 15g
Qian Cao Gen (Radix Rubiae Cordifoliae) 15g
Huo Xue Teng (Caulis seu Radix Schisandrae) 15g
Huang Qi (Radix Astragali seu Hedysari) 10g
Xiang Fu (Rhizoma Cyperi Rotundi) 10g
Qing Pi (Pericarpium Citri Reticulatae Viride) 10g
Chen Pi (Pericarpium Citri Reticulatae) 10g
Chi Shao (Radix Paeoniae Rubra) 6g
San Leng (Rhizoma Sparganii Stoloniferi) 6g
E Zhu (Rhizoma Curcumae) 6g
Ling Xiao Hua (Flos Campsitis) 6g
Si Gua Luo (Fasciculus Vascularis Luffae) 6g
Jiang Can ‡ (Bombyx Batryticatus) 6g

Explanation
- *Huang Qi* (Radix Astragali seu Hedysari), *Dan Shen* (Radix Salviae Miltiorrhizae), *Ze Lan* (Herba Lycopi Lucidi), *Chi Shao* (Radix Paeoniae Rubra), *Xiang Fu* (Rhizoma Cyperi Rotundi), *Qing Pi* (Pericarpium Citri Reticulatae Viride), *Huo Xue Teng* (Caulis seu Radix Schisandrae), and *Chen Pi* (Pericarpium Citri

Reticulatae) augment Qi and invigorate the Blood, regulate Qi and transform Blood stasis.
- *Ling Xiao Hua* (Flos Campsitis), *Qian Cao Gen* (Radix Rubiae Cordifoliae) and *Si Gua Luo* (Fasciculus Vascularis Luffae) cool the Blood and free the network vessels.
- *San Leng* (Rhizoma Sparganii Stoloniferi) and *E Zhu* (Rhizoma Curcumae) transform Blood stasis and reduce erythema.
- *Jiang Can* ‡ (Bombyx Batryticatus) dissipates Wind and alleviates itching.

WIND-DRYNESS DUE TO BLOOD DEFICIENCY

This pattern occurs in the chronic phase of all types of psoriasis and in patients with a weak constitution. It is characterized by thin, pale red or dark red lesions distributed in numerous patches throughout the body. Lesions are covered by large quantities of dry silvery-white scales that peel off in layers. Old lesions tend to remain fixed in size and position and new lesions seldom appear. Accompanying symptoms and signs include itching of varying intensity, a lusterless facial complexion and lassitude, or dizziness, insomnia and poor appetite. The tongue body is pale with a scant coating or no coating; the pulse is wiry and thready, or deep and thready.

Treatment principle

Nourish the Blood and harmonize the Ying level, augment Qi and dispel Wind.

Prescription
YANG XUE QU FENG TANG JIA JIAN
Decoction for Nourishing the Blood and Dispelling Wind, with modifications

Huang Qi (Radix Astragali seu Hedysari) 10g
Dang Shen (Radix Codonopsitis Pilosulae) 10g
Dang Gui (Radix Angelicae Sinensis) 10g
Huo Ma Ren (Semen Cannabis Sativae) 10g
Xuan Shen (Radix Scrophulariae Ningpoensis) 12g
Bai Shao (Radix Paeoniae Lactiflorae) 12g
Shu Di Huang (Radix Rehmanniae Glutinosae Conquita) 12g
Ji Xue Teng (Caulis Spatholobi) 12g
Mai Men Dong (Radix Ophiopogonis Japonici) 12g
Bai Xian Pi (Cortex Dictamni Dasycarpi Radicis) 15g
Bai Zhi (Radix Angelicae Dahuricae) 6g
Bai Ji Li (Fructus Tribuli Terrestris) 6g

Explanation
- *Huang Qi* (Radix Astragali seu Hedysari), *Dang Shen* (Radix Codonopsitis Pilosulae), *Dang Gui* (Radix Angelicae Sinensis), *Bai Shao* (Radix Paeoniae Lactiflorae), *Shu Di Huang* (Radix Rehmanniae Glutinosae

Conquita), and *Ji Xue Teng* (Caulis Spatholobi) augment Qi, nourish the Blood and harmonize the Ying level.

- *Huo Ma Ren* (Semen Cannabis Sativae), *Xuan Shen* (Radix Scrophulariae Ningpoensis) and *Mai Men Dong* (Radix Ophiopogonis Japonici) nourish Yin and moisten Dryness.
- *Bai Xian Pi* (Cortex Dictamni Dasycarpi Radicis) relieves Toxicity and alleviates itching.
- *Bai Zhi* (Radix Angelicae Dahuricae) and *Bai Ji Li* (Fructus Tribuli Terrestris) disperse Wind and alleviate itching.

BLOOD-DRYNESS DUE TO DAMAGE TO YIN

In this pattern, the disease tends to linger with persistent lesions distributed over the trunk and limbs. The lesions are dark red, brownish-red or pale red and appear in various shapes, but mostly present as patches or rings. They are dry, crack easily and are covered by a thick or thin layer of dry silvery-white scale that is difficult to peel off. Itching may be slight or severe. Accompanying symptoms and signs include dry throat and lips, a feverish sensation in the chest, palms and soles or in the palms alone, a dry mouth, thirst without a desire for drinks, and constipation. The tongue body is dry and red with a thin, dry, yellow coating; the pulse is wiry and thready, or thready and rapid.

Treatment principle
Enrich Yin and moisten Dryness, clear Heat and expel Wind.

Prescription
YANG XUE RUN FU TANG JIA JIAN
Decoction for Nourishing the Blood and Moistening the Skin, with modifications

Dang Gui (Radix Angelicac Sinensis) 10g
Dan Shen (Radix Salviae Miltiorrhizae) 10g
Mu Dan Pi (Cortex Moutan Radicis) 10g
Chi Shao (Radix Paeoniae Rubra) 10g
He Shou Wu (Radix Polygoni Multiflori) 12g
Sheng Di Huang (Radix Rehmanniae Glutinosae) 12g
Shu Di Huang (Radix Rehmanniae Glutinosae Conquita) 12g
Bei Dou Gen (Rhizoma Menispermi) 12g
Tian Men Dong (Radix Asparagi Cochinchinensis) 12g
Mai Men Dong (Radix Ophiopogonis Japonici) 12g
Chong Lou (Rhizoma Paridis) 15g
Bai Xian Pi (Cortex Dictamni Dasycarpi Radicis) 15g
Bai Ji Li (Fructus Tribuli Terrestris) 15g

Explanation
- *Dang Gui* (Radix Angelicae Sinensis), *He Shou Wu* (Radix Polygoni Multiflori), *Sheng Di Huang* (Radix Rehmanniae Glutinosae), *Shu Di Huang* (Radix

Rehmanniae Glutinosae Conquita), *Tian Men Dong* (Radix Asparagi Cochinchinensis), and *Mai Men Dong* (Radix Ophiopogonis Japonici) enrich Yin and moisten Dryness.
- *Dan Shen* (Radix Salviae Miltiorrhizae), *Mu Dan Pi* (Cortex Moutan Radicis) and *Chi Shao* (Radix Paeoniae Rubra) clear Heat and cool the Blood.
- *Chong Lou* (Rhizoma Paridis), *Bai Xian Pi* (Cortex Dictamni Dasycarpi Radicis), *Bei Dou Gen* (Rhizoma Menispermi), and *Bai Ji Li* (Fructus Tribuli Terrestris) dissipate Wind and alleviate itching, clear Heat and relieve Toxicity.

DAMP-HEAT

This pattern occurs in flexural psoriasis. Eruptions appear most frequently in skin folds (the axillae, the popliteal and antecubital fossae, the submammary region, the inguinal groove, the perineum, and the genital region). Lesions are red or light red on a thin base and often coalesce into large patches with local moisture or exudation and a small amount of thin scaling. Accompanying symptoms and signs include slight itching, a dry mouth without thirst, generalized fever, and lassitude. The tongue body is red with a yellow coating that may be greasy at the root; the pulse is slippery and rapid.

Treatment principle
Clear Heat and benefit the movement of Dampness, cool the Blood and relieve Toxicity.

Prescription
XIAO YIN ER HAO TANG JIA JIAN
No. 2 Decoction for Dispersing Psoriasis, with modifications

Chao Long Dan Cao (Radix Gentianae Scabrae, stir-fried) 6g
Ku Shen (Radix Sophorae Flavescentis) 6g
Huang Qin (Radix Scutellariae Baicalensis) 6g
Cang Zhu (Rhizoma Atractylodis) 6g
Fu Ling (Sclerotium Poriae Cocos) 10g
Ze Xie (Rhizoma Alismatis Orientalis) 10g
Bi Xie (Rhizoma Dioscoreae Hypoglaucae seu Septemlobae) 10g
Bei Dou Gen (Rhizoma Menispermi) 10g
Chong Lou (Rhizoma Paridis) 15g
Tu Fu Ling (Rhizoma Smilacis Glabrae) 15g
Mu Dan Pi (Cortex Moutan Radicis) 12g

Explanation
- *Chao Long Dan Cao* (Radix Gentianae Scabrae, stir-fried) and *Huang Qin* (Radix Scutellariae Baicalensis) clear Heat from the Liver and drain Fire.
- *Tu Fu Ling* (Rhizoma Smilacis Glabrae), *Chong Lou* (Rhizoma Paridis) and *Bei Dou Gen* (Rhizoma Menispermi) clear Heat and relieve Toxicity.

- *Ku Shen* (Radix Sophorae Flavescentis), *Cang Zhu* (Rhizoma Atractylodis), *Fu Ling* (Sclerotium Poriae Cocos), *Ze Xie* (Rhizoma Alismatis Orientalis), and *Bi Xie* (Rhizoma Dioscoreae Hypoglaucae seu Septemlobae) clear Heat and dry Dampness.
- *Mu Dan Pi* (Cortex Moutan Radicis) cools the Blood and reduces erythema.

DISHARMONY OF THE CHONG AND REN VESSELS

In this pattern, lesions are closely related to menstruation, pregnancy and childbirth. The condition may appear at any time but can be aggravated before menstruation or postpartum; in some patients, it may appear after menstruation. Lesions manifest as bright red or pale red widely distributed papules and plaques covered by silvery-white scales. Accompanying symptoms and signs include slight itching, irritability, dry mouth, dizziness, aching in the lower back, and general malaise. The tongue body is red or pale red with a thin coating; the pulse is slippery and rapid, or deep and thready.

Treatment principle
Regulate and contain the Chong and Ren vessels.

Prescription
ER XIAN TANG JIA JIAN
Two Immortals Decoction, with modifications

Xian Mao (Rhizoma Curculiginis Orchioidis) 6g
Huang Bai (Cortex Phellodendri) 6g
Zhi Mu (Rhizoma Anemarrhenae Asphodeloidis) 6g
Yin Yang Huo (Herba Epimedii) 12g
Ba Ji Tian (Radix Morindae Officinalis) 12g
Tu Si Zi (Semen Cuscutae) 12g
Sheng Di Huang (Radix Rehmanniae Glutinosae) 12g
Shu Di Huang (Radix Rehmanniae Glutinosae Conquita) 12g
Dang Gui (Radix Angelicae Sinensis) 10g
Nü Zhen Zi (Fructus Ligustri Lucidi) 15g
Han Lian Cao (Herba Ecliptae Prostratae) 15g

Explanation
- *Xian Mao* (Rhizoma Curculiginis Orchioidis), *Yin Yang Huo* (Herba Epimedii), *Ba Ji Tian* (Radix Morindae Officinalis), and *Tu Si Zi* (Semen Cuscutae) warm Yang and boost the Kidneys.
- *Dang Gui* (Radix Angelicae Sinensis), *Sheng Di Huang* (Radix Rehmanniae Glutinosae), *Shu Di Huang* (Radix Rehmanniae Glutinosae Conquita), *Nü Zhen Zi* (Fructus Ligustri Lucidi), and *Han Lian Cao* (Herba Ecliptae Prostratae) enrich Yin and nourish the Blood.
- *Huang Bai* (Cortex Phellodendri) and *Zhi Mu* (Rhizoma Anemarrhenae Asphodeloidis) clear Deficiency-Heat in the Lower Burner.

WIND-DAMP BI SYNDROME

This pattern is encountered with psoriatic arthritis. Typical manifestations of psoriasis such as erythema, papules, silvery-white scales and Auspitz's sign (punctate bleeding) are accompanied by other symptoms such as pain and swelling of the joints with difficulty in extension and flexion. The joints affected are mostly small joints, especially the distal joints of the fingers and toes. The tongue body is red with a yellow and greasy coating; the pulse is wiry and rapid, or slippery and rapid.

Treatment principle
Dispel Dampness and dissipate Wind, relieve Toxicity and free the network vessels.

Prescription
DU HUO JI SHENG TANG JIA JIAN
Pubescent Angelica Root and Mistletoe Decoction, with modifications

Qiang Huo (Rhizoma et Radix Notopterygii) 10g
Du Huo (Radix Angelicae Pubescentis) 10g
Fang Feng (Radix Ledebouriellae Divaricatae) 10g
Qin Jiao (Radix Gentianae Macrophyllae) 10g
Sang Ji Sheng (Ramulus Loranthi) 12g
Bi Xie (Rhizoma Dioscoreae Hypoglaucae seu Septemlobae) 12g
Xi Xian Cao (Herba Siegesbeckiae) 12g
Tou Gu Cao (Herba Speranskiae seu Impatientis) 12g
Jiang Can ‡ (Bombyx Batryticatus) 12g
Luo Shi Teng (Caulis Trachelospermi Jasminoidis) 15g
Ban Zhi Lian (Herba Scutellariae Barbatae) 15g
Gui Jian Yu (Lignum Suberalatum Euonymi) 15g
Wu Jia Pi (Cortex Acanthopanacis Gracilistyli Radicis) 6g
Hai Tong Pi (Cortex Erythrinae) 6g
Sang Ji Sheng (Ramulus Loranthi) 6g

Explanation
- *Qiang Huo* (Rhizoma et Radix Notopterygii), *Du Huo* (Radix Angelicae Pubescentis), *Fang Feng* (Radix Ledebouriellae Divaricatae), *Sang Ji Sheng* (Ramulus Loranthi), and *Qin Jiao* (Radix Gentianae Macrophyllae) dissipate Wind and disperse swelling.
- *Wu Jia Pi* (Cortex Acanthopanacis Gracilistyli Radicis), *Hai Tong Pi* (Cortex Erythrinae), *Sang Ji Sheng* (Ramulus Loranthi), *Tou Gu Cao* (Herba Speranskiae seu Impatientis), and *Jiang Can* ‡ (Bombyx Batryticatus) dispel Dampness and free Bi syndrome.
- *Xi Xian Cao* (Herba Siegesbeckiae), *Bi Xie* (Rhizoma Dioscoreae Hypoglaucae seu Septemlobae) and *Luo Shi Teng* (Caulis Trachelospermi Jasminoidis) eliminate Dampness and dissipate Cold, free the network vessels and alleviate pain.
- *Gui Jian Yu* (Lignum Suberalatum Euonymi) invigorates the Blood and frees the network vessels.

- *Ban Zhi Lian* (Herba Scutellariae Barbatae) relieves Toxicity and reduces erythema.

INSUFFICIENCY OF THE LIVER AND KIDNEYS

This is a chronic, persistent and recurrent condition that develops into psoriatic arthritis. The appearance of skin lesions associated with ordinary psoriasis is accompanied by arthralgia that gradually worsens with deformity of the joints, destruction of the bones and limitation of movement in the affected joints. Accompanying symptoms and signs include aching and pain in the lower back and knees. The tongue body is pale red or dark red with a scant coating or no coating; the pulse is deep and slippery, or thready and weak.

Treatment principle
Supplement the Liver and Kidneys, dispel Wind and eliminate Dampness.

Prescription
JIAN BU HU QIAN WAN JIA JIAN
Steady Gait Hidden Tiger Pill, with modifications

Shu Di Huang (Radix Rehmanniae Glutinosae Conquita) 12g
Shan Zhu Yu (Fructus Corni Officinalis) 12g
Xu Duan (Radix Dipsaci) 12g
Chao Du Zhong (Cortex Eucommiae Ulmoidis, stir-fried) 12g
Mu Gua (Fructus Chaenomelis) 10g
Gui Ban* (Plastrum Testudinis) 10g, decocted for 30 minutes before adding the other ingredients
Jiang Can‡ (Bombyx Batryticatus) 10g
Shen Jin Cao (Herba Lycopodii Japonici) 10g
Xi Xian Cao (Herba Siegesbeckiae) 10g
Gou Ji (Rhizoma Cibotii Barometz) 15g
Tu Fu Ling (Rhizoma Smilacis Glabrae) 15g

Explanation
- *Shu Di Huang* (Radix Rehmanniae Glutinosae Conquita), *Shan Zhu Yu* (Fructus Corni Officinalis), *Gui Ban** (Plastrum Testudinis), *Chao Du Zhong* (Cortex Eucommiae Ulmoidis, stir-fried), and *Xu Duan* (Radix Dipsaci) enrich the Liver and supplement the Kidneys.
- *Mu Gua* (Fructus Chaenomelis), *Shen Jin Cao* (Herba Lycopodii Japonici), *Xi Xian Cao* (Herba Siegesbeckiae), and *Gou Ji* (Rhizoma Cibotii Barometz) expel Wind and eliminate Dampness.
- *Tu Fu Ling* (Rhizoma Smilacis Glabrae) and *Jiang Can‡* (Bombyx Batryticatus) relieve Toxicity and reduce lesions, dredge Wind and alleviate itching.

ACCUMULATION OF TOXINS DUE TO DAMP-HEAT

This pattern, which is seen with pustular psoriasis, is characterized by acute onset and manifests as large erythematous patches spreading rapidly throughout the body. A dense distribution of recurrent crops of thin-walled pustules ranging in size from 2-5 mm appears on the erythema. Pustules coalesce after rupture, with crusts and scales then forming on the surface. Maceration is evident in the skin folds with the formation of purulent crusts. The nails are also affected, resulting in breaking, separation, thickening, or opaqueness of the nail plate. Accompanying symptoms and signs include raging fever, irritability, thirst, reddening of the face, swollen and painful joints, constipation, and reddish urine. This can be a life-threatening disorder. The tongue body is red with a yellow and greasy coating; the pulse is wiry and slippery, or wiry and rapid.

Treatment principle
Dispel Dampness and clear Heat, cool the Blood and relieve Toxicity.

Prescription
KE YIN YI HAO JIA JIAN
No. 1 Prescription for Restraining Psoriasis, with modifications

Bei Dou Gen (Rhizoma Menispermi) 12g
Sheng Di Huang (Radix Rehmanniae Glutinosae) 12g
Mu Dan Pi (Cortex Moutan Radicis) 12g
Chong Lou (Rhizoma Paridis) 12g
Ye Ju Hua (Flos Chrysanthemi Indici) 12g
Shi Gao‡ (Gypsum Fibrosum) 15g, decocted for 30 minutes before adding the other ingredients
Pu Gong Ying (Herba Taraxaci cum Radice) 15g
Zi Hua Di Ding (Herba Violae Yedoensitis) 15g
Ze Xie (Rhizoma Alismatis Orientalis) 10g
Huang Qin (Radix Scutellariae Baicalensis) 10g
Chao Long Dan Cao (Radix Gentianae Scabrae, stir-fried) 10g
Che Qian Zi (Semen Plantaginis) 10g, wrapped

Explanation
- *Bei Dou Gen* (Rhizoma Menispermi), *Chong Lou* (Rhizoma Paridis), *Ye Ju Hua* (Flos Chrysanthemi Indici), *Pu Gong Ying* (Herba Taraxaci cum Radice), and *Zi Hua Di Ding* (Herba Violae Yedoensitis) clear Heat and relieve Toxicity.
- *Sheng Di Huang* (Radix Rehmanniae Glutinosae) and *Mu Dan Pi* (Cortex Moutan Radicis) cool the Blood and reduce erythema.
- *Huang Qin* (Radix Scutellariae Baicalensis) and *Chao Long Dan Cao* (Radix Gentianae Scabrae, stir-fried) clear Heat from the Liver and drain Fire.
- *Shi Gao‡* (Gypsum Fibrosum), *Che Qian Zi* (Semen Plantaginis) and *Ze Xie* (Rhizoma Alismatis Orientalis) clear Heat and benefit the movement of Dampness.

SPLEEN DEFICIENCY WITH RESIDUAL TOXINS

After treatment of generalized pustular psoriasis, the erythema fades or turns dull red or reddish-brown with most pustules disappearing. Crusts form on the few pustules remaining or the occasional new lesions. There is an obvious reduction in scaling. Accompanying symptoms and signs include lassitude, fatigued limbs, reduced appetite, and loose stools. The tongue body is red with a yellow coating that is greasy at the root; the pulse is soggy or slippery.

Treatment principle

Fortify the Spleen and eliminate Dampness, clear and relieve residual Toxicity.

Prescription

CHU SHI WEI LING TANG JIA JIAN

Poria Five Decoction for Eliminating Dampness and Calming the Stomach, with modifications

Chao Bai Zhu (Rhizoma Atractylodis Macrocephalae, stir-fried) 10g
Cang Zhu (Rhizoma Atractylodis) 10g
Hou Po (Cortex Magnoliae Officinalis) 10g
Chen Pi (Pericarpium Citri Reticulatae) 10g
Jiao Zhi Zi (Fructus Gardeniae Jasminoidis, scorch-fried) 10g
Huang Qin (Radix Scutellariae Baicalensis) 10g
Fu Ling (Sclerotium Poriae Cocos) 12g
Ze Xie (Rhizoma Alismatis Orientalis) 12g
Chong Lou (Rhizoma Paridis) 15g
Ban Zhi Lian (Herba Scutellariae Barbatae) 15g
Tu Fu Ling (Rhizoma Smilacis Glabrae) 15g
Yi Yi Ren (Semen Coicis Lachryma-jobi) 15g

Explanation

- Cang Zhu (Rhizoma Atractylodis), Chao Long Dan Cao (Radix Gentianae Scabrae, stir-fried), Chao Bai Zhu (Rhizoma Atractylodis Macrocephalae, stir-fried), Hou Po (Cortex Magnoliae Officinalis), and Chen Pi (Pericarpium Citri Reticulatae) dry Dampness and support the Spleen.
- Fu Ling (Sclerotium Poriae Cocos), Ze Xie (Rhizoma Alismatis Orientalis) and Yi Yi Ren (Semen Coicis Lachryma-jobi) transform Dampness and boost the Stomach.
- Chong Lou (Rhizoma Paridis), Ban Zhi Lian (Herba Scutellariae Barbatae) and Tu Fu Ling (Rhizoma Smilacis Glabrae) clear Heat and relieve Toxicity.
- Huang Qin (Radix Scutellariae Baicalensis) and Jiao Zhi Zi (Fructus Gardeniae Jasminoidis, scorch-fried) relieve Toxicity and reduce erythema.

HEAT TOXINS DAMAGING THE YING LEVEL

This pattern occurs in erythrodermic psoriasis. Diffuse deep red or purplish-red erythema spreads rapidly throughout the body including the face. Lesions feel hot on contact and blanch under pressure. They are slightly swollen and covered by layers of scale that constantly peel off. Accompanying symptoms and signs include raging fever, aversion to cold, irritability, thirst, listlessness, and lassitude. The tongue body is red or crimson with scant moisture and a thin or clean coating; the pulse is wiry and rapid, or slippery and rapid.

Treatment principle

Cool the Blood and relieve Toxicity, clear Heat from the Ying level and reduce erythema.

Prescription

LING YANG HUA BAN TANG JIA JIAN

Antelope Horn Decoction for Transforming Macules, with modifications

Ling Yang Jiao Fen ‡ (Cornu Antelopis, powdered) 0.6g, infused in the prepared decoction
Sheng Di Huang (Radix Rehmanniae Glutinosae) 30-45g
Jin Yin Hua (Flos Lonicerae) 15-30g
Zi Cao (Radix Arnebiae seu Lithospermi) 15-30g
Bai Hua She She Cao (Herba Hedyotidis Diffusae) 15-30g
Mu Dan Pi (Cortex Moutan Radicis) 10g
Chi Shao (Radix Paeoniae Rubra) 10g
Xuan Shen (Radix Scrophulariae Ningpoensis) 10g
Nan Sha Shen (Radix Adenophorae) 10g
Lian Qiao (Fructus Forsythiae Suspensae) 10g
Huang Qin (Radix Scutellariae Baicalensis) 6g
Huang Lian (Rhizoma Coptidis) 6g
Zhi Mu (Rhizoma Anemarrhenae Asphodeloidis) 6g
Shi Gao ‡ (Gypsum Fibrosum) 30g, decocted for 30 minutes before adding the other ingredients

Explanation

- Ling Yang Jiao Fen ‡ (Cornu Antelopis, powdered) clears Heat from the Liver and reduces fever.
- Zhi Mu (Rhizoma Anemarrhenae Asphodeloidis), Shi Gao ‡ (Gypsum Fibrosum), Xuan Shen (Radix Scrophulariae Ningpoensis), and Nan Sha Shen (Radix Adenophorae) clear Heat from Qi level and cool the Ying level.
- Sheng Di Huang (Radix Rehmanniae Glutinosae), Mu Dan Pi (Cortex Moutan Radicis), Chi Shao (Radix Paeoniae Rubra), and Zi Cao (Radix Arnebiae seu Lithospermi) cool the Blood and relieve Toxicity.
- Huang Qin (Radix Scutellariae Baicalensis) and Huang Lian (Rhizoma Coptidis) drain Fire with cold and bitterness.

- *Bai Hua She She Cao* (Herba Hedyotidis Diffusae), *Jin Yin Hua* (Flos Lonicerae) and *Lian Qiao* (Fructus Forsythiae Suspensae) clear Heat and relieve Toxicity.

General modifications

1. For lesions located mainly on the limbs, add *Jiang Huang* (Rhizoma Curcumae Longae) and *Sang Zhi* (Ramulus Mori Albae).
2. For lesions located mainly on the trunk, add *Chai Hu* (Radix Bupleuri) and *Yu Jin* (Radix Curcumae).
3. For lesions located mainly on the lumbosacral region, add *Chao Du Zhong* (Cortex Eucommiae Ulmoidis, stir-fried) and *Xi Xian Cao* (Herba Siegesbeckiae).
4. For lesions located mainly on the scalp, add *Ju Hua* (Flos Chrysanthemi Morifolii) and *Sang Ye* (Folium Mori Albae).
5. For psoriatic arthritis, add *Lao Guan Cao* (Herba Erodii seu Geranii), *Ji Xue Teng* (Caulis Spatholobi) and *Gui Zhi* (Ramulus Cinnamomi Cassiae).
6. For pustular lesions, add *Bai Hua She She Cao* (Herba Hedyotidis Diffusae) and *Chong Lou* (Rhizoma Paridis).
7. For erythroderma, add *Lü Dou Yi* (Testa Phaseoli Radiati), *Shui Niu Jiao* ‡ (Cornu Bubali) and *Gui Ban** (Plastrum Testudinis).
8. For female patients, clinical experience indicates that adding *Zi Bei Chi* ‡ (Concha Mauritiae), *Ye Jiao Teng* (Caulis Polygoni Multiflori), *He Huan Pi* (Cortex Albizziae Julibrissin), and *He Huan Hua* (Flos Albizziae Julibrissin) enhances effectiveness.
9. For male patients, clinical experience indicates that adding *Gui Ban Jiao** (Gelatinum Plastri Testudinis) and *Gou Qi Zi* (Fructus Lycii) enhances effectiveness.

PATENT HERBAL MEDICINES

- For the active phase, take *Pi Fu Bing Xue Du Wan* (Skin Disease Blood Toxicity Pill) 10 pills, twice a day.
- For the quiescent phase, take *Yin Le Wan* (Psoriasis Happiness Pill) 6g twice a day or *Lu Sun Pian* (Asparagus Tablet) five tablets twice a day.
- For psoriatic arthritis, take *Lei Gong Teng Pian* (Thunder God Vine Tablet) two tablets three times a day or *Lu Sun Pian* (Asparagus Tablet) five tablets twice a day.
- For predominance of Blood-Heat, take *Fu Fang Kang Yin Ji* (Compound Anti-Psoriasis Preparation) 6g twice a day.

EXTERNAL TREATMENT

- For guttate psoriasis or extensive plaque psoriasis at the initial stage, apply non-irritating ointments such as *Qin Bai Gao* (Scutellaria and Phellodendron Paste), *Zi Lian Gao* (Gromwell Root and Coptis Paste) and *Qing Liang Gao* (Cool Clearing Paste) twice a day to the affected area.
- For stubborn eruptions with relatively profuse scaling, wash the affected area first with *Cang Fu Shui Xi Ji* (Atractylodes and Broom Cypress Wash Preparation) or *Lu Lu Tong Shui Xi Ji* (Sweetgum Fruit Wash Preparation) once a day. Then apply *Pu Lian Gao* (Universal Coptis Paste) or *Hei Dou Liu You Ruan Gao* (Black Soybean and Vaseline® Ointment).

ACUPUNCTURE

Selection of points according to pattern identification

Blood-Heat
Prescription 1: BL-18 Ganshu and BL-23 Shenshu.
Prescription 2: BL-12 Fengmen, BL-18 Ganshu and BL-23 Shenshu.
Prescription 3: BL-15 Xinshu, BL-18 Ganshu and BL-23 Shenshu.
Technique: Use the three groups of points alternately and apply the reducing method. Treat once every other day for two months.

Wind-Dryness due to Blood Deficiency
Prescription 1: BL-17 Geshu and BL-19 Danshu.
Prescription 2: BL-12 Fengmen, BL-17 Geshu and BL-19 Danshu.
Prescription 3: BL-13 Feishu, BL-19 Danshu and BL-20 Pishu.
Technique: Use the three groups of points alternately and apply the reinforcing method. Treat once every other day for two months.

Selection of points according to location of the disease

- For lesions on the scalp and arms, select LI-4 Hegu, LI-11 Quchi, TB-6 Zhigou, and GB-20 Fengchi.
- For lesions on the trunk or buttocks or in the genital region, select SP-6 Sanyinjiao, SP-10 Xuehai and GB-34 Yanglingquan.
- For lesions on the lower limbs, select SP-10 Xuehai, SP-6 Sanyinjiao and ST-36 Zusanli.
- For generalized lesions, select GV-14 Dazhui, LI-11 Quchi, SP-10 Xuehai, and SP-6 Sanyinjiao.

Technique: Use the reducing method in the acute phase and the reinforcing method in the chronic phase. Treat once every other day for one month in the acute phase and for three months in the chronic phase.

Explanation
- Front-*mu* points are combined with back-*shu* points according to three main principles:

- If the disease is mainly due to Blood Deficiency, BL-17 Geshu, BL-20 Pishu, BL-13 Feishu, and BL-19 Danshu are used to nourish and invigorate the Blood.
  - If the disease is mainly due to Blood-Heat, BL-15 Xinshu, BL-23 Shenshu, BL-12 Fengmen, BL-18 Ganshu, and GV-14 Dazhui are used to clear Heat and cool the Blood.
  - If the disease is mainly due to Blood stasis, BL-17 Geshu and BL-23 Shenshu are used to invigorate the Blood and free the network vessels.
- In addition, GB-20 Fengchi, LI-11 Quchi, LI-4 Hegu, and TB-6 Zhigou dissipate Wind and alleviate itching.
- SP-6 Sanyinjiao, SP-10 Xuehai, GB-34 Yanglingquan, and ST-36 Zusanli fortify the Spleen and nourish the Blood, expel Wind and alleviate itching.

ACUPUNCTURE COMBINED WITH CUPPING THERAPY
Points: GV-14 Dazhui, GV-13 Taodao, BL-18 Ganshu, and BL-20 Pishu.
Technique: Use the reducing method. Remove the needles after obtaining Qi and immediately apply flash-cupping (see page 62). Retain the cups for five to ten minutes. Treat once every other day for two months.

MOXIBUSTION
Points: Ashi points (sites of stubborn, thick plaques).
Technique: Peel some fresh garlic, pound it to a pulp and place on the Ashi points. Position moxa cones 1.5cm apart and light until local heat, itching and burning pain reach the patient's tolerance level. Treat once every other day.

PRICKING TO BLEED TREATMENT
Prescription 1
Main points: Ear Apex, Helix$_2$ and Helix$_6$.

Auxiliary points
- For lesions on the back, add GV-14 Dazhui and Jianjiagangshang (located at the midpoint of the superior scapular spine, bilateral).
- For lesions on the head, add GV-20 Baihui and EX-HN-1 Sishencong. [ii]

Prescription 2
Point: BL-40 Weizhong.

Technique
Use the prescriptions alternately. After sterilization of the local area, prick with a three-edged needle to cause a small amount of bleeding or until the subcutaneous area turns bluish-purple. Treat once every two to three days. A course consists of six treatment sessions.

PRICKING TO BLEED COMBINED WITH CUPPING THERAPY
Main points: GV-14 Dazhui and GV-13 Taodao.

Auxiliary points
- For lesions on the upper limbs, add Jianjiagang (located at the midpoint of the scapular spine, bilateral) and LI-15 Jianyu.
- For lesions on the lumbosacral region, add BL-23 Shenshu, GB-30 Huantiao, SP-10 Xuehai, ST-34 Liangqiu, and GB-34 Yanglingquan.
- For lesions on the head and face, add EX-HN-14 Yiming,[iii] SI-19 Tinggong, GV-20 Baihui, and EX-HN-1 Sishencong. [ii]

Technique
Prick the points with a small three-edged needle and follow up immediately with application of the flash-cupping method. Remove the cup when there is slight bleeding. Treat once every two days. Do not use cupping on the head.

Clinical notes

- Treatment for this disease falls into three different categories:
1. Focus on treating the Blood by cooling the Blood and relieving Toxicity for Blood-Heat patterns, by enriching Yin and moistening Dryness for Blood-Dryness patterns, and by transforming Blood stasis and relieving Toxicity for Blood stasis patterns.
2. Treat according to the different patterns listed above.
3. Treat according to the different periods of the disease by expelling pathogenic factors during the active or progressive phase, by simultaneously expelling pathogenic factors and supplementing Vital Qi (Zheng Qi) during the regressive phase, and by supporting Vital Qi and consolidating the Root or enriching Yin and protecting Body Fluids during the quiescent phase.
- In terms of external treatment, wash preparations are effective in removing scales and alleviating itching and are used for widely distributed lesions. Ointments have good permeability and are effective in dispersing erythema; they are therefore used for

---

[ii] M-HN-1 according to the system employed by the Shanghai College of Traditional Chinese Medicine.
[iii] M-HN-13 according to the system employed by the Shanghai College of Traditional Chinese Medicine.

circumscribed or persistent lesions. Diluted, lower-concentration medications tend to work better; ingredients should have a mild action without being dry so as to prevent irritation of the skin and the occurrence of secondary erythroderma.

- Acupuncture and moxibustion therapy is very effective as an auxiliary method for alleviating itching.
- In China, for certain types of psoriasis which require hospital admission such as generalized pustular psoriasis and erythrodermic psoriasis or severe complications such as psoriatic arthritis, TCM treatment will usually be given in conjunction with treatment by Western medicine.

Advice for the patient

- Try to build up bodily strength and avoid infection of the upper respiratory tract.
- Reduce intake of meat and fatty food and eat more fresh vegetables and fruit.
- Avoid spicy food and alcohol.
- Avoid stress and excessive fatigue.

Case histories

Case 1

Patient
Female, aged 40.

Clinical manifestations
One month previously, a rash had appeared on the patient's trunk and limbs without a predisposing cause; the rash was itchy and covered by silvery-white scales. The condition gradually worsened. The patient was given a steroid cream for external use (whose name she had forgotten) in a hospital clinic, but no obvious effect was achieved. Red plaques of varying size covered by silvery-white scales had now spread over the trunk and limbs; the patient felt itchy and suffered from discomfort in the throat. Appetite, urine and stool were normal. The tongue body was red with a white coating; the pulse was rapid.

Diagnosis
Plaque psoriasis (*bai bi*), progressive phase.

Pattern identification
Blood-Heat

Treatment principle
Cool and invigorate the Blood, clear Heat and relieve Toxicity.

Prescription
LIANG XUE HUO XUE TANG
Decoction for Cooling and Invigorating the Blood

Zi Cao (Radix Arnebiae seu Lithospermi) 15g

Qian Cao Gen (Radix Rubiae Cordifoliae) 15g
Ban Lan Gen (Radix Isatidis seu Baphicacanthi) 30g
Da Qing Ye (Folium Isatidis seu Baphicacanthi) 30g
Tu Fu Ling (Rhizoma Smilacis Glabrae) 30g
Huai Hua (Flos Sophorae Japonicae) 30g
Shan Dou Gen (Radix Sophorae Tonkinensis) 10g
Xuan Shen (Radix Scrophulariae Ningpoensis) 15g
Gua Jin Deng (Calyx Physalis Alkekengi) 10g
Tian Hua Fen (Radix Trichosanthis) 15g
Bai Xian Pi (Cortex Dictamni Dasycarpi Radicis) 30g
Gan Di Huang (Radix Rehmanniae Glutinosae Exsiccata) 15g
Chi Shao (Radix Paeoniae Rubra) 15g
Jin Yin Hua (Flos Lonicerae) 15g
Yi Yi Ren (Semen Coicis Lachryma-jobi) 30g
Ling Yang Jiao Fen‡ (Cornu Antelopis, powdered) 0.6g, infused in the prepared decoction

One bag a day was used to prepare a decoction, taken twice a day.

Outcome
After 21 bags, the skin lesions had completely disappeared, leaving pigmented spots; the throat discomfort had also been relieved. The patient was told to continue with the prescription for another 14 bags to consolidate the improvement.

Discussion
This formula for cooling and invigorating the Blood is the result of clinical experience gained over more than 40 years; it is very effective in the treatment of Blood-Heat patterns of psoriasis. The clinical manifestations of recent skin rash, throat discomfort, itching, a red tongue body, and a rapid pulse are all characteristic of patterns of internally exuberant Blood-Heat. Thus, the treatment principle of cooling and invigorating the Blood and clearing Heat and relieving Toxicity was applied.

In the prescription, *Zi Cao* (Radix Arnebiae seu Lithospermi), *Qian Cao Gen* (Radix Rubiae Cordifoliae), *Gan Di Huang* (Radix Rehmanniae Glutinosae Exsiccata) and *Chi Shao* (Radix Paeoniae Rubra) cool and invigorate the Blood; *Ban Lan Gen* (Radix Isatidis seu Baphicacanthi), *Da Qing Ye* (Folium Isatidis seu Baphicacanthi), *Huai Hua* (Flos Sophorae Japonicae), *Shan Dou Gen* (Radix Sophorae Tonkinensis), *Gua Jin Deng* (Calyx Physalis Alkekengi), *Bai Xian Pi* (Cortex Dictamni Dasycarpi Radicis), and *Jin Yin Hua* (Flos Lonicerae) clear Heat and relieve Toxicity; *Xuan Shen* (Radix Scrophulariae Ningpoensis) and *Tian Hua Fen* (Radix Trichosanthis) benefit the throat and relieve Toxicity; and *Yi Yi Ren* (Semen Coicis Lachryma-jobi) and *Tu Fu Ling* (Rhizoma Smilacis Glabrae) eliminate Dampness and relieve Toxicity. These ingredients were combined with powdered *Ling Yang Jiao*‡ (Cornu Antelopis) to cool the Blood and calm the Spirit. [1]

Case 2
Patient
Male, aged 17.

Clinical manifestations
Three years previously, plaques had appeared on the patient's trunk and limbs; the plaques were itchy and became covered by

silvery-white scales. Despite treatment in other clinics, the plaques gradually increased in number. The patient felt discomfort in the throat and caught colds easily. Appetite, urine and stool were normal. Examination revealed pale red, coin-shaped infiltrative plaques distributed over the trunk and limbs and covered by silvery-white scales. Plaques were densely distributed on the back, buttocks and thighs. The tongue body was pale with a thin white coating; the pulse was deep.

Diagnosis
Plaque psoriasis (*bai bi*), quiescent phase.

Pattern identification
Blood-Dryness.

Treatment principle
Nourish and invigorate the Blood, clear Heat and relieve Toxicity.

Prescription ingredients
Sheng Di Huang (Radix Rehmanniae Glutinosae) 15g
Shu Di Huang (Radix Rehmanniae Glutinosae Conquita) 15g
Chi Shao (Radix Paeoniae Rubra) 15g
Bai Shao (Radix Paeoniae Lactiflorae) 15g
Dang Gui (Radix Angelicae Sinensis) 15g
Chuan Xiong (Rhizoma Ligustici Chuanxiong) 10g
Hong Hua (Flos Carthami Tinctorii) 10g
Ban Lan Gen (Radix Isatidis seu Baphicacanthi) 30g
Da Qing Ye (Folium Isatidis seu Baphicacanthi) 30g
Zi Cao (Radix Arnebiae seu Lithospermi) 15g
Qian Cao Gen (Radix Rubiae Cordifoliae) 15g
Shan Dou Gen (Radix Sophorae Tonkinensis) 10g
Xuan Shen (Radix Scrophulariae Ningpoensis) 15g
Tian Hua Fen (Radix Trichosanthis) 15g
Tu Fu Ling (Rhizoma Smilacis Glabrae) 30g
Yi Yi Ren (Semen Coicis Lachryma-jobi) 30g
Ye Jiao Teng (Caulis Polygoni Multiflori) 30g

One bag a day was used to prepare a decoction, taken twice a day.

External treatment
Pu Lian Gao (Universal Coptis Paste) was applied twice a day to the affected areas.

Outcome
After 14 bags of the decoction, the patient no longer felt discomfort in the throat, and some of the lesions were beginning to disappear from the center. After another 42 bags of the decoction and external application of *Pu Lian Gao* (Universal Coptis Paste) for the same period, the plaques had disappeared completely, leaving pigmented patches.

Discussion
The Blood-Dryness pattern often occurs in the quiescent phase of psoriasis and is difficult to treat because of its enduring condition. This pattern often manifests as pale red lesions without severe itching, a pale tongue body with a thin white coating, and a deep pulse.

Zhang Zhili generally follows the treatment principle of nourishing and invigorating the Blood, clearing Heat and relieving Toxicity in treating this type of psoriasis. In this particular case, *Si Wu Tang* (Four Agents Decoction), composed of *Dang Gui* (Radix Angelicae Sinensis), *Sheng Di Huang* (Radix Rehmanniae Glutinosae), *Shu Di Huang* (Radix Rehmanniae Glutinosae Conquita), *Chuan Xiong* (Rhizoma Ligustici Chuanxiong), and *Bai Shao* (Radix Paeoniae Lactiflorae), was combined with *Hong Hua* (Flos Carthami Tinctorii), *Zi Cao* (Radix Arnebiae seu Lithospermi), *Qian Cao Gen* (Radix Rubiae Cordifoliae), *Chi Shao* (Radix Paeoniae Rubra), and *Ye Jiao Teng* (Caulis Polygoni Multiflori) to nourish and invigorate the Blood; with *Ban Lan Gen* (Radix Isatidis seu Baphicacanthi) and *Da Qing Ye* (Folium Isatidis seu Baphicacanthi) to clear Heat and relieve Toxicity; and with *Shan Dou Gen* (Radix Sophorae Tonkinensis), *Xuan Shen* (Radix Scrophulariae Ningpoensis) and *Tian Hua Fen* (Radix Trichosanthis) as key herbs for treating discomfort of the throat and common colds.

In Dr. Zhang's experience, this prescription has proven very effective in treating psoriasis manifesting with recurrent colds and a sore dry throat. *Tu Fu Ling* (Rhizoma Smilacis Glabrae) and *Yi Yi Ren* (Semen Coicis Lachryma-jobi) were added to the prescription to eliminate Dampness and relieve Toxicity in order to get rid of all the pathogenic factors. Having established that the prescription was having an effect after the first 14 bags, the patient was asked to continue the prescription in order to consolidate the improvement and eventually achieve a cure of this obstinate condition. [2]

Case 3
Patient
Female, aged 49.

Clinical manifestations
Plaques had initially appeared on the patient's scalp 18 years previously. These plaques were covered by silvery-white scales and the condition was diagnosed as psoriasis. Although the patient had undergone different types of treatment in the intervening period, the condition constantly recurred. The plaques gradually developed to become generalized and itchy. Examination revealed the patient's head to be covered by silvery-white scales. Large, thick, dark red plaques were found on the lumbar region, back and both thighs. The tongue body was dull purple with a white coating; the pulse was deep and moderate.

Diagnosis
Chronic plaque psoriasis (*bai bi*) with involvement of the scalp, quiescent phase.

Pattern identification
Blood stasis.

Treatment principle
Invigorate the Blood and transform Blood stasis, eliminate Dampness and relieve Toxicity.

Prescription ingredients
Tao Ren (Semen Persicae) 10g
Hong Hua (Flos Carthami Tinctorii) 10g
San Leng (Rhizoma Sparganii Stoloniferi) 10g
E Zhu (Rhizoma Curcumae) 10g
Zi Cao (Radix Arnebiae seu Lithospermi) 15g
Qian Cao Gen (Radix Rubiae Cordifoliae) 15g

Ban Lan Gen (Radix Isatidis seu Baphicacanthi) 30g
Da Qing Ye (Folium Isatidis seu Baphicacanthi) 30g
Tu Fu Ling (Rhizoma Smilacis Glabrae) 30g
Huai Hua (Flos Sophorae Japonicae) 30g
Sheng Di Huang (Radix Rehmanniae Glutinosae) 15g
Bai Xian Pi (Cortex Dictamni Dasycarpi Radicis) 30g
Ku Shen (Radix Sophorae Flavescentis) 15g

One bag a day was used to prepare a decoction, taken twice a day.

External treatment
5% salicylic acid cream.

Second visit
After 28 bags of the decoction, the skin lesions became thinner, papular eruptions were seen within some of the thicker, dark red plaques, and the amount of silvery-white scales had decreased. The prescription was modified by the addition of *Yi Yi Ren* (Semen Coicis Lachryma-jobi) 30g and *Zhi Ke* (Fructus Citri Aurantii) 10g.

Outcome
After 28 bags of the modified prescription and continued application of the cream, the large lesions had disappeared, leaving patches of pigmentation. The patient was asked to continue the modified prescription for another 14 days to consolidate the improvement.

Discussion
The Blood stasis pattern is often seen in patients with obstinate psoriasis. In this particular case, the condition had persisted for 18 years. The key to treating this pattern is to follow the principle of invigorating the Blood and transforming Blood stasis, eliminating Dampness and relieving Toxicity.

In treating this case, Dr. Zhang used *Tao Ren* (Semen Persicae), *Hong Hua* (Flos Carthami Tinctorii), *San Leng* (Rhizoma Sparganii Stoloniferi), *E Zhu* (Rhizoma Curcumae), *Zi Cao* (Radix Arnebiae seu Lithospermi), *Qian Cao Gen* (Radix Rubiae Cordifoliae), *Sheng Di Huang* (Radix Rehmanniae Glutinosae), and *Huai Hua* (Flos Sophorae Japonicae) to invigorate and cool the Blood and transform Blood stasis; *Tu Fu Ling* (Rhizoma Smilacis Glabrae), *Bai Xian Pi* (Cortex Dictamni Dasycarpi Radicis) and *Ku Shen* (Radix Sophorae Flavescentis) to eliminate Dampness; and *Ban Lan Gen* (Radix Isatidis seu Baphicacanthi) and *Da Qing Ye* (Folium Isatidis seu Baphicacanthi) to clear Heat and relieve Toxicity.

After the patient had taken 28 bags of the decoction, the lesions had started to become thinner, and *Yi Yi Ren* (Semen Coicis Lachryma-jobi) and *Zhi Ke* (Fructus Citri Aurantii) were added to eliminate Dampness and harmonize the Stomach to achieve the goal of dispelling pathogenic factors without damaging Vital Qi (Zheng Qi) in the Stomach. This is an example of the principle of safeguarding Stomach Qi in the treatment of obstinate diseases.[3]

Case 4
Patient
Female, aged 31.

Clinical manifestations
The patient had suffered from red plaques distributed over the scalp, trunk and limbs for irregular periods during the six months prior to the consultation; these plaques were covered by silvery-white scales. The patient usually had irregular periods; new plaques appeared before menstruation. Accompanying symptoms and signs included itching, a bitter taste in the mouth, dry throat, poor appetite, abdominal distension, lack of strength in the limbs, and clear, thin and profuse white vaginal discharge which became more pronounced after eating raw or cold food.

Examination revealed bright red infiltrative papules and plaques of varying size distributed over the scalp, trunk and limbs and covered by silvery-white scales. The plaques were dense in the scalp. The tongue body was red with a thin yellow coating; the pulse was wiry and rapid.

Diagnosis
Plaque psoriasis (*bai bi*), progressive phase.

Pattern identification
Disharmony of the Chong and Ren vessels, Qi and Blood stagnation, internal retention of Damp-Heat.

Treatment principle
Regulate and harmonize the Chong and Ren vessels, invigorate and nourish the Blood, regulate the Spleen and eliminate Dampness.

Prescription ingredients
Dan Shen (Radix Salviae Miltiorrhizae) 15g
Chi Shao (Radix Paeoniae Rubra) 15g
Dang Gui (Radix Angelicae Sinensis) 10g
Xiang Fu (Rhizoma Cyperi Rotundi) 10g
Yi Mu Cao (Herba Leonuri Heterophylli) 10g
Bai Zhu (Rhizoma Atractylodis Macrocephalae) 10g
Zhi Ke (Fructus Citri Aurantii) 10g
Yi Yi Ren (Semen Coicis Lachryma-jobi) 30g
Chi Shi Zhi‡ (Halloysitum Rubrum) 30g
Hou Po (Cortex Magnoliae Officinalis) 10g
Tu Fu Ling (Rhizoma Smilacis Glabrae) 30g
Zi Cao (Radix Arnebiae seu Lithospermi) 15g
Ban Lan Gen (Radix Isatidis seu Baphicacanthi) 30g

One bag a day was used to prepare a decoction, taken twice a day.

External treatment ingredients
Ce Bai Ye (Cacumen Biotae Orientalis) 100g
Ku Shen (Radix Sophorae Flavescentis) 80g
Chu Shi Zi (Fructus Broussonetiae) 50g
Zao Jiao Ci (Spina Gleditsiae Sinensis) 25g

The ingredients were added to 3000ml of cold water and decocted for 20 minutes. The liquid was then used to wash the affected areas twice a day. After washing, 5% *Hei Dou Liu You Ruan Gao* (Black Soybean and Vaseline® Ointment) and 5% salicylic acid cream were applied alternately.

Second visit
After 14 bags of the prescription, the white vaginal discharge was much less profuse. No new plaques had appeared and

itching had subsided. The patient was asked to take another 14 bags of the decoction and to continue with the external ointments.

Outcome

After the second batch of the decoction, the papules had become paler in color and much fewer in number; the infiltrative plaques were thinner, and the white vaginal discharge had almost stopped. Periods were more regular than before and the appetite had improved. The abdominal distension and lack of strength in the limbs had been relieved. The prescription was modified by removing *Chi Shi Zhi*‡ (Halloysitum Rubrum) and adding *Tao Ren* (Semen Persicae) 10g, *Hong Hua* (Flos Carthami Tinctorii) 10g, *Ye Jiao Teng* (Caulis Polygoni Multiflori) 30g, and *Ji Xue Teng* (Caulis Spatholobi) 15g. After taking the decoction for another 30 days, the papules disappeared completely.

Discussion

Lesions in this pattern of psoriasis are often characterized by eczematoid changes in the axillary fossae, the submammary region and the perineum. Plaques at these sites are less hyperkeratotic than at other sites, and most patients identified with this pattern experience severe itching often accompanied by abdominal distension, a bitter taste in the mouth, a dry throat, poor appetite, and profuse white, or clear and thin, or yellow and smelly vaginal discharge. The tongue body is usually red with a yellow and greasy coating; the pulse is wiry, slippery and rapid.

In the prescription, *Bai Zhu* (Rhizoma Atractylodis Macrocephalae), *Zhi Ke* (Fructus Citri Aurantii), *Yi Yi Ren* (Semen Coicis Lachryma-jobi), *Tu Fu Ling* (Rhizoma Smilacis Glabrae), and *Chi Shi Zhi*‡ (Halloysitum Rubrum) clear Heat from the Spleen, eliminate Dampness and relieve Toxicity; *Zi Cao* (Radix Arnebiae seu Lithospermi) and *Ban Lan Gen* (Radix Isatidis seu Baphicacanthi) cool the Blood and relieve Toxicity; *Dang Gui* (Radix Angelicae Sinensis) and *Yi Mu Cao* (Herba Leonuri Heterophylli) regulate and nourish the Blood and regulate menstruation; *Dan Shen* (Radix Salviae Miltiorrhizae) and *Chi Shao* (Radix Paeoniae Rubra) cool and invigorate the Blood, regulate the Blood and break up Blood stasis; and *Xiang Fu* (Rhizoma Cyperi Rotundi) and *Hou Po* (Cortex Magnoliae Officinalis) move Qi and harmonize the Spleen.

In the modified prescription, *Tao Ren* (Semen Persicae) and *Hong Hua* (Flos Carthami Tinctorii) were added to consolidate the improvement by invigorating and cooling the Blood, and *Ye Jiao Teng* (Caulis Polygoni Multiflori) and *Ji Xue Teng* (Caulis Spatholobi) were added to regulate and harmonize Yin and Yang as well as to invigorate the Blood and free the channels. [4]

Literature excerpts

In *Wai Ke Zheng Zhi Quan Shu: Bai Bi* [A Compendium of External Symptoms and Treatment: White Crust], it says: "The skin is dry and itchy with whitish plaques. Scales appear and the skin gradually becomes dry with bleeding and painful fissuring on the limbs and trunk. The skin is thick and itchy between the fingers. This condition often occurs in thin people with Blood Deficiency. *Sheng Xue Run Fu Yin* (Beverage for Generating Blood and Moistening the Skin) should be taken internally and combined with pork fat for external use."

In *Zhao Bing Nan Lin Chuang Jing Yan Ji* [A Collection of Zhao Bingnan's Clinical Experiences], it says: "The initial stage of erythroderma in psoriasis is characterized by generalized redness, inflammation and swelling, aversion to cold, fever, and dry skin with scales. This is due to Damp transforming into Heat. Retention of Damp-Heat results in Fire flowing to the Xue level to cause Blood-Heat and Blood-Dryness, leading to reddening of the skin and desquamation.

"*Zi Cao* (Radix Arnebiae seu Lithospermi), *Mu Dan Pi* (Cortex Moutan Radicis), *Qian Cao Gen* (Radix Rubiae Cordifoliae), and *Chi Shao* (Radix Paeoniae Rubra) are therefore used to clear Heat, benefit the movement of Dampness and cool and invigorate the Blood on account of their sweet and cold or bitter and cold properties. *Hong Hua* (Flos Carthami Tinctorii) invigorates the Blood with warmth and acridity.

"*Huang Bai* (Cortex Phellodendri), *Huang Qin* (Radix Scutellariae Baicalensis), *Tu Fu Ling* (Rhizoma Smilacis Glabrae), *Ze Xie* (Rhizoma Alismatis Orientalis), *Che Qian Zi* (Semen Plantaginis), *Bai Xian Pi* (Cortex Dictamni Dasycarpi Radicis), *Yin Chen Hao* (Herba Artemisiae Scopariae), *Yi Yi Ren* (Semen Coicis Lachryma-jobi), and *Mu Tong** (Caulis Mutong) are used to clear Heat and benefit the movement of Dampness. Meanwhile, *Sheng Di Huang* (Radix Rehmanniae Glutinosae) is added to clear Heat and cool the Blood, enrich Yin and moisten the skin.

"In the final stage of the disease, Heat begins to subside, Yin-Liquids are depleted, and both Qi and Blood are damaged. Therefore, *Dang Gui* (Radix Angelicae Sinensis), *Huang Qi* (Radix Astragali seu Hedysari), *Sheng Di Huang* (Radix Rehmanniae Glutinosae), and *Shu Di Huang* (Radix Rehmanniae Glutinosae Conquita) are used to supplement and nourish the Blood, nourish Yin and moisten the skin."

Modern clinical experience

TREATMENT ACCORDING TO PATTERN IDENTIFICATION

1. **Zhou** divided psoriasis into three patterns. [5]
- **Blood-Heat**

Treatment principle
Clear Heat and cool the Blood.

Prescription ingredients
Shan Dou Gen (Radix Sophorae Tonkinensis) 15g

Jin Yin Hua (Flos Lonicerae) 15g
Bai Xian Pi (Cortex Dictamni Dasycarpi Radicis) 10g
Mu Dan Pi (Cortex Moutan Radicis) 10g
Huang Qin (Radix Scutellariae Baicalensis) 10g
Chan Tui‡ (Periostracum Cicadae) 10g
Shi Gao‡ (Gypsum Fibrosum) 10g, decocted for
   30 minutes before adding the other ingredients
Gan Cao (Radix Glycyrrhizae) 10g
Ban Lan Gen (Radix Isatidis seu Baphicacanthi) 15g
Dang Gui (Radix Angelicae Sinensis) 15g
Fu Ling (Sclerotium Poriae Cocos) 15g

- **Blood Deficiency**

Treatment principle
Regulate and supplement the Liver and Kidneys, nourish the Blood and dispel Wind.

Prescription ingredients

Shu Di Huang (Radix Rehmanniae Glutinosae Conquita) 20g
Bai Xian Pi (Cortex Dictamni Dasycarpi Radicis) 10g
Tian Men Dong (Radix Asparagi Cochinchinensis) 10g
Mai Men Dong (Radix Ophiopogonis Japonici) 10g
Tian Hua Fen (Radix Trichosanthis) 10g
Wei Ling Xian (Radix Clematidis) 10g
Bai Mao Gen (Rhizoma Imperatae Cylindricae) 10g
Xia Ku Cao (Spica Prunellae Vulgaris) 10g
Chuan Xiong (Rhizoma Ligustici Chuanxiong) 10g
Gan Cao (Radix Glycyrrhizae) 10g
Dang Gui (Radix Angelicae Sinensis) 15g
Dang Shen (Radix Codonopsitis Pilosulae) 15g
Huang Qi (Radix Astragali seu Hedysari) 15g

- **Blood-Dryness**

Treatment principle
Cool the Blood, generate Body Fluids and moisten Dryness.

Prescription ingredients

Xuan Shen (Radix Scrophulariae Ningpoensis) 15g
Yu Zhu (Rhizoma Polygonati Odorati) 15g
Bai Shao (Radix Paeoniae Lactiflorae) 15g
Ji Xue Teng (Caulis Spatholobi) 15g
Dang Gui (Radix Angelicae Sinensis) 15g
Zhi Mu (Rhizoma Anemarrhenae Asphodeloidis) 10g
Chi Shao (Radix Paeoniae Rubra) 10g
Chan Tui‡ (Periostracum Cicadae) 10g
Bai Zhi (Radix Angelicae Dahuricae) 10g
Tao Ren (Semen Persicae) 10g
Dang Shen (Radix Codonopsitis Pilosulae) 10g
Gan Cao (Radix Glycyrrhizae) 10g

In all cases, one bag a day was used to prepare a decoction, taken twice a day.

2. **Zhang** also divided psoriasis into three patterns for treatment during both the progressive and quiescent phases of the condition.[6]

- **Blood-Heat**

Treatment principle
Cool the Blood, clear Heat and relieve Toxicity

Prescription ingredients

Wu Jia Pi (Cortex Acanthopanacis Gracilistyli Radicis) 10g
Zhi Zi (Fructus Gardeniae Jasminoidis) 10g
Zi Cao (Radix Arnebiae seu Lithospermi) 10g
Bai Mao Gen (Rhizoma Imperatae Cylindricae) 15g
Mu Dan Pi (Cortex Moutan Radicis) 10g
Chi Shao (Radix Paeoniae Rubra) 10g
Sheng Di Huang (Radix Rehmanniae Glutinosae) 10g
Tu Fu Ling (Rhizoma Smilacis Glabrae) 15g
Bai Hua She She Cao (Herba Hedyotidis Diffusae) 30g
Da Qing Ye (Folium Isatidis seu Baphicacanthi) 30g
Ban Lan Gen (Radix Isatidis seu Baphicacanthi) 30g

- **Blood-Dryness**

Treatment principle
Nourish the Blood, enrich Yin and moisten the skin.

Prescription ingredients

Dang Gui (Radix Angelicae Sinensis) 10g
Chi Shao (Radix Paeoniae Rubra) 10g
Bai Shao (Radix Paeoniae Lactiflorae) 10g
Sheng Di Huang (Radix Rehmanniae Glutinosae) 10g
Chuan Xiong (Rhizoma Ligustici Chuanxiong) 10g
Ji Xue Teng (Caulis Spatholobi) 15g
Dan Shen (Radix Salviae Miltiorrhizae) 10g
Mai Men Dong (Radix Ophiopogonis Japonici) 10g
Tian Men Dong (Radix Asparagi Cochinchinensis) 10g
He Shou Wu (Radix Polygoni Multiflori) 15g
Feng Fang‡ (Nidus Vespae) 6g
Bai Hua She She Cao (Herba Hedyotidis Diffusae) 30g
Huang Qin (Radix Scutellariae Baicalensis) 10g

- **Blood stasis**

Treatment principle
Invigorate the Blood, transform Blood stasis and move Qi.

Prescription ingredients

Dang Gui (Radix Angelicae Sinensis) 10g
Tao Ren (Semen Persicae) 10g
Hong Hua (Flos Carthami Tinctorii) 10g
San Leng (Rhizoma Sparganii Stoloniferi) 10g
E Zhu (Rhizoma Curcumae) 10g
Ji Xue Teng (Caulis Spatholobi) 15g
Gui Jian Yu (Lignum Suberalatum Euonymi) 10g
Long Gu‡ (Os Draconis) 15g

Mu Li‡ (Concha Ostreae) 15g
Zhen Zhu Mu‡ (Concha Margaritifera) 30g
Zhi Ke (Fructus Citri Aurantii) 10g
Bai Xian Pi (Cortex Dictamni Dasycarpi Radicis) 30g
Bai Hua She She Cao (Herba Hedyotidis Diffusae) 30g

In all cases, one bag a day was used to prepare a decoction, taken twice a day.

3. **Chen** proposed treatments based on pattern identification combined with disease differentiation. [7]

- **Blood-Heat due to exuberant Wind**

This pattern is often seen in the progressive phase of the disease, and should be treated by cooling the Blood and dispelling Wind.

Prescription
TU HUAI YIN JIA JIAN
Glabrous Green Briar and Pagoda Tree Flower Beverage, with modifications

Tu Fu Ling (Rhizoma Smilacis Glabrae) 15g
Huai Hua (Flos Sophorae Japonicae) 15g
Sheng Di Huang (Radix Rehmanniae Glutinosae) 30g
Mu Dan Pi (Cortex Moutan Radicis) 15g
Bai Xian Pi (Cortex Dictamni Dasycarpi Radicis) 15g
Ku Shen (Radix Sophorae Flavescentis) 10g
Bai Mao Gen (Rhizoma Imperatae Cylindricae) 30g
Zi Cao (Radix Arnebiae seu Lithospermi) 15g
Qian Cao Gen (Radix Rubiae Cordifoliae) 15g

- **Blood-Dryness due to Wind-Heat**

This pattern is often seen in the quiescent or regressive phases and should be treated by nourishing the Blood and enriching Yin, dispelling Wind and moistening Dryness.

Prescription
ZI YIN YANG YIN TANG JIA JIAN
Decoction for Enriching and Nourishing Yin, with modifications

Dang Gui (Radix Angelicae Sinensis) 10g
Sheng Di Huang (Radix Rehmanniae Glutinosae) 15g
Chuan Xiong (Rhizoma Ligustici Chuanxiong) 10g
Bai Shao (Radix Paeoniae Lactiflorae) 15g
Bei Sha Shen (Radix Glehniae Littoralis) 10g
Xuan Shen (Radix Scrophulariae Ningpoensis) 10g
Bai Xian Pi (Cortex Dictamni Dasycarpi Radicis) 15g
Ku Shen (Radix Sophorae Flavescentis) 10g

- **Heat Toxins mixed with Dampness**

This pattern corresponds to pustular psoriasis and should be treated by clearing Heat, relieving Toxicity and benefiting the movement of Dampness.

Prescription
WU WEI XIAO DU YIN HE YIN CHEN HAO TANG JIA JIAN
Five-Ingredient Beverage for Dispersing Toxicity Combined With Oriental Wormwood Decoction, with modifications

Zi Hua Di Ding (Herba Violae Yedoensitis) 15g
Ye Ju Hua (Flos Chrysanthemi Indici) 10g
Pu Gong Ying (Herba Taraxaci cum Radice) 10g
Lian Qiao (Fructus Forsythiae Suspensae) 10g
Tian Kui Zi (Tuber Semiaquilegiae) 10g
Yin Chen Hao (Herba Artemisiae Scopariae) 10g
Chao Zhi Zi (Fructus Gardeniae Jasminoidis, stir-fried) 10g
Bi Xie (Rhizoma Dioscoreae Hypoglaucae seu Septemlobae) 10g
Che Qian Zi (Semen Plantaginis) 15g
Ze Xie (Rhizoma Alismatis Orientalis) 15g

- **Wind-Damp obstructing the network vessels**

This pattern corresponds to psoriatic arthritis and should be treated by dispelling Wind and eliminating Dampness, invigorating the Blood and freeing the network vessels.

Prescription
DU HUO JI SHENG TANG JIA JIAN
Pubescent Angelica Root and Mistletoe Decoction, with modifications

Du Huo (Radix Angelicae Pubescentis) 10g
Sang Ji Sheng (Ramulus Loranthi) 10g
Bai Zhu (Rhizoma Atractylodis Macrocephalae) 10g
Fu Ling (Sclerotium Poriae Cocos) 10g
Dang Gui (Radix Angelicae Sinensis) 10g
Chuan Xiong (Rhizoma Ligustici Chuanxiong) 15g
Sang Zhi (Ramulus Mori Albae) 15g
Bai Shao (Radix Paeoniae Lactiflorae) 10g
Dan Shen (Radix Salviae Miltiorrhizae) 10g
Ji Xue Teng (Caulis Spatholobi) 15g

- **Exuberant Heat damaging Yin**

This pattern corresponds to erythrodermic psoriasis and should be treated by clearing Heat from the Ying level and cooling the Blood, nourishing the Blood and moistening Dryness.

Prescription
QING YING TANG HE ZENG YE TANG JIA JIAN
Decoction for Clearing Heat from the Ying Level Combined With Decoction for Increasing Body Fluids, with modifications

Ling Yang Jiao Fen‡ (Cornu Antelopis, powdered) 0.6g, infused in the prepared decoction
Sheng Di Huang (Radix Rehmanniae Glutinosae) 15g

Jin Yin Hua Tan (Flos Lonicerae Carbonisatus) 10g
Xuan Shen (Radix Scrophulariae Ningpoensis) 10g
Mu Dan Pi (Cortex Moutan Radicis) 10g
Mai Men Dong (Radix Ophiopogonis Japonici) 15g
Lian Qiao (Fructus Forsythiae Suspensae) 10g
Bai Mao Gen (Rhizoma Imperatae Cylindricae) 30g
Zi Cao (Radix Arnebiae seu Lithospermi) 15g
Qian Cao Gen (Radix Rubiae Cordifoliae) 15g

TREATMENT ACCORDING TO DISEASE PHASE

1. **Liu** treated patients who had been in the progressive or quiescent phase of the disease for periods ranging from two months to three years. [8]

- **Progressive phase**

Treatment principle
Clear Heat and relieve Toxicity, dissipate Wind and alleviate itching.

Prescription ingredients
Jin Yin Hua (Flos Lonicerae) 15g
Chan Tui ‡ (Periostracum Cicadae) 15g
Da Qing Ye (Folium Isatidis seu Baphicacanthi) 15g
Qin Jiao (Radix Gentianae Macrophyllae) 12g
Fang Feng (Radix Ledebouriellae Divaricatae) 12g
Chong Lou (Rhizoma Paridis) 12g
Jing Jie (Herba Schizonepetae Tenuifoliae) 12g
San Leng (Rhizoma Sparganii Stoloniferi) 12g
Zao Jiao Ci (Spina Gleditsiae Sinensis) 12g
Zi Cao (Radix Arnebiae seu Lithospermi) 12g
Chi Shao (Radix Paeoniae Rubra) 12g
Bai Zhu (Rhizoma Atractylodis Macrocephalae) 12g
Huang Qi (Radix Astragali seu Hedysari) 12g
Bai Ji Li (Fructus Tribuli Terrestris) 30g
Cang Er Zi (Fructus Xanthii Sibirici) 30g
Bai Hua She She Cao (Herba Hedyotidis Diffusae) 30g
Quan Xie ‡ (Buthus Martensi) 8g
Jiang Can ‡ (Bombyx Batryticatus) 10g

- **Quiescent phase**

Treatment principle
Invigorate the Blood and transform stasis, augment Qi and free the network vessels.

Prescription ingredients
Shu Di Huang (Radix Rehmanniae Glutinosae Conquita) 15g
Fang Feng (Radix Ledebouriellae Divaricatae) 15g
Bai Fu Zi (Rhizoma Typhonii Gigantei) 15g
Ban Lan Gen (Radix Isatidis seu Baphicacanthi) 15g
Zi Cao (Radix Arnebiae seu Lithospermi) 15g
Cao Dou Kou (Semen Alpiniae Katsumadai) 15g
Bai Xian Pi (Cortex Dictamni Dasycarpi Radicis) 15g

Mai Men Dong (Radix Ophiopogonis Japonici) 15g
Zi He Che ‡ (Placenta Hominis) 15g
Ji Xue Teng (Caulis Spatholobi) 15g
Ren Shen (Radix Ginseng) 15g
Tian Men Dong (Radix Asparagi Cochinchinensis) 20g
Shan Dou Gen (Radix Sophorae Tonkinensis) 20g
Ren Dong Teng (Caulis Lonicerae Japonicae) 20g
Huang Qi (Radix Astragali seu Hedysari) 20g
Tu Fu Ling (Rhizoma Smilacis Glabrae) 30g
Hong Hua (Flos Carthami Tinctorii) 10g
Gan Cao (Radix Glycyrrhizae) 10g

In both prescriptions, the ingredients were first decocted in 550ml of water and cooked until there was 400ml of water left; 200ml of the decoction was then drained off. Another 100ml of water was added and the decoction was cooked a second time until 150ml was left, which was mixed with the liquid from the first decoction and set aside for oral administration. The residue was cooked a third time with 400ml of water to prepare a decoction for external use, first for steaming and then for washing. Results were seen after one month of treatment.

2. **Wang** treated patients in the progressive, quiescent and regressive phases. [9]

- **Progressive phase**

Treatment principle
Cool the Blood and dispel Wind, clear Heat and relieve Toxicity.

Prescription ingredients
Sheng Di Huang (Radix Rehmanniae Glutinosae) 30g
Sang Ye (Folium Mori Albae) 15g
Chi Shao (Radix Paeoniae Rubra) 15g
Mu Dan Pi (Cortex Moutan Radicis) 15g
Dang Gui (Radix Angelicae Sinensis) 15g
Bai Xian Pi (Cortex Dictamni Dasycarpi Radicis) 15g
Ku Shen (Radix Sophorae Flavescentis) 15g
Di Fu Zi (Fructus Kochiae Scopariae) 15g
Cang Er Zi (Fructus Xanthii Sibirici) 15g
Wu Shao She ‡ (Zaocys Dhumnades) 10g
Gan Cao (Radix Glycyrrhizae) 6g

- **Quiescent and regressive phases**

Treatment principle
Nourish the Blood, dispel Wind and moisten Dryness

Prescription ingredients
Sheng Di Huang (Radix Rehmanniae Glutinosae) 30g
Shu Di Huang (Radix Rehmanniae Glutinosae Conquita) 30g
He Shou Wu (Radix Polygoni Multiflori) 15g
Bai Shao (Radix Paeoniae Lactiflorae) 15g

Chi Shao (Radix Paeoniae Rubra) 15g
Ku Shen (Radix Sophorae Flavescentis) 15g
Bai Xian Pi (Cortex Dictamni Dasycarpi Radicis) 15g
Gui Zhi (Ramulus Cinnamomi Cassiae) 12g
Tu Si Zi (Semen Cuscutae) 12g

Two bags of the ingredients were used every three days. On the first two days, one bag a day was used to prepare a decoction taken twice a day. The ingredients were then decocted again on the third day for use as an external wash for the affected areas. One month of treatment made up a course. Around 60 percent of patients needed one course, with the remainder requiring two courses.

SPECIAL PRESCRIPTIONS

1. **Lin** used *Lei Gong Teng Pian* (Thunder God Vine Tablet) to treat 78 patients who had been suffering from plaque psoriasis for a time span ranging from two weeks to 40 years; for ten patients this was the first episode. Treatment consisted of oral administration of two tablets of *Lei Gong Teng Pian* (Thunder God Vine Tablet) three times daily for one to three months. While under treatment, 18 patients suffered from irregular periods or amenorrhea, one male patient developed hyposexuality and 20 patients developed other symptoms including irritation of the digestive tract, dry eyes and hyperpigmentation. Of the 40 patients who recovered from their psoriasis, 29 suffered recurrence within 2-12 months. They were again treated with *Lei Gong Teng Pian* (Thunder God Vine Tablet) for a similar period with good results without any increase in the dosage. [10]

2. **Wei** used *Wu She Qu Feng Tang* (Black-Tail Snake Decoction for Expelling Wind) to treat psoriasis. [11]

Prescription ingredients

Wu Shao She ‡ (Zaocys Dhumnades) 12g
Chan Tui ‡ (Periostracum Cicadae) 12g
Bai Zhi (Radix Angelicae Dahuricae) 12g
Jin Yin Hua (Flos Lonicerae) 12g
Jing Jie (Herba Schizonepetae Tenuifoliae) 9g
Fang Feng (Radix Ledebouriellae Divaricatae) 9g
Qiang Huo (Rhizoma et Radix Notopterygii) 9g
Huang Qin (Radix Scutellariae Baicalensis) 9g
Lian Qiao (Fructus Forsythiae Suspensae) 9g
Gan Cao (Radix Glycyrrhizae) 9g
Huang Lian (Rhizoma Coptidis) 6g

One bag a day was used to prepare a decoction, taken twice a day. Ten days of treatment made up a course. Good results were seen after four courses.

3. **Yu** prepared *Jie Du Xiao Feng Wan* (Pill for Relieving Toxicity and Dispersing Wind) to treat psoriasis. [12]

Prescription ingredients

Jin Yin Hua (Flos Lonicerae) 15g
Bai Xian Pi (Cortex Dictamni Dasycarpi Radicis) 30g
Tu Fu Ling (Rhizoma Smilacis Glabrae) 15g
Chong Lou (Rhizoma Paridis) 15g
Ba Qia (Rhizoma Smilacis Chinensis) 10g
Sheng Di Huang (Radix Rehmanniae Glutinosae) 15g
Mu Dan Pi (Cortex Moutan Radicis) 10g
Zi Cao (Radix Arnebiae seu Lithospermi) 10g
Da Huang (Radix et Rhizoma Rhei) 6g
Huai Hua (Flos Sophorae Japonicae) 15g
Da Qing Ye (Folium Isatidis seu Baphicacanthi) 30g
Ban Lan Gen (Radix Isatidis seu Baphicacanthi) 30g
Jing Jie (Herba Schizonepetae Tenuifoliae) 10g
Fang Feng (Radix Ledebouriellae Divaricatae) 10g
Cang Er Zi (Fructus Xanthii Sibirici) 6g
Chan Tui ‡ (Periostracum Cicadae) 6g
Wu Shao She ‡ (Zaocys Dhumnades) 10g
Quan Xie ‡ (Buthus Martensi) 5g
Gan Cao (Radix Glycyrrhizae) 6g
Wu Mei (Fructus Pruni Mume) 10g

The ingredients were ground into a powder and mixed with water to make the pills. Ten grams of pills were taken three times a day. For enduring diseases with thick scaling, patients were also given 6g twice a day of *Er Hao Xiao Yong Wan* (No. 2 Pill for Dispersing *Yong* Abscesses), prepared with *Wu Gong* ‡ (Scolopendra Subspinipes), *Quan Xie* ‡ (Buthus Martensi), *Chan Tui* ‡ (Periostracum Cicadae) and *Jiang Can* ‡ (Bombyx Batryticatus). *Mo Feng Gao* (Fashionable Paste) was recommended for external application. Results were seen after one month of treatment.

4. **Su** prepared a series of pills for treating psoriasis with the ingredients varying according to the pattern. [13]

Basic prescription
XIAO YIN LING
Marvelous Pill for Dispersing Psoriasis

Dang Gui (Radix Angelicae Sinensis) 10g
Sheng Di Huang (Radix Rehmanniae Glutinosae) 10g
Chuan Xiong (Rhizoma Ligustici Chuanxiong) 10g
Mu Dan Pi (Cortex Moutan Radicis) 10g
Bai Hua She She Cao (Herba Hedyotidis Diffusae) 30g
Huang Qin (Radix Scutellariae Baicalensis) 6g
Bai Xian Pi (Cortex Dictamni Dasycarpi Radicis) 30g
Bai Ji Li (Fructus Tribuli Terrestris) 15g
Zao Jiao Ci (Spina Gleditsiae Sinensis) 10g
Gan Cao (Radix Glycyrrhizae) 6g

Modifications

1. For Blood-Heat patterns, *Jin Yin Hua* (Flos Lonicerae) 15g, *Lian Qiao* (Fructus Forsythiae Suspensae)

15g and *Tu Fu Ling* (Rhizoma Smilacis Glabrae) 15g were added.

2. For Blood stasis patterns, *San Leng* (Rhizoma Sparganii Stoloniferi) 10g, *E Zhu* (Rhizoma Curcumae) 10g, *Hong Hua* (Flos Carthami Tinctorii) 10g, and *Ji Xue Teng* (Caulis Spatholobi) 15g were added.

3 For Blood-Dryness patterns, *He Shou Wu* (Radix Polygoni Multiflori) 15g, *Mai Men Dong* (Radix Ophiopogonis Japonici) 10g, *Tian Men Dong* (Radix Asparagi Cochinchinensis) 10g, and *Xuan Shen* (Radix Scrophulariae Ningpoensis) 10g were added.

These ingredients were processed with water into tiny pills, which were put into balls containing 100 pills and weighing 6-7g in total. One ball of pills was taken twice a day for two months.

5. **Wang** reported on the treatment of psoriasis with a classical formula. [14]

Treatment principle
Invigorate the Blood and transform Blood stasis, relieve Toxicity and free the network vessels.

Prescription
XUE FU ZHU YU TANG JIA WEI
Decoction for Expelling Stasis from the House of Blood, with additions

Sheng Di Huang (Radix Rehmanniae Glutinosae) 12g
Dang Gui (Radix Angelicae Sinensis) 12g
Chi Shao (Radix Paeoniae Rubra) 12g
Dan Shen (Radix Salviae Miltiorrhizae) 12g
Chuan Xiong (Rhizoma Ligustici Chuanxiong) 9g
Tao Ren (Semen Persicae) 9g
Hong Hua (Flos Carthami Tinctorii) 9g
Niu Xi (Radix Achyranthis Bidentatae) 9g
San Leng (Rhizoma Sparganii Stoloniferi) 9g
E Zhu (Rhizoma Curcumae) 9g
Zhi Ke (Fructus Citri Aurantii) 9g
Chan Tui ‡ (Periostracum Cicadae) 9g
Wu Shao She ‡ (Zaocys Dhumnades) 9g
Chai Hu (Radix Bupleuri) 6g
Jie Geng (Radix Platycodi Grandiflori) 6g
Gan Cao (Radix Glycyrrhizae) 6g

Modifications
1. *Qin Jiao* (Radix Gentianae Macrophyllae) 12g, *Qiang Huo* (Rhizoma et Radix Notopterygii) 9g, *Du Huo* (Radix Angelicae Pubescentis) 9g, and *Ji Xue Teng* (Caulis Spatholobi) 15g were added for joint pain.
2. *Huang Qin* (Radix Scutellariae Baicalensis) 9g, *Huang Bai* (Cortex Phellodendri) 9g and *Huang Lian* (Rhizoma Coptidis) 6g were added for fever.

One bag a day was used to prepare a decoction, taken twice a day. Results were seen between one and two months.

6. **Liu** also reported on the treatment of psoriasis with a classical formula. [15]

Treatment principle
Cool and invigorate the Blood, clear Heat and relieve Toxicity.

Prescription
LIANG XUE JIE DU TANG
Decoction for Cooling the Blood and Relieving Toxicity

Sheng Di Huang (Radix Rehmanniae Glutinosae) 30g
Tu Fu Ling (Rhizoma Smilacis Glabrae) 30g
Chong Lou (Rhizoma Paridis) 30g
Chi Shao (Radix Paeoniae Rubra) 12g
Mu Dan Pi (Cortex Moutan Radicis) 12g
Bai Mao Gen (Rhizoma Imperatae Cylindricae) 15g
Bai Xian Pi (Cortex Dictamni Dasycarpi Radicis) 15g
Ban Zhi Lian (Herba Scutellariae Barbatae) 15g
Hu Zhang (Radix et Rhizoma Polygoni Cuspidati) 15g
Bai Hua She She Cao (Herba Hedyotidis Diffusae) 15g
Gan Cao (Radix Glycyrrhizae) 10g
Wei Ling Xian (Radix Clematidis) 10g

Modifications
1. For patients in the progressive phase with obvious erythema, *Shi Gao* ‡ (Gypsum Fibrosum) and *Zhi Mu* (Rhizoma Anemarrhenae Asphodeloidis) were added.
2. For lichenified lesions, *Dan Shen* (Radix Salviae Miltiorrhizae), *San Leng* (Rhizoma Sparganii Stoloniferi) and *E Zhu* (Rhizoma Curcumae) were added.
3. For pale erythema, *Dang Gui* (Radix Angelicae Sinensis) and *He Shou Wu* (Radix Polygoni Multiflori) were added.
4. For sore throat, *Xuan Shen* (Radix Scrophulariae Ningpoensis) and *Ban Lan Gen* (Radix Isatidis seu Baphicacanthi) were added.
5. For severe pruritus, *Ku Shen* (Radix Sophorae Flavescentis) and *Bai Ji Li* (Fructus Tribuli Terrestris) were added.
6. For constipation, *Da Qing Ye* (Folium Isatidis seu Baphicacanthi) was added.

One bag a day was used to prepare a decoction, taken twice a day. On average, results were seen after two months.

7. **Zhan** reported on a combination of internal and external treatment. [16]

Treatment principle
Cool and invigorate the Blood, clear Heat and relieve Toxicity.

Internal treatment prescription
BAI BI TANG
Psoriasis Decoction

Bai Hua She She Cao (Herba Hedyotidis Diffusae) 20g
Da Qing Ye (Folium Isatidis seu Baphicacanthi) 20g
Jin Yin Hua (Flos Lonicerae) 30g
Fang Feng (Radix Ledebouriellae Divaricatae) 30g
Lian Qiao (Fructus Forsythiae Suspensae) 10g
Sheng Di Huang (Radix Rehmanniae Glutinosae) 10g
Mu Dan Pi (Cortex Moutan Radicis) 10g
Bai Mao Gen (Rhizoma Imperatae Cylindricae) 10g

One bag a day was used to prepare a decoction, taken twice a day.

External treatment prescription
NIU PI XUAN XI JI
Psoriasis Wash Preparation

Mu Dan Pi (Cortex Moutan Radicis) 50g
Bai Xian Pi (Cortex Dictamni Dasycarpi Radicis) 50g
Di Gu Pi (Cortex Lycii Radicis) 50g
Sang Bai Pi (Cortex Mori Albae Radicis) 100g
Ku Shen (Radix Sophorae Flavescentis) 30g

The ingredients were added to 1000ml of water and boiled down to a concentrated decoction of 250ml, which was then mixed with 5 liters of water for use as a wash once a day. After the wash, a cold cream containing the steroid betamethasone dipropionate was applied to the affected area in some patients. Results were seen after one month of treatment.

ERYTHRODERMIC PSORIASIS

Chen combined a variety of treatment methods to treat this serious condition. [17]

i. **Internal treatment**

Treatment principle
Clear Heat, cool the Blood and relieve Toxicity.

Prescription ingredients

Shui Niu Jiao ‡ (Cornu Bubali) 30g, decocted for 30 minutes before adding the other ingredients
Sheng Di Huang (Radix Rehmanniae Glutinosae) 15g
Chi Shao (Radix Paeoniae Rubra) 10g
Mu Dan Pi (Cortex Moutan Radicis) 10g
Gou Gan Cai (Herba Diclipterae Chinensis) 6g
Tu Fu Ling (Rhizoma Smilacis Glabrae) 15g
Zi Cao (Radix Arnebiae seu Lithospermi) 15g
Shan Yao (Radix Dioscoreae Oppositae) 15g
Bai Ji Li (Fructus Tribuli Terrestris) 15g
Gan Cao (Radix Glycyrrhizae) 6g

ii. **Intravenous infusion** with 20-30ml of *Dan Shen Zhu She Ye* (Red Sage Root Injection) mixed with 500ml of 5 percent glucose, given once a day.

iii. Separate, daily **oral intake** of 1-1.5mg of *Lei Gong Teng Duo Dai* (Thunder God Vine Multiple Glycoside).

iv. **External wash**

Prescription
XIAO FAN XI FANG
Mirabilitum and Alumen Lotion

Mang Xiao ‡ (Mirabilitum) 15g
Ming Fan ‡ (Alumen) 15g
Di Yu (Radix Sanguisorbae Officinalis) 60g
Ce Bai Ye (Cacumen Biotae Orientalis) 60g
Jing Jie Sui (Spica Schizonepetae Tenuifoliae) 30g
Wang Bu Liu Xing (Semen Vaccariae Segetalis) 30g
Zi Hua Di Ding (Herba Violae Yedoensitis) 50g
Xu Chang Qing (Radix Cynanchi Paniculati) 50g

These ingredients were used to prepare a decoction for use warm as an external wash.

v. **Other external application**
Local application of 5-10% *Liu Huang Ruan Gao* (Sulfur Ointment) and *Pu Lian Gao* (Universal Coptis Paste).

Results indicated a significant reduction in the severity of the disease after 29-150 days of treatment.

COMBINED TREATMENT WITH TCM AND WESTERN MEDICINE

1. **Jing** formulated his own prescription to treat guttate psoriasis induced by infection. [18]

Treatment principle
Warm Yang, invigorate the Blood and transform Blood stasis

Prescription ingredients

*Fu Zi** (Radix Lateralis Aconiti Carmichaeli Praeparata) 6g
Rou Gui (Cortex Cinnamomi Cassiae) 10g
Rou Cong Rong (Herba Cistanches Deserticolae) 10g
San Qi (Radix Notoginseng) 15g
*Pao Chuan Shan Jia** (Squama Manitis Pentadactylae, blast-fried) 10g
Dang Gui (Radix Angelicae Sinensis) 15g
Chuan Xiong (Rhizoma Ligustici Chuanxiong) 10g
Tao Ren (Semen Persicae) 10g
Hong Hua (Flos Carthami Tinctorii) 10g
Chen Pi (Pericarpium Citri Reticulatae) 6g
Gan Cao (Radix Glycyrrhizae) 6g

One bag a day was used to prepare a decoction, taken twice a day until the lesions disappeared.

Western medicine
An intramuscular injection of 480mg of penicillin was given three times a day until the lesions disappeared and

the antistreptolysin O test and white blood cell count became normal. For severe cases, penicillin was administered intravenously.

After the lesions had disappeared, treatment continued with honey pills to warm Yang, invigorate the Blood and transform Blood stasis prepared with the above ingredients. Each pill contained 9g and two pills were taken three times a day for three weeks. Follow-up visits indicated that 16 of the 100 patients experienced recurrence within 3-5 years, 27 within 5-7 years, 28 within 7-10 years and 29 had experienced no recurrence after 10 years.

2. **Li** treated two groups of patients with psoriasis with different methods. [19]

- In a group treated with Western medicine only, 146 patients were given 8mg of chlorphenamine (chlorpheniramine) maleate and 0.3g of spiramycin taken orally three times daily, an intravenous infusion of 5 percent glucose with 2.5g of vitamin C once a day, and external application of 1:10000 dichlorodiethyl sulfide ointment once a day.

- In a group of 247 patients treated with TCM and Western medicine, the Western treatment described

above was supplemented with a decoction prepared with the following ingredients:

Jin Yin Hua (Flos Lonicerae) 10g
Niu Bang Zi (Fructus Arctii Lappae) 10g
Dang Gui (Radix Angelicae Sinensis) 15g
Shu Di Huang (Radix Rehmanniae Glutinosae Conquita) 10g
Chi Shao (Radix Paeoniae Rubra) 10g
Dan Shen (Radix Salviae Miltiorrhizae) 15g
Ji Xue Teng (Caulis Spatholobi) 30g
Di Fu Zi (Fructus Kochiae Scopariae) 10g
Bai Xian Pi (Cortex Dictamni Dasycarpi Radicis) 15g
Bai Hua She She Cao (Herba Hedyotidis Diffusae) 30g

One bag a day was used to prepare a decoction, taken twice a day.

A course of treatment lasted twenty days for both groups. Patients followed the treatment for two courses. In the combined treatment group, 24 patients recovered after one course of treatment and 138 after two courses (66 percent); in the Western medicine treatment group, nine patients recovered after one course of treatment and 74 after two courses (57 percent).

Palmoplantar pustulosis
掌跖脓疱病

This is a chronic recurrent disease occurring on the palms and soles and manifesting as small, deep, sterile pustules appearing periodically on an erythematous base, often accompanied by keratinization and desquamation.

Clinical manifestations

- Women are more likely to be affected than men, with the highest rate of incidence seen in the 30 to 50 age range.
- The disease mainly occurs on the palms and soles, in a symmetrical distribution, with the soles being affected more often, especially in the plantar arch.
- At the initial stage, small vesicles appear on an erythematous base, rapidly evolving into sterile 3-10 mm pustules of varying colors, usually yellow or brown. After five to seven days, the fluid in the pustules is absorbed, the pustules dry up and desquamation follows. After a certain time, crops of

pustules will reappear.

- Palmoplantar pustulosis may be triggered or exacerbated by various external stimuli (such as washing with soap or the external application of irritant medications), by profuse sweating in summer, by mental stress, or in the premenstrual period.

Differential diagnosis

Acrodermatitis continua

This condition occurs unilaterally following mild trauma and generally only involves the extremity of a finger or toe. After the superficial vesicles or pustules ulcerate, a bright red erosive surface appears with a little exudation or crusting or the lesions may dry up spontaneously, with crust formation and desquamation. New pustules often appear as the old ones heal. Nail fold infection and pathological changes in the nail may be accompanying symptoms.

Tinea manuum and tinea pedis

Tinea manuum is usually asymmetrical, mainly involving the center of the palm and the palmar aspect of the fingers. Small transparent pinpoint vesicles appear, quickly rupturing with a little exudate. They soon dry up to be covered with layers of white scale. Tinea pedis may involve the soles, which are covered by diffuse white scale. In another variant, vesicles evolve on the sole, collecting under the thick surface. Fungal culture is usually positive.

Pompholyx

At the initial stage, lesions manifest as a sudden eruption of deep-seated domed vesicles, 1-5 mm in diameter, raised slightly above the skin surface. Vesicles are filled with a clear fluid, which may occasionally turn turbid. Scaling and peeling follow drying of the vesicles. There is usually symmetrical involvement of the palms and, less frequently, the soles.

Etiology and pathology

- Exuberant Heat Toxins result from accumulated Damp-Heat transforming into Toxins in an enduring illness. Invasion by external Toxic pathogenic factors can also lead to Damp Toxins binding with Heat and generating exuberant Heat Toxins. These Damp Toxins are caused by an invasion of Dampness as a result of living in a humid place, being caught in the rain or working in water for a long period.

- Dietary irregularities can damage the transformation and transportation function of the Spleen, leading to Spleen Deficiency and exuberant Dampness. Dampness retained over a long period generates Heat. The Spleen governs the four limbs so that if Damp-Heat accumulates internally, it moves outward to the skin and flesh of the hands and feet.

- Enduring illnesses result in Deficiency and impair the ability of Vital Qi (Zheng Qi) to overcome pathogenic factors. Damp-Heat then accumulates and binds and moves outward to the fleshy exterior, causing recurrent and persistent pustules that are difficult to treat.

- Inadvertent intake of toxic materia medica containing metals or minerals or metal poisoning from other sources produces Fire Toxins, which move along the channels and network vessels to the palms and soles, eventually resulting in deep pustules.

Pattern identification and treatment

INTERNAL TREATMENT

EXUBERANT HEAT TOXINS

Clusters of vesicles and pustules of various sizes appear on the palms and soles, especially in the plantar arch; there are more pustules than vesicles in this type, which has a rapid onset. Lesions may be erosive and painful after rupture; for lesions on the soles, this can result in difficulty in walking. Accompanying symptoms and signs include general malaise, fever, aversion to cold, and thirst. The tongue body is deep crimson with a scant coating; the pulse is rapid.

Treatment principle

Clear Heat and relieve Toxicity, transform Dampness and drain Fire.

Prescription

QING WEN BAI DU YIN JIA JIAN
Beverage for Clearing Scourge and Vanquishing Toxicity, with modifications

Ban Lan Gen (Radix Isatidis seu Baphicacanthi) 6g
Chao Huang Qin (Radix Scutellariae Baicalensis, stir-fried) 6g
Chao Huang Lian (Rhizoma Coptidis, stir-fried) 6g
Jiao Zhi Zi (Fructus Gardeniae Jasminoidis, scorch-fried) 6g
Sheng Ma (Rhizoma Cimicifugae) 6g
Jin Yin Hua (Flos Lonicerae) 12g
Lian Qiao (Fructus Forsythiae Suspensae) 12g
Da Qing Ye (Folium Isatidis seu Baphicacanthi) 12g
Lü Dou Yi (Testa Phaseoli Radiati) 12g
Yi Yi Ren (Semen Coicis Lachryma-jobi) 15g
Chi Shao (Radix Paeoniae Rubra) 15g
Chi Xiao Dou (Semen Phaseoli Calcarati) 15g
Huang Bai (Cortex Phellodendri) 10g
Hua Shi‡ (Talcum) 10g
Ze Xie (Rhizoma Alismatis Orientalis) 10g

Explanation

- *Chao Huang Lian* (Rhizoma Coptidis, stir-fried), *Chao Huang Qin* (Radix Scutellariae Baicalensis, stir-fried), *Huang Bai* (Cortex Phellodendri), and *Jiao Zhi Zi* (Fructus Gardeniae Jasminoidis, scorch-fried) drain Fire with cold and bitterness.

- *Ban Lan Gen* (Radix Isatidis seu Baphicacanthi), *Da Qing Ye* (Folium Isatidis seu Baphicacanthi), *Lü Dou Yi* (Testa Phaseoli Radiati), *Jin Yin Hua* (Flos Lonicerae), and *Lian Qiao* (Fructus Forsythiae Suspensae) clear Heat and relieve Toxicity.

- *Hua Shi*‡ (Talcum), *Ze Xie* (Rhizoma Alismatis Orientalis), *Chi Xiao Dou* (Semen Phaseoli Calcarati), *Yi Yi Ren* (Semen Coicis Lachryma-jobi), and *Chi Shao* (Radix Paeoniae Rubra) clear Heat and transform Dampness, invigorate the Blood and disperse swelling.

- *Sheng Ma* (Rhizoma Cimicifugae) bears Yang upward (to protect Spleen Yang in view of the bitter and cold ingredients used) and relieves Toxicity.

DAMP-HEAT DUE TO SPLEEN DEFICIENCY

Eruptions in this pattern occur mainly on the soles, appearing less often on the palms. Lesions manifest as clusters of thick-walled vesicles and pustules, which may coalesce, with exudation and relatively severe erosion after rupture; in this type, there are more vesicles than pustules. Onset is slow and there are no obvious systemic symptoms. The tongue body is red with a thin yellow or yellow and greasy coating; the pulse is soggy and rapid.

Treatment principle
Clear Heat and transform Dampness, augment Qi and support the Spleen.

Prescription
ER MIAO WAN JIA WEI
Mysterious Two Pill, with additions

Cang Zhu (Rhizoma Atractylodis) 10g
Chen Pi (Pericarpium Citri Reticulatae) 10g
Chao Huang Bai (Cortex Phellodendri, stir-fried) 10g
Huang Qi (Radix Astragali seu Hedysari) 15g
Dang Shen (Radix Codonopsitis Pilosulae) 15g
Shan Yao (Radix Dioscoreae Oppositae) 15g
Yi Yi Ren (Semen Coicis Lachryma-jobi) 15g
Ren Dong Teng (Caulis Lonicerae Japonicae) 12g
Pu Gong Ying (Herba Taraxaci cum Radice) 12g
Ma Chi Xian (Herba Portulacae Oleraceae) 12g
Chi Fu Ling (Sclerotium Poriae Cocos Rubrae) 18g
Ze Xie (Rhizoma Alismatis Orientalis) 18g
Huang Qin (Radix Scutellariae Baicalensis) 18g

Explanation
- *Cang Zhu* (Rhizoma Atractylodis), *Huang Qi* (Radix Astragali seu Hedysari), *Dang Shen* (Radix Codonopsitis Pilosulae), *Shan Yao* (Radix Dioscoreae Oppositae), and *Chen Pi* (Pericarpium Citri Reticulatae) augment Qi and support the Spleen, transform Dampness and disperse eruptions.
- *Pu Gong Ying* (Herba Taraxaci cum Radice), *Ma Chi Xian* (Herba Portulacae Oleraceae), *Huang Qin* (Radix Scutellariae Baicalensis), and *Ren Dong Teng* (Caulis Lonicerae Japonicae) relieve Toxicity and free the network vessels.
- *Chi Fu Ling* (Sclerotium Poriae Cocos Rubrae), *Chao Huang Bai* (Cortex Phellodendri, stir-fried), *Ze Xie* (Rhizoma Alismatis Orientalis), and *Yi Yi Ren* (Semen Coicis Lachryma-jobi) benefit the movement of Dampness and clear Heat.

ATTACK BY METAL OR MINERAL TOXINS

In this pattern, eruptions mainly involve the palms and soles, but in some cases characteristic psoriasis plaques may be present on the dorsum of the foot, the lower leg, the knee, the dorsum of the hand, and the elbow. Lesions are characterized by dull red pustules, hyperkeratosis and bran-like scales, accompanied by moderate or severe pruritus. The tongue body is red with a scant or completely peeled coating; the pulse is thready and rapid.

Treatment principle
Clear and relieve Fire Toxins, protect the Heart and alleviate itching.

Prescription
HUANG LIAN JIE DU TANG JIA JIAN
Coptis Decoction for Relieving Toxicity, with modifications

Chao Huang Lian (Rhizoma Coptidis, stir-fried) 6g
Jiao Zhi Zi (Fructus Gardeniae Jasminoidis, scorch-fried) 6g
Lian Qiao Xin (Semen Forsythiae Suspensae) 6g
Lü Dou Yi (Testa Phaseoli Radiati) 30g
Xuan Shen (Radix Scrophulariae Ningpoensis) 12g
*Shi Hu** (Herba Dendrobii) 12g
Mai Men Dong (Radix Ophiopogonis Japonici) 12g
Gan Cao (Radix Glycyrrhizae) 12g
Chao Huang Qin (Radix Scutellariae Baicalensis, stir-fried) 10g
Hu Po‡ (Succinum) 6g
Deng Xin Cao (Medulla Junci Effusi) 6g

Explanation
- *Chao Huang Qin* (Radix Scutellariae Baicalensis, stir-fried), *Chao Huang Lian* (Rhizoma Coptidis, stir-fried) and *Jiao Zhi Zi* (Fructus Gardeniae Jasminoidis, scorch-fried) drain Fire with cold and bitterness.
- *Xuan Shen* (Radix Scrophulariae Ningpoensis), *Mai Men Dong* (Radix Ophiopogonis Japonici), *Shi Hu** (Herba Dendrobii), *Gan Cao* (Radix Glycyrrhizae), and *Lian Qiao Xin* (Semen Forsythiae Suspensae) nourish Yin and clear Heat, relieve Toxicity and protect the Heart.
- *Lü Dou Yi* (Testa Phaseoli Radiati), *Hu Po‡* (Succinum) and *Deng Xin Cao* (Medulla Junci Effusi) protect the Heart and ward off pathogenic factors.

RESIDUAL TOXINS

This pattern occurs when the condition is continuous or chronic with relapses. The remission phase varies in length; in the exacerbation phase, lesions appear every three to five days. The tongue body is red with a scant or completely peeled coating; the pulse is deep and thready.

Treatment principle
Nourish Yin and augment Qi, clear Heat and relieve Toxicity.

Prescription

WU WEI XIAO DU YIN JIA JIAN

Five-Ingredient Beverage for Dispersing Toxicity, with modifications

Pu Gong Ying (Herba Taraxaci cum Radice) 12g
Zi Hua Di Ding (Herba Violae Yedoensitis) 12g
Fu Ling Pi (Cortex Poriae Cocos) 12g
Lian Qiao (Fructus Forsythiae Suspensae) 12g
Nan Sha Shen (Radix Adenophorae) 15g
Shi Hu* (Herba Dendrobii) 15g
Tai Zi Shen (Radix Pseudostellariae Heterophyllae) 15g
Shu Di Huang (Radix Rehmanniae Glutinosae Conquita) 15g
Shan Yao (Radix Dioscoreae Oppositae) 15g
Dang Gui (Radix Angelicae Sinensis) 10g
Bai Shao (Radix Paeoniae Lactiflorae) 10g
Gan Cao (Radix Glycyrrhizae) 10g
Zhe Bei Mu (Bulbus Fritillariae Thunbergii) 10g
Yi Yi Ren (Semen Coicis Lachryma-jobi) 30g
Bai Hua She She Cao (Herba Hedyotidis Diffusae) 30g

Explanation

- Pu Gong Ying (Herba Taraxaci cum Radice), Zi Hua Di Ding (Herba Violae Yedoensitis), Bai Hua She She Cao (Herba Hedyotidis Diffusae), and Lian Qiao (Fructus Forsythiae Suspensae) clear Heat and relieve Toxicity.
- Nan Sha Shen (Radix Adenophorae), Zhe Bei Mu (Bulbus Fritillariae Thunbergii), Tai Zi Shen (Radix Pseudostellariae Heterophyllae), Shi Hu* (Herba Dendrobii), Shan Yao (Radix Dioscoreae Oppositae), and Gan Cao (Radix Glycyrrhizae) augment Qi and nourish Yin.
- Dang Gui (Radix Angelicae Sinensis), Bai Shao (Radix Paeoniae Lactiflorae) and Shu Di Huang (Radix Rehmanniae Glutinosae Conquita) supplement Blood to support Vital Qi (Zheng Qi).
- Fu Ling Pi (Cortex Poriae Cocos) and Yi Yi Ren (Semen Coicis Lachryma-jobi) fortify the Spleen to transform Dampness.

PATENT HERBAL MEDICINES

- For residual Toxins, take Huo Xue Xiao Yan Wan (Pill for Invigorating the Blood and Dispersing Inflammation) 3g twice a day.
- For exuberant Heat Toxins, take Long Dan Xie Gan Wan (Chinese Gentian Pill for Draining the Liver) 6g twice a day.

EXTERNAL TREATMENT

- For numerous vesicles and pustules, apply Cang Fu Shui Xi Ji (Atractylodes and Broom Cypress Wash Preparation) or Pi Yan Xi Ji (Dermatitis Wash Prepa- ration) as a wet compress or a soak for 15 minutes two or three times a day.
- For painful lesions with exudation and erosion, mix Shi Zhen Fen (Eczema Powder) or Qing Dai San (Indigo Powder) to a paste with vegetable oil and apply once a day to the affected area until the lesions heal.

ACUPUNCTURE

Points

- For lesions on the sole, select GB-34 Yanglingquan, SP-6 Sanyinjiao, and ST-40 Fenglong.
- For lesions on the palm, select TB-6 Zhigou, LI-4 Hegu and PC-6 Neiguan.

Technique: Apply the reducing method and retain the needles for 30 minutes after obtaining Qi. Treat once a day. A course consists of ten treatment sessions.

Explanation

- SP-6 Sanyinjiao and ST-40 Fenglong fortify the Spleen and transform Dampness.
- GB-34 Yanglingquan, TB-6 Zhigou, LI-4 Hegu, and PC-6 Neiguan drain Fire, clear Heat and relieve Toxicity.

MOXIBUSTION

Point: Ashi points (the sites of pustules on the palm or sole).

Technique: Ignite a moxa stick and use the sparrow-pecking method over the lesions for five to ten minutes. Treat once a day. A course consists of ten treatment sessions.

Clinical notes

- This disease is recalcitrant to treatment, and can persist for years with unexplained remissions and exacerbations.
- In internal treatment, differentiation should be made according to the relative severity of the Heat Toxins, with treatment focusing on the Heart. It is also important to distinguish whether Damp-Heat is acute or chronic and treat accordingly, with the focus on the Spleen.
- Externally, a wet compress or soak prepared with Chinese materia medica can achieve good results. Use mild external medications, thus avoiding irritation of the skin and helping the lesions to heal more quickly.
- Patients with tonsillitis or rhinitis should be treated promptly to eliminate infectious foci.
- Avoid exposure to toxic metals.

Case history

Patient
Male, aged 40.

Clinical manifestations
The patient had pustules on both soles, causing pain and making walking difficult. Some of the pustules had dried up and desquamation had occurred. The tongue body was red with a thin yellow coating; the pulse was thready and rapid.

Pattern identification
Damp-Heat pouring down, transforming into Fire and Toxins.

Treatment principle
Clear Heat and relieve Toxicity, fortify the Spleen and benefit the movement of Dampness.

Prescription ingredients
Ma Chi Xian (Herba Portulacae Oleraceae) 30g
Pu Gong Ying (Herba Taraxaci cum Radice) 15g
Ren Dong Teng (Caulis Lonicerae Japonicae) 12g
Huang Qin (Radix Scutellariae Baicalensis) 9g
Chi Shao (Radix Paeoniae Rubra) 9g
Ze Xie (Rhizoma Alismatis Orientalis) 9g
Che Qian Zi (Semen Plantaginis) 9g
Liu Yi San (Six-To-One Powder) 9g, wrapped
Huang Bai (Cortex Phellodendri) 9g
Cang Zhu (Rhizoma Atractylodis) 9g
Tong Cao (Medulla Tetrapanacis Papyriferi) 3g

One bag a day was used to prepare a decoction, taken twice a day.

External treatment
A decoction was prepared with *Cang Er Zi* (Fructus Xanthii Sibirici) 15g, *Lu Gan Shi* (Calamina) 15g and *Ming Fan* ‡ (Alumen) 9g as a wash for the feet.

Second visit
After five days, most of the pustules had subsided, although some new ones had appeared. The patient had afternoon fever (38°C) and a poor appetite.

Treatment principle
Fortify the Spleen and benefit the movement of Dampness, clear and relieve residual Toxicity.

Prescription ingredients
Cang Zhu (Rhizoma Atractylodis) 9g
Chen Pi (Pericarpium Citri Reticulatae) 9g
Zhu Ling (Sclerotium Polypori Umbellati) 9g
Ze Xie (Rhizoma Alismatis Orientalis) 9g
Liu Yi San (Six-To-One Powder) 9g, wrapped
Huang Qin (Radix Scutellariae Baicalensis) 9g
Bi Xie (Rhizoma Dioscoreae Hypoglaucae seu Septemlobae) 9g
Ma Chi Xian (Herba Portulacae Oleraceae) 30g
Pu Gong Ying (Herba Taraxaci cum Radice) 15g
Ren Dong Teng (Caulis Lonicerae Japonicae) 15g

The external treatment continued as before.

Third visit
After another five days, the symptoms of fever and poor appetite had been relieved, but a number of new pustules had appeared, resulting in distension and pain, and still making walking difficult.

Treatment principle
Clear Heat and relieve Toxicity with the secondary consideration of regulating Dampness.

Prescription ingredients
Ma Wei Lian (Radix Thalictri) 10g
Huang Qin (Radix Scutellariae Baicalensis) 9g
Lian Qiao (Fructus Forsythiae Suspensae) 9g
Fu Ling (Sclerotium Poriae Cocos) 9g
Ze Xie (Rhizoma Alismatis Orientalis) 9g
Liu Yi San (Six-To-One Powder) 9g
Er Miao Wan (Mysterious Two Pill) 9g
Ma Chi Xian (Herba Portulacae Oleraceae) 15g
Pu Gong Ying (Herba Taraxaci cum Radice) 15g
Ren Dong Teng (Caulis Lonicerae Japonicae) 15g

Outcome
After ten bags of the new prescription, all the symptoms and lesions had disappeared. [20]

Literature excerpt

According to *Xu Lü He Wai Ke Yi An Yi Hua Ji* [A Collection of Xu Lühe's Medical Records on External Diseases], "The following ingredients can be used to treat palmoplantar pustulosis: *Li Lu* (Radix et Rhizoma Veratri), which is bitter, cold and toxic, kills Worms; *Ku Shen* (Radix Sophorae Flavescentis), which is very bitter and cold, dispels Wind and kills Worms; *Ku Fan* ‡ (Alumen Praeparatum), which is salty, sour, cold, and astringent, dries Dampness and kills Worms; and *Xiong Huang* * (Realgar), which is acrid, warm and toxic, repels foulness and kills Worms. When these ingredients are mixed together with *Huang Lian Ruan Gao* (Coptis Ointment) as the excipient, they are very effective in dispelling Wind, drying Dampness, clearing Heat, relieving Toxicity, and killing Worms."

Modern clinical experience

COMBINED INTERNAL AND EXTERNAL TREATMENT

1. **Liu** treated palmoplantar pustulosis with *Bi Xie Shen Shi Tang Jia Jian* (Yam Rhizome Decoction for Percolating Dampness, with modifications). [21]

Prescription ingredients
Bi Xie (Rhizoma Dioscoreae Hypoglaucae seu Septemlobae) 15g
Yi Yi Ren (Semen Coicis Lachryma-jobi) 30g

Ze Xie (Rhizoma Alismatis Orientalis) 12g
Huang Bai (Cortex Phellodendri) 10g
Fu Ling (Sclerotium Poriae Cocos) 10g
Mu Dan Pi (Cortex Moutan Radicis) 10g
Hua Shi ‡ (Talcum) 10g
Tong Cao (Medulla Tetrapanacis Papyriferi) 10g

One bag a day was used to prepare a decoction, taken twice a day. The residue was decocted a third time to prepare a soak for the affected area. Results were seen after 50 days.

2. **Zhou** treated 16 patients with *Ying Xian Tang* (Dandelion and Purslane Decoction).[22]

Prescription ingredients

Pu Gong Ying (Herba Taraxaci cum Radice) 30g
Ma Chi Xian (Herba Portulacae Oleraceae) 30g
Tu Fu Ling (Rhizoma Smilacis Glabrae) 30g
Ku Shen (Radix Sophorae Flavescentis) 30g
Bai Xian Pi (Cortex Dictamni Dasycarpi Radicis) 10g
Chong Lou (Rhizoma Paridis) 10g
Huai Hua (Flos Sophorae Japonicae) 20g

One bag a day was used to prepare a decoction, taken twice a day. The residue was decocted a third time to prepare a soak for the affected area. Patients took the medication for six days and then had a one-day break. Results were assessed after three months.

EXTERNAL TREATMENT

Man devised his own external formula for treating palmoplantar pustulosis. [23]

Prescription
SHEN BAI SAN HUANG TANG
Three Yellows Decoction with Flavescent Sophora Root and Pulsatilla Root

Ku Shen (Radix Sophorae Flavescentis) 30g
She Chuang Zi (Fructus Cnidii Monnieri) 30g
Huang Bai (Cortex Phellodendri) 30g
Huang Qi (Radix Astragali seu Hedysari) 30g
Huang Jing (Rhizoma Polygonati) 30g
Bai Tou Weng (Radix Pulsatillae Chinensis) 30g
Fu Ling (Sclerotium Poriae Cocos) 30g
Dang Gui (Radix Angelicae Sinensis) 20g
Ku Fan ‡ (Alumen Praeparatum) 20g

The ingredients were decocted in 2000ml of water over a strong heat for 10 minutes and then over a mild heat for another 20 minutes. The decoction was used to soak the affected area for 20 minutes twice a day. Results were seen after eight weeks.

Acrodermatitis continua
连续性肢端皮炎

This is a rare, chronic, recurrent, aseptic, and pustular skin disease that occurs on the fingers and toes after minor trauma or infection. In TCM, it is also known as *xuan zhi gan* (chancrous digit sore).

Clinical manifestations

- This disease generally only involves the extremity of a finger or toe; it does not usually extend above the wrist or ankle.
- At the initial stage, lesions manifest as 0.5-2.0 mm superficial vesicles or pustules, which may become confluent. After ulceration, a bright red erosive surface appears with a little exudation or crusting; alternatively, the lesions may dry up spontaneously, with crust formation and desquamation. New pustules often appear as the old ones heal.
- In chronic cases, the disease may affect the finger or toe nails, causing deformity, thickening or separation.
- The disease develops slowly; it is recurrent and difficult to cure.
- Acrodermatitis may progress to generalized psoriasis, particularly in the elderly.

Differential diagnosis

Palmoplantar pustulosis
Sterile pustules mainly appear in a symmetrical distribution in the center of the palms and soles or on the major and minor thenar eminences.

Pyogenic paronychia (whitlow)
The tissue around the nail appears swollen and inflamed. The swelling then spreads and abscesses form around the fingernail or toenail. The end of the finger or toe turns red and can swell up to a considerable size. In some cases, an abscess forms along the edge of the nail, which may then eventually come off.

Frostbite

Lesions mainly involve exposed parts of the body such as the fingers and toes. Immediately after injury due to exposure to cold, symptoms initially appear as pallor of the skin, a sensation of freezing cold and pain, followed by numbness in the affected area. In moderate cases, vesicles appear at the initial stage and then dry up to form black crusts. In serious cases, the local skin color changes from pale white to blue and then to black. Swelling and blisters occur around the lesions, accompanied by severe pain. Necrotic tissue finally separates and the lesions heal slowly.

Etiology and pathology

- Acrodermatitis continua is caused internally by Damp-Heat in the Spleen and Stomach and externally by seasonal Heat Toxins. When both internal and external causes are involved, Damp, Heat and Toxins bind together, making the disease difficult to treat.

- Where Yang pathogenic factors are retained for a long period, they may transform into Fire and Toxins, which settle in the exterior, especially in the extremities. When Heat prevails, recurrent pustules occur with erosion and maceration of the area; the condition then becomes persistent.

- The Spleen governs the four limbs. Overindulgence in sweet and fatty foods or excessive consumption of alcohol or coffee damages the transformation and transportation function of the Spleen and Stomach, leading to accumulation of Damp-Heat in the Spleen. Damp-Heat subsequently transforms into Toxins and moves along the channels and network vessels to the extremities, causing pustules on the fingers and toes with erosion.

Pattern identification and treatment

INTERNAL TREATMENT

HEAT TOXINS

Lesions manifest as clusters of pustules on the finger or toe with inflammation and swelling; exudation of fluid or pus occurs after rupture. The periungual region is swollen; if the disease persists, the nail may separate, thicken or become deformed. Itching may be present, accompanied by a sensation of burning heat and pain. Other symptoms include fever, dry throat and thirst, constipation, and yellow or reddish urine. The tongue body is red with a thin yellow coating; the pulse is surging and rapid.

Treatment principle
Clear Heat and relieve Toxicity.

Prescription
NEI SHU HUANG LIAN TANG JIA JIAN
Coptis Decoction for Dredging the Interior, with modifications

Chao Huang Lian (Rhizoma Coptidis, stir-fried) 6g
Jiao Zhi Zi (Fructus Gardeniae Jasminoidis, scorch-fried) 6g
Chao Huang Qin (Radix Scutellariae Baicalensis, stir-fried) 10g
Chao Huang Bai (Cortex Phellodendri, stir-fried) 10g
Chi Fu Ling (Sclerotium Poriae Cocos Rubrae) 10g
Jiang Huang (Rhizoma Curcumae Longae) 10g
Ren Dong Teng (Caulis Lonicerae Japonicae) 15g
Ma Bian Cao (Herba cum Radice Verbenae) 15g
Bai Jiang Cao (Herba cum Radice Patriniae) 15g
Chi Xiao Dou (Semen Phaseoli Calcarati) 30g

Explanation

- *Chao Huang Qin* (Radix Scutellariae Baicalensis, stir-fried), *Chao Huang Lian* (Rhizoma Coptidis, stir-fried), *Chao Huang Bai* (Cortex Phellodendri, stir-fried), and *Jiao Zhi Zi* (Fructus Gardeniae Jasminoidis, scorch-fried) drain Fire, dry Dampness and relieve Toxicity with cold and bitterness.

- *Ren Dong Teng* (Caulis Lonicerae Japonicae), *Bai Jiang Cao* (Herba cum Radice Patriniae) and *Ma Bian Cao* (Herba cum Radice Verbenae) relieve Toxicity and free the network vessels.

- *Chi Fu Ling* (Sclerotium Poriae Cocos Rubrae), *Chi Xiao Dou* (Semen Phaseoli Calcarati) and *Jiang Huang* (Rhizoma Curcumae Longae) transform Dampness and disperse swelling.

DAMP-HEAT

The skin on the finger or toe is inflamed and ulcerated with exudation of pus. Pustules and vesicles are interspersed on the skin and are recurrent. There may be slight local itching and pain. Accompanying symptoms and signs include lassitude, poor appetite and abdominal distension. The tongue body is red with a yellow and slightly greasy coating; the pulse is soggy and rapid.

Treatment principle
Clear Heat and transform Dampness, invigorate the network vessels and relieve Toxicity.

Prescription
WU LING SAN JIA JIAN
Poria Five Powder, with modifications

Bai Zhu (Rhizoma Atractylodis Macrocephalae) 6g
Cang Zhu (Rhizoma Atractylodis) 6g
Chao Long Dan Cao (Radix Gentianae Scabrae, stir-fried) 6g
Jin Yin Hua (Flos Lonicerae) 15g

Zhu Ling (Sclerotium Polypori Umbellati) 10g
Ze Xie (Rhizoma Alismatis Orientalis) 10g
Fu Ling Pi (Cortex Poriae Cocos) 10g
Tian Hua Fen (Radix Trichosanthis) 10g
Rou Gui (Cortex Cinnamomi Cassiae) 6g
Chao Huang Lian (Rhizoma Coptidis, stir-fried) 3g
Jiao Zhi Zi (Fructus Gardeniae Jasminoidis, scorch-fried) 3g
Si Gua Luo (Fasciculus Vascularis Luffae) 3g
Ju Luo (Retinervus Fructus Citri Reticulatae) 3g
Dan Shen (Radix Salviae Miltiorrhizae) 30g
Chi Xiao Dou (Semen Phaseoli Calcarati) 30g

Explanation

- *Fu Ling Pi* (Cortex Poriae Cocos), *Ze Xie* (Rhizoma Alismatis Orientalis), *Chi Xiao Dou* (Semen Phaseoli Calcarati), *Zhu Ling* (Sclerotium Polypori Umbellati), *Bai Zhu* (Rhizoma Atractylodis Macrocephalae), and *Cang Zhu* (Rhizoma Atractylodis) clear Heat and transform Dampness, invigorate the Blood and disperse swelling.

- *Jin Yin Hua* (Flos Lonicerae), *Chao Huang Lian* (Rhizoma Coptidis, stir-fried), *Jiao Zhi Zi* (Fructus Gardeniae Jasminoidis, scorch-fried), and *Chao Long Dan Cao* (Radix Gentianae Scabrae, stir-fried) drain Fire with cold and bitterness.

- *Chi Xiao Dou* (Semen Phaseoli Calcarati), *Dan Shen* (Radix Salviae Miltiorrhizae), *Ju Luo* (Retinervus Fructus Citri Reticulatae), and *Si Gua Luo* (Fasciculus Vascularis Luffae) invigorate the Blood and free the network vessels.

- *Tian Hua Fen* (Radix Trichosanthis) clears Heat, relieves Toxicity and expels pus.

- *Rou Gui* (Cortex Cinnamomi Cassiae) prevents damage to the Stomach by ingredients with bitter and cold properties and assists *Bai Zhu* (Rhizoma Atractylodis Macrocephalae) and *Cang Zhu* (Rhizoma Atractylodis) to overcome Dampness and expel pathogenic factors.

General modifications

Channel conductors can be added according to the site of the lesions:

1. For lesions on the thumb (the Lung channel of Hand-Taiyin), add *Jie Geng* (Radix Platycodi Grandiflori), *Sheng Ma* (Rhizoma Cimicifugae), *Cong Bai* (Bulbus Allii Fistulosi), and *Bai Zhi* (Radix Angelicae Dahuricae).
2. For lesions on the index finger (the Large Intestine channel of Hand-Yangming), add *Bai Zhi* (Radix Angelicae Dahuricae), *Sheng Ma* (Rhizoma Cimicifugae) and *Shi Gao*‡ (Gypsum Fibrosum).
3. For lesions on the middle finger (the Pericardium channel of Hand-Jueyin), add *Chai Hu* (Radix Bupleuri) and *Mu Dan Pi* (Cortex Moutan Radicis).

4. For lesions on the lateral side of the ring finger (the Triple Burner channel of Hand-Shaoyang), add *Lian Qiao* (Fructus Forsythiae Suspensae) and *Chai Hu* (Radix Bupleuri).
5. For lesions on the medial side of the little finger (the Heart channel of Hand-Shaoyin), add *Huang Lian* (Rhizoma Coptidis) and *Xi Xin** (Herba cum Radice Asari).
6. For lesions on the lateral side of the little finger (the Small Intestine channel of Hand-Taiyang), add *Gao Ben* (Rhizoma et Radix Ligustici) and *Huang Bai* (Cortex Phellodendri).
7. For lesions on the sole (the Kidney channel of Foot-Shaoyin), add *Qiang Huo* (Rhizoma seu Radix Notopterygii), *Zhi Mu* (Rhizoma Anemarrhenae Asphodeloidis), *Rou Gui* (Cortex Cinnamomi Cassiae), and *Xi Xin** (Herba cum Radice Asari).
8. For lesions on the big toe (the Liver channel of Foot-Jueyin), add *Qing Pi* (Pericarpium Citri Reticulatae Viride), *Wu Zhu Yu* (Fructus Evodiae Rutaecarpae), *Chuan Xiong* (Rhizoma Ligustici Chuanxiong), and *Chai Hu* (Radix Bupleuri).
9. For lesions on the second toe (the Stomach channel of Foot-Yangming), add *Bai Zhi* (Radix Angelicae Dahuricae), *Sheng Ma* (Rhizoma Cimicifugae), *Shi Gao*‡ (Gypsum Fibrosum), *Ge Gen* (Radix Puerariae), *Cang Zhu* (Rhizoma Atractylodis), and *Bai Shao* (Radix Paeoniae Lactiflorae).
10. For lesions on the little toe and the lateral side of the fourth toe (the Gallbladder channel of Foot-Shaoyang), add *Chai Hu* (Radix Bupleuri) and *Qing Pi* (Pericarpium Citri Reticulatae Viride).
11. For lesions on the lateral side of the little toe (the Bladder channel of Foot-Taiyang), add *Qiang Huo* (Rhizoma seu Radix Notopterygii).
12. For recurrent pustules, add *Ban Zhi Lian* (Herba Scutellariae Barbatae), *Long Kui* (Herba Solani Nigri), *Bai Hua She She Cao* (Herba Hedyotidis Diffusae), and *Tu Fu Ling* (Rhizoma Smilacis Glabrae).

PATENT HERBAL MEDICINES

- For mild cases, oral administration of one of the following is recommended – *San Huang Wan* (Three Yellows Pill), *Qing Jie Pian* (Clearing and Relieving Tablet) or *Long Dan Xie Gan Wan* (Chinese Gentian Pill for Draining the Liver) 6g, twice a day.
- For severe cases, patients in China would be given *Xing Xiao Wan* (Awakening and Dispersing Pill) 6g twice a day or *Xi Huang Xing Xiao Wan* (Western Bovine Bezoar Awakening and Dispersing Pill) 6g twice a day. In those countries where use of these pills is not permitted, *Xiao Bai Du Gao* (Minor Toxicity-Vanquishing Syrup) 15g twice a day, dissolved in warm water, may be substituted.

EXTERNAL TREATMENT

For multiple vesicles or pustules, first use *Cang Fu Shui Xi Ji* (Atractylodes and Broom Cypress Wash Preparation) or *Lu Lu Tong Shui Xi Ji* (Sweetgum Fruit Wash Preparation) as a soak or wet compress for 15 minutes once a day. Then apply *Yu Lu Gao* (Jade Dew Ointment) or *Qu Shi San* (Powder for Dispelling Dampness) mixed with vegetable oil.

ACUPUNCTURE
Points
- For lesions on the hand, select PC-6 Neiguan, LI-11 Quchi and TB-5 Waiguan.
- For lesions on the foot, select ST-36 Zusanli, GB-34 Yanglingquan and SP-6 Sanyinjiao.

Technique: Apply the reducing method and retain the needles for 30 minutes after obtaining Qi. During this period, manipulate the needles three to five times. Treat once a day. A course consists of ten treatment sessions.

Explanation
- PC-6 Neiguan, LI-11 Quchi and TB-5 Waiguan drain Fire, clear Heat and relieve Toxicity.
- ST-36 Zusanli, GB-34 Yanglingquan and SP-6 Sanyinjiao clear Heat, eliminate Dampness and relieve Toxicity.

EAR ACUPUNCTURE
Points: Spleen, Heart, Ear-Shenmen, Adrenal Gland, and Finger (or Toe).
Technique: Retain the needles for 30 minutes. During this period, manipulate the needles three to five times. Treat once every other day. A course consists of seven treatment sessions.

Clinical notes

- In treating this disease, TCM focuses on the Spleen.

At the initial stage, the main cause is Damp-Heat transforming into Toxins. The treatment principle should be based on draining Fire with cold and bitterness. If the disease persists, this indicates binding of Dampness and Heat with Dampness predominating. The treatment principle should be based on clearing Heat and transforming Dampness. It is also important to add channel conductors for lesions at the extremities of the limbs.

- Treat promptly so that lesions will dry up and form crusts as quickly as possible.
- This disease tends to recur, and it is therefore necessary to continue with the medication for two to three months to consolidate the cure.

Advice for the patient

- Keep the affected area clean, dry and free from infection.
- Follow a light diet, rich in nutrition (such as soybean products).
- Do not break pustules by pricking or use force to remove crusts.

Literature excerpt

In *Wai Ke Mi Lu* [Secret Records of External Diseases], it says: "Skin sores on the toes are extremely difficult to treat. The Spleen governs the four limbs; this means that, although the sores appear next to the twelve Jing-Well points, it is not correct to treat the local area only, since these sores have their origin in Damp-Heat in the Spleen. In summer, Damp-Heat is dominant and everything erodes easily. In treating this disease, the focus should be placed on transforming Damp-Heat. At the same time, treatment of the Stomach should not be neglected since the Spleen and Stomach are closely related to each other."

Erythroderma (exfoliative dermatitis)
红皮病(剥脱性皮炎)

This is an acute and possibly life-threatening skin disease characterized by generalized diffuse reddening of the skin and recurrent large patches of desquamation. The white, silvery or light brown desquamation can be bran-like or scaly and dry or oily.

Erythroderma is a secondary process of skin reaction, manifesting as the generalized spreading of a skin or systemic disease. The main causes of erythroderma include eczema (contact, seborrheic or atopic), psoriasis, lymphoma, and drug eruption.

In TCM, this disease is also known as *tuo pi chuang* (sloughing skin sore).

Clinical manifestations

- This disease has an acute onset and develops from pre-existing diseases. It is more common in men than women and mainly affects the middle-aged and elderly.
- Lesions of the skin and mucosa are of two different types:
1. The exfoliative dermatitis type has a rapid onset and is accompanied by obvious systemic symptoms. It manifests principally as generalized diffuse reddening of the skin, swelling and exudation, being particularly marked in the skin folds and the joint flexures, and is complicated by mucosal lesions such as conjunctivitis, marginal blepharitis, cheilitis, angular stomatitis, and erosion of the vulva, urethra and anus. Scaling and exfoliation may be profuse and continuous.
2. The erythrodermic type manifests principally as diffuse reddening and infiltration of the skin with relatively mild exfoliation, and severe pruritus. Scratch marks, bloody crusts, exfoliative strips, and secondary infection are also possible. There is also loss of heat and transdermal loss of fluid and protein with the potential for major systemic upset.
- Some degree of scalp and body hair loss is likely.
- Atrophy, opaqueness, pitting, longitudinal ridges, and deformity of the nail may occur.
- Two-thirds of cases have varying degrees of enlargement of the lymph nodes.
- One-third to two-thirds of cases have enlargement of the liver and/or spleen. Incidence is even higher in patients with allergic drug reactions.
- Cardiac failure and hypothermia are additional complications, especially in the elderly. Skin or respiratory infections are also possible.

Etiology and pathology

Exuberant Heart-Fire complicated by an invasion of Wind-Heat leads to transformation into Toxins. Heat Toxins gradually enter the Ying and Xue levels to consume Body Fluids, thus depriving the skin and flesh of nourishment.

Pattern identification and treatment

INTERNAL TREATMENT

QI AND XUE LEVELS BOTH ABLAZE
Pathogenic Heat in the Qi level has not yet been released, but pathogenic Heat in the Ying and Xue levels has already become exuberant. This pattern occurs in the initial and intermediate acute stages of both the erythrodermic and exfoliative dermatitis types. The skin is red, swollen and inflamed, with profuse and continuous exfoliation of scales. Accompanying symptoms and signs include raging fever, irritability and restlessness, and thirst with a desire for drinks. The tongue body is red or crimson with a yellow and slightly dry coating; the pulse is rapid.

Treatment principle
Clear Heat from the Qi Level and cool the Xue level, relieve Toxicity and transform Dampness.

Prescription
YU NÜ JIAN JIA JIAN
Jade Lady Brew, with modifications

Shi Gao ‡ (Gypsum Fibrosum) 30-60g, decocted for 30 minutes before adding the other ingredients
Chao Zhi Mu (Rhizoma Anemarrhenae Asphodeloidis, stir-fried) 10g
Chao Mu Dan Pi (Cortex Moutan Radicis, stir-fried) 10g
Chi Shao (Radix Paeoniae Rubra) 10g
Chao Huang Qin (Radix Scutellariae Baicalensis, stir-fried) 10g
Xuan Shen (Radix Scrophulariae Ningpoensis) 15g
Nan Sha Shen (Radix Adenophorae) 15g
Mai Men Dong (Radix Ophiopogonis Japonici) 15g
Sheng Di Huang (Radix Rehmanniae Glutinosae) 15g
Ban Lan Gen (Radix Isatidis seu Baphicacanthi) 12g
Di Gu Pi (Cortex Lycii Radicis) 12g
Pu Gong Ying (Herba Taraxaci cum Radice) 12g

Explanation
- *Shi Gao* ‡ (Gypsum Fibrosum) and *Chao Zhi Mu* (Rhizoma Anemarrhenae Asphodeloidis, stir-fried) clear Heat from the Qi level and reduce fever.
- *Chao Mu Dan Pi* (Cortex Moutan Radicis, stir-fried), *Chi Shao* (Radix Paeoniae Rubra) and *Sheng Di Huang* (Radix Rehmanniae Glutinosae) cool the Blood and reduce erythema.
- *Nan Sha Shen* (Radix Adenophorae), *Xuan Shen* (Radix Scrophulariae Ningpoensis), *Mai Men Dong* (Radix Ophiopogonis Japonici), and *Di Gu Pi* (Cortex Lycii Radicis) nourish Yin and clear Heat.
- *Ban Lan Gen* (Radix Isatidis seu Baphicacanthi), *Pu Gong Ying* (Herba Taraxaci cum Radice) and *Chao Huang Qin* (Radix Scutellariae Baicalensis, stir-fried) drain Fire and relieve Toxicity.

HEAT SCORCHING THE YING AND XUE LEVELS
This pattern occurs in the later acute stage of both the erythrodermic and exfoliative dermatitis types. The skin is

inflamed or dark red with ecchymosis (occasionally cyanotic) and exfoliation of bran-like scale. In severe cases, hair loss or nail deformity may occur. Accompanying symptoms and signs include fever, dry mouth and lips, and possibly mental confusion and delirium due to Heat entering the Pericardium. The tongue body is red with a scant coating or no coating; the pulse is thready and rapid.

Treatment principle
Clear Heat from the Ying level and cool the Xue level, relieve Toxicity and protect Yin.

Prescription
QING YING TANG JIA JIAN
Decoction for Clearing Heat from the Ying level, with modifications

Shui Niu Jiao‡ (Cornu Bubali) 15-30g, decocted for 30 minutes before adding the other ingredients
Xian Di Huang (Radix Rehmanniae Glutinosae Recens) 30-45g
Xian Bai Mao Gen (Rhizoma Imperatae Cylindricae Recens) 30-45g
Shi Gao‡ (Gypsum Fibrosum) 30-45g, decocted for 30 minutes before adding the other ingredients
Mai Men Dong (Radix Ophiopogonis Japonici) 12g
Tian Men Dong (Radix Asparagi Cochinchinensis) 12g
Jin Yin Hua (Flos Lonicerae) 12g
Xuan Shen (Radix Scrophulariae Ningpoensis) 12g
Lü Dou Yi (Testa Phaseoli Radiati) 15g
Chao Mu Dan Pi (Cortex Moutan Radicis, stir-fried) 10g
Zi Cao (Radix Arnebiae seu Lithospermi) 10g
Hong Hua (Flos Carthami Tinctorii) 10g
Shan Yao (Radix Dioscoreae Oppositae) 30g

Explanation
- *Shi Gao*‡ (Gypsum Fibrosum), *Shan Yao* (Radix Dioscoreae Oppositae) and *Xian Bai Mao Gen* (Rhizoma Imperatae Cylindricae Recens) clear Heat from the Qi level and reduce fever.
- *Mai Men Dong* (Radix Ophiopogonis Japonici), *Tian Men Dong* (Radix Asparagi Cochinchinensis), *Xuan Shen* (Radix Scrophulariae Ningpoensis), and *Xian Di Huang* (Radix Rehmanniae Glutinosae Recens) enrich Yin and protect Body Fluids.
- *Jin Yin Hua* (Flos Lonicerae), *Lü Dou Yi* (Testa Phaseoli Radiati) and *Shui Niu Jiao*‡ (Cornu Bubali) clear Heat from the Ying level and relieve Toxicity.
- *Chao Mu Dan Pi* (Cortex Moutan Radicis, stir-fried), *Zi Cao* (Radix Arnebiae seu Lithospermi) and *Hong Hua* (Flos Carthami Tinctorii) cool the Blood and relieve Toxicity.

DEPLETION OF QI AND BLOOD
This pattern is seen in the recovery phase of both types with depletion of Qi and Blood. It manifests as dry, pale red skin, with exposure of red, tender flesh after peeling of the skin, particularly in the hands and feet. Accompanying symptoms and signs include thirst, dry eyes, itching, and constipation. The tongue body is red with a scant coating; the pulse is deficient and thready.

Treatment principle
Augment Qi and nourish Yin, support Vital Qi (Zheng Qi) and fortify the Spleen.

Prescription
ZI ZAO YANG RONG TANG JIA JIAN
Decoction for Enriching Dryness and Nourishing the Ying Level, with modifications

Dang Gui (Radix Angelicae Sinensis) 10g
Huang Qi (Radix Astragali seu Hedysari) 10g
Sheng Di Huang (Radix Rehmanniae Glutinosae) 10g
Shu Di Huang (Radix Rehmanniae Glutinosae Conquita) 10g
Chao Bai Shao (Radix Paeoniae Lactiflorae, stir-fried) 12g
Mai Men Dong (Radix Ophiopogonis Japonici) 12g
Nan Sha Shen (Radix Adenophorae) 12g
Xuan Shen (Radix Scrophulariae Ningpoensis) 12g
Fu Ling (Sclerotium Poriae Cocos) 6g
Gan Cao (Radix Glycyrrhizae) 6g
Bai Zhu (Rhizoma Atractylodis Macrocephalae) 6g
Tian Men Dong (Radix Asparagi Cochinchinensis) 15g
*Shi Hu** (Herba Dendrobii) 15g
Shan Yao (Radix Dioscoreae Oppositae) 30g

Explanation
- *Huang Qi* (Radix Astragali seu Hedysari), *Nan Sha Shen* (Radix Adenophorae), *Mai Men Dong* (Radix Ophiopogonis Japonici), *Tian Men Dong* (Radix Asparagi Cochinchinensis), *Xuan Shen* (Radix Scrophulariae Ningpoensis), and *Shi Hu** (Herba Dendrobii) augment Qi and nourish Yin.
- *Sheng Di Huang* (Radix Rehmanniae Glutinosae), *Shu Di Huang* (Radix Rehmanniae Glutinosae Conquita), *Chao Bai Shao* (Radix Paeoniae Lactiflorae, stir-fried), and *Dang Gui* (Radix Angelicae Sinensis) nourish the Blood and moisten Dryness.
- *Fu Ling* (Sclerotium Poriae Cocos), *Shan Yao* (Radix Dioscoreae Oppositae), *Bai Zhu* (Rhizoma Atractylodis Macrocephalae), and *Gan Cao* (Radix Glycyrrhizae) support the Spleen with warmth and sweetness, consolidate the Root and ward off pathogenic factors.

General modifications
1. For constipation, add *Da Huang* (Radix et Rhizoma Rhei), 5 minutes before the end of the decoction process, *Huo Ma Ren* (Semen Cannabis Sativae) and *Yu Li Ren* (Semen Pruni).

2. For severe pruritus, add *Bai Xian Pi* (Cortex Dictamni Dasycarpi Radicis), *Ku Shen* (Radix Sophorae Flavescentis) and *Gou Teng* (Ramulus Uncariae cum Uncis).

3. For hyperactivity of Heat Toxins, add *Huang Lian* (Rhizoma Coptidis) and *Huang Bai* (Cortex Phellodendri).

4. For damage to Yin and consumption of Body Fluids, add *Shi Hu** (Herba Dendrobii), *Yu Zhu* (Rhizoma Polygonati Odorati) and *Tian Hua Fen* (Radix Trichosanthis).

5. For high fever with delirium or Heat Toxins entering the interior, add *Ren Gong Niu Huang Fen* ‡ (Calculus Bovis Syntheticus, powdered), taken separately.

6. For rapid breathing with cough, add *Yu Xing Cao* (Herba Houttuyniae Cordatae), *Bai Mao Gen* (Rhizoma Imperatae Cylindricae), *Zhu Li* (Succus Bambusae), and *Fa Ban Xia* (Rhizoma Pinelliae Ternatae Praeparata).

7. Where the condition is caused by eczema, add *Long Dan Cao* (Radix Gentianae Scabrae), *Tong Cao* (Medulla Tetrapanacis Papyriferi), *Che Qian Zi* (Semen Plantaginis), and *Ze Xie* (Rhizoma Alismatis Orientalis) in the acute stage, and add *Chen Pi* (Pericarpium Citri Reticulatae), *Chao Bai Zhu* (Rhizoma Atractylodis Macrocephalae, stir-fried), *Fu Ling* (Sclerotium Poriae Cocos), and *Shan Yao* (Rhizoma Dioscoreae Oppositae) in the recovery phase.

8. Where the condition is caused by psoriasis or pityriasis rubra pilaris add *Tu Fu Ling* (Rhizoma Smilacis Glabrae) and *Chong Lou* (Rhizoma Paridis).

EMPIRICAL FORMULAE

ACCUMULATION OF HEAT TOXINS

Prescription
HUA BAN JIE DU TANG JIA JIAN
Decoction for Transforming Erythema and Relieving Toxicity, with modifications

Shi Gao ‡ (Gypsum Fibrosum) 15-30g, decocted for 30 minutes before adding the other ingredients
Zhi Mu (Rhizoma Anemarrhenae Asphodeloidis) 10g
Xuan Shen (Radix Scrophulariae Ningpoensis) 10g
Lian Qiao (Fructus Forsythiae Suspensae) 10g
Zi Cao (Radix Arnebiae seu Lithospermi) 10g
Sheng Ma (Rhizoma Cimicifugae) 6g
Huang Qin (Radix Scutellariae Baicalensis) 6g
Niu Bang Zi (Fructus Arctii Lappae) 12g
Da Qing Ye (Folium Isatidis seu Baphicacanthi) 12g
Gan Cao (Radix Glycyrrhizae) 3g

HEAT TOXINS COMPLICATED BY DAMPNESS

Prescription
QING WEN BAI DU YIN JIA JIAN
Beverage for Clearing Scourge and Vanquishing Toxicity, with modifications

Shi Gao ‡ (Gypsum Fibrosum) 15-30g, decocted for 30 minutes before adding the other ingredients
Zhi Mu (Rhizoma Anemarrhenae Asphodeloidis) 6g
Huang Qin (Radix Scutellariae Baicalensis) 6g
Zhi Zi (Fructus Gardeniae Jasminoidis) 6g
Sheng Di Huang (Radix Rehmanniae Glutinosae) 10g
Chi Shao (Radix Paeoniae Rubra) 10g
Jin Yin Hua (Flos Lonicerae) 10g
Yin Chen Hao (Herba Artemisiae Scopariae) 10g
Zhu Ling (Sclerotium Polypori Umbellati) 10g
Fu Ling (Sclerotium Poriae Cocos) 10g
Da Huang (Radix et Rhizoma Rhei) 3g
Gan Cao (Radix Glycyrrhizae) 3g

SEVERE HEAT DAMAGING YIN

Prescription
ZENG YE TANG JIA JIAN
Decoction for Increasing Body Fluids, with modifications

Xian Di Huang (Radix Rehmanniae Glutinosae Recens) 15g
Xuan Shen (Radix Scrophulariae Ningpoensis) 10g
Mai Men Dong (Radix Ophiopogonis Japonici) 10g
*Shi Hu** (Herba Dendrobii) 10g
Zhi Mu (Rhizoma Anemarrhenae Asphodeloidis) 6g
Tian Hua Fen (Radix Trichosanthis) 6g
Shi Gao ‡ (Gypsum Fibrosum) 15-30g, decocted for 30 minutes before adding the other ingredients
Gan Cao (Radix Glycyrrhizae) 3g

INITIAL STAGE

Prescription
JIE DU LIANG XUE TANG JIA JIAN
Decoction for Relieving Toxicity and Cooling the Blood, with modifications

Shui Niu Jiao ‡ (Cornu Bubali) 15-30g, decocted for 30 minutes before adding the other ingredients
Sheng Di Huang Tan (Radix Rehmanniae Glutinosae Carbonisata) 15g
Jin Yin Hua Tan (Flos Lonicerae Carbonisata) 15g
Lian Zi Xin (Plumula Nelumbinis Nuciferae) 6g
Bai Mao Gen (Rhizoma Imperatae Cylindricae) 30g
Tian Hua Fen (Radix Trichosanthis) 10g
Zi Hua Di Ding (Herba Violae Yedoensitis) 10g
Zhi Zi (Fructus Gardeniae Jasminoidis) 10g
Chong Lou (Rhizoma Paridis) 10g

Gan Cao (Radix Glycyrrhizae) 10g

Huang Lian (Rhizoma Coptidis) 6g

Shi Gao‡ (Gypsum Fibrosum) 15g, decocted for 30 minutes before adding the other ingredients

RECOVERY STAGE

Prescription
JIE DU YANG YIN TANG JIA JIAN
Decoction for Relieving Toxicity and Nourishing Yin, with modifications

Xi Yang Shen* (Radix Panacis Quinquefolii) 10g

Nan Sha Shen (Radix Adenophorae) 12g

Bei Sha Shen (Radix Glehniae Littoralis) 12g

Shi Hu* (Herba Dendrobii) 12g

Xuan Shen (Radix Scrophulariae Ningpoensis) 12g

Fo Shou (Fructus Citri Sarcodactylis) 10g

Huang Qi (Radix Astragali seu Hedysari) 10g

Gan Di Huang (Rhizoma Rehmanniae Glutinosae Exsiccata) 15g

Dan Shen (Radix Salviae Miltiorrhizae) 12g

Jin Yin Hua (Flos Lonicerae) 12g

Tian Men Dong (Radix Asparagi Cochinchinensis) 12g

Mai Men Dong (Radix Ophiopogonis Japonici) 12g

Yu Zhu (Rhizoma Polygonati Odorati) 12g

Pu Gong Ying (Herba Taraxaci cum Radice) 12g

EXTERNAL TREATMENT
- For itching in the early stages of the disease, apply *San Shi Shui* (Three Stones Lotion) two or three times a day.
- For dry and reddened skin with desquamation, apply *Gan Cao You* (Licorice Oil) or *Zi Cao You* (Gromwell Root Oil).
- For damp exudation, use *Qing Dai San* (Indigo Powder) mixed with vegetable oil.

Clinical notes

- Treatment of this disease requires hospitalization. Experience in China suggests that treatment results are improved when a combination of TCM and Western medicine is employed. Prompt administration of an appropriate quantity of topical steroids (and systemic steroids in severe cases) and provision of supportive treatment (maintenance of a warm room temperature and monitoring of bodily functions) is important.
- At the initial stage, TCM treatment should be based on the principle of clearing Heat from the Qi level and cooling the Xue level with the focus on the Lungs and Stomach; in the later stages, it should be based on the principle of nourishing Yin and moistening Dryness with the focus on the Liver and Kidneys.
- If the condition is critical, treat as for conditions with pathogenic Heat transmitted to the Pericardium.

Advice for the patient/carer

- Patients should be kept in separate rooms in order to prevent cross-infection.
- Disinfect the room and bedding regularly and keep the patient warm.
- Pay attention to oral hygiene and keep the lesions clean in order to prevent infection.

Literature excerpt

In *Xu Lü He Wai Ke Yi An Yi Hua Ji* [A Collection of Xu Lühe's Medical Records on External Diseases], the author explains: "Since this disease appears suddenly and develops rapidly, it is necessary to use large dosages of ingredients to clear Heat and relieve Toxicity in order to bring it under control. I often use *Huang Lian Jie Du Tang* (Coptis Decoction for Relieving Toxicity) with the addition of *Jin Yin Hua* (Flos Lonicerae), *Lian Qiao* (Fructus Forsythiae Suspensae), *Liu Yi San* (Six-To-One Powder), *Xian Di Huang* (Radix Rehmanniae Glutinosae Recens), *Mu Dan Pi* (Cortex Moutan Radicis), *Ye Ju Hua* (Flos Chrysanthemi Indici), and *Lü Dou Yi* (Testa Phaseoli Radiati). For severe itching, add *Di Fu Zi* (Fructus Kochiae Scopariae) and *Bai Xian Pi* (Cortex Dictamni Dasycarpi Radicis); for a crimson tongue body, add *Shui Niu Jiao*‡ (Cornu Bubali) and *Xuan Shen* (Radix Scrophulariae Ningpoensis); for exuberant Heat Toxins, add *Zi Cao* (Radix Arnebiae seu Lithospermi) and *Da Qing Ye* (Folium Isatidis seu Baphicacanthi); for a yellow facial complexion, add *Yin Chen Hao* (Herba Artemisiae Scopariae); for inhibited urination, add *Che Qian Zi* (Semen Plantaginis) and *Hua Shi*‡ (Talcum); for purulent infection, add *Zi Hua Di Ding* (Herba Violae Yedoensitis) and *Ban Bian Lian* (Herba Lobeliae Chinensis cum Radice); and for damage to Body Fluids, add *Xi Yang Shen** (Radix Panacis Quinquefolii), *Mai Men Dong* (Radix Ophiopogonis Japonici) and *Shi Hu** (Herba Dendrobii)."

Pityriasis rosea
玫瑰糠疹

Pityriasis rosea is a common, benign, self-limited, inflammatory skin disease of unknown etiology. It is often preceded by the appearance of a herald patch – a single, red, oval or round plaque measuring from 2 to 10 cm – followed by a number of similar, smaller plaques.

In TCM, pityriasis rosea is also known as *feng re chuang* (Wind-Heat sore).

Clinical manifestations

- Pityriasis rosea usually involves the trunk and proximal extremities.
- It tends to affect children and young adults, occurring principally in colder weather.
- Skin lesions generally manifest initially in the axillary region or the lower abdomen as a herald patch, followed after one or two weeks by clusters of oval plaques appearing on the trunk and other regions, most commonly on the lower abdomen.
- Lesions commence as pale red, yellowish-brown or reddish-brown oval plaques, gradually turning rosy. Individuals with pigmented skin may exhibit hyperpigmented lesions. The plaques have a discrete distribution and are covered by a thin layer of bran-like scales. A fine scale often remains within the border of the plaque, resulting in a characteristic "collarette" ring of scale.
- The longitudinal axis of the plaques tends to be oriented along the skin lines (along the lines of the ribs for lesions on the chest and back).
- Itching of varying intensity is often an accompanying symptom.
- The disease usually clears spontaneously within one to two months.
- Recurrence is rare.

Differential diagnosis

Tinea corporis
The herald patch of pityriasis rosea is sometimes confused with tinea corporis, where lesions manifest as circular, semicircular or concentric patches with distinct borders. The central area heals as the lesions spread outward; the advancing border may have papules or vesicles. Thin, fine scaling may sometimes be noted.

Itching may be a prominent feature. The condition is exacerbated in summer and alleviated in winter.

Pityriasis versicolor
Lesions start with multiple small macules, which soon enlarge to round or oval patches covered by a layer of fine scaling. Lesions may be pale white, pale red, yellowish-brown, or dark brown, tending to be paler in dark or tanned skin and darker in untanned skin. This condition occurs mainly in adults (generally young adults) in summer or in hot and humid climates. Itching is usually slight.

Guttate psoriasis
This disease occurs most frequently in adolescents and young adults and is characterized by the sudden onset on the trunk or limbs of numerous uniform, small, round, symmetrically distributed plaques, which resemble drops of wax on the skin. Lesions become larger after the acute phase and the disease may develop into chronic plaque psoriasis.

Etiology and pathology

- The main factors are Blood-Heat accumulating internally and external contraction of Wind-Heat. When these internal and external pathogenic factors combine, they are retained in the skin and flesh, obstructing the interstices (*cou li*) and causing the disease. If Heat overflows in the channels and network vessels, erythema results; if Wind leads to Blood-Dryness, the skin and flesh are undernourished, and scaling results; if Wind flows backward and forward between the skin and interstices (*cou li*), itching results.
- Externally-contracted Wind-Heat or sweating at a time when there is an invasion of Wind leads to retention of these external pathogenic factors in the skin and flesh, thus blocking the interstices (*cou li*). If the pathogenic factors are not dissipated, they will transform into Heat, which consumes Yin and Blood. The skin is therefore deprived of nourishment and moisture.
- Intake of too much sweet, fatty, spicy, or fried food, or irritability and restlessness and disorders of the five emotions can lead to Blood-Heat accumulating internally. If this is complicated by an invasion of external Wind, Wind and Heat will fight, thus giving rise to the disease.

- Insufficiency of Lung Yin and impairment of the transformation of Qi results in the Body Fluids not being disseminated correctly to nourish the skin and flesh. This additionally leads to the internal generation of Yin-Fire (depletion of Yin giving rise to hyperactivity of Deficiency-Fire) with Spleen-Damp and Lung-Dryness, thus also depriving the skin of nourishment. As a consequence, the skin becomes itchy and scaling is profuse.

Pattern identification and treatment

INTERNAL TREATMENT

WIND-HEAT

This pattern is marked by acute onset with eruptions involving the trunk and upper limbs; the herald patch is mostly located in the axillary or hypochondriac regions. This is followed by the appearance of a few to numerous large, pale red or bright red, round or oval papules that tend to coalesce into plaques. The surface is usually covered by bran-like scales. Itching is moderate to severe. Accompanying symptoms and signs prior to and after appearance of the eruptions include slight fever, sore throat, a slight cough, and thirst with a desire for drinks. The tongue body is slightly red with a thin yellow coating or a scant coating; the pulse is floating and rapid.

Treatment principle
Dredge Wind and clear Heat.

Prescription
YIN QIAO SAN JIA JIAN
Honeysuckle and Forsythia Powder, with modifications

Jin Yin Hua (Flos Lonicerae) 15g
Lü Dou Yi (Testa Phaseoli Radiati) 15g
Chao Niu Bang Zi (Fructus Arctii Lappae, stir-fried) 6g
Jie Geng (Radix Platycodi Grandiflori) 6g
Jing Jie (Herba Schizonepetae Tenuifoliae) 6g
Fang Feng (Radix Ledebouriellae Divaricatae) 6g
Gan Cao (Radix Glycyrrhizae) 6g
Sheng Di Huang (Radix Rehmanniae Glutinosae) 10g
Chao Mu Dan Pi (Cortex Moutan Radicis, stir-fried) 10g
Lian Qiao (Fructus Forsythiae Suspensae) 10g
Da Qing Ye (Folium Isatidis seu Baphicacanthi) 10g
Nan Sha Shen (Radix Adenophorae) 12g

Explanation
- *Jing Jie* (Herba Schizonepetae Tenuifoliae), *Fang Feng* (Radix Ledebouriellae Divaricatae), *Jie Geng* (Radix Platycodi Grandiflori), and *Chao Niu Bang Zi* (Fructus Arctii Lappae, stir-fried) dredge Wind and alleviate itching.

- *Sheng Di Huang* (Radix Rehmanniae Glutinosae) and *Chao Mu Dan Pi* (Cortex Moutan Radicis, stir-fried) cool the Blood and reduce erythema.
- *Jin Yin Hua* (Flos Lonicerae), *Lü Dou Yi* (Testa Phaseoli Radiati), *Lian Qiao* (Fructus Forsythiae Suspensae), and *Da Qing Ye* (Folium Isatidis seu Baphicacanthi) clear Heat and relieve Toxicity.
- *Nan Sha Shen* (Radix Adenophorae) and *Gan Cao* (Radix Glycyrrhizae) enrich Yin and moisten Dryness.

BLOOD-HEAT

This is a pattern of short duration. Skin eruptions mainly involve the trunk, particularly the chest and abdomen. Lesions manifest as red, round or oval papular patches, usually 2-5 cm in diameter and rarely larger. The color becomes deeper on contact with warmth or in the afternoon. A ring of fine, tissue paper-like scale ("collarette" scale) is evident in the center of the patches. Patients may experience a sensation of slight itching or occasional short bursts of stabbing pain. Accompanying symptoms and signs include impatience, restlessness, irritability, a quick temper, difficulty in getting to sleep, and short voidings of yellow urine. The tongue body is red with a scant coating; the pulse is thready and rapid.

Treatment principle
Cool the Blood and disperse Wind.

Prescription
LIANG XUE XIAO FENG SAN JIA JIAN
Powder for Cooling the Blood and Dispersing Wind, with modifications

Sheng Di Huang (Radix Rehmanniae Glutinosae) 18g
Zi Cao (Radix Arnebiae seu Lithospermi) 12g
Chao Huai Hua (Flos Sophorae Japonicae, stir-fried) 12g
Chao Mu Dan Pi (Cortex Moutan Radicis, stir-fried) 10g
Chi Shao (Radix Paeoniae Rubra) 10g
Qian Cao Gen (Radix Rubiae Cordifoliae) 10g
Huang Qin (Radix Scutellariae Baicalensis) 10g
Jiao Zhi Zi (Fructus Gardeniae Jasminoidis, scorch-fried) 6g
Jing Jie Tan (Herba Schizonepetae Tenuifoliae Carbonisata) 6g
Fang Feng (Radix Ledebouriellae Divaricatae) 6g
Sang Bai Pi (Cortex Mori Albae Radicis) 6g
Hong Hua (Flos Carthami Tinctorii) 6g
Ling Xiao Hua (Flos Campsitis) 6g

Explanation
- *Sheng Di Huang* (Radix Rehmanniae Glutinosae), *Chao Mu Dan Pi* (Cortex Moutan Radicis, stir-fried), *Chi Shao* (Radix Paeoniae Rubra), *Hong Hua* (Flos Carthami Tinctorii), and *Ling Xiao Hua* (Flos Campsitis) cool the Blood and reduce erythema.

- *Chao Huai Hua* (Flos Sophorae Japonicae, stir-fried), *Zi Cao* (Radix Arnebiae seu Lithospermi), *Qian Cao Gen* (Radix Rubiae Cordifoliae), and *Huang Qin* (Radix Scutellariae Baicalensis) cool the Blood and relieve Toxicity.
- *Jing Jie Tan* (Herba Schizonepetae Tenuifoliae Carbonisata), *Fang Feng* (Radix Ledebouriellae Divaricatae), *Jiao Zhi Zi* (Fructus Gardeniae Jasminoidis, scorch-fried), and *Sang Bai Pi* (Cortex Mori Albae Radicis) drain the Lungs and clear Heat, dissipate Wind and alleviate itching.

BLOOD-DRYNESS

This pattern is usually of longer duration and is more difficult to treat. Skin lesions mainly involve the lower abdomen, lumbosacral region and thighs, manifesting as brown or pale brown, round or oval papules with irregular margins, covered by relatively large amounts of fine bran-like scales. The skin is dry with occasional slight lichenification; scant exudate and mild erosion may be present. Itching is severe. Accompanying symptoms and signs include a slightly dry and sore throat, poor appetite, a sensation of distension and discomfort in the epigastrium and abdomen, dry mouth with little desire for drinks, and inhibited voidings of reddish urine. The tongue body is red with a scant coating or no coating; the pulse is thready and rapid.

Treatment principle
Enrich Yin and moisten Dryness.

Prescription
ZI YIN CHU SHI TANG JIA JIAN
Decoction for Enriching Yin and Eliminating Dampness, with modifications

Nan Sha Shen (Radix Adenophorae) 30g
Bei Sha Shen (Radix Glehniae Littoralis) 30g
Xuan Shen (Radix Scrophulariae Ningpoensis) 12g
*Shi Hu** (Herba Dendrobii) 12g
Yi Yi Ren (Semen Coicis Lachryma-jobi) 12g
Bai Zhu (Rhizoma Atractylodis Macrocephalae) 12g
Dang Gui (Radix Angelicae Sinensis) 10g
Ze Xie (Rhizoma Alismatis Orientalis) 10g
Chao Bai Shao (Radix Paeoniae Lactiflorae, stir-fried) 10g
Dan Shen (Radix Salviae Miltiorrhizae) 10g
Bai Xian Pi (Cortex Dictamni Dasycarpi Radicis) 15g
Sheng Di Huang (Radix Rehmanniae Glutinosae) 15g
Gan Cao (Radix Glycyrrhizae) 6g

Explanation
- *Nan Sha Shen* (Radix Adenophorae), *Bei Sha Shen* (Radix Glehniae Littoralis), *Xuan Shen* (Radix Scrophulariae Ningpoensis), and *Shi Hu** (Herba Dendrobii) enrich Yin and moisten Dryness.

- *Yi Yi Ren* (Semen Coicis Lachryma-jobi), *Bai Zhu* (Rhizoma Atractylodis Macrocephalae), *Ze Xie* (Rhizoma Alismatis Orientalis), and *Gan Cao* (Radix Glycyrrhizae) fortify the Spleen and transform Dampness.
- *Dang Gui* (Radix Angelicae Sinensis), *Chao Bai Shao* (Radix Paeoniae Lactiflorae, stir-fried), *Sheng Di Huang* (Radix Rehmanniae Glutinosae), and *Dan Shen* (Radix Salviae Miltiorrhizae) nourish and invigorate the Blood.
- *Bai Xian Pi* (Cortex Dictamni Dasycarpi Radicis) relieves Toxicity and alleviates itching.

General modifications
1. For eruptions on the lower abdomen and the medial aspect of the thighs, add *Chao Du Zhong* (Cortex Eucommiae Ulmoidis, stir-fried), *Sang Ji Sheng* (Ramulus Loranthi) and *Yi Yi Ren* (Semen Coicis Lachryma-jobi).
2. For eruptions in the axillary and hypochondriac regions, add *Chai Hu* (Radix Bupleuri) and *Qing Hao* (Herba Artemisiae Chinghao).
3. For constipation, add *Chao Zhi Ke* (Fructus Citri Aurantii, stir-fried), *Da Huang* (Radix et Rhizoma Rhei), *Huo Ma Ren* (Semen Cannabis Sativae), and *Jie Geng* (Radix Platycodi Grandiflori).
4. For loose stools, add *Shan Yao* (Radix Dioscoreae Oppositae) and *Cang Zhu* (Rhizoma Atractylodis).
5. For severe pruritus, add *Gou Teng* (Ramulus Uncariae cum Uncis), *Di Fu Zi* (Fructus Kochiae Scopariae) and *Ku Shen* (Radix Sophorae Flavescentis).
6. For attacks lasting more than 4-6 weeks, add *Chao Huai Hua* (Flos Sophorae Japonicae, stir-fried), *Yi Mu Cao* (Herba Leonuri Heterophylli), *Chi Xiao Dou* (Semen Phaseoli Calcarati), and *Dan Shen* (Radix Salviae Miltiorrhizae).

EXTERNAL TREATMENT
- For generalized lesions with confluent erythema and papules, apply one of *San Huang Xi Ji* (Three Yellows Wash Preparation), *San Shi Shui* (Three Stones Lotion) or 5-10% *Liu Huang Ruan Gao* (Sulfur Ointment) once or twice a day.
- For generalized lesions with slight or severe itching, apply *Qing Liang Fen* (Cool Clearing Powder) to the affected area two or three times a day.

ACUPUNCTURE

Selection of points on the affected channels
Main points: LI-4 Hegu, GB-20 Fengchi and SP-10 Xuehai.
Auxiliary points: GV-14 Dazhui, LI-11 Quchi and ST-36 Zusanli.

Technique: Apply the reducing method for bright red eruptions and the reinforcing method for pale red eruptions. Retain the needles for 30 minutes after obtaining Qi. Treat once a day. A course consists of ten treatment sessions.

Empirical points
Points: TB-13 Naohui, SI-16 Tianchuang and BL-21 Weishu (all bilateral).
Technique: Apply the even method and retain the needles for 15 minutes after obtaining Qi. Treat once a day. A course consists of ten treatment sessions.

Explanation
- SI-16 Tianchuang, LI-4 Hegu and GB-20 Fengchi dissipate Wind and alleviate itching.
- GV-14 Dazhui and LI-11 Quchi eliminate Wind and clear Heat.
- SP-10 Xuehai and TB-13 Naohui nourish the Blood and moisten the skin, cool the Blood and reduce erythema.
- ST-36 Zusanli and BL-21 Weishu fortify the Spleen and transform Dampness.

EAR ACUPUNCTURE
Points: Lung, Heart, Liver, and Subcortex.
Technique: Retain the needles for 30 minutes. Treat once every two days. A course consists of ten treatment sessions.

PRICKING TO BLEED COMBINED WITH CUPPING THERAPY
Point: GV-14 Dazhui.
Technique: Prick the point with a three-edged needle and then use fire-cupping for three to five minutes so that a small amount of blood appears. Treat once every three days. A course consists of five treatment sessions.

Clinical notes

This disease should either be treated according to the principle of dredging Wind and releasing the exterior or cooling the Blood and reducing erythema. *Zi Cao* (Radix Arnebiae seu Lithospermi) is a particularly useful herb in this respect (see also Modern clinical experience).

Advice for the patient

- Avoid eating spicy or other irritating food or applying strongly-irritant medication such as coal tar or turpentine oil on the lesions during an attack.
- In spring and autumn, keep out of draughts after a shower or bath and avoid sweating, thus preventing the body being invaded by Wind-Heat. Reduce the frequency of hot showers or baths during an attack.

Literature excerpt

In *Dong Tian Ao Zhi (Wai Ke Mi Lu)* [Secret Records of External Diseases], it says: "*Feng re chuang* (Wind-Heat sores) often occur on the limbs, chest and hypochondrium. Initially they manifest as intolerably itchy pimples; itching is often temporarily relieved by scratching. However, prolonged scratching may result in ulceration or bleeding. The disease is caused by the conflict between internal Heat in the Lung channel and externally-contracted Wind-Heat; Wind and Heat stimulate each other in the skin and hair to cause the disease. Some doctors prescribe *Fang Feng Tong Sheng San* (Ledebouriella Powder that Sagely Unblocks), but others prefer external applications."

Modern clinical experience

1. **Zhao** decocted *Zi Cao* (Radix Arnebiae seu Lithospermi) 30g and *Gan Cao* (Radix Glycyrrhizae) 30g in 250ml of water until there was 200ml of liquid left, taken twice a day in 100ml portions. The residue of the decoction was used to rub the affected areas gently. In most cases, results were seen after ten days of treatment. [24]

2. **Ma** treated pityriasis rosea with *Liang Xue Xiao Ban Tang* (Decoction for Cooling the Blood and Dispersing Erythema). [25]

Prescription ingredients
Sheng Di Huang (Radix Rehmanniae Glutinosae) 15g
Huai Hua (Flos Sophorae Japonicae) 15g
Zi Cao (Radix Arnebiae seu Lithospermi) 15g
Bai Xian Pi (Cortex Dictamni Dasycarpi Radicis) 15g
Chi Shao (Radix Paeoniae Rubra) 10g
Mu Dan Pi (Cortex Moutan Radicis) 10g
Di Fu Zi (Fructus Kochiae Scopariae) 10g
Fang Feng (Radix Ledebouriellae Divaricatae) 10g
Bai Ji Li (Fructus Tribuli Terrestris) 10g
Bai Mao Gen (Rhizoma Imperatae Cylindricae) 20g
Gan Cao (Radix Glycyrrhizae) 6g

Modifications
1. For severe itching, *Ku Shen* (Radix Sophorae Flavescentis) and *Chan Tui*‡ (Periostracum Cicadae) were added.
2. For irritability and thirst, *Dan Shen* (Radix Salviae Miltiorrhizae) and *Tian Hua Fen* (Radix Trichosanthis) were added.

3. For a prolonged attack, *Ji Xue Teng* (Caulis Spatholobi) and *Ye Jiao Teng* (Caulis Polygoni Multiflori) were added.

One bag a day was used to prepare a decoction, taken twice a day for four weeks.

Pityriasis alba
白色糠疹

Pityriasis alba (previously known as pityriasis simplex) often occurs on the faces of children and young adults, particularly those who are atopic. Skin lesions present as dry, superficial, desquamative, hypopigmented macules or patches.

In TCM, this disease is also known as *chui hua xuan* (blown blossom tinea).

Clinical manifestations

• Pityriasis alba is more common in spring, but becomes most obvious in summer when the affected skin does not tan.

• Incidence is higher among children; the condition usually resolves by early adulthood.

• The disease generally involves the face, particularly the area around the mouth, and the chin, cheeks and forehead. Less commonly, pityriasis alba affects other locations, such as the neck, shoulder, upper arm, or thigh.

• Lesions usually manifest as white or pale pink patches of varying size (generally up to 2cm in diameter, although they may be larger, especially on the trunk) and with indistinct borders. Their surface is usually covered by fine dry scales.

• Slight itching may occur with very dry lesions.

Differential diagnosis

Vitiligo
Vitiligo is more common in adolescents and young adults and less likely in children. Lesions manifest as circumscribed depigmented patches with sharply demarcated though irregular borders and may spread throughout the body. There is no scale.

Pityriasis versicolor
Pityriasis alba on the shoulders and arms may be confused with pityriasis versicolor, where lesions start with multiple small macules, which soon enlarge to round or oval patches covered by a layer of fine scaling. Lesions may be pale white, pale red, yellowish-brown or dark brown, tending to be paler in dark or tanned skin and darker in untanned skin. Pityriasis versicolor is very rare on the face.

Etiology and pathology

• Yang Qi moves outward in spring, with Heat from the Lungs and Stomach rising to warm the face. If there is an invasion of external Wind at this time, Wind and Yang-Heat tend to fight each other and are retained in the skin and interstices (*cou li*), thus giving rise to the disease.

• Impairment of the transformation and transportation function of the Spleen due to dietary irregularities or Worm accumulation in children eventually results in binding of Damp-Heat. If these pathogenic factors ascend to the face, pityriasis alba can occur.

Pattern identification and treatment

INTERNAL TREATMENT

WIND-HEAT ATTACKING THE SKIN
Pale pink or white patches covered by bran-like scales appear on the face, sometimes accompanied by slight itching. The tongue body is red with a thin white coating; the pulse is rapid.

Treatment principle
Dredge Wind and clear Heat, harmonize the Stomach and alleviate itching.

Prescription
XIAO FENG SAN JIA JIAN
Powder for Dispersing Wind, with modifications

Jing Jie (Herba Schizonepetae Tenuifoliae) 10g
Chao Niu Bang Zi (Fructus Arctii Lappae, stir-fried) 10g
Ju Hua (Flos Chrysanthemi Morifolii) 10g

Fu Ping (Herba Spirodelae Polyrrhizae) 10g
Lian Qiao (Fructus Forsythiae Suspensae) 10g
Mu Dan Pi (Cortex Moutan Radicis) 10g
Sheng Di Huang (Radix Rehmanniae Glutinosae) 15g
Bai Mao Gen (Rhizoma Imperatae Cylindricae) 30g
Chan Tui ‡ (Periostracum Cicadae) 6g
Huang Qin (Radix Scutellariae Baicalensis) 4.5g
Jiao Zhi Zi (Fructus Gardeniae Jasminoidis, scorch-fried) 4.5g

Explanation

- *Jing Jie* (Herba Schizonepetae Tenuifoliae), *Chao Niu Bang Zi* (Fructus Arctii Lappae, stir-fried), *Ju Hua* (Flos Chrysanthemi Morifolii), *Fu Ping* (Herba Spirodelae Polyrrhizae), and *Chan Tui* ‡ (Periostracum Cicadae) clear and diffuse Lung-Heat, disperse Wind and alleviate itching.
- *Sheng Di Huang* (Radix Rehmanniae Glutinosae), *Mu Dan Pi* (Cortex Moutan Radicis) and *Bai Mao Gen* (Rhizoma Imperatae Cylindricae) cool the Blood and clear Heat.
- *Lian Qiao* (Fructus Forsythiae Suspensae), *Huang Qin* (Radix Scutellariae Baicalensis) and *Jiao Zhi Zi* (Fructus Gardeniae Jasminoidis, scorch-fried) clear residual Heat from the Heart and Lung channels.

IMPAIRMENT OF THE SPLEEN'S TRANSFORMATION AND TRANSPORTATION FUNCTION

This pattern presents as white macules on the face with white scales after scratching. Accompanying symptoms and signs include poor appetite and epigastric discomfort. The tongue body is red with a scant coating; the pulse is moderate and rapid.

Treatment principle

Fortify the Spleen, harmonize the Stomach and kill Worms.

Prescription

XIANG SHA LIU JUN ZI TANG JIA JIAN

Six Gentlemen Decoction with Aucklandia and Amomum, with modifications

*Mu Xiang** (Radix Aucklandiae Lappae) 10g
Chao Bai Zhu (Rhizoma Atractylodis Macrocephalae, stir-fried) 10g

Dang Shen (Radix Codonopsitis Pilosulae) 10g
Fu Ling (Sclerotium Poriae Cocos) 10g
Sha Ren (Fructus Amomi) 6g
Fang Feng (Radix Ledebouriellae Divaricatae) 6g
Jing Jie (Herba Schizonepetae Tenuifoliae) 6g
Shi Jun Zi (Fructus Quisqualis Indicae) 6g
*Bing Lang** (Semen Arecae Catechu) 6g
Chan Tui ‡ (Periostracum Cicadae) 4.5g

Explanation

- *Dang Shen* (Radix Codonopsitis Pilosulae), *Fu Ling* (Sclerotium Poriae Cocos), *Sha Ren* (Fructus Amomi), *Chao Bai Zhu* (Rhizoma Atractylodis Macrocephalae, stir-fried), and *Mu Xiang** (Radix Aucklandiae Lappae) support the Spleen and harmonize the Stomach.
- *Jing Jie* (Herba Schizonepetae Tenuifoliae), *Fang Feng* (Radix Ledebouriellae Divaricatae) and *Chan Tui* ‡ (Periostracum Cicadae) dredge Wind and alleviate itching.
- *Bing Lang** (Semen Arecae Catechu) and *Shi Jun Zi* (Fructus Quisqualis Indicae) kill Worms and disperse food accumulation.

EXTERNAL TREATMENT

- For pale macules at the initial stage, apply *Pu Xuan Shui* (Universal Tinea Lotion), *Ku Shen Jiu* (Flavescent Sophora Root Wine) or *San Huang Xi Ji* (Three Yellows Wash Preparation) to the affected area once or twice a day.
- For dry lesions with scales and slight itching, apply *Run Ji Gao* (Flesh-Moistening Paste) or *Sheng Ji Bai Yu Gao* (White Jade Paste for Generating Flesh) to the affected area two or three times a day.

Clinical notes

- The key treatment for this disease is to dredge Wind, clear Heat from the Lungs and diffuse Lung Qi.
- Materia medica for expelling Worms can be added for children, if required.

Advice for the patient

Avoid spicy food during an attack.

Pityriasis rubra pilaris
毛发红糠疹

This is a rare chronic inflammatory skin disease of unknown cause. There are two types – a childhood type, which may recur regularly, and a more common adult type, which may begin in the late teens or early twenties.

In TCM, this skin disorder is also known as *hu niao ci* (fox's prickles).

Clinical manifestations

- Pityriasis rubra pilaris occurs mainly in children and young people, but may also affect middle-aged people.
- The disease begins with redness and bran-like scaling of the scalp and face and subsequently develops to involve the trunk and limbs, especially the extensor aspects. The entire body may be involved in a severe case, which can closely resemble erythroderma.
- Lesions manifest as pink or red pinpoint to 0.5mm follicular, keratotic papules; moving the hand over the skin feels like rubbing against a file. As the papules increase in number, they merge into large red plaques covered by grayish-white scale.
- Some areas of skin may be spared by the plaques, although red plugged follicles are likely to be evident in these areas.
- The skin on the palms and soles becomes thick, yellow and keratinized with fissuring. Follicular plugging within plaques is particularly noticeable on the dorsum of the fingers. The finger and toe nails may become rough and thickened.
- The disease generally resolves spontaneously after one or two years, but may recur.

Differential diagnosis

Psoriasis
Lesions are characterized by plaques of various shapes and sizes, covered by silvery-white scales. Bleeding points appear when the scales are removed (Auspitz's sign). Psoriasis does not manifest with follicular plugging within the plaques or in otherwise uninvolved areas nor does it have the thickening of the palms and soles characteristic of pityriasis rubra pilaris.

Lichen planus
Lesions present as intensely pruritic purplish-red flat-topped polygonal papules with a shiny wax-like surface.

A lacy white pattern of lines (Wickham's striae) may be seen on the lesions and in the buccal mucosa.

Etiology and pathology

- Where invasion of Wind-Heat complicates a situation of Heat in the Blood, Blood-Heat accumulates in the skin and flesh to cause the disease.
- Spleen Deficiency will result in failure of the Spleen's transportation function and Qi Deficiency in the Middle Burner. Where there is exterior Deficiency, external pathogenic factors can take advantage and invade to cause disharmony between Qi and Blood. The Essence of food and water will therefore not be distributed properly, and the skin and flesh will lack normal nourishment. As a result, clusters of small prickles will appear on the skin.
- Enduring diseases damage Yin and consume Body Fluids, thus generating Deficiency-Heat. The Lungs are therefore impaired in their function of diffusing Qi and the skin is consequently deprived of its normal warmth. This results in dull red, dry skin and the presence of red or purple spots resembling prickles.

Pattern identification and treatment

INTERNAL TREATMENT

WIND-HEAT SETTLING IN THE SKIN
This pattern is characterized by acute onset and rapid spread of the lesions. Infiltrative erythema appears initially on the scalp and face, subsequently spreading to the trunk and extensor aspect of the limbs. The skin is inflamed and covered by white bran-like scales. Accompanying symptoms and signs include itching and dry withered hair on the scalp. The tongue body is red with a thin yellow coating; the pulse is floating and rapid.

Treatment principle
Dredge Wind and clear Heat, dissipate pathogenic factors and alleviate itching.

Prescription
JING FANG BAI DU SAN JIA JIAN
Schizonepeta and Ledebouriella Powder for Vanquishing Toxicity, with modifications

Jing Jie (Herba Schizonepetae Tenuifoliae) 10g

Fang Feng (Radix Ledebouriellae Divaricatae) 10g
Chi Shao (Radix Paeoniae Rubra) 10g
Bai Shao (Radix Paeoniae Lactiflorae) 10g
Bai Xian Pi (Cortex Dictamni Dasycarpi Radicis) 10g
Chuan Xiong (Rhizoma Ligustici Chuanxiong) 10g
Bai Ji Li (Fructus Tribuli Terrestris) 10g
Dang Gui (Radix Angelicae Sinensis) 12g
Sheng Di Huang (Radix Rehmanniae Glutinosae) 12g
Chan Tui‡ (Periostracum Cicadae) 6g
Ku Shen (Radix Sophorae Flavescentis) 6g

Explanation

- *Jing Jie* (Herba Schizonepetae Tenuifoliae), *Fang Feng* (Radix Ledebouriellae Divaricatae), *Bai Ji Li* (Fructus Tribuli Terrestris), and *Chan Tui*‡ (Periostracum Cicadae) dredge Wind and clear Heat, dissipate the Blood and alleviate itching.
- *Sheng Di Huang* (Radix Rehmanniae Glutinosae), *Chi Shao* (Radix Paeoniae Rubra), *Bai Shao* (Radix Paeoniae Lactiflorae), *Dang Gui* (Radix Angelicae Sinensis), and *Chuan Xiong* (Rhizoma Ligustici Chuanxiong) invigorate the Blood and soften the skin.
- *Bai Xian Pi* (Cortex Dictamni Dasycarpi Radicis) and *Ku Shen* (Radix Sophorae Flavescentis) relieve Toxicity and transform Dampness, expel Wind and alleviate itching.

SPLEEN AND STOMACH DEFICIENCY

This pattern manifests as dry pink skin on the trunk and limbs with fine bran-like scales that tend to be shed in layers, keratinization or dry cracking of the palms and soles, and thickening of the finger and toe nails. Accompanying symptoms and signs include scant sweating and dry mouth and lips. The tongue body is red with a white or slightly yellow coating; the pulse is wiry, faint and moderate.

Treatment principle

Fortify the Spleen and harmonize the Stomach, nourish the Blood and moisten the skin.

Prescription
BA ZHEN TANG JIA JIAN
Eight Treasure Decoction, with modifications

Dang Shen (Radix Codonopsitis Pilosulae) 15g
Shan Yao (Radix Dioscoreae Oppositae) 15g
Dan Shen (Radix Salviae Miltiorrhizae) 15g
Ji Xue Teng (Caulis Spatholobi) 15g
Gan Di Huang (Rhizoma Rehmanniae Glutinosae Exsiccata) 12g
Chao Bai Shao (Radix Paeoniae Lactiflorae, stir-fried) 12g
Chen Pi (Pericarpium Citri Reticulatae) 12g
Nan Sha Shen (Radix Adenophorae) 12g
Dang Gui (Radix Angelicae Sinensis) 12g

Bai Zhu (Rhizoma Atractylodis Macrocephalae) 12g
Gan Cao (Radix Glycyrrhizae) 12g
He Shou Wu (Radix Polygoni Multiflori) 10g
Yi Yi Ren (Semen Coicis Lachryma-jobi) 30g

Explanation

- *Dang Shen* (Radix Codonopsitis Pilosulae), *Bai Zhu* (Rhizoma Atractylodis Macrocephalae), *Gan Cao* (Radix Glycyrrhizae), *Chen Pi* (Pericarpium Citri Reticulatae), and *Shan Yao* (Radix Dioscoreae Oppositae) augment Qi and support the Spleen.
- *Dang Gui* (Radix Angelicae Sinensis), *Gan Di Huang* (Rhizoma Rehmanniae Glutinosae Exsiccata) and *Chao Bai Shao* (Radix Paeoniae Lactiflorae, stir-fried) nourish the Blood and moisten Dryness.
- *He Shou Wu* (Radix Polygoni Multiflori), *Nan Sha Shen* (Radix Adenophorae) and *Yi Yi Ren* (Semen Coicis Lachryma-jobi) enrich Yin and moisten the skin.
- *Dan Shen* (Radix Salviae Miltiorrhizae) and *Ji Xue Teng* (Caulis Spatholobi) invigorate the Blood and free the network vessels.

DEPLETION OF QI AND BLOOD

This pattern manifests as reddening of the skin of the trunk and limbs, a covering of bran-like scales, itching that worsens at night, and dry mouth and lips. The tongue body is red with a thin or scant coating; the pulse is thready and rapid.

Treatment principle

Augment Qi and nourish Yin, invigorate the Blood and dissipate Blood stasis.

Prescription
ZENG YE TANG JIA JIAN
Decoction for Increasing Body Fluids, with modifications

Nan Sha Shen (Radix Adenophorae) 30g
Sheng Di Huang (Radix Rehmanniae Glutinosae) 15g
Xuan Shen (Radix Scrophulariae Ningpoensis) 15g
*Shi Hu** (Herba Dendrobii) 15g
Tian Hua Fen (Radix Trichosanthis) 10g
Zi Cao (Radix Arnebiae seu Lithospermi) 10g
Hu Zhang (Radix et Rhizoma Polygoni Cuspidati) 10g
Dan Shen (Radix Salviae Miltiorrhizae) 10g
Hong Hua (Flos Carthami Tinctorii) 6g
Jie Geng (Radix Platycodi Grandiflori) 6g
Shan Yao (Radix Dioscoreae Oppositae) 12g
Chao Bai Bian Dou (Semen Dolichoris Lablab, stir-fried) 12g
Yu Zhu (Rhizoma Polygonati Odorati) 12g

Explanation

- *Nan Sha Shen* (Radix Adenophorae), *Xuan Shen* (Radix Scrophulariae Ningpoensis), *Shi Hu** (Herba

Dendrobii), *Yu Zhu* (Rhizoma Polygonati Odorati), *Shan Yao* (Radix Dioscoreae Oppositae), *Chao Bai Bian Dou* (Semen Dolichoris Lablab, stir-fried), and *Sheng Di Huang* (Radix Rehmanniae Glutinosae) augment Qi and nourish Yin, increase Body Fluids and moisten the skin.

- *Zi Cao* (Radix Arnebiae seu Lithospermi), *Hong Hua* (Flos Carthami Tinctorii), *Tian Hua Fen* (Radix Trichosanthis), *Dan Shen* (Radix Salviae Miltiorrhizae), *Hu Zhang* (Radix et Rhizoma Polygoni Cuspidati), and *Jie Geng* (Radix Platycodi Grandiflori) invigorate the Blood and transform Blood stasis, free the network vessels and alleviate itching.

PATENT HERBAL MEDICINES

- Take *Cang Zhu Gao* (Concentrated Atractylodes Syrup) 10ml three times a day.
- Take *Di Long Pian* (Earthworm Tablet) 1.5g (five tablets) two or three times a day.
- Take *Dan Shen Pian* (Red Sage Root Tablet) 6g two or three times a day.

EXTERNAL TREATMENT

- For dry, prickly lesions, apply *Qin Bai Gao* (Scutellaria and Phellodendron Paste) twice a day.
- For widespread, dry, rough, and lichenified lesions, mix equal amounts of *Dan Huang You* (Egg Yolk Oil) and *Gan Cao You* (Licorice Oil) and apply the mixture to the affected area twice a day.

Clinical notes

The disease has a long duration with an irregular pattern of development and intermittent remission and exacerbation. Skin lesions may disappear spontaneously but tend to recur, especially in summer.

Advice for the patient

Do not wash the affected areas with soap. Avoid taking frequent baths; once a week is sufficient.

Case histories

Case 1

Patient
Male, aged 13.

Clinical manifestations
Three weeks previously, the patient had begun to suffer from a flushed face, desquamation which was particularly obvious on the scalp, dry and cracked palms and soles, and itching. The tongue was red and bare; the pulse was thready and slippery.

Pattern identification
Heat in the Blood generating Wind, which in turn had generated Dryness.

Treatment principle
Cool the Blood and clear Heat, enrich Yin and moisten Dryness.

Prescription ingredients
Sheng Di Huang (Radix Rehmanniae Glutinosae) 30g
Mu Dan Pi (Cortex Moutan Radicis) 9g
Huang Qin (Radix Scutellariae Baicalensis) 9g
Xuan Shen (Radix Scrophulariae Ningpoensis) 9g
Shi Hu* (Herba Dendrobii) 9g
Tian Hua Fen (Radix Trichosanthis) 9g
Bai Ji Li (Fructus Tribuli Terrestris) 9g
Zi Cao (Radix Arnebiae seu Lithospermi) 15g
Da Qing Ye (Folium Isatidis seu Baphicacanthi) 15g
Qian Cao Gen (Radix Rubiae Cordifoliae) 12g
Mai Men Dong (Radix Ophiopogonis Japonici) 6g

One bag a day was used to prepare a decoction, taken twice a day.

Second visit
After drinking three bags of this prescription, the patient was also given *Jia Wei Cang Zhu Gao* (Concentrated Atractylodes Syrup, with additions). The syrup was prepared by decocting *Cang Zhu* (Rhizoma Atractylodis) 300g, *Dang Gui* (Radix Angelicae Sinensis) 9g and *Bai Ji Li* (Fructus Tribuli Terrestris) 9g three times, concentrating the liquid into a paste and mixing with 250g of honey. One tablespoonful was taken twice a day. Meanwhile, *Xin Wu Yu Gao* (New Five-Jade Paste) was used externally. [iv]

Outcome
After two months of treatment, the skin lesions, itching and cracking were significantly reduced. The patient was asked to continue with the decoction and external application for another two weeks to consolidate the improvement. The lesions disappeared completely leaving slight pigmentation, which the patient chose not to have treated. [26]

Case 2
Patient
Male, aged 2.

Clinical manifestations
The patient had been diagnosed with pityriasis rubra pilaris one month previously in a hospital clinic, but treatment had not brought any obvious improvement. Physical examination revealed red macules and papules on the head, face, neck, trunk, and extensor aspects of the limbs with large amounts

---

[iv] In those countries where the use of certain ingredients contained in this paste are not permitted, it can be replaced by *Pu Lian Gao* (Universal Coptis Paste).

of scaling. Small follicular papules had coalesced, presenting a "chicken skin" appearance and giving a prickly feeling like touching the surface of a file. Removal of scale from the surface of the papules revealed a horny core in the opening of the follicle. Infiltration and redness were noted around the base of the follicles. The skin was dry and tight. Accompanying symptoms and signs included irritability and restlessness, shortness of breath and no desire to speak. The tongue body was red with a slightly greasy coating; the pulse was soggy and slightly rapid.

Pattern identification

Spleen and Stomach Deficiency, Dampness predominating over Heat.

Treatment principle

Supplement Qi in the Middle Burner, fortify the Spleen and eliminate Dampness, relieve Toxicity and alleviate itching, dredge Wind and moisten Dryness.

Prescription
SAN DOU YIN

Three Bean Beverage

Lü Dou (Semen Phaseoli Radiati) 20g
Hei Da Dou (Semen Glycines Atrum) 20g
Chi Xiao Dou (Semen Phaseoli Calcarati) 20g
Bai Zhu (Rhizoma Atractylodis Macrocephalae) 6g
Fu Ling (Sclerotium Poriae Cocos) 6g
Bai Xian Pi (Cortex Dictamni Dasycarpi Radicis) 10g
Ku Shen (Radix Sophorae Flavescentis) 6g

Mu Dan Pi (Cortex Moutan Radicis) 6g
Sheng Di Huang (Radix Rehmanniae Glutinosae) 6g
Che Qian Zi (Semen Plantaginis) 10g
Ze Xie (Rhizoma Alismatis Orientalis) 10g

Outcome

After ten bags, the skin lesions had clearly shrunk. After 20 bags, all the symptoms disappeared. A follow-up visit three months later showed no recurrence.[27]

Literature excerpt

In *Wai Ke Jing Yan Xuan* [Selected Experiences in the Treatment of External Diseases], it says: "The main focus of treatment of *hu niao ci* (fox's prickles) is based on the principle that the Lungs govern the skin and hairs. For hard, red papules with dry skin and desquamation, use *Sheng Di Huang* (Radix Rehmanniae Glutinosae), *Nan Sha Shen* (Radix Adenophorae) and *Tian Hua Fen* (Radix Trichosanthis) to nourish Yin, generate Body Fluids and moisten the Lungs; use *Bai Hua She She Cao* (Herba Hedyotidis Diffusae), *Zi Cao* (Radix Arnebiae seu Lithospermi) and *Tu Fu Ling* (Rhizoma Smilacis Glabrae) to clear Heat and relieve Toxicity; and use *Ji Xue Teng* (Caulis Spatholobi), *Hu Zhang* (Radix et Rhizoma Polygoni Cuspidati) and *Cha Shu Gen* (Radix Camelliae Sinensis) to harmonize the Ying level and invigorate the Blood."

Parapsoriasis (chronic superficial dermatitis)
副银屑病

This is a relatively rare skin disease characterized by erythema, papules, infiltration, and desquamation with little or no itching. The disease is chronic and difficult to cure. Although it has some resemblance to psoriasis, it is in fact unrelated and many Western dermatologists now prefer the term chronic superficial dermatitis.

Clinical manifestations

- This disease occurs most often in middle-aged people, affecting males more than females.
- It involves the trunk and limbs, principally the abdomen, buttocks and thighs, but does not affect the mucosa.
- Skin eruptions are characterized by pale red, yellowish-red or purplish-brown patches or plaques with clearly-demarcated margins and covered by a small amount of scale. Lesions, which vary in number, may be small with a finger-like shape or larger and asymmetrical with a round, oval or irregular shape.

- There are no obvious subjective symptoms apart from slight itching.

- Lesions may persist for a long time, with aggravation in winter and remission in summer. In some cases, lichenoid hypertrophic or atrophic changes may appear resembling those present in poikiloderma (reticulate hyperpigmentation, telangiectasia and atrophy); in such instances, the disease may develop into cutaneous T-cell lymphoma (previously known as mycosis fungoides).

Differential diagnosis

Psoriasis
Scaling is much larger, thicker and more pronounced in plaque psoriasis than in chronic superficial dermatitis. The lesions of chronic superficial dermatitis are typically more asymmetrical than those of psoriasis and, once established, tend not to change in size.

Pityriasis rosea
In pityriasis rosea, a herald patch generally precedes the rash. Lesions, which commence as pale red, yellowish-brown or reddish-brown oval plaques before gradually turning rosy, are usually confined to the trunk and proximal extremities; they tend to be oriented along skin lines. Lesions are covered by a thin layer of bran-like scales. A "collarette" ring of fine scale often remains within the border of the lesions.

Nummular eczema
The lesions of nummular eczema mainly involve the limbs, but may also occur on the dorsum of the hands, the buttocks and the trunk. Lesions manifest as very itchy, sharply demarcated, coin-shaped plaques 1-5 cm in diameter formed from the confluence of densely distributed red papules or vesicles. In contrast, once established, the lesions of chronic superficial dermatitis tend not to change in size.

Tinea corporis
The lesions of tinea corporis develop from grouped red papules or papulovesicles, gradually increasing in number and size and spreading outward to form single or multiple sharply circumscribed circular, semicircular or concentric erythema. Thin, fine scaling may sometimes be noted. By contrast, the lesions of chronic superficial dermatitis tend not to change in size.

Etiology and pathology

Spleen Deficiency and depletion of Yin leads to retention of Heat in the Xue level, which moves outward to affect the skin and flesh. Blood stasis due to Qi and Yin Deficiency leads to accumulation of static Heat in the skin and flesh.

Pattern identification and treatment

INTERNAL TREATMENT

QI AND YIN DEFICIENCY
Lesions mainly appear on the neck, trunk and lower legs and manifest as sharply delineated reddish or purplish-brown small strips or large patches. The disease goes through a slow evolution from infiltration to lichenification. In some cases, cutaneous T-cell lymphoma may develop. Accompanying symptoms and signs include emaciation, dizziness, and dry mouth with a desire for drinks. The tongue has stasis marks with a peeling coating; the pulse is slippery and rapid.

Treatment principle
Augment Qi and nourish Yin, clear Heat and invigorate the Blood.

Prescription
SHA SHEN MAI DONG YIN JIA JIAN
Adenophora and Ophiopogon Beverage, with modifications

Sheng Di Huang (Radix Rehmanniae Glutinosae) 60g
Huang Qi (Radix Astragali seu Hedysari) 30g
Dang Shen (Radix Codonopsitis Pilosulae) 30g
Mai Men Dong (Radix Ophiopogonis Japonici) 30g
Nan Sha Shen (Radix Adenophorae) 30g
Bai Hua She She Cao (Herba Hedyotidis Diffusae) 30g
Dan Shen (Radix Salviae Miltiorrhizae) 30g
Chi Shao (Radix Paeoniae Rubra) 30g
Bai Mao Gen (Rhizoma Imperatae Cylindricae) 30g
Jin Yin Hua (Flos Lonicerae) 15g
Tian Men Dong (Radix Asparagi Cochinchinensis) 15g
Mu Dan Pi (Cortex Moutan Radicis) 15g
Yu Zhu (Rhizoma Polygonati Odorati) 12g

Explanation
- *Sheng Di Huang* (Radix Rehmanniae Glutinosae), *Mai Men Dong* (Radix Ophiopogonis Japonici), *Tian Men Dong* (Radix Asparagi Cochinchinensis), *Nan Sha Shen* (Radix Adenophorae), *Yu Zhu* (Rhizoma Polygonati Odorati), *Huang Qi* (Radix Astragali seu Hedysari), and *Dang Shen* (Radix Codonopsitis Pilosulae) augment Qi and nourish Yin.

- *Dan Shen* (Radix Salviae Miltiorrhizae), *Chi Shao* (Radix Paeoniae Rubra), *Bai Mao Gen* (Rhizoma Imperatae Cylindricae), and *Mu Dan Pi* (Cortex Moutan Radicis) cool and invigorate the Blood, clear Heat and disperse erythema.

- *Jin Yin Hua* (Flos Lonicerae) and *Bai Hua She She Cao* (Herba Hedyotidis Diffusae) clear Heat and relieve Toxicity.

EXTERNAL TREATMENT
- For patches of dryish, itchy lesions, apply *Hei Dou Liu You Ruan Gao* (Black Soybean and Vaseline® Ointment) once or twice a day.

- For widespread lesions with slight itching, apply *Qin Bai Gao* (Scutellaria and Phellodendron Paste) or *Huang Lian Ruan Gao* (Coptis Ointment) once or twice a day.

Clinical notes

- This disease is obstinate and difficult to cure. It is therefore important to persist with the treatment until results are achieved.
- At the initial stage, treatment should be based on the principle of cooling the Blood, relieving Toxicity and dispersing erythema; in the latter stages, treatment should be based on the principle of enriching Yin and protecting Body Fluids, augmenting Qi and supporting the Spleen.
- Cutaneous T-cell lymphoma may develop from larger plaques; patients with this type of plaque should be referred to a doctor of Western medicine for a biopsy to confirm the diagnosis.

Modern clinical experience

Ma Shaoyao considered parapsoriasis to be due to Yin Deficiency and internal Heat. [28]

Treatment principle
Nourish Yin and clear Heat, relieve Toxicity and free the network vessels.

Prescription
DI XUAN MAI DONG TANG
Rehmannia, Scrophularia and Ophiopogon Decoction

Sheng Di Huang (Radix Rehmanniae Glutinosae) 12g
Mai Men Dong (Radix Ophiopogonis Japonici) 12g
Xuan Shen (Radix Scrophulariae Ningpoensis) 12g
Di Gu Pi (Cortex Lycii Radicis) 12g
Bai Hua She She Cao (Herba Hedyotidis Diffusae) 30g
Tu Fu Ling (Rhizoma Smilacis Glabrae) 30g
Ji Xue Teng (Caulis Spatholobi) 30g
Hu Zhang (Radix et Rhizoma Polygoni Cuspidati) 15g
Ren Dong Teng (Caulis Lonicerae Japonicae) 15g
Shan Zha (Fructus Crataegi) 9g
Ji Xing Zi (Semen Impatientis Balsaminae) 9g

One bag a day was used to prepare a decoction, taken twice a day.

After one month of treatment, 70 percent of the lesions had disappeared, with the rest disappearing after another month. A follow-up visit four and half years later indicated no recurrence of the disease.

Pityriasis lichenoides
苔癣样糠疹

This is a relatively rare skin disease that occurs in two forms – a chronic type similar to guttate psoriasis and an acute type which heals with scarring.

Clinical manifestations

Pityriasis lichenoides chronica
- This disease occurs most frequently during puberty, affecting males more than females.
- Lesions generally appear on the trunk and limbs.
- Skin eruptions are characterized by pale red or reddish-brown pinpoint to 5mm macules or maculopapules with slight infiltration but no tendency to coalesce. Lesions are covered by a thin layer of fine, adherent scaling. They resolve after several weeks, leaving temporary pigmentation. New lesions may continue to appear afterwards.
- There are no subjective symptoms apart from slight itching.

- The disease progresses slowly and may resolve spontaneously after 6-12 months. In a few cases, the disease may last for several years, but the patient's general health is not affected.

Acute varioliform lichenoid pityriasis
- This disease may occur in people of any age, but is more frequent in young people.
- Lesions are widespread, but mainly involve the trunk and the flexor aspects of the limbs. The mucosa of the mouth and genitals may also be involved.
- Skin eruptions are polymorphic, manifesting as pale red or reddish-brown, round, 2-10 mm papules or papulovesicles. Hemorrhagic necrosis, crusting or scaling tends to occur. Slightly depressed varioliform scars are left when lesions heal. The simultaneous presence of lesions at different stages is characteristic of this disease because of the recurrence of crops of lesions.
- There are no obvious subjective symptoms.

- The disease is usually characterized by sudden onset and short duration and frequently resolves spontaneously within a period of several weeks to six months. However, it may become chronic, with crops of lesions recurring in subsequent months or years.

Differential diagnosis

Psoriasis
Pityriasis lichenoides chronica resembles guttate psoriasis, but the lesions in pityriasis lichenoides are covered by a thin layer of fine scaling.

Pityriasis rosea
In pityriasis rosea, a herald patch generally precedes the rash. Lesions, which commence as pale red, yellowish-brown or reddish-brown oval plaques before gradually turning rosy, are usually confined to the trunk and proximal extremities; they tend to be oriented along skin lines. Lesions are covered by a thin layer of bran-like scales. A "collarette" ring of fine scale often remains within the border of the lesions.

Varicella (chickenpox)
The acute form of lichenoid pityriasis needs to be differentiated from varicella (chickenpox), where skin eruptions begin on the trunk and spread to the face, scalp and limbs. Eruptions occur in successive crops passing through the stages of macule, papule, vesicle, and pustule. The lesions finally dry out and form crusts which separate, usually without scarring. Rarely in severe cases, necrosis occurs around the vesicles; hemorrhagic necrosis and scarring are much more common in the acute form of lichenoid pityriasis.

Etiology and pathology

- External pathogenic Wind and Cold may settle in the skin and flesh to influence the normal diffusion of Qi by the Lungs and Spleen. These pathogenic factors then obstruct the channels and network vessels and stagnate in the skin and interstices (*cou li*), depriving the skin and flesh of nourishment.
- In situations of Qi Deficiency and Blood stasis, static Heat accumulates and binds in the skin and flesh to generate Heat Toxins.

Pattern identification and treatment

INTERNAL TREATMENT

WIND-COLD
This pattern occurs in pityriasis lichenoides chronica.

Lesions manifest as discrete, pinpoint to 5mm pale red or reddish-brown circular scaly macules or papules. Accompanying symptoms and signs include fear of cold and lassitude. The tongue body is pale with a thin white coating; the pulse is floating and rapid.

Treatment principle
Expel Wind and dissipate Cold, and harmonize the Ying and Wei levels.

Prescription
MA HUANG GUI ZHI GE BAN TANG JIA JIAN
Ephedra and Cinnamon Twig Half-and-Half Decoction, with modifications

Ma Huang* (Herba Ephedrae) 3g
Gui Zhi (Ramulus Cinnamomi Cassiae) 6g
Xing Ren (Semen Pruni Armeniacae) 10g
Bai Shao (Radix Paeoniae Lactiflorae) 10g
Dang Gui (Radix Angelicae Sinensis) 10g
Gan Cao (Radix Glycyrrhizae) 10g
Di Fu Zi (Fructus Kochiae Scopariae) 15g
Bai Xian Pi (Cortex Dictamni Dasycarpi Radicis) 15g
Chi Xiao Dou (Semen Phaseoli Calcarati) 15g
Sheng Jiang (Rhizoma Zingiberis Officinalis Recens) 10g
Da Zao (Fructus Ziziphi Jujubae) 15g

Explanation
- *Ma Huang** (Herba Ephedrae), *Gui Zhi* (Ramulus Cinnamomi Cassiae), *Xing Ren* (Semen Pruni Armeniacae), *Bai Shao* (Radix Paeoniae Lactiflorae), *Sheng Jiang* (Rhizoma Zingiberis Officinalis Recens), *Da Zao* (Fructus Ziziphi Jujubae), and *Gan Cao* (Radix Glycyrrhizae) expel Wind and dissipate Cold, and harmonize the Ying and Wei levels.
- *Dang Gui* (Radix Angelicae Sinensis) invigorates the Blood and disperses eruptions.
- *Bai Xian Pi* (Cortex Dictamni Dasycarpi Radicis), *Chi Xiao Dou* (Semen Phaseoli Calcarati) and *Di Fu Zi* (Fructus Kochiae Scopariae) expel Wind and disperse erythema, invigorate the Blood and alleviate itching.

HEAT TOXINS
This pattern occurs in acute varioliform lichenoid pityriasis and manifests as widespread, generalized pale red or reddish-brown lesions in the form of papules, papulovesicles, hemorrhagic papules, or papular pustules; lesions may be restricted to one of these types or several types may appear simultaneously. Accompanying symptoms and signs include fever, lassitude, and aching and painful joints. The tongue body is red with a yellow, greasy coating; the pulse is rapid.

Treatment principle
Clear Heat and relieve Toxicity, cool the Blood and dispel Blood stasis.

Prescription
XI JIAO DI HUANG TANG JIA JIAN
Rhinoceros Horn and Rehmannia Decoction, with modifications

Lü Dou Yi (Testa Phaseoli Radiati) 30g
Chi Shao (Radix Paeoniae Rubra) 30g
Xuan Shen (Radix Scrophulariae Ningpoensis) 30g
Zhi Mu (Rhizoma Anemarrhenae Asphodeloidis) 30g
Dan Shen (Radix Salviae Miltiorrhizae) 30g
Qing Hao (Herba Artemisiae Chinghao) 30g, added
  5 minutes before the end of the decoction process
Pu Gong Ying (Herba Taraxaci cum Radice) 30g
Sheng Di Huang (Radix Rehmanniae Glutinosae) 60g
Zhi Mu (Rhizoma Anemarrhenae Asphodeloidis) 12g
Qin Jiao (Radix Gentianae Macrophyllae) 15g

Explanation
- *Lü Dou Yi* (Testa Phaseoli Radiati) cools the Blood and clears Heat from the Ying level.
- *Pu Gong Ying* (Herba Taraxaci cum Radice), *Qing Hao* (Herba Artemisiae Chinghao) and *Zhi Mu* (Rhizoma Anemarrhenae Asphodeloidis) clear Heat and relieve Toxicity.
- *Chi Shao* (Radix Paeoniae Rubra), *Dan Shen* (Radix Salviae Miltiorrhizae) and *Sheng Di Huang* (Radix Rehmanniae Glutinosae) clear Heat and cool the Blood, transform Blood stasis and reduce eruptions.
- *Xuan Shen* (Radix Scrophulariae Ningpoensis) and *Qin Jiao* (Radix Gentianae Macrophyllae) nourish Yin and clear Heat.

EXTERNAL TREATMENT
- For patches of dryish, itchy lesions, apply *Hei Dou Liu You Ruan Gao* (Black Soybean and Vaseline® Ointment) once or twice a day.
- For widespread lesions with slight itching, apply *Qin Bai Gao* (Scutellaria and Phellodendron Paste) or *Huang Lian Ruan Gao* (Coptis Ointment) once or twice a day.

Clinical notes

Although some cases may resolve spontaneously within 6-12 months, these diseases are generally obstinate and difficult to cure. It is therefore important to continue with the treatment until results are achieved.

Modern clinical experience

PITYRIASIS LICHENOIDES CHRONICA
Xia Han treated chronic pityriasis lichenoides with *Liang Xue Qu Feng Tang* (Decoction for Cooling the Blood and Dispelling Wind). [28]

Treatment principle
Dispel Wind and eliminate Dampness, cool the Blood and relieve Toxicity.

Prescription ingredients
Sheng Di Huang (Radix Rehmanniae Glutinosae) 12g
Bai Ji Li (Fructus Tribuli Terrestris) 12g
Fu Ling Pi (Cortex Poriae Cocos) 12g
Mu Dan Pi (Cortex Moutan Radicis) 9g
Huang Qin (Radix Scutellariae Baicalensis) 9g
Huai Hua (Flos Sophorae Japonicae) 9g
Zi Cao (Radix Arnebiae seu Lithospermi) 9g
Da Qing Ye (Folium Isatidis seu Baphicacanthi) 15g
Yi Yi Ren (Semen Coicis Lachryma-jobi) 15g
Gan Cao (Radix Glycyrrhizae) 5g

For slight itching, *Zhen Zhu Mu* ‡ (Concha Margaritifera) 30g, *Ci Shi* ‡ (Magnetitum) 30g and *Shu Qu Cao* (Herba Gnaphalii Affinis) 15g were added. Results were seen after two weeks.

ACUTE VARIOLIFORM LICHENOID PITYRIASIS

1. **Gu Bohua** treated the acute (Heat Toxin) type of pityriasis lichenoides with *Di Xuan Qin Lian Tang* (Rehmannia, Scrophularia, Scutellaria, and Picrorhiza Decoction). [28]

Prescription ingredients
Sheng Di Huang (Radix Rehmanniae Glutinosae) 30g
Xuan Shen (Radix Scrophulariae Ningpoensis) 9g
Huang Qin (Radix Scutellariae Baicalensis) 9g
Zhi Mu (Rhizoma Anemarrhenae Asphodeloidis) 9g
Mu Dan Pi (Cortex Moutan Radicis) 9g
Shui Niu Jiao ‡ (Cornu Bubali) 15g, decocted for
  30 minutes before adding the other ingredients
Hu Huang Lian (Rhizoma Picrorhizae Scrophularii-florae) 6g
Dan Zhu Ye (Herba Lophatheri Gracilis) 6g
Gan Cao (Radix Glycyrrhizae) 6g

One bag a day was used to prepare a decoction, taken twice a day. Clinical observation of a number of cases indicated that the condition resolved after four months of treatment on average.

2. **Zhao** formulated his own prescription to treat this disease. [29]

Prescription ingredients
Ban Lan Gen (Radix Isatidis seu Baphicacanthi) 30g
Tu Fu Ling (Rhizoma Smilacis Glabrae) 30g
Bai Mao Gen (Rhizoma Imperatae Cylindricae) 30g
Da Qing Ye (Folium Isatidis seu Baphicacanthi) 15g

Ye Ju Hua (Flos Chrysanthemi Indici) 15g
Zi Cao (Radix Arnebiae seu Lithospermi) 10g
Lian Qiao (Fructus Forsythiae Suspensae) 10g
Mu Dan Pi (Cortex Moutan Radicis) 10g
Chi Shao (Radix Paeoniae Rubra) 10g

Modifications

1. For bright red lesions that did not blanch under pressure, *Sheng Di Huang Tan* (Radix Rehmanniae Glutinosae Carbonisata) and *Jin Yin Hua Tan* (Flos Lonicerae Carbonisata) were added.
2. For dark red lesions that did not blanch under pres-

sure, *Dan Shen* (Radix Salviae Miltiorrhizae) and *Ji Xue Teng* (Caulis Spatholobi) were added.
3. For constipation, *Zhi Zi* (Fructus Gardeniae Jasminoidis) and *Da Huang* (Radix et Rhizoma Rhei) were added.
4. For sore throat, *Shan Dou Gen* (Radix Sophorae Tonkinensis) was added.

One bag a day was used to prepare a decoction, taken twice a day. It took four to seven days for the prescription to start to have an effect, and three to eight weeks for lesions to fully resolve.

Lichen planus
扁平苔癣

Lichen planus is an acute or chronic inflammatory disease of the skin and mucous membranes of unknown etiology. Genetic factors and liver disease (especially hepatitis C-related) may be implicated. Eruptions similar to lichen planus may occur due to certain drugs, infections and the graft-versus-host reaction: these are referred to as lichenoid reactions to distinguish them from lichen planus.

In TCM, this disease is also known as *zi dian feng* (purple patch Wind).

Clinical manifestations

- The disease may occur at any age, although it is rare in children under 5. Two-thirds of cases occur in individuals between the ages of 30 and 60.
- Eruptions usually involve the flexor surfaces of the wrists and forearms, and the lower legs around and above the ankles; it is rare for the whole body to be affected. The buccal mucosa, the lips and tongue, the glans penis, or the labia may also be involved.
- Lesions manifest as intensely pruritic 2-10 mm flat-topped shiny papules with an irregular, sharply defined angulated border. They are generally red or pink initially, subsequently turning purplish-red, dull red or reddish-brown. The surface is waxy when observed obliquely.
- The surface of the lesions exhibits a lacy white pattern of lines (Wickham's striae).
- Lesions that persist, most frequently on the shins, may develop into confluent hypertrophic plaques. These lesions can become hyperkeratotic with a coarse surface covered by scales.

- Mucous membranes are involved in 40-60% of individuals, commonly manifesting as grayish-white papules or Wickham's striae on the buccal mucosa, lips, tongue, and glans penis.
- Nail dystrophy may occur.
- Lesions on the scalp can result in patchy scarring alopecia.
- Lichen planus usually disappears within one to two years leaving pigmentation; recurrences are frequent. The hyperkeratotic variant on the lower legs may last for many years.

Differential diagnosis

GENERALIZED LICHEN PLANUS

Guttate psoriasis
Guttate psoriasis is characterized by the sudden onset of numerous uniform, small, round, symmetrically distributed plaques, which resemble drops of wax on the skin. Lesions are usually more widespread than those of lichen planus, occurring on the trunk as well as the limbs. Wickham's striae are absent and the mucosae are not involved.

Lichenoid drug eruptions
Lichenoid eruptions can be caused by drugs. However, involvement of the buccal mucosa is rare.

HYPERTROPHIC LICHEN PLANUS

Lichen simplex chronicus (neurodermatitis)
Lichen simplex chronicus generally involves the nape of the neck, the elbows and the knees, but may also spread

to the limbs, the areas around the eyes and the sacro-coccygeal region. Lesions manifest as reddish-brown plaques of various sizes with rough skin and deepened skin creases in the affected area. Lichenification is likely if the lesions persist. The mucosae are not involved.

Psoriasis
Psoriasis usually involves the extensor aspect of the limbs, especially the extensor aspect of the elbows and knees, but sometimes spreads to affect the whole body. The nails and scalp may also be involved. Lesions manifest as erythematous papules covered by silvery-white scales. If the scales are removed, bleeding points appear (Auspitz's sign).

Nodular prurigo
Initially the skin lesions are pale red papules. These develop into hemispherical nodules up to 30mm in diameter involving the upper and lower limbs. They have a rough surface area, without the flat tops characteristic of lichen planus, and are reddish-brown or grayish-brown in color. Excoriated bloody crusting is present.

ORAL LICHEN PLANUS

Pemphigus vulgaris
Oral lesions in pemphigus tend to appear before other manifestations and to be erosive, which is much rarer in oral lichen planus. The characteristic lacy white pattern of lines (Wickham's striae) is absent in pemphigus.

Oral candidiasis (thrush)
Lesions may appear in any part of the mouth, but are more common on the tongue, the cheeks, the soft palate, and the floor of the mouth. In the affected area, lesions manifest as adherent, milky-white, velvety membranes that resemble clotted milk. If they are removed by force, the base is red and tends to bleed. Wickham's striae are absent.

Etiology and pathology

- If external Wind-Heat that has settled in the fleshy exterior is retained there for a long period, it can transform into further Heat and obstruct the skin and flesh, resulting in Qi stagnation and Blood stasis. Movement of Qi in the channels is inhibited, depriving the skin of proper nourishment and giving rise to dry skin and itching.
- Wind and Damp accumulate and bind in the skin and interstices (*cou li*), stagnating to form lesions that usually manifest as hard purplish-red papules or maculopapules accompanied by intense itching.
- Wind, Damp and Heat pathogenic factors, retained over a long period and not dispersed, will cause Qi

stagnation and Blood stasis and deprive the skin and flesh of nourishment, resulting in skin eruptions. If the eruptions cannot be cured relatively quickly, the affected area may become hypertrophic.

- An improper diet can impair the normal functions of the Spleen and Stomach and generate internal Damp-Heat. If the body is attacked by external Wind, then Damp, Heat and Wind will combine to obstruct the skin and flesh and stagnate in the channels and network vessels, resulting in the disease.
- Spleen Deficiency leads to impairment of the transformation and transportation function and can produce internal Damp-Heat, which may steam and ascend to the mouth, manifesting as bad breath and ulceration and erosion of the mouth and tongue, or descend to the lower body, manifesting as a variety of skin eruptions or genital ulceration.
- Yin Deficiency of the Liver and Kidneys will lead to insufficient Essence and Blood resulting externally in the skin being deprived of moisture and nourishment, consequently becoming dry with desquamation and itching, and internally in a shortage of Yin-Liquids, thus giving rise to recurrent, non-healing mouth and tongue sores.

Pattern identification and treatment

INTERNAL TREATMENT

BINDING OF WIND-HEAT
This pattern has an acute onset with generalized red smooth flat-topped papules and maculopapules in a discrete or clustered distribution; in a few patients, lesions may also include vesicles or bullae. Itching is severe. The tongue body is red with a scant coating; the pulse is floating and rapid.

Treatment principle
Dredge Wind, clear Heat and free the network vessels.

Prescription
XIAO FENG SAN JIA JIAN
Powder for Dispersing Wind, with modifications

Shi Gao‡ (Gypsum Fibrosum) 15g, decocted for 30 minutes before adding the other ingredients
Sheng Di Huang (Radix Rehmanniae Glutinosae) 15g
Jing Jie (Herba Schizonepetae Tenuifoliae) 6g
Ku Shen (Radix Sophorae Flavescentis) 6g
Chan Tui‡ (Periostracum Cicadae) 6g
Chao Niu Bang Zi (Fructus Arctii Lappae, stir-fried) 10g
Dang Gui (Radix Angelicae Sinensis) 10g
Fang Feng (Radix Ledebouriellae Divaricatae) 10g
Di Fu Zi (Fructus Kochiae Scopariae) 10g

Yi Yi Ren (Semen Coicis Lachryma-jobi) 12g
Dan Shen (Radix Salviae Miltiorrhizae) 12g
Si Gua Luo (Fasciculus Vascularis Luffae) 4.5g
Cang Er Zi (Fructus Xanthii Sibirici) 3g
Xu Chang Qing (Radix Cynanchi Paniculati) 3g

Explanation

- *Shi Gao* ‡ (Gypsum Fibrosum) thrusts Heat outward with coolness and acridity.
- *Sheng Di Huang* (Radix Rehmanniae Glutinosae), *Dan Shen* (Radix Salviae Miltiorrhizae) and *Dang Gui* (Radix Angelicae Sinensis) invigorate the Blood and free the network vessels, cool the Blood and reduce erythema.
- *Chao Niu Bang Zi* (Fructus Arctii Lappae, stir-fried), *Fang Feng* (Radix Ledebouriellae Divaricatae), *Jing Jie* (Herba Schizonepetae Tenuifoliae), and *Chan Tui* ‡ (Periostracum Cicadae) dredge Wind and clear Heat.
- *Xu Chang Qing* (Radix Cynanchi Paniculati), *Di Fu Zi* (Fructus Kochiae Scopariae), *Cang Er Zi* (Fructus Xanthii Sibirici), and *Ku Shen* (Radix Sophorae Flavescentis) percolate Dampness and clear Heat, alleviate itching and dissipate lumps.
- *Yi Yi Ren* (Semen Coicis Lachryma-jobi) and *Si Gua Luo* (Fasciculus Vascularis Luffae) transform Dampness and free the network vessels.

ACCUMULATION AND BINDING OF WIND AND DAMPNESS

Skin eruptions are characterized by itchy purplish-red maculopapules that become confluent to form linear bands or plaques. The surface of the lesions is smooth, shiny and wax-like. Some female patients may experience chronic leukorrhea. The tongue body is pale red, swollen and tender with a thin white or slightly greasy coating; the pulse is soggy and moderate.

Treatment principle

Dispel Wind and benefit the movement of Dampness, invigorate the Blood and free the network vessels.

Prescription

DA FANG FENG TANG JIA JIAN
Major Ledebouriella Decoction, with modifications

Fang Feng (Radix Ledebouriellae Divaricatae) 10g
Qiang Huo (Rhizoma et Radix Notopterygii) 10g
Jiang Can ‡ (Bombyx Batryticatus) 10g
Chi Shao (Radix Paeoniae Rubra) 10g
Dang Shen (Radix Codonopsitis Pilosulae) 12g
Bai Zhu (Rhizoma Atractylodis Macrocephalae) 12g
Bai Xian Pi (Cortex Dictamni Dasycarpi Radicis) 12g
Dan Shen (Radix Salviae Miltiorrhizae) 15g
Lu Lu Tong (Fructus Liquidambaris) 15g
Chuan Xiong (Rhizoma Ligustici Chuanxiong) 6g
Fu Pen Zi (Fructus Rubi Chingii) 6g

Explanation

- *Fang Feng* (Radix Ledebouriellae Divaricatae), *Qiang Huo* (Rhizoma et Radix Notopterygii), *Chuan Xiong* (Rhizoma Ligustici Chuanxiong), and *Jiang Can* ‡ (Bombyx Batryticatus) expel Wind and overcome Dampness, alleviate itching and disperse eruptions.
- *Dang Shen* (Radix Codonopsitis Pilosulae) and *Bai Zhu* (Rhizoma Atractylodis Macrocephalae) augment Qi and support the Spleen, consolidate the Root and fortify the Middle Burner.
- *Dan Shen* (Radix Salviae Miltiorrhizae), *Chi Shao* (Radix Paeoniae Rubra) and *Fu Pen Zi* (Fructus Rubi Chingii) warm Yang and invigorate the Blood, dissipate lumps and alleviate itching.
- *Bai Xian Pi* (Cortex Dictamni Dasycarpi Radicis) and *Lu Lu Tong* (Fructus Liquidambaris) free the network vessels and alleviate itching.

BLOOD STASIS IN THE CHANNELS AND VESSELS

This pattern is of prolonged duration. The dull purple, dull red or reddish-brown lesions are hypertrophic, coarse and lichenified, and covered by a small amount of scales. Itching is intense and incessant. The tongue body is dark red or has stasis marks with a scant coating; the pulse is deep and choppy.

Treatment principle

Invigorate the Blood and free the network vessels, soften hardness and alleviate itching.

Prescription

TONG JING ZHU YU TANG JIA JIAN
Decoction for Freeing the Channels and Expelling Blood Stasis, with modifications

Sheng Di Huang (Radix Rehmanniae Glutinosae) 30g
Tao Ren (Semen Persicae) 10g
Hong Hua (Flos Carthami Tinctorii) 10g
E Zhu (Rhizoma Curcumae) 10g
Xu Chang Qing (Radix Cynanchi Paniculati) 10g
Bai Zhi (Radix Angelicae Dahuricae) 10g
Lian Qiao (Fructus Forsythiae Suspensae) 10g
Fang Feng (Radix Ledebouriellae Divaricatae) 10g
Niu Xi (Radix Achyranthis Bidentatae) 10g
Di Long ‡ (Lumbricus) 10g
Dang Gui (Radix Angelicae Sinensis) 12g
He Shou Wu (Radix Polygoni Multiflori) 12g
Dan Shen (Radix Salviae Miltiorrhizae) 12g
Bai Ji Li (Fructus Tribuli Terrestris) 12g
Jie Geng (Radix Platycodi Grandiflori) 6g

Explanation

- *Tao Ren* (Semen Persicae), *Hong Hua* (Flos Carthami Tinctorii), *E Zhu* (Rhizoma Curcumae), *Dan Shen*

(Radix Salviae Miltiorrhizae), *Niu Xi* (Radix Achyranthis Bidentatae), and *Dang Gui* (Radix Angelicae Sinensis) transform Blood stasis and free the network vessels, soften hardness and dissipate lumps.

- *Xu Chang Qing* (Radix Cynanchi Paniculati), *Fang Feng* (Radix Ledebouriellae Divaricatae) and *Bai Ji Li* (Fructus Tribuli Terrestris) arrest Wind and alleviate itching.
- *He Shou Wu* (Radix Polygoni Multiflori) and *Sheng Di Huang* (Radix Rehmanniae Glutinosae) nourish the Blood and moisten Dryness.
- *Bai Zhi* (Radix Angelicae Dahuricae), *Lian Qiao* (Fructus Forsythiae Suspensae), *Di Long* ‡ (Lumbricus), and *Jie Geng* (Radix Platycodi Grandiflori) soften the skin and disperse eruptions, free the network vessels and alleviate itching.

DAMP-HEAT DUE TO SPLEEN DEFICIENCY

This is a chronic pattern, manifesting as grayish-white maculopapules or blisters on the buccal mucosa and genitals, possibly accompanied by erosion or ulceration of varying severity. The tongue body is pale red with a thin white coating; the pulse is deficient and thready.

Treatment principle
Support the Spleen and transform Dampness, clear Heat and relieve Toxicity.

Prescription
SHEN LING BAI ZHU SAN JIA JIAN
Ginseng, Poria and White Atractylodes Powder, with modifications

Dang Shen (Radix Codonopsitis Pilosulae) 10g
Bai Zhu (Rhizoma Atractylodis Macrocephalae) 10g
Fu Ling (Sclerotium Poriae Cocos) 10g
Chen Pi (Pericarpium Citri Reticulatae) 10g
Chao Bai Bian Dou (Semen Dolichoris Lablab, stir-fried) 15g
Dan Shen (Radix Salviae Miltiorrhizae) 15g
Huo Xue Teng (Caulis seu Radix Schisandrae) 15g
Ren Dong Teng (Caulis Lonicerae Japonicae) 15g
Shan Yao (Radix Dioscoreae Oppositae) 30g
Chi Xiao Dou (Semen Phaseoli Calcarati) 30g
Chao Huang Bai (Cortex Phellodendri, stir-fried) 6g
Sheng Ma (Rhizoma Cimicifugae) 6g
Sha Ren (Fructus Amomi) 6g, added 5 minutes before the end of the decoction process
Chao Long Dan Cao (Radix Gentianae Scabrae, stir-fried) 6g

Explanation
- *Dang Shen* (Radix Codonopsitis Pilosulae), *Fu Ling* (Sclerotium Poriae Cocos), *Bai Zhu* (Rhizoma Atractylodis Macrocephalae), *Shan Yao* (Radix Dioscoreae Oppositae), *Chao Bai Bian Dou* (Semen Doli-

choris Lablab, stir-fried), and *Chen Pi* (Pericarpium Citri Reticulatae) augment Qi and support the Spleen, transform Dampness and clear Heat.
- *Dan Shen* (Radix Salviae Miltiorrhizae), *Huo Xue Teng* (Caulis seu Radix Schisandrae), *Ren Dong Teng* (Caulis Lonicerae Japonicae), and *Chi Xiao Dou* (Semen Phaseoli Calcarati) relieve Toxicity and free the network vessels, transform Dampness and clear Heat.
- *Chao Huang Bai* (Cortex Phellodendri, stir-fried) and *Chao Long Dan Cao* (Radix Gentianae Scabrae, stir-fried) clear Heat and relieve Toxicity.
- *Sheng Ma* (Rhizoma Cimicifugae) and *Sha Ren* (Fructus Amomi) bear Yang upward and regulate Qi in order to send clear Yang Qi upward and turbid Yin downward, which benefits the process of recovery.

YIN DEFICIENCY OF THE LIVER AND KIDNEYS

Lesions generally manifest as milky white reticular striae or maculopapules on the lips, buccal mucosa, tongue, and gums; erosion occurs in severe cases. Accompanying symptoms and signs include dizziness, dry eyes, poor vision, and generalized fatigue. The tongue body is red with a scant coating or no coating; the pulse is deep and thready.

Treatment principle
Nourish the Liver and boost the Kidneys, enrich Yin and bear Fire downward.

Prescription
MAI WEI DI HUANG TANG JIA JIAN
Ophiopogon and Rehmannia Decoction, with modifications

Gan Di Huang (Radix Rehmanniae Glutinosae Exsiccata) 10g
Shan Zhu Yu (Fructus Corni Officinalis) 10g
Fu Ling (Sclerotium Poriae Cocos) 10g
Chao Mu Dan Pi (Cortex Moutan Radicis, stir-fried) 10g
Mai Men Dong (Radix Ophiopogonis Japonici) 12g
Tian Men Dong (Radix Asparagi Cochinchinensis) 12g
*Shi Hu** (Herba Dendrobii) 12g
Gou Qi Zi (Fructus Lycii) 12g
Xuan Shen (Radix Scrophulariae Ningpoensis) 15g
Nan Sha Shen (Radix Adenophorae) 12g
Huang Bai (Cortex Phellodendri) 15g
Huang Qi (Radix Astragali seu Hedysari) 6g
Sheng Ma (Rhizoma Cimicifugae) 6g

Explanation
- *Gan Di Huang* (Radix Rehmanniae Glutinosae Exsiccata), *Shan Zhu Yu* (Fructus Corni Officinalis), *Gou Qi Zi* (Fructus Lycii), *Shi Hu** (Herba Dendrobii), and *Nan Sha Shen* (Radix Adenophorae) enrich the Liver and supplement the Kidneys.

- *Huang Bai* (Cortex Phellodendri), *Chao Mu Dan Pi* (Cortex Moutan Radicis, stir-fried), *Mai Men Dong* (Radix Ophiopogonis Japonici), *Tian Men Dong* (Radix Asparagi Cochinchinensis), and *Xuan Shen* (Radix Scrophulariae Ningpoensis) enrich Yin and bear Fire downward.
- *Fu Ling* (Sclerotium Poriae Cocos) and *Sheng Ma* (Rhizoma Cimicifugae) bear Yang upward and transform Dampness.
- *Huang Qi* (Radix Astragali seu Hedysari) supports the Spleen and augments Qi while reinforcing the effect of the formula in enriching the Liver and supplementing the Kidneys.

General modifications

1. For relatively severe conditions involving the buccal mucosa, add *Jin Lian Hua* (Flos Trollii), *Jin Que Hua* (Flos Caraganae Sinicae) and *Jin Guo Lan* (Tuber Tinosporae); or add *Er Dong Gao* (Asparagus and Ophiopogon Syrup) or *Yin Hua Tang* (Honeysuckle Decoction). The latter two preparations may be taken at the same time if the condition is extremely severe.
2. For severe itching, add *Chan Tui*‡ (Periostracum Cicadae) and *Jiang Can*‡ (Bombyx Batryticatus).
3. For lesions principally in the genital region, add *Chao Du Zhong* (Cortex Eucommiae Ulmoidis, stir-fried) and *Chao Long Dan Cao* (Radix Gentianae Scabrae, stir-fried).
4. For bullous lesions, add *Zi Cao* (Radix Arnebiae seu Lithospermi), *Bi Xie* (Rhizoma Dioscoreae Hypoglaucae seu Septemlobae), *Cang Zhu* (Rhizoma Atractylodis) and *Hong Hua* (Flos Carthami Tinctorii).

EXTERNAL TREATMENT

- For lesions in the mouth with erosion, use *Xi Gua Shuang Pen Ji* (Watermelon Frost Spray Preparation) three to five times a day as an insufflation for the affected area.
- For lesions in the vulva with erosion, wash the affected area with *Lu Lu Tong Shui Xi Ji* (Sweetgum Fruit Wash Preparation) once or twice a day and then apply *Gan Cao You* (Licorice Oil) and *Qu Shi San* (Powder for Dispelling Dampness).
- For itchy skin lesions, wash the area with *Bai Bu Ding* (Stemona Root Tincture) or *Lu Hu Xi Ji* (Calamine and Giant Knotweed Wash Preparation) twice a day.
- For hypertrophic eruptions, apply *Gan Cao You* (Licorice Oil), *Huang Lian Ruan Gao* (Coptis Ointment) or *Hei Bu Yao Gao* (Black Cloth Medicated Paste) to the affected area twice a day.

ACUPUNCTURE
Points

- For involvement of the upper limbs, select LU-9 Taiyuan, LU-7 Lieque, LI-4 Hegu, LI-10 Shousanli, and LI-11 Quchi.
- For involvement of the lower limbs, select GB-31 Fengshi, BL-40 Weizhong, ST-36 Zusanli, BL-57 Chengshan, and KI-3 Taixi.

Technique: Apply the even method at all points. Treat once every two days. A course consists of seven to ten treatment sessions.

Explanation
This group of points includes both local and distal points on the affected channels:

- LI-10 Shousanli, ST-36 Zusanli, LI-11 Quchi, LI-4 Hegu, and BL-57 Chengshan support the Spleen and fortify the Stomach, transform Dampness and free the network vessels.
- LU-9 Taiyuan, LU-7 Lieque, GB-31 Fengshi, BL-40 Weizhong, and KI-3 Taixi transform Blood stasis and invigorate the Blood, disperse eruptions and alleviate itching.

EAR ACUPUNCTURE
Points: Spleen, Heart, Kidney, and Endocrine.
Technique: Retain the needles for 15-30 minutes. Treat once every two days. A course consists of seven to ten treatment sessions.

Clinical notes

- Treatment for lichen planus is usually determined by the areas involved:
  - dispel Dampness and transform Blood stasis if the lesions involve the skin
  - nourish Yin and clear Heat if the condition involves the mucous membranes of the mouth
  - enrich the Liver and boost the Kidneys if the mucous membranes of the genitals are involved
- Although no completely satisfactory therapies have yet been found, many reports indicate that long-term application of TCM treatment can lead to some improvement in symptoms, and even to a complete resolution in some cases
- The incidence of squamous cell carcinoma in individuals with oral lichen planus is in the region of 5%.

Advice for the patient

Cut down on smoking, alcohol and intake of stimulating food.

Case histories

Case 1

Patient
Female, aged 23.

Clinical manifestations
The patient had been suffering from lichen planus for two years. Lesions manifested as pale red, pinhead, flat-topped papules densely distributed in a linear arrangement along the right arm accompanied by itching and slight lichenification. The papules extended on the radial side of the right arm and hand from 4cm above the elbow joint via the wrist joint to LU-11 Shaoshang. The nail of the thumb was incomplete on the lateral side.

Points
LU-9 Taiyuan, LU-7 Lieque, LI-4 Hegu, LI-10 Shousanli, and LI-11 Quchi.

Technique
Treatment took place once every two days with three of the five points being selected each time.

Outcome
After three treatment sessions, the eruptions were no longer itchy. After eight treatment sessions, the eruptions above the elbow joint had disappeared completely. A few eruptions still remained around the styloid process of the radius after 40 treatment sessions. A follow-up visit two years later revealed no recurrence. [30]

Case 2

Patient
Male, aged 50.

Clinical manifestations
The patient had suffered from generalized lichen planus with purple plaques and itching for five years. In the previous two months, the patient had been working on the repair of a boiler. Strenuous work in a high-temperature environment had resulted in profuse sweating, which had aggravated the condition. Sleep was badly disturbed by increased skin eruptions and intense itching.

Examination revealed a generalized discrete distribution of 5-10 mm purple lesions, some of which had fused into slightly elevated plaques. Scratch marks were evident, particularly on the legs, chest and abdomen. There were also a few vesicles and bloody blisters. The tongue body was red with a thin yellow coating; the pulse was wiry and slippery.

Pattern identification
Wind, Damp and Heat pathogenic factors binding in the skin and flesh. Long-term retention of external Wind resulted in transformation into Heat, which had been complicated by external contraction of Damp-Heat.

Treatment principle
Cool the Blood, clear Heat and dispel Dampness, arrest Wind and alleviate itching.

Prescription ingredients
Sheng Di Huang (Radix Rehmanniae Glutinosae) 30g
Mu Dan Pi (Cortex Moutan Radicis) 10g
Chi Shao (Radix Paeoniae Rubra) 10g
Jin Yin Hua (Flos Lonicerae) 10g
Lian Qiao (Fructus Forsythiae Suspensae) 10g
Bai Zhi (Radix Angelicae Dahuricae) 10g
Qiang Huo (Rhizoma et Radix Notopterygii) 10g
Bai Xian Pi (Cortex Dictamni Dasycarpi Radicis) 12g

One bag a day was used to prepare a decoction, taken twice a day.

Second visit
After the patient had followed this prescription for a fortnight, the vesicles and bloody blisters had disappeared leaving crusts; purple lesions were still discretely distributed over the body and itching remained intense. This suggested that Dampness had been eliminated, but that some Heat was retained and Wind had not been expelled from the skin and flesh.

Treatment principle
Arrest Wind, clear Heat and alleviate itching.

Prescription
WU SHE QU FENG TANG
Black-Tail Snail Decoction for Expelling Wind

Wu Shao She ‡ (Zaocys Dhumnades) 10g
Jing Jie (Herba Schizonepetae Tenuifoliae) 10g
Fang Feng (Radix Ledebouriellae Divaricatae) 10g
Qiang Huo (Rhizoma et Radix Notopterygii) 10g
Bai Zhi (Radix Angelicae Dahuricae) 10g
Huang Qin (Radix Scutellariae Baicalensis) 10g
Jin Yin Hua (Flos Lonicerae) 10g
Lian Qiao (Fructus Forsythiae Suspensae) 10g
Chan Tui ‡ (Periostracum Cicadae) 6g
Huang Lian (Rhizoma Coptidis) 6g
Gan Cao (Radix Glycyrrhizae) 6g

Third visit
After following this prescription for another fortnight, the itching sensation was gradually alleviated and most purple patches had flattened and turned darker in color. The prescription was modified by adding *Chi Shao* (Radix Paeoniae Rubra) 10g and *Hong Hua* (Flos Carthami Tinctorii) 6g and removing *Huang Lian* (Rhizoma Coptidis), *Qiang Huo* (Rhizoma et Radix Notopterygii) and *Lian Qiao* (Fructus Forsythiae Suspensae).

Outcome
This prescription was taken for a little over a month until the eruption disappeared completely. A follow-up visit a year and a half later found no recurrence. [31]

Literature excerpts

In *Zhu Ren Kang Lin Chuang Jin Yan Ji* [A Collection of Zhu Renkang's Clinical Experiences], it says: "Lichen planus falls into the category of *zi dian feng* (purple patch Wind) in TCM. It is caused by accumulation of Wind-Damp, which transforms into Toxins when retained for a prolonged period; these Toxins are obstructed in the skin and interstices (*cou li*) and lead to Qi stagnation and Blood stasis. This disease should therefore be treated by arresting Wind, drying Dampness, clearing Heat, and relieving Toxicity. *Wu Shao She*‡ (Zaocys Dhumnades) and *Chan Tui*‡ (Periostracum Cicadae) are the chief ingredients for arresting Wind and transforming Toxicity. They are assisted by *Jing Jie* (Herba Schizonepetae Tenuifoliae), *Fang Feng* (Radix Ledebouriellae Divaricatae), *Qiang Huo* (Rhizoma et Radix Notopterygii), and *Bai Zhi* (Radix Angelicae Dahuricae) with their functions of expelling Wind and alleviating itching; and supported by *Huang Lian* (Rhizoma Coptidis), *Huang Qin* (Radix Scutellariae Baicalensis), *Jin Yin Hua* (Flos Lonicerae), *Lian Qiao* (Fructus Forsythiae Suspensae), and *Gan Cao* (Radix Glycyrrhizae) with their functions of clearing Heat and relieving Toxicity. Materia medica with the functions of invigorating the Blood and transforming Blood stasis such as *Tao Ren* (Semen Persicae), *Hong Hua* (Flos Carthami Tinctorii) and *Qian Cao Gen* (Radix Rubiae Cordifoliae) may be added to invigorate the Blood and disperse Wind."

In *Xu Lü He Wai Ke Yi An Yi Hua Ji* [A Collection of Xu Lühe's Medical Records on External Diseases], the author explains: "Densely distributed papules with coarse and thickened skin like moss can be considered as caused by Blood-Dryness generating Wind. Use *Qu Feng Huan Ji Wan* (Pill for Dispelling Wind and Regenerating the Flesh) to moisten Dryness and dispel Wind. Alternate application to the affected area of *Ku Lian Pi Gao* (Chinaberry Bark Paste) and *Xing Ren Gao* (Apricot Kernel Paste) will achieve the effect of moistening Dryness and dispelling Wind because *Ku Lian Pi* (Cortex Meliae Radicis) clears Heat with cold and bitterness and *Xing Ren* (Semen Pruni Armeniacae) diffuses congestion and moistens Dryness."

Modern clinical experience

TREATMENT ACCORDING TO PATTERN IDENTIFICATION

Li identified three patterns for the treatment of lichen planus. [32]

- **Accumulation of Wind, Dampness and Heat**

Treatment principle
Clear Heat and eliminate Dampness.

Prescription ingredients
Ban Lan Gen (Radix Isatidis seu Baphicacanthi) 20g

Huang Qin (Radix Scutellariae Baicalensis) 9g
Zhi Zi (Fructus Gardeniae Jasminoidis) 9g
Bai Xian Pi (Cortex Dictamni Dasycarpi Radicis) 9g
Di Fu Zi (Fructus Kochiae Scopariae) 9g
Chan Tui‡ (Periostracum Cicadae) 9g
Jiang Can‡ (Bombyx Batryticatus) 9g
Sang Zhi (Ramulus Mori Albae) 9g
Ju Hua (Flos Chrysanthemi Morifolii) 9g
Mu Zei (Herba Equiseti Hiemalis) 9g
Cang Er Zi (Fructus Xanthii Sibirici) 9g
Ze Xie (Rhizoma Alismatis Orientalis) 9g
Dang Gui (Radix Angelicae Sinensis) 9g

- **Qi stagnation and Blood stasis**

Treatment principle
Invigorate the Blood and transform Blood stasis.

Prescription ingredients
Huang Qi (Radix Astragali seu Hedysari) 20g
Sheng Di Huang (Radix Rehmanniae Glutinosae) 20g
Shu Di Huang (Radix Rehmanniae Glutinosae Conquita) 20g
Ji Xue Teng (Caulis Spatholobi) 12g
Tao Ren (Semen Persicae) 9g
Hong Hua (Flos Carthami Tinctorii) 9g
Bai Shao (Radix Paeoniae Lactiflorae) 9g
Chuan Xiong (Rhizoma Ligustici Chuanxiong) 9g
Dang Gui (Radix Angelicae Sinensis) 9g
Xiang Fu (Rhizoma Cyperi Rotundi) 9g
Bai Ji Li (Fructus Tribuli Terrestris) 9g
Gan Cao (Radix Glycyrrhizae) 6g

- **Steaming of Damp-Heat** (manifesting in the mouth)

Treatment principle
Fortify the Spleen and benefit the movement of Dampness.

Prescription ingredients
Sheng Di Huang (Radix Rehmanniae Glutinosae) 20g
Xuan Shen (Radix Scrophulariae Ningpoensis) 20g
Dan Zhu Ye (Herba Lophatheri Gracilis) 6g
Tong Cao (Medulla Tetrapanacis Papyriferi) 6g
Chen Pi (Pericarpium Citri Reticulatae) 9g
Huang Lian (Rhizoma Coptidis) 9g
Fu Ling (Sclerotium Poriae Cocos) 12g
Yi Yi Ren (Semen Coicis Lachryma-jobi) 12g
Fa Ban Xia (Rhizoma Pinelliae Ternatae Praeparata) 12g
Gan Cao (Radix Glycyrrhizae) 6g

One bag a day of the ingredients was used to prepare a decoction, taken twice a day. Results were seen after two weeks of treatment.

References

1. Zhang Zhili, *Zhang Zhi Li Pi Fu Bing Lin Chuang Jing Yan Ji Yao* [A Collection of Zhang Zhili's Clinical Experiences in the Treatment of Skin Diseases] (Beijing: China Medical Science and Technology Publishing House, 2001), 264.

2. Zhang Zhili, *Zhang Zhi Li Pi Fu Bing Lin Chuang Jing Yan Ji Yao*, 265.

3. Zhang Zhili, *Zhang Zhi Li Pi Fu Bing Lin Chuang Jing Yan Ji Yao*, 266.

4. Zhang Zhili, *Zhang Zhi Li Pi Fu Bing Lin Chuang Jing Yan Ji Yao*, 267.

5. Zhou Xiaoling, *Zhong Yao Zhi Liao Yin Xie Bing 95 Li* [Treatment of 95 Cases of Psoriasis with Traditional Chinese Medicine], *Liao Ning Zhong Yi Za Zhi* [Liaoning Journal of Traditional Chinese Medicine] 25, 1 (1998): 26.

6. Zhang Xiaowei, *Cong Xue Lun Zhi Xun Chang Xing Yin Xie Bing 86 Li Liao Xiao Guan Cha* [Survey of the Effectiveness of Treatment of 86 Cases of Psoriasis by Treating the Blood], *Bei Jing Zhong Yi* [Beijing Journal of Traditional Chinese Medicine] 5 (1998): 35.

7. Chen Liang, *Yin Xie Bing De Zhong Yi Zheng Zhi* [Diagnosis and Treatment of Psoriasis with Traditional Chinese Medicine], *Shi Yong Zhong Xi Yi Jie He Za Zhi* [Practical Journal of Integrated TCM and Western Medicine] 11, 2 (1998): 175.

8. Liu Yan, *Zhong Yi Zhi Liao Yin Xie Bing 285 Li Liao Xiao Guan Cha* [Observation of the Effectiveness of Treatment of 285 Cases of Psoriasis with Traditional Chinese Medicine], *Pi Fu Bing Yu Xing Bing* [Journal of Skin Diseases and Venereal Diseases] 21, 4 (1999): 25-26.

9. Wang Zhaozi, *Zhong Yao Zhi Liao Yin Xie Bing 210 Li Liao Xiao Guan Cha* [Observation of the Effectiveness of Treatment of 210 Cases of Psoriasis with Chinese Materia Medica], *Pi Fu Bing Yu Xing Bing* [Journal of Skin Diseases and Venereal Diseases] 20, 2 (1998): 31.

10. Lin Chun'ai, *Lei Gong Teng Pian Zhi Liao Xun Chang Xing Yin Xie Bing 78 Li* [Treatment of 78 Cases of Psoriasis Vulgaris with *Lei Gong Teng Pian* (Thunder God Vine Tablet)], *Zhong Guo Pi Fu Xing Bing Xue Za Zhi* [Chinese Journal of Dermatology and Venereology] 9, 3 (1995): 175.

11. Wei Feng, *Wu Shi Qu Feng Tang Zhi Liao Xun Chang Xing Yin Xie Bing 100 Li* [Treatment of 100 Cases of Psoriasis Vulgaris with *Wu She Qu Feng Tang* (Black-Tail Snake Decoction for Expelling Wind)], *Shan Dong Zhong Yi Za Zhi* [Shandong Journal of Traditional Chinese Medicine] 14, 4 (1995): 163-4.

12. Yu Xijiang, *Jie Du Xiao Feng Wan Zhi Liao Yin Xie Bing 826 Li* [Treatment of 826 Cases of Psoriasis with *Jie Du Xiao Feng Wan* (Pill for Relieving Toxicity and Dispersing Wind)], *Shan Dong Zhong Yi Za Zhi* [Shandong Journal of Traditional Chinese Medicine] 15, 1 (1996): 17-18.

13. Su Yongsheng, *Zhong Yao Xiao Yin Ling Xi Lie Zhi Liao Xun Chang Xing Yin Xie Bing 108 Li Liao Xiao Guan Cha* [Survey of the Effectiveness of Treatment of 108 Cases of Psoriasis with the *Xiao Yin Ling* (Marvelous Pill for Dispersing Psoriasis) Series], *Shi Yong Zhong Xi Yi Jie He Za Zhi* [Practical Journal of Integrated TCM and Western

Medicine] 11, 4 (1998): 363-4.

14. Wang Peimao, *Xue Fu Zhu Yu Tang Jia Wei Zhi Liao Yin Xie Bing 23 Li* [Treatment of 23 Cases of Psoriasis with Augmented *Xue Fu Zhu Yu Tang* (Decoction for Expelling Stasis from the House of Blood)], *Si Chuan Zhong Yi* [Sichuan Journal of Traditional Chinese Medicine] 11 (1994): 42.

15. Liu Wenjing, *Liang Xue Jie Du Tang Zhi Liao Xun Chang Xing Yin Xie Bing 106 Li* [Treatment of 106 Cases of Psoriasis Vulgaris with *Liang Xue Jie Du Tang* (Decoction for Cooling the Blood and Relieving Toxicity)], *Shan Dong Zhong Yi Za Zhi* [Shandong Journal of Traditional Chinese Medicine] 16, 1 (1997): 16-17.

16. Zhan Zhaoxin, *Bai Bi Tang He Niu Pi Xuan Xi Ji Zhi Liao Yin Xie Bing 265 Li* [Treatment of 265 Cases of Psoriasis with *Bai Bi Tang* (Psoriasis Decoction) Combined with *Niu Pi Xuan Xi Ji* (Psoriasis Wash Preparation)], *Liao Ning Zhong Yi Za Zhi* [Liaoning Journal of Traditional Chinese Medicine] 25, 7 (1998): 315.

17. Chen Hanzhang, *Zong He Zhi Liao Hong Pi Bing Xing Yin Xie Bing 10 Li Lin Chuang Bao Dao* [Clinical Report on the Complex Treatment of 10 Cases of Erythrodermic Psoriasis], *Xin Zhong Yi* [New Journal of Traditional Chinese Medicine] 29, 10 (1997): 39.

18. Jing Xiamin, *Zhong Xi Yi Jie He Zhi Liao Yin Xie Bing 100 Li Liao Xiao Guan Cha* [Observation of the Effectiveness of Treatment of 100 Cases of Psoriasis with a Combination of TCM and Western Medicine], *Shan Xi Zhong Yi* [Shanxi Journal of Traditional Chinese Medicine] 11, 5 (1995): 27.

19. Li Huang, *Zhong Xi Yi Jie He Zhi Liao Yin Xie Bing 247 Li* [Treatment of 247 Cases of Psoriasis with a Combination of TCM and Western Medicine], *Shi Yong Zhong Xi Yi Jie He Za Zhi* [Practical Journal of Integrated TCM and Western Medicine] 11, 1 (1998): 80.

20. Traditional Chinese Medicine Research Academy: Beijing Guang'anmen Hospital, *Zhu Ren Kang Lin Chuang Jing Yan Ji* [A Collection of Zhu Renkang's Clinical Experiences] (Beijing: People's Medical Publishing House, 1979), 222.

21. Liu Jinxing, *Bi Xie Shen Shi Tang Jia Jian Zhi Liao Zhang Zhi Nong Pao Bing 55 Li* [Treatment of 55 Cases of Palmoplantar Pustulosis with Modified *Bi Xie Shen Shi Tang* (Yam Rhizome Decoction for Percolating Dampness)], *Shan Dong Zhong Yi Za Zhi* [Shandong Journal of Traditional Chinese Medicine] 14, 4 (1995): 164.

22. Zhou Chunying, *Ying Xian Tang Zhi Liao Zhang Zhi Nong Pao Bing De Liao Xiao Guan Cha* [Clinical Observation of the Treatment of Palmoplantar Pustulosis with *Ying Xian Tang* (Dandelion and Purslane Decoction)], *Zhong Hua Pi Fu Ke Za Zhi* [Chinese Journal of Dermatology] 19, 3 (1986): 165-6.

23. Man Lijun, *Shen Bai San Huang Tang Zhi Liao Zhang Zhi Nong Pao Bing* [Treatment of Palmoplantar Pustulosis with *Shen Bai San Huang Tang* (Three Yellows Decoction with Flavescent Sophora Root and Pulsatilla Root)], *Lin Chuang Pi Fu Ke Za Zhi* [Journal of Clinical Dermatology] 27, 3

(1998): 207.

24. Zhao Lixin, *Zi Cao Tang Zhi Liao Mei Gui Kang Zhen 131 Li* [Treatment of 131 Cases of Pityriasis Rosea with *Zi Cao Tang* (Gromwell Root Decoction)], *Zhe Jiang Zhong Yi Za Zhi* [Zhejiang Journal of Traditional Chinese Medicine] 32, 12 (1997): 557.

25. Ma Yuguo, *Liang Xue Xiao Ban Tang Zhi Liao Mei Gui Kang Zhen 147 Li* [Treatment of 147 Cases of Pityriasis Rosea with *Liang Xue Xiao Ban Tang* (Decoction for Cooling the Blood and Dispersing Erythema)], *Zong He Lin Chuang Yi Xue* [Journal of Clinical Medicine] 12, 6 (1996): 283.

26. Traditional Chinese Medicine Research Academy: Beijing Guang'anmen Hospital, *Zhu Ren Kang Lin Chuang Jing Yan Ji*, 224.

27. Zhou Jingfang, *Zi Ni San Dou Yin Zhi Liao Mao Fa Hong Kang Zhen Yi Li* [Treatment of One Case of Pityriasis Rubra Pilaris with the Self-Prepared *San Dou Yin* (Three Bean Decoction)], *Yun Nan Zhong Yi Za Zhi* [Yunnan Journal of Traditional Chinese Medicine] 15, 1 (1994): 27.

28. Hu Ximing (ed.), *Zhong Guo Zhong Yi Mi Fang Da Quan* [Compendium of Secret Prescriptions of Traditional Chinese Medicine] (Shanghai: Wen Hui Publishing House, 1991), 297-9.

29. Zhao Qingli, *Zhong Cao Yao Zhi Liao Ji Xing Dou Chuang Yang Tai Xuan Yang Kang Zhen Jiu Li* [Treatment of Nine Cases of Acute Varioliform Lichenoid Pityriasis with Chinese Materia Medica], *Zhong Hua Pi Fu Ke Za Zhi* [Chinese Journal of Dermatology] 31, 6 (1998): 388-9.

30. Cai Weili, *Zhen Ci Zhi Liao Xian Zhuang Bian Ping Tai Xian Yi Li* [Acupuncture Treatment of One Case of Linear Lichen Planus], *Xin Zhong Yi* [New Journal of Traditional Chinese Medicine] 19, 7 (1987): 39.

31. Traditional Chinese Medicine Research Academy, *Zhong Guo Zhong Yi Yan Jiu Yuan Zhong Yi Shuo Shi Yan Jiu Sheng Lun Wen Ji* [A Collection of Research Theses from TCM Master's Degree Students at the Chinese TCM Research Academy] (Beijing: People's Medical Publishing House, 1997), 456.

32. Li Wenwei, *Bian Zhi Bian Ping Tai Xian 22 Li* [Differential Treatment of 22 Cases of Lichen Planus], *Liao Ning Zhong Yi Za Zhi* [Liaoning Journal of Traditional Chinese Medicine] 11, 9 (1987): 29.

Urticaria and related disorders

The pathogenesis of urticaria and related disorders depends on the release of chemical mediators, the most important of which is histamine. Histamine is contained in the granules of mast cells, large cells in the connective tissue. Degranulation of mast cells occurs through a variety of immunologic and non-immunologic mechanisms, resulting in the release of histamine into the surrounding tissue and the systemic circulation. Histamine release causes vasodilatation resulting in erythema. Contraction of the endothelial cells lining blood vessels opens up spaces between these cells and permits the leakage of intravascular fluid into the surrounding tissues. This causes edema of tissues and wheal formation.

Type I hypersensitivity reactions probably cause most cases of acute urticaria. In this type of reaction, antigens attach to immunoglobulin E (IgE) antibodies bound to the cell membrane. This process results in a series of intracellular reactions which cause mast cell degranulation and histamine release. The response usually occurs within minutes, although may occasionally be delayed.

A less common immunologic reaction, type III hypersensitivity (immune complex-mediated reaction), may also be responsible for some cases of urticaria. In this case, insoluble antigen-antibody complexes are deposited in the walls of small vessels, often those in the skin. Activation of complement occurs, with subsequent release of histamine from the mast cell.

However, it is also important to remember that non-immunologic mechanisms may be responsible for urticaria, especially the "physical" urticarias, when mediators such as opioid drugs, strawberries and shellfish react with the surface of mast cells, resulting in degranulation.

TCM recognizes that the causes of urticarial disorders are complex and varied. They include internal factors such as constitutional insufficiency, Deficiency of Qi and Blood, weakness of Wei Qi (Defensive Qi), or emotional disturbances, and external factors such as invasion by pathogenic Wind or Worms, attack by external Toxins such as substances contained in hair dye or cosmetics, or overintake of spicy and greasy food or seafood, which may transform into Heat and generate internal Wind.

Where external factors predominate, the disease has acute onset and evolves rapidly; where internal factors predominate, the disease will be chronic with frequent recurrences.

Urticaria
荨麻疹

Urticaria (also known as nettle rash or hives) is a common distinctive reaction pattern, characterized by transient, edematous, usually pruritic, wheals of varying sizes and shapes. Most cases of urticaria are an acute reaction, lasting for a few hours or more. However, a minority of patients have chronic urticaria, where the duration of the disease, rather than individual wheals themselves, lasts for more than six weeks. Acute urticaria may be triggered by an allergen in foods, pollen or medical drugs. Allergens may also be the provoking factor in chronic urticaria, but in many cases no cause can be found.

In TCM, this condition is also known as *yin zhen* (dormant papules) or *feng yin zhen* (Wind dormant papules), so named because lesions come and go quickly like wind without leaving marks on the skin.

Clinical manifestations

- Urticaria may occur on any part of the body. Involvement of the throat constitutes an acute medical emergency.
- The disorder may affect people of any age.

- Skin lesions mainly manifest as bright red, pink or milky-white wheals of various shapes, sizes and configurations. Wheals may present with a discrete distribution or form confluent plaques.

- Wheals may manifest at any time, appearing and disappearing swiftly, typically lasting from a few hours to less than a day. New lesions appear as old ones resolve. When they disappear, they usually leave no marks or scars.

- Appearance of the wheals often triggers intense itching. In severe cases, the urticarial rash may involve the whole body and may be accompanied by mucosal involvement; this results in nausea and vomiting, abdominal pain and diarrhea, swelling of the throat (angioedema), and lower respiratory symptoms such as oppression in the chest or dyspnea.

Differential diagnosis

Papular urticaria
Despite the nomenclature, papular urticaria is not a variant of urticaria: rather it represents a reaction to insect bites, possibly of allergic etiology. Papular urticaria is more common in children and usually involves the trunk and limbs. Lesions manifest as short wheals capped by small vesicles. They characteristically occur in irregular lines and clusters and may last for up to two weeks. Scratching may result in some lesions becoming infected and impetiginized.

Erythema multiforme
This disease commonly involves the dorsum of the hands and feet, the palms and soles, and the extensor surfaces of the arm and leg. Lesions take a variety of forms including erythema, papulovesicles, wheals, and vesicles. The typical lesion is circular with a red, slightly raised border and a dark red or purple slightly depressed central area with a small vesicle (also known as a "target" or "iris" lesion). Each episode of erythema multiforme lasts approximately one month, far longer than the few hours typical of urticaria.

Etiology and pathology

The etiology and pathology of urticaria is complex and varied.

Invasion of pathogenic Wind
Invasion of pathogenic Wind is often combined with pathogenic Cold or Heat. When Wind passes through the skin and flesh, it triggers intense itching.

- Wind and Heat settling in the skin and flesh and fighting one another results in disharmony of the Ying and Wei levels; lesions are red due to exuberant Heat obstructing the channels and network vessels.

- After an external invasion of Wind-Cold, these pathogenic factors accumulate in the skin and flesh and block the interstices (*cou li*). Lesions are pale or white due to stagnation in the network vessels.

Emotional factors
Mental stress, anxiety and other emotional factors are considered as causative factors because they can impair the functioning of the Zang-Fu organs, upset the balance of Yin and Yang and lead to disharmony between the Ying and Wei levels. Emotional disturbances and irritability can result in accumulated Heat in the Heart channel, which then transforms into Fire, leading to exuberant Heat in the Blood; this in turn can cause accumulation and obstruction of the channels and network vessels and bring on the symptoms of the disease.

Damage to the Spleen and Stomach
- Excessive intake of fish, seafood or spicy food impairs the transformation and transportation function of the Spleen and Stomach. Dampness accumulates internally and transforms into Heat, when can then stir Wind. When these pathogenic factors cannot be drained internally or thrust outward through the exterior, they are retained in the skin and interstices (*cou li*), thus inducing the disease.

- An unhygienic diet and the generation of Worms results in Worm accumulation damaging the Spleen and Stomach, leading to internal generation of Damp-Heat, which steams to the skin and flesh.

Qi and Blood Deficiency
Underlying constitutional weakness or weakness after a prolonged illness can result in insufficiency of Qi and Blood. When Qi is insufficient, Wei Qi (Defensive Qi) is impaired in its function of consolidating the exterior, and so pathogenic Wind can take advantage of this deficiency and invade the body. When Blood is insufficient, Deficiency-Wind is generated internally, thus depriving the skin and flesh of nourishment and giving rise to itchy skin.

Other factors
Other causative factors include the bites of poisonous insects, contact with pollen, parasitic infestation, and intake of certain medications. Stagnation of Heat Toxins subsequently sets the Ying level ablaze.

Invasion by external factors results in acute urticaria, whereas internal Wind leads to chronic urticaria. If the Manifestations are predominant, the disease has a rapid onset; if the Root is predominant, it recurs frequently and persists for a long time.

A Deficiency pattern is caused by Qi and Blood Deficiency generating Wind, whereas an Excess pattern results from exuberant Heart-Fire with Heat in the

Blood generating Wind, or disharmony of the channels and network vessels leading to Blood stasis generating Wind. A Deficiency-Excess complex is usually the consequence of weakness of Wei Qi (Defensive Qi) or disharmony of the Chong and Ren vessels complicated by an invasion of external Wind. In these circumstances, the disease tends to recur frequently.

Itching is caused by Wind wandering through the skin and flesh; invasion of external Wind results in intense intermittent itching, whereas internal Wind gives rise to constant itching that varies in intensity. Since itching is often the result of a combination of internal and external Wind, its intensity and persistence varies from individual to individual and even between different bouts in the same individual.

Pattern identification and treatment

INTERNAL TREATMENT

WIND AND HEAT FIGHTING ONE ANOTHER

In this pattern with acute onset, red wheals coalesce into plaques of varying configuration. Palpation produces a sensation of burning heat; itching is intense, usually alleviated by cold and aggravated by warmth. Accompanying symptoms and signs include slight fever, aversion to wind, irritability, thirst, and hyperemia of the throat. The tongue body is red with a thin yellow coating or a scant coating; the pulse is floating and rapid.

Treatment principle
Dredge Wind and clear Heat.

Prescription
YIN QIAO SAN JIA JIAN
Honeysuckle and Forsythia Powder, with modifications

Jin Yin Hua (Flos Lonicerae) 12g
Lian Qiao (Fructus Forsythiae Suspensae) 12g
Sheng Di Huang (Radix Rehmanniae Glutinosae) 12g
Chao Niu Bang Zi (Fructus Arctii Lappae, stir-fried) 10g
Da Qing Ye (Folium Isatidis seu Baphicacanthi) 10g
Mu Dan Pi (Cortex Moutan Radicis) 10g
Jing Jie (Herba Schizonepetae Tenuifoliae) 6g
Fang Feng (Radix Ledebouriellae Divaricatae) 6g
Gan Cao (Radix Glycyrrhizae) 6g
Chan Tui‡ (Periostracum Cicadae) 6g

Explanation
- *Jin Yin Hua* (Flos Lonicerae), *Lian Qiao* (Fructus Forsythiae Suspensae) and *Da Qing Ye* (Folium Isatidis seu Baphicacanthi) dissipate Wind-Heat.
- *Sheng Di Huang* (Radix Rehmanniae Glutinosae) and *Mu Dan Pi* (Cortex Moutan Radicis) clear Heat and cool the Blood.

- *Chao Niu Bang Zi* (Fructus Arctii Lappae, stir-fried), *Jing Jie* (Herba Schizonepetae Tenuifoliae), *Fang Feng* (Radix Ledebouriellae Divaricatae), *Gan Cao* (Radix Glycyrrhizae), and *Chan Tui*‡ (Periostracum Cicadae) dissipate Wind and alleviate itching.

Modifications
1. For lesions becoming confluent to form large patches throughout the body, add *Zhi Mu* (Rhizoma Anemarrhenae Asphodeloidis) and *Shi Gao*‡ (Gypsum Fibrosum).
2. For pronounced irritability and thirst, add *Huang Lian* (Rhizoma Coptidis), *Dan Zhu Ye* (Herba Lophatheri Gracilis) and *Mai Men Dong* (Radix Ophiopogonis Japonici).
3. For raised and persistent lesions, add *Dong Gua Pi* (Epicarpium Benincasae Hispidae) and *Tong Cao* (Medulla Tetrapanacis Papyriferi).
4. For intense itching, add *Bai Xian Pi* (Cortex Dictamni Dasycarpi Radicis).

WIND-COLD FETTERING THE EXTERIOR

In this acute onset pattern, wheals are pink or porcelain white in color. Wheals and itching are worse on exposure to wind or contact with cold water but improve on exposure to warmth. Accompanying symptoms and signs include aversion to wind, fear of cold and absence of thirst. The tongue body is pale with a thin white coating; the pulse is floating and tight.

Treatment principle
Dredge Wind and dissipate Cold.

Prescription
MA HUANG TANG JIA JIAN
Ephedra Decoction, with modifications

*Zhi Ma Huang** (Herba Ephedrae, mix-fried with honey) 6g
Gui Zhi (Ramulus Cinnamomi Cassiae) 6g
Chao Bai Zhu (Rhizoma Atractylodis Macrocephalae, stir-fried) 10g
Xing Ren (Semen Pruni Armeniacae) 10g
Qiang Huo (Rhizoma et Radix Notopterygii) 10g
Dang Shen (Radix Codonopsitis Pilosulae) 10g
Zi Su Ye (Folium Perillae Frutescentis) 10g
Da Zao (Fructus Ziziphi Jujubae) 20g
Sheng Jiang (Rhizoma Zingiberis Officinalis Recens) 10g

Explanation
- *Zhi Ma Huang** (Herba Ephedrae, mix-fried with honey), *Gui Zhi* (Ramulus Cinnamomi Cassiae), *Da Zao* (Fructus Ziziphi Jujubae), and *Sheng Jiang* (Rhizoma Zingiberis Officinalis Recens) harmonize the Ying and Wei levels.
- *Chao Bai Zhu* (Rhizoma Atractylodis Macrocephalae, stir-fried) and *Dang Shen* (Radix Codonopsitis Pilosulae)

support the Spleen and augment Qi.

- *Xing Ren* (Semen Pruni Armeniacae), *Qiang Huo* (Rhizoma et Radix Notopterygii) and *Zi Su Ye* (Folium Perillae Frutescentis) dissipate Wind-Cold.

Modification

For generalized lesions, add *Chuan Xiong* (Rhizoma Ligustici Chuanxiong) and *Chi Shao* (Radix Paeoniae Rubra).

RETENTION OF HEAT IN THE HEART CHANNEL

This acute pattern manifests as inflamed wheals with a sensation of burning heat and prickly itching. After scratching, wheals evolve rapidly into linear, scar-like marks and coalesce into patches. Itching is usually more intense at night. Accompanying symptoms and signs include irritability, insomnia and erosion of the mouth and tongue. The tongue body is red with a dark red tip and a scant coating; the pulse is thready and rapid or slippery and rapid.

Treatment principle

Clear Heat from the Heart and cool the Blood, quiet the Spirit and alleviate itching.

Prescription
LIAN ZI QING XIN YIN JIA JIAN

Lotus Seed Beverage for Clearing Heat from the Heart, with modifications

Lian Zi (Semen Nelumbinis Nuciferae) 12g
Di Gu Pi (Cortex Lycii Radicis) 12g
Mai Men Dong (Radix Ophiopogonis Japonici) 12g
Chai Hu (Radix Bupleuri) 6g
Huang Qin (Radix Scutellariae Baicalensis) 6g
Huang Lian (Rhizoma Coptidis) 6g
Dang Shen (Radix Codonopsitis Pilosulae) 10g
Huang Qi (Radix Astragali seu Hedysari) 10g
Gan Cao (Radix Glycyrrhizae) 10g
Tong Cao (Medulla Tetrapanacis Papyriferi) 10g
Dan Zhu Ye (Herba Lophatheri Gracilis) 10g

Explanation

- *Lian Zi* (Semen Nelumbinis Nuciferae), *Dang Shen* (Radix Codonopsitis Pilosulae), *Huang Qi* (Radix Astragali seu Hedysari), and *Gan Cao* (Radix Glycyrrhizae) augment Qi and consolidate the exterior.
- *Di Gu Pi* (Cortex Lycii Radicis), *Mai Men Dong* (Radix Ophiopogonis Japonici) and *Huang Lian* (Rhizoma Coptidis) enrich Yin and reduce Heat.
- *Chai Hu* (Radix Bupleuri) and *Huang Qin* (Radix Scutellariae Baicalensis) free the skin and interstices (*cou li*).
- *Tong Cao* (Medulla Tetrapanacis Papyriferi) and *Dan Zhu Ye* (Herba Lophatheri Gracilis) clear Heat from the Heart and guide out reddish urine to direct Heat downward.

Modifications

1. For lesions coalescing to form large patches, add *Ze Xie* (Rhizoma Alismatis Orientalis) and *Dong Gua Pi* (Epicarpium Benincasae Hispidae).
2. For itching, add *Bai Ji Li* (Fructus Tribuli Terrestris) and *Zhen Zhu Mu* (Concha Margaritifera).

HEAT TOXINS SETTING THE YING LEVEL ABLAZE

Large, red wheals appear suddenly and may spread throughout the body, becoming confluent in some cases. Itching is severe. Accompanying symptoms and signs include raging fever and aversion to cold, thirst with a desire for cold drinks, red face and eyes, irritability and disquiet, constipation, and short voidings of reddish urine. The tongue body is red with a yellow or dry yellow coating; the pulse is surging and rapid.

Treatment principle

Clear Heat from the Ying level and cool the Blood, relieve Toxicity and alleviate itching.

Prescription
PI YAN TANG JIA JIAN

Dermatitis Decoction, with modifications

Sheng Di Huang (Radix Rehmanniae Glutinosae) 10g
Chao Mu Dan Pi (Cortex Moutan Radicis, stir-fried) 10g
Chi Shao (Radix Paeoniae Rubra) 10g
Chao Zhi Mu (Rhizoma Anemarrhenae Asphodeloidis, stir-fried) 10g
Lian Qiao (Fructus Forsythiae Suspensae) 10g
Shi Gao ‡ (Gypsum Fibrosum) 15g
Jin Yin Hua (Flos Lonicerae) 12g
Lü Dou Yi (Cortex Phaseoli Radiati) 12g
Xuan Shen (Radix Scrophulariae Ningpoensis) 9g
Bei Sha Shen (Radix Glehniae Littoralis) 9g
Gan Cao (Radix Glycyrrhizae) 9g
Chi Xiao Dou (Semen Phaseoli Calcarati) 30g

Explanation

- *Sheng Di Huang* (Radix Rehmanniae Glutinosae), *Chao Mu Dan Pi* (Cortex Moutan Radicis, stir-fried) and *Chi Shao* (Radix Paeoniae Rubra) cool and invigorate the Blood.
- *Chao Zhi Mu* (Rhizoma Anemarrhenae Asphodeloidis, stir-fried), *Shi Gao* ‡ (Gypsum Fibrosum), *Xuan Shen* (Radix Scrophulariae Ningpoensis), and *Bei Sha Shen* (Radix Glehniae Littoralis) clear Heat from the Qi level and cool the Ying level.
- *Lian Qiao* (Fructus Forsythiae Suspensae), *Jin Yin Hua* (Flos Lonicerae), *Lü Dou Yi* (Cortex Phaseoli Radiati), *Gan Cao* (Radix Glycyrrhizae), and *Chi Xiao Dou* (Semen Phaseoli Calcarati) clear Heat and relieve Toxicity, invigorate the Blood and reduce erythema.

DISHARMONY OF THE SPLEEN AND STOMACH

Wheals are pale red or flesh-colored, cloud-like in shape. Accompanying symptoms and signs include epigastric and abdominal discomfort or pain, diarrhea, nausea and vomiting, and a poor appetite. The tongue body is pale red with a thin white coating or a scant coating; the pulse is moderate, or deep and weak.

Treatment principle

Fortify the Spleen and harmonize the Stomach, dispel Wind and alleviate itching.

Prescription
ZHI ZHU TANG JIA JIAN

Immature Bitter Orange and White Atractylodes Decoction, with modifications

Chao Zhi Shi (Fructus Immaturus Citri Aurantii, stir-fried) 6g
Sha Ren (Fructus Amomi) 6g, added 5 minutes before the end of the decoction process
Chen Pi (Pericarpium Citri Reticulatae) 6g
Jing Jie (Herba Schizonepetae Tenuifoliae) 6g
Fang Feng (Radix Ledebouriellae Divaricatae) 6g
Chao Bai Zhu (Rhizoma Atractylodis Macrocephalae, stir-fried) 10g
Zhi Xiang Fu (Rhizoma Cyperi Rotundi, mix-fried with alcohol) 10g
Wu Yao (Radix Linderae Strychnifoliae) 10g
*Mu Xiang** (Radix Aucklandiae Lappae) 10g
Gan Cao (Radix Glycyrrhizae) 4.5g
Da Zao (Fructus Ziziphi Jujubae) 15g
Sheng Jiang (Rhizoma Zingiberis Officinalis Recens) 10g

Explanation

- *Chao Zhi Shi* (Fructus Immaturus Citri Aurantii, stir-fried), *Chen Pi* (Pericarpium Citri Reticulatae), *Wu Yao* (Radix Linderae Strychnifoliae), *Mu Xiang** (Radix Aucklandiae Lappae), and *Zhi Xiang Fu* (Rhizoma Cyperi Rotundi, mix-fried with alcohol) loosen the Middle Burner and regulate Qi.
- *Sha Ren* (Fructus Amomi), *Jing Jie* (Herba Schizonepetae Tenuifoliae) and *Fang Feng* (Radix Ledebouriellae Divaricatae) dissipate Wind and alleviate itching.
- *Chao Bai Zhu* (Rhizoma Atractylodis Macrocephalae, stir-fried), *Gan Cao* (Radix Glycyrrhizae), *Da Zao* (Fructus Ziziphi Jujubae), and *Sheng Jiang* (Rhizoma Zingiberis Officinalis Recens) fortify the Spleen and harmonize the Stomach.

WORM ACCUMULATION DAMAGING THE SPLEEN

This pattern mainly affects children. Wheals and itching occur at irregular intervals. Children are usually very thin with a sallow complexion, or suffer from facial pityriasis alba (Worm macules), or have pain in the umbilical region. They may also be partial to certain foods or have a preference for snacks or they may bite their nails. Some children have dental caries. The tongue body is pale red with a thin white coating; the pulse is weak or soggy.

Treatment principle

Fortify the Spleen and disperse accumulation, kill Worms and alleviate itching.

Prescription
XIANG SHA LIU JUN ZI TANG JIA JIAN

Six Gentlemen Decoction with Aucklandia and Amomum, with modifications

Xiang Fu (Rhizoma Cyperi Rotundi) 6g
Sha Ren (Fructus Amomi) 6g, added 5 minutes before the end of the decoction process
Jiang Ban Xia (Rhizoma Pinelliae Ternatae, processed with ginger) 6g
Wu Mei (Fructus Pruni Mume) 6g
Dang Shen (Radix Codonopsitis Pilosulae) 10g
Bai Zhu (Rhizoma Atractylodis Macrocephalae) 10g
Chen Pi (Pericarpium Citri Reticulatae) 10g
Fu Ling (Sclerotium Poriae Cocos) 10g
Shen Qu (Massa Fermentata) 10g
Shan Zha (Fructus Crataegi) 12g
Shi Jun Zi (Fructus Quisqualis Indicae) 12g
Nan Gua Zi (Semen Cucurbitae Moschatae) 12g
Gan Cao (Radix Glycyrrhizae) 4.5g

Explanation

- *Jiang Ban Xia* (Rhizoma Pinelliae Ternatae, processed with ginger), *Dang Shen* (Radix Codonopsitis Pilosulae), *Bai Zhu* (Rhizoma Atractylodis Macrocephalae), *Chen Pi* (Pericarpium Citri Reticulatae), and *Fu Ling* (Sclerotium Poriae Cocos) fortify the Spleen and harmonize the Stomach.
- *Xiang Fu* (Rhizoma Cyperi Rotundi) regulates Qi and disperses accumulation.
- *Wu Mei* (Fructus Pruni Mume), *Shen Qu* (Massa Fermentata), *Shan Zha* (Fructus Crataegi), *Shi Jun Zi* (Fructus Quisqualis Indicae), and *Nan Gua Zi* (Semen Cucurbitae Moschatae) disperse accumulation and kill Worms.
- *Sha Ren* (Fructus Amomi) and *Gan Cao* (Radix Glycyrrhizae) dredge Wind and alleviate itching.
- *Sha Ren* (Fructus Amomi) is very effective in treating urticaria due to disharmony of the Stomach and Intestines.

WEI QI (DEFENSIVE QI) FAILING TO CONSOLIDATE THE EXTERIOR

Skin lesions vary in size from pinpoint to 3 mm. Wheals rarely become confluent. However, groups of wheals may appear if there is exposure to wind when sweating, or aversion to cold due to exterior Deficiency. Itching is intense and incessant. Accompanying symptoms and signs include aversion to wind and spontaneous sweating. The tongue body is pale red with a thin white coating or a scant coating; the pulse is deep and thready.

Treatment principle
Consolidate the exterior and keep out Wind.

Prescription
YU PING FENG SAN JIA JIAN
Jade Screen Powder, with modifications

Huang Qi (Radix Astragali seu Hedysari) 15g
Fang Feng (Radix Ledebouriellae Divaricatae) 10g
Tu Chao Bai Zhu (Rhizoma Atractylodis Macrocephalae, stir-fried with earth) 6g
Gui Zhi (Ramulus Cinnamomi Cassiae) 6g
Chao Bai Shao (Radix Paeoniae Lactiflorae, stir-fried) 6g
Lian Qiao (Fructus Forsythiae Suspensae) 6g
Chi Xiao Dou (Semen Phaseoli Calcarati) 30g
Yi Mu Cao (Herba Leonuri Heterophylli) 12g
Long Gu‡ (Os Draconis) 15g
Mu Li‡ (Concha Ostreae) 15g
Wu Wei Zi (Fructus Schisandrae) 4.5g

Explanation
* *Huang Qi* (Radix Astragali seu Hedysari), *Fang Feng* (Radix Ledebouriellae Divaricatae) and *Tu Chao Bai Zhu* (Rhizoma Atractylodis Macrocephalae, stir-fried with earth) augment Qi and consolidate the exterior.
* *Chao Bai Shao* (Radix Paeoniae Lactiflorae, stir-fried), *Long Gu*‡ (Os Draconis), *Mu Li*‡ (Concha Ostreae), and *Wu Wei Zi* (Fructus Schisandrae) generate Body Fluids and consolidate the exterior.
* *Gui Zhi* (Ramulus Cinnamomi Cassiae), *Lian Qiao* (Fructus Forsythiae Suspensae), *Chi Xiao Dou* (Semen Phaseoli Calcarati), and *Yi Mu Cao* (Herba Leonuri Heterophylli) invigorate the Blood and alleviate itching. This is in accordance with the principle that "to treat Wind, first treat the Blood. If the Blood is circulating smoothly, Wind will be eliminated."

Modification
For spontaneous sweating, add *Fu Xiao Mai* (Fructus Tritici Aestivi Levis) and *Ma Huang Gen* (Radix Ephedrae).

DEFICIENCY OF QI AND BLOOD
Wheals are pale red or flesh-colored, appearing frequently and lingering for months or years, increasing in severity with fatigue. Accompanying symptoms and signs include dizziness, a pale complexion, mental exhaustion, lassitude, and insomnia. The tongue body is pale red with a thin white coating or a scant coating; the pulse is thready and moderate.

Treatment principle
Augment Qi and nourish the Blood.

Prescription
BA ZHEN TANG JIA JIAN
Eight Treasure Decoction, with modifications

Dang Shen (Radix Codonopsitis Pilosulae) 10g
Bai Zhu (Rhizoma Atractylodis Macrocephalae) 10g
Dang Gui (Radix Angelicae Sinensis) 10g
Chao Bai Shao (Radix Paeoniae Lactiflorae, stir-fried) 10g
Fu Ling (Sclerotium Poriae Cocos) 12g
Sheng Di Huang (Radix Rehmanniae Glutinosae) 12g
Shu Di Huang (Radix Rehmanniae Glutinosae Conquita) 12g
Chai Hu (Radix Bupleuri) 6g
Gan Cao (Radix Glycyrrhizae) 6g
Huang Qin (Radix Scutellariae Baicalensis) 6g
E Jiao‡ (Gelatinum Corii Asini) 15g, melted in the prepared decoction

Explanation
* *Dang Shen* (Radix Codonopsitis Pilosulae), *Bai Zhu* (Rhizoma Atractylodis Macrocephalae), *Fu Ling* (Sclerotium Poriae Cocos), and *Gan Cao* (Radix Glycyrrhizae) augment Qi and support the Spleen.
* *Dang Gui* (Radix Angelicae Sinensis), *Chao Bai Shao* (Radix Paeoniae Lactiflorae, stir-fried), *Shu Di Huang* (Radix Rehmanniae Glutinosae Conquita), *Sheng Di Huang* (Radix Rehmanniae Glutinosae), and *E Jiao*‡ (Gelatinum Corii Asini) enrich Yin and supplement the Blood.
* *Chai Hu* (Radix Bupleuri) and *Huang Qin* (Radix Scutellariae Baicalensis) free the exterior and interior.
* Since *E Jiao*‡ (Gelatinum Corii Asini) is also effective in consolidating and astringing the exterior, it is often employed for Deficiency-type urticaria.

DISHARMONY OF THE CHONG AND REN VESSELS
Pale red wheals mainly appear on the lower abdomen, the lumbosacral region and the thighs. They generally become pronounced prior to menstruation, fading gradually thereafter. Accompanying symptoms and signs include menstrual irregularities and abdominal pain during menstruation. The tongue body is normal or pale red with a thin white coating or a scant coating; the pulse is wiry and thready or wiry and slippery.

Treatment principle
Regulate the Chong and Ren vessels.

Prescription
ER XIAN TANG JIA JIAN
Two Immortals Decoction, with modifications

Xian Mao (Rhizoma Curculiginis Orchioidis) 6g
Dang Gui (Radix Angelicae Sinensis) 6g
Chuan Xiong (Rhizoma Ligustici Chuanxiong) 6g
Yin Yang Huo (Herba Epimedii) 12g
Sheng Di Huang (Radix Rehmanniae Glutinosae) 12g

Shu Di Huang (Radix Rehmanniae Glutinosae Conquita) 12g
Tu Si Zi (Semen Cuscutae) 12g
Gou Qi Zi (Fructus Lycii) 12g
Nü Zhen Zi (Fructus Ligustri Lucidi) 12g
Han Lian Cao (Herba Ecliptae Prostratae) 12g
Chao Mu Dan Pi (Cortex Moutan Radicis, stir-fried) 10g
Yi Mu Cao (Herba Leonuri Heterophylli) 10g
Yan Hu Suo (Rhizoma Corydalis Yanhusuo) 10g

Explanation

- *Xian Mao* (Rhizoma Curculiginis Orchioidis), *Yin Yang Huo* (Herba Epimedii), *Shu Di Huang* (Radix Rehmanniae Glutinosae Conquita), and *Tu Si Zi* (Semen Cuscutae) warm Yang and boost the Kidneys, and regulate the Chong and Ren vessels.
- *Dang Gui* (Radix Angelicae Sinensis), *Chuan Xiong* (Rhizoma Ligustici Chuanxiong), *Yi Mu Cao* (Herba Leonuri Heterophylli), and *Yan Hu Suo* (Rhizoma Corydalis Yanhusuo) regulate menstruation and alleviate pain.
- *Gou Qi Zi* (Fructus Lycii), *Nü Zhen Zi* (Fructus Ligustri Lucidi), *Han Lian Cao* (Herba Ecliptae Prostratae), *Chao Mu Dan Pi* (Cortex Moutan Radicis, stir-fried), and *Sheng Di Huang* (Radix Rehmanniae Glutinosae) enrich Yin and reduce erythema.

BLOOD STASIS IN THE CHANNELS AND NETWORK VESSELS

Wheals are dull red or purplish-red and mainly involve the waist and the watch-strap area of the wrist. Accompanying symptoms and signs include a dark complexion, purplish-blue lips and a dry mouth with no desire to drink. The tongue body is dull purple or has stasis marks and a scant coating; the pulse is thready and rough.

Treatment principle

Regulate Qi, invigorate the Blood, and free the channels and network vessels.

Prescription

TONG JING ZHU YU TANG JIA JIAN

Decoction for Freeing the Channels and Expelling Blood Stasis, with modifications

Tao Ren (Semen Persicae) 6g
Chi Shao (Radix Paeoniae Rubra) 6g
Chuan Xiong (Rhizoma Ligustici Chuanxiong) 6g
Di Long ‡ (Lumbricus) 6g
Zao Jiao Ci (Spina Gleditsiae Sinensis) 10g
San Qi (Radix Notoginseng) 10g
Jing Jie (Herba Schizonepetae Tenuifoliae) 10g
Fang Feng (Radix Ledebouriellae Divaricatae) 10g
Dang Gui (Radix Angelicae Sinensis) 12g
Bai Ji Li (Fructus Tribuli Terrestris) 12g
Wu Yao (Radix Linderae Strychnifoliae) 4.5g

Xiang Fu (Rhizoma Cyperi Rotundi) 4.5g
Qing Pi (Pericarpium Citri Reticulatae Viride) 4.5g

Explanation

- *Tao Ren* (Semen Persicae), *Chi Shao* (Radix Paeoniae Rubra), *Di Long* ‡ (Lumbricus), *Zao Jiao Ci* (Spina Gleditsiae Sinensis), and *San Qi* (Radix Notoginseng) transform Blood stasis and dissipate lumps, free the network vessels and alleviate itching.
- *Chuan Xiong* (Rhizoma Ligustici Chuanxiong), *Wu Yao* (Radix Linderae Strychnifoliae), *Xiang Fu* (Rhizoma Cyperi Rotundi), and *Qing Pi* (Pericarpium Citri Reticulatae Viride) regulate Qi and invigorate the Blood.
- *Bai Ji Li* (Fructus Tribuli Terrestris) dispels Wind and alleviates itching.
- *Jing Jie* (Herba Schizonepetae Tenuifoliae), *Fang Feng* (Radix Ledebouriellae Divaricatae) and *Dang Gui* (Radix Angelicae Sinensis) invigorate the Blood and dissipate Wind to reinforce the effect of *Zao Jiao Ci* (Spina Gleditsiae Sinensis) and *San Qi* (Radix Notoginseng) in alleviating itching.

Modification

Where lesions are a brighter red, add *Sheng Di Huang* (Radix Rehmanniae Glutinosae) and *Mu Dan Pi* (Cortex Moutan Radicis).

PATENT HERBAL MEDICINES

- For Wind-Heat patterns, take *Tuo Min Wan Yi Hao* (Desensitization Pill No. 1) 3-5g two or three times a day with warm, boiled water.
- For patterns of Wei Qi (Defensive Qi) failing to consolidate the exterior, take *Tuo Min Wan Er Hao* (Desensitization Pill No. 2) 3-5g two or three times a day with warm, boiled water.

EXTERNAL TREATMENT

- For extensive skin eruptions and intense itching, prepare a decoction with three to five of the following ingredients – *Chu Tao Ye* (Folium Broussonetiae) 50g, *Ku Shen* (Radix Sophorae Flavescentis) 200g, *Wei Ling Xian* (Radix Clematidis) 50g, *Zhang Mu* (Lignum Cinnamomi Camphorae) 200g, *Cang Er Zi* (Fructus Xanthii Sibirici) 30g, *Fu Ping* (Herba Spirodelae Polyrrhizae) 30g, *Lu Lu Tong* (Fructus Liquidambaris) 30g, *Xiang Fu* (Rhizoma Cyperi Rotundi) 30g, *Wu Zhu Yu* (Fructus Evodiae Rutaecarpae) 10g, and *Bai Bu* (Radix Stemonae) 50g – and use as a wash for the affected area once or twice a day.
- For extensive lesions with a sensation of burning heat and prickly itching, rub *Bai Bu Ding* (Stemona Root Tincture) on the affected area two or three times a day.

ACUPUNCTURE

Selection of points on the affected channels

- For Wind invading the Yang channels, select GV-14 Dazhui, SP-10 Xuehai and ST-36 Zusanli.
- For Damp invading the Spleen channel, select BL-20 Pishu, LI-11 Quchi and ST-36 Zusanli.
- For involvement of the Liver channel as a result of Blood-Dryness generating Wind, select SP-6 Sanyinjiao, SP-10 Xuehai and LR-2 Xingjian.

Selection of adjacent points

- For wheals on the head and face, select TB-23 Sizhukong, LI-20 Yingxiang and GB-20 Fengchi.
- For wheals on the abdomen, select CV-12 Zhongwan.
- For wheals in the lumbar region, select BL-13 Feishu and BL-23 Shenshu.
- For wheals on the legs, select ST-32 Futu, GB-31 Fengshi, ST-36 Zusanli, and BL-40 Weizhong.

Selection of points according to etiology

- For wheals due to pathogenic Wind-Heat, select GV-14 Dazhui, GB-20 Fengchi, GV-20 Baihui, and BL-40 Weizhong.
- For wheals caused by disharmony of the Spleen and Stomach, select BL-25 Dachangshu, CV-12 Zhongwan, LI-4 Hegu, and ST-36 Zusanli.

Technique

Apply the reinforcing method for a Deficiency pattern and the reducing method for an Excess pattern. Retain the needles for 10-15 minutes after obtaining Qi. Treat once a day or every other day. A course consists of ten treatment sessions.

Empirical points

Prescription 1: GV-14 Dazhui.
Main condition treated: Acute urticaria.
Technique: Insert the needle to a depth of 0.3-0.5 cun and apply the reducing method, rotating the needle in large amplitude. The needle is not retained. Treat once a day.

Prescription 2: BL-25 Dachangshu.
Main condition treated: Chronic urticaria.
Technique: Insert the needle to a depth of 0.8-1.2 cun and apply the reinforcing method. Retain the needles for 30 minutes after obtaining Qi; during this period, manipulate the needle three to five times. Treat once a day.

Explanation

The points chosen above are based on five treatment principles:

- GV-14 Dazhui, SP-10 Xuehai, GB-20 Fengchi, GB-31 Fengshi, and GV-20 Baihui dissipate Wind and alleviate itching.
- SP-10 Xuehai, LR-2 Xingjian and BL-40 Weizhong invigorate the Blood and free the network vessels.
- CV-12 Zhongwan, BL-23 Shenshu, BL-13 Feishu, SP-6 Sanyinjiao, ST-36 Zusanli, LI-4 Hegu, and BL-25 Dachangshu harmonize the functions of the Zang-Fu organs.
- LI-20 Yingxiang, TB-23 Sizhukong and ST-32 Futu free the channels and network vessels, and diffuse the Qi and Wei levels.
- BL-20 Pishu and LI-11 Quchi fortify the Spleen and eliminate Dampness

COMBINATION OF FILIFORM NEEDLING AND PRICKING TO BLEED THERAPY

Points: GV-14 Dazhui, TB-10 Tianjing, SP-10 Xuehai, GB-39 Xuanzhong, LI-11 Quchi, PC-3 Quze, and BL-40 Weizhong.
Main conditions treated: Chronic urticaria, cholinergic urticaria and cold urticaria.
Technique: Apply the even method to the points and retain the needles for five minutes after obtaining Qi. After the needles are withdrawn, apply electro-acupuncture at PC-3 Quze and BL-40 Weizhong, briefly inserting and withdrawing the needles, then press to cause a little bleeding. Treat once a day.

MOXIBUSTION

Points: LI-4 Hegu, TB-4 Yangchi, LI-11 Quchi, LR-2 Xingjian, ST-36 Zusanli, SP-10 Xuehai, and SP-6 Sanyinjiao.
Main conditions treated: Chronic urticaria and cold urticaria.
Technique: Place a slice of fresh ginger on each point and employ indirect moxibustion with three to five moxa cones. Treat once a day.

EAR ACUPUNCTURE

Main points: Lung and Urticaria.
Auxiliary points

- For cold urticaria, add Brain Point, Occiput and Sympathetic Nerve.
- For urticaria due to Wind-Heat, add Heart and Liver.
- For cholinergic urticaria, add Sympathetic Nerve, Adrenal Gland and Allergy Point.

Technique

Apply the reducing method to these points. Retain the needles for 30 minutes. Treat once a day.

ELECTRO-ACUPUNCTURE AT EAR POINTS

Points: Areas corresponding to the sites of the urticarial lesions (one needle for each site).
Technique: After inserting the needles, apply electro-acupuncture up to the patient's tolerance level. Retain the needles for three to five minutes. Treat once a day.

EAR ACUPUNCTURE WITH SEEDS

Points: Lung, Adrenal Gland, Ear-Shenmen, Endocrine, Allergy Point, and points corresponding to the sites of urticarial lesions.

Technique: Select three or four points each time and attach *Wang Bu Liu Xing* (Semen Vaccariae Segetalis) seeds to them with adhesive tape. Ask the patient to press the seeds for one minute three to five times a day. Change the seeds every three days.

EAR ACUPUNCTURE WITH EMBEDDING OF NEEDLES

Points: Lung, Adrenal Gland, Ear-Shenmen, and points corresponding to the sites of urticarial lesions.

Technique: Insert thumbtack needles into two or three points after routine sterilization. Attach the needles with adhesive tape and retain for one hour in acute cases and up to 72 hours in chronic cases. The treatment can be repeated after an interval of three to four days.

CUPPING THERAPY

Point: Ashi point (where wheals are most densely distributed).

Technique: Wrap *Fang Feng* (Radix Ledebouriellae Divaricatae) 10g and *Xu Chang Qing* (Radix Cynanchi Paniculati) 10g, or *Xu Chang Qing* (Radix Cynanchi Paniculati) 15g, *Ku Shen* (Radix Sophorae Flavescentis) 15g and *Wu Mei* (Fructus Pruni Mume) 15g, in a cloth and decoct in boiling water for 30 minutes. Place a bamboo cup in the decoction and boil for another three to five minutes. Take the cup out and place over the Ashi point quickly while it is still hot. Keep the cup on the point for five to ten minutes. Treat once a day or every two days. Great care should be taken not to scald the patient.

POINT LASER THERAPY

Main point: LI-11 Quchi.

Auxiliary points

- For Wind-Cold fettering the exterior, add ST-36 Zusanli.
- For insufficiency of Yin and Blood, add SP-6 Sanyinjiao and ST-36 Zusanli.
- For disharmony of the Chong and Ren vessels, add SP-6 Sanyinjiao and SP-10 Xuehai.

Technique

Expose each point to a helium-neon laser for one minute. Treat once a day.

Clinical notes

- Urticaria is caused by a variety of factors and can be treated by many methods. As the etiology of this disease is complicated, a single method will not usually achieve a good result. An effective option is to treat Deficiency and Excess at the same time with hot and cold materia medica.
- At onset and in the acute stage, treatment should focus on expelling pathogenic factors; for chronic or recurrent urticaria, treatment should focus on supporting Vital Qi (Zheng Qi).
- For an enduring illness, the emphasis should be put on treating the Kidneys and the network vessels in addition to routine treatment.
- Both acupuncture and cupping therapy are effective in alleviating itching.

Advice for the patient

- Try to identify factors that trigger the disease, such as fish, seafood, nuts, spicy food, alcohol, pollen, feathers, or fur, and avoid ingestion or contact. Any medications which appear to set off the disease should also be avoided.
- If the disease is caused by parasites, treat by expelling or destroying the parasites.
- Increase or decrease the amount of clothing worn in accordance with weather conditions. If onset of the disease is associated with stimulation by cold or heat, it is better to try to adjust the body gradually to the stimulating factor.

Case histories

Case 1

Patient
Female, aged 19.

Clinical manifestations
Three days previously the patient was exposed to strong winds when returning home after swimming. Almost immediately, itchy dark red wheals appeared all over her body; lesions were aggravated by exposure to wind. The patient also began to develop a temperature. Accompanying symptoms and signs included aversion to cold, dry stools and constipation, slightly yellow urine, fatigue, and lack of appetite. However, her general mood had not been affected.

Examination revealed a temperature of 39.6°C and generalized itchy urticarial lesions which had coalesced into plaques that blanched on pressure. The tongue was normal with a thin white coating; the pulse was wiry, slippery and slightly rapid.

Diagnosis
Acute urticaria (*feng yin zhen*).

Pattern identification
Internal Heat complicated by external contraction of Wind-Cold.

Treatment principle

Clear Heat and cool the Blood, dissipate Wind and alleviate itching.

Prescription ingredients

Da Qing Ye (Folium Isatidis seu Baphicacanthi) 30g

Shi Gao‡ (Gypsum Fibrosum) 30g

Ma Huang* (Herba Ephedrae) 5g

Jiu Zhi Da Huang (Radix et Rhizoma Rhei, processed with alcohol) 15g

Zi Cao (Radix Arnebiae seu Lithospermi) 25g

Qian Cao Gen (Radix Rubiae Cordifoliae) 15g

Sheng Di Huang (Radix Rehmanniae Glutinosae) 30g

Bai Mao Gen (Rhizoma Imperatae Cylindricae) 30g

Chi Shao (Radix Paeoniae Rubra) 15g

Bai Xian Pi (Cortex Dictamni Dasycarpi Radicis) 30g

Ku Shen (Radix Sophorae Flavescentis) 25g

Bo He (Herba Menthae Haplocalycis) 15g, added 5 minutes before the end of the decoction process

One bag was used to prepare a decoction, taken twice a day.

Further visits

After one bag of the decoction, the temperature had returned to normal, the skin was less red, itching had diminished, bowel movements were normal, and appetite had improved. The prescription was modified by removing Ma Huang* (Herba Ephedrae), Bai Xian Pi (Cortex Dictamni Dasycarpi Radicis) and Ku Shen (Radix Sophorae Flavescentis), and adding Mu Dan Pi (Cortex Moutan Radicis) 15g and Xuan Shen (Radix Scrophulariae Ningpoensis) 15g.

After drinking another three bags of the decoction, itching had stopped and most of the lesions had disappeared, although a small amount of diffuse erythema remained on the trunk. The treatment principle was amended to include nourishing Yin and cooling the Blood and the second prescription modified by removing Shi Gao‡ (Gypsum Fibrosum), Da Huang (Radix et Rhizoma Rhei) and Bo He (Herba Menthae Haplocalycis) and adding Di Fu Zi (Fructus Kochiae Scopariae) 15g and Huang Qin (Radix Scutellariae Baicalensis) 15g.

Outcome

After drinking another three bags of the decoction, the patient was able to go swimming again without any recurrence of the condition.

Discussion

The symptoms of fatigue, lack of appetite, dry stools and constipation, and slightly yellow urine indicated stagnation of Heat. The patient had swum in cold water and so was open to an attack of Wind-Cold after coming out of the water. The generalized dark red wheals clearly indicated that Heat had already scorched Yin-Blood. Therefore, a small dose of Ma Huang* (Herba Ephedrae) was used to open the pores with warmth and acridity.

Bo He (Herba Menthae Haplocalycis) was used to release the exterior and dispel pathogenic factors with coolness and acridity; Chi Shao (Radix Paeoniae Rubra), Zi Cao (Radix Arnebiae seu Lithospermi), Qian Cao Gen (Radix Rubiae Cordifoliae), Sheng Di Huang (Radix Rehmanniae Glutinosae), and Bai Mao Gen (Rhizoma Imperatae Cylindricae) to cool and invigorate the Blood; Da Qing Ye (Folium Isatidis seu Baphicacanthi) and Shi Gao‡ (Gypsum Fibrosum) to clear Heat and transform Blood stasis; Bai Xian Pi (Cortex Dictamni Dasycarpi Radicis) and Ku Shen (Radix Sophorae Flavescentis) to clear Heat, dispel Dampness and alleviate itching; and Jiu Zhi Da Huang (Radix et Rhizoma Rhei, processed with alcohol) to free the interior and guide out stagnant Heat. The overall formula thus released both the exterior and the interior.

One bag of the decoction returned the temperature to normal, freed the bowels, released pathogenic factors from the exterior, and reduced Heat in the interior. However, Heat had still not been cleared from the Xue level, which required the addition of materia medica for cooling and invigorating the Blood and for clearing Heat and transforming Blood stasis. [1]

Case 2

Patient

Female, aged 40.

Clinical manifestations

The patient had been suffering from chronic urticaria for more than ten years. The disease would manifest as flat, pale red eruptions each time that the patient became overtired or during menstruation. Itching was severe, becoming more intense at night. Accompanying symptoms and signs included a lusterless facial complexion, irritability and insomnia, heat in the palms and soles, fatigue, shortness of breath, dry mouth, and constipation. The current outbreak of the disease had lasted three months. Itchy eruptions followed scratching of the skin. The tongue body was dry and pale red with a thin white coating; the pulse was wiry and thready.

Diagnosis

Chronic urticaria (yin zhen).

Pattern identification

This was a stubborn pattern with Yin and Qi Deficiency and latent Wind due to Blood-Dryness.

Prescription ingredients

He Shou Wu (Radix Polygoni Multiflori) 30g

Can Sha‡ (Excrementum Bombycis Mori) 30g

Dang Gui (Radix Angelicae Sinensis) 15g

Dang Shen (Radix Codonopsitis Pilosulae) 15g

Bai Xian Pi (Cortex Dictamni Dasycarpi Radicis) 15g

Mu Dan Pi (Cortex Moutan Radicis) 15g

Bai Wei (Radix Cynanchi Atrati) 15g

Wu Shao She‡ (Zaocys Dhumnades) 15g

Jiang Can‡ (Bombyx Batryticatus) 15g

Huang Qi (Radix Astragali seu Hedysari) 20g

Hei Zhi Ma (Semen Sesami Indici) 25g

One bag a day was used to prepare a decoction, taken twice a day.

Subsequent visits

After six days of drinking a decoction prepared with the above ingredients, the eruption was receding, the itching was less severe, the constipation had disappeared, and the patient could sleep better. However, the condition was not yet stabilized. The prescription was modified by removing Hei Zhi Ma (Semen Sesami Indici) and a further 20 bags prescribed.

Although the symptoms had basically disappeared, the disease continued to recur in a mild form during menstruation. *Chuan Xiong* (Rhizoma Ligustici Chuanxiong), *Chi Shao* (Radix Paeoniae Rubra), *Bai Shao* (Radix Paeoniae Lactiflorae), and *Shu Di Huang* (Radix Rehmanniae Glutinosae Praeparata) were added to the original prescription to be taken for one week before the period.

After a further three months, the urticaria no longer appeared during menstruation and had not recurred by the time of a follow-up visit six months later. [2]

Case 3
Patient
Male, aged 37.

Clinical manifestations
Three years previously, the patient began to suffer from generalized pruritus and intermittent eruptions after exposure to wind. He attended the outpatient department of a Western medicine hospital, where he was prescribed a course of antihistamines without any obvious effect on his condition. Eruptions had now begun to recur more frequently with accompanying symptoms and signs of itching, aversion to wind, profuse sweating, poor appetite, and disturbed sleep. Examination revealed dry skin and pink urticarial plaques distributed over the trunk and limbs. The tongue body was pale with tooth marks at the margins and a thin white coating; the pulse was floating.

Diagnosis
Chronic urticaria (*yin zhen*).

Pattern identification
Blood Deficiency depriving the skin of nourishment with Wind-Cold fettering the exterior.

Treatment principle
Nourish the Blood, dredge Wind and dissipate Cold.

Prescription ingredients
Wu Jia Pi (Cortex Acanthopanacis Gracilistyli Radicis) 6g
Sang Bai Pi (Cortex Mori Albae Radicis) 15g
Dong Gua Pi (Epicarpium Benincasae Hispidae) 15g
Da Fu Pi (Pericarpium Arecae Catechu) 15g
Bai Xian Pi (Cortex Dictamni Dasycarpi Radicis) 30g
Fu Ling Pi (Cortex Poriae Cocos) 15g
Gui Zhi (Ramulus Cinnamomi Cassiae) 10g
Gan Jiang (Rhizoma Zingiberis Officinalis) 6g
Fu Ping (Herba Spirodelae Polyrrhizae) 10g
Jiang Can ‡ (Bombyx Batryticatus) 10g
Chan Tui ‡ (Periostracum Cicadae) 10g
Ye Jiao Teng (Caulis Polygoni Multiflori) 30g
Dang Gui (Radix Angelicae Sinensis) 10g
Chen Pi (Pericarpium Citri Reticulatae) 10g

One bag a day was used to prepare a decoction, taken twice a day.

Outcome
After drinking 14 bags of the decoction, itching was considerably alleviated and after another 14 bags, the lesions were reduced. The condition resolved after another 28 bags.

Discussion
Since the patient had been suffering from a recurring condition for three years, Yin-Blood had been damaged, as was evident from the tongue and pulse conditions. Insufficiency of Yin-Blood resulted in lack of nourishment of the skin and flesh, whereas Wind-Cold fettering the exterior meant that the defensive exterior was not consolidated and profuse sweating could result. The treatment principle followed was that of nourishing the Blood and dredging Wind with a modified prescription based on *Duo Pi Yin* (Many-Peel Beverage).

In the prescription, *Wu Jia Pi* (Cortex Acanthopanacis Gracilistyli Radicis), *Da Fu Pi* (Pericarpium Arecae Catechu), *Bai Xian Pi* (Cortex Dictamni Dasycarpi Radicis), and *Chen Pi* (Pericarpium Citri Reticulatae) dispel Wind and dissipate Cold; *Dong Gua Pi* (Epicarpium Benincasae Hispidae) and *Fu Ling Pi* (Cortex Poriae Cocos) benefit the movement of water and disperse swelling; *Sang Bai Pi* (Cortex Mori Albae Radicis) clears Heat and diffuses the Lungs and when combined with *Gui Zhi* (Ramulus Cinnamomi Cassiae), *Gan Jiang* (Rhizoma Zingiberis Officinalis), *Ye Jiao Teng* (Caulis Polygoni Multiflori), and *Dang Gui* (Radix Angelicae Sinensis) nourishes the Blood and dissipates Cold; *Fu Ping* (Herba Spirodelae Polyrrhizae), *Chan Tui* ‡ (Periostracum Cicadae) and *Jiang Can* ‡ (Bombyx Batryticatus) are important materia medica for dispelling Wind and alleviating itching. [3]

Case 4
Patient
Female, aged 34.

Clinical manifestations
Eight years ago, the patient started to suffer from itchy skin after exposure to wind postpartum. This was followed by the intermittent appearance of wheals of various sizes with increasingly intense itching. The condition, which was worsened by exposure to cold, made sleeping difficult and led to loss of appetite; itching was unbearable at times. The patient's constitution became weaker over the years. Accompanying symptoms and signs included dizziness, blurred vision, fear of cold, aversion to wind, and sweating brought on by exertion.

Examination revealed emaciation and weakness, dry skin and numerous 1-2 cm urticarial plaques on the limbs and abdomen, slightly elevated above the skin surface. The tongue body was pale with tooth marks at the margins and a thin white coating; the pulse was deep and thready.

Diagnosis
Chronic urticaria (*feng yin zhen*).

Pattern identification
Blood Deficiency depriving the skin of nourishment combined with looseness of the interstices (*cou li*), complicated by external invasion of Wind-Cold.

Treatment principle
Nourish the Blood, dredge Wind and dissipate Cold, augment Qi, consolidate the exterior and alleviate itching.

Prescription ingredients
Dang Gui (Radix Angelicae Sinensis) 10g

Shu Di Huang (Radix Rehmanniae Glutinosae Conquita) 10g
Bai Shao (Radix Paeoniae Lactiflorae) 10g
Ye Jiao Teng (Caulis Polygoni Multiflori) 30g
Huang Qi (Radix Astragali seu Hedysari) 15g
Bai Zhu (Rhizoma Atractylodis Macrocephalae) 10g
Fang Feng (Radix Ledebouriellae Divaricatae) 10g
Fu Ping (Herba Spirodelae Polyrrhizae) 10g
Gui Zhi (Ramulus Cinnamomi Cassiae) 10g
Gan Jiang (Rhizoma Zingiberis Officinalis) 10g
Jiang Can‡ (Bombyx Batryticatus) 10g
Bai Xian Pi (Cortex Dictamni Dasycarpi Radicis) 30g

One bag a day was used to prepare a decoction, taken twice a day.

Outcome
After drinking seven bags of the decoction, itching was alleviated; after another seven bags, most of the wheals had disappeared and the patient felt that her mood was better. The prescription was modified by replacing *Fang Feng* (Radix Ledebouriellae Divaricatae) and *Fu Ping* (Herba Spirodelae Polyrrhizae) by *Fu Ling* (Sclerotium Poriae Cocos) 10g and *Ku Shen* (Radix Sophorae Flavescentis) 15g. After two more 14-day courses, the condition had resolved and had not recurred by the time of a follow-up visit two years later. [4]

Case 5
Patient
Male, aged 31.

Clinical manifestations
The patient had been suffering from wheals all over the body for 14 years. Eruptions were worse in spring and autumn. Itching was intermittent. Although antihistamines improved the condition, it would flare up again as soon as the medication was stopped. The condition had worsened considerably in the past three days. Accompanying symptoms and signs included abdominal pain, loose stools and diarrhea, and oppression in the chest.

Examination revealed slightly raised wheals of various shapes and sizes on the trunk and limbs; some of the wheals had become confluent. Scratch marks with bloody crusts were also evident. The tongue body was pale red with a white coating; the pulse was rapid.

Diagnosis
Acute flare-ups of chronic urticaria.

Pattern identification
External contraction of pathogenic Wind with looseness of the interstices (*cou li*).

Treatment principle
Dredge Wind and alleviate itching.

Prescription ingredients
Ma Huang* (Herba Ephedrae) 4.5g
Jing Jie (Herba Schizonepetae Tenuifoliae) 9g
Fang Feng (Radix Ledebouriellae Divaricatae) 9g
Xing Ren (Semen Pruni Armeniacae) 9g
Bai Xian Pi (Cortex Dictamni Dasycarpi Radicis) 15g
Di Fu Zi (Fructus Kochiae Scopariae) 12g
Jiang Can‡ (Bombyx Batryticatus) 9g

Sang Bai Pi (Cortex Mori Albae Radicis) 10g
Qin Jiao (Radix Gentianae Macrophyllae) 15g
Jin Yin Hua (Flos Lonicerae) 20g
Yin Chen Hao (Herba Artemisiae Scopariae) 15g
Si Gua Luo (Fasciculus Vascularis Luffae) 15g

One bag a day was used to prepare a decoction, taken twice a day.

Outcome
After 34 bags of the decoction, the lesions had been reduced in size and number and itching was less. The patient continued to drink the decoction for another month until lesions and itching disappeared. A follow-up letter after six months indicated that the condition had not recurred.

Discussion
This condition was a Wind-Cold pattern of a chronic disease with acute flare-ups. It was treated by a modified combination of *Ma Huang Tang* (Ephedra Decoction) and *Jing Fang Tang* (Schizonepeta and Ledebouriella Decoction). By dispelling the pathogenic factors responsible, further flare-ups were prevented. [5]

Modern clinical experience

TREATMENT BASED ON PATTERN IDENTIFICATION

1. **Gao** identified four different patterns in a group of 106 patients. [6]

- **Wind-Heat**

Prescription
SAN FENG QING RE YIN JIA JIAN
Beverage for Dissipating Wind and Clearing Heat, with modifications

Jin Yin Hua (Flos Lonicerae) 20g
Bai Xian Pi (Cortex Dictamni Dasycarpi Radicis) 20g
Sheng Di Huang (Radix Rehmanniae Glutinosae) 20g
Chan Tui‡ (Periostracum Cicadae) 15g
Niu Bang Zi (Fructus Arctii Lappae) 15g
Fu Ping (Herba Spirodelae Polyrrhizae) 15g
Chi Shao (Radix Paeoniae Rubra) 15g
Lian Qiao (Fructus Forsythiae Suspensae) 15g
Jie Geng (Radix Platycodi Grandiflori) 10g
Jing Jie Sui (Spica Schizonepetae Tenuifoliae) 10g
Gan Cao (Radix Glycyrrhizae) 10g

- **Damp-Heat**

Prescription
FANG FENG TONG SHENG SAN JIA JIAN
Ledebouriella Powder that Sagely Unblocks, with modifications

Fang Feng (Radix Ledebouriellae Divaricatae) 15g
Ma Huang* (Herba Ephedrae) 15g
Dang Gui (Radix Angelicae Sinensis) 15g
Bai Shao (Radix Paeoniae Lactiflorae) 15g

Zhi Zi (Fructus Gardeniae Jasminoidis) 15g
Huang Qin (Radix Scutellariae Baicalensis) 15g
Shi Gao‡ (Gypsum Fibrosum) 50g
Jing Jie (Herba Schizonepetae Tenuifoliae) 20g
Lian Qiao (Fructus Forsythiae Suspensae) 20g
Bo He (Herba Menthae Haplocalycis) 20g
Jie Geng (Radix Platycodi Grandiflori) 20g
Hua Shi‡ (Talcum) 20g
Gan Cao (Radix Glycyrrhizae) 10g

- **Wind-Cold**

Prescription
QU FENG SAN HAN YIN JIA JIAN
Beverage for Dispelling Wind and Dissipating Cold,
with modifications

Ma Huang* (Herba Ephedrae) 15g
Qiang Huo (Rhizoma et Radix Notopterygii) 15g
Jie Geng (Radix Platycodi Grandiflori) 15g
Jing Jie (Herba Schizonepetae Tenuifoliae) 20g
Fang Feng (Radix Ledebouriellae Divaricatae) 20g
Dang Gui (Radix Angelicae Sinensis) 20g
Bai Zhi (Radix Angelicae Dahuricae) 20g
Fu Ping (Herba Spirodelae Polyrrhizae) 25g
Di Fu Zi (Fructus Kochiae Scopariae) 25g
Bai Xian Pi (Cortex Dictamni Dasycarpi Radicis) 25g

- **Qi and Blood Deficiency**

Prescription
DANG GUI YIN ZI JIA JIAN
Chinese Angelica Root Drink, with modifications

Dang Gui (Radix Angelicae Sinensis) 25g
Sheng Di Huang (Radix Rehmanniae Glutinosae) 25g
Chuan Xiong (Rhizoma Ligustici Chuanxiong) 20g
Huang Qi (Radix Astragali seu Hedysari) 20g
Dang Shen (Radix Codonopsitis Pilosulae) 20g
Bai Ji Li (Fructus Tribuli Terrestris) 20g
Quan Xie‡ (Buthus Martensi) 20g
Fu Ping (Herba Spirodelae Polyrrhizae) 20g
Bai Zhu (Rhizoma Atractylodis Macrocephalae) 15g
He Shou Wu (Radix Polygoni Multiflori) 15g
Jing Jie (Herba Schizonepetae Tenuifoliae) 15g
Fang Feng (Radix Ledebouriellae Divaricatae) 15g

2. **Ding** also identified four different patterns. [7]

- **Wind-Cold**

Prescription ingredients
Ma Huang* (Herba Ephedrae) 10g
Xing Ren (Semen Pruni Armeniacae) 10g
Gan Cao (Radix Glycyrrhizae) 10g
Jing Jie (Herba Schizonepetae Tenuifoliae) 10g
Fang Feng (Radix Ledebouriellae Divaricatae) 10g
Chan Tui‡ (Periostracum Cicadae) 10g

Gui Zhi (Ramulus Cinnamomi Cassiae) 12g
Bai Xian Pi (Cortex Dictamni Dasycarpi Radicis) 30g
Di Fu Zi (Fructus Kochiae Scopariae) 30g
Xu Chang Qing (Radix Cynanchi Paniculati) 30g

- **Wind-Heat**

Prescription ingredients

Jin Yin Hua (Flos Lonicerae) 30g
Sheng Di Huang (Radix Rehmanniae Glutinosae) 30g
Bai Xian Pi (Cortex Dictamni Dasycarpi Radicis) 30g
Lian Qiao (Fructus Forsythiae Suspensae) 15g
Ju Hua (Flos Chrysanthemi Morifolii) 15g
Huang Qin (Radix Scutellariae Baicalensis) 15g
Fang Feng (Radix Ledebouriellae Divaricatae) 10g
Chi Shao (Radix Paeoniae Rubra) 10g
Jing Jie (Herba Schizonepetae Tenuifoliae) 10g
Chan Tui‡ (Periostracum Cicadae) 10g
Gan Cao (Radix Glycyrrhizae) 10g
Mu Dan Pi (Cortex Moutan Radicis) 12g

- **Stomach-Heat**

Prescription ingredients

Jin Yin Hua (Flos Lonicerae) 20g
Jing Jie (Herba Schizonepetae Tenuifoliae) 10g
Fang Feng (Radix Ledebouriellae Divaricatae) 10g
Hou Po (Cortex Magnoliae Officinalis) 10g
Zhi Shi (Fructus Immaturus Citri Aurantii) 10g
Shi Gao‡ (Gypsum Fibrosum) 30g
Di Fu Zi (Fructus Kochiae Scopariae) 30g
Huang Qin (Radix Scutellariae Baicalensis) 15g
Ku Shen (Radix Sophorae Flavescentis) 15g
Tao Ren (Semen Persicae) 6g
Hong Hua (Flos Carthami Tinctorii) 6g
Da Huang (Radix et Rhizoma Rhei) 6g

- **Blood Deficiency**

Prescription ingredients

Dang Gui (Radix Angelicae Sinensis) 15g
He Shou Wu (Radix Polygoni Multiflori) 15g
Di Fu Zi (Fructus Kochiae Scopariae) 15g
Bai Xian Pi (Cortex Dictamni Dasycarpi Radicis) 15g
Sheng Di Huang (Radix Rehmanniae Glutinosae) 20g
Huang Qi (Radix Astragali seu Hedysari) 30g
Chuan Xiong (Rhizoma Ligustici Chuanxiong) 10g
Fang Feng (Radix Ledebouriellae Divaricatae) 10g

3. **Zheng** reported on the identification of three
patterns involving the Blood. [8]

- **Blood Deficiency complicated by invasion of Wind**

Prescription ingredients

Chi Shao (Radix Paeoniae Rubra) 12g
Bai Shao (Radix Paeoniae Lactiflorae) 12g

Sheng Di Huang (Radix Rehmanniae Glutinosae) 12g
Dang Gui (Radix Angelicae Sinensis) 12g
Xing Ren (Semen Pruni Armeniacae) 12g
*Ma Huang** (Herba Ephedrae) 15g
Lian Qiao (Fructus Forsythiae Suspensae) 15g
Huang Qi (Radix Astragali seu Hedysari) 18g
Chuan Xiong (Rhizoma Ligustici Chuanxiong) 9g
Fang Feng (Radix Ledebouriellae Divaricatae) 9g
Chi Xiao Dou (Semen Phaseoli Calcarati) 30g
Gan Cao (Radix Glycyrrhizae) 3g

- **Blood-Heat complicated by invasion of Wind**

Prescription ingredients

Fu Ping (Herba Spirodelae Polyrrhizae) 9g
Fang Feng (Radix Ledebouriellae Divaricatae) 9g
Jing Jie (Herba Schizonepetae Tenuifoliae) 9g
Sheng Di Huang (Radix Rehmanniae Glutinosae) 18g
Chi Shao (Radix Paeoniae Rubra) 18g
Mu Dan Pi (Cortex Moutan Radicis) 12g
Fang Feng (Radix Ledebouriellae Divaricatae) 9g
Gui Zhi (Ramulus Cinnamomi Cassiae) 9g
Sheng Jiang (Rhizoma Zingiberis Officinalis Recens) 9g
Zhi Gan Cao (Radix Glycyrrhizae, mix-fried with honey) 6g

- **Deficiency of the Middle Burner complicated by invasion of Wind-Cold**

Prescription ingredients

Huang Qi (Radix Astragali seu Hedysari) 30g
Gui Zhi (Ramulus Cinnamomi Cassiae) 9g
Sheng Jiang (Rhizoma Zingiberis Officinalis Recens) 9g
Sheng Ma (Rhizoma Cimicifugae) 9g
Bai Shao (Radix Paeoniae Lactiflorae) 18g
Zhi Gan Cao (Radix Glycyrrhizae, mix-fried with honey) 6g
Da Zao (Fructus Ziziphi Jujubae) 12g
Dang Gui (Radix Angelicae Sinensis) 12g
Ge Gen (Radix Puerariae) 12g
Yi Tang (Saccharum Granorum) 30g

For Deficiency patterns, the writer used *Dang Gui Bu Xue Tang* (Chinese Angelica Root Decoction for Supplementing the Blood) as an essential formula for augmenting Qi and nourishing the Blood to extinguish Wind.

4. **Han** divided chronic urticaria cases into two groups based on pattern identification. [9]

- **Insufficiency of Yin-Blood leading to Wind-Dryness due to Blood Deficiency**

Treatment principle
Enrich Yin and nourish the Blood, moisten Dryness and dispel Wind to alleviate itching.

Prescription ingredients

Sheng Di Huang (Radix Rehmanniae Glutinosae) 15g

Shu Di Huang (Radix Rehmanniae Glutinosae Conquita) 15g
Mai Men Dong (Radix Ophiopogonis Japonici) 10g
Dang Gui (Radix Angelicae Sinensis) 10g
He Shou Wu (Radix Polygoni Multiflori) 15g
Bai Ji Li (Fructus Tribuli Terrestris) 15g
Fu Ping (Herba Spirodelae Polyrrhizae) 6g
Fang Feng (Radix Ledebouriellae Divaricatae) 6g
Huang Qi (Radix Astragali seu Hedysari) 15g

- **Spleen and Lung Deficiency complicated by Wind-Cold fettering the exterior**

Treatment principle
Fortify the Spleen and boost the Lungs, dispel Wind and dissipate Cold to alleviate itching.

Prescription ingredients

Bai Zhu (Rhizoma Atractylodis Macrocephalae) 10g
Fu Ling (Sclerotium Poriae Cocos) 10g
Bei Sha Shen (Radix Glehniae Littoralis) 10g
Huang Qi (Radix Astragali seu Hedysari) 15g
Sang Bai Pi (Cortex Mori Albae Radicis) 15g
Di Gu Pi (Cortex Lycii Radicis) 15g
Gan Jiang (Rhizoma Zingiberis Officinalis) 6g
Gui Zhi (Ramulus Cinnamomi Cassiae) 6g
Fang Feng (Radix Ledebouriellae Divaricatae) 6g

An intracutaneous test on allergens in 96 other patients produced a positive reaction in 73 cases. Shellfish, seafood and chillis had the highest positive rate.

5. **Chen** also varied the treatment of chronic urticaria according to pattern identification. [10]

- **Wind-Dryness due to Blood Deficiency**

Treatment principle
Nourish the Blood and dispel Wind.

Prescription
DANG GUI YIN ZI JIA JIAN
Chinese Angelica Root Drink, with modifications

Dang Gui (Radix Angelicae Sinensis) 6-10g
Chuan Xiong (Rhizoma Ligustici Chuanxiong) 6-10g
Shu Di Huang (Radix Rehmanniae Glutinosae Conquita) 20-30g
Huang Qi (Radix Astragali seu Hedysari) 20-30g
Chi Shao (Radix Paeoniae Rubra) 10-15g
He Shou Wu (Radix Polygoni Multiflori) 10-15g
Huang Qin (Radix Scutellariae Baicalensis) 10-15g
Bai Ji Li (Fructus Tribuli Terrestris) 10-20g
Jing Jie (Herba Schizonepetae Tenuifoliae) 10g
Fang Feng (Radix Ledebouriellae Divaricatae) 10g

- **Wind-Damp-Heat**

Treatment principle
Dispel Wind, clear Heat and eliminate Dampness.

Prescription
HUO TAN MU YIN JIA JIAN
Chinese Smartweed Beverage, with modifications

Huo Tan Mu (Herba Polygoni Chinensis) 15-30g
Shi Wei (Folium Pyrrosiae) 15-30g
Yin Chen Hao (Herba Artemisiae Scopariae) 15-20g
Bai Ji Li (Fructus Tribuli Terrestris) 10-20g
Chan Tui‡ (Periostracum Cicadae) 10g
Ku Shen (Radix Sophorae Flavescentis) 10g
Huang Qin (Radix Scutellariae Baicalensis) 10-15g
Di Fu Zi (Fructus Kochiae Scopariae) 10-15g
Bai Hua She She Cao (Herba Hedyotidis Diffusae) 20-30g
Huang Jing Ye (Folium Viticis Negundinis) 20-30g
Huang Jing Gen (Radix Viticis Negundinis) 20-30g

- **Kidney Deficiency**

Treatment principle
Boost the Kidneys, dispel Wind and relieve Toxicity.

Prescription
LIU WEI DI HUANG WAN JIA JIAN
Six-Ingredient Rehmannia Pill, with modifications

Shu Di Huang (Radix Rehmanniae Glutinosae Conquita) 30g
Shan Zhu Yu (Fructus Corni Officinalis) 10-15g
Shan Yao (Radix Dioscoreae Oppositae) 10-15g
Mu Dan Pi (Cortex Moutan Radicis) 10-15g
Zhu Ling (Sclerotium Polypori Umbellati) 12g
Ba Qia (Rhizoma Smilacis Chinensis) 20-30g
Bai Ji Li (Fructus Tribuli Terrestris) 10-20g
Fang Feng (Radix Ledebouriellae Divaricatae) 10-20g

Modifications to Kidney Deficiency prescription
1. For predominance of Kidney Yin Deficiency, *Zhi Mu* (Rhizoma Anemarrhenae Asphodeloidis) and *Huang Bai* (Cortex Phellodendri) were added and *Sheng Di Huang* (Radix Rehmanniae Glutinosae) was used to replace *Shu Di Huang* (Radix Rehmanniac Glutinosae Conquita).
2. For predominance of Kidney Yang Deficiency, *Yin Yang Huo* (Herba Epimedii), *Xian Mao* (Rhizoma Curculiginis Orchioidis), *Rou Gui* (Cortex Cinnamomi Cassiae), and *Gu Sui Bu* (Rhizoma Drynariae) were added.

For each pattern, one bag a day was used to prepare a decoction, taken twice a day. The course of treatment lasted four weeks, at the end of which most patients had responded.

SPECIAL PRESCRIPTIONS

ACUTE URTICARIA

1. **Wang** treated acute urticaria due to Wind-Heat with his own formulation. [11]

Prescription
KANG QIAN TANG
Anti-Urticaria Decoction

Jing Jie (Herba Schizonepetae Tenuifoliae) 10g
Fang Feng (Radix Ledebouriellae Divaricatae) 10g
Mu Dan Pi (Cortex Moutan Radicis) 10g
Chi Shao (Radix Paeoniae Rubra) 10g
Lian Qiao (Fructus Forsythiae Suspensae) 10g
Sheng Di Huang (Radix Rehmanniae Glutinosae) 15g
Chao Suan Zao Ren (Semen Ziziphi Spinosae, stir-fried) 15g
Jin Yin Hua (Flos Lonicerae) 20g
Ye Jiao Teng (Caulis Polygoni Multiflori) 20g
Bai Xian Pi (Cortex Dictamni Dasycarpi Radicis) 12g
Bai Ji Li (Fructus Tribuli Terrestris) 12g
Chan Tui‡ (Periostracum Cicadae) 9g
Gan Cao (Radix Glycyrrhizae) 6g

Modifications
1. For intense itching, *Jiang Can*‡ (Bombyx Batryticatus) 9g was added.
2. For constipation, *Da Huang* (Radix et Rhizoma Rhei) 6g was added.
3. For loose stools, *Fu Ling* (Sclerotium Poriae Cocos) 15g was added.

One bag a day was used to prepare a decoction, taken twice a day. Results were seen within two to nine days of treatment.

2. **Ma** also prepared his own prescription to treat acute urticaria due to Wind-Heat. [12]

Prescription
XIAO ZHEN ZHI YANG TANG
Decoction for Dispersing Eruptions and Alleviating Itching

Di Fu Zi (Fructus Kochiae Scopariae) 30g
Jin Yin Hua (Flos Lonicerae) 30g
Jing Jie (Herba Schizonepetae Tenuifoliae) 15g
Fang Feng (Radix Ledebouriellae Divaricatae) 15g
Niu Bang Zi (Fructus Arctii Lappae) 15g
Chan Tui‡ (Periostracum Cicadae) 15g
Fu Ping (Herba Spirodelae Polyrrhizae) 15g
Tao Ren (Semen Persicae) 15g
Dang Gui (Radix Angelicae Sinensis) 15g
Bo He (Herba Menthae Haplocalycis) 10g
Hong Hua (Flos Carthami Tinctorii) 10g
Chuan Xiong (Rhizoma Ligustici Chuanxiong) 10g
Gan Cao (Radix Glycyrrhizae) 10g

Modification
For Damp-Heat signs, *Ku Shen* (Radix Sophorae Flavescentis) 10g and *Bai Xian Pi* (Cortex Dictamni Dasycarpi Radicis) 15g were added.

3. **Chen** treated urticaria with his own formulation. [13]

Prescription
GU BEN CHU FENG TANG
Decoction for Consolidating the Root and Eliminating Wind

Huang Qi (Radix Astragali seu Hedysari) 30g
Bai Zhu (Rhizoma Atractylodis Macrocephalae) 20g
Fu Ling (Sclerotium Poriae Cocos) 25g
Dang Gui (Radix Angelicae Sinensis) 25g
Chuan Xiong (Rhizoma Ligustici Chuanxiong) 15g
Gui Zhi (Ramulus Cinnamomi Cassiae) 10g
Di Fu Zi (Fructus Kochiae Scopariae) 10g
She Chuang Zi (Fructus Cnidii Monnieri) 10g
Fang Feng (Radix Ledebouriellae Divaricatae) 9g
Sheng Jiang (Rhizoma Zingiberis Officinalis Recens) 12g
Da Zao (Fructus Ziziphi Jujubae) 15g

One bag a day was used to prepare a decoction, taken in the morning and evening. Results were better if the patient sweated slightly after drinking the decoction. Acute cases began to respond after two to four bags, chronic cases after seven to ten bags.

4. **Fang** reported on the following formulation. [14]

Prescription
TONG XIE SHU FENG TANG
Decoction for Freeing the Bowels, Discharging Heat and Dredging Wind

Da Huang (Radix et Rhizoma Rhei) 10g
Jing Jie (Herba Schizonepetae Tenuifoliae) 10g
Zhi Zi (Fructus Gardeniae Jasminoidis) 10g
Mu Dan Pi (Cortex Moutan Radicis) 10g
Gan Cao (Radix Glycyrrhizae) 15-30g
Bai Ji Li (Fructus Tribuli Terrestris) 10-20g
Yi Yi Ren (Semen Coicis Lachryma-jobi) 20g
Chi Shao (Radix Paeoniae Rubra) 10-15g
Ye Jiao Teng (Caulis Polygoni Multiflori) 20-30g

During the treatment, patients were advised to abstain from spicy, fatty, sweet, and rich food. Out of 53 patients receiving this treatment, only three failed to respond. The time required for eruptions and itching to disappear varied from seven days to three months.

5. **Ye** reported on his treatment of acute urticaria. [15]

Prescription
ZHI ZHU CHI DOU YIN
Bitter Orange, White Atractylodes and Aduki Bean Beverage

Chao Bai Zhu (Rhizoma Atractylodis Macrocephalae, stir-fried) 10g
Chao Zhi Ke (Fructus Citri Aurantii, stir-fried) 10g

Chan Tui ‡ (Periostracum Cicadae) 10g
Chi Shao (Radix Paeoniae Rubra) 10g
Fang Feng (Radix Ledebouriellae Divaricatae) 10g
Jing Jie (Herba Schizonepetae Tenuifoliae) 10g
Fu Ling Pi (Cortex Poriae Cocos) 12g
Chi Xiao Dou (Semen Phaseoli Calcarati) 12g
Dong Gua Pi (Epicarpium Benincasae Hispidae) 12g

Modifications
1. For Qi Deficiency, *Huang Qi* (Radix Astragali seu Hedysari) and *Dang Shen* (Radix Codonopsitis Pilosulae) were added.
2. For Heat signs, *Jin Yin Hua* (Flos Lonicerae) and *Lian Qiao* (Fructus Forsythiae Suspensae) were added.
3. For obvious Cold signs, *Ma Huang** (Herba Ephedrae) and *Gui Zhi* (Ramulus Cinnamomi Cassiae) were added.
4. For Dampness, *Hou Po* (Cortex Magnoliae Officinalis) and *Yi Yi Ren* (Semen Coicis Lachryma-jobi) were added.
5. For severe itching, *Di Fu Zi* (Fructus Kochiae Scopariae), *She Chuang Zi* (Fructus Cnidii Monnieri) and *Qian Li Guang* (Herba Senecionis Scandentis) were added.

CHRONIC URTICARIA

1. **Lü** treated chronic urticaria with a modified formula. [16]

Prescription
BU YANG HUAN WU TANG JIA JIAN
Five-Returning Decoction for Supplementing Yang, with modifications

Huang Qi (Radix Astragali seu Hedysari) 20g
Chi Shao (Radix Paeoniae Rubra) 15g
Dang Gui (Radix Angelicae Sinensis) 15g
Di Long ‡ (Lumbricus) 10g
Tao Ren (Semen Persicae) 10g
Hong Hua (Flos Carthami Tinctorii) 10g
Chuan Xiong (Rhizoma Ligustici Chuanxiong) 10g
Jing Jie (Herba Schizonepetae Tenuifoliae) 10g
Fang Feng (Radix Ledebouriellae Divaricatae) 10g
Quan Xie ‡ (Buthus Martensi) 10g

Modifications
1. If the condition worsened on exposure to cold, *Gui Zhi* (Ramulus Cinnamomi Cassiae) 10g was added.
2. If the condition worsened on exposure to heat, *Mu Dan Pi* (Cortex Moutan Radicis) 10g and *Sheng Di Huang* (Radix Rehmanniae Glutinosae) 10g were added.
3. For conditions complicated by Damp-Heat, *Huang Qin* (Radix Scutellariae Baicalensis) 10g, *Ku Shen* (Radix Sophorae Flavescentis) 10g, *Bai Xian Pi* (Cortex Dictamni Dasycarpi Radicis) 10g, and *Tu Fu Ling* (Rhizoma Smilacis Glabrae) 15g were added.

4. For intestinal worms, *Shi Jun Zi* (Fructus Quisqualis Indicae) 10g and *Bing Lang** (Semen Arecae Catechu) 10g were added.
5. If the condition had persisted for a long time and was severe, *Chuan Shan Jia** (Squama Manitis Pentadactylae) 10g, *Zao Jiao Ci* (Spina Gleditsiae Sinensis) 10g and *Wu Shao She‡* (Zaocys Dhumnades) 10g were added.

2. **Ying** proposed the following treatment for chronic urticaria. [17]

Prescription
XIAO ZHEN TANG
Decoction for Dispersing Eruptions

Dang Gui (Radix Angelicae Sinensis) 10g
Chi Shao (Radix Paeoniae Rubra) 10g
Chuan Xiong (Rhizoma Ligustici Chuanxiong) 8g
Chan Tui‡ (Periostracum Cicadae) 8g
Sheng Di Huang (Radix Rehmanniae Glutinosae) 12g
Huang Qi (Radix Astragali seu Hedysari) 5g
She Tui‡ (Exuviae Serpentis) 6g
Fang Feng (Radix Ledebouriellae Divaricatae) 6g
Gan Cao (Radix Glycyrrhizae) 5g

Modifications
1. For intense itching, *Di Fu Zi* (Fructus Kochiae Scopariae) 20g was added.
2. For persistent, non-healing cases, *Jiang Can‡* (Bombyx Batryticatus) 10g was added.

One bag a day was used to prepare a decoction, taken three times a day (morning, lunchtime and evening). Seven days constituted a course of treatment and one or two courses were needed to see results.

3. **Zhao** used *Dang Gui Yin Zi* (Chinese Angelica Root Drink) to treat chronic urticaria. [18]

Prescription ingredients

Dang Gui (Radix Angelicae Sinensis) 18g
Sheng Di Huang (Radix Rehmanniae Glutinosae) 12g
Chuan Xiong (Rhizoma Ligustici Chuanxiong) 12g
Zhi Huang Qi (Radix Astragali seu Hedysari, mix-fried with honey) 30g
Bai Ji Li (Fructus Tribuli Terrestris) 15g
Zhi He Shou Wu (Radix Polygoni Multiflori Praeparata) 15g
Chi Shao (Radix Paeoniae Rubra) 10g
Jing Jie (Herba Schizonepetae Tenuifoliae) 10g
Fang Feng (Radix Ledebouriellae Divaricatae) 10g
Gan Cao (Radix Glycyrrhizae) 6g

Modifications
1. For exuberant Wind, *Chan Tui‡* (Periostracum Cicadae) and *Hei Zhi Ma* (Semen Sesami Indici) were added.
2. For exuberant Heat, *Jin Yin Hua* (Flos Lonicerae), *Pu Gong Ying* (Herba Taraxaci cum Radice) and *Zi Hua Di Ding* (Herba Violae Yedoensitis) were added.
3. For severe Dampness, *Cang Zhu* (Rhizoma Atractylodis) and *Ze Xie* (Rhizoma Alismatis Orientalis) were added.
4. For Yin depletion, *Yu Zhu* (Rhizoma Polygonati Odorati) and *Gou Qi Zi* (Fructus Lycii) were added.
5. For Qi and Blood Deficiency, *Tai Zi Shen* (Radix Pseudostellariae Heterophyllae) was added and *Shu Di Huang* (Radix Rehmanniae Glutinosae Conquita) was used instead of *Sheng Di Huang* (Radix Rehmanniae Glutinosae).

A course of treatment lasted two weeks. Three out of 52 patients failed to respond to treatment after two courses.

4. **Liu** proposed internal treatment accompanied by a steam-wash to treat chronic urticaria. [19]

Prescription
TUO MIN XIAO ZHEN TANG
Desensitization Decoction for Dispersing Eruptions

Jing Jie (Herba Schizonepetae Tenuifoliae) 12g
Fang Feng (Radix Ledebouriellae Divaricatae) 12g
Chi Shao (Radix Paeoniae Rubra) 12g
Di Fu Zi (Fructus Kochiae Scopariae) 12g
Jiang Can‡ (Bombyx Batryticatus) 12g
Dang Gui (Radix Angelicae Sinensis) 12g
Fu Ping (Herba Spirodelae Polyrrhizae) 20g
Sheng Di Huang (Radix Rehmanniae Glutinosae) 20g
Bai Xian Pi (Cortex Dictamni Dasycarpi Radicis) 20g
Chan Tui‡ (Periostracum Cicadae) 10g
Mu Dan Pi (Cortex Moutan Radicis) 15g
Long Gu‡ (Os Draconis) 15g, decocted for 30 minutes before adding the other ingredients
Mu Li‡ (Concha Ostreae) 30g, decocted for 30 minutes before adding the other ingredients

One bag a day was used to prepare a decoction, taken twice a day. A course consisted of seven days of treatment.

Internal treatment was accompanied by a decoction prepared for steam-washing the affected area twice a day with the following ingredients:

Ku Shen (Radix Sophorae Flavescentis) 30g
Di Fu Zi (Fructus Kochiae Scopariae) 30g
She Chuang Zi (Fructus Cnidii Monnieri) 30g

Results were seen after four weeks.

5. **Jin** reported on his treatment of chronic urticaria. [20]

Prescription
XIAO ZHEN YIN
Beverage for Dispersing Eruptions

*Ma Huang** (Herba Ephedrae) 10g
Dang Gui (Radix Angelicae Sinensis) 12g

Fang Feng (Radix Ledebouriellae Divaricatae) 12g
Huang Qin (Radix Scutellariae Baicalensis) 12g
Gan Cao (Radix Glycyrrhizae) 12g
Wu Shao She‡ (Zaocys Dhumnades) 15g
Di Fu Zi (Fructus Kochiae Scopariae) 15g
Jing Jie (Herba Schizonepetae Tenuifoliae) 15g
Mu Dan Pi (Cortex Moutan Radicis) 15g
Bai Shao (Radix Paeoniae Lactiflorae) 15g
Bai Ji Li (Fructus Tribuli Terrestris) 18g
Sheng Di Huang (Radix Rehmanniae Glutinosae) 18g
Xuan Shen (Radix Scrophulariae Ningpoensis) 18g

Modifications

1. For predominance of Wind-Cold, *Gui Zhi* (Ramulus Cinnamomi Cassiae) 10g was added and *Huang Qin* (Radix Scutellariae Baicalensis) removed.
2. For predominance of Wind-Heat, *Zhi Zi* (Fructus Gardeniae Jasminoidis) 12g and *Ju Hua* (Flos Chrysanthemi Morifolii) 10g were added.
3. For older patients with a weak constitution, *He Shou Wu* (Radix Polygoni Multiflori) 15g and *Huang Qi* (Radix Astragali seu Hedysari) 15g were added.
4. For exuberant Wind, *Chan Tui*‡ (Periostracum Cicadae) 6g was added.

COMBINED TCM AND WESTERN MEDICINE

1. **Liu** established three treatment groups. [21]
- The first group of 96 patients was treated with TCM and Western medicine.

TCM treatment consisted of the application of a medicated paste to acupuncture points.

Paste ingredients

Chuan Xiong (Rhizoma Ligustici Chuanxiong) 30g
Qiang Huo (Rhizoma et Radix Notopterygii) 30g
Di Long‡ (Lumbricus) 10g
Rou Gui (Cortex Cinnamomi Cassiae) 10g

Modifications

1. For Wind-Cold patterns, *Ma Huang** (Herba Ephedrae) 10g and *Xi Xin* (Herba cum Radice Asari) 10g were added.
2. For Wind-Heat patterns, *Huang Qin* (Radix Scutellariae Baicalensis) 10g and *Jin Yin Hua* (Flos Lonicerae) 20g were added.
3. For insufficiency of Yin-Blood, *Huang Qi* (Radix Astragali seu Hedysari) 15g and *Dang Gui* (Radix Angelicae Sinensis) 15g were added.

The ingredients were ground into a fine powder and sieved through an 80-mesh screen. For each treatment, 16-24g of the mixture (a reduced amount for children) was mixed into a paste with an appropriate quantity of mature vinegar and divided into eight slices for application to GB-31 Fengshi, LI-11 Quchi, BL-17 Geshu, and SP-10 Xuehai (all bilateral). The slices were attached to the point by adhesive tape for 24 hours and the treatment given once every three days. A course consisted of five treatment sessions.

For the **Western medicine treatment**, patients were given the antihistamine diphenhydramine 25mg via oral administration for 15 days.

- The second group of 36 patients was treated according to pattern identification:

- **Wind-Cold**

Prescription
MA HUANG FANG
Zhao Bingnan's Ephedra Formula

*Ma Huang** (Herba Ephedrae) 3g
Xing Ren (Semen Pruni Armeniacae) 6g
Gan Jiang (Rhizoma Zingiberis Officinalis) 3g
Fu Ping (Herba Spirodelae Polyrrhizae) 3g
Bai Xian Pi (Cortex Dictamni Dasycarpi Radicis) 15g
Chen Pi (Pericarpium Citri Reticulatae) 9g
Mu Dan Pi (Cortex Moutan Radicis) 9g
Dan Shen (Radix Salviae Miltiorrhizae) 15g
Jiang Can‡ (Bombyx Batryticatus) 9g

- **Wind-Heat**

Prescription
SANG JU YIN
Mulberry Leaf and Chrysanthemum Beverage

Sang Ye (Folium Mori Albae) 9g
Ju Hua (Flos Chrysanthemi Morifolii) 9g
Xing Ren (Semen Pruni Armeniacae) 9g
Jie Geng (Radix Platycodi Grandiflori) 9g
Gan Cao (Radix Glycyrrhizae) 3g
Bo He (Herba Menthae Haplocalycis) 3g
Lian Qiao (Fructus Forsythiae Suspensae) 9g
Lu Gen (Rhizoma Phragmitis Communis) 12g

- **Insufficiency of Yin-Blood**

Prescription
DANG GUI YIN ZI
Chinese Angelica Root Drink

Dang Gui (Radix Angelicae Sinensis) 15g
Sheng Di Huang (Radix Rehmanniae Glutinosae) 12g
Bai Shao (Radix Paeoniae Lactiflorae) 9g
Chuan Xiong (Rhizoma Ligustici Chuanxiong) 9g
He Shou Wu (Radix Polygoni Multiflori) 15g
Jing Jie (Herba Schizonepetae Tenuifoliae) 6g
Fang Feng (Radix Ledebouriellae Divaricatae) 6g
Bai Ji Li (Fructus Tribuli Terrestris) 15g
Huang Qi (Radix Astragali seu Hedysari) 12g
Gan Cao (Radix Glycyrrhizae) 9g

For each pattern, one bag a day was used to prepare a

decoction, taken twice a day. A course of treatment consisted of 15 days.

- The third group of 36 patients was given the same Western medication as the first group, but without any TCM treatment.

Clinical results in the first group were significantly better than those of the second and third groups.

2. **Huang** divided 78 patients at random into two groups. [22]

- A comparison group of 38 patients was prescribed 60mg of terfenadine and 150 mg of ranitidine for oral administration three times per day for 14 days. Once the wheals were brought under control, the medication was reduced to once a day for seven days, and then to once every two days for another week.
- The other group of 40 patients was treated with Chinese materia medica in addition to the Western medication.
  - For Wei Qi (Defensive Qi) failing to consolidate the exterior, a prescription based on *Yu Ping Feng San* (Jade Screen Powder) was used.
  - For internal Heat due to Yin Deficiency, a prescription based on *Liu Wei Di Huang Wan* (Six-Ingredient Rehmannia Pill) was used.
  - For Damp-Heat patterns, a prescription based on *Tu Ling Yin Chen Tang* (Glabrous Green Briar and Oriental Wormwood Decoction) was used.

Results for the TCM/Western medicine group were better than those for the control group.

OTHER TREATMENT METHODS

1. Combination of Chinese materia medica and acupuncture

Wu treated acute urticaria by combining internal treatment with acupuncture. [23]

Internal prescription ingredients

Dang Gui (Radix Angelicae Sinensis) 15g
Huang Qi (Radix Astragali seu Hedysari) 15g
Chi Shao (Radix Paeoniae Rubra) 15g
Di Long ‡ (Lumbricus) 15g
Dan Shen (Radix Salviae Miltiorrhizae) 20g

Jiang Can ‡ (Bombyx Batryticatus) 6g
Bo He (Herba Menthae Haplocalycis) 6g
Fang Feng (Radix Ledebouriellae Divaricatae) 10g
Niu Bang Zi (Fructus Arctii Lappae) 10g
Di Fu Zi (Fructus Kochiae Scopariae) 12g

One bag a day was used to prepare a decoction, taken twice a day.

Acupuncture point prescription

Main points: PC-6 Neiguan, GB-20 Fengchi and ST-36 Zusanli.

Auxiliary points

- For intense itching, HT-7 Shenmen was added.
- For severe Heat, Ear Apex was added.
- For severe Cold, GV-14 Dazhui was added.
- For Qi and Blood Deficiency, SP-10 Xuehai was added.

Technique: The points were needled with the even method, with the needles being retained for 20 minutes. Treatment was given once a day. A course consisted of five treatment sessions.

2. Acupuncture treatment of acute urticaria

Wu treated acute urticaria by needling LI-11 Quchi and SP-10 Xuehai (both bilateral). The needles were retained for 15-30 minutes after obtaining Qi and manipulated every two to three minutes. Treatment was given once a day and seven days made up a course. Seven out of 85 patients failed to respond to this treatment. [24]

3. Acupuncture plus cupping therapy

Gu treated urticaria with a combination of acupuncture and cupping therapy. [25]

Main point: CV-8 Shenque.

Auxiliary points: LI-11 Quchi and SP-10 Xuehai; for stubborn cases, GV-14 Dazhui, BL-13 Feishu, BL-20 Pishu, BL-18 Ganshu, ST-36 Zusanli, and SP-6 Sanyinjiao were added.

Technique: Two or three auxiliary points were used for each treatment session, with cupping therapy applied to all the points needled. Treatment was given once a day and ten days made up a course.

Cold urticaria
寒冷性荨麻疹

Urticaria can be caused by physical stimuli with attacks generally lasting less than an hour. Dermographism is the commonest form of physical urticaria. Other types include cold urticaria, where wheals develop after exposure to cold; cholinergic urticaria caused by strenuous exercise, heat or anxiety; and solar urticaria occurring after exposure to the sun. Delayed pressure urticaria is rarer and takes longer to appear than the other physical urticarias, manifesting as deep swellings occurring up to six hours after physical stimulus and lasting for up to three days. This chapter discusses cold urticaria and dermographism.

In cold urticaria, patients develop wheals in areas exposed to the cold. Infection or emotional stress may be predisposing factors.

Clinical manifestations

- Skin eruptions mainly occur on exposed areas, such as the face and limbs. In severe cases, the mouth, tongue and throat will also be involved, with the condition manifesting as mucosal angioedema.
- Wheals are pale red and become more apparent on exposure to cold water or a sudden drop in air temperature.
- Accompanying symptoms include cold limbs, abdominal pain or joint pain.
- The diagnosis may be confirmed by immersing a limb in cold water or placing an ice cube against the skin.

Etiology and pathology

When Yang Qi is depleted or Deficient, Wei Qi is impaired in its defensive function. A sudden invasion of Wind-Cold results in retention of pathogenic factors in the skin and flesh, thus causing urticaria.

Pattern identification and treatment

INTERNAL TREATMENT

SPLEEN YANG DEFICIENCY

Wheals usually occur on the limbs, worsening on contact with cold and alleviating on contact with heat. The tongue body is pale with a scant coating; the pulse is soggy and thready.

Treatment principle
Augment Qi and warm Yang.

Prescription
ZAI ZAO SAN JIA JIAN
Renewal Powder, with modifications

Gan Jiang (Rhizoma Zingiberis Officinalis) 10g
Gui Zhi (Ramulus Cinnamomi Cassiae) 10g
Bai Shao (Radix Paeoniae Lactiflorae) 10g
Dang Shen (Radix Codonopsitis Pilosulae) 10g
Qiang Huo (Rhizoma et Radix Notopterygii) 10g
Fang Feng (Radix Ledebouriellae Divaricatae) 12g
Huang Qi (Radix Astragali seu Hedysari) 12g
Zi Su Ye (Folium Perillae Frutescentis) 10g
Chuan Xiong (Rhizoma Ligustici Chuanxiong) 6g
Zhi Gan Cao (Radix Glycyrrhizae, mix-fried with honey) 6g
Sheng Jiang (Rhizoma Zingiberis Officinalis Recens) 10g

Explanation

- *Gan Jiang* (Rhizoma Zingiberis Officinalis), *Gui Zhi* (Ramulus Cinnamomi Cassiae) and *Zi Su Ye* (Folium Perillae Frutescentis) warm Yang and dissipate Cold.
- *Bai Shao* (Radix Paeoniae Lactiflorae), *Dang Shen* (Radix Codonopsitis Pilosulae), *Huang Qi* (Radix Astragali seu Hedysari), *Gan Cao* (Radix Glycyrrhizae), and *Sheng Jiang* (Rhizoma Zingiberis Officinalis Recens) augment Qi and support the Spleen.
- *Qiang Huo* (Rhizoma et Radix Notopterygii), *Fang Feng* (Radix Ledebouriellae Divaricatae) and *Chuan Xiong* (Rhizoma Ligustici Chuanxiong) dispel Wind and alleviate itching.

KIDNEY YANG DEFICIENCY

Wheals usually occur in winter and persist for a long time. Accompanying symptoms and signs include a pale facial complexion, cold limbs and fatigue. The tongue body is pale with a scant coating; the pulse is deep and thready.

Treatment principle
Warm the Kidneys and consolidate the exterior.

Prescription
YOU GUI YIN JIA JIAN
Restoring the Right [Kidney Yang] Beverage, with modifications

Fu Pen Zi (Fructus Rubi Chingii) 12g
Shu Di Huang (Radix Rehmanniae Glutinosae Conquita) 12g
Fu Shen (Sclerotium Poriae Cocos cum Ligno Hospite) 12g
Shan Zhu Yu (Fructus Corni Officinalis) 12g

Shan Yao (Radix Dioscoreae Oppositae) 10g
Gou Qi Zi (Fructus Lycii) 10g
Lu Jiao‡ (Cornu Cervi) 10g
Rou Gui (Cortex Cinnamomi Cassiae) 6g
Huang Qi (Radix Astragali seu Hedysari) 15g
Xu Chang Qing (Radix Cynanchi Paniculati) 30g

Explanation

- *Fu Pen Zi* (Fructus Rubi Chingii), *Lu Jiao*‡ (Cornu Cervi), *Rou Gui* (Cortex Cinnamomi Cassiae), *Huang Qi* (Radix Astragali seu Hedysari), and *Xu Chang Qing* (Radix Cynanchi Paniculati) augment Qi and warm the Kidneys, dissipate Cold and alleviate itching.

- *Shu Di Huang* (Radix Rehmanniae Glutinosae Conquita), *Shan Zhu Yu* (Fructus Corni Officinalis), *Fu Shen* (Sclerotium Poriae Cocos cum Ligno Hospite), *Shan Yao* (Radix Dioscoreae Oppositae), and *Gou Qi Zi* (Fructus Lycii) emolliate the Liver and enrich the Kidneys to prevent acrid and hot materia medica damaging Yin.

General modifications

1. For intense itching, add *Bai Ji Li* (Fructus Tribuli Terrestris) and *Di Long*‡ (Lumbricus).
2. For disharmony of the Chong and Ren vessels, add *Xian Mao* (Rhizoma Curculiginis Orchioidis) and *Yin Yang Huo* (Herba Epimedii).
3. For insomnia and profuse dreaming, add *Ye Jiao Teng* (Caulis Polygoni Multiflori), *Zhen Zhu Mu*‡ (Concha Margaritifera) and *Mu Li*‡ (Concha Ostreae).

PATENT HERBAL MEDICINES AND OTHER INTERNAL TREATMENT

- For Deficiency of the Spleen and Kidneys, take both *Shen Ling Bai Zhu Wan* (Ginseng, Poria and White Atractylodes Pill) and *Jin Kui Shen Qi Wan* (Kidney Qi Pill from the Golden Cabinet), 6g of each twice a day.
- Once the disease has been stabilized, take *Ren Shen Gu Ben Wan* (Ginseng Pill for Consolidating the Root) 6g twice a day to consolidate the improvement.
- Take *Er Shi Yi Hao Tang Jiang* (Syrup No. 21), made by covering 500g of *Xu Chang Qing* (Radix Cynanchi Paniculati) with six times the amount of water and decocting down to 1000ml. Add a little sugar to the prepared decoction. Drink 15-20ml of the decoction two or three times a day.

MOXIBUSTION

Main point: GV-14 Dazhui.
Auxiliary points: ST-36 Zusanli and BL-23 Shenshu.
Technique: Apply moxibustion with a moxa stick for five to ten minutes once a day. A course consists of seven treatment sessions.

Point functions: Moxibustion at these points warms Yang and consolidates the exterior.
Indications: Moxibustion can be applied as supplementary therapy if the condition recurs often.

Clinical notes

This disease possesses hereditary characteristics and responds slowly to treatment.

Advice for the patient

Try to avoid contact with cold water or intake of cold drinks during the treatment.

Literature excerpt

According to *Xu Yi Hou Pi Fu Bing Lin Chuang Jing Yan Ji Yao* [A Summary of Xu Yihou's Clinical Experiences in the Treatment of Skin Diseases]: "Insufficiency of Yuan Qi (Original Qi) impairs the functioning of Wei Qi (Defensive Qi), thus allowing external pathogenic factors to invade. *Si Jun Zi Tang* (Four Gentlemen Decoction) is therefore used as the basis of a prescription for augmenting Qi with warmth and sweetness. *Huang Qi* (Radix Astragali seu Hedysari) and *Fang Feng* (Radix Ledebouriellae Divaricatae) are added to augment Wei Qi and consolidate the exterior; *E Jiao*‡ (Gelatinum Corii Asini) is added to supplement and nourish the Blood; *Chen Pi* (Pericarpium Citri Reticulatae), *Mu Xiang** (Radix Aucklandiae Lappae) and *Wu Yao* (Radix Linderae Strychnifoliae) are added to regulate Spleen Qi and prevent the accumulation of Dampness as well as to assist *Huang Qi* (Radix Astragali seu Hedysari) and *E Jiao*‡ (Gelatinum Corii Asini) to supplement without causing stagnation; in this way, the body will become strong enough to drive out the pathogenic factors. *Yi Mu Cao* (Herba Leonuri Heterophylli) is also needed to invigorate the Blood in accordance with the principle that 'to treat Wind, first treat the Blood. If the Blood is circulating smoothly, Wind will be eliminated.' Although treatment of this disease should focus on augmenting Qi with sweet and warm materia medica, the stress should also be put on strengthening Wei Qi (Defensive Qi) and regulating the Spleen and Stomach, which can therefore be considered as another principle for the treatment of cold urticaria."

Modern clinical experience

Si modified *Yang He Tang* (Harmonious Yang Decoction) to treat cold urticaria. [26]

Prescription ingredients

Ma Huang* (Herba Ephedrae) 5g

Pao Jiang (Rhizoma Zingiberis Officinalis Praeparata) 5g

Hong Hua (Flos Carthami Tinctorii) 10g

Bai Jie Zi (Semen Sinapis Albae) 10g

Shu Di Huang (Radix Rehmanniae Glutinosae Conquita) 12g

Gui Zhi (Ramulus Cinnamomi Cassiae) 12g

Lu Jiao Shuang‡ (Cornu Cervi Degelatinatum) 15g

Jing Jie (Herba Schizonepetae Tenuifoliae) 15g

Fang Feng (Radix Ledebouriellae Divaricatae) 15g

Huang Qi (Radix Astragali seu Hedysari) 18g

Zhi Gan Cao (Radix Glycyrrhizae, mix-fried with honey) 6g

Modifications

1. For aching and cold pain in the lumbar region, cold limbs and chills, *Fu Zi** (Radix Lateralis Aconiti Carmichaeli Praeparata) 10g and *Gou Ji** (Rhizoma Cibotii Barometz) 15g were added.

2. For cyanosis of the extremities, *Sang Zhi* (Ramulus Mori Albae) 10g and *Dan Shen* (Radix Salviae Miltiorrhizae) 12g were added.

3. For relatively severe itching, *Wu Shao She* ‡ (Zaocys Dhumnades) 15g and *Quan Xie* ‡ (Buthus Martensi) 5g were added.

Dermographism
人工性荨麻疹

In dermographism, mast cells in the skin release additional histamine after rubbing or scratching. The condition can be reproduced in the clinic by stroking the skin of the back with a blunt object.

Clinical manifestations

- The condition may occur at any age.
- Wheals usually appear at a location that has recently been rubbed or scratched or in areas under pressure from tight garments or belts.
- Rubbing or scratching produces linear wheals with itching and a sensation of burning heat.
- Wheals generally fade in 15 to 60 minutes.

Etiology and pathology

The prerequisite condition for this disease is a weak constitution and looseness of the interstices (*cou li*). If external Wind takes advantage of this weakness to invade, it is retained in the skin and flesh to result in Blood-Heat. Over time, Blood-Heat causes the Blood to coagulate and stagnate in the vessels and the disease develops.

Pattern identification and treatment

INTERNAL TREATMENT

BLOOD-HEAT

A linear wheal appears shortly after the skin is scratched, with the wheal following the path made by the scratch. A sensation of burning heat and prickly itching is experienced. Accompanying symptoms and signs include erosion of the mouth and tongue, or two menstrual periods within one month. The tongue body is red with a scant coating; the pulse is thready and rapid.

Treatment principle
Cool the Blood and disperse Wind.

Prescription
LIANG XUE XIAO FENG SAN JIA JIAN
Powder for Cooling the Blood and Dispersing Wind, with modifications

Sheng Di Huang (Radix Rehmanniae Glutinosae) 30g

Shi Gao ‡ (Gypsum Fibrosum) 30g

Dang Gui (Radix Angelicae Sinensis) 10g

Bai Ji Li (Fructus Tribuli Terrestris) 10g

Zi Cao (Radix Arnebiae seu Lithospermi) 10g

Chi Shao (Radix Paeoniae Rubra) 10g

Xuan Shen (Radix Scrophulariae Ningpoensis) 10g

Zhi Mu (Rhizoma Anemarrhenae Asphodeloidis) 10g

Jing Jie (Herba Schizonepetae Tenuifoliae) 6g

Chan Tui ‡ (Periostracum Cicadae) 6g

Tao Ren (Semen Persicae) 6g

Hong Hua (Flos Carthami Tinctorii) 6g

Gan Cao (Radix Glycyrrhizae) 6g

Explanation

- *Sheng Di Huang* (Radix Rehmanniae Glutinosae), *Shi Gao* ‡ (Gypsum Fibrosum), *Zi Cao* (Radix Arnebiae seu Lithospermi), *Chi Shao* (Radix Paeoniae Rubra), *Xuan Shen* (Radix Scrophulariae Ningpoensis), and *Zhi Mu* (Rhizoma Anemarrhenae Asphodeloidis) clear Heat from the Qi level and cool the Blood.

- *Bai Ji Li* (Fructus Tribuli Terrestris), *Jing Jie* (Herba Schizonepetae Tenuifoliae) and *Chan Tui*‡ (Periostracum Cicadae) dredge Wind and alleviate itching.
- *Dang Gui* (Radix Angelicae Sinensis), *Gan Cao* (Radix Glycyrrhizae), and small doses of *Tao Ren* (Semen Persicae) and *Hong Hua* (Flos Carthami Tinctorii) reduce erythema and balance the effect of the Blood-cooling ingredients, while assisting *Bai Ji Li* (Fructus Tribuli Terrestris), *Jing Jie* (Herba Schizonepetae Tenuifoliae) and *Chan Tui*‡ (Periostracum Cicadae) to alleviate itching.

WIND-HEAT

Itching is marked, especially at night when the body is exposed to heat. Discrete, raised, linear wheals appear after scratching. The tongue body is red with a thin yellow coating; the pulse is thready and rapid.

Treatment principle
Dredge Wind and clear Heat.

Prescription
WU SHE QU FENG TANG JIA JIAN
Black-Tail Snake Decoction for Expelling Wind, with modifications

Xu Chang Qing (Radix Cynanchi Paniculati) 10g
Jing Jie (Herba Schizonepetae Tenuifoliae) 10g
Fang Feng (Radix Ledebouriellae Divaricatae) 10g
Qiang Huo (Rhizoma et Radix Notopterygii) 10g
Lian Qiao (Fructus Forsythiae Suspensae) 10g
Chan Tui‡ (Periostracum Cicadae) 6g
Ku Shen (Radix Sophorae Flavescentis) 6g
Huang Qin (Radix Scutellariae Baicalensis) 6g
Huang Lian (Rhizoma Coptidis) 6g
Gan Cao (Radix Glycyrrhizae) 3g

Explanation
- *Xu Chang Qing* (Radix Cynanchi Paniculati), *Jing Jie* (Herba Schizonepetae Tenuifoliae), *Fang Feng* (Radix Ledebouriellae Divaricatae), *Qiang Huo* (Rhizoma et Radix Notopterygii), *Chan Tui*‡ (Periostracum Cicadae), and *Ku Shen* (Radix Sophorae Flavescentis) arrest Wind and dissipate pathogenic factors, disperse Wind and alleviate itching.
- *Lian Qiao* (Fructus Forsythiae Suspensae), *Huang Qin* (Radix Scutellariae Baicalensis), *Huang Lian* (Rhizoma Coptidis), and *Gan Cao* (Radix Glycyrrhizae) drain Fire with bitterness and acridity, relieve Toxicity and clear Heat.

BLOOD STASIS

Lesions in this pattern tend to last longer than in the other two patterns. Scratching or just stroking the skin may lead immediately to raised red wheals. The tongue body is dark red; the pulse is thready and choppy.

Treatment principle
Invigorate the Blood and dispel Wind.

Prescription
TAO HONG SI WU TANG JIA JIAN
Peach Kernel and Safflower Four Agents Decoction, with modifications

Dang Gui Wei (Extremitas Radicis Angelicae Sinensis) 10g
Chi Shao (Radix Paeoniae Rubra) 10g
Tao Ren (Semen Persicae) 10g
Hong Hua (Flos Carthami Tinctorii) 10g
Jing Jie (Herba Schizonepetae Tenuifoliae) 10g
Fang Feng (Radix Ledebouriellae Divaricatae) 10g
Jin Yin Hua (Flos Lonicerae) 10g
Mu Dan Pi (Cortex Moutan Radicis) 6g
Chan Tui‡ (Periostracum Cicadae) 6g
Wu Wei Zi (Fructus Schisandrae) 6g
Qian Cao Gen (Radix Rubiae Cordifoliae) 6g

Explanation
- *Dang Gui Wei* (Extremitas Radicis Angelicae Sinensis), *Chi Shao* (Radix Paeoniae Rubra), *Tao Ren* (Semen Persicae), *Hong Hua* (Flos Carthami Tinctorii), *Mu Dan Pi* (Cortex Moutan Radicis), and *Qian Cao Gen* (Radix Rubiae Cordifoliae) invigorate the Blood and transform Blood stasis, cool the Blood and reduce erythema.
- *Jing Jie* (Herba Schizonepetae Tenuifoliae), *Fang Feng* (Radix Ledebouriellae Divaricatae) and *Chan Tui*‡ (Periostracum Cicadae) dissipate Wind and alleviate itching.
- *Jin Yin Hua* (Flos Lonicerae) and *Wu Wei Zi* (Fructus Schisandrae) relieve Toxicity and clear Heat, while promoting contraction of the sweat pores.

Modifications to this prescription
1. Where the condition is complicated by Wind-Cold, add *Zi Su Ye* (Folium Perillae Frutescentis) and *Gui Zhi* (Ramulus Cinnamomi Cassiae).
2. Where the condition is complicated by Wind-Dryness, add *He Shou Wu* (Radix Polygoni Multiflori) and *Gou Qi Zi* (Fructus Lycii).
3. Where the condition is complicated by severe Dampness, add *Hou Po* (Cortex Magnoliae Officinalis), *Che Qian Zi* (Semen Plantaginis) and *Ze Xie* (Rhizoma Alismatis Orientalis).
4. For Blood Deficiency, add *Huang Qi* (Radix Astragali seu Hedysari) and *E Jiao*‡ (Gelatinum Corii Asini).
5. For Qi Deficiency, add *Huang Qi* (Radix Astragali seu Hedysari) and *Dang Shen* (Radix Codonopsitis Pilosulae).
6. For Spleen Deficiency, add *Bai Zhu* (Rhizoma Atractylodis Macrocephalae) and *Fu Ling* (Sclerotium Poriae Cocos).
7. For intense itching, add *Xu Chang Qing* (Radix Cynanchi Paniculati) and *Ye Jiao Teng* (Caulis Polygoni Multiflori).

8. For disharmony of the Chong and Ren vessels, add *Xian Mao* (Rhizoma Curculiginis Orchioidis) and *Yin Yang Huo* (Herba Epimedii).
9. For a Cold-Heat complex, add *Huang Lian* (Rhizoma Coptidis) and *Gan Jiang* (Rhizoma Zingiberis Officinalis).

EAR ACUPUNCTURE
Main point: Heart.
Auxiliary points: Liver, Endocrine and Sympathetic Nerve.
Technique: Retain the needles for 30 minutes. Treat once every two days.

Case history

Patient
Male, aged 40.

Clinical manifestations
For the previous ten years, the patient had experienced recurrent bouts of itching; scratching produced large patches of intermittent erythema that was worse in the morning and evening and was especially bad during winter nights. Internal administration of corticosteroids and antihistamines proved ineffective. Accompanying symptoms and signs included fatigue, poor appetite, insomnia, profuse dreaming, mental confusion, palpitations, and night sweating. Examination revealed scratch marks with bloody crusts distributed over the trunk and limbs; in some places, the skin had become rough and lichenified. The tongue body was pale with a white coating; the pulse was moderate.

Pattern identification
Weakness of Wei Qi (Defensive Qi) due to Heart and Spleen Deficiency.

Treatment principle
Nourish the Blood and quiet the Spirit, augment Qi and consolidate the exterior.

Prescription ingredients
Huang Qi (Radix Astragali seu Hedysari) 10g
Sheng Di Huang (Radix Rehmanniae Glutinosae) 10g
Bai Shao (Radix Paeoniae Lactiflorae) 15g
Mai Men Dong (Radix Ophiopogonis Japonici) 10g
Ye Jiao Teng (Caulis Polygoni Multiflori) 30g
Zhen Zhu Mu‡ (Concha Margaritifera) 30g

Gou Teng (Ramulus Uncariae cum Uncis) 10g
Bai Ji Li (Fructus Tribuli Terrestris) 30g
Wu Jia Pi (Cortex Acanthopanacis Gracilistyli Radicis) 10g
Sang Bai Pi (Cortex Mori Albae Radicis) 15g
Di Gu Pi (Cortex Lycii Radicis) 15g
Chi Fu Ling (Sclerotium Poriae Cocos Rubrae) 15g
Dong Gua Pi (Epicarpium Benincasae Hispidae) 15g
Bai Xian Pi (Cortex Dictamni Dasycarpi Radicis) 30g
Gan Jiang (Rhizoma Zingiberis Officinalis) 10g
Jiang Can‡ (Bombyx Batryticatus) 10g

One bag a day was used to prepare a decoction, taken twice a day.

Outcome
After seven bags of the decoction, itching was reduced and attacks occurred less frequently; small red wheals still arose after scratching. After another seven bags, sleep had improved and palpitations and night sweating had moderated. The patient was given another 14 bags, after which itching and lesions had disappeared. [27]

Modern clinical experience

Cai used *Xiao Zhen Tang* (Decoction for Dispersing Eruptions) to treat dermographism. [28]

Prescription ingredients

Huang Qi (Radix Astragali seu Hedysari) 20-40g
Bai Zhu (Rhizoma Atractylodis Macrocephalae) 15g
He Shou Wu (Radix Polygoni Multiflori) 15g
Fang Feng (Radix Ledebouriellae Divaricatae) 10g
Lian Qiao (Fructus Forsythiae Suspensae) 10g
Bai Ji Li (Fructus Tribuli Terrestris) 10g
Ku Shen (Radix Sophorae Flavescentis) 10g
*Ma Huang** (Herba Ephedrae) 5g
Chi Xiao Dou (Semen Phaseoli Calcarati) 30g
Chan Tui‡ (Periostracum Cicadae) 6g
Gan Cao (Radix Glycyrrhizae) 3g

One bag a day was used to prepare a decoction, drunk twice a day. Five days made up a course of treatment. Of the 138 patients receiving treatment, 48 (34.8 percent) recovered completely, 83 (60.1 percent) showed varying degrees of improvement and 7 (5.1 percent) showed no improvement after two courses.

Angioedema
血管性水肿

Angioedema (also known as angioneurotic edema) is an acute or chronic urticaria-like swelling in the subcutaneous tissue of the skin and mucosa and submucosal layers of the respiratory and gastrointestinal tracts. It may occur simultaneously with urticaria, but the deeper edematous reaction produces a more diffuse swelling.

In TCM, angioedema is also known as *chi bai you feng* (red and white wandering Wind).

Clinical manifestations

- Lesions usually occur on the lips, eyelids, palms, soles, limbs, trunk, and genitalia. In severe cases, they may involve the mouth, throat and larynx.
- Lesions generally manifest as circumscribed edema with ill-defined borders and a tight, shiny, uniform pink or flesh-colored surface that is non-pitting on pressure.
- The disease usually attacks suddenly and produces subjective feelings of local distension, fullness, numbness, and burning pain. Itching is not as pronounced as in urticaria.
- If the throat is involved, there may be dyspnea or, in severe cases, asphyxia.

Differential diagnosis

Facial erysipelas
Skin lesions are preceded by a prodromal phase of fever, chills and malaise. Lesions manifest as localized bright red edematous erythema with irregular, sharply demarcated and rapidly expanding borders. The surface of the lesions is tense, shiny and hot. The condition is usually accompanied by sensations of moderate to severe itching, burning, tenderness, and pain.

Etiology and pathology

Qi Deficiency of the Spleen and Lungs
Qi Deficiency of the Spleen causes accumulation of Dampness in the skin and flesh; impairment of the function of the Lungs results in damage to the functional activities of Qi and looseness of the interstices (*cou li*), making the exterior vulnerable to attack by pathogenic factors. If Wind and Cold invade and meet Dampness in the skin and flesh, they will fight with one another to produce pale swollen lesions.

Dryness-Heat in the Spleen and Lungs
When Dryness-Heat in the Spleen and Lungs, usually due to intake of fish, seafood, spicy, or fried food and certain medications, encounters Dryness transformed from external Wind-Heat, they combine to attack the skin and interstices (*cou li*), leading to redness and swelling.

Pattern identification and treatment

INTERNAL TREATMENT

QI DEFICIENCY OF THE SPLEEN AND LUNGS WITH WIND AND COLD FIGHTING ONE ANOTHER
The lips, eyelids or limbs suddenly become swollen. Local skin is tight and shiny and is pale or a normal color. The swelling does not pit or change color when pressed. This condition may last for several days before disappearing. Accompanying symptoms and signs include slight aversion to wind and cold, absence of sweating, shortness of breath, lassitude, and poor appetite. The tongue body is pale with a thin white coating; the pulse is soggy and thready, or moderate.

Treatment principle
Supplement the Lungs and boost the Spleen, dredge Wind and dissipate Cold.

Prescription
BU ZHONG YI QI TANG HE BU FEI TANG JIA JIAN
Decoction for Supplementing the Middle and Augmenting Qi Combined With Decoction for Supplementing the Lungs, with modifications

Huang Qi (Radix Astragali seu Hedysari) 10g
Dang Shen (Radix Codonopsitis Pilosulae) 10g
Shu Di Huang (Radix Rehmanniae Glutinosae Conquita) 10g
Bai Zhu (Rhizoma Atractylodis Macrocephalae) 10g
Dang Gui (Radix Angelicae Sinensis) 10g
Sheng Ma (Rhizoma Cimicifugae) 6g
Chai Hu (Radix Bupleuri) 6g
Wu Wei Zi (Fructus Schisandrae) 6g
Gan Cao (Radix Glycyrrhizae) 6g
Chen Pi (Pericarpium Citri Reticulatae) 6g
Chan Tui‡ (Periostracum Cicadae) 6g

Explanation
- *Huang Qi* (Radix Astragali seu Hedysari), *Bai Zhu* (Rhizoma Atractylodis Macrocephalae), *Dang Shen* (Radix Codonopsitis Pilosulae), *Chai Hu* (Radix

Bupleuri), and *Sheng Ma* (Rhizoma Cimicifugae) bear Yang upward and augment Qi, and support the Spleen to transform Dampness with warmth and sweetness.

- *Shu Di Huang* (Radix Rehmanniae Glutinosae Conquita) and *Dang Gui* (Radix Angelicae Sinensis) nourish the Blood and emolliate the Liver.

- *Chen Pi* (Pericarpium Citri Reticulatae) and *Chan Tui*‡ (Periostracum Cicadae) dissipate Heat and alleviate itching.

- *Wu Wei Zi* (Fructus Schisandrae) and *Gan Cao* (Radix Glycyrrhizae) supplement Lung Qi.

DRYNESS-HEAT IN THE SPLEEN AND LUNGS WITH STAGNATION OF WIND-HEAT

Lesions mainly involve the lips and eyelids, but may spread to the entire face in severe cases. The cloud-like swellings have no clearly demarcated margins. The skin is hot and pale red and may become paler under pressure although the swelling does not pit. This pattern usually has a rapid onset and disappears relatively quickly. Accompanying symptoms and signs include dry mouth with a desire for drinks, generalized fever and yellow urine. The tongue body is red with a thin yellow coating; the pulse is rapid or slippery and rapid.

Treatment principle
Clear Heat from the Spleen and moisten the Lungs, disperse Wind and dissipate Heat.

Prescription
SI WU XIAO FENG SAN JIA JIAN
Four Agents Powder for Dispersing Wind, with modifications

Dang Gui (Radix Angelicae Sinensis) 10g
Chao Bai Shao (Radix Paeoniae Lactiflorae, stir-fried) 10g
Sheng Di Huang (Radix Rehmanniae Glutinosae) 10g
Jing Jie (Herba Schizonepetae Tenuifoliae) 6g
Chai Hu (Radix Bupleuri) 6g
Chan Tui‡ (Periostracum Cicadae) 6g
Huang Qin (Radix Scutellariae Baicalensis) 6g
Fu Ping (Herba Spirodelae Polyrrhizae) 12g
Shi Gao‡ (Gypsum Fibrosum) 12g
Bai Mao Gen (Rhizoma Imperatae Cylindricae) 30g

Explanation
- *Dang Gui* (Radix Angelicae Sinensis), *Chao Bai Shao* (Radix Paeoniae Lactiflorae, stir-fried) and *Sheng Di Huang* (Radix Rehmanniae Glutinosae) nourish Yin and moisten Dryness.

- *Jing Jie* (Herba Schizonepetae Tenuifoliae), *Chai Hu* (Radix Bupleuri), *Chan Tui*‡ (Periostracum Cicadae),

and *Fu Ping* (Herba Spirodelae Polyrrhizae) dissipate Wind and alleviate itching.

- *Huang Qin* (Radix Scutellariae Baicalensis), *Shi Gao*‡ (Gypsum Fibrosum) and *Bai Mao Gen* (Rhizoma Imperatae Cylindricae) clear Heat from the Qi level and reduce fever to enrich Yin and moisten Dryness.

EXTERNAL TREATMENT
- For local swelling, mix *Ru Yi Jin Huang San* (Agreeable Golden Yellow Powder) or *Ru Bing San* (Ice-Like Powder) with cold boiled water and apply to the affected areas.

- For local swelling and itching, apply *Lu Hu Xi Ji* (Calamine and Giant Knotweed Wash Preparation) or *San Huang Xi Ji* (Three Yellows Wash Preparation) externally to the lesions.

ACUPUNCTURE

Selection of points according to the affected area
Points
- For lesions on the eyelids, select ST-2 Sibai, GB-14 Yangbai and EX-HN-5 Taiyang.[i]

- For lesions on the lips, select ST-4 Dicang, GV-26 Shuigou, CV-24 Chengjiang, LI-11 Quchi, and LI-4 Hegu.

- For lesions in the genital region, select CV-3 Zhongji and CV-9 Shuifen.

Technique: Use the reducing method and retain the needles for 30 minutes after obtaining Qi. Manipulate the needles three to five times during this time. Treat once a day. A course consists of five treatment sessions.

Selection of adjacent points
Points: CV-17 Danzhong and LI-4 Hegu.
Technique: After obtaining Qi at CV-17 Danzhong, point the needle tip toward CV-22 Tiantu and manipulate the needle gently for three to five minutes before withdrawing it. Needle LI-4 Hegu with the reducing method and retain the needle for 30 minutes. Treat once a day. A course consists of three treatment sessions.
Indications: This method is indicated for laryngeal edema as a result of its effectiveness in relieving suffocation.

Explanation
Most of the points selected are local points since they produce good results in dredging Wind, dispersing swelling, freeing the network vessels, and alleviating itching.

EAR ACUPUNCTURE
Points: Lung, Heart, Subcortex, and sites of urticarial lesions.

---

[i] M-HN-9 according to the system employed by the Shanghai College of Traditional Chinese Medicine.

Technique: Apply the reducing method and retain the needles for 30 minutes after obtaining Qi; during this period, manipulate the needles three to five times. Treat once a day. A course consists of five treatment sessions.

PRICKING TO BLEED METHOD
Point: Ashi point (red and swollen area of the lips).
Technique: After routine sterilization of the Ashi point, prick the area repeatedly with three to five short filiform needles bundled together until there is slight exudation or bleeding. Treat once every two days. A course consists of three treatment sessions.

Clinical notes

- This disease is frequently related to pathogenic Wind and Spleen-Damp. The treatment principle should therefore concentrate on dredging Wind and dispersing swelling as well as on supporting the Spleen and transforming Dampness; combining these two approaches will produce a better result.
- For acute emergency symptoms such as laryngeal edema, the patient should be referred immediately to a Western medicine doctor for treatment, which may require parenteral administration of epinephrine, corticosteroids and antihistamine.

Advice for the patient

Keep to a light diet and avoid intake of seafood and known allergens.

Modern clinical experience

Shi treated chronic angioedema with a prescription based on *Si Wu Tang* (Four Agents Decoction).[29]

Prescription ingredients

Sheng Di Huang (Radix Rehmanniae Glutinosae) 10g
Dang Gui (Radix Angelicae Sinensis) 10g
Bai Shao (Radix Paeoniae Lactiflorae) 10g
Chuan Xiong (Rhizoma Ligustici Chuanxiong) 10g

Modifications

1. For Blood-Heat patterns, *Chao Mu Dan Pi* (Cortex Moutan Radicis, stir-fried) 10g and *Chao Huang Qin* (Radix Scutellariae Baicalensis, stir-fried) 10g were added.
2. For pruritus, *Di Fu Zi* (Fructus Kochiae Scopariae) 10g and *Bai Xian Pi* (Cortex Dictamni Dasycarpi Radicis) 10g were added.
3. For fever, *Jin Yin Hua* (Flos Lonicerae) 10g, *Zhi Zi* (Fructus Gardeniae Jasminoidis) 10g and *Pu Gong Ying* (Herba Taraxaci cum Radice) 10g were added.
4. For exuberant Dampness, *Fu Ling* (Sclerotium Poriae Cocos) 10g, *Yi Yi Ren* (Semen Coicis Lachryma-jobi) 10g, *Pei Lan* (Herba Eupatorii Fortunei) 10g, and *Ze Xie* (Rhizoma Alismatis Orientalis) 10g were added.

One bag a day was used to prepare a decoction, which was drunk twice a day. A course of treatment consisted of ten bags; most patients recovered after two or three courses.

References

1. Beijing Hospital of Traditional Chinese Medicine, *Zhao Bing Nan Lin Chuang Jing Yan Ji* [A Collection of Zhao Bingnan's Clinical Experiences] (Beijing: People's Medical Publishing House, 1975), 183.
2. Shi Yuguang and Shan Shujian (eds.), *Dang Dai Ming Yi Lin Zheng Jing Hua: Pi Fu Bing Zhuan Ji – Li Shou Shan An* [A Selection of Clinical Experiences of Famous Contemporary Practitioners: Skin Disease Specialists – Li Shoushan's Cases] (Beijing: Traditional Chinese Medicine Publishing House, 1992), 11.
3. Zhang Zhili, *Zhang Zhi Li Pi Fu Bing Lin Chuang Jing Yan Ji Yao* [A Collection of Zhang Zhili's Clinical Experiences in the Treatment of Skin Diseases] (Beijing: China Medical Science and Technology Publishing House, 2001), 252.
4. An Jiafeng and Zhang Peng, *Zhang Zhi Li Pi Fu Bing Yi An Xuan Cui* [A Collection of Zhang Zhili's Skin Disease Cases] (Beijing: People's Medical Publishing House, 1994), 146.
5. Beijing Hospital of Traditional Chinese Medicine, *Zhao Bing Nan Lin Chuang Jing Yan Ji*, 181.
6. Gao Zongkui, *Zhong Yi Bian Zheng Zhi Liao Qian Ma Zhen 106 Li Liao Xiao Guan Cha* [Survey of Treatment of 106 Cases of Urticaria Based on TCM Pattern Identification], *Pi Fu Xing Bing Xue Za Zhi* [Journal of Dermatology and Venereology] 4, 2 (1998): 36-37.
7. Ding Huazhong, *Bian Zheng Zhi Liao Qian Ma Zhen 46 Li* [Treatment of 46 Cases of Urticaria Based on Pattern Identification], *Guang Xi Zhong Yi Yao* [Guangxi Journal of Traditional Chinese Medicine and Materia Medica] 20, 6 (1997): 86.
8. Zheng Weiqin, *Lao Zhong Yi Zhou Bai Chuan Zhi Liao Qian Ma Zhen Jing Yan Zong Jie* [Experiences of Senior TCM Doctor Zhou Baichuan in the Treatment of Urticaria], *Yun Nan Zhong Yi Zhong Yao Za Zhi* [Yunnan Journal of Traditional Chinese Medicine and Materia Medica] 18, 2 (1997): 32-33.
9. Han Bing, *32 Li Man Xing Qian Ma Zhen Zhong Yi Bian Zheng Lun Zhi – Fu 96 Li Bian Tai Fan Ying Yuan Ce Ding Fen Xi* [Discussion of Treatment of 32 Cases of Chronic Urticaria Based on Pattern Identification with an Appendix Analyzing Allergies in 96 Cases], *Bei Jing Zhong Yi* [Beijing Journal of Traditional Chinese Medicine] 3 (1998): 20.
10. Chen Hanzhang, *Zhong Yao Zhi Liao Man Xing Qian Ma*

Zhen 54 Li [Treatment of 54 Cases of Chronic Urticaria with Chinese Materia Medica], *Xin Zhong Yi* [New Journal of Traditional Chinese Medicine] 1 (1997): 42.

11. Wang Yuzhen, *Kang Qian Tang Zhi Liao Feng Re Xing Ji Xing Qian Ma Zhen 60 Li* [Treatment of 60 Cases of Acute Urticaria due to Wind-Heat with *Kang Qian Tang* (Anti-Urticaria Decoction)], *He Bei Zhong Yi* [Hebei Journal of Traditional Chinese Medicine] 17, 3 (1995): 40.

12. Ma Xiang, *Xiao Zhen Zhi Yang Tang Zhi Liao Feng Re Xing Qian Ma Zhen 36 Li* [Treatment of 36 Cases of Urticaria due to Wind-Heat with *Xiao Zhen Zhi Yang Tang* (Decoction for Dispersing Eruptions and Alleviating Itching)], *Zhong Hua Shi Yong Zhong Xi Yi Za Zhi* [Chinese Journal of Practical Integrated TCM and Western Medicine] 12, 5 (1999): 869.

13. Chen Jinguang, *Zi Ni Gu Ben Chu Feng Tang Zhi Liao Qian Ma Zhen 105 Li Liao Xiao Bao Gao* [Report on the Effectiveness of Treatment of 105 Cases of Urticaria with the Empirical Prescription *Gu Ben Chu Feng Tang* (Decoction for Consolidating the Root and Eliminating Wind)], *Shan Xi Zhong Yi Xue Yuan Xue Bao* [Journal of Shanxi College of Traditional Chinese Medicine] 19, 3 (1996): 23.

14. Fang Xiangming, *Tong Xie Shu Feng Tang Zhi Liao Qian Ma Zhen* [Treatment of Urticaria with *Tong Xie Shu Feng Tang* (Decoction for Freeing the Bowels, Discharging Heat and Dredging Wind)], *Hu Bei Zhong Yi Za Zhi* [Hubei Journal of Traditional Chinese Medicine] 19, 3 (1997): 40.

15. Ye Fei, *Zhi Zhu Chi Dou Yin Zhi Liao Qian Ma Zhen 46 Li* [Treatment of 46 Cases of Urticaria with *Zhi Zhu Chi Dou Yin* (Bitter Orange, White Atractylodes and Aduki Bean Beverage)], *Yun Nan Zhong Yi Zhong Yao Za Zhi* [Yunnan Journal of Traditional Chinese Medicine and Materia Medica] 20, 5 (1999): 31.

16. Lü Fuquan, *Bu Yang Huan Wu Tang Jia Jian Zhi Liao Man Xing Qian Ma Zhen 36 Li* [Treatment of 36 Cases of Chronic Urticaria with Modified *Bu Yang Huan Wu Tang* (Five-Returning Decoction for Supplementing Yang)], *Tian Jin Zhong Yi* [Tianjin Journal of Traditional Chinese Medicine] 15, 3 (1998): 113.

17. Ying Dansong, *Xiao Zhen Tang Zhi Liao Man Xing Qian Ma Zhen 36 Li* [Treatment of 36 Cases of Chronic Urticaria with *Xiao Zhen Tang* (Decoction for Dispersing Eruptions)], *Zhong Guo Zhong Yi Yao Xin Xi Za Zhi* [Traditional Chinese Medicine and Materia Medica Information Bulletin] 6, 7 (1999): 61.

18. Zhao Dongri, *Dang Gui Yin Zi Zhi Liao Man Xing Qian Ma Zhen 70 Li* [Treatment of 70 Cases of Chronic Urticaria with *Dang Gui Yin Zi* (Chinese Angelica Root Drink)], *Zhe Jiang Zhong Yi Za Zhi* [Zhejiang Journal of Traditional Chinese Medicine] 34, 6 (1999): 243.

19. Liu Xingxin, *Tuo Min Xiao Zhen Tang Zhi Liao Wan Gu Xing Qian Ma Zhen 38 Li* [Treatment of 38 Cases of Stubborn Urticaria with *Tuo Min Xiao Zhen Tang* (Desensitization Decoction for Dispersing Eruptions)], *Si Chuan Zhong Yi* [Sichuan Journal of Traditional Chinese Medicine] 12 (1996): 47.

20. Jin Zhidao, *Xiao Zhen Yin Zhi Liao Wan Gu Xing Qian Ma Zhen* [Treatment of Stubborn Urticaria with *Xiao Zhen Yin* (Beverage for Dispersing Eruptions)], *Hu Bei Zhong Yi Za Zhi* [Hubei Journal of Traditional Chinese Medicine] 18, 6 (1996): 26.

21. Liu Tianji, *Zhong Xi Yi Jie He Zhi Liao Man Xing Qian Ma Zhen 96 Li* [Treatment of 96 Cases of Chronic Urticaria with a Combination of TCM and Western Medicine], *Zhong Guo Zhong Xi Yi Jie He Za Zhi* [Journal of Integrated TCM and Western Medicine] 16, 3 (1996): 159.

22. Huang Yongjing, *Zhong Xi Yi Jie He Zhi Liao Man Xing Qian Ma Zhen 40 Li Yuan Jin Qi Liao Xiao Guan Cha* [Survey of the Immediate and Delayed Effect of Treatment of 40 Cases of Chronic Urticaria with a Combination of TCM and Western Medicine], *Xin Zhong Yi* [New Journal of Traditional Chinese Medicine] 30, 6 (1998): 43.

23. Wu Qiyu, *Yao Zhen He Yong Zhi Liao Qian Ma Zhen 20 Li* [Treatment of 20 Cases of Urticaria with Chinese Materia Medica and Acupuncture], *Si Chuan Zhong Yi* [Sichuan Journal of Traditional Chinese Medicine] 15, 10 (1997): 34.

24. Wu Fengwei, *Zhen Ci Zhi Liao Ji Xing Qian Ma Zhen 85 Li* [Treatment of 85 Cases of Acute Urticaria with Acupuncture], *Shan Dong Zhong Yi Za Zhi* [Shandong Journal of Traditional Chinese Medicine] 18, 5 (1999): 218.

25. Gu Ruipu, *Zhen Ci Ba Guan Zhi Liao Qian Ma Zhen 40 Li* [Treatment of 40 Cases of Urticaria with Acupuncture and Cupping Therapy], *Xin Jiang Zhong Yi Yao* [Xinjiang Journal of Traditional Chinese Medicine and Materia Medica] 2 (1996): 24.

26. Si Zaihe, *Bian Tong Yang He Tang Zhi Liao Han Leng Xing Qian Ma Zhen 50 Li* [Treatment of 50 Cases of Cold Urticaria with Modified *Yang He Tang* (Harmonious Yang Decoction)], *Guang Xi Zhong Yi* [Guangxi Journal of Traditional Chinese Medicine] 14, 1 (1992): 16.

27. An Jiafeng and Zhang Peng, *Zhang Zhi Li Pi Fu Bing Yi An Xuan Cui*, 147.

28. Cai Wenmo, *Xiao Zhen Tang Zhi Liao Pi Fu Hua Hen Zheng 138 Li* [Treatment of 138 Cases of Dermographism with *Xiao Zhen Tang* (Decoction for Dispersing Eruptions)], *Fu Jian Zhong Yi Yao* [Fujian Journal of Traditional Chinese Medicine and Materia Medica] 6, 3 (1995): 49.

29. Shi Mingzhi, *Si Wu Tang Zhi Liao Xue Guan Shen Jing Xing Shui Zhong 20 Li* [Treatment of 20 Cases of Angioedema with *Si Wu Tang* (Four Agents Decoction)], *Guang Xi Zhong Yi Yao* [Guangxi Journal of Traditional Chinese Medicine and Materia Medica] 19, 1 (1996): 14.

Sebaceous and sweat gland disorders

Sebaceous glands are associated with the hair follicles, lying between the follicle and the epidermis. They are most numerous on the scalp, face, chest, and back. Sebaceous glands produce sebum, which is discharged into the hair follicle and functions to lubricate the skin and hair and act as a mild bactericide. These glands are dormant in children, but become active at puberty when they are stimulated by androgenic hormones.

Sweat glands are tightly coiled glands lying deep in the dermis. Sweat secreted by the glands reaches the surface of the skin through the sweat ducts. In total, the body has two to three million eccrine sweat glands, which are most numerous on the palms, soles, axillae, and forehead.

These sweat glands are important for regulating body temperature and up to 10 liters a day of sweat may be excreted.

Apocrine sweat glands are larger than eccrine glands and open into the hair follicles. They are mostly found around the axillae, nipples and perineum. Sweat produced by these glands is odorless, with an odor only developing after being acted upon by bacteria on the skin.

In TCM, etiological analysis generally starts with the nature of the disease – diseases of the sebaceous glands are usually related to the Lungs and Spleen, diseases of the sweat glands to disharmony between the Ying and Wei levels or retention of Heat in the Spleen channel.

Acne
痤疮

Acne is a disorder of the hair follicle sebaceous glands, consisting of non-inflammatory lesions (open and closed comedones) and inflammatory lesions (papules, pustules and nodules). Many factors are responsible for the development of acne – sebum excretion, androgenic hormones, occlusion of sebaceous gland pores, and infection with *Propionibacterium acnes*. The development of acne is also influenced by genetic factors, gastrointestinal function, environmental factors, cosmetics, and emotional factors.

Acne is essentially due to excessive activity of the sebaceous glands, which are most numerous in the skin of the face, chest and back. During puberty, these glands grow rapidly and keratin may block the opening. Where partially dried keratinous matter blocks the opening of the sebaceous glands, comedones (whiteheads or blackheads) appear. In more serious cases, sebum trapped in the glands leaks around the pilosebaceous unit and may become infected by bacteria, resulting in papules, pustules, nodules, or cysts.

In TCM, acne is known as *fei feng fen ci* (Lung-Wind powder prickles). This name is derived from the starch-colored fluid that can be squeezed out of the thorn-like papular or pustular eruptions characteristic of acne and the attribution of the disease to the Lungs.

Clinical manifestations

- Acne is common among adolescents and young adults, usually starting between the ages of 12 and 14 and peaking between the ages of 16 and 19; females are normally affected earlier than males. Although acne generally disappears once puberty and growth are over, it may persist into adulthood. It may reappear in adult life after hormone treatment for other disorders; in some women, acne may be exacerbated in the premenstrual phase.

- Lesions generally appear on the face (especially the forehead, cheeks and chin), the chest, the back, and the interscapular area. Involvement is symmetrical.

- At the initial stage, lesions manifest as open comedones (blackheads), caused by keratin and sebum plugging the pilosebaceous orifice, or closed comedones (whiteheads), small white or grayish papules caused by occlusion of the follicle opening. As the disease develops, lesions may evolve into inflammatory papules or pustules.

- In a few cases, mostly in males, papules may develop into red or dark red nodules or cysts, which are located deeper in the skin than papules, but may still raise the skin slightly. The surface of large cysts is fluctuant when palpated. Atrophic and pitted scarring may occur where lesions are deep.

- Acne is often complicated by increased sebaceous activity on the face and scalp, manifesting as an oily complexion with enlarged follicles and a greasy scalp.

- Subjective symptoms are rare in most cases except for the emotional stress caused by the appearance of the lesions.

Differential diagnosis

Rosacea
This condition affects middle-aged people most commonly. Lesions manifest initially as erythema and capillary dilatation (telangiectasia) on the forehead, cheeks, nose, chin, and around the eyes, with papules, pustules and nodules appearing later. There are no comedones and no other areas of the body are involved.

Perioral dermatitis
This disorder occurs most frequently in women in the 20-40 age group. Eruptions usually start around the mouth, but may also involve the areas around the nose and eyes. Lesions mainly manifest as erythema, pinpoint papules, papulovesicles or pustules, with some scaling. There are no comedones and no other areas of the body are involved.

Hidradenitis suppurativa
This disorder is more common in young or middle-aged women, and is worse in the obese. Lesions usually occur in the axillae, the groin, the area under the female breast, and the anogenital region. There are no comedones.

Etiology and pathology

- Underlying Heat in the Blood is the main internal factor responsible for the onset of the disease, whereas improper diet and invasion by external pathogenic factors are the main external causes; Blood stasis and binding of Phlegm result in complications and aggravation of the condition.

- A tendency toward exuberance of constitutional Yang-Heat during adolescence (when the body is growing rapidly) gradually warms up the Ying and Xue levels. Blood-Heat moves out to the exterior and congests the vessels, resulting in stagnation of Qi and Blood.

- Spicy food has a hot, Yang nature and transforms into Heat if too much is eaten over a long period. Overindulgence in fishy and fatty foods impairs the transformation and transportation function of the Middle Burner and generates Fire and Heat from prolonged accumulation. Fire and Heat tend to steam upward to affect the face, giving rise to small red eruptions.

- General poor health resulting in repeated contraction of pathogenic Wind-Heat or washing in cold water resulting in binding of Blood-Heat gradually leads to clusters of inflamed lesions or blackheads.

- Stagnation of Qi and Blood in the channels and network vessels due to persistent illness or emotional disturbance, or Blood stasis and binding of Phlegm due to prolonged accumulation of Heat in the Lungs and Stomach, which transforms into Damp and generates Phlegm, will result in widespread eruptions or the formation of nodules and cysts.

Pattern identification and treatment

INTERNAL TREATMENT

ACCUMULATION OF HEAT IN THE LUNGS
This pattern arises when Heat in the Lung channel is complicated by external contraction of pathogenic Wind, which causes the retention of Lung-Heat in the skin and flesh. Lesions are distributed over the cheeks and forehead and around the nose, manifesting as discrete pinpoint to 2mm red or pale red papules; in severe cases, lesions may involve the chest and back. Blackheads may be seen on some lesions. Pressure may produce excretion of a plug of greasy matter or thick, yellow purulent discharge. The skin looks oily and shiny. Accompanying symptoms include a dry mouth and nose, a red tongue body with a thin yellow coating, and a floating pulse.

Treatment principle
Clear Heat from the Lungs.

Prescription
PI PA QING FEI YIN JIA JIAN
Loquat Beverage for Clearing Heat from the Lungs, with modifications

Pi Pa Ye (Folium Eriobotryae Japonicae) 10g
Jiao Zhi Zi (Fructus Gardeniae Jasminoidis, scorch-fried) 10g

Lian Qiao (Fructus Forsythiae Suspensae) 10g
Chi Shao (Radix Paeoniae Rubra) 10g
Sang Bai Pi (Cortex Mori Albae Radicis) 10g
Huang Qin (Radix Scutellariae Baicalensis) 6g
Chao Mu Dan Pi (Cortex Moutan Radicis, stir-fried) 6g
Hong Hua (Flos Carthami Tinctorii) 6g
Ling Xiao Hua (Flos Campsitis) 6g
Sheng Di Huang (Radix Rehmanniae Glutinosae) 12g
Jin Yin Hua (Flos Lonicerae) 12g
Dong Gua Pi (Epicarpium Benincasae Hispidae) 12g
Dong Gua Ren (Semen Benincasae Hispidae) 12g

Explanation

- *Pi Pa Ye* (Folium Eriobotryae Japonicae), *Jiao Zhi Zi* (Fructus Gardeniae Jasminoidis, scorch-fried), *Sang Bai Pi* (Cortex Mori Albae Radicis), *Huang Qin* (Radix Scutellariae Baicalensis), and *Lian Qiao* (Fructus Forsythiae Suspensae) clear and diffuse Heat retained in the Lungs.
- *Chao Mu Dan Pi* (Cortex Moutan Radicis, stir-fried), *Chi Shao* (Radix Paeoniae Rubra), *Hong Hua* (Flos Carthami Tinctorii), *Ling Xiao Hua* (Flos Campsitis), *Sheng Di Huang* (Radix Rehmanniae Glutinosae), and *Jin Yin Hua* (Flos Lonicerae) cool and invigorate the Blood and reduce erythema.
- *Dong Gua Pi* (Epicarpium Benincasae Hispidae) and *Dong Gua Ren* (Semen Benincasae Hispidae) transform Dampness and moisten the skin.

ACCUMULATION OF HEAT IN THE STOMACH

Stomach-Heat arises from accumulated Heat in the Spleen and Stomach caused by overindulgence in spicy, fatty and fried foods, with Heat then being retained in the skin and flesh. Lesions are similar to those in the Lung-Heat pattern, except that they are mainly distributed around the mouth. Accompanying symptoms and signs include bad breath, aversion to heat, thirst with a desire for cold drinks, constipation, and dark yellow urine. The tongue body is red with a thin yellow or thick and greasy coating; the pulse is slippery and rapid.

Treatment principle
Clear Heat from the Yangming channel.

Prescription
TIAO WEI CHENG QI TANG
Decoction for Regulating the Stomach and Sustaining Qi

Jiu Zhi Da Huang (Radix et Rhizoma Rhei, processed with wine) 12g
Zhi Gan Cao (Radix Glycyrrhizae, mix-fried with honey) 6g
Mang Xiao‡ (Mirabilitum) 12g, infused in the decoction

Explanation

- *Jiu Zhi Da Huang* (Radix et Rhizoma Rhei, processed with wine) clears the Fu organs and drains Heat.

- *Mang Xiao*‡ (Mirabilitum) flushes out accumulation and guides out stagnation.
- *Zhi Gan Cao* (Radix Glycyrrhizae, mix-fried with honey) moderates and harmonizes the properties of the other ingredients to reduce the rate of draining.

BLOOD-HEAT

Internal damage due to emotional disturbances leads to Qi Depression, eventually transforming into Heat. Latent Heat in the Ying and Xue levels finally results in acne. Lesions manifest as 1-2 mm red papules on the face, concentrated around the nose and mouth and between the eyebrows, accompanied by telangiectasia, tidal reddening of the face and a sensation of scorching heat. For women, papules normally increase before and after menstruation. Accompanying symptoms include dry stools and yellow or reddish urine. The tongue tip is red with a thin yellow coating; the pulse is thready, slippery and rapid.

Treatment principle
Cool the Blood and clear Heat, transform stasis and reduce erythema.

Prescription
TAO HONG SI WU TANG HE LIANG XUE WU HUA TANG JIA JIAN
Peach Kernel and Safflower Four Agents Decoction Combined With Five Flowers Decoction for Cooling the Blood, with modifications

Tao Ren (Semen Persicae) 6g
Hong Hua (Flos Carthami Tinctorii) 6g
Ling Xiao Hua (Flos Campsitis) 6g
Chuan Xiong (Rhizoma Ligustici Chuanxiong) 6g
Chao Mu Dan Pi (Cortex Moutan Radicis, stir-fried) 10g
Sheng Di Huang (Radix Rehmanniae Glutinosae) 10g
Chi Shao (Radix Paeoniae Rubra) 10g
Jin Yin Hua (Flos Lonicerae) 10g
Chao Huai Hua (Flos Sophorae Japonicae, stir-fried) 10g
Ji Guan Hua (Flos Celosiae Cristatae) 10g
Shi Gao‡ (Gypsum Fibrosum) 12g
Huang Qin (Radix Scutellariae Baicalensis) 6g

Explanation

- *Sheng Di Huang* (Radix Rehmanniae Glutinosae), *Chao Mu Dan Pi* (Cortex Moutan Radicis, stir-fried), *Chi Shao* (Radix Paeoniae Rubra), *Ling Xiao Hua* (Flos Campsitis), and *Chao Huai Hua* (Flos Sophorae Japonicae, stir-fried) cool the Blood and clear Heat.
- *Tao Ren* (Semen Persicae), *Chuan Xiong* (Rhizoma Ligustici Chuanxiong), *Hong Hua* (Flos Carthami Tinctorii), and *Ji Guan Hua* (Flos Celosiae Cristatae) transform Blood stasis and reduce erythema.
- *Jin Yin Hua* (Flos Lonicerae), *Shi Gao*‡ (Gypsum Fibrosum) and *Huang Qin* (Radix Scutellariae Baicalensis)

clear Heat in the Stomach to help reduce redness on the face.

STAGNATION OF QI AND BLOOD

This pattern presents as red or dark red eruptions on the face that persist for several years. In women, eruptions are usually aggravated during menstruation and are alleviated after periods. Accompanying symptoms and signs due to disharmony of the Chong and Ren vessels may include menstrual irregularities, menstrual clots and abdominal pain. In men, the complexion may be dark red or purplish-red. The tongue body is dark red or has stasis marks; the pulse is deep, thready and rough.

Treatment principle

Move Qi and regulate the Blood, relieve Toxicity and dissipate lumps.

Prescription

LIANG XUE QING FEI YIN JIA JIAN

Beverage for Cooling the Blood and Clearing Heat from the Lungs, with modifications

Sheng Di Huang (Radix Rehmanniae Glutinosae) 30g
Jin Yin Hua (Flos Lonicerae) 30g
Yin Chen Hao (Herba Artemisiae Scopariae) 30g
Bai Hua She She Cao (Herba Hedyotidis Diffusae) 30g
Chao Mu Dan Pi (Cortex Moutan Radicis, stir-fried) 10g
Huang Qin (Radix Scutellariae Baicalensis) 10g
Chi Shao (Radix Paeoniae Rubra) 10g
Tao Ren (Semen Persicae) 10g
Yi Mu Cao (Herba Leonuri Heterophylli) 12g
Zhe Bei Mu (Bulbus Fritillariae Thunbergii) 12g
Lian Qiao (Fructus Forsythiae Suspensae) 12g
Zi Hua Di Ding (Herba Violae Yedoensitis) 12g
Chao Zhi Mu (Rhizoma Anemarrhenae Asphodeloidis, stir-fried) 6g
Pi Pa Ye (Folium Eriobotryae Japonicae) 6g

Explanation

- *Sheng Di Huang* (Radix Rehmanniae Glutinosae), *Chao Mu Dan Pi* (Cortex Moutan Radicis, stir-fried), *Chao Zhi Mu* (Rhizoma Anemarrhenae Asphodeloidis, stir-fried), *Chi Shao* (Radix Paeoniae Rubra), *Tao Ren* (Semen Persicae), and *Yi Mu Cao* (Herba Leonuri Heterophylli) cool and invigorate the Blood, regulate menstruation and improve the complexion.

- *Jin Yin Hua* (Flos Lonicerae), *Huang Qin* (Radix Scutellariae Baicalensis), *Yin Chen Hao* (Herba Artemisiae Scopariae), *Bai Hua She She Cao* (Herba Hedyotidis Diffusae), *Zi Hua Di Ding* (Herba Violae Yedoensitis), and *Pi Pa Ye* (Folium Eriobotryae Japonicae) clear Heat and relieve Toxicity, clear and diffuse Heat from the Lungs.

- *Zhe Bei Mu* (Bulbus Fritillariae Thunbergii) and *Lian Qiao* (Fructus Forsythiae Suspensae) soften hardness

and dissipate lumps, draw out Toxicity from the interior and expel pus.

BLOOD STASIS AND BINDING OF PHLEGM

This pattern manifests as repeated and persistent eruptions on the cheeks and lower jaw, gradually enlarging into 3-5 mm or larger, unevenly protruding, purplish-red lumps that feel soft on palpation, with excretion of pus and blood or sticky yellow matter on pressure. Scars form after rupture. The tongue body is pale red with a slippery and greasy coating; the pulse is soggy and slippery.

Treatment principle

Invigorate the Blood and transform Blood stasis, disperse Phlegm and soften hardness.

Prescription

HAI ZAO YU HU TANG JIA JIAN

Sargassum Jade Flask Decoction, with modifications

Hai Zao (Herba Sargassi) 10g
Zhe Bei Mu (Bulbus Fritillariae Thunbergii) 10g
Chen Pi (Pericarpium Citri Reticulatae) 10g
Kun Bu (Thallus Laminariae seu Eckloniae) 10g
Fa Ban Xia (Rhizoma Pinelliae Ternatae Praeparata) 10g
Lian Qiao (Fructus Forsythiae Suspensae) 12g
Xia Ku Cao (Spica Prunellae Vulgaris) 12g
Long Gu ‡ (Os Draconis) 12g
Mu Li ‡ (Concha Ostreae) 12g
Dang Gui (Radix Angelicae Sinensis) 6g
Chuan Xiong (Rhizoma Ligustici Chuanxiong) 6g
Qing Pi (Pericarpium Citri Reticulatae Viride) 6g
Ju He (Semen Citri Reticulatae) 10g

Explanation

- *Hai Zao* (Herba Sargassi), *Kun Bu* (Thallus Laminariae seu Eckloniae), *Lian Qiao* (Fructus Forsythiae Suspensae), *Fa Ban Xia* (Rhizoma Pinelliae Ternatae Praeparata), *Zhe Bei Mu* (Bulbus Fritillariae Thunbergii), *Xia Ku Cao* (Spica Prunellae Vulgaris), *Long Gu* ‡ (Os Draconis), *Mu Li* ‡ (Concha Ostreae), and *Ju He* (Semen Citri Reticulatae) disperse Phlegm and soften hardness, eliminate pus and dissipate lumps.

- *Chen Pi* (Pericarpium Citri Reticulatae), *Qing Pi* (Pericarpium Citri Reticulatae Viride), *Dang Gui* (Radix Angelicae Sinensis), and *Chuan Xiong* (Rhizoma Ligustici Chuanxiong) invigorate the Blood and transform Blood stasis, regulate Qi and free the network vessels.

General modifications

1. For a persistent red complexion, add *Ji Guan Hua* (Flos Celosiae Cristatae), *Mei Gui Hua* (Flos Rosae Rugosae), *Shi Gao* ‡ (Gypsum Fibrosum), and *Han Shui Shi* ‡ (Calcitum).

2. For severe abscesses with distending pain, add *Pu Gong Ying* (Herba Taraxaci cum Radice), *Zi Hua Di Ding* (Herba Violae Yedoensitis), *Chong Lou* (Rhizoma Paridis), and *Hu Zhang* (Radix et Rhizoma Polygoni Cuspidati).
3. For constipation, add *Chao Zhi Ke* (Fructus Citri Aurantii, stir-fried), *Shu Da Huang* (Radix et Rhizoma Rhei Conquitum) and *Fan Xie Ye* (Folium Sennae).
4. For severe nodules and cysts, add *Huang Yao Zi* (Rhizoma Dioscoreae Bulbiferae), *Tu Bei Mu* (Tuber Bolbostemmatis), *Zao Jiao Ci* (Spina Gleditsiae Sinensis), *Kun Bu* (Thallus Laminariae seu Eckloniae), and *Jiang Can* ‡ (Bombyx Batryticatus).
5. For menstrual irregularities or increased severity of eruption prior to periods, add *Yi Mu Cao* (Herba Leonuri Heterophylli), *Wu Yao* (Radix Linderae Strychnifoliae), *Xiang Fu* (Rhizoma Cyperi Rotundi), *Yin Yang Huo* (Herba Epimedii), *Chao Bai Shao* (Radix Paeoniae Lactiflorae, stir-fried), and *Dang Gui* (Radix Angelicae Sinensis).
6. For very oily or greasy skin, add *Wu Wei Zi* (Fructus Schisandrae), *Yin Chen Hao* (Herba Artemisiae Scopariae) and *Hu Zhang* (Radix et Rhizoma Polygoni Cuspidati).

EXTERNAL TREATMENT
- For lesions manifesting mainly as papules with a few pustules, apply *San Huang Xi Ji* (Three Yellows Wash Preparation) or *Cuo Chuang Xi Ji* (Acne Wash Preparation) to the affected area.
- For lesions manifesting mainly as nodules, cysts and scars, apply *Hei Bu Yao Gao* (Black Cloth Medicated Paste), *Du Jiao Lian Gao* (Giant Typhonium Paste) or *Si Huang Gao* (Four Yellows Paste) to the affected area.

ACUPUNCTURE
Selection of points based on pattern identification
- For Heat in the Lung channel, select GV-14 Dazhui and BL-20 Pishu.
- For Heat in the Spleen and Stomach, select ST-36 Zusanli and LI-4 Hegu.
- For disharmony of the Chong and Ren vessels, select SP-6 Sanyinjiao and BL-23 Shenshu.

Selection of points on the affected channels
LI-11 Quchi, LI-4 Hegu, SP-6 Sanyinjiao, BL-2 Cuanzhu,ⁱ and LI-20 Yingxiang.

Selection of adjacent points
EX-HN-5 Taiyang,ii BL-2 Cuanzhu,i LI-20 Yingxiang, SI-18 Quanliao, EX-HN-3 Yintang,iii and ST-6 Jiache.

Technique
Apply the even method for all points and retain the needles for 30 minutes. Treat once a day. A course consists of seven treatment sessions.

Explanation
- GV-14 Dazhui, LI-4 Hegu and BL-2 Cuanzhuⁱ clear and diffuse Heat from the Lungs.
- LI-11 Quchi, ST-36 Zusanli, BL-20 Pishu, ST-6 Jiache, and LI-20 Yingxiang clear Heat and transform Dampness.
- BL-23 Shenshu and SP-6 Sanyinjiao regulate the Chong and Ren vessels.
- The adjacent points cool the Blood and reduce redness, dissipate Wind and alleviate itching.

EAR ACUPUNCTURE
Selection of points based on disease differentiation
Main points: Lung and Kidney (both bilateral).
Auxiliary points
- For pustules, add Heart.
- For constipation, add Large Intestine.
- For greasy skin, add Spleen.
- For painful periods, add Liver and Endocrine.

Empirical points
Points: Lung (bilateral), Ear-Shenmen, Sympathetic Nerve, Endocrine, and Subcortex.
Technique: Retain the needles for 30 minutes. Treat once every two days. A course consists of ten treatment sessions.

EAR ACUPUNCTURE WITH SEEDS
Points: Endocrine, Subcortex, Lung, Heart, and Stomach.
Technique: Attach *Wang Bu Liu Xing* (Semen Vaccariae Segetalis) seeds to the points with adhesive tape and ask the patient to press the seeds gently for one minute each day. Change the seeds once every five days. A course consists of seven treatment sessions (35 days).

PRICKING TO BLEED METHOD
Points: BL-13 Feishu (bilateral) and GV-14 Dazhui.
Technique: After routine sterilization, prick the points with a small gauge three-edged needle to cause slight

ⁱ Also known as Zanzhu.
ii M-HN-9 according to the system employed by the Shanghai College of Traditional Chinese Medicine.
iii M-HN-3 according to the system employed by the Shanghai College of Traditional Chinese Medicine.

bleeding. Treat once every three days. A course consists of five treatment sessions.

PRICKING METHOD
Points: BL-12 Fengmen, BL-13 Feishu (bilateral, since the disease is closely related to the Lungs), BL-14 Jueyinshu, BL-15 Xinshu, BL-17 Geshu, BL-18 Ganshu, BL-19 Danshu, BL-20 Pishu, BL-21 Weishu, BL-22 Sanjiaoshu, BL-23 Shenshu, and BL-24 Qihaishu.
Technique: After routine sterilization, prick five to seven of the points with a three-edged needle in each treatment session; alternate with the other points in the following treatment sessions. Treat once every three days. A course consists of seven treatment sessions.

PRICKING AND CUPPING
Main points: BL-14 Dazhui, GV-4 Mingmen, GV-8 Jinsuo, GV-9 Zhiyang, GV-11 Shendao, and GV-12 Shenzhu.
Auxiliary points: Blood Pressure-Lowering Groove on the back of the ear and Hot Point on the ear.
Technique: After routine sterilization, prick the main points with a three-edged needle to cause slight bleeding. Apply cupping over these points immediately, keeping the cups in place for five minutes. Prick the auxiliary points to cause slight bleeding; no cupping is applied afterwards. Treat once every three days. A course consists of seven treatment sessions.

Clinical notes

- Acne is a common skin disease among younger people and tends to recur during treatment. The treatment principle should therefore include regulating menstruation for women and regulating the gastrointestinal function for men.
- External treatment and acupuncture can be used to assist in the dispersal and elimination of lesions and to shorten the course of treatment.

Advice for the patient

- Cut down on intake of fatty and sweet food and eat more vegetables and fruit in order to regulate the digestive function.
- Wash the face frequently with warm water or apply a wet compress; do not rub the skin or press the spots with the hands.
- Squeezing the lesions may leave permanent pitted scarring.
- Steroid, bromide or iodine medication is contraindicated.

Case histories

Case 1

Patient
Male, aged 20.

Clinical manifestations
The patient had been healthy throughout his childhood and adolescence. At the age of 18, red papules and open comedones (blackheads) started to appear on the face. In the following year, successive crops of increasingly severe red papules and pustules appeared. Lesions of different sizes were distributed over the forehead and chin and around the nose. Comedones were noted in the center of some of the papules, which were most densely concentrated around the nose. The patient's face was very greasy. He was keen on sports, had a good appetite and tended to eat large amounts. Accompanying symptoms and signs included dry mouth and dry and smelly stools, with bowel movements only once every few days. The tongue body was red with a thin yellow coating; the pulse was wiry and slippery.

Pattern identification
Heat accumulating in the Lungs and Stomach with external contraction of pathogenic Toxins.

Treatment principle
Clear Heat from the Lungs and Stomach and relieve Toxicity.

Prescription
YIN QIAO SAN JIA JIAN
Honeysuckle and Forsythia Powder

Jin Yin Hua (Flos Lonicerae) 15g
Lian Qiao (Fructus Forsythiae Suspensae) 15g
Pu Gong Ying (Herba Taraxaci cum Radice) 30g
Zi Hua Di Ding (Herba Violae Yedoensitis) 15g
Sang Bai Pi (Cortex Mori Albae Radicis) 15g
Huang Qin (Radix Scutellariae Baicalensis) 10g
Zhi Zi (Fructus Gardeniae Jasminoidis) 10g
Chi Shao (Radix Paeoniae Rubra) 10g
Mu Dan Pi (Cortex Moutan Radicis) 10g
Sheng Di Huang (Radix Rehmanniae Glutinosae) 30g
Gua Lou (Fructus Trichosanthis) 15g
Shu Da Huang (Radix et Rhizoma Rhei Conquitum) 10g
Ye Ju Hua (Flos Chrysanthemi Indici) 15g
Di Gu Pi (Cortex Lycii Radicis) 15g

One bag a day was used to prepare a decoction, taken twice a day.

Second visit
After 14 bags of the prescription, stool was passed once a day and the dry mouth was relieved. No new red papules had appeared. The pustules had disappeared but the oily secretion was still pronounced. Numerous open and closed comedones also remained. The patient was told to continue with the prescription for another 28 days.

In addition, *Liu Lei Xi Ji* (Sulfur and Resorcinol Wash

Preparation) and *Lü Liu Ding* (Chloramphenicol Salicylate Tincture) were applied externally once a day. [iv]

Third visit
The red papules had disappeared completely, leaving pale pigmented spots. The skin was still greasy and slightly red on both sides of the nose. The prescription was modified by removing *Gua Lou* (Fructus Trichosanthis) and *Shu Da Huang* (Radix et Rhizoma Rhei Conquitum) and adding *Mei Gui Hua* (Flos Rosae Rugosae) 10g, *Ji Guan Hua* (Flos Celosiae Cristatae) 10g and *Ling Xiao Hua* (Flos Campsitis) 10g. The patient followed the revised prescription for one month to consolidate the improvement. The external wash prescription was changed to washing the face with alkaline soap three times a day. The patient was also advised not to eat deep-fried food and sweet food.

Outcome
At the end of the course, the condition had resolved.

Discussion
Zhang Zhili considers that acne is closely related to Damp-Heat in the Lungs and Stomach. This is a typical case of Heat accumulating in the Lungs and Stomach. The patient was young, strong and full of energy, with the result that Yang-Heat tended to be exuberant.

In the prescription, *Sang Bai Pi* (Cortex Mori Albae Radicis), *Di Gu Pi* (Cortex Lycii Radicis), *Huang Qin* (Radix Scutellariae Baicalensis), and *Zhi Zi* (Fructus Gardeniae Jasminoidis) clear Heat in the Lungs and Stomach; *Jin Yin Hua* (Flos Lonicerae), *Lian Qiao* (Fructus Forsythiae Suspensae), *Pu Gong Ying* (Herba Taraxaci cum Radice), *Zi Hua Di Ding* (Herba Violae Yedoensitis), and *Ye Ju Hua* (Flos Chrysanthemi Indici) clear Heat and relieve Toxicity; *Shu Da Huang* (Radix et Rhizoma Rhei Conquitum) and *Gua Lou* (Fructus Trichosanthis) clear Excess-Heat in the Stomach; and *Chi Shao* (Radix Paeoniae Rubra), *Mu Dan Pi* (Cortex Moutan Radicis) and *Sheng Di Huang* (Radix Rehmanniae Glutinosae) cool the Blood and relieve Toxicity. The whole prescription achieved the effect of clearing Heat accumulated in the Lungs and Stomach. *Mei Gui Hua* (Flos Rosae Rugosae), *Ji Guan Hua* (Flos Celosiae Cristatae) and *Ling Xiao Hua* (Flos Campsitis) were used later to treat oily skin due to exuberant Stomach-Fire. [1]

Case 2
Patient
Male, aged 21.

Clinical manifestations
Papules started to appear on the patient's face at the age of 16 with intermittent exacerbation and alleviation. The papules gradually increased in number and turned redder, some of them becoming confluent. When the papules burst, a white secretion came out. The patient was diagnosed with cystic acne with secondary inflammation.

Examination revealed closed comedones, papules and pustules of different sizes concentrated on the forehead and both cheeks. A number of hard nodules 10mm in diameter were noted on various parts of the face. Some of the nodules were mobile and discharged a white plug when squeezed. The patient's face was very greasy. Accompanying symptoms and signs included dry mouth and a liking for cold drinks. Stool and urine were normal. The tongue body was red with a white and greasy coating; the pulse was wiry and slippery.

Pattern identification
Damp-Heat in the Lungs and Stomach, external contraction of pathogenic Toxins, Blood-Heat accumulating and binding.

Treatment principle
Clear Damp-Heat in the Lungs and Stomach, cool the Blood and relieve Toxicity, soften hardness and dissipate lumps.

Prescription ingredients
Sang Bai Pi (Cortex Mori Albae Radicis) 15g
Di Gu Pi (Cortex Lycii Radicis) 15g
Huang Qin (Radix Scutellariae Baicalensis) 15g
Zhi Zi (Fructus Gardeniae Jasminoidis) 10g
Huang Lian (Rhizoma Coptidis) 10g
Ye Ju Hua (Flos Chrysanthemi Indici) 15g
Ji Guan Hua (Flos Celosiae Cristatae) 10g
Jin Yin Hua (Flos Lonicerae) 15g
Lian Qiao (Fructus Forsythiae Suspensae) 15g
Pu Gong Ying (Herba Taraxaci cum Radice) 15g
Zi Hua Di Ding (Herba Violae Yedoensitis) 10g
Chi Shao (Radix Paeoniae Rubra) 10g
Mu Dan Pi (Cortex Moutan Radicis) 10g
Xia Ku Cao (Spica Prunellae Vulgaris) 15g
Che Qian Zi (Semen Plantaginis) 15g
Yi Yi Ren (Semen Coicis Lachryma-jobi) 30g

One bag a day was used to prepare a decoction, taken twice a day.

External treatment
The patient was also told to apply *Liu Lei Xi Ji* (Sulfur and Resorcinol Wash Preparation)[v] externally to the papules and pustules once a day. For the hard nodules, a mixture of equal proportions of *Hei Bu Yao Gao* (Black Cloth Medicated Paste) and *Hua Du San Gao* (Powder Paste for Transforming Toxicity) was prepared for application twice a day. [vi]

Second visit
After three days, the skin lesions had improved, and some of the papules and pustules had begun to subside. The patient was told to continue the prescription and the external applications for another seven days. The hard nodules and cystic area began to shrink and flatten. He was told to continue for another four days.

[iv] These preparations are usually only available through a registered pharmacist or registered doctor.

[v] This preparation is usually only available through a registered pharmacist or registered doctor.

[vi] In those countries where the use of certain ingredients contained in this powder paste are not permitted, it can be replaced by *Fu Rong Gao* (Cotton Rose Flower Paste) combined with *Da Bai Du Gao* (Major Toxicity-Vanquishing Syrup).

Third visit

After 14 bags overall, most of the lesions were flat and no new papules had appeared; the oily secretion was disappearing and the cysts were smaller. The tongue body was dark red with a white coating; the pulse was wiry and slippery. The prescription was modified by removing *Ji Guan Hua* (Flos Celosiae Cristatae) and *Huang Qin* (Rhizoma Coptidis) and adding *Dan Shen* (Radix Salviae Miltiorrhizae) 15g and *Hong Hua* (Flos Carthami Tinctorii) 15g. The external application continued as before.

Outcome

After 14 bags of the amended prescription, the skin lesions had disappeared completely, leaving pale pigmented spots and shallow scarring.

Discussion

The patient in this case had a liking for cold drinks, which caused Damp-Heat in the Lungs and Stomach. This was complicated by external contraction of pathogenic Toxins resulting in Blood-Heat accumulating and binding. Since the disease was in the acute stage manifesting as red papules, pustules and cysts, *Sang Bai Pi* (Cortex Mori Albae Radicis), *Di Gu Pi* (Cortex Lycii Radicis) and *Huang Qin* (Radix Scutellariae Baicalensis) were used initially to clear Lung-Heat, and *Huang Lian* (Rhizoma Coptidis) and *Zhi Zi* (Fructus Gardeniae Jasminoidis) to clear Stomach-Heat; *Zhi Zi* (Fructus Gardeniae Jasminoidis) was also included to clear exuberant Fire in the Triple Burner; *Jin Yin Hua* (Flos Lonicerae), *Lian Qiao* (Fructus Forsythiae Suspensae), *Pu Gong Ying* (Herba Taraxaci cum Radice), *Ye Ju Hua* (Flos Chrysanthemi Indici), and *Zi Hua Di Ding* (Herba Violae Yedoensitis) clear Heat and relieve Toxicity; *Chi Shao* (Radix Paeoniae Rubra), *Mu Dan Pi* (Cortex Moutan Radicis) and *Xia Ku Cao* (Spica Prunellae Vulgaris) cool the Blood, relieve Toxicity and soften hardness; *Che Qian Zi* (Semen Plantaginis) and *Yi Yi Ren* (Semen Coicis Lachryma-jobi) clear and drain Damp-Heat; and *Ji Guan Hua* (Flos Celosiae Cristatae) cools the Blood and clears Heat. The subsequent addition of *Dan Shen* (Radix Salviae Miltiorrhizae) and *Hong Hua* (Flos Carthami Tinctorii) was made to regulate Qi and invigorate the Blood, soften hardness and dissipate lumps to treat the hard nodules and cysts left when the inflammation subsided. [2]

Case 3
Patient
Female, aged 18.

Clinical manifestations

Red papules appeared on the patient's face when she was 15 and gradually became worse. The patient was diagnosed with acne by a number of hospitals but treatment with Western medicines was never successful. Three months previously after the patient had gone to a beauty salon, the red papules worsened significantly, with some of them turning into pustules. The papules were distributed symmetrically over the face, being particularly obvious on the cheeks; most of them manifested as closed comedones surrounded by a red border. They were painful to the touch. Accompanying symptoms and signs included a painful, red and hot face, dry stools, irritability and restlessness, and early and profuse periods. The tongue was red with a white and greasy coating; the pulse was wiry, slippery and rapid.

Pattern identification

Heat Toxins binding and accumulating in the skin.

Prescription ingredients

Jin Yin Hua (Flos Lonicerae) 15g
Lian Qiao (Fructus Forsythiae Suspensae) 15g
Pu Gong Ying (Herba Taraxaci cum Radice) 30g
Zi Hua Di Ding (Herba Violae Yedoensitis) 10g
Sang Bai Pi (Cortex Mori Albae Radicis) 15g
Di Gu Pi (Cortex Lycii Radicis) 15g
Huang Qin (Radix Scutellariae Baicalensis) 10g
Zhi Zi (Fructus Gardeniae Jasminoidis) 10g
Sheng Di Huang (Radix Rehmanniae Glutinosae) 30g
Chi Shao (Radix Paeoniae Rubra) 15g
Mu Dan Pi (Cortex Moutan Radicis) 15g
Gua Lou (Fructus Trichosanthis) 15g
Shu Da Huang (Radix et Rhizoma Rhei Conquitum) 10g
Yi Mu Cao (Herba Leonuri Heterophylli) 10g
Ye Ju Hua (Flos Chrysanthemi Indici) 15g
Xia Ku Cao (Spica Prunellae Vulgaris) 15g
Ling Yang Jiao Fen ‡ (Cornu Antelopis, powdered) 0.6g, infused in the prepared decoction

One bag a day was used to prepare a decoction, taken twice a day.

Second visit

After 14 bags, the pustules had disappeared completely. The red papules had become paler and the irritability had disappeared, but the patient still suffered from dry stools. A few new red papules had appeared. The prescription was modified by removing *Lian Qiao* (Fructus Forsythiae Suspensae) and *Jin Yin Hua* (Flos Lonicerae) and adding *Mei Gui Hua* (Flos Rosae Rugosae) 10g and *Huai Hua* (Flos Sophorae Japonicae) 30g.

Outcome

After 14 bags of the amended prescription, all the papules had disappeared, leaving pale pigmented spots. The menstrual flow was lighter and the stool was normal. The tongue body was red with a white coating; the pulse was wiry and slippery. The patient was prescribed *Lian Qiao Bai Du Wan* (Forsythia Pill for Vanquishing Toxicity) 6g, twice a day, and *Dang Gui Ku Shen Wan* (Chinese Angelica Root and Flavescent Sophora Root Pill) 9g, twice a day, for one month to consolidate the improvement.

Discussion

As stated in the discussion of Case 1 above, Dr. Zhang considers that Damp-Heat in the Lungs and Stomach is part of the etiology of all cases of acne and therefore materia medica for clearing Damp-Heat in the Lungs and Stomach should be included in the treatment. In this prescription, *Sang Bai Pi* (Cortex Mori Albae Radicis), *Di Gu Pi* (Cortex Lycii Radicis), *Huang Qin* (Radix Scutellariae Baicalensis), and *Zhi Zi* (Fructus Gardeniae Jasminoidis) serve this purpose. In addition, *Jin Yin Hua* (Flos Lonicerae), *Lian Qiao* (Fructus Forsythiae Suspensae), *Pu Gong Ying* (Herba Taraxaci cum Radice), *Zi Hua Di*

Ding (Herba Violae Yedoensitis), and *Ye Ju Hua* (Flos Chrysanthemi Indici) clear Heat and relieve Toxicity; and *Gua Lou* (Fructus Trichosanthis) and *Shu Da Huang* (Radix et Rhizoma Rhei Conquitum) clear Excess-Heat in the Stomach. In addition, because the patient presented with a red and hot face, red papules with pustules, and pain due to Heat Toxins accumulating and binding, *Sheng Di Huang* (Radix Rehmanniae Glutinosae), *Chi Shao* (Radix Paeoniae Rubra), *Mu Dan Pi* (Cortex Moutan Radicis), and *Ling Yang Jiao Fen* ‡ (Cornu Antelopis, powdered) were included to cool the Blood and relieve Toxicity. *Xia Ku Cao* (Spica Prunellae Vulgaris) was used to dissipate lumps and *Yi Mu Cao* (Herba Leonuri Heterophylli) to regulate and harmonize the Chong and Ren vessels. *Mei Gui Hua* (Flos Rosae Rugosae) and *Huai Hua* (Flos Sophorae Japonicae) were added to guide the other ingredients upward and assist in elimination of the lesions. [3]

Modern clinical experience

TREATMENT BASED ON PATTERN IDENTIFICATION

1. **Li** identified four patterns. [4]

- **Accumulation of Heat in the Lungs and Stomach**

Prescription
PI PA QING FEI YIN JIA JIAN
Loquat Beverage for Clearing Heat from the Lungs, with modifications

Pi Pa Ye (Folium Eriobotryae Japonicae) 10g
Sang Bai Pi (Cortex Mori Albae Radicis) 10g
Huang Qin (Radix Scutellariae Baicalensis) 10g
Zhi Zi (Fructus Gardeniae Jasminoidis) 10g
Mu Dan Pi (Cortex Moutan Radicis) 10g
Che Qian Cao (Herba Plantaginis) 10g
Bai Mao Gen (Rhizoma Imperatae Cylindricae) 30g
Shi Gao ‡ (Gypsum Fibrosum) 30g, decocted for
  30 minutes before adding the other ingredients

- **Exuberant Heat Toxins**

Prescription
WU WEI XIAO DU YIN JIA JIAN
Five-Ingredient Beverage for Dispersing Toxicity, with modifications

Jin Yin Hua (Flos Lonicerae) 15g
Lian Qiao (Fructus Forsythiae Suspensae) 15g
Pu Gong Ying (Herba Taraxaci cum Radice) 15g
Zi Hua Di Ding (Herba Violae Yedoensitis) 15g
Ye Ju Hua (Flos Chrysanthemi Indici) 10g
Pi Pa Ye (Folium Eriobotryae Japonicae) 10g
Zhi Zi (Fructus Gardeniae Jasminoidis) 10g
Xuan Shen (Radix Scrophulariae Ningpoensis) 10g
Huang Qin (Radix Scutellariae Baicalensis) 10g

- **Disharmony of the Chong and Ren vessels**

Prescription
SI WU TANG HE PI PA QING FEI YIN JIA JIAN
Four Agents Decoction Combined With Loquat Beverage for Clearing Heat from the Lungs, with modifications

Sheng Di Huang (Radix Rehmanniae Glutinosae) 10g
Chi Shao (Radix Paeoniae Rubra) 10g
Bai Shao (Radix Paeoniae Lactiflorae) 10g
Dang Gui (Radix Angelicae Sinensis) 10g
Chuan Xiong (Rhizoma Ligustici Chuanxiong) 10g
Nü Zhen Zi (Fructus Ligustri Lucidi) 10g
Han Lian Cao (Herba Ecliptae Prostratae) 10g
Di Gu Pi (Cortex Lycii Radicis) 10g
Pi Pa Ye (Folium Eriobotryae Japonicae) 10g

- **Blood stasis and Phlegm congealing**

Prescription
TAO HONG SI WU TANG HE ER CHEN TANG JIA JIAN
Peach Kernel and Safflower Four Agents Decoction Combined With Two Matured Ingredients Decoction, with modifications

Dang Gui (Radix Angelicae Sinensis) 10g
Chi Shao (Radix Paeoniae Rubra) 10g
Tao Ren (Semen Persicae) 10g
Hong Hua (Flos Carthami Tinctorii) 10g
Sheng Di Huang (Radix Rehmanniae Glutinosae) 10g
Chuan Xiong (Rhizoma Ligustici Chuanxiong) 10g
Xiang Fu (Rhizoma Cyperi Rotundi) 10g
Fa Ban Xia (Rhizoma Pinelliae Ternatae Praeparata) 10g
Chen Pi (Pericarpium Citri Reticulatae) 10g
Fu Ling (Sclerotium Poriae Cocos) 10g
Jiang Can ‡ (Bombyx Batryticatus) 10g
Xia Ku Cao (Spica Prunellae Vulgaris) 10g
Lian Qiao (Fructus Forsythiae Suspensae) 10g

With all patterns, one bag a day of the ingredients was decocted twice for oral administration and then a third time for use as a cold, wet compress on the affected area. A course of treatment lasted for two weeks. Results were seen after two courses.

2. **Yu** also identified four patterns for the treatment of acne. [5]

- **Liver Depression and Blood stasis**

Prescription ingredients
Chai Hu (Radix Bupleuri) 10g
Zhi Zi (Fructus Gardeniae Jasminoidis) 10g
Dang Gui (Radix Angelicae Sinensis) 6g
Chi Shao (Radix Paeoniae Rubra) 6g
Hong Hua (Flos Carthami Tinctorii) 6g

Huang Qin (Radix Scutellariae Baicalensis) 10g
Bo He (Herba Menthae Haplocalycis) 3g, added 5 minutes before the end of the decoction process
Chen Pi (Pericarpium Citri Reticulatae) 10g
E Zhu (Rhizoma Curcumae) 6g
Chuan Xiong (Rhizoma Ligustici Chuanxiong) 6g
Gan Cao (Radix Glycyrrhizae) 6g

- **Lung-Heat complicated by invasion of Wind**

Prescription ingredients

Jing Jie (Herba Schizonepetae Tenuifoliae) 10g
Fang Feng (Radix Ledebouriellae Divaricatae) 10g
Bai Zhi (Radix Angelicae Dahuricae) 6g
Jie Geng (Radix Platycodi Grandiflori) 6g
Chuan Xiong (Rhizoma Ligustici Chuanxiong) 10g
Huang Qin (Radix Scutellariae Baicalensis) 10g
Zhi Zi (Fructus Gardeniae Jasminoidis) 10g
Lian Qiao (Fructus Forsythiae Suspensae) 10g
Bo He (Herba Menthae Haplocalycis) 3g, added 5 minutes before the end of the decoction process
Huang Lian (Rhizoma Coptidis) 6g
Gan Cao (Radix Glycyrrhizae) 6g

- **Accumulation of Heat Toxins**

Prescription ingredients

Jin Yin Hua (Flos Lonicerae) 15g
Tian Hua Fen (Radix Trichosanthis) 10g
Zhe Bei Mu (Bulbus Fritillariae Thunbergii) 6g
Dang Gui Wei (Extremitas Radicis Angelicae Sinensis) 10g
Chi Shao (Radix Paeoniae Rubra) 10g
Ze Xie (Rhizoma Alismatis Orientalis) 15g
*Chuan Shan Jia** (Squama Manitis Pentadactylae) 10g
Ru Xiang (Gummi Olibanum) 6g
Mo Yao (Myrrha) 6g
Fang Feng (Radix Ledebouriellae Divaricatae) 6g
Gan Cao (Radix Glycyrrhizae) 6g

- **Deficiency of Vital Qi (Zheng Qi) complicated by Blood stasis and accumulation of Toxins**

Prescription ingredients

Huang Qi (Radix Astragali seu Hedysari) 15g
Gui Zhi (Ramulus Cinnamomi Cassiae) 6g
Dang Gui (Radix Angelicae Sinensis) 10g
Chi Shao (Radix Paeoniae Rubra) 10g
*Chuan Shan Jia** (Squama Manitis Pentadactylae) 10g
Ru Xiang (Gummi Olibanum) 6g
Mo Yao (Myrrha) 6g
Bai Zhi (Radix Angelicae Dahuricae) 6g
Zhe Bei Mu (Bulbus Fritillariae Thunbergii) 6g
Gan Cao (Radix Glycyrrhizae) 6g

With all patterns, one bag a day was used to prepare a decoction, taken twice a day. A course of treatment lasted five to seven days. Results were seen after four courses.

3. **Zha** divided the disease into three patterns. [6]

- **Wind-Heat in the Lung channel**

Treatment principle
Dredge Wind, diffuse the Lungs and clear Heat.

Prescription
PI PA QING FEI YIN JIA JIAN
Loquat Beverage for Clearing Heat from the Lungs, with modifications

Pi Pa Ye (Folium Eriobotryae Japonicae) 10g
Sang Bai Pi (Cortex Mori Albae Radicis) 10g
Huang Qin (Radix Scutellariae Baicalensis) 10g
Lian Qiao (Fructus Forsythiae Suspensae) 10g
Mu Dan Pi (Cortex Moutan Radicis) 10g
Sheng Di Huang (Radix Rehmanniae Glutinosae) 10g
Di Gu Pi (Cortex Lycii Radicis) 10g
Gan Cao (Radix Glycyrrhizae) 6g

- **Accumulation and binding of Damp-Heat**

Treatment principle
Clear Heat, transform Dampness and regulate the functions of the Fu organs.

Prescription
YIN CHEN HAO TANG JIA JIAN
Oriental Wormwood Decoction, with modifications

Yin Chen Hao (Herba Artemisiae Scopariae) 10g
Yi Yi Ren (Semen Coicis Lachryma-jobi) 15g
Dang Gui (Radix Angelicae Sinensis) 10g
Ku Shen (Radix Sophorae Flavescentis) 15g
Zhi Zi (Fructus Gardeniae Jasminoidis) 10g
Huang Bai (Cortex Phellodendri) 10g
Ye Ju Hua (Flos Chrysanthemi Indici) 10g
Ji Guan Hua (Flos Celosiae Cristatae) 10g
Jie Geng (Radix Platycodi Grandiflori) 3g
Zi Hua Di Ding (Herba Violae Yedoensitis) 10g
Chen Pi (Pericarpium Citri Reticulatae) 10g
Gan Cao (Radix Glycyrrhizae) 6g

- **Phlegm-Damp congealing and binding**

Treatment principle
Fortify the Spleen, transform Phlegm and eliminate Dampness.

Prescription
SHEN LING BAI ZHU SAN JIA JIAN
Ginseng, Poria and White Atractylodes Powder, with modifications

Bai Zhu (Rhizoma Atractylodis Macrocephalae) 10g
Fu Ling (Sclerotium Poriae Cocos) 10g

Yi Yi Ren (Semen Coicis Lachryma-jobi) 20g

Sha Ren (Fructus Amomi) 6g, added 5 minutes before
  the end of the decoction process

Shan Yao (Radix Dioscoreae Oppositae) 15g

Jie Geng (Radix Platycodi Grandiflori) 3g

Xia Ku Cao (Spica Prunellae Vulgaris) 6g

Hai Zao (Herba Sargassi) 10g

Mu Li‡ (Concha Ostreae) 15g

Chen Pi (Pericarpium Citri Reticulatae) 10g

Lian Qiao (Fructus Forsythiae Suspensae) 10g

Ban Xia (Rhizoma Pinelliae Ternatae) 6g

With all patterns, one bag a day was used to prepare a
decoction, taken twice a day for one month.

BASIC FORMULAE MODIFIED IN ACCORDANCE WITH SYMPTOMS

1. **Sun** formulated the following basic prescription to
invigorate the Blood and clear Heat from the Lungs. [7]

Prescription ingredients

Chuan Xiong (Rhizoma Ligustici Chuanxiong) 5-10g

Hu Zhang (Radix et Rhizoma Polygoni Cuspidati) 15g

Shan Zha (Fructus Crataegi) 15-30g

Tu Da Huang (Radix Rumicis Madaio) 10g

Sang Ye (Folium Mori Albae) 10g

Sang Bai Pi (Cortex Mori Albae Radicis) 10g

Chan Tui‡ (Periostracum Cicadae) 10g

Huang Qin (Radix Scutellariae Baicalensis) 5g

Shi Gao‡ (Gypsum Fibrosum) 15g, decocted for
  30 minutes before adding the other ingredients

Huang Lian (Rhizoma Coptidis) 3g

Bai Hua She She Cao (Herba Hedyotidis Diffusae) 30g

Modifications

1. For white comedones, *Qiang Huo* (Rhizoma et Radix
   Notopterygii) 3g, *Yi Yi Ren* (Semen Coicis Lachryma-
   jobi) 15g and *Fu Ling* (Sclerotium Poriae Cocos) 10g
   were added.
2. For red papules, *Chi Shao* (Radix Paeoniae Rubra)
   10g, *Mu Dan Pi* (Cortex Moutan Radicis) 10g and
   Dan Shen (Radix Salviae Miltiorrhizae) 10g were
   added.
3. For pustules, *Bai Jiang Cao* (Herba Patriniae cum
   Radice) 15g and *Shu Da Huang* (Radix et Rhizoma
   Rhei Conquitum) 10g were added.
4. For nodules and cysts, *Tao Ren* (Semen Persicae) 10g
   and *Hong Hua* (Flos Carthami Tinctorii) 5g were
   added.
5. For pale residual pigmentation, *Gan Cao* (Radix Glycyrrhizae) 3g and *Bai Zhi* (Radix Angelicae Dahuricae) 10g were added.

One bag a day was used to prepare a decoction, taken
twice a day. Initial results were seen after 15 days.

2. **Ou** treated acne with a basic formula and modified it
according to the pattern involved. [8]

Basic prescription
AN CHUANG JING TANG
Acne-Cleansing Decoction

Bai Hua She She Cao (Herba Hedyotidis Diffusae) 20g

Jin Yin Hua (Flos Lonicerae) 15g

Ban Bian Lian (Herba Lobeliae Chinensis cum Radice) 15g

Pu Gong Ying (Herba Taraxaci cum Radice) 15g

Zhe Bei Mu (Bulbus Fritillariae Thunbergii) 15g

Zao Jiao Ci (Spina Gleditsiae Sinensis) 15g

Hai Zao (Herba Sargassi) 12g

Mo Yao (Myrrha) 10g

Xuan Shen (Radix Scrophulariae Ningpoensis) 30g

Modifications

1. For Blood-Dryness due to Wind-Heat, *Bo He* (Herba
   Menthae Haplocalycis) 6g, *Lian Qiao* (Fructus Forsythiae Suspensae) 10g, *Zi Cao* (Radix Arnebiae seu
   Lithospermi) 10g, and *Chan Tui*‡ (Periostracum Cicadae) 10g were added.
2. For exuberant Heat Toxins, *Huang Lian* (Rhizoma
   Coptidis) 10g, *Da Huang* (Radix et Rhizoma Rhei)
   10g, *Yi Yi Ren* (Semen Coicis Lachryma-jobi) 15g,
   and *Dong Gua Ren* (Semen Benincasae Hispidae) 15g
   were added.
3. For Blood stasis and binding of Phlegm, *Bai Jie Zi*
   (Semen Sinapis Albae) 10g, *San Qi* (Radix Notoginseng) 6g, *Wu Gong*‡ (Scolopendra Subspinipes) 3g,
   and *Quan Xie*‡ (Buthus Martensi) 3g were added.
4. For internal accumulation of Phlegm-Damp and
   turbid Dampness, *She Chuang Zi* (Fructus Cnidii
   Monnieri) 6g, *Bai Jie Zi* (Semen Sinapis Albae) 10g,
   Shan Zha (Fructus Crataegi) 10g, and *Ku Shen* (Radix
   Sophorae Flavescentis) 10g were added.
5. For Phlegm congealing and Blood stasis due to
   insufficiency of Qi and Blood, *Huang Qi* (Radix
   Astragali seu Hedysari) 15g, *Dang Shen* (Radix Codonopsitis Pilosulae) 10g, *Dang Gui* (Radix Angelicae
   Sinensis) 10g, and *San Qi* (Radix Notoginseng) 6g
   were added.

One bag a day was used to prepare a decoction, taken
twice a day.

External prescription
AN CHUANG JING TU MO JI
Mask Preparation for Cleansing Acne

Huang Lian (Rhizoma Coptidis)

Da Huang (Radix et Rhizoma Rhei)

Mo Yao (Myrrha)

Zao Jiao Ci (Spina Gleditsiae Sinensis)

San Qi (Radix Notoginseng)

Liquid extracts of these herbs were added to polyvinyl alcohol or other base substances. The mask was applied to the face every evening and washed off the following morning. Results were seen after 7 to 15 days.

3. Guo formulated a basic prescription to clear Damp-Heat from the Lungs and Stomach. [9]

Prescription ingredients

Pi Pa Ye (Folium Eriobotryae Japonicae) 10g
Sang Bai Pi (Cortex Mori Albae Radicis) 10g
Huang Qin (Radix Scutellariae Baicalensis) 10g
Zhi Zi (Fructus Gardeniae Jasminoidis) 10g
Chi Shao (Radix Paeoniae Rubra) 10g
Ku Shen (Radix Sophorae Flavescentis) 10g
Ye Ju Hua (Flos Chrysanthemi Indici) 8g
Huang Lian (Rhizoma Coptidis) 6g
Bai Mao Gen (Rhizoma Imperatae Cylindricae) 30g
Huai Hua (Flos Sophorae Japonicae) 15g

Modifications

1. For constipation, *Da Huang* (Radix et Rhizoma Rhei) 6g was added 10 minutes before the end of the decoction process.
2. For severe infection, *Pu Gong Ying* (Herba Taraxaci cum Radice) 15g and *Zi Hua Di Ding* (Herba Violae Yedoensitis) 15g were added.
3. For cysts, *Xia Ku Cao* (Spica Prunellae Vulgaris) 15g and *Zhe Bei Mu* (Bulbus Fritillariae Thunbergii) 10g were added.
4. For seborrhea, *Yi Yi Ren* (Semen Coicis Lachryma-jobi) 15g, *Zhi Ke* (Fructus Citri Aurantii) 10g and *Bai Zhu* (Rhizoma Atractylodis Macrocephalae) 10g were added.

One bag a day was used to prepare a decoction, taken twice a day. Results were seen after 15 days.

4. Li formulated a basic prescription to clear Heat and dry Dampness. [10]

Prescription ingredients

Huang Bai (Cortex Phellodendri) 15g
Cang Zhu (Rhizoma Atractylodis) 15g
Yi Yi Ren (Semen Coicis Lachryma-jobi) 50g
Jin Yin Hua (Flos Lonicerae) 50g
Pu Gong Ying (Herba Taraxaci cum Radice) 50g
Lian Qiao (Fructus Forsythiae Suspensae) 25g

Modifications

1. For aggravation of lesions prior to menstruation, *Chai Hu* (Radix Bupleuri) 15g, *Dang Gui* (Radix Angelicae Sinensis) 15g, *Mu Dan Pi* (Cortex Moutan Radicis) 10g, and *Sheng Di Huang* (Radix Rehmanniae Glutinosae) 25g were added.
2. For constipation, *Da Huang* (Radix et Rhizoma Rhei)

5g and *Huang Qin* (Radix Scutellariae Baicalensis) 15g were added.
3. For itching on the face, *Fang Feng* (Radix Ledebouriellae Divaricatae) 15g, *Chi Shao* (Radix Paeoniae Rubra) 10g and *Dan Shen* (Radix Salviae Miltiorrhizae) 30g were added.

One bag was used to prepare a decoction, taken twice a day. Results were seen between 7 and 28 days.

SPECIAL PRESCRIPTIONS

1. Zhang reported on his treatment of facial acne in women. [11]

Prescription
QING GAN DA YU TANG
Decoction for Clearing Heat from the Liver and Driving Out Depression

Chen Pi (Pericarpium Citri Reticulatae) 6g
Ju Hua (Flos Chrysanthemi Morifolii) 10g
Mu Dan Pi (Cortex Moutan Radicis) 10g
Zhi Zi (Fructus Gardeniae Jasminoidis) 10g
Chai Hu (Radix Bupleuri) 10g
Dang Gui (Radix Angelicae Sinensis) 12g
Bai Shao (Radix Paeoniae Lactiflorae) 12g
Bai Zhu (Rhizoma Atractylodis Macrocephalae) 12g
Fu Ling (Sclerotium Poriae Cocos) 12g
Gan Cao (Radix Glycyrrhizae) 5g
Sheng Jiang (Rhizoma Zingiberis Officinalis Recens) 3g
Bo He (Herba Menthae Haplocalycis) 3g, added 5 minutes before the end of the decoction process

One bag a day was used to prepare a decoction, taken twice a day. Fourteen days made up a course of treatment. Results were seen after one to two courses.

2. Liu formulated an empirical prescription to treat acne. [12]

Prescription
KE CUO TANG
Overcoming Acne Decoction

Pi Pa Ye (Folium Eriobotryae Japonicae) 10g
Ku Shen (Radix Sophorae Flavescentis) 10g
Dan Shen (Radix Salviae Miltiorrhizae) 10g
Lian Qiao (Fructus Forsythiae Suspensae) 20g
Jin Yin Hua (Flos Lonicerae) 20g
Chan Tui ‡ (Periostracum Cicadae) 6g
Tian Hua Fen (Radix Trichosanthis) 6g
Chi Shao (Radix Paeoniae Rubra) 12g
Pu Gong Ying (Herba Taraxaci cum Radice) 15g

One bag a day was used to prepare a decoction, taken twice a day. Seven days made up a course of treatment. Results were seen after three courses.

COMBINATION OF INTERNAL AND EXTERNAL TREATMENTS

1. **Xu** combined internal treatment with external application of a powder. [13]

Prescription
SI WU LIANG XUE QING FEI YIN
Four Agents Beverage for Cooling the Blood and Clearing Heat from the Lungs

Sheng Di Huang (Radix Rehmanniae Glutinosae) 15g
Chi Shao (Radix Paeoniae Rubra) 15g
Dang Gui (Radix Angelicae Sinensis) 10g
Mu Dan Pi (Cortex Moutan Radicis) 10g
Chuan Xiong (Rhizoma Ligustici Chuanxiong) 10g
Huang Qin (Radix Scutellariae Baicalensis) 10g
Zhi Zi (Fructus Gardeniae Jasminoidis) 10g
Da Huang (Radix et Rhizoma Rhei) 10g
Bai Ji Li (Fructus Tribuli Terrestris) 10g
Bai Zhi (Radix Angelicae Dahuricae) 12g
Sang Bai Pi (Cortex Mori Albae Radicis) 12g
Shi Gao ‡ (Gypsum Fibrosum) 30g, decocted for
   30 minutes before adding the other ingredients
Gan Cao (Radix Glycyrrhizae) 6g

One bag a day was used to prepare a decoction, taken twice a day.

External treatment
For cysts and/or nodules, *Dian Dao San* (Reversal Powder), made by grinding equal amounts of *Da Huang* (Radix et Rhizoma Rhei) and *Liu Huang* ‡ (Sulphur) to a fine powder and mixing with cool boiled water or tea, was applied to the affected area twice a day for three months.

2. **Gao** combined internal treatment with a topical application. [14]

Internal prescription
QING FEI QU CUO YIN
Beverage for Clearing Heat from the Lungs and Dispelling Acne

Pi Pa Ye (Folium Eriobotryae Japonicae) 12g
Sheng Di Huang (Radix Rehmanniae Glutinosae) 12g
Zhe Bei Mu (Bulbus Fritillariae Thunbergii) 12g
Sang Bai Pi (Cortex Mori Albae Radicis) 10g
Huang Qin (Radix Scutellariae Baicalensis) 10g
Mu Dan Pi (Cortex Moutan Radicis) 10g
Jie Geng (Radix Platycodi Grandiflori) 10g
Yi Yi Ren (Semen Coicis Lachryma-jobi) 20g
Ban Lan Gen (Radix Isatidis seu Baphicacanthi) 15g
Pu Gong Ying (Herba Taraxaci cum Radice) 15g

One bag a day was used to prepare a decoction, taken twice a day. Ten days made up a course of treatment.

External application
XIAO CUO YE
Dispersing Acne Liquid

Da Huang (Radix et Rhizoma Rhei)
Zi Hua Di Ding (Herba Violae Yedoensitis)
Chi Shao (Radix Paeoniae Rubra)
Huang Lian (Rhizoma Coptidis)
Zhi Zi (Fructus Gardeniae Jasminoidis)

The ingredients were ground together into a fine powder in a proportion of 2:2:2:1:1. Then, 100g of the powder was added to 500ml of 75 percent ethanol and left to steep for two weeks before being filtered prior to application. The greasy surface of the acne was first washed with warm water before the medicated liquid was spread over the affected area with a cotton bud three times a day. Results were seen after ten days.

3. **Wu** employed a combination of internal treatment and an external steam-wash. [15]

Prescription
XIAO CUO TANG
Dispersing Acne Decoction

Sheng Di Huang (Radix Rehmanniae Glutinosae) 30g
Bai Hua She She Cao (Herba Hedyotidis Diffusae) 30g
Hu Zhang (Radix et Rhizoma Polygoni Cuspidati) 30g
Dan Shen (Radix Salviae Miltiorrhizae) 30g
Xuan Shen (Radix Scrophulariae Ningpoensis) 9g
Tu Da Huang (Radix Rumicis Madaio) 9g
Mai Men Dong (Radix Ophiopogonis Japonici) 9g
Zhi Mu (Rhizoma Anemarrhenae Asphodeloidis) 9g
Huang Bai (Cortex Phellodendri) 9g
Sang Bai Pi (Cortex Mori Albae Radicis) 15g
Di Gu Pi (Cortex Lycii Radicis) 15g
Shan Zha (Fructus Crataegi) 15g
Gan Cao (Radix Glycyrrhizae) 3g

One bag a day of the ingredients was decocted three times. The first two decoctions were mixed to be taken half in the morning and evening; the third decoction was used externally, initially hot to steam the affected area and then warm as a wash for 20-30 minutes every evening. The area was patted dry afterwards. Results were seen after one to three months of treatment.

EXTERNAL TREATMENT
Huang used an external treatment for facial acne. [16]

Prescription
KU SHEN SHOU WU HE JI
Flavescent Sophora Root and Fleeceflower Mixture

He Shou Wu (Radix Polygoni Multiflori) 50g
Ku Shen (Radix Sophorae Flavescentis) 50g

Dang Gui (Radix Angelicae Sinensis) 50g
Bai Zhi (Radix Angelicae Dahuricae) 50g
Bai Cu (Acetum Album) 500ml

The ingredients were placed in a glass bottle, which was sealed and decocted in a double boiler for one hour. The bottle was opened on the following day and the liquid applied twice a day to the affected area with a cotton bud. A course of treatment lasted for 20 days. The liquid could also be used for a second course, at full strength or diluted. Results were seen after one to two courses.

ACUPUNCTURE TREATMENT

1. **Li** combined filiform and three-edged needles. [17]
Points: BL-12 Fengmen, BL-13 Feishu, ST-9 Renying, and ST-36 Zusanli (all bilateral).

Technique

- BL-12 Fengmen and BL-13 Feishu were pricked with a three-edged needle to cause bleeding once every two days.
- Filiform needles were used at ST-9 Renying and ST-36 Zusanli and the even method was applied. The needling sensation at ST-9 Renying was sent upward to the face. The needles were retained for 30 minutes and manipulated two or three times during this period.

Treatment was given once a day and six days' treatment made up a course. There was a break of one or two days between courses. Best results were seen after five courses.

2. **Yan** used filiform needling only. [18]
Points: CV-24 Chengjiang, GB-20 Fengchi, ST-9 Renying, EX-HN-3 Yintang,[vii] EX-HN-5 Taiyang,[viii] ST-10 Shuitu, and SI-17 Tianrong.
Technique: ST-9 Renying and ST-10 Shuitu were needled perpendicularly to send the needling sensation to the chest. No manipulation was performed at these two points. The other points were needled routinely. The needles were retained for 20 minutes. Treatment was given once a day; ten days made up a course. Results were seen after three courses.

EAR ACUPUNCTURE

1. **Yang** performed ear acupuncture with embedding of needles. [19]
Main points: Subcortex, Endocrine, Adrenal Gland or Kidney, and Sympathetic Nerve.

Auxiliary points

- For acne on the nose, Nose was added.
- For acne on the forehead, Forehead was added.
- For acne on the cheeks, Cheek was added.
- For Lung-Heat and Blood-Heat patterns, Lung was added.
- For patterns of Damp-Heat in the Stomach and Intestines, Liver and Stomach were added.
- For Phlegm-Damp due to Spleen Deficiency, Spleen and Stomach were added.

Technique: The main points were used in every treatment, with auxiliary points being selected in accordance with the site of the lesions. The needles were embedded in the points and changed every three to five days. The patients were asked to press the needles several times a day. Treatment continued for two months.

2. **Li** performed ear acupuncture with seeds. [20]
Main points: Shenmen, Lung, Endocrine, Subcortex, Adrenal Gland, and Heart.

Auxiliary points

- For Stomach-Heat patterns, Spleen and Stomach were added.
- For Lung-Heat patterns, Lower Rectum was added.
- For Blood-Heat due to Liver Depression, Uterus and Ovary were added.

Technique
Wang Bu Liu Xing (Semen Vaccariae Segetalis) seeds were attached to the points on one ear with adhesive plaster or tape. Patients were told to press the seeds for two minutes, three times a day. The seeds were changed every three to five days. One ear was treated each time in alternation. A course of treatment lasted three months.

TREATMENT ACCORDING TO THE MENSTRUAL CYCLE

1. **Deng** varied treatment depending on the stage of the menstrual cycle. [21]

- He started the treatment on the fifth or sixth day of the cycle, when ovarian follicle maturation for ovulation can be promoted.

Treatment principle
Augment Qi and nourish the Blood, supplement the Liver and Kidneys and regulate menstruation, supported by clearing Heat and relieving Toxicity.

[vii] M-HN-3 according to the system employed by the Shanghai College of Traditional Chinese Medicine.
[viii] M-HN-9 according to the system employed by the Shanghai College of Traditional Chinese Medicine.

Prescription
SHI QUAN DA BU TANG JIA JIAN
Perfect Major Supplementation Decoction, with modifications

Huang Qi (Radix Astragali seu Hedysari) 15g
Dang Shen (Radix Codonopsitis Pilosulae) 15g
Bai Zhu (Rhizoma Atractylodis Macrocephalae) 10g
Fu Ling (Sclerotium Poriae Cocos) 10g
Dang Gui (Radix Angelicae Sinensis) 10g
Zi He Che‡ (Placenta Hominis) 10g
Bai Shao (Radix Paeoniae Lactiflorae) 10g
Shu Di Huang (Radix Rehmanniae Glutinosae Conquita) 10g
Rou Gui (Cortex Cinnamomi Cassiae) 6g
Chuan Xiong (Rhizoma Ligustici Chuanxiong) 6g
Zhi Gan Cao (Radix Glycyrrhizae, mix-fried with honey) 6g
Pu Gong Ying (Herba Taraxaci cum Radice) 30g

Modifications
1. For delayed menstruation with scant menstrual flow, Xiang Fu (Rhizoma Cyperi Rotundi) 6g was added.
2. For pronounced Yang Deficiency, Fu Zi* (Radix Lateralis Aconiti Carmichaeli Praeparata) 3g was added.
3. For pronounced Yin Deficiency, Rou Gui (Cortex Cinnamomi Cassiae) and Chuan Xiong (Rhizoma Ligustici Chuanxiong) were removed and Shu Di Huang (Radix Rehmanniae Glutinosae Conquita) was replaced by Sheng Di Huang (Radix Rehmanniae Glutinosae) 10g.

• Between periods and after ovulation, the treatment principle focused on regulating and supplementing the Spleen and Kidneys to maintain the functions of the corpus luteum. The prescription was also based on Shi Quan Da Bu Tang (Perfect Major Supplementation Decoction), but the dosages of Dang Shen (Radix Codonopsitis Pilosulae) and Huang Qi (Radix Astragali seu Hedysari) were increased to 30g and Shan Yao (Radix Dioscoreae Oppositae) 30g, Ba Ji Tian (Radix Morindae Officinalis) 10g, Tu Si Zi (Semen Cuscutae) 10g, Nü Zhen Zi (Fructus Ligustri Lucidi) 10g, and Yin Yang Huo (Herba Epimedii) 10g were added.

• Seven days before menstruation, the prescription was changed.

Treatment principle
Dredge the Liver and harmonize the Spleen, regulate Qi and invigorate the Blood, and free menstruation.

Prescription
XIAO YAO SAN JIA JIAN
Free Wanderer Powder, with modifications

Chai Hu (Radix Bupleuri) 30g
Dang Gui (Radix Angelicae Sinensis) 30g
Fu Ling (Sclerotium Poriae Cocos) 30g
Bai Shao (Radix Paeoniae Lactiflorae) 30g
Bai Zhu (Rhizoma Atractylodis Macrocephalae) 30g
Zhi Gan Cao (Radix Glycyrrhizae, mix-fried with honey) 15g
Dan Shen (Radix Salviae Miltiorrhizae) 15g
Niu Xi (Radix Achyranthis Bidentatae) 15g
Tao Ren (Semen Persicae) 15g
Hong Hua (Flos Carthami Tinctorii) 6g
Yan Hu Suo (Rhizoma Corydalis Yanhusuo) 6g

Results were seen after three months' treatment.

2. **Lin** based treatment on pattern identification with modifications depending on the stage of the menstrual cycle. [22]

• For Kidney Deficiency and Liver Depression patterns, he based the prescription on Zuo Gui Yin (Restoring the Left [Kidney Yin] Beverage) on its own or combined with Xiao Yao San (Free Wanderer Powder).

• For effulgent Yin Deficiency-Fire patterns, he based the prescription on Zhi Bai Di Huang Wan (Anemarrhena, Phellodendron and Rehmannia Pill).

• For patterns of Qi and Blood Deficiency, he based the prescription on Ba Zhen Tang (Eight Treasure Decoction).

• For patterns of Excess Heat in the Liver channel, he based the prescription on Long Dan Xie Gan Tang (Chinese Gentian Decoction for Draining the Liver).

Modifications to the above prescriptions were made depending on the stage of the menstrual cycle:

1. In the later stage of the cycle or after bleeding following involution of the corpus luteum, he added herbs for enriching and supplementing Kidney Yin and regulating and nourishing the Chong and Ren vessels such as Shan Zhu Yu (Fructus Corni Officinalis), Tu Si Zi (Semen Cuscutae), Nü Zhen Zi (Fructus Ligustri Lucidi), and Han Lian Cao (Herba Ecliptae Prostratae).

2. Prior to or during ovulation, he added herbs for invigorating the Blood and promoting ovulation such as Dan Shen (Radix Salviae Miltiorrhizae), Tao Ren (Semen Persicae) and Liu Ji Nu (Herba Artemisiae Anomalae).

3. After ovulation, he added herbs for supplementing the Kidneys, regulating the Chong and Ren vessels, and fortifying the functions of the corpus luteum such as Ba Ji Tian (Radix Morindae Officinalis), Xian Mao (Rhizoma Curculiginis Orchioidis) and Yin Yang Huo (Herba Epimedii).

One menstrual cycle was taken as a course of treatment. Results were seen at the earliest after one course and at the latest after six courses.

3. **Zhu** applied acupuncture treatment to female patients in accordance with the menstrual cycle. [23]

Main points: GV-11 Shendao, GV-10 Lingtai and GV-9 Zhiyang.

Auxiliary points

- For lesions on the forehead, BL-13 Feishu was added.
- For involvement of the cheeks and alae nasi, BL-21 Weishu was added.
- For lesions on the chin, BL-23 Shenshu was added.
- For aggravation of lesions prior to menstruation, BL-18 Ganshu was added.

Technique

After routine sterilization, a no. 28 filiform needle, 4 cun in length, was inserted at GV-11 Shendao to a depth of 0.2 cun; the needle was then moved gently subcutaneously downward through GV-10 Lingtai to join GV-9 Zhiyang. The needle was rotated in large amplitude, but without lifting or thrusting. The other points were needled obliquely to a depth of 0.5-0.8 cun. All the needles were retained for 20 minutes.

This treatment was started 12 to 15 days after termination of menstruation and was given once a day for six to nine days for three successive cycles. Patients with amenorrhea were given the treatment for nine days and then, after a break of 20 days, for another nine days, also for three successive cycles.

Rosacea
酒渣鼻

Rosacea is a chronic inflammatory condition involving the nose, cheeks, forehead, and chin. It may be exacerbated by emotional factors, gastrointestinal or endocrine dysfunction, alcohol or strong tea, overindulgence in spicy food or excessively hot or cold food, or exposure to the sun or other heat sources. Rosacea tends to be seen more often in individuals who flush easily, for example after eating spicy food or in response to embarrassment.

In TCM, rosacea is known as *jiu zha bi* (drinker's nose) or *bi chi* (red nose).

Clinical manifestations

- Rosacea occurs most frequently in middle-aged individuals (30 to 50 years old), women more often than men, but also affects young adults and the elderly. Alcohol may exacerbate the condition, but does not cause the disease.
- Lesions normally involve the nose, chin, cheeks, and forehead, sparing the periorbital area.
- At the initial stage, temporary flushing and erythema interspersed with discrete inflamed pinhead papules and pustules appear. As the condition develops, the erythema does not fade and dilatation of the capillaries (telangiectasia) occurs.
- Chronic and deep inflammation of the nose may lead to rhinophyma (irreversible hypertrophy), more particularly in men.
- Lymphedema may occur below the eyes and on the forehead.
- Accompanying symptoms and signs affecting the eyes include mild conjunctivitis with soreness and lacrimation. Blepharitis, and less commonly keratitis, may also occur.

Differential diagnosis

Acne

This condition begins in adolescence, whereas rosacea usually appears later. It presents with comedones (blackheads or whiteheads, both of which are absent in rosacea) or with papules, pustules or nodules. The diffuse erythema or telangiectasia characteristic of rosacea is not present in acne. Lesions in acne can also appear on the chest and back.

Perioral dermatitis

This skin disorder occurs most frequently in women in the 20-40 age group. Eruptions usually start around the mouth, but may also involve the areas around the nose and eyes. Lesions mainly manifest as erythema, pinpoint papules, papulovesicles, and pustules, with some scaling but without flushing.

Folliculitis

Typical body sites affected include the face, scalp, thighs, axillae, and inguinal area. The primary lesion is a papule or pustule with a central hair, which may not always be seen. A gridlike pattern of multiple red papules and/or pustules on hair-bearing areas of the body occurs. Rosacea has more pronounced flushing and erythema and is restricted to the face.

Other conditions

Rosacea should also be differentiated from seborrheic eczema, contact dermatitis and photosensitive eruptions, but these conditions lack the pustules characteristic of rosacea and are usually more scaly.

Etiology and pathology

- Prevalence of Yang Qi in the Lung channel may transform into Heat if it is retained for a long period. This Heat, once formed, may fight with the Blood, and, since the Lungs open into the nose, Blood-Heat will enter the nose, which will gradually redden, thus giving rise to the condition.
- Indulgence in pungent or spicy food generates Heat, which transforms into Fire. Where Heat and Fire steam along the channels, they may overfill the network vessels, manifesting as tidal reddening of the nose.
- Cold invading the face due to Wind-Cold settling in the skin or washing the face with cold water can lead to Blood stasis, because Cold is characterized by a tendency to congeal. The nose may initially become red, before turning purple and finally dull red.

Pattern identification and treatment

INTERNAL TREATMENT

ACCUMULATION OF HEAT IN THE LUNGS AND STOMACH

The skin on the nose and cheeks reddens persistently, gradually forming diffuse erythema, which flushes, turning redder on exposure to heat. Accompanying symptoms and signs include dry mouth and thirst with a desire for drinks, and oily and shiny skin. The tongue body is red with a yellow coating; the pulse is rapid.

Treatment principle

Clear and drain accumulated Heat from the Lungs and Stomach.

Prescription

PI PA QING FEI YIN JIA JIAN

Loquat Beverage for Clearing Heat from the Lungs, with modifications

Zhi Pi Pa Ye (Folium Eriobotryae Japonicae, mix-fried with honey) 10g

Huang Qin (Radix Scutellariae Baicalensis) 10g
Di Gu Pi (Cortex Lycii Radicis) 10g
Sang Bai Pi (Cortex Mori Albae Radicis) 12g
Chao Mu Dan Pi (Cortex Moutan Radicis, stir-fried) 6g
Chao Zhi Mu (Rhizoma Anemarrhenae Asphodeloidis, stir-fried) 6g
Gan Cao (Radix Glycyrrhizae) 6g
Hong Hua (Flos Carthami Tinctorii) 4.5g
Jiu Zhi Da Huang (Radix et Rhizoma Rhei, mix-fried with wine) 3g
Shi Gao ‡ (Gypsum Fibrosum) 15g, decocted for 30 minutes before adding the other ingredients

Explanation

- *Zhi Pi Pa Ye* (Folium Eriobotryae Japonicae, mix-fried with honey), *Huang Qin* (Radix Scutellariae Baicalensis), *Di Gu Pi* (Cortex Lycii Radicis), *Shi Gao*‡ (Gypsum Fibrosum), *Chao Zhi Mu* (Rhizoma Anemarrhenae Asphodeloidis, stir-fried), and *Sang Bai Pi* (Cortex Mori Albae Radicis) clear and drain accumulated Heat from the Lungs and Stomach.
- *Hong Hua* (Flos Carthami Tinctorii), *Jiu Zhi Da Huang* (Radix et Rhizoma Rhei, mix-fried with wine) and *Chao Mu Dan Pi* (Cortex Moutan Radicis, stir-fried) cool the Blood and transform stasis, relieve Toxicity and reduce erythema.
- *Gan Cao* (Radix Glycyrrhizae) harmonizes the Middle Burner and relieves Toxicity.

CONGESTION OF BLOOD-HEAT

This pattern manifests as persistent dark red erythematous skin with telangiectasia and pinpoint or slightly larger red papules and pustules on the tip of the nose, the cheeks and the forehead. Accompanying symptoms and signs include dry stools and yellow urine. The tongue body is red with a thin yellow coating; the pulse is slippery and rapid, or wiry and rapid.

Treatment principle

Cool the Blood and clear Heat from the Lungs.

Prescription

LIANG XUE QING FEI YIN JIA JIAN

Beverage for Cooling the Blood and Clearing Heat from the Lungs, with modifications

Sheng Di Huang (Radix Rehmanniae Glutinosae) 12g
Huang Qin (Radix Scutellariae Baicalensis) 12g
Shi Gao ‡ (Gypsum Fibrosum) 12g, decocted for 30 minutes before adding the other ingredients
Chao Mu Dan Pi (Cortex Moutan Radicis, stir-fried) 10g
Chi Shao (Radix Paeoniae Rubra) 10g
Sang Bai Pi (Cortex Mori Albae Radicis) 10g
Pi Pa Ye (Folium Eriobotryae Japonicae) 10g
Gan Cao (Radix Glycyrrhizae) 6g

Jiao Zhi Zi (Fructus Gardeniae Jasminoidis, scorch-fried) 4.5g
Bai Mao Gen (Rhizoma Imperatae Cylindricae) 30g

Explanation

- *Sheng Di Huang* (Radix Rehmanniae Glutinosae), *Chao Mu Dan Pi* (Cortex Moutan Radicis, stir-fried), *Chi Shao* (Radix Paeoniae Rubra), and *Bai Mao Gen* (Rhizoma Imperatae Cylindricae) cool and invigorate the Blood and reduce erythema.
- *Pi Pa Ye* (Folium Eriobotryae Japonicae), *Sang Bai Pi* (Cortex Mori Albae Radicis), *Huang Qin* (Radix Scutellariae Baicalensis), *Shi Gao‡* (Gypsum Fibrosum), *Gan Cao* (Radix Glycyrrhizae), and *Jiao Zhi Zi* (Fructus Gardeniae Jasminoidis, scorch-fried) clear and drain accumulated Heat from the Lungs and Stomach.
- Eruptions on the nose due to retained Heat will be eliminated when Heat is cleared from the Blood and the functions of the Stomach are freed.

BLOOD STASIS

This pattern manifests as persistent dark red or purplish-red erythema on the nose with thickening of the skin and rhinophyma. The tongue body is dull red or has stasis macules; the pulse is wiry and rough.

Treatment principle

Invigorate the Blood and transform Blood stasis.

Prescription

TONG QIAO HUO XUE TANG JIA JIAN

Decoction for Freeing the Orifices and Invigorating the Blood, with modifications

Dang Gui Wei (Extremitas Radicis Angelicae Sinensis) 10g
Chi Shao (Radix Paeoniae Rubra) 10g
Tao Ren (Semen Persicae) 10g
Hong Hua (Flos Carthami Tinctorii) 10g
Bai Zhi (Radix Angelicae Dahuricae) 6g
Chuan Xiong (Rhizoma Ligustici Chuanxiong) 6g
Sheng Di Huang (Radix Rehmanniae Glutinosae) 12g
Chao Mu Dan Pi (Cortex Moutan Radicis, stir-fried) 12g
Ling Xiao Hua (Flos Campsitis) 9g
Huai Hua (Flos Sophorae Japonicae) 9g
Sheng Ma (Rhizoma Cimicifugae) 3g
Jiu Zhi Da Huang (Radix et Rhizoma Rhei, mix-fried with wine) 3g

Explanation

- *Dang Gui Wei* (Extremitas Radicis Angelicae Sinensis), *Chi Shao* (Radix Paeoniae Rubra), *Tao Ren* (Semen Persicae), *Hong Hua* (Flos Carthami Tinctorii), *Bai Zhi* (Radix Angelicae Dahuricae), and *Chuan Xiong* (Rhizoma Ligustici Chuanxiong) transform Blood stasis and dissipate lumps, free the network vessels and reduce erythema.

- *Sheng Di Huang* (Radix Rehmanniae Glutinosae), *Mu Dan Pi* (Cortex Moutan Radicis), *Ling Xiao Hua* (Flos Campsitis), and *Huai Hua* (Flos Sophorae Japonicae) cool the Blood and reduce eruptions.
- *Sheng Ma* (Rhizoma Cimicifugae) bears Yang upward and relieves Toxicity, directing the effect of the other ingredients to the affected area.
- *Jiu Da Huang* (Radix et Rhizoma Rhei, mix-fried with wine) drains Heat from the Fu organs, relieves Toxicity and dissipates lumps.

General modifications

1. For pustules, add *Pu Gong Ying* (Herba Taraxaci cum Radice), *Jin Yin Hua* (Flos Lonicerae) and *Zi Hua Di Ding* (Herba Violae Yedoensitis).
2. For pronounced erythema, add *Bai Hua She She Cao* (Herba Hedyotidis Diffusae) and *Chong Lou* (Rhizoma Paridis).
3. For constipation, add *Chao Zhi Ke* (Fructus Citri Aurantii, stir-fried), *Hou Po* (Cortex Magnoliae Officinalis) and *Chao Huang Lian* (Rhizoma Coptidis, stir-fried).
4. For flushing due to alcohol, add *Zhi Zi* (Fructus Gardeniae Jasminoidis), *Ge Hua* (Flos Puerariae) and *Ku Shen* (Radix Sophorae Flavescentis).
5. For exacerbation of eruptions prior to menstruation, add *Yi Mu Cao* (Herba Leonuri Heterophylli) or take *Si Zhi Xiang Fu Wan* (Quadruply Processed Cyperus Pill) with the decoction.

PATENT HERBAL MEDICINES

- Where erythema, papules and pustules are the principal lesions, take *Zhi Zi Qin Hua Wan* (Gardenia, Scutellaria and Trichosanthes Root Pill) 4.5-6g, twice a day, or *Ling Xiao Hua San* (Campsis Flower Powder) 6-10g, twice a day in an infusion or a decoction.
- For the early stage of rhinophyma, take *Da Huang Zhe Chong Wan* (Rhubarb and Wingless Cockroach Pill) 6-10g, two or three times a day.

EXTERNAL TREATMENT

- For papules, pustules and erythema, grind equal proportions of *Ming Fan‡* (Alumen), *Liu Huang‡* (Sulphur) and *Ru Xiang* (Gummi Olibanum) into a fine powder, mix with cold boiled water or tea and apply to the affected area; alternatively, *Dian Dao San* (Reversal Powder) can be applied with the same procedure.
- For papules, pustules, erythema, and mild rhinophyma, apply *Si Huang Gao* (Four Yellows Paste), *Huang Lian Ruan Gao* (Coptis Ointment) or *Fu Rong Gao* (Cotton Rose Flower Paste) to the affected area.

ACUPUNCTURE

Selection of points on the affected channels
Main points: GV-25 Suliao, GV-23 Shangxing and GV-14 Dazhui.
Auxiliary points: BL-12 Fengmen, BL-13 Feishu and LI-20 Yingxiang.

Selection of adjacent points
Main points: EX-HN-3 Yintang,[ix] LI-20 Yingxiang and GV-25 Suliao.
Auxiliary points: LI-19 Kouheliao and SI-18 Quanliao.

Technique
Apply the even method at all points. Retain the needles for 30 minutes. When withdrawing the needles, allow GV-25 Suliao to bleed a little. Treat once every two days. A course consists of ten treatment sessions.

Explanation
- GV-25 Suliao, LI-20 Yingxiang, EX-HN-3 Yintang, LI-19 Kouheliao, and SI-18 Quanliao clear Heat from the Lungs and Stomach.
- GV-14 Dazhui, BL-12 Fengmen and BL-13 Feishu dredge and dissipate Wind-Heat.
- GV-23 Shangxing inhibits secretion of sebum and improves greasy skin.

EAR ACUPUNCTURE
Points: External Nose, Lung, Endocrine, and Adrenal Gland.
Technique: Apply the reducing method and retain the needles for 30 minutes. Treat once a day. A course consists of ten treatment sessions.

PRICKING TO BLEED METHOD
Points: LI-20 Yingxiang (bilateral), GV-25 Suliao and LU-11 Shaoshang.
Technique: Prick the points with a small gauge three-edged needle to cause slight bleeding. Treat once every three days. A course consists of seven treatment sessions.

POINT LASER THERAPY
Points: ST-2 Sibai, GV-25 Suliao, LI-20 Yingxiang, and SI-18 Quanliao.
Technique: Apply a helium-neon laser to the affected area for 10-15 minutes once every two days. A course consists of ten treatment sessions.

Clinical notes

- TCM treatment of rosacea focuses on clearing Heat from the Lungs and cooling the Blood at the initial stage of the disease and on transforming Blood stasis and dissipating lumps in the later stages.
- Acupuncture treatment and external application can reduce and disperse lesions, thus shortening the course of the disease.
- For hyperplasia of nasal skin (rhinophyma), consideration should be given to referring to a doctor of Western medicine for cryotherapy or laser or plastic surgery.

Advice for the patient

- Avoid irritating food in order to regulate the gastro-intestinal function; giving up smoking and drinking helps significantly.
- Avoid secondary infection of the nose; wash the face with lukewarm water.
- The nose and face should be washed in lukewarm water and dried before the application of external medication.
- Since eruptions on the nose are particularly noticeable and are likely to make the patient extremely sensitive, especially where there is rhinophyma, medical practitioners, family members and friends should be especially attentive and try to reassure the patient.

Case history

Patient
Female, aged 38.

Clinical manifestations
Flushing had initially appeared on the patient's cheeks and the tip of her nose five years previously; the condition gradually developed, with papules and pustules of various sizes subsequently appearing on an erythematous base. Various treatments had not brought a cure. Flushing was localized to the paranasal areas and the cheeks with obvious telangiectasia. Red papules 1-2 mm in diameter were found in these areas, which were covered by an oily secretion. The patient also experienced slight itching. Accompanying symptoms and signs included irritability and impatience, thirst and a liking for cold drinks, dry stools with bowel movements once every few days, and yellow urine. The tongue body was red with a thin white coating; the pulse was wiry and slippery.

Pattern identification
Accumulation of Heat in the Lungs and Stomach with binding of Blood-Heat.

Treatment principle
Clear Heat from the Lungs and Stomach, cool and transform the Blood.

[ix] M-HN-3 according to the system employed by the Shanghai College of Traditional Chinese Medicine.

Prescription ingredients

Sang Bai Pi (Cortex Mori Albae Radicis) 15g
Di Gu Pi (Cortex Lycii Radicis) 15g
Huang Qin (Radix Scutellariae Baicalensis) 15g
Huang Lian (Rhizoma Coptidis) 10g
Shi Gao‡ (Gypsum Fibrosum) 30g, decocted for 30 minutes
   before adding the other ingredients
Zhi Zi (Fructus Gardeniae Jasminoidis) 10g
Jin Yin Hua (Flos Lonicerae) 10g
Mei Gui Hua (Flos Rosae Rugosae) 10g
Ji Guan Hua (Flos Celosiae Cristatae) 10g
Huai Hua (Flos Sophorae Japonicae) 30g
Ye Ju Hua (Flos Chrysanthemi Indici) 15g
Sheng Di Huang (Radix Rehmanniae Glutinosae) 30g
Chi Shao (Radix Paeoniae Rubra) 15g
Dan Shen (Radix Salviae Miltiorrhizae) 15g
Xiang Fu (Rhizoma Cyperi Rotundi) 10g
Gua Lou (Fructus Trichosanthis) 30g
Yi Mu Cao (Herba Leonuri Heterophylli) 10g

One bag a day was used to prepare a decoction, taken twice a day.

External application

Liu Lei Xi Ji (Sulfur and Resorcinol Wash Preparation) applied every evening and 1% metronidazole cream (metronidazole 0.4g, 10% sulfur ointment 20g and silica gel 20g) applied every morning.ˣ

Second visit

After 14 bags, the flushing was diminishing, the papules and pustules were decreasing in number and the itching had improved. The patient was told to continue the prescription for another 14 bags.

Third visit

The erythema had disappeared. The prescription was changed to *Lian Qiao Bai Du Wan* (Forsythia Pill for Vanquishing Toxicity) 6g, twice a day, and *Jia Wei Xiao Yao Wan* (Augmented Free Wanderer Pill) 6g, twice a day, with the objective of cooling the Blood, relieving Toxicity and regulating and harmonizing the Chong and Ren vessels in order to consolidate the overall improvement.

Outcome

After one month, the flushing, papules and oily secretion had disappeared completely. Stool and urine were normal.

Discussion

Rosacea is caused by internal steaming of Blood-Heat in the Lung channel accompanied by Wind-Cold restricting the exterior, thus leading to Blood stasis and stagnation. The treatment principle is to clear accumulated Heat in the Lungs and Stomach and cool and transform the Blood. In the prescription, *Sang Bai Pi* (Cortex Mori Albae Radicis), *Di Gu Pi* (Cortex Lycii Radicis), *Huang Qin* (Radix Scutellariae Baicalensis), *Huang Lian* (Rhizoma Coptidis), *Zhi Zi* (Fructus Gardeniae Jasminoidis), and *Shi Gao*‡ (Gypsum Fibrosum), clear Heat from the Lungs and Stomach; *Mei Gui Hua* (Flos Rosae

Rugosae), *Jin Yin Hua* (Flos Lonicerae), *Ji Guan Hua* (Flos Celosiae Cristatae), *Huai Hua* (Flos Sophorae Japonicae), *Ye Ju Hua* (Flos Chrysanthemi Indici), and *Sheng Di Huang* (Radix Rehmanniae) cool and transform the Blood and clear Heat; *Chi Shao* (Radix Paeoniae Rubra), *Dan Shen* (Radix Salviae Miltiorrhizae), *Xiang Fu* (Rhizoma Cyperi Rotundi), and *Yi Mu Cao* (Herba Leonuri Heterophylli) regulate Qi, transform the Blood, dissipate Blood stasis, and regulate and harmonize the Chong and Ren vessels; and *Gua Lou* (Fructus Trichosanthis) softens hardness and dissipates lumps, disperses and guides out accumulation, and frees the bowels. [24]

Literature excerpt

In *Feng Shi Jin Nang Mi Lu* [Feng's Secret Records of the Best Counsels], it says: "The Lungs, the uppermost Zang organ, are so fragile that they are averse to both Cold and Heat. For this reason, somebody who has a fondness for alcohol is predisposed to rosacea and the nose may turn red due to the steaming of Heat from alcohol. A red nose may turn purplish-black if Blood-Heat encounters Cold and congeals, thus impairing the ejection of filth. The treatment varies according to pattern identification. If the disease is related to loss of Blood, warm Yang and supplement the Blood; if it is caused by Heat in the Blood, clear Heat and regulate the Blood; for Cold congealing, transform stagnation and generate flesh with *Si Wu Tang* (Four Agents Decoction) plus *Jiu Huang Qin* (Radix Scutellariae Baicalensis, stir-fried in wine) and *Jiu Hong Hua* (Flos Carthami Tinctorii, stir-fried in wine); for Qi Deficiency, add *Huang Qi* (Radix Astragali seu Hedysari), steeped in wine, in order to move Qi."

Modern clinical experience

COMBINED INTERNAL AND EXTERNAL TREATMENT

Zeng treated rosacea with a combination of internal and external treatments. [25]

Internal treatment prescription
QING ZHEN TANG JIA WEI
Cimicifuga and Atractylodes Decoction, with additions

Sheng Ma (Rhizoma Cimicifugae) 15g
Cang Zhu (Rhizoma Atractylodis) 15g
He Ye (Folium Nclumbinis Nuciferae) 15g

Modifications
1. For reddening of the skin at the tip of the nose, *Pi Pa Ye* (Folium Eriobotryae Japonicae) 10g and *Xin Yi Hua* (Flos Magnoliae) 10g were added.

ˣ These preparations are usually only available through a registered pharmacist or registered doctor.

2. For profuse pustules, *Zhi Zi* (Fructus Gardeniae Jasminoidis) 10g and *Jin Yin Hua* (Flos Lonicerae) 15g were added.
3. For constipation, *Da Huang* (Radix et Rhizoma Rhei) 5-10g was added 5 minutes before the end of the decoction process.
4. For indigestion, *Jiao Shan Zha* (Fructus Crataegi, scorch-fried) 15-20g and *Chao Chen Pi* (Pericarpium Citri Reticulatae, stir-fried) 10g were added.
5. For thickened lesions, *Chi Shao* (Radix Paeoniae Rubra) 10g and *Dan Shen* (Radix Salviae Miltiorrhizae) 10g were added.

One bag a day was used to prepare a decoction, taken twice a day. A course of treatment consisted of six bags of herbs plus a break of one day.

External treatment
Dian Dao San (Reversal Powder) mixed with *Bai Bu Ding* (Stemona Root Tincture) was applied to the affected area twice a day. Results were seen after four weeks.

ACUPUNCTURE
Chen combined three-edged and filiform needling to treat rosacea. [26]

Three-edged needling
After sterilization of the affected areas, a three-edged needle was used to prick LU-11 Shaoshang and the inflamed areas of the nose and alae nasi to induce slight bleeding. When the bleeding stopped, the area was cleaned with dry, sterilized cotton wool. This treatment was given once every two days.

Filiform needling
Points: LI-20 Yingxiang, LI-11 Quchi, LI-4 Hegu, and ST-36 Zusanli.
Technique: After obtaining Qi, the even method was employed, with the needling sensation directed toward the affected area. Treatment was given once a day.

A course of treatment lasted ten days with a break of five days between courses. Results were seen after three courses.

COMBINED TREATMENT WITH TCM AND WESTERN MEDICINE
Cheng recommended TCM internal treatment with a combined TCM/Western medicine external application. [27]

Internal prescription
LIANG XUE SI WU TANG JIA WEI
Four Agents Decoction for Cooling the Blood, with additions

Dang Gui (Radix Angelicae Sinensis) 15g
Chi Shao (Radix Paeoniae Rubra) 15g
Huang Qin (Radix Scutellariae Baicalensis) 15g
Chuan Xiong (Rhizoma Ligustici Chuanxiong) 15g
Hong Hua (Flos Carthami Tinctorii) 15g
Mu Dan Pi (Cortex Moutan Radicis) 15g
Sheng Di Huang (Radix Rehmanniae Glutinosae) 20g
Mei Gui Hua (Flos Rosae Rugosae) 20g
Ji Guan Hua (Flos Celosiae Cristatae) 20g

One bag a day was used to prepare a decoction, taken twice a day. Ten bags made up a course.

External prescription
XIAO ZHA SAN
Dispersing Rosacea Powder [xi]

Liu Huang‡ (Sulphur) 15g
Da Huang (Radix et Rhizoma Rhei) 15g
Duan Shi Gao‡ (Gypsum Fibrosum Calcinatum) 15g
Huang Qin (Radix Scutellariae Baicalensis) 10g
Zhi Zi (Fructus Gardeniae Jasminoidis) 10g
Qing Dai (Indigo Naturalis) 10g
Xin Yi Hua (Flos Magnoliae) 10g
Metronidazole 4g
Prednisone 50mg
Alficetin powder 3g

The ingredients were ground into a powder. For each application, 1-2g was mixed to a paste with liquid honey; 0.5ml of laurocapram was then added to enhance transdermal absorption and the medication applied to the lesion twice a day for 20 days (equivalent to two courses of the internal treatment).

[xi] The Western drugs included in this external formula will normally only be available on prescription from a registered doctor or registered pharmacist.

Pyoderma faciale
面部脓皮病

This disease is a variant of cystic acne which affects adult women and is confined to the face. It is caused by Gram-positive organisms. Delay in treatment will result in scarring once the lesion heals.

In TCM, pyoderma faciale is also known as *mian fa du* (Toxic facial eruption).

Clinical manifestations

- Pyoderma faciale usually affects women from the teens to the fifth decade.
- The condition starts with the sudden appearance on the face of pustules and cysts up to 1 cm or more in diameter. Lesions, which may be isolated or densely distributed forming plaques, are surrounded by bright red or purplish-red erythema and are located mostly on the central portion of the cheeks.
- Lesions are red and inflamed, painful and hard. Comedones are usually absent.
- Lesions may link with each other through sinus tracts; the yellowish-green pus they contain can be squeezed out by pressure.
- Scars usually form after the lesions heal.

Differential diagnosis

Acne
This condition is characterized by blackheads (open comedones) or whiteheads (closed comedones) or the two in combination, with inflammation leading to the formation of pustules, nodules or cysts. Lesions may appear on the back and upper chest in addition to the facial area.

Etiology and pathology

Wind-Heat Toxins
Looseness of the interstices (*cou li*) means that Wei Qi (Defensive Qi) is not strong enough to defend the body against external invasion. As a result, Wind-Heat invades and settles in the Yangming channel, attacking upward into the face to cause the disease.

Damp-Heat Toxins
Improper diet or overindulgence in fatty, sweet and rich foods leads to Heat accumulating in the Spleen and Stomach and transforming into Toxins. Alternatively, after Damp pathogenic factors have accumulated inside the body over a long period, they transform into Heat and turn Toxic, attacking upward along the channels to the facial region.

Pattern identification and treatment

INTERNAL TREATMENT

WIND-HEAT TOXINS
Pustules with solid walls and surrounding areola are present in the affected area. Pressure on the lesions will cause exudation of yellowish-green pus. Accompanying symptoms and signs include itching and pain, fever, aversion to cold, thirst with a desire for cold drinks, irritability and irascibility, constipation, and short voidings of reddish urine. The tongue body is red with a yellow coating; the pulse is wiry and rapid.

Treatment principle
Dissipate Wind and clear Heat, relieve Toxicity and cool the Blood.

Prescription
JING FANG BAI DU SAN JIA JIAN
Schizonepeta and Ledebouriella Powder for Vanquishing Toxicity, with modifications

Jing Jie (Herba Schizonepetae Tenuifoliae) 10g
Fang Feng (Radix Ledebouriellae Divaricatae) 10g
Qiang Huo (Rhizoma et Radix Notopterygii) 10g
Jie Geng (Radix Platycodi Grandiflori) 10g
Mu Dan Pi (Cortex Moutan Radicis) 10g
Lian Qiao (Fructus Forsythiae Suspensae) 10g
Bai Zhi (Radix Angelicae Dahuricae) 10g
Gan Cao (Radix Glycyrrhizae) 10g
Di Yu (Radix Sanguisorbae Officinalis) 10g

Explanation
- This prescription is designed to keep Toxicity under control.
- *Jing Jie* (Herba Schizonepetae Tenuifoliae), *Fang Feng* (Radix Ledebouriellae Divaricatae) and *Qiang Huo* (Rhizoma et Radix Notopterygii) dredge Wind and clear Heat.
- *Jie Geng* (Radix Platycodi Grandiflori), *Mu Dan Pi* (Cortex Moutan Radicis) and *Bai Zhi* (Radix Angelicae Dahuricae) invigorate and cool the Blood.
- *Lian Qiao* (Fructus Forsythiae Suspensae), *Gan Cao* (Radix Glycyrrhizae) and *Di Yu* (Radix Sanguisorbae Officinalis) cool the Blood and relieve Toxicity.

DAMP-HEAT TOXINS

Pustules and cysts grow in clusters surrounded by erythema. Lesions link with each other through sinus tracts, from which yellowish-green pus oozes. Accompanying symptoms and signs include high fever and aversion to cold, constipation, and reddish urine. The tongue body is red with a scant coating; the pulse is rapid.

Treatment principle

Clear Heat and eliminate Dampness, relieve Toxicity and expel pus.

Prescription
JIE DU PAI NONG TANG JIA JIAN
Decoction for Relieving Toxicity and Expelling Pus, with modifications

Jin Yin Hua (Flos Lonicerae Japonicae) 15g
Chao Niu Bang Zi (Fructus Arctii Lappae, stir-fried) 10g
Zao Jiao Ci (Spina Gleditsiae Sinensis) 10g
Chuan Xiong (Rhizoma Ligustici Chuanxiong) 10g
Huang Qin (Radix Scutellariae Baicalensis) 10g
Jiao Zhi Zi (Fructus Gardeniae Jasminoidis, scorch-fried) 10g
Bai Zhi (Radix Angelicae Dahuricae) 10g
Zhe Bei Mu (Bulbus Fritillariae Thunbergii) 10g
Huang Lian (Rhizoma Coptidis) 6g
Shan Ci Gu (Pseudobulbus Shancigu) 6g

Explanation

- *Jin Yin Hua* (Flos Lonicerae), *Huang Qin* (Radix Scutellariae Baicalensis), *Huang Lian* (Rhizoma Coptidis), and *Jiao Zhi Zi* (Fructus Gardeniae Jasminoidis, scorch-fried) clear Heat and relieve Toxicity.
- *Zao Jiao Ci* (Spina Gleditsiae Sinensis), *Chuan Xiong* (Rhizoma Ligustici Chuanxiong), *Bai Zhi* (Radix Angelicae Dahuricae), and *Zhe Bei Mu* (Bulbus Fritillariae Thunbergii) expel pus and dissipate nodules; *Bai Zhi* (Radix Angelicae Dahuricae) also dries Dampness.
- *Chao Niu Bang Zi* (Fructus Arctii Lappae, stir-fried) dredges Wind and disperses swelling.
- *Shan Ci Gu* (Pseudobulbus Shancigu) transforms Toxicity and dissipates nodules.

EXTERNAL TREATMENT

- In the initial stage before rupture of the lesions, prepare a decoction of *Bai Ji* (Rhizoma Bletillae Striatae) 10g, *Jin Yin Hua* (Flos Lonicerae) 10g, *Pu Gong Ying* (Herba Taraxaci cum Radice) 15g, and *Huang Bai* (Cortex Phellodendri) 15g and apply it to the affected area as a wet compress. Follow the treatment two or three times a day, for 30-45 minutes each time.
- After the pustules or cysts have ruptured, insert a medicated thread processed with *Huang Lian Gan Ru Gao* (Coptis, Calamine and Frankincense Paste) into the lesion. Then apply *Hua Du Gao* (Transforming Toxicity Paste) on top. The treatment is given once a day. [xii,xiii]

Clinical notes

- Internal treatment for this disease should follow the principle of correct differentiation between Wind-Heat Toxins and Damp-Heat Toxins:
  - For Wind-Heat, follow the principle of dissipating Wind and clearing Heat, relieving Toxicity and dispersing swelling to alleviate pain by using ingredients such as *Jing Jie* (Herba Schizonepetae Tenuifoliae), *Fang Feng* (Radix Ledebouriellae Divaricatae), *Qiang Huo* (Rhizoma et Radix Notopterygii), and *Niu Bang Zi* (Fructus Arctii Lappae).
  - For Damp-Heat, use ingredients such as *Zhi Zi* (Fructus Gardeniae Jasminoidis), *Huang Qin* (Radix Scutellariae Baicalensis), *Zhe Bei Mu* (Bulbus Fritillariae Thunbergii), and *Huang Lian* (Rhizoma Coptidis).
- In the author's experience, consideration must also be given throughout the treatment to supporting Vital Qi (Zheng Qi) and transforming Blood stasis. Ingredients recommended for this purpose include *Huang Qi* (Radix Astragali seu Hedysari), *Dang Shen* (Radix Codonopsitis Pilosulae), *Sheng Ma* (Rhizoma Cimicifugae), *Dan Shen* (Radix Salviae Miltiorrhizae), and *Tao Ren* (Semen Persicae).
- Surgical incision or drainage should be avoided.
- If signs of septicemia, such as rigors or circulatory collapse, appear while treating the disease with TCM, the patient should be referred immediately to a doctor of Western medicine.
- Appropriate and timely treatment can help to achieve complete healing of the lesions; otherwise, they may persist for months.

[xii] Medicated thread involves the application of highly absorbent paper (mulberry or silk floss paper) twisted into a thread and coated with a medicated paste. This is then inserted into sinus tracts, fistulae or abscesses to drain pus, expel putridity and generate flesh.
[xiii] In the author's experience, this is the only effective TCM external treatment at this stage of the disease. This method has therefore been included to indicate how treatment would be carried out in China; in other countries, the use of some of the ingredients contained in the preparation may not be permitted.

Advice for the patient

- Keep the affected area clean.
- Patients should be warned not to squeeze the lesions themselves.

Literature excerpt

In *Chuang Yang Jing Yan Quan Shu* [A Complete Manual of Experience in the Treatment of Sores], it says: "*Mian fa du* (Toxic facial eruption) usually occurs as a result of overindulgence in sex, which allows Wind to take advantage of Deficiency to enter the channels and network vessels leading to Deficiency of the Yangming channels. Eruptions often involve the face, sometimes with boils. Patients are anxious to finish the treatment as quickly as possible. If they consult a physician with mediocre treatment skills, they may be treated by external application of toxic medications, or by moxibustion, puncturing by needles or incision with a knife. If patients with this condition do not stop having sexual intercourse after rupture of the lesions, or if they expose themselves to Wind, Cold or other strong Toxic pathogenic factors, the Toxic factors will interact with each other and make the condition worse. The face is the confluence of the Yang channels. It is forbidden to use any kind of method involving fire or knives or toxic medications. It is also the place where the ears, eyes, mouth, and nose are located, and is different from the four limbs. If insufficient attention is paid, the patient's life will be at risk."

Perioral dermatitis
口周皮炎

Perioral dermatitis generally presents as a papular eruption around the mouth, either with undetermined cause or as a result of use of strong topical fluorinated steroids.

Clinical manifestations

- This condition occurs most frequently in women in the 20-40 age group.
- Eruptions usually start around the mouth in the nasolabial folds or the chin, but may also involve the areas around the nose and eyes.
- Lesions mainly manifest as erythema, pinpoint papules, papulovesicles and pustules, and scaling; these lesions may exacerbate on exposure to sunshine or after intake of hot or cold food or drinks.
- Itching or a sensation of burning heat may be felt.
- Persistent eruptions may last for months or years. Relapse is rare.

Differential diagnosis

Acne

This skin disorder is common among adolescents and young adults, and may flare up before menstruation. Eruptions generally appear on the face, especially the forehead, cheeks and chin, but may also involve the chest and back. Lesions may manifest as open comedones (blackheads) or closed comedones (whiteheads), or as inflammatory papules and pustules. The features of perioral dermatitis do not include comedones.

Rosacea

This condition most commonly affects middle-aged individuals. Lesions have a wider distribution than those of perioral dermatitis and can also involve the cheeks and forehead. At the initial stage of rosacea, temporary flushing and erythema appear interspersed with discrete inflamed pinhead papules and pustules. As the condition develops, the erythema persists and telangiectasia occurs. Perioral dermatitis lacks the flushing characteristic of rosacea.

Seborrheic eczema

This condition most commonly affects young and middle-aged individuals. The main sites of involvement are areas of the skin with abundant sebaceous activity. The disease often starts on the scalp and may involve the eyebrows, nasolabial folds, axillae, groins, and sub-mammary area. Chronic blepharitis and otitis externa may be associated. Lesions initially manifest as yellowish-red or pale red erythema, with papulovesicles subsequently appearing; there is exudation after scratching.

Etiology and pathology

- A partiality for spicy or oily foods leads to internal accumulation of Damp-Heat in the Spleen and

Stomach, which then harasses upward along the channels.

- Retention of Heat in the Lungs and Spleen, when complicated by an external invasion of Wind pathogenic factors, obstructs the skin and interstices (*cou li*).

Pattern identification and treatment

INTERNAL TREATMENT

RETENTION OF HEAT IN THE LUNGS AND SPLEEN

A dense distribution of red papules and papulovesicles of different sizes appears on an erythematous base in the perioral area; a few pustules may also manifest on the cheeks. Accompanying symptoms and signs include dry mouth with a desire for drinks, and dry stools. The tongue body is red with a scant coating; the pulse is floating and rapid.

Treatment principle
Diffuse the Lungs and clear Heat from the Spleen, cool the Blood and alleviate itching.

Prescription
LIANG XUE WU HUA TANG JIA JIAN
Five Flowers Decoction for Cooling the Blood, with modifications

Hong Hua (Flos Carthami Tinctorii) 6g
Ling Xiao Hua (Flos Campsitis) 6g
Jiao Zhi Zi (Fructus Gardeniae Jasminoidis, scorch-fried) 6g
Chao Huang Qin (Radix Scutellariae Baicalensis, stir-fried) 6g
Jin Yin Hua (Flos Lonicerae) 12g
Qing Hao (Herba Artemisiae Chinghao) 12g, added 5 minutes from the end of the decoction process
Shi Gao‡ (Gypsum Fibrosum) 12g, decocted for 30 minutes before adding the other ingredients
Sheng Di Huang (Radix Rehmanniae Glutinosae) 12g
Sheng Ma (Rhizoma Cimicifugae) 4.5g
Da Huang (Radix et Rhizoma Rhei) 3g, added 5 minutes from the end of the decoction process

Explanation
- *Chao Huang Qin* (Radix Scutellariae Baicalensis, stir-fried), *Qing Hao* (Herba Artemisiae Chinghao), *Shi Gao* ‡ (Gypsum Fibrosum), *Sheng Di Huang* (Radix Rehmanniae Glutinosae), and *Da Huang* (Radix et Rhizoma Rhei) diffuse the Lungs and clear Heat from the Spleen.
- *Hong Hua* (Flos Carthami Tinctorii), *Ling Xiao Hua* (Flos Campsitis), *Jin Yin Hua* (Flos Lonicerae), and *Sheng Ma* (Rhizoma Cimicifugae) cool the Blood and alleviate itching.

- *Jiao Zhi Zi* (Fructus Gardeniae Jasminoidis, scorch-fried) drains Fire with cold and bitterness to clear residual Heat from the Lungs and Spleen.

EXCESS-FIRE IN THE SPLEEN AND STOMACH

Persistent papules and pustules and stubborn erythema appear around the mouth, often accompanied by bran-like scaling. The tongue body is red with a thin yellow coating; the pulse is soggy and rapid.

Treatment principle
Clear Heat from the Spleen and Stomach, drain Fire and transform Dampness.

Prescription
XIE HUANG SAN JIA JIAN
Yellow-Draining Powder, with modifications

Huo Xiang (Herba Agastaches seu Pogostemi) 12g
Pei Lan (Herba Eupatorii Fortunei) 12g
Huang Qin (Radix Scutellariae Baicalensis) 12g
Sheng Di Huang (Radix Rehmanniae Glutinosae) 12g
Shi Gao‡ (Gypsum Fibrosum) 15-30g, decocted for 30 minutes before adding the other ingredients
Huang Lian (Rhizoma Coptidis) 6g
Sheng Ma (Rhizoma Cimicifugae) 6g
Fang Feng (Radix Ledebouriellae Divaricatae) 6g
Jiao Zhi Zi (Fructus Gardeniae Jasminoidis, scorch-fried) 10g
Pu Gong Ying (Herba Taraxaci cum Radice) 10g
Xuan Shen (Radix Scrophulariae Ningpoensis) 10g
Yi Yi Ren (Semen Coicis Lachryma-jobi) 15g

Explanation
- *Huo Xiang* (Herba Agastaches seu Pogostemi), *Pei Lan* (Herba Eupatorii Fortunei), *Huang Qin* (Radix Scutellariae Baicalensis), *Shi Gao*‡ (Gypsum Fibrosum), *Huang Lian* (Rhizoma Coptidis), and *Jiao Zhi Zi* (Fructus Gardeniae Jasminoidis, scorch-fried) clear Heat from the Spleen and Stomach and drain Fire.
- *Sheng Di Huang* (Radix Rehmanniae Glutinosae) and *Xuan Shen* (Radix Scrophulariae Ningpoensis) enrich Yin and clear Heat.
- *Sheng Ma* (Rhizoma Cimicifugae) and *Fang Feng* (Radix Ledebouriellae Divaricatae) dissipate Wind and alleviate itching.
- *Pu Gong Ying* (Herba Taraxaci cum Radice) and *Yi Yi Ren* (Semen Coicis Lachryma-jobi) transform Dampness and relieve Toxicity.

General modifications
1. For predominance of Dampness, add *Chao Huai Hua* (Flos Sophorae Japonicae, stir-fried), *Shan Zha* (Fructus Crataegi) and *Chi Xiao Dou* (Semen Phaseoli Calcarati).

2. For predominance of Wind, add *Bai Fu Zi* (Rhizoma Typhonii Gigantei), *Qiang Huo* (Rhizoma et Radix Notopterygii) and *Sang Ye* (Folium Mori Albae).
3. For constipation, add *Chao Zhi Ke* (Fructus Citri Aurantii, stir-fried) and *Shu Da Huang* (Radix et Rhizoma Rhei Conquitum).

EXTERNAL TREATMENT

If lesions manifest mainly as papules and papulovesicles, mix *Yue Shi San* (Borax Powder) with warm boiled water and apply to the affected areas two or three times a day for 7-10 days.

Clinical notes

- Since lesions manifest around the mouth, treatment should focus on clearing Heat from the Spleen and transforming Dampness, dissipating Wind and alleviating itching.
- As this disease occurs on the face, materia medica of a mild or bland nature such as *Peng Sha* ‡ (Borax) or *Xuan Ming Fen* ‡ (Mirabilitum Depuratum) should be used for external medications.

Advice for the patient

- Avoid oily or spicy food.
- Keep bowel movements regular.

Literature excerpt

In *Xu Yi Hou Pi Fu Bing Lin Chuang Jing Yan Ji Yao* [A Summary of Xu Yihou's Clinical Experiences in the Treatment of Skin Diseases], the author states: "Persistent papules, papulovesicles and pustules and stubborn erythema appear with bran-like scaling in the perioral area in some young and middle-aged people. The main cause is Excess-Fire in the Spleen and Stomach harassing upward. Since the Spleen opens into the mouth and its bloom is in the lips, this Fire moves along the Spleen channel to the area around the mouth to manifest as skin eruptions. Use of *Xie Huang San* (Yellow-Draining Powder) plus *Huang Qin* (Radix Scutellariae Baicalensis) and *Jing Jie* (Herba Schizonepetae Tenuifoliae) is recommended. This prescription has clearing and dissipating functions, and transforms Dampness and eliminates Heat, allowing the eruptions to be brought under control."

Seborrhea
皮脂溢

Seborrhea is a marked increase in secretion of the sebaceous glands as a result of dysfunction of these glands. The clinical manifestations include greasy, shining hair and skin, and a greasy scalp, or, where there is pityrosporum infection, dry skin and profuse scaling.

In TCM, this condition is known as *bai xie feng* (white scaling Wind).

Clinical manifestations

Seborrhoea oleosa

- The skin on the scalp, face and nose is oily or greasy, as is the hair. The opening of the pilosebaceous ducts is dilated and oozes a soft white greasy substance on pressure.
- The condition is most severe between the ages of 20 and 40; it then becomes milder.
- Acne and seborrheic alopecia are common complications.

Seborrhoea sicca (dandruff)

- This condition is closely related to pityrosporum infection of the scalp.
- Tiny gray or white bran-like scales fall from the scalp on combing or scratching.
- Scales regenerate rapidly after shampooing.
- The scalp feels itchy.

Differential diagnosis

Psoriasis of the scalp

The scalp is bright red or dark red and is covered by layers of silvery-white scale. The hair may form matted bundles in the area of the skin lesions, which often spread beyond the hairline. Areas of scaling may be interspersed with normal skin. Similar lesions may also be present on other parts of the body. Lesions are frequently exacerbated in winter and alleviated in summer.

Seborrheic eczema

Seborrheic eczema is a chronic inflammatory condition mainly affecting hair-bearing areas of the head and body. An itchy red or yellowish-red scaly or exudative erythematous eruption affects the scalp and scalp margins, the sides of the nose, the eyebrows, and the ears. The presternal and interscapular areas and body flexures may also be involved. On the scalp, the condition may be accompanied by marked dandruff.

Etiology and pathology

- Frequent intake of fried food can lead to exuberant Heat in the skin and interstices (*cou li*); if this is complicated by pathogenic Wind invading the hair follicles, retained Heat will transform into Dryness. The skin and flesh will therefore be deprived of nourishment, resulting in dry, itchy skin and persistent desquamation of white scale.

- If Damp-Heat which is obstructed internally is complicated by an invasion of Wind, the three pathogenic factors accumulate and steam upward along the channels to the face, manifesting as greasy, shiny skin and oily scale.

Pattern identification and treatment

INTERNAL TREATMENT

WIND, HEAT AND DRYNESS IN THE FLESH

Large quantities of fine dry white or grayish-white scale accumulate in the scalp before being shed; the process is continuous with scale being constantly regenerated. Scaling may decrease temporarily after washing the hair. The scalp is itchy. The tongue body is red with a thin coating; the pulse is rapid.

Treatment principle

Cool the Blood and clear Heat, disperse Wind and alleviate itching.

Prescription
LIANG XUE XIAO FENG SAN JIA JIAN

Powder for Cooling the Blood and Dispersing Wind, with modifications

Jing Jie (Herba Schizonepetae Tenuifoliae) 3g
Bai Fu Zi (Rhizoma Typhonii Gigantei) 3g
Qiang Huo (Rhizoma et Radix Notopterygii) 6g
Fang Feng (Radix Ledebouriellae Divaricatae) 12g
Ze Xie (Rhizoma Alismatis Orientalis) 12g
Ju Hua (Flos Chrysanthemi Morifolii) 12g
Gou Teng (Ramulus Uncariae cum Uncis) 12g

Chuan Xiong (Rhizoma Ligustici Chuanxiong) 4.5g
Cang Er Zi (Fructus Xanthii Sibirici) 4.5g
Yi Yi Ren (Semen Coicis Lachryma-jobi) 30g
Sheng Di Huang (Radix Rehmanniae Glutinosae) 15g
Dong Gua Ren (Semen Benincasae Hispidae) 15g
Chao Mu Dan Pi (Cortex Moutan Radicis, stir-fried) 15g

Explanation

- *Sheng Di Huang* (Radix Rehmanniae Glutinosae), *Dong Gua Ren* (Semen Benincasae Hispidae), *Chao Mu Dan Pi* (Cortex Moutan Radicis, stir-fried), and *Ju Hua* (Flos Chrysanthemi Morifolii) clear Heat and cool the Blood, moisten Dryness and alleviate itching.

- *Jing Jie* (Herba Schizonepetae Tenuifoliae), *Bai Fu Zi* (Rhizoma Typhonii Gigantei), *Qiang Huo* (Rhizoma et Radix Notopterygii), *Fang Feng* (Radix Ledebouriellae Divaricatae), *Gou Teng* (Ramulus Uncariae cum Uncis), *Chuan Xiong* (Rhizoma Ligustici Chuanxiong), and *Cang Er Zi* (Fructus Xanthii Sibirici) dredge Wind and clear Heat, free the network vessels and alleviate itching.

- *Ze Xie* (Rhizoma Alismatis Orientalis) and *Yi Yi Ren* (Semen Coicis Lachryma-jobi) bear turbidity downward and eliminate Dampness.

ACCUMULATION AND STEAMING OF DAMP-HEAT

Dilated openings of the pilosebaceous ducts can be seen on the scalp and face, which are oily and shining and covered by greasy sebum or some scaling; washing does not get rid of the grease. Slight itching may be experienced. The tongue body is red with a thin coating; the pulse is slippery and rapid.

Treatment principle

Clear Heat and eliminate Dampness, dissipate Wind and alleviate itching.

Prescription
QU FENG HUAN JI SAN JIA JIAN

Powder for Dispelling Wind and Regenerating the Flesh, with modifications

Xi Xian Cao (Herba Siegesbeckiae) 6g
Ku Shen (Radix Sophorae Flavescentis) 6g
Cang Zhu (Rhizoma Atractylodis) 6g
Chuan Xiong (Rhizoma Ligustici Chuanxiong) 6g
Dang Gui (Radix Angelicae Sinensis) 10-12g
Chi Fu Ling (Sclerotium Poriae Cocos Rubrae) 10-12g
Hei Zhi Ma (Semen Sesami Indici) 10-12g
He Shou Wu (Radix Polygoni Multiflori) 10-12g
Chong Wei Zi (Semen Leonuri Heterophylli) 15g
Ju Hua (Flos Chrysanthemi Morifolii) 15g
Shan Zha (Fructus Crataegi) 15g

Hu Zhang (Radix et Rhizoma Polygoni Cuspidati) 15g
Yin Chen Hao (Herba Artemisiae Scopariae) 15g

Explanation

- *Xi Xian Cao* (Herba Siegesbeckiae), *Ku Shen* (Radix Sophorae Flavescentis), *Cang Zhu* (Rhizoma Atractylodis), *Chuan Xiong* (Rhizoma Ligustici Chuanxiong), *Chi Fu Ling* (Sclerotium Poriae Cocos Rubrae), *Yin Chen Hao* (Herba Artemisiae Scopariae), and *Ju Hua* (Flos Chrysanthemi Morifolii) dissipate Wind and alleviate itching, clear Heat and eliminate Dampness.
- *Dang Gui* (Radix Angelicae Sinensis), *He Shou Wu* (Radix Polygoni Multiflori), *Chong Wei Zi* (Semen Leonuri Heterophylli), *Shan Zha* (Fructus Crataegi), and *Hu Zhang* (Radix et Rhizoma Polygoni Cuspidati) nourish the Blood and emolliate the Liver, extinguish Wind and alleviate itching.
- *Hei Zhi Ma* (Semen Sesami Indici) enriches Yin and moistens Dryness to counteract Dryness produced by the other ingredients.

General modifications

1. For profuse scaling, add *Man Jing Zi* (Fructus Viticis), *Wang Bu Liu Xing* (Semen Vaccariae Segetalis) and *Bi Xie* (Rhizoma Dioscoreae Hypoglaucae seu Septemlobae).
2. For intense itching, add *Bai Ji Li* (Fructus Tribuli Terrestris), *Tian Ma** (Rhizoma Gastrodiae Elatae) and *Shi Chang Pu* (Rhizoma Acori Graminei).
3. For very oily or greasy skin, add *Wu Wei Zi* (Fructus Schisandrae), *Bai Hua She She Cao* (Herba Hedyotidis Diffusae) and *Qing Hao* (Herba Artemisiae Chinghao).

EXTERNAL TREATMENT

- In the greasy type of seborrhea, for involvement of the scalp, apply *Bai Xie Feng Ding* (Seborrhea Tincture) three times a day; for involvement of the face, apply *Yu Ji San* (Jade Flesh Powder) twice a day; and for involvement of the neck, apply *Bing Liu San* (Borneol and Sulfur Powder) twice a day.
- For Wind, Heat and Dryness in the flesh, grind equal quantities of *Zi Cao* (Radix Arnebiae seu Lithospermi) and *Dang Gui* (Radix Angelicae Sinensis) into a fine powder and mix into a paste with sesame oil for application to the affected area twice a day; alternatively, apply *Run Ji Gao* (Flesh-Moistening Paste).
- For accumulation and steaming of Damp-Heat, apply *Bai Xie Feng Ding* (Seborrhea Tincture) to the affected area twice a day.
- For dry skin and profuse white scales due to Heat in the flesh, apply *Hua Jiao You* (Chinese Prickly Ash Oil) or *Shan Dou Gen You Ji* (Subprostrate Sophora Root Oil Preparation) to the affected area twice a day.

- For an oily or greasy face or greasy scaling, decoct *Cang Er Zi* (Fructus Xanthii Sibirici) 30g and *Guan Zhong** (Rhizoma Dryopteris Crassirhizomae) 30g for use as an external wash once a day.
- For a greasy scalp with layers of scaling, shampoo with *Cang Fu Shui Xi Ji* (Atractylodes and Broom Cypress Wash Preparation), *Tou Gu Cao Shui Xi Ji* (Speranskia Wash Preparation), *Shan Dou Gen Shui Xi Ji* (Subprostrate Sophora Root Wash Preparation), or *Zhi Yi Xi Fang* (Seborrhea Wash Formula) three times a week.

ACUPUNCTURE

Points: GB-20 Fengchi, GV-16 Fengfu, BL-57 Chengshan, BL-20 Pishu, BL-21 Weishu, BL-18 Ganshu, and BL-19 Danshu.
Technique: Apply the reducing method to all the points, and use the pricking method on BL-19 Danshu. Retain the needles for 30 minutes. Treat once every two days. A course consists of five treatment sessions.

Explanation

- GB-20 Fengchi and GV-16 Fengfu dissipate Wind and alleviate itching.
- BL-20 Pishu, BL-21 Weishu and BL-18 Ganshu clear and transform Damp-Heat in the Spleen and Stomach.
- BL-57 Chengshan and BL-19 Danshu clear Heat and drain Toxicity.
- Once Damp-Heat is dispelled and Wind-Heat eliminated, scaling on the face and scalp and itching can be relieved.

EAR ACUPUNCTURE

Points: Spleen, Stomach and Endocrine.
Technique: Retain the needles for 30 minutes. Treat once every two days. A course consists of ten treatment sessions.

Clinical notes

- Treat dry seborrhea by focusing on the Heart and Lungs, according to the principle of cooling the Blood and dissipating Wind to alleviate itching.
- Treat damp seborrhea by focusing on the Spleen and Stomach, according to the principle of eliminating Dampness, dissipating Wind and freeing the Fu organs to alleviate itching.
- Some cases are chronic, possibly leading to hair loss. However, if patients persist with the treatment, improvement or total alleviation of the condition is possible.

Advice for the patient

- Cut down on spicy, fatty and sweet foods, and avoid ginger, garlic, alcohol, and strong tea; increase intake of vegetables, fruit and soybean products.
- Do not wash the hair or face too frequently; use medicinal soap with sulfur rather than strongly alkaline soap.

Literature excerpt

In *Wai Ke Zheng Zong* [An Orthodox Manual of External Diseases], it says: "*Bai xie feng* (white scaling Wind) usually occurs on the scalp, face, ear, and neck. It manifests initially with slight itching, but as it persists, white scales start to pile up and be shed continuously. The disease is caused by internal Heat and external Wind transforming into Wind-Heat. It can therefore be treated initially with *Xiao Feng San* (Powder for Dispersing Wind) or *Yu Ji San* (Jade Flesh Powder) and subsequently by *Dang Gui Gao* (Chinese Angelica Root Paste) to moisten the skin."

Modern clinical experience

SPECIAL PRESCRIPTIONS

1. **Cheng** reported on internal treatment of 40 patients with seborrhea. [28]

Prescription
DA CHAI HU TANG JIA JIAN
Major Bupleurum Decoction, with modifications

Chai Hu (Radix Bupleuri) 12g
Zhi Shi (Fructus Immaturus Citri Aurantii) 12g

Huang Qin (Radix Scutellariae Baicalensis) 12g
Da Huang (Radix et Rhizoma Rhei) 6-12g, added
　5 minutes before the end of the decoction process
Bai Shao (Radix Paeoniae Lactiflorae) 30g
Shan Zha (Fructus Crataegi) 30g
Bai Hua She She Cao (Herba Hedyotidis Diffusae) 30g
Shi Gao‡ (Gypsum Fibrosum) 30g, decocted for
　30 minutes before adding the other ingredients
Gan Cao (Radix Glycyrrhizae) 6g

One bag a day was used to prepare a decoction, taken twice a day. Generally, the condition started to improve after one to two weeks.

2. **Bao** described Zhong Yitang's experience in combining internal and external treatments. [29]

Internal prescription ingredients

Zhi Shou Wu (Radix Polygoni Multiflori Praeparata) 25g
Dang Gui (Radix Angelicae Sinensis) 25g
Dan Shen (Radix Salviae Miltiorrhizae) 20g
Bai Xian Pi (Cortex Dictamni Dasycarpi Radicis) 15g
Huang Qin (Radix Scutellariae Baicalensis) 15g
Xing Ren (Semen Pruni Armeniacae) 15g
Gan Cao (Radix Glycyrrhizae) 3g
Sheng Ma (Rhizoma Cimicifugae) 10g

One bag a day was used to prepare a decoction, taken twice a day.

External prescription ingredients

He Ye (Folium Nelumbinis Nuciferae) 15g
Bai Zhi (Radix Angelicae Dahuricae) 10g
Shan Zha (Fructus Crataegi) 30g
Xing Ren (Semen Pruni Armeniacae) 25g

The ingredients were used to prepare a wash for use once a day. Results were seen after four weeks.

Hyperhidrosis
多汗症

Hyperhidrosis is the secretion of abnormal quantities of sweat due to functional disorders such as emotional stress and to organic disorders such as endocrine dysfunction (for example, in carcinoid syndrome, diabetes mellitus and Cushing's syndrome) or nervous system diseases affecting the preoptic hypothalamus such as cerebral tumors or cerebrovascular accident. Generalized hyperhidrosis may also be a feature of menopausal hot flushes, lymphomas and opiate withdrawal. Localized hyperhidrosis usually affects young adults.

In TCM, hyperhidrosis is known as *duo han* (profuse sweating).

Clinical manifestations

- Hyperhidrosis is more common in young people, particularly young men. It is usually more marked during the day, stopping during sleep.

- Profuse local sweating involves the palms, soles, forehead, axillae, and genitals symmetrically, with sweating in the palms and soles being the most common.
- In mild cases, the condition manifests as obvious sweating in certain areas, but in more marked cases, pearls of sweat emerge continuously, especially at times of excitement. In severe cases, profuse sweating can lead to dyshidrotic features such as blisters, erosions or hyperkeratosis, which may make walking difficult if the soles are affected. Other consequences include the foul smell produced by bacteria acting on stale sweat, or secondary fungal infection.

Differential diagnosis

Bromhidrosis

Bromhidrosis is hyperhidrosis with a foul smell, which is stronger in summer and may not be evident at all in winter. Bromhidrosis mainly involves the axillae, the umbilicus, the genitals, and the toes.

Chromhidrosis

In chromhidrosis, the secretion of sweat colored as a result of biological activity causes staining of the clothes with which it comes into contact. The condition mainly involves the axillae and scrotum.

Etiology and pathology

- Excessive intake of spicy food, alcohol or coffee can lead to steaming of Yang Heat internally, forcing Body Fluids out of the skin, manifesting as profuse sweating.
- Internal damage caused by emotional disturbances can result in Liver Qi Depression, which then transforms into Fire, causing steaming of Body Fluids to produce sweating. Over a long period, Qi Depression associated with emotional disturbances can either transform directly into Heart-Fire or indirectly where Heart-Fire is transmitted from Liver-Fire.
- Loss of Blood or Essence, or enduring cough due to pulmonary consumption causes depletion of and damage to Yin-Blood, which results in Yin Deficiency generating internal Heat. Exuberant Deficiency-Fire impedes Yin-Liquids from being stored, leading to profuse sweating.
- Profuse sweating may also be caused by weakness of Yang Qi, which fails to consolidate the defensive exterior and secure the interstices (*cou li*), giving rise to disharmony between the Ying and Wei levels; hence the sweat drains away with Qi. Deficiency of

Heart Yang resulting in failure to consolidate the defensive exterior and Deficiency of Kidney Yang, which impairs the storage function, also lead to profuse sweating.
- Overindulgence in raw, cold, fatty, or sweet foods and alcohol or eating at irregular mealtimes can damage the Spleen and Stomach. The Spleen's transformation and transportation function is impaired and Damp is generated internally, obstructing the normal movement of Qi. As a result, Damp moves to the skin to be discharged as sweat instead of being distributed by Spleen Qi. However, exuberant Damp arising in this way produces different types of sweat in terms of etiology and location:
  1. The head is the confluence of the Yang channels. Profuse sweating on the forehead with no sweating on other parts of the body is due to Damp-Heat steaming upward to the head to create heat.
  2. Profuse sweating involving the hands and feet is related to Damp in the Spleen and Stomach steaming to the extremities.
  3. Sweating in the genital region, also known as Yin sweat, is due to Damp-Heat in the Lower Burner.
  4. Yang Deficiency of the Spleen and Stomach due to Cold in the Middle Burner means that Spleen Qi is too weak to control Body Fluids, and Water and Dampness overflow throughout the body to cause profuse cold sweating.

  Although both Damp-Heat and Cold-Damp can be responsible for profuse sweating, Damp-Heat is the more common cause.
- In the elderly, impaired circulation of Qi and Blood, Blood stasis due to Qi Deficiency, or obstruction of the channels and vessels can cause profuse sweating on one side of the body or the upper or lower half of the body.
- Insufficiency of Qi and Blood complicated internally by Cold congealing results in Qi and Blood not circulating smoothly and may lead to obstruction of the channels and network vessels to cause profuse sweating.

Pattern identification and treatment

INTERNAL TREATMENT

STEAMING OF INTERNAL HEAT

HEAT IN THE STOMACH CHANNEL

If profuse sweating is seen on the forehead during a meal, it is caused by Heat in the Yangming channel. The tongue body is red with a thin and white or thin and yellow coating; the pulse is slippery.

Treatment principle
Clear the Stomach and drain Heat.

Prescription
BAI HU TANG JIA JIAN
White Tiger Decoction, with modifications

Shi Gao‡ (Gypsum Fibrosum) 15-30g, decocted for 30 minutes before adding the other ingredients
Chao Zhi Mu (Rhizoma Anemarrhenae Asphodeloidis, stir-fried) 6g
Gan Cao (Radix Glycyrrhizae) 6g
Jiao Zhi Zi (Fructus Gardeniae Jasminoidis, scorch-fried) 6g
Chao Huang Qin (Radix Scutellariae Baicalensis, stir-fried) 6g
Shan Yao (Radix Dioscoreae Oppositae) 15g
Xuan Shen (Radix Scrophulariae Ningpoensis) 12g
*Shi Hu** (Herba Dendrobii) 12g

Explanation
- *Shi Gao*‡ (Gypsum Fibrosum), *Chao Zhi Mu* (Rhizoma Anemarrhenae Asphodeloidis, stir-fried), *Gan Cao* (Radix Glycyrrhizae), *Jiao Zhi Zi* (Fructus Gardeniae Jasminoidis, scorch-fried), *Shi Hu** (Herba Dendrobii), and *Shan Yao* (Radix Dioscoreae Oppositae) clear the Stomach and drain Heat.
- *Xuan Shen* (Radix Scrophulariae Ningpoensis) clears Deficiency-Heat from the Kidney channel, whereas *Chao Huang Qin* (Radix Scutellariae Baicalensis, stir-fried) drains Excess-Heat from the Lung channel. Once Heat in the Kidney and Lung channels has been cleared, it is easier to drain Heat from the Stomach channel.

LIVER DEPRESSION TRANSFORMING INTO FIRE
Profuse sweating has a sudden onset and is accompanied by impatience and irascibility. The side margins of the tongue are red and the tongue has a thin white coating; the pulse is wiry.

Treatment principle
Clear Heat from the Liver and drain Fire.

Prescription
DANG GUI LONG HUI WAN JIA JIAN
Angelica, Gentian and Aloe Pill, with modifications

Chao Long Dan Cao (Radix Gentianae Scabrae, stir-fried) 6g
Jiao Zhi Zi (Fructus Gardeniae Jasminoidis, scorch-fried) 6g
Chao Huang Lian (Rhizoma Coptidis, stir-fried) 6g
Chao Huang Bai (Cortex Phellodendri, stir-fried) 10g
Chao Huang Qin (Radix Scutellariae Baicalensis, stir-fried) 10g
Chao Bai Shao (Radix Paeoniae Lactiflorae, stir-fried) 10g
Dang Gui (Radix Angelicae Sinensis) 10g
Chai Hu (Radix Bupleuri) 4.5g
Qing Dai (Indigo Naturalis) 4.5g

Explanation
- *Chao Long Dan Cao* (Radix Gentianae Scabrae, stir-fried), *Chai Hu* (Radix Bupleuri), *Jiao Zhi Zi* (Fructus Gardeniae Jasminoidis, scorch-fried), *Chao Bai Shao* (Radix Paeoniae Lactiflorae, stir-fried), and *Dang Gui* (Radix Angelicae Sinensis) clear Heat from the Liver and drain Fire.
- *Chao Huang Lian* (Rhizoma Coptidis, stir-fried) clears Fire from the Heart.
- *Chao Huang Qin* (Radix Scutellariae Baicalensis, stir-fried) clears Fire from the Lungs.
- *Chao Huang Bai* (Cortex Phellodendri, stir-fried) clears Fire from the Kidneys.
- *Qing Dai* (Indigo Naturalis) clears and drains Fire from the Liver and Lungs.
- Clearing Fire from the Zang organs will calm impatience and irascibility and constrain sweating.

HEART-FIRE
Profuse sweating is accompanied by emotional stress and irritability. The tip of the tongue is red; the pulse is thready and rapid.

Treatment principle
Clear Heat from the Heart and drain Fire.

Prescription
QING XIN LIAN ZI TANG JIA JIAN
Lotus Seed Decoction for Clearing Heat from the Heart, with modifications

Huang Qin (Radix Scutellariae Baicalensis) 10g
Mai Men Dong (Radix Ophiopogonis Japonici) 10g
Di Gu Pi (Cortex Lycii Radicis) 10g
Gan Cao (Radix Glycyrrhizae) 10g
Lian Zi (Semen Nelumbinis Nuciferae) 12g
Fu Ling (Sclerotium Poriae Cocos) 12g
Huang Qi (Radix Astragali seu Hedysari) 12g
Dang Shen (Radix Codonopsitis Pilosulae) 12g
Deng Xin Cao (Medulla Junci Effusi) 5g
Che Qian Zi (Semen Plantaginis) 15g, wrapped

Explanation
- *Huang Qi* (Radix Astragali seu Hedysari), *Dang Shen* (Radix Codonopsitis Pilosulae) and *Gan Cao* (Radix Glycyrrhizae) augment Qi and consolidate the exterior to prevent the fluid of the Heart (sweat) from being drained to the exterior.
- *Mai Men Dong* (Radix Ophiopogonis Japonici), *Di Gu Pi* (Cortex Lycii Radicis), *Lian Zi* (Semen Nelumbinis Nuciferae), and *Deng Xin Cao* (Medulla Junci Effusi) nourish Yin and clear Heat from the Heart, drain Fire and constrain sweating.
- *Fu Ling* (Sclerotium Poriae Cocos) quiets the Heart.

- *Huang Qin* (Radix Scutellariae Baicalensis) clears Heat from the Lungs, thus assisting *Huang Qi* (Radix Astragali seu Hedysari) and *Dang Shen* (Radix Codonopsitis Pilosulae) to consolidate the exterior.
- *Che Qian Zi* (Semen Plantaginis) guides Heat downward to drain Heart-Fire through urination.

INTERNAL HEAT DUE TO YIN DEFICIENCY

Profuse sweating occurs simultaneously with a feverish sensation in the palms and soles, dry throat and reddening of the cheeks. The tongue body is red with a scant coating; the pulse is thready.

Treatment principle
Nourish Yin and clear Heat.

Prescription
MAI WEI DI HUANG WAN JIA JIAN
Ophiopogon and Rehmannia Pill, with modifications

Mai Men Dong (Radix Ophiopogonis Japonici) 12g
Gan Di Huang (Radix Rehmanniae Glutinosae Exsiccata) 12g
Shan Zhu Yu (Fructus Corni Officinalis) 12g
Fu Ling (Sclerotium Poriae Cocos) 10g
Ze Xie (Rhizoma Alismatis Orientalis) 10g
Di Gu Pi (Cortex Lycii Radicis) 10g
Chao Mu Dan Pi (Cortex Moutan Radicis, stir-fried) 10g
Shan Yao (Radix Dioscoreae Oppositae) 15g
Wu Wei Zi (Fructus Schisandrae) 6g
Duan Long Gu‡ (Os Draconis Calcinatum) 30g
Duan Mu Li‡ (Concha Ostreae Calcinata) 30g
Shi Jue Ming‡ (Concha Haliotidis) 30g

Explanation
- *Mai Men Dong* (Radix Ophiopogonis Japonici), *Wu Wei Zi* (Fructus Schisandrae), *Gan Di Huang* (Radix Rehmanniae Glutinosae Exsiccata), *Shan Zhu Yu* (Fructus Corni Officinalis), *Di Gu Pi* (Cortex Lycii Radicis), and *Chao Mu Dan Pi* (Cortex Moutan Radicis, stir-fried) nourish Yin and clear Heat.
- *Fu Ling* (Sclerotium Poriae Cocos), *Shan Yao* (Radix Dioscoreae Oppositae) and *Ze Xie* (Rhizoma Alismatis Orientalis) support the Spleen and transform Dampness.
- *Duan Long Gu‡* (Os Draconis Calcinatum), *Duan Mu Li‡* (Concha Ostreae Calcinata) and *Shi Jue Ming‡* (Concha Haliotidis) constrain sweating and astringe Body Fluids.

YANG DEFICIENCY

YANG DEFICIENCY FAILING TO CONSOLIDATE THE DEFENSIVE EXTERIOR

Profuse sweating is induced by exertion with accompanying symptoms and signs of aversion to wind, mental fatigue and cold limbs. The tongue body is pale with a thin white coating; the pulse is floating.

Treatment principle
Regulate the Ying and Wei levels, consolidate the exterior and constrain sweating.

Prescription
GUI ZHI TANG JIA JIAN
Cinnamon Twig Decoction, with modifications

Gui Zhi (Ramulus Cinnamomi Cassiae) 6g
Gan Cao (Radix Glycyrrhizae) 6g
Chao Bai Shao (Radix Paeoniae Lactiflorae, stir-fried) 12g
Huang Qi (Radix Astragali seu Hedysari) 12g
Duan Long Gu‡ (Os Draconis Calcinatum) 12g
Duan Mu Li‡ (Concha Ostreae Calcinata) 12g
Dang Shen (Radix Codonopsitis Pilosulae) 12g
Bai Zhu (Rhizoma Atractylodis Macrocephalae) 12g
*Ma Huang** (Herba Ephedrae) 4.5g
Da Zao (Fructus Ziziphi Jujubae) 15g

Explanation
- *Gui Zhi* (Ramulus Cinnamomi Cassiae), *Gan Cao* (Radix Glycyrrhizae), *Chao Bai Shao* (Radix Paeoniae Lactiflorae, stir-fried), *Ma Huang** (Herba Ephedrae), and *Da Zao* (Fructus Ziziphi Jujubae) regulate the Ying and Wei levels.
- *Huang Qi* (Radix Astragali seu Hedysari), *Duan Long Gu‡* (Os Draconis Calcinatum), *Duan Mu Li‡* (Concha Ostreae Calcinata), *Dang Shen* (Radix Codonopsitis Pilosulae), and *Bai Zhu* (Rhizoma Atractylodis Macrocephalae) augment Qi and consolidate the exterior to constrain sweating.

HEART YANG DEFICIENCY

There is persistent perspiration on exposure to wind, complicated by palpitations and insomnia. The tongue body is pale and enlarged with a thin white coating; the pulse is deep.

Treatment principle
Augment Qi and warm Yang.

Prescription
SHEN FU TANG JIA JIAN
Ginseng and Aconite Decoction, with modifications

Dang Shen (Radix Codonopsitis Pilosulae) 10g
Mai Men Dong (Radix Ophiopogonis Japonici) 10g
Gan Cao (Radix Glycyrrhizae) 10g
Sheng Di Huang (Radix Rehmanniae Glutinosae) 10g
Di Gu Pi (Cortex Lycii Radicis) 10g
Fu Pen Zi (Fructus Rubi Chingii) 12g
Huang Qi (Radix Astragali seu Hedysari) 6g
Dang Gui (Radix Angelicae Sinensis) 6g
Wu Wei Zi (Fructus Schisandrae) 4.5g

Explanation

- *Dang Shen* (Radix Codonopsitis Pilosulae), *Fu Pen Zi* (Fructus Rubi Chingii), *Huang Qi* (Radix Astragali seu Hedysari), *Dang Gui* (Radix Angelicae Sinensis), and *Wu Wei Zi* (Fructus Schisandrae) augment Qi, warm Yang and constrain sweating.

- *Mai Men Dong* (Radix Ophiopogonis Japonici), *Gan Cao* (Radix Glycyrrhizae), *Sheng Di Huang* (Radix Rehmanniae Glutinosae), and *Di Gu Pi* (Cortex Lycii Radicis) nourish Yin and clear Heat to prevent Deficiency-Heat crossing to the exterior.

YANG DEFICIENCY OF THE HEART AND KIDNEYS

Profuse sweating only involves the axillae and sweating increases as the weather gets colder. Accompanying symptoms and signs include aversion to cold and cold limbs. The tongue body is pale with a white coating; the pulse is deep.

Treatment principle

Support Vital Qi (Zheng Qi) and reinforce Yang.

Prescription
YOU GUI YIN JIA JIAN

Restoring the Right [Kidney Yang] Beverage, with modifications

Fu Pen Zi (Fructus Rubi Chingii) 10-15g
Shan Zhu Yu (Fructus Corni Officinalis) 10g
Chao Du Zhong (Cortex Eucommiae Ulmoidis, stir-fried) 10g
Shu Di Huang (Radix Rehmanniae Glutinosae Conquita) 10g
Gou Qi Zi (Fructus Lycii) 10g
Shan Yao (Radix Dioscoreae Oppositae) 15g
Gan Cao (Radix Glycyrrhizae) 4.5g
Rou Gui (Cortex Cinnamomi Cassiae) 4.5g

Explanation

- *Fu Pen Zi* (Fructus Rubi Chingii), *Shan Zhu Yu* (Fructus Corni Officinalis), *Chao Du Zhong* (Cortex Eucommiae Ulmoidis, stir-fried), *Shu Di Huang* (Radix Rehmanniae Glutinosae Conquita), *Gou Qi Zi* (Fructus Lycii), and *Rou Gui* (Cortex Cinnamomi Cassiae) support Vital Qi (Zheng Qi), reinforce Yang, and enrich and supplement the Liver and Kidneys.

- *Shan Yao* (Radix Dioscoreae Oppositae) and *Gan Cao* (Radix Glycyrrhizae) support the Spleen and consolidate the Root.

STEAMING OF DAMP-HEAT

DAMP-HEAT STEAMING UPWARD

Profuse sweating on the head is accompanied by generalized fever. The tongue body is pale red with a thick greasy yellow coating; the pulse is soggy and rapid.

Treatment principle

Clear the Spleen and drain Heat.

Prescription
XIE HUANG SAN JIA JIAN

Yellow-Draining Powder, with modifications

Huo Xiang (Herba Agastaches seu Pogostemi) 10g
Pei Lan (Herba Eupatorii Fortunei) 10g
Fu Ling (Sclerotium Poriae Cocos) 10g
Shi Gao ‡ (Gypsum Fibrosum) 15g, decocted for
   30 minutes before adding the other ingredients
Jiao Zhi Zi (Fructus Gardeniae Jasminoidis, scorch-fried) 6g
Chao Huang Lian (Rhizoma Coptidis, stir-fried) 6g
Chao Huang Qin (Radix Scutellariae Baicalensis, stir-fried) 6g
Sheng Ma (Rhizoma Cimicifugae) 6g
Ze Xie (Rhizoma Alismatis Orientalis) 12g

Explanation

- *Huo Xiang* (Herba Agastaches seu Pogostemi), *Pei Lan* (Herba Eupatorii Fortunei), *Shi Gao* ‡ (Gypsum Fibrosum), *Jiao Zhi Zi* (Fructus Gardeniae Jasminoidis, scorch-fried), *Chao Huang Lian* (Rhizoma Coptidis, stir-fried), and *Chao Huang Qin* (Radix Scutellariae Baicalensis, stir-fried) clear the Spleen and drain Heat, and aromatically transform turbidity.

- *Fu Ling* (Sclerotium Poriae Cocos) and *Ze Xie* (Rhizoma Alismatis Orientalis) percolate Dampness and promote urination so that Heat can be eliminated with the urine.

- *Sheng Ma* (Rhizoma Cimicifugae) bears the clear upward and the turbid downward, and conducts the other materia medica to the affected area.

DAMP-HEAT FLOWING TO THE EXTREMITIES

Incessant, profuse perspiration occurs on the hands and feet. The tongue body is red with a thin yellow coating; the pulse is wiry and rapid.

Treatment principle

Clear Heat and dry Dampness.

Prescription
QING PI YIN JIA JIAN

Beverage for Clearing Heat from the Spleen, with modifications

Chai Hu (Radix Bupleuri) 6g
Huang Qin (Radix Scutellariae Baicalensis) 6g
Hou Po (Cortex Magnoliae Officinalis) 6g
Fa Ban Xia (Rhizoma Pinelliae Ternatae Praeparata) 6g
Bai Zhu (Rhizoma Atractylodis Macrocephalae) 12g
Shi Gao ‡ (Gypsum Fibrosum) 12g, decocted for
   30 minutes before adding the other ingredients
Chao Niu Bang Zi (Fructus Arctii Lappae, stir-fried) 12g

Chao Zhi Mu (Rhizoma Anemarrhenae Asphodeloidis, stir-fried) 3g

Chao Huang Lian (Rhizoma Coptidis, stir-fried) 3g

Explanation

* *Chai Hu* (Radix Bupleuri), *Huang Qin* (Radix Scutellariae Baicalensis), *Shi Gao*‡ (Gypsum Fibrosum), *Chao Zhi Mu* (Rhizoma Anemarrhenae Asphodeloidis, stir-fried), and *Chao Huang Lian* (Rhizoma Coptidis, stir-fried) clear Excess-Heat from the Heart and Spleen.
* *Hou Po* (Cortex Magnoliae Officinalis), *Fa Ban Xia* (Rhizoma Pinelliae Ternatae Praeparata) and *Bai Zhu* (Rhizoma Atractylodis Macrocephalae) aromatically arouse the Spleen, dry Dampness and dispel sweat.
* *Chao Niu Bang Zi* (Fructus Arctii Lappae, stir-fried) clears and diffuses Heat from the Lungs to release pathogenic factors from the exterior.

DAMP-HEAT POURING DOWN

Profuse sweating in the scrotum or groin makes clothing damp and sticky. The tongue body is red with a yellow and greasy coating; the pulse is wiry and rapid.

Treatment principle

Clear Heat from the Liver and drain Fire.

Prescription

LONG DAN XIE GAN TANG JIA JIAN

Chinese Gentian Decoction for Draining the Liver, with modifications

Chao Long Dan Cao (Radix Gentianae Scabrae, stir-fried) 6g
Jiao Zhi Zi (Fructus Gardeniae Jasminoidis, scorch-fried) 6g
Chai Hu (Radix Bupleuri) 6g
Huang Qin (Radix Scutellariae Baicalensis) 6g
Ze Xie (Rhizoma Alismatis Orientalis) 12g
Chao Bai Shao (Radix Paeoniae Lactiflorae, stir-fried) 12g
Chao Du Zhong (Cortex Eucommiae Ulmoidis, stir-fried) 12g
Fu Ling (Sclerotium Poriae Cocos) 12g
Che Qian Zi (Semen Plantaginis) 15g, wrapped

Explanation

* *Chao Long Dan Cao* (Radix Gentianae Scabrae, stir-fried), *Jiao Zhi Zi* (Fructus Gardeniae Jasminoidis, scorch-fried), *Chai Hu* (Radix Bupleuri), *Huang Qin* (Radix Scutellariae Baicalensis), *Fu Ling* (Sclerotium Poriae Cocos), *Ze Xie* (Rhizoma Alismatis Orientalis), and *Che Qian Zi* (Semen Plantaginis) clear Heat from the Liver and drain Fire.
* *Chao Bai Shao* (Radix Paeoniae Lactiflorae, stir-fried) constrains Yin and stops sweating with sourness and bitterness.
* *Chao Du Zhong* (Cortex Eucommiae Ulmoidis, stir-fried) supplements the Kidneys and constrains sweating.
* This prescription contains more ingredients for

draining Heat than for supplementing Deficiency. For Excess patterns of profuse sweating in the scrotum, draining Heat is the main treatment principle.

IMPAIRED MOVEMENT OF QI AND BLOOD

QI STAGNATION AND BLOOD STASIS

Sweat like raindrops involves one side of the body (hyperhidrosis lateralis) or the upper or lower half of the body. This pattern occurs mostly in elderly people with a weak constitution. The tongue body is pale and dull with a white coating; the pulse is weak.

Treatment principle

Augment Qi and supplement the Blood.

Prescription

SHI QUAN DA BU TANG JIA JIAN

Perfect Major Supplementation Decoction, with modifications

Huang Qi (Radix Astragali seu Hedysari) 10g
Dang Shen (Radix Codonopsitis Pilosulae) 10g
Fu Ling (Sclerotium Poriae Cocos) 10g
Bai Zhu (Rhizoma Atractylodis Macrocephalae) 10g
Chen Pi (Pericarpium Citri Reticulatae) 10g
Dang Gui (Radix Angelicae Sinensis) 12g
Chi Shao (Radix Paeoniae Rubra) 12g
Bai Shao (Radix Paeoniae Lactiflorae) 12g
Shu Di Huang (Radix Rehmanniae Glutinosae Conquita) 12g
Chuan Xiong (Rhizoma Ligustici Chuanxiong) 4.5g
Dan Shen (Radix Salviae Miltiorrhizae) 4.5g
Hong Hua (Flos Carthami Tinctorii) 4.5g

Explanation

* *Huang Qi* (Radix Astragali seu Hedysari), *Dang Shen* (Radix Codonopsitis Pilosulae), *Fu Ling* (Sclerotium Poriae Cocos), *Bai Zhu* (Rhizoma Atractylodis Macrocephalae), *Dang Gui* (Radix Angelicae Sinensis), *Chi Shao* (Radix Paeoniae Rubra), *Bai Shao* (Radix Paeoniae Lactiflorae), and *Shu Di Huang* (Radix Rehmanniae Glutinosae Conquita) augment Qi and supplement the Blood, consolidate the exterior and astringe sweating.
* *Chen Pi* (Pericarpium Citri Reticulatae) regulates Qi.
* *Chuan Xiong* (Rhizoma Ligustici Chuanxiong), *Dan Shen* (Radix Salviae Miltiorrhizae) and *Hong Hua* (Flos Carthami Tinctorii) invigorate the Blood, free the network vessels and dredge the interstices (*cou li*) to promote harmony between the Ying and Wei levels.

INSUFFICIENCY OF QI AND BLOOD

Sweat like raindrops can appear on any part of the body, with the condition alternating between exacerbation and alleviation. The tongue body is dark with stasis marks and a thin white coating; the pulse is rough.

Treatment principle
Regulate Qi and invigorate the Blood.

Prescription
FU YUAN HUO XUE TANG JIA JIAN
Decoction for Reviving the Origin by Invigorating the Blood, with modifications

Jiu Dang Gui (Radix Angelicae Sinensis, processed with wine) 10g
Chao Bai Shao (Radix Paeoniae Lactiflorae, stir-fried) 10g
Gan Di Huang (Radix Rehmanniae Glutinosae Exsiccata) 10g
Tian Hua Fen (Radix Trichosanthis) 10g
Shu Da Huang (Radix et Rhizoma Rhei Conquitum) 6g
Chao Zhi Ke (Fructus Citri Aurantii, stir-fried) 6g
Chai Hu (Radix Bupleuri) 6g
Gan Cao (Radix Glycyrrhizae) 6g
Dan Shen (Radix Salviae Miltiorrhizae) 12g
Yi Mu Cao (Herba Leonuri Heterophylli) 12g

Explanation
- *Jiu Dang Gui* (Radix Angelicae Sinensis, processed with wine), *Chao Bai Shao* (Radix Paeoniae Lactiflorae, stir-fried), *Gan Di Huang* (Radix Rehmanniae Glutinosae Exsiccata), *Chai Hu* (Radix Bupleuri), *Dan Shen* (Radix Salviae Miltiorrhizae), *Gan Cao* (Radix Glycyrrhizae), and *Yi Mu Cao* (Herba Leonuri Heterophylli) regulate Qi and invigorate the Blood.
- *Shu Da Huang* (Radix et Rhizoma Rhei Conquitum) and *Chao Zhi Ke* (Fructus Citri Aurantii, stir-fried) free the Fu organs and drain Heat.
- *Tian Hua Fen* (Radix Trichosanthis) generates Body Fluids and alleviates thirst, thus supplementing Deficiency arising from the discharge of sweat.

PATENT HERBAL MEDICINES
- For profuse sweating on the forehead, take *E Han Fang* (Forehead Sweating Formula) 6g twice a day.
- For profuse sweating in the scrotum, take *An Shen Wan* (Quieting the Kidney Pill) 6g, twice a day.

EXTERNAL TREATMENT
- For generalized profuse sweating, grind *Ma Huang Gen** (Radix Ephedrae) 20g, *Mu Li*‡ (Concha Ostreae) 20g, *Long Gu*‡ (Os Draconis) 15g, and *Chi Shi Zhi*‡ (Halloysitum Rubrum) 15g to a fine powder and apply to the affected area once a day.
- For profuse sweating of the hands and feet, use *Ge Gen Shui Xi Ji* (Kudzu Vine Root Wash Preparation)

as a soak for the affected areas once a day; alternatively, apply *Mu Fan Dan* (Oyster, Alum and Minium Powder) three times a day externally.

ACUPUNCTURE
Points
- For generalized profuse sweating, select LI-4 Hegu, SI-3 Houxi, KI-7 Fuliu, and LU-10 Yuji.
- For profuse sweating on one side of the face, select Dazhi (located on the line joining EX-HN-14 Yiming[xiv] and GB-20 Fengchi at a distance of one-third of the line from GB-20 Fengchi).
- For profuse sweating on the head, neck and face, select GV-14 Dazhui, LI-4 Hegu and KI-7 Fuliu.
- For profuse sweating of the hands and feet, select LI-4 Hegu, KI-7 Fuliu and HT-6 Yinxi.

Technique: Apply the reinforcing method for Deficiency patterns and the reducing method for Excess patterns. Treat once a day. A course consists of ten treatment sessions.

Explanation
- LU-10 Yuji and SI-3 Houxi harmonize Qi and Blood.
- KI-7 Fuliu and LI-4 Hegu augment Qi and constrain sweating.
- HT-6 Yinxi, GV-14 Dazhui and Dazhi enrich Yin and clear Heat.

EAR ACUPUNCTURE
Points: Heart, Kidney, Lung, Ear-Shenmen, Sympathetic Nerve, Subcortex, and Blood Pressure-Reducing Groove.
Technique: Retain the needles for 30 minutes and manipulate them five times during this period. Treat once every two days. A course consists of ten treatment sessions.

EAR ACUPUNCTURE WITH SEEDS
Points: Heart, Kidney and Stomach.
Technique: Attach *Wang Bu Liu Xing* (Semen Vaccariae Segetalis) seeds to the points with adhesive tape. Ask the patient to press the seeds for one minute several times a day. Change the seeds every five days.

NEEDLE EMBEDDING
Body points: LU-10 Yuji and KI-7 Fuliu.
Ear points: Heart, Kidney, Stomach, and Lung.
Technique: After routine sterilization, insert the intradermal needles into the points and attach them with adhesive tape. Ask the patient to press the points for three to five minutes three or four times a day. Keep the needles in place for one week, then repeat the procedure.

[xiv]M-HN-13 according to the system employed by the Shanghai College of Traditional Chinese Medicine.

UMBILICAL THERAPY

Grind *Wu Bei Zi* ‡ (Galla Rhois Chinensis) or *He Shou Wu* (Radix Polygoni Multiflori) to a fine powder and mix to a paste with warm boiled water. Apply the mixture to the umbilicus and cover with sterilized gauze. Remove the following morning.

Clinical notes

- Hyperhidrosis is generally treated from the interior by clearing Heat and draining Fire for Excess patterns, and augmenting Qi and constraining sweating for Deficiency patterns.
- For elderly people with hyperhidrosis lateralis due to disharmony of Qi and Blood causing Qi stagnation and Blood stasis, appropriate care should be given to prevent Wind-stroke.
- The prognosis for most cases is good if the primary disease can be treated promptly and correctly. However, cases with oily or pearly sweating or continuous heavy sweating or cases of hyperhidrosis with asthma and a sensation of fullness in the chest are more stubborn.

Advice for the patient

- Avoid spicy food and alcohol.
- Patients with profuse sweating due to emotional disturbances transforming into Fire should be advised to avoid stressful situations and to balance activity and rest.
- Patients with profuse sweating of the feet must wash the feet and change shoes and socks regularly to prevent secondary infection by tinea pedis (athlete's foot) or plantar warts (verrucae plantaris). If possible, wear shoes that let the air in.

Bromhidrosis
臭汗症

Bromhidrosis is hyperhidrosis with a foul smell, caused by bacterial decomposition of apocrine secretions.

In TCM, bromhidrosis is also known as *hu chou* (foxy smell).

Clinical manifestations

- Bromhidrosis is seen most commonly in the young, with women more affected than men.
- The disease mainly involves the axillae, the umbilicus, the genitals, and the toes.
- The foul smell is stronger in summer and may not be evident at all in winter.
- The smell is strongest during adolescence and fades or disappears as individuals get older.
- Sweat may stain clothing.

Differential diagnosis

Chromhidrosis

Rather than sending out a foul smell, this disease manifests only as the secretion of sweat colored as a result of biological activity. This sweat causes staining of the clothes with which it comes into contact.

Etiology and pathology

- Sweating with a foul smell emanating from the axillae due to the expulsion of turbid Qi is often hereditary.
- Excessive intake of spicy, fried, fatty, greasy, sweet, or rich foods or alcohol causes Damp-Heat to accumulate internally. If this happens in a person who wears too many clothes in summer and who washes infrequently, the movement of Body Fluids will be inhibited and there will be disharmony between Qi and Blood. Accumulated Damp-Heat will be transformed into turbid Qi, which steams and moves to the exterior, where it causes a foul stench.
- In the axillae, there are numerous apertures in the skin creases. Turbid Qi follows the sweat out of the pores, thus giving rise to a fetid smell.

Pattern identification and treatment

INTERNAL TREATMENT

INTERNAL ACCUMULATION OF FOUL TURBIDITY

There is usually a family history of this illness, which normally affects adolescents. The foul smell, which emanates from the axillae, breast areolae, umbilical area, groin, or genitals, is stronger in summer or during sweating. Where there are visible brown apertures in the axillae, the sweat is fetid and yellow, leaving yellow marks on clothing; in these cases, there may also be soft wax in the ear. Tongue and pulse are normal, since the Zang-Fu organs have not been affected.

Treatment principle
Aromatically repel foulness.

Prescription
WU XIANG WAN JIA JIAN
Five Fragrance Pill, with modifications

Huo Xiang (Herba Agastaches seu Pogostemi) 12g
Ding Xiang (Flos Caryophylli) 4.5g
*Mu Xiang** (Radix Aucklandiae Lappae) 4.5g
Xiang Fu (Rhizoma Cyperi Rotundi) 4.5g
Xiang Ru (Herba Elshotziae seu Moslae) 6g
Bai Zhi (Radix Angelicae Dahuricae) 10g
Dang Gui (Radix Angelicae Sinensis) 10g
Da Fu Pi (Pericarpium Arecae Catechu) 10g
Fu Ling (Sclerotium Poriae Cocos) 15g
Bi Xie (Rhizoma Dioscoreae Hypoglaucae seu Septemlobae) 5g
Chai Hu (Radix Bupleuri) 6g
Huang Qin (Radix Scutellariae Baicalensis) 6g

Explanation
• *Huo Xiang* (Herba Agastaches seu Pogostemi), *Ding Xiang* (Flos Caryophylli), *Mu Xiang** (Radix Aucklandiae Lappae), *Xiang Fu* (Rhizoma Cyperi Rotundi), *Xiang Ru* (Herba Elshotziae seu Moslae), and *Bai Zhi* (Radix Angelicae Dahuricae) aromatically repel foulness.
• *Dang Gui* (Radix Angelicae Sinensis), *Chai Hu* (Radix Bupleuri) and *Huang Qin* (Radix Scutellariae Baicalensis) harmonize the exterior and interior to clear internal Heat and dissipate external pathogenic factors.
• *Da Fu Pi* (Pericarpium Arecae Catechu), *Fu Ling* (Sclerotium Poriae Cocos) and *Bi Xie* (Rhizoma Dioscoreae Hypoglaucae seu Septemlobae) clear Heat and transform Dampness; turbidity will be cleared once Dampness is eliminated.

STEAMING OF DAMP-HEAT
This pattern does not involve a family history of the illness, but also tends to occur in summer. Profuse sweating, usually in the axillae, gives off a faint foul smell and stains clothing yellow. The smell may fade temporarily or disappear after washing. The tongue body is red with a yellow and slightly greasy coating; the pulse is slippery and rapid.

Treatment principle
Clear Heat, benefit the movement of Dampness and aromatically transform turbidity.

Prescription
GAN LU XIAO DU DAN JIA JIAN
Sweet Dew Special Pill for Dispersing Toxicity, with modifications

Yin Chen Hao (Herba Artemisiae Scopariae) 30g
Huo Xiang (Herba Agastaches seu Pogostemi) 12g
Lian Qiao (Fructus Forsythiae Suspensae) 12g
Hua Shi ‡ (Talcum) 12g, wrapped in *He Ye* (Folium Nelumbinis Nuciferae) for decoction
Shi Chang Pu (Rhizoma Acori Graminei) 6g
Chuan Bei Mu (Bulbus Fritillariae Cirrhosae) 6g
Tong Cao (Medulla Tetrapanacis Papyriferi) 6g
Pei Lan (Herba Eupatorii Fortunei) 10g
Gan Song (Rhizoma Nardostachydis) 10g

Explanation
• *Yin Chen Hao* (Herba Artemisiae Scopariae), *Hua Shi* ‡ (Talcum) and *Tong Cao* (Medulla Tetrapanacis Papyriferi) clear Heat and benefit the movement of Dampness.
• *Lian Qiao* (Fructus Forsythiae Suspensae) clears Heat from the Heart and relieves Toxicity.
• *Shi Chang Pu* (Rhizoma Acori Graminei) frees the orifices of the Heart.
• *Chuan Bei Mu* (Bulbus Fritillariae Cirrhosae) transforms Phlegm and dissipates lumps.
• *Huo Xiang* (Herba Agastaches seu Pogostemi), *Pei Lan* (Herba Eupatorii Fortunei) and *Gan Song* (Rhizoma Nardostachydis) aromatically transform turbidity.

EXTERNAL TREATMENT
• Grind *Ku Fan* ‡ (Alumen Praeparatum) 30g, *Hai Ge Ke* ‡ (Concha Meretricis seu Cyclinae) 15g and *Zhang Nao* (Camphora) 15g to a fine powder and apply to the affected area three times a day.
• Grind *Ding Xiang* (Flos Caryophylli) 30g and *Bing Pian** (Borneolum) 6g to a powder and apply to the affected area once a day for two weeks.
• When sweat on the hands and feet, axillae and scrotum gives off a foul smell, wash these areas three times a day with a warm decoction of *Ge Gen Shui Xi Ji* (Kudzu Vine Root Wash Preparation) or *Bai Zhi Shui Xi Ji* (White Angelica Root Wash Preparation), then apply *Fei Zi Fen* (Miliaria Powder), *Gu Yue Fen* (Ancient Moon Powder) or *Qu Shi San* (Powder for Dispelling Dampness).

ACUPUNCTURE

Selection of points on the affected channels
Points: LR-2 Xingjian and HT-9 Shaochong.
Technique: Apply the reducing method and retain the needles for 30 minutes after obtaining Qi; during this

period, manipulate the needles three to five times. Treat once a day. A course consists of ten treatment sessions.

Explanation

LR-2 Xingjian and HT-9 Shaochong quiet the Heart and Spirit, dredge the Liver and relieve Depression.

Empirical points

Main point: Yexia (located in the axilla, generally close to HT-1 Jiquan; gentle pressure indicates an obvious tender point. Care should be taken to avoid the blood vessels).

Auxiliary points: Tuiqian 4 (located on the lower quarter of the medial aspect of the anterior tibia, close to SP-6 Sanyinjiao) and Shoubei 1 (located on the central part of the dorsal muscles of the thumb, close to LI-4 Hegu).

Technique: Apply the reducing method and retain the needles for 30 minutes after obtaining Qi; during this period, manipulate the needles three to five times. Treat once a day. A course consists of ten treatment sessions.

MOXIBUSTION

Mix 10g of cornstarch with a little water. Shave the axillary hair and spread the starch liquid over the axilla. After six or seven days, some pinpoint black spots will appear; these are the central points of the apocrine ducts. Apply direct moxibustion to these spots with three to four rice grain-sized moxa cones. Treat once every two days. A course consists of five treatment sessions.

Clinical notes

Bromhidrosis is best treated externally with medications to constrain sweating and eliminate the foul smell. Internal treatment can repel foulness and turbidity to improve the overall effect of treatment. Although there is some response to treatment, it is difficult to treat the root cause.

Advice for the patient

- Cut down on or cut out strongly irritating food from the diet and give up smoking and alcohol.
- Wash frequently and try to keep potentially sweaty areas dry afterwards.
- Patients with foul-smelling, sweaty feet should wear shoes that let the air in.
- In most cases, the foul smell will diminish or disappear as the patient gets older.

Modern clinical experience

Ruan Shijun treated bromhidrosis with *Fang Ji Huang Qi Tang* (Stephania and Astragalus Decoction) plus *Gan Jiang* (Rhizoma Zingiberis Officinalis) 9g and *Da Zao* (Fructus Ziziphi Jujubae) 20g. *Cang Zhu* (Rhizoma Atractylodis) 10g, *Che Qian Cao* (Herba Plantaginis) 15g and *Che Qian Zi* (Semen Plantaginis) 15g were added for severe Dampness; *Fu Ling Pi* (Cortex Poriae Cocos) 10g and *Ze Xie* (Rhizoma Alismatis Orientalis) 15g for pronounced Spleen Deficiency; and *Yin Chen Hao* (Herba Artemisiae Scopariae) 20g and *Jiao Zhi Zi* (Fructus Gardeniae Jasminoidis, scorch-fried) 20g for accompanying obesity. Results were seen after two months to six and a half months. [30]

Chromhidrosis
色汗症

Chromhidrosis is the secretion of colored sweat stained by pigment-yielding bacteria. This sweat may appear as blue, green, red, purple, brown, or black, but is most commonly yellow, which is the condition described in this section.

Clinical manifestations

- Yellow sweat affects people of all ages.
- The condition mainly involves the axillae and scrotum.

- Yellow sweat may stain clothing.
- Accompanying symptoms in some cases include twitching of the muscles, generalized pain, irritability and restlessness, and difficulty in urination.

Etiology and pathology

- Where cases of Damp-Heat in the Spleen and Stomach accompanied by sweating are complicated by invasion of the body by water while taking a shower, wading through water or being caught in the rain, Water-Qi enters the interstices (*cou li*) via the sweat pores and Water-Cold is trapped in the flesh, impairing the diffusion of Wei Qi (Defensive Qi). Heat accumulated internally is trapped by Water-Cold; Damp and Heat obstruct each other and move to the skin where they steam out through the interstices (*cou li*) and combine with sweat. Since yellow is the color associated with the Spleen, the sweat appears yellow.

- Disharmony of the Ying and Wei levels due to Deficiency of the exterior, invasion of water and Dampness or steaming of Damp-Heat can all lead to yellow sweat.
- Damp-Heat pouring down in the Liver Channel can lead to excessive moisture in the scrotum, resulting in yellow sweat in that area.

Pattern identification and treatment

INTERNAL TREATMENT

STEAMING OF DAMP-HEAT
This pattern manifests as yellow sweat complicated by edema, with fever and thirst after sweating. The tongue coating is yellow and greasy; the pulse is deep and slow.

Treatment principle
Transform water and Dampness with warmth, consolidate the exterior and support Yang.

Prescription
HUANG QI SHAO YAO GUI ZHI KU JIU TANG JIA JIAN
Astragalus, Peony, Cinnamon Twig, and Vinegar Decoction, with modifications

Huang Qi (Radix Astragali seu Hedysari) 15g
Chao Bai Shao (Radix Paeoniae Lactiflorae, stir-fried) 10g
Gui Zhi (Ramulus Cinnamomi Cassiae) 10g
Yin Chen Hao (Herba Artemisiae Scopariae) 12g
Jiao Zhi Zi (Fructus Gardeniae Jasminoidis, scorch-fried) 12g
Che Qian Zi (Semen Plantaginis) 12g

Decoct in a mixture of vinegar and water in the proportions 1:6 and drink warm.

Explanation
- *Gui Zhi* (Ramulus Cinnamomi Cassiae) and *Yin Chen Hao* (Herba Artemisiae Scopariae) transform water and Dampness.
- *Huang Qi* (Radix Astragali seu Hedysari) and *Chao Bai Shao* (Radix Paeoniae Lactiflorae, stir-fried) consolidate the exterior and support Yang.
- *Jiao Zhi Zi* (Fructus Gardeniae Jasminoidis, scorch-

fried) clears Damp-Heat in the Triple Burner.
- *Che Qian Zi* (Semen Plantaginis), when used in combination with vinegar, frees Lin syndrome and promotes urination to drain Damp-Heat via urination.

DISHARMONY OF THE YING AND WEI LEVELS
This pattern manifests as yellow sweat complicated by generalized pain, twitching of the muscles, irritability and restlessness, cold legs, and difficulty in urination. The tongue coating is white; the pulse is deep.

Treatment principle
Augment Qi and move Yang, regulate and harmonize the Ying and Wei levels.

Prescription
GUI ZHI JIA HUANG QI TANG JIA JIAN
Cinnamon Twig Plus Astragalus Decoction, with modifications

Gui Zhi (Ramulus Cinnamomi Cassiae) 10g
Chao Bai Shao (Radix Paeoniae Lactiflorae, stir-fried) 10g
Huang Qi (Radix Astragali seu Hedysari) 12g
Fang Feng (Radix Ledebouriellae Divaricatae) 12g
Gan Cao (Radix Glycyrrhizae) 12g
Da Zao (Fructus Ziziphi Jujubae) 15g
Jie Geng (Radix Platycodi Grandiflori) 6g
Sang Bai Pi (Cortex Mori Albae Radicis) 6g
Duan Mu Li ‡ (Concha Ostreae Calcinata) 15g

Explanation
- *Huang Qi* (Radix Astragali seu Hedysari) and *Chao Bai Shao* (Radix Paeoniae Lactiflorae, stir-fried) consolidate the exterior and support Yang.
- *Gui Zhi* (Ramulus Cinnamomi Cassiae), *Fang Feng* (Radix Ledebouriellae Divaricatae), *Gan Cao* (Radix Glycyrrhizae), *Da Zao* (Fructus Ziziphi Jujubae), and *Jie Geng* (Radix Platycodi Grandiflori) regulate and harmonize the Ying and Wei levels.
- *Sang Bai Pi* (Cortex Mori Albae Radicis) diffuses the Lungs and clears Heat.
- *Duan Mu Li* ‡ (Concha Ostreae Calcinata) subdues Yang and constrains sweating.

DAMP-HEAT POURING DOWN
This pattern manifests as incessant sweating in the scrotum staining clothing yellow and is accompanied by itching, a smell of urine, and an unbearable sensation of burning heat when wearing thick or tight clothing. The tongue body is red with a thin, yellow and slightly greasy coating; the pulse is wiry and rapid.

Treatment principle
Clear Liver-Fire and dispel Damp-Heat.

Prescription

LONG DAN XIE GAN TANG JIA JIAN

Chinese Gentian Decoction for Draining the Liver, with modifications

Chao Long Dan Cao (Radix Gentianae Scabrae, stir-fried) 6g
Jiao Zhi Zi (Fructus Gardeniae Jasminoidis, scorch-fried) 6g
Chai Hu (Radix Bupleuri) 6g
Dang Gui (Radix Angelicae Sinensis) 6g
Ze Xie (Rhizoma Alismatis Orientalis) 12g
Chi Fu Ling (Sclerotium Poriae Cocos Rubrae) 12g
Chi Xiao Dou (Semen Phaseoli Calcarati) 12g
Ren Dong Teng (Caulis Lonicerae Japonicae) 12g
Qing Pi (Pericarpium Citri Reticulatae Viride) 4.5g
Xiao Hui Xiang (Fructus Foeniculi Vulgaris) 4.5g
Chao Du Zhong (Cortex Eucommiae Ulmoidis, stir-fried) 10g
She Chuang Zi (Fructus Cnidii Monnieri) 10g.

Explanation

- *Chao Long Dan Cao* (Radix Gentianae Scabrae, stir-fried), *Jiao Zhi Zi* (Fructus Gardeniae Jasminoidis, scorch-fried), *Chai Hu* (Radix Bupleuri), *Ze Xie* (Rhizoma Alismatis Orientalis), and *Chi Fu Ling* (Sclerotium Poriae Cocos Rubrae) clear Heat from the Liver and drain Fire.

- *Dang Gui* (Radix Angelicae Sinensis), *Chi Xiao Dou* (Semen Phaseoli Calcarati), *Ren Dong Teng* (Caulis Lonicerae Japonicae), and *Qing Pi* (Pericarpium Citri Reticulatae Viride) invigorate the Blood, free the network vessels and expel Damp-Heat.

- *Xiao Hui Xiang* (Fructus Foeniculi Vulgaris) warms Yang and dissipates Cold.

- *Chao Du Zhong* (Cortex Eucommiae Ulmoidis, stir-fried) and *She Chuang Zi* (Fructus Cnidii Monnieri) supplement the Kidneys and constrain sweating, kill parasites and alleviate itching.

EXTERNAL TREATMENT

For yellow sweat in the axillae or the scrotum, apply *Mu Fan Dan* (Oyster, Alum and Minium Powder) to the affected area once or twice a day.

Advice for the patient

- Cut down on spicy and fried foods, spring onions and garlic, and alcohol.

- When hot and sweaty, wash or shower with warm rather than cold water.

Miliaria rubra (prickly heat)
痱子

Miliaria rubra develops as a result of exposure to hot and humid weather conditions (such as those found in the tropics), which cause profuse perspiration. Occlusion of the intradermal part of the sweat gland ducts leads to blockage of the ducts; retention of sweat may cause these ducts to rupture. As a consequence, there is superficial inflammatory reaction centered on the sweat glands.

In TCM, miliaria rubra is also known as *han zhen* (sweat papules).

Clinical manifestations

- Miliaria rubra mostly occurs during scorching-hot summer weather and is more likely to affect children or obese individuals.

- It mainly involves areas covered by clothing, or those parts of the body which are prone to sweating; it does not affect the palms or soles.

- Lesions manifest as papules or small, thin-walled, superficial pinpoint vesicles, surrounded by an erythematous halo. They are slightly shiny and break easily when rubbed. Thin, fine scaling is noted after the vesicles dry up. Lesions may also be capped by pinpoint sterile pustules.

- Lesions in patients with severe or recurrent miliaria rubra manifest as red papules 1-3 mm in size that penetrate deeper layers of tissue.

- Patients experience a slight burning sensation and a prickly itchy feeling.

- If lesions are extensive, they may lead to tropical anhidrotic asthenia or heat exhaustion with accompanying systemic symptoms such as lassitude, poor appetite, fatigue and somnolence, dizziness, and headache.

Differential diagnosis

Miliaria alba

This condition is often seen in patients with Warm-Damp diseases. Fever and sweating cause transparent vesicles to appear white rather than red. Other symptoms are similar to miliaria rubra.

Drug eruption

Patients have a history of taking certain medications. There is often a sudden onset of morbilliform (measles-like) or scarlatiniform (scarlet fever-like) rashes unrelated to seasonal factors.

Etiology and pathology

- In summer, when the weather is hot, pathogenic Summerheat can invade the exterior to block the *cou li* (interstices) and obstruct the sweat pores, resulting in sweat being unable to diffuse and disperse and eventually resulting in miliaria rubra.
- When the weather is hot, the body is hot and sweaty. Taking a cold bath or shower or getting caught in cold rain will result in closure of the sweat pores and the body being steeped in hot sweat.
- Wearing thick clothing when working in a high-temperature environment will result in the body sweating. Damp and Heat mix together, leading to Heat in the Lungs and Damp in the Spleen and the appearance of miliaria rubra.

Pattern identification and treatment

INTERNAL TREATMENT

SUMMERHEAT-DAMP INVADING THE EXTERIOR

The condition manifests as densely distributed miliaria rubra papules or papulovesicles with prickly itching or pain. The urine is reddish-yellow. The tongue body is red with a scant coating; the pulse is floating and rapid.

Treatment principle

Clear Summerheat and drain Dampness, relieve Toxicity and alleviate itching.

Prescription

QING SHU TANG JIA JIAN

Decoction for Clearing Summerheat, with modifications

Qing Hao (Herba Artemisiae Chinghao) 15g
Xian Huo Xiang (Herba Agastaches seu Pogostemi Recens) 15g
Xian Pei Lan (Herba Eupatorii Fortunei Recens) 15g
Liu Yi San (Six-To-One Powder) 15g, wrapped in *He Ye* (Folium Nelumbinis Nuciferae)
Lü Dou Yi (Testa Phaseoli Radiati) 12g
Jin Yin Hua (Flos Lonicerae) 12g
Chi Fu Ling (Sclerotium Poriae Cocos Rubrae) 10g

Nan Sha Shen (Radix Adenophorae) 10g
Deng Xin Cao (Medulla Junci Effusi) 9g
Xi Gua Pi (Epicarpium Citrulli Vulgaris) 30g
Dong Gua Pi (Epicarpium Benincasae Hispidae) 30g

Explanation

- *Xian Huo Xiang* (Herba Agastaches seu Pogostemi Recens), *Xian Pei Lan* (Herba Eupatorii Fortunei Recens) and *Qing Hao* (Herba Artemisiae Chinghao) clear Summerheat and aromatically transform turbidity to flush out Dampness.
- *Liu Yi San* (Six-To-One Powder), *Chi Fu Ling* (Sclerotium Poriae Cocos Rubrae) and *Deng Xin Cao* (Medulla Junci Effusi) clear Heat by guiding it out through the urine.
- *Nan Sha Shen* (Radix Adenophorae), *Lü Dou Yi* (Testa Phaseoli Radiati), *Jin Yin Hua* (Flos Lonicerae), *Xi Gua Pi* (Epicarpium Citrulli Vulgaris), and *Dong Gua Pi* (Epicarpium Benincasae Hispidae) relieve Toxicity and alleviate itching.

PATENT HERBAL MEDICINES

Drink *Jin Yin Hua Lu* (Honeysuckle Flower Distillate) or *Di Gu Pi Lu* (Wolfberry Root Bark Distillate) as a tea.

EXTERNAL TREATMENT

- For lesions mainly manifesting as red papules and papulovesicles, use *San Huang Xi Ji* (Three Yellows Wash Preparation) or *Lu Hu Shui Xi Ji* (Calamine and Giant Knotweed Wash Preparation) as a wet compress or wash. External application to the affected area of *Qing Liang Fen* (Cool Clearing Powder), *Fei Zi Fen* (Miliaria Powder) or *Qing Liang Fei Zi Fen* (Cool Clearing Miliaria Powder) is also effective.
- If the lesions are toxic and purulent, mix *Yu Lu San* (Jade Dew Powder) or *Qing Dai San* (Indigo Powder) into a paste with vegetable oil and apply to the affected area once or twice a day.

ACUPUNCTURE

Points: LI-11 Quchi, LI-4 Hegu and SP-10 Xuehai.
Technique: Apply the reducing method and retain the needles for 15 minutes. Treat once a day. A course consists of seven treatment sessions.

Explanation

LI-11 Quchi, LI-4 Hegu and SP-10 Xuehai are used together to dredge Wind and alleviate itching, flush out Summerheat and eliminate miliaria.

EAR ACUPUNCTURE

Points: Lung, Adrenal Gland, Occiput, Ear-Shenmen, and Heart.

Technique: Retain the needles in the points for 15 minutes. Treat once a day. A course consists of seven treatment sessions.

EAR PRESSURE
Points: Heart, Lung, Heat Boils (located in the upper portion of the central scaphoid fossa), and Ear-Shenmen.
Technique: Attach *Wang Bu Liu Xing* (Semen Vaccariae Segetalis) seeds to the points with adhesive tape. The seeds should be changed every other day. A course consists of five treatment sessions. Patients should be reminded to stimulate each seed for one minute, three to five times a day.

Clinical notes

- Internal treatment for miliaria rubra should follow the principles of clearing Summerheat and draining Dampness, relieving Toxicity and alleviating itching; external treatment should focus on releasing the flesh with coolness and acridity.
- If Toxicity is present, add materia medica for transforming Dampness and relieving Toxicity.

Advice for the patient

- Wash frequently with lukewarm water; keep the skin clean and dry.
- Wear loose clothing; change underwear regularly if miliaria is present in those areas.
- Avoid scratching the skin.

- Avoid working in sunshine in scorching heat. Have cooling and refreshing drinks such as *Suan Mei Tang* (Sweet-Sour Plum Juice).

Literature excerpts

In *Yi Xue Ru Men* [Elementary Medicine], it says: "Miliaria rubra occurs as a result of Dampness caused by sweating. In mild cases, the rash spreads densely over the skin with lesions resembling millet seeds. Treat with an external wash using a decoction prepared with *Qing Hao* (Herba Artemisiae Chinghao) or *Zao Ye* (Folium Ziziphi Jujubae). In severe cases with heat leading to profuse sweating and a dense distribution of sores, soak a piece of soft cloth in the decoction before application. If sores form because lesions rupture after rubbing, prepare a decoction with *Huang Bai* (Cortex Phellodendri) 15g, *Zao Ye* (Folium Ziziphi Jujubae) 15g and *Bing Pian* (Borneolum) 3g and use as an external wash."

According to *Wai Ke Zheng Zong* [An Orthodox Manual of External Diseases]: "Miliaria rubra spreads densely over the skin with millet seed-sized spots capped with points like prickles. Patients experience pain, itching and a generalized prickling sensation. The condition develops because of blockage of the sweat pores due to an invasion of Wind when there is Heat in the body. Treat internally with *Xiao Feng San* (Powder for Dispersing Wind) and externally with a wash using *Ku Shen Tang* (Flavescent Sophora Root Decoction). For severe conditions with a particularly dense distribution of sores, *E Huang San* (Light Yellow Powder) can be applied externally with a silk cloth."

Hidradenitis suppurativa
化脓性汗腺炎

Hidradenitis suppurativa is a chronic suppurative inflammatory condition which may result either from formation of a keratin plug in the skin follicles or from occlusion of apocrine sweat ducts. Secretions trapped in the glands become infected with bacteria; infection extends into the surrounding tissues, causing subcutaneous induration, inflammation, abscess formation, and the development of discharging fistulae.

In TCM, this condition is also known as *ye yong* (armpit *yong* abscess).

Clinical manifestations

- Hidradenitis suppurativa is more common in young or middle-aged women, and is worse in the obese.
- Lesions usually occur in the axillae, the groin, the area under the female breast, and the anogenital region.
- The lesion starts with a tender red subcutaneous nodule, which gradually enlarges; further lesions develop. The overlying skin finally ruptures and a small amount of

purulent fluid is discharged. Fistulae may form; if the disease involves the perineum, anal fistulae may occur.

- The condition is generally persistent and recurrent, and frequently results in induration and scarring at the sites of lesions.
- Patients experience local pain.
- On occasions, there may be systemic symptoms such as fever.

Differential diagnosis

Acne
Acne is common among adolescents and young adults; in some women, it may be exacerbated in the premenstrual phase. Eruptions generally appear on the face, especially the forehead, cheeks and chin, but may also involve the chest and back. Lesions may manifest as open comedones (blackheads) or closed comedones (whiteheads), or as inflammatory papules and pustules. The features of hidradenitis suppurativa do not include comedones.

Furuncles
Furuncles (boils) can affect any hair-bearing site and are common on the neck as well as the axillae and groin. Lesions manifest initially as papules, later growing bigger and firmer and becoming red. In two to three days, an abscess will form with a central necrotic core. It crusts and heals within one to two weeks.

Carbuncles
Where several furuncles join together to form a carbuncle, a swollen, painful, suppurating area will be formed with discharge of pus from different points. Common sites for carbuncles include the back of the neck, the upper and lower back, the buttocks, and the lateral thighs.

Etiology and pathology

- Qi and Blood stagnation in the Liver and Spleen channels due to emotional factors such as anxiety, worry and anger lead to obstruction in the axillae, resulting in the formation of hard nodules.
- If sores or ulcers on the arms become infected, Toxins and pathogenic factors can flow along the channels to the axillae resulting in the appearance of nodules.

Pattern identification and treatment

INTERNAL TREATMENT

QI STAGNATION IN THE LIVER AND SPLEEN CHANNELS
Hard nodules of various sizes grow in quick succession

in the axillae and external genitals in cord-like bands or patches. The white or pale red lesions are tender on pressure. The tongue body is dark red with a thin white coating; the pulse is wiry and rough.

Treatment principle
Soothe the Liver and regulate the Spleen, transform Phlegm and dissipate nodules.

Prescription
XIANG BEI YANG RONG TANG JIA JIAN
Cyperus and Fritillaria Decoction for Nourishing Ying Qi, with modifications

Zhi Xiang Fu (Rhizoma Cyperi Rotundi, processed) 10g
Zhe Bei Mu (Bulbus Fritillariae Thunbergii) 10g
Chi Shao (Radix Paeoniae Rubra) 10g
Bai Shao (Radix Paeoniae Lactiflorae) 10g
Jiang Can‡ (Bombyx Batryticatus) 10g
Tian Hua Fen (Radix Trichosanthis) 10g
Qing Pi (Pericarpium Citri Reticulatae Viride) 10g
Chen Pi (Pericarpium Citri Reticulatae) 10g
Dang Shen (Radix Codonopsitis Pilosulae) 6g
Fu Ling (Sclerotium Poriae Cocos) 6g
Jie Geng (Radix Platycodi Grandiflori) 6g
Chuan Xiong (Rhizoma Ligustici Chuanxiong) 6g
Shu Di Huang (Radix Rehmanniae Glutinosae Conquita) 10g
Bai Zhu (Rhizoma Atractylodis Macrocephalae) 10g
Dang Gui (Radix Angelicae Sinensis) 10g
Xia Ku Cao (Spica Prunellae Vulgaris) 15g
Ju He (Semen Citri Reticulatae) 15g

Explanation
- This prescription is recommended for the initial stage of the condition, as it will help to disperse swelling and alleviate pain.
- *Zhi Xiang Fu* (Rhizoma Cyperi Rotundi, processed), *Qing Pi* (Pericarpium Citri Reticulatae Viride), *Chen Pi* (Pericarpium Citri Reticulatae), *Ju He* (Semen Citri Reticulatae), and *Chuan Xiong* (Rhizoma Ligustici Chuanxiong) soothe the Liver and regulate Qi.
- *Zhe Bei Mu* (Bulbus Fritillariae Thunbergii), *Jiang Can*‡ (Bombyx Batryticatus), *Xia Ku Cao* (Spica Prunellae Vulgaris), *Jie Geng* (Radix Platycodi Grandiflori), and *Fu Ling* (Sclerotium Poriae Cocos) transform Phlegm and dissipate nodules.
- *Tian Hua Fen* (Radix Trichosanthis) eliminates swelling and expels pus.
- *Chi Shao* (Radix Paeoniae Rubra) and *Bai Shao* (Radix Paeoniae Lactiflorae) act in combination to nourish and invigorate the Blood.
- *Dang Shen* (Radix Codonopsitis Pilosulae), *Shu Di Huang* (Radix Rehmanniae Glutinosae Conquita), *Bai Zhu* (Rhizoma Atractylodis Macrocephalae), and *Dang Gui* (Radix Angelicae Sinensis) support the

Spleen and emolliate the Liver and are often used at the initial stage of this condition to disperse swelling and alleviate pain.

FORMATION OF PUS DUE TO INFECTION BY TOXINS

The hard nodules enlarge and feel fluctuant on pressure; the local skin is red and inflamed. Accompanying symptoms and signs include high fever or low-grade fever, and severe pain, which worsens at night since Vital Qi Deficiency impairs the drawing out of Toxins. The tongue body is red with a scant coating. The pulse is wiry and rapid.

Treatment principle

Draw out pathogenic factors from the interior and expel pus, regulate Qi and dissipate nodules.

Prescription
TUO LI PAI NONG TANG JIA JIAN

Decoction for Drawing Out Pathogenic Factors from the Interior and Expelling Pus, with modifications

Dang Gui (Radix Angelicae Sinensis) 15g
Huang Qi (Radix Astragali seu Hedysari) 30g
Fu Ling (Sclerotium Poriae Cocos) 12g
Zhe Bei Mu (Bulbus Fritillariae Thunbergii) 12g
Bai Zhu (Rhizoma Atractylodis Macrocephalae) 10g
Lian Qiao (Fructus Forsythiae Suspensae) 10g
Jin Yin Hua (Flos Lonicerae) 10g
Chen Pi (Pericarpium Citri Reticulatae) 10g
Bai Zhi (Radix Angelicae Dahuricae) 10g
Chuan Xiong (Rhizoma Ligustici Chuanxiong) 10g
Zi Hua Di Ding (Herba Violae Yedoensitis) 10g

Explanation

- *Dang Gui* (Radix Angelicae Sinensis), *Bai Zhu* (Rhizoma Atractylodis Macrocephalae), *Huang Qi* (Radix Astragali seu Hedysari), *Fu Ling* (Sclerotium Poriae Cocos), and *Chen Pi* (Pericarpium Citri Reticulatae) augment Qi and draw out Toxins.
- *Chuan Xiong* (Rhizoma Ligustici Chuanxiong), *Zhe Bei Mu* (Bulbus Fritillariae Thunbergii), *Lian Qiao* (Fructus Forsythiae Suspensae), and *Bai Zhi* (Radix Angelicae Dahuricae) draw out pathogenic factors from the interior and expel pus.
- *Jin Yin Hua* (Flos Lonicerae) and *Zi Hua Di Ding* (Herba Violae Yedoensitis) clear Heat and relieve Toxicity.

RESIDUAL PUS AND TOXINS

The lesion has ruptured and pus has been discharged, but the sinus tract remains unhealed. The peripheral area of the lesion still feels hard. Patients may also present with other symptoms and signs such as shortness of breath, lassitude and poor appetite. The tongue body is pale red with a thin white coating. The pulse is thready and weak.

Treatment principle

Support Vital Qi (Zheng Qi) and consolidate the Root, expel pus and generate flesh.

Prescription
BA ZHEN SAN JIA JIAN

Eight Treasure Powder, with modifications

Dang Gui (Radix Angelicae Sinensis) 10g
Chao Bai Shao (Radix Paeoniae Lactiflorae, stir-fried) 10g
Gan Di Huang (Radix Rehmanniae Glutinosae Exsiccata) 10g
Huang Qi (Radix Astragali seu Hedysari) 12g
Dang Shen (Radix Codonopsitis Pilosulae) 12g
Fu Ling (Sclerotium Poriae Cocos) 12g
Tu Chao Bai Zhu (Rhizoma Atractylodis Macrocephalae, stir-fried with earth) 12g
Zhi Xiang Fu (Rhizoma Cyperi Rotundi, processed) 15g
Zhe Bei Mu (Bulbus Fritillariae Thunbergii) 15g
Ju He (Semen Citri Reticulatae) 15g
Jiang Can ‡ (Bombyx Batryticatus) 10g

Explanation

- *Dang Shen* (Radix Codonopsitis Pilosulae), *Huang Qi* (Radix Astragali seu Hedysari) and *Gan Di Huang* (Radix Rehmanniae Glutinosae Exsiccata) augment Qi, supplement the Blood, support Vital Qi (Zheng Qi) and expel Toxins to generate flesh.
- *Tu Chao Bai Zhu* (Rhizoma Atractylodis Macrocephalae, stir-fried with earth) and *Fu Ling* (Sclerotium Poriae Cocos) regulate the Spleen and benefit the movement of Dampness to help *Dang Shen* (Radix Codonopsitis Pilosulae) augment Qi and supplement the Spleen.
- *Dang Gui* (Radix Angelicae Sinensis) and *Chao Bai Shao* (Radix Paeoniae Lactiflorae, stir-fried) nourish the Blood and harmonize Ying Qi (Nutritive Qi) to help *Gan Di Huang* (Radix Rehmanniae Glutinosae Exsiccata) supplement and enrich the Blood.
- *Xiang Fu* (Rhizoma Cyperi Rotundi), *Zhe Bei Mu* (Bulbus Fritillariae Thunbergii), *Ju He* (Semen Citri Reticulatae), and *Jiang Can* ‡ (Bombyx Batryticatus) transform Phlegm and dissipate nodules to eliminate the remaining hardness.

General modifications

1. For ruptured lesions that do not heal, add *Bai Lian* (Radix Ampelopsis Japonicae).
2. For persistent hardness around the lesions after rupture, take *Nei Xiao Luo Li Wan* (Scrofula Internal Dispersion Pill) or *San Jie Ling* (Efficacious Remedy for Dissipating Nodules) with the decoction.

EXTERNAL TREATMENT

Before rupture of lesions

- Mash *Chong He Gao* (Harmonious Flow Paste) with a handful of *Cong Bai* (Bulbus Allii Fistulosi) and apply directly to the lesions once a day.
- Alternatively, mix *Zi Se Xiao Zhong Fen* (Purple Powder for Dispersing Swelling) with vinegar into a thick paste. Apply directly to the affected area two or three times a day.

After rupture of lesions

- If the area around the nodules remains hard after rupture, mix *Ding Gui San* (Clove and Cinnamon Powder) with *Xia Ku Cao Gao* (Prunella Paste) for external application. Change the dressing once every three to five days.
- Alternatively, apply *Tie Gu San Gao* (Iron Hoop Powder Paste) directly to the affected area two or three times per day until the hardness disappears.

Clinical notes

- If the lesions are located in the axillae, treatment at the initial stage should follow the principle of regulating Qi and transforming Phlegm, invigorating the Blood and dissipating nodules. This type of management will help the lesions disappear spontaneously before the formation of pus or ulceration and the period of treatment required will be shorter. Early treatment is therefore of great importance.
- External application of *Chong He Gao* (Harmonious Flow Paste) is very effective in helping promotion of internal absorption and dispersal of the lesions.
- If a hard nodule remains after the lesions heal, dissolve 15g of *Xiao Bai Du Gao* (Minor Toxicity-Vanquishing Syrup) in warm boiled water twice a day and drink.
- Early management of the lesion will help it disappear spontaneously; healing will take longer once pus appears. Even if hard nodules remain non-transformed locally after the lesions heal, treatment should continue with materia medica for transforming Phlegm and dissipating nodules to bring about the complete disappearance of the hard nodules and prevent recurrence of the condition.

Advice for the patient

- Pay attention to hygiene of the affected areas.
- Wear cotton underwear and loose-fitting clothes to avoid clothing sticking to the skin.
- Do not squeeze the nodule, as this can spread the toxins.

Literature excerpt

According to *Wai Ke Zheng Zong* [An Orthodox Manual of External Diseases], "*Ye yong* (armpit *yong* abscess) grows in the armpits without any change in skin color; it is characterized by a diffuse swelling without a head, accompanied by persistent pain. Subsequent symptoms include chills and fever. The abscess develops because of Blood stagnation in the Liver channel and Qi congealing in the Spleen channel. The lesion is difficult to disperse and pus will collect. *Chai Hu Qing Gan Tang* (Bupleurum Decoction for Clearing the Liver) is recommended if the lesion has not ruptured. If rupture has already taken place, use *Shi Quan Da Bu Tang* (Perfect Major Supplementation Decoction), modified by removing *Rou Gui* (Cortex Cinnamomi Cassiae) and adding *Xiang Fu* (Rhizoma Cyperi Rotundi) and *Chen Pi* (Pericarpium Citri Reticulatae). Incise the lesion if the condition is acute. Use warming and supplementing medications in the initial and late stages; cold or cool medications are contraindicated."

References

1. Zhang Zhili, *Zhang Zhi Li Pi Fu Bing Lin Chuang Jing Yan Ji Yao* [A Collection of Zhang Zhili's Clinical Experiences in the Treatment of Skin Diseases] (Beijing: China Medical Science and Technology Publishing House, 2001), 253.
2. An Jiafeng and Zhang Fan, *Zhang Zhi Li Pi Fu Bing Yi An Xuan Cui* [A Collection of Zhang Zhili's Skin Disease Cases] (Beijing: People's Medical Publishing House, 1994), 222.
3. Zhang Zhili, *Zhang Zhi Li Pi Fu Bing Lin Chuang Jing Yan Ji Yao*, 254.
4. Li Zheng, *Bian Zheng Fen Xing Zhi Liao Xun Chang Xing Cuo Chuang 136 Li Liao Xiao Guan Cha* [Clinical Observation of the Effectiveness of Pattern Identification in the Treatment of 136 Cases of Acne Vulgaris], *Zhong Guo Pi Fu Xing Bing Xue Za Zhi* [Chinese Journal of Dermatology and Venereology] 11, 5 (1997): 294.
5. Yu Ling, *Zhong Yi Yao Bian Zheng Zhi Liao Cuo Chuang 38 Li* [Pattern Identification in the Treatment of 38 Cases of Acne with Traditional Chinese Medicine and Materia Medica], *Yun Nan Zhong Yi Zhong Yao Za Zhi* [Yunnan Journal of Traditional Chinese Medicine and Materia Medica] 19, 5 (1998): 15-16.
6. Zha Xiuming, *Cuo Chuang 70 Li De Zhong Bian Zheng Zhi Liao* [Pattern Identification in the Treatment of 70 Cases of Acne], *Bei Jing Zhong Yi* [Beijing Journal of Traditional

Chinese Medicine] 4 (1999): 54.

7. Sun Zhenhe, *Huo Xue Qing Fei Fa Zhi Liao Cuo Chuang 45 Li* [Treatment of 45 Cases of Acne by Invigorating the Blood and Clearing Heat from the Lungs], *Jiang Su Zhong Yi* [Jiangsu Journal of Traditional Chinese Medicine] 18, 5 (1997): 27.

8. Ou Zuhui, *Zhong Yi Bian Zheng Shi Zhi Jia An Chuang Jing Tu Mo Ji Wai Yong Zhi Liao Cuo Chuang 89 Li Liao Xiao Guan Cha* [Clinical Observation of TCM Pattern Identification Plus External Application of *An Chuang Jing Tu Mo Ji* (Mask Preparation for Cleansing Acne) in the Treatment of 89 Cases of Acne], *Zhong Guo Pi Fu Xing Bing Xue Za Zhi* [Chinese Journal of Dermatology and Venereology] 11, 3 (1997): 171.

9. Guo Meihua, *Qing Chu Fei Wei Shi Re Fa Zhi Liao Xun Chang Xing Cuo Chuang 32 Li* [Treatment of 32 Cases of Acne Vulgaris with the Method of Clearing Damp-Heat from the Lungs and Stomach], *Jiang Su Zhong Yi* [Jiangsu Journal of Traditional Chinese Medicine] 18, 11 (1997): 24.

10. Li Zhishun, *Qing Re Zao Shi Fa Zhi Liao Cuo Chuang 50 Li* [Treatment of 50 Cases of Acne with the Method of Clearing Heat and Drying Dampness], *Shan Xi Zhong Yi* [Shanxi Journal of Traditional Chinese Medicine] 12, 6 (1996): 26.

11. Zhang Peisong, *Qing Gan Da Yu Tang Zhi Liao Fu Nü Mian Bu Cuo Chuang 30 Li* [Treatment of 30 Cases of Facial Acne in Women with *Qing Gan Da Yu Tang* (Decoction for Clearing Heat from the Liver and Driving Out Depression)], *Xin Zhong Yi* [New Journal of Traditional Chinese Medicine] 30, 3 (1998): 45.

12. Liu Chunling, *Zi Ni Ke Cuo Tang Zhi Liao Cuo Chuang 56 Li* [Treatment of 56 Cases of Acne with the Empirical Prescription *Ke Cuo Tang* (Overcoming Acne Decoction)], *Zhong Guo Pi Fu Xing Bing Xue Za Zhi* [Chinese Journal of Dermatology and Venereology] 12, 5 (1998): 308.

13. Xu Jinxiu, *Si Wu Liang Xue Qing Fei Yin Zhi Liao Mian Bu Xun Chang Cuo Chuang* [Treatment of Facial Acne Vulgaris with *Si Wu Liang Xue Qing Fei Yin* (Four Agents Beverage for Cooling the Blood and Clearing Heat from the Lungs)], *Shan Dong Zhong Yi Za Zhi* [Shandong Journal of Traditional Chinese Medicine] 17, 8 (1998): 353.

14. Gao Huailan, *Nei Fu Wai Yong Zhong Yao Zhi Liao Xun Chang Xing Cuo Chuang 80 Li* [Treatment of 80 Cases of Acne Vulgaris with Chinese Materia Medica for Internal and External Usage], *Beng Bu Yi Xue Yuan Xue Bao* [Journal of Bengbu Medical College] 23, 6 (1998): 439.

15. Wu Shengli, *Xiao Cuo Tang Zhi Liao Cuo Chuang 100 Li Lin Chuang Guan Cha* [Clinical Observation of the Treatment of 100 Cases of Acne with *Xiao Cuo Tang* (Dispersing Acne Decoction)], *Xin Jiang Zhong Yi Yao* [Xinjiang Journal of Traditional Chinese Medicine and Materia Medica] 17, 3 (1997): 21-22.

16. Huang Heqing, *Ku Shen Shou Wu He Ji Wai Cha Zhi Liao Mian Bu Cuo Chuang 34 Li* [Treatment of 34 Cases of Facial Acne with External Application of *Ku Shen Shou Wu He Ji* (Flavescent Sophora Root and Fleeceflower Mixture)], *Zhong Yi Wai Zhi Za Zhi* [Journal of Traditional Chinese Medicine External Treatments] 6, 2 (1997): 27.

17. Li Hongqin, *Zhen Ci Zhi Liao Xun Chang Xing Cuo Chuang 42 Li* [Acupuncture Treatment of 42 Cases of Acne Vul-

garis], *Zhong Guo Zhen Jiu* [Chinese Journal of Acupuncture and Moxibustion] 18, 3 (1998): 166.

18. Yan Jinfang, *Zhen Ci Zhi Liao Xun Chang Cuo Chuang 36 Li* [Acupuncture Treatment of 36 Cases of Acne Vulgaris], *Zhong Guo Zhen Jiu* [Chinese Journal of Acupuncture and Moxibustion] 17, 3 (1997): 185.

19. Yang Heikun, *Er Zhen Zhi Liao Xun Chang Cuo Chuang 30 Li* [Treatment of 30 Cases of Acne Vulgaris with Ear Acupuncture], *Jiang Su Zhong Yi* [Jiangsu Journal of Traditional Chinese Medicine] 20, 7 (1999): 41.

20. Li Yang, *Er Xue Tian Ya Yao Zi Fa Zhi Liao Fen Ci* [Treatment of Acne with Ear Acupressure], *Xin Jiang Zhong Yi Yao* [Xinjiang Journal of Traditional Chinese Medicine and Materia Medica] 4 (1993): 20.

21. Deng Weimin, *An Yue Jing Zhou Qi Bian Zheng Yong Yao Zhi Liao Mian Bu Cuo Chuang 78 Li* [Treatment of 78 Cases of Facial Acne Based on Pattern Identification According to the Menstrual Cycle], *Zhe Jiang Zhong Yi Za Zhi* [Zhejiang Journal of Traditional Chinese Medicine] 33, 10 (1998): 454.

22. Lin Shanru, *Tiao Jing Zhi Liao Mian Bu Cuo Chuang 30 Li Lin Chuang Guan Cha* [Clinical Observation of the Treatment of 30 Cases of Facial Acne by Regulating Menstruation], *Shi Yong Zhong Xi Yi Jie He Za Zhi* [Practical Journal of Integrated TCM and Western Medicine] 11, 1 (1998): 84.

23. Zhu Tao, *Zhou Qi Zhen Ci Fa Zhi Liao Nü Xing Cuo Chuang 85 Li* [Acupuncture Treatment Based on the Menstrual Cycle for 85 Cases of Acne in Women], *Zhong Yuan Yi Kan* [Central Plains Medical Publications] 25, 2 (1998): 48.

24. An Jiafeng and Zhang Fan, *Zhang Zhi Li Pi Fu Bing Yi An Xuan Cui*, 224.

25. Zeng Zhaoxun, *Qing Zhen Tang Jia Wei Zhi Liao Jiu Zha Bi 80 Li* [Treatment of 80 Cases of Rosacea with Augmented *Qing Zhen Tang* (Cimicifuga and Atractylodes Decoction)], *Zhong Guo Yi Xue Mei Xue Mei Rong Za Zhi* [Chinese Journal of Medical Aesthetics and Cosmetology] 4, 3 (1995): 154.

26. Chen Weiyu, *Zhen Ci Zhi Liao Jiu Zha Bi 28 Li* [Acupuncture Treatment of 28 Cases of Rosacea], *Zhong Guo Zhen Jiu* [Chinese Journal of Acupuncture and Moxibustion] 18, 9 (1998): 534.

27. Cheng Zhen, *Zhong Xi Yi Jie He Zhi Liao Jiu Zha Bi De Liao Xiao Guan Cha* [Clinical Observation of the Treatment of Rosacea with a Combination of TCM and Western Medicine], *Zhong Guo Mei Rong Yi Xue* [Chinese Journal of Cosmetology] 8, 3 (1999): 164-165.

28. Cheng Xiaochun, *Da Chai Hu Tang Jia Jian Zhi Liao Pi Zhi Yi Chu Zheng 40 Li* [Treatment of 40 Cases of Seborrhea with Modified *Da Chai Hu Tang* (Major Bupleurum Decoction)], *Si Chuan Zhong Yi* [Sichuan Journal of Traditional Chinese Medicine] 15, 11 (1997): 49.

29. Bao Xueyan, *Zhong Yi Tang Zhi Liao Bai Xie Feng Jing Yan* [Zhong Yitang's Experiences in the Treatment of Seborrhea], *Zhe Jiang Zhong Yi Za Zhi* [Zhejiang Journal of Traditional Chinese Medicine] 28, 12 (1993): 535.

30. Wei Juxian, *Zhong Yi Ming Fang Ying Yong Jin Zhan: Ruan Shi Jun* [Advanced Applications of Famous TCM Formulae: Ruan Shijun] (Beijing: China Science and Technology Publishing House, 1999), 475.

Erythema and blood vessel disorders

This chapter discusses two categories of disorders affecting the cutaneous blood vessels – erythema and vascular diseases.

ERYTHEMA

The arteries, veins and capillaries of the skin are known as cutaneous blood vessels. Erythema is redness of the skin caused by dilatation of the cutaneous blood vessels and hyperemia in the local skin area; it is present in all inflammatory skin conditions. It may be localized, as for example with a fixed drug eruption, liver disease or rheumatoid arthritis; or it may be generalized, as in other types of drug eruption, bacterial or viral infections, connective tissue diseases, or underlying malignancy. Reactive erythemas such as erythema multiforme and erythema nodosum are characterized by inflammation around the blood vessels as a reaction to infection, drugs or systemic diseases.

According to TCM, there are two types of erythema – Yang erythema and Yin erythema – and five main causes of this type of lesion. This explanation applies to all the various skin disorders with erythema as a feature.

Yang-type erythema

- Erythema due to Blood-Heat and Wind-Dryness is caused by irritability, anxiety or other emotional problems, dietary irregularities, and external pathogenic Wind and Dryness-Heat settling in the skin and flesh. The combination of internal and external pathogenic factors results in Heat congesting in the Blood vessels to lead to erythema.

- External contraction of Wind and Heat pathogenic factors complicating Blood-Heat and internal accumulation of Dampness causes disharmony of the Ying and Wei levels leading to erythema.

- Dietary irregularities damage the Spleen and Stomach, leading to accumulation of Dampness, which subsequently transforms into Heat. Heat stagnates in the Blood vessels and obstructs the channels and network vessels resulting in erythema due to Qi stagnation and Blood stasis.

Yin-type erythema

- Dietary irregularities, disharmony of Cold and Warmth, irritability and excessive thought and pre-occupation, or improper nourishment after an illness damage Spleen Qi, meaning that it is no longer able to control and contain the Blood, which therefore fails to return to the channels and spills out to form erythema.

- Erythema due to effulgent Yin Deficiency-Fire is caused by constitutional insufficiency or Fire due to damage to the five emotions. Fire consumes and scorches Yin-Blood, leading to disharmony of the Yin network vessels. In addition, exposure to strong sun causes retention of Heat Toxins in the skin and interstices (*cou li*); these Toxins scorch Yin-Blood causing obstruction of the channels and network vessels.

VASCULAR SKIN DISEASES

Diseases affecting the structure of the cutaneous blood vessels are known as vascular skin diseases. Insufficiency of arterial blood supply can cause skin atrophy or gangrene (as in Raynaud's disease); poor venous return may give rise to cutaneous dysfunction, manifesting as edema, stasis eczema or ulceration (as in venous leg ulcers); and damage to the capillaries is one of the causes of purpura (as in small vessel vasculitis). Dysfunction of the cutaneous blood vessels is often revealed by skin discoloration, pallor, flushing, or edema.

In terms of etiology, TCM identifies three causes of vascular diseases:

- Debilitation of Spleen and Kidney Yang impairs circulation in the Blood vessels so that the extremities become cyanotic and icy cold, with ulceration in serious cases.

- Invasion by Cold pathogenic factors leads to Qi stagnation and Blood stasis and causes obstruction of the channels and network vessels.

- A weak constitution, congenital insufficiency, or Heat Toxins from heavy smoking and drinking can all lead to Deficiency of the Zang-Fu organs.

Erythema multiforme
多形红斑

Erythema multiforme is an acute inflammatory skin disease, commonly associated with herpes simplex or mycoplasm infections. However, it can also be caused by a variety of other factors including bacteria, fungi and viruses, drugs such as sulfonamides, barbiturates and salicylates, or contact allergens, X-ray therapy and physical agents, or by certain systemic diseases such as lupus erythematosus or malignant lymphoma. Menstruation, pregnancy or exposure to cold may also trigger attacks. No cause can be found in approximately half of cases.

In TCM, this condition is also known as *mao yan chuang* (cat's eye sore), so named because the typical lesion resembles a cat's eye.

Clinical manifestations

- Erythema multiforme usually manifests with symmetrical involvement of the dorsum of the hands and feet (and sometimes also the palms and soles), the extensor surfaces of the arm and leg, and more rarely the face and neck.

- The disease occurs most frequently in early spring and late autumn, but sometimes also in winter.

- Lesions take a variety of forms including papules, maculopapules, vesicles, or bullae. The typical lesion, measuring 1-3 cm in diameter, has a red, slightly raised border and a dark red or purple slightly depressed central area with a small vesicle (also known as a "target" or "iris" lesion). Lesions, usually numerous, are scattered or clustered. In severe conditions, the lips and oral cavity may become eroded and ulcerated.

- At the initial stage, accompanying symptoms and signs include headache, lassitude and reduced appetite. High fever and aching and painful joints occur in severe, generalized conditions.

- Each episode of erythema multiforme lasts approximately one month, and recurrences are fairly common. Lesions heal without scarring, but frequently with hypopigmentation or hyperpigmentation.

Differential diagnosis

Pemphigus vulgaris
Flaccid easily-ruptured vesicles and bullae of different sizes appear on the skin surface. Application of slight pressure may cause the vesicles to move (Nikolsky's sign is positive). Pemphigus vulgaris usually involves the trunk, limb flexures, scalp, and oral mucosa, where it may be confused with a severe manifestation of erythema multiforme.

Chilblains and frostbite
Lesions usually appear on the hand, foot, ear, or tip of the nose. The affected area feels cold and exhibits edematous erythema. Frostbite is also characterized by vesicles and gangrene. However, neither of these conditions has the typical target lesion.

Urticaria
In urticaria, the wheals can appear in an annular form, sometimes resembling the initial lesions of erythema multiforme. However, in erythema multiforme, the lesions last for longer than the few hours typical of urticaria, are a deeper red color, usually develop into the classic target lesions, and, unlike urticaria, may involve the mucous membrane.

Etiology and pathology

- Internal factors include Damp-Heat accumulating in the Spleen and Lungs; the main external factors are Wind, Heat and Cold. In addition, Toxins may invade the interior to bind with Damp-Heat and lead to an acute onset of the disease. If Heat Toxins enter the Ying level, this can give rise to a severe condition.

- In early spring and late autumn, Wind and Cold pathogenic factors are likely to be encountered. In these seasons, Yang Qi is insufficient and cannot circulate adequately to reach the extremities of the limbs, resulting in the body and limbs feeling cold. If at the same time Cold pathogenic factors are exuberant, the circulation of Qi and Blood is inhibited and they are obstructed in the skin and flesh, resulting in lesions.

- The Spleen likes Dryness and loathes Dampness. Indulgence in fatty, sweet, spicy, or rich foods damages the Spleen and Stomach and impairs the Spleen in its transformation and transportation function. Accumulation of Dampness generates Heat, which combines to produce Damp-Heat; this in turn spreads to the skin and flesh to cause the disease.

- Congenital sensitivity to drug Toxins or Blood-Heat transforming into Toxins results in these Toxins disturbing the Ying and Xue levels. Heat Toxins attack internally and also move outward to attack the skin, resulting in erythema and papules. Heat Toxins may also bind with Damp-Heat, causing Damp-Heat to spread to the exterior, leading to herpes and other diseases that are precursors of erythema multiforme.

Pattern identification and treatment

INTERNAL TREATMENT

DAMP-HEAT RETAINED IN THE SKIN

This pattern manifests as a discrete distribution of numerous red target lesions of various sizes on the hands and feet, forearms and legs. Erosive lesions may appear on the oral mucosa, lips or genital region in severe cases. Accompanying symptoms and signs include fever, headache, lassitude, poor appetite, constipation, and yellow or reddish urine. The tongue body is red with a thin coating at the front and a greasy coating toward the root; the pulse is slippery and rapid, or soggy.

Treatment principle
Clear Heat and benefit the movement of Dampness.

Prescription
QING JI SHEN SHI TANG JIA JIAN
Decoction for Clearing Heat from the Flesh and Percolating Dampness, with modifications

Cang Zhu (Rhizoma Atractylodis) 6g
Chai Hu (Radix Bupleuri) 6g
Huang Lian (Rhizoma Coptidis) 6g
Jiao Zhi Zi (Fructus Gardeniae Jasminoidis, scorch-fried) 6g
Sheng Ma (Rhizoma Cimicifugae) 6g
Hou Po (Cortex Magnoliae Officinalis) 10g
Chen Pi (Pericarpium Citri Reticulatae) 10g
Ze Xie (Rhizoma Alismatis Orientalis) 10g
Ze Lan (Herba Lycopi Lucidi) 10g
Dan Shen (Radix Salviae Miltiorrhizae) 10g
Chi Xiao Dou (Semen Phaseoli Calcarati) 15g
Yi Yi Ren (Semen Coicis Lachryma-jobi) 15g
Fu Ling (Sclerotium Poriae Cocos) 12g
Hong Hua (Flos Carthami Tinctorii) 4.5g

Explanation
- *Cang Zhu* (Rhizoma Atractylodis), *Ze Xie* (Rhizoma Alismatis Orientalis), *Fu Ling* (Sclerotium Poriae Cocos), *Yi Yi Ren* (Semen Coicis Lachryma-jobi), *Chen Pi* (Pericarpium Citri Reticulatae), and *Hou Po* (Cortex Magnoliae Officinalis) fortify the Spleen and dry Dampness.
- *Yi Yi Ren* (Semen Coicis Lachryma-jobi) and *Chi Xiao Dou* (Semen Phaseoli Calcarati) invigorate the Blood and disperse swelling.
- *Huang Lian* (Rhizoma Coptidis) and *Jiao Zhi Zi* (Fructus Gardeniae Jasminoidis, scorch-fried) clear Heat and relieve Toxicity.
- *Hong Hua* (Flos Carthami Tinctorii), *Ze Lan* (Herba Lycopi Lucidi) and *Dan Shen* (Radix Salviae Miltiorrhizae) transform Blood stasis and reduce eruptions.
- *Chai Hu* (Radix Bupleuri) and *Sheng Ma* (Rhizoma Cimicifugae) relieve Toxicity and bear Yang upward.

BINDING OF COLD-DAMP
This pattern manifests as purplish-red or dull red target lesions on the hands and feet interspersed with a few vesicles. Lesions are exacerbated by cold and alleviated by warmth. Accompanying signs include cold limbs. The tongue body is pale red with a thin white coating at the front and a slightly greasy coating toward the root; the pulse is deep and tight, or wiry and tight.

Treatment principle
Dissipate Cold and dispel Dampness, warm the channels and free the network vessels.

Prescription
DANG GUI SI NI TANG JIA JIAN
Chinese Angelica Root Counterflow Cold Decoction, with modifications

Dang Gui (Radix Angelicae Sinensis) 10g
Gui Zhi (Ramulus Cinnamomi Cassiae) 10g
Chi Shao (Radix Paeoniae Rubra) 10g
Bai Shao (Radix Paeoniae Lactiflorae) 10g
Huo Xue Teng (Caulis seu Radix Schisandrae) 15g
Ji Xue Teng (Caulis Spatholobi) 15g
Shi Nan Teng (Caulis Photiniae) 15g
Qiang Huo (Rhizoma et Radix Notopterygii) 6g
Xin Yi Hua (Flos Magnoliae) 6g
Gan Jiang (Rhizoma Zingiberis Officinalis) 6g
Zhi Gan Cao (Radix Glycyrrhizae, mix-fried with honey) 4.5g
*Chuan Shan Jia** (Squama Manitis Pentadactylae) 4.5g
Da Zao (Fructus Ziziphi Jujubae) 15g

Explanation
- *Gui Zhi* (Ramulus Cinnamomi Cassiae), *Qiang Huo* (Rhizoma et Radix Notopterygii), *Xin Yi Hua* (Flos Magnoliae), *Gan Jiang* (Rhizoma Zingiberis Officinalis), *Zhi Gan Cao* (Radix Glycyrrhizae, mix-fried with honey), and *Da Zao* (Fructus Ziziphi Jujubae) warm Yang and dissipate Cold.
- *Dang Gui* (Radix Angelicae Sinensis), *Chi Shao* (Radix Paeoniae Rubra), *Bai Shao* (Radix Paeoniae Lactiflorae), *Huo Xue Teng* (Caulis Schisandrae), *Ji Xue Teng* (Caulis Spatholobi), *Shi Nan Teng* (Caulis Photiniae), and *Chuan Shan Jia** (Squama Manitis Pentadactylae) invigorate the Blood and free the network vessels.

HEAT TOXINS INVADING THE YING LEVEL
This pattern manifests as large patches of edematous erythema, ecchymoses, vesicles or bloody blisters on the

skin surface, or as severe erosion of the nasal and oral cavities. Accompanying symptoms and signs include fever, headache, lassitude, and painful joints. The tongue body is crimson with a scant coating; the pulse is thready and rapid, or slippery and rapid.

Treatment principle
Clear Heat from the Ying level and cool the Blood, relieve Toxicity and dispel Dampness.

Prescription
XI JIAO DI HUANG TANG JIA JIAN
Rhinoceros Horn and Rehmannia Decoction, with modifications

Shui Niu Jiao ‡ (Cornu Bubali) 15-30g
Mu Dan Pi (Cortex Moutan Radicis) 10g
Sheng Di Huang Tan (Radix Rehmanniae Glutinosae Carbonisata) 15g
Yin Hua Tan (Flos Lonicerae Carbonisata) 15g
Lian Qiao (Fructus Forsythiae Suspensae) 15g
Shi Hu* (Herba Dendrobii) 15g
Zi Cao (Radix Arnebiae seu Lithospermi) 12g
Nan Sha Shen (Radix Adenophorae) 30g
Yi Yi Ren (Semen Coicis Lachryma-jobi) 30g
Hong Hua (Flos Carthami Tinctorii) 6g
Ling Xiao Hua (Flos Campsitis) 6g
Gan Cao (Radix Glycyrrhizae) 6g

Explanation
- *Shui Niu Jiao* ‡ (Cornu Bubali), *Sheng Di Huang Tan* (Radix Rehmanniae Glutinosae Carbonisata), *Yin Hua Tan* (Flos Lonicerae Carbonisata), and *Lian Qiao* (Fructus Forsythiae Suspensae) clear Heat from the Ying level and cool the Blood, relieve Toxicity and reduce erythema.
- *Mu Dan Pi* (Cortex Moutan Radicis), *Zi Cao* (Radix Arnebiae seu Lithospermi), *Hong Hua* (Flos Carthami Tinctorii), and *Ling Xiao Hua* (Flos Campsitis) invigorate and cool the Blood.
- *Nan Sha Shen* (Radix Adenophorae), *Yi Yi Ren* (Semen Coicis Lachryma-jobi), *Shi Hu** (Herba Dendrobii), and *Gan Cao* (Radix Glycyrrhizae) nourish Yin and transform Dampness.

General modifications
1. For predominance of Wind-Heat, add *Chao Niu Bang Zi* (Fructus Arctii Lappae, stir-fried), *Fang Feng* (Radix Ledebouriellae Divaricatae), *Jie Geng* (Radix Platycodi Grandiflori), and *Jiang Can* ‡ (Bombyx Batryticatus).
2. For predominance of Wind-Cold, add *Cong Bai* (Bulbus Allii Fistulosi), *Jiang Huang* (Rhizoma Curcumae Longae) and *Jiu Xiang Chong* ‡ (Aspongopus).
3. For predominance of Cold-Damp, add *Qin Jiao* (Radix Gentianae Macrophyllae), *Du Huo* (Radix Angelicae Pubescentis), *Mu Gua* (Fructus Chaenomelis), and *Tong Cao* (Medulla Tetrapanacis Papyriferi).
4. For predominance of Blood-Heat, add *Qian Cao Gen* (Radix Rubiae Cordifoliae) and *Bai Mao Gen* (Rhizoma Imperatae Cylindricae).
5. For raging fever, add *Ling Yang Jiao** (Cornu Antelopis) and *Shi Gao* ‡ (Gypsum Fibrosum).
6. For painful joints, add *Xi Xian Cao* (Herba Siegesbeckiae), *Gui Jian Yu* (Lignum Suberalatum Euonymi), *Sang Ji Sheng* (Ramulus Loranthi), and *Lao Guan Cao* (Herba Erodii seu Geranii).
7. For cold hands and feet, add *Wu Zhu Yu* (Fructus Evodiae Rutaecarpae), *Gan Jiang* (Rhizoma Zingiberis Officinalis) and *Rou Gui* (Cortex Cinnamomi Cassiae).
8. For recurrent attacks due to Deficiency of Vital Qi (Zheng Qi), add *Huang Qi* (Radix Astragali seu Hedysari) and *Dang Shen* (Radix Codonopsitis Pilosulae).

EXTERNAL TREATMENT
- For inflammation and itching, apply *Lu Hu Xi Ji* (Calamine and Giant Knotweed Wash Preparation).
- For numerous vesicles with exudation on rupture, prepare a decoction with *Di Yu* (Radix Sanguisorbae Officinalis) 30g and *Guan Zhong** (Rhizoma Dryopteris Crassirhizomae) 30g and apply as a wet compress for 30 minutes twice a day.
- For lesions manifesting with papulovesicles or as target lesions, apply *Zi Se Xiao Zhong Gao* (Purple Paste for Dispersing Swelling) to the affected area once or twice a day.
- For localized dull purple patches and cold limbs, prepare a compress with *Jiao Ai Tang* (Chinese Prickly Ash and Mugwort Decoction):

Hua Jiao (Pericarpium Zanthoxyli) 15g
Ai Ye (Folium Artemisiae Argyi) 15g
Hong Hua (Flos Carthami Tinctorii) 15g
Gui Zhi (Ramulus Cinnamomi Cassiae) 15g
Tou Gu Cao (Herba Speranskiae seu Impatientis) 30g
Wang Bu Liu Xing (Semen Vaccariae Segetalis) 30g

Soak the ingredients in 800ml of water for 30 minutes, then boil for 20 minutes. Allow the decoction to cool before applying as a wet compress to the affected areas for 15 minutes, two or three times a day. Follow this with application of *Zi Se Xiao Zhong Gao* (Purple Paste for Dispersing Swelling).

- For erosion of the oral cavity, use *Qing Guo Shui Xi Ji* (Chinese Olive Wash Preparation) as a mouthwash and then use *Xi Gua Shuang Pen Ji* (Watermelon Frost Spray Preparation) as an insufflation for the affected area three to five times a day.

ACUPUNCTURE

Points

- For involvement of the upper limbs, select TB-5 Waiguan, LI-11 Quchi and LI-4 Hegu.
- For involvement of the lower limbs, select ST-36 Zusanli, GB-34 Yanglingquan and ST-41 Jiexi.

Technique: Apply the reducing method and retain the needles for 30 minutes after obtaining Qi. Manipulate the needles three to five times during this period. Treat once a day. A course consists of seven treatment sessions.

Explanation

- TB-5 Waiguan, LI-11 Quchi and LI-4 Hegu move Qi, cool the Blood and free the network vessels.
- ST-36 Zusanli, GB-34 Yanglingquan and ST-41 Jiexi fortify the Spleen, eliminate Dampness and invigorate the Blood.

EAR ACUPUNCTURE

Points: Lung, Spleen, Kidney, and Endocrine.
Technique: Retain the needles for 15 minutes. Treat once a day. A course consists of seven treatment sessions.

Clinical notes

TCM treatment of erythema multiforme is based on the type of skin eruption and the season:

- Red, swollen or painful lesions should be treated according to the principle of transforming Dampness and invigorating Blood to relieve Toxicity.
- For frequent attacks in autumn and winter, treat according to the principle of augmenting Qi and warming Yang, invigorating the Blood and freeing the network vessels.

Advice for the patient

- If occurrence of the disease is associated with a medication (for example, sulfonamides, penicillin, barbiturates, or NSAIDs), stop taking it immediately.
- For severe cases, keep the lesions clean, change the sheets every day and pay attention to hygiene of the eyes, nose, mouth, anus, and genitals.

Case history

Patient
Female, aged 15.

Clinical manifestations
Two patches of erythema multiforme had appeared on the cheeks in winter five years previously; these patches disappeared after about one month. Since then, they had recurred on the face and the dorsum of the hand every autumn and winter, sometimes appearing two or three times a year.

Examination revealed multiple, round, dark red, 1-2 cm maculopapular plaques on the dorsum of the hands. Target-like lesions were located in the center of the plaques. The tongue body was pale with a thin white coating; the pulse was wiry and thready.

Pattern identification
Binding of Cold-Damp.

Treatment principle
Dissipate Cold and dispel Dampness, warm the channels and free the network vessels.

Prescription ingredients

Sheng Ma (Rhizoma Cimicifugae) 9g
Qiang Huo (Rhizoma et Radix Notopterygii) 9g
Fang Feng (Radix Ledebouriellae Divaricatae) 9g
Dang Gui (Radix Angelicae Sinensis) 9g
Hong Hua (Flos Carthami Tinctorii) 9g
Chi Shao (Radix Paeoniae Rubra) 9g
Lian Qiao (Fructus Forsythiae Suspensae) 9g
Bai Zhi (Radix Angelicae Dahuricae) 6g
Gan Cao (Radix Glycyrrhizae) 6g

One bag a day was used to prepare a decoction, taken twice a day.

Second visit
After five bags, most of the lesions on the dorsum of the hands had disappeared. However, the patient complained of poor appetite, for which *Chen Pi* (Pericarpium Citri Reticulatae) 9g and *Fu Ling* (Sclerotium Poriae Cocos) 9g were added to the previous prescription.

Outcome
After five bags of the revised prescription, the eruptions had disappeared completely. In a follow-up visit eighteen months later, the patient said that two more attacks had occurred in the previous year, but eruptions had disappeared after taking two bags of the second prescription. [1]

Literature excerpt

In *Yi Zong Jin Jian: Wai Ke Xin Fa Yao Jue* [The Golden Mirror of Medicine: Essential Methods for the Treatment of External Diseases], it says: "*Mao yan chuang* (cat's eye sores) usually involve the face and the body. They are caused by retention of Damp-Heat in the Spleen channel over a long period, complicated by congealing of external Cold. At the initial stage, lesions look like cat's eyes, shiny and glistening but without bleeding. Pain and itching occur occasionally. To treat, prescribe oral administration of *Qing Ji Shen Shi Tang* (Decoction for Clearing Heat from the Flesh and Percolating Dampness) and external application of *Miao Tie San* (Wondrous Adhering Powder)."

Modern clinical experience

Reports on the use of TCM to treat erythema multiforme include treatment with Chinese materia medica and treatment of cold-type erythema multiforme by TCM alone and in combination with Western medicine.

TREATMENT WITH CHINESE MATERIA MEDICA

1. **Shen** formulated his own prescription to treat erythema multiforme. [2]

Prescription
SHENG MA LIAN YI TANG
Bugbane, Forsythia and Coix Seed Decoction

Sheng Ma (Rhizoma Cimicifugae) 10g
Lian Qiao (Fructus Forsythiae Suspensae) 10g
Dan Shen (Radix Salviae Miltiorrhizae) 10g
Zi Su Ye (Folium Perillae Frutescentis) 10g
Yi Yi Ren (Semen Coicis Lachryma-jobi) 20g
Xu Chang Qing (Radix Cynanchi Paniculati) 15g
Di Fu Zi (Fructus Kochiae Scopariae) 15g
Bai Xian Pi (Cortex Dictamni Dasycarpi Radicis) 15g
Gan Cao (Radix Glycyrrhizae) 4g

One bag a day was used to prepare a decoction, taken three times a day. Four days made up a course of treatment. Results were seen within a range of one to three courses. If patients suffered a relapse in subsequent months, they were treated again with the same prescription.

2. **Li** also formulated an empirical prescription. [3]

Prescription
XIAO BAN HE JI
Dispersing Erythema Mixture

Cang Zhu (Rhizoma Atractylodis) 15g
Ku Shen (Radix Sophorae Flavescentis) 15g
Zhi Mu (Rhizoma Anemarrhenae Asphodeloidis) 10g
Jing Jie (Herba Schizonepetae Tenuifoliae) 10g
Fang Feng (Radix Ledebouriellae Divaricatae) 10g
Dang Gui (Radix Angelicae Sinensis) 10g
Chao Niu Bang Zi (Fructus Arctii Lappae, stir-fried) 10g
Chan Tui‡ (Periostracum Cicadae) 10g
Wei Ling Xian (Radix Clematidis) 10g
Duan Shi Gao‡ (Gypsum Fibrosum Calcinatum) 12g
Sheng Di Huang (Radix Rehmanniae Glutinosae) 12g
Jin Yin Hua (Flos Lonicerae) 12g
He Shou Wu (Radix Polygoni Multiflori) 12g
Huang Bai (Cortex Phellodendri) 8g
Huang Lian (Rhizoma Coptidis) 8g
Shi Chang Pu (Rhizoma Acori Graminei) 6g
Gan Cao (Radix Glycyrrhizae) 3g

One bag a day was used to prepare a decoction, taken warm twice a day. The mixture was used without modification, except for patients with fever, when Western antipyretics and antibiotics were prescribed. Results were seen within a range of five to twenty-five days.

TREATMENT OF COLD PATTERNS OF ERYTHEMA MULTIFORME

1. **Lu** treated 40 patients with Cold patterns of erythema multiforme. [4]

Prescription
GUI ZHI HONG HUA TANG
Cinnamon Twig and Safflower Decoction

Gui Zhi (Ramulus Cinnamomi Cassiae) 9g
Hong Hua (Flos Carthami Tinctorii) 9g
Niu Xi (Radix Achyranthis Bidentatae) 9g
Dang Gui (Radix Angelicae Sinensis) 9g
Chi Shao (Radix Paeoniae Rubra) 9g
Wei Ling Xian (Radix Clematidis) 9g
Gan Jiang (Rhizoma Zingiberis Officinalis) 6g
Gan Cao (Radix Glycyrrhizae) 6g
Xi Xin* (Herba cum Radice Asari) 3g
Ma Huang* (Herba Ephedrae) 3g
Ji Xue Teng (Caulis Spatholobi) 15g

For severe internal Cold, the prescription was modified by adding Fu Zi* (Radix Lateralis Aconiti Carmichaeli Praeparata) 10g.

One bag a day was used to prepare a decoction, taken twice a day. Results were evaluated after one course of two weeks' treatment. Half of the patients had recovered and the rest showed varying degrees of improvement.

2. **Zhong** considered that Cold-type erythema multiforme was caused by retention of external Wind-Cold in the skin and flesh, leading to disharmony between the Ying and Wei levels, Qi stagnation and Blood stasis. [5]

Treatment principle
Warm the channels to dissipate Cold, invigorate the Blood to transform Blood stasis.

Prescription ingredients

Fu Zi* (Radix Lateralis Aconiti Carmichaeli Praeparata) 10g
Gui Zhi (Ramulus Cinnamomi Cassiae) 10g
Ma Huang* (Herba Ephedrae) 10g
Tao Ren (Semen Persicae) 10g
Hong Hua (Flos Carthami Tinctorii) 10g
Chuan Xiong (Rhizoma Ligustici Chuanxiong) 10g
Di Fu Zi (Fructus Kochiae Scopariae) 20g
Xi Xin* (Herba cum Radice Asari) 5g
Gan Cao (Radix Glycyrrhizae) 5g

Modifications
1. For involvement of the upper limbs, *Jiang Huang* (Rhizoma Curcumae Longae) was added.
2. For involvement of the lower limbs, *Niu Xi* (Radix Achyranthis Bidentatae) was added.
3. For erosive lesions, *Gan Cao You* (Licorice Oil) was applied externally twice a day.

Dosages were halved for children. One bag a day was used to prepare a decoction, taken twice a day. Five bags constituted a course. Results were seen after two courses.

3. Bao treated this pattern of erythema multiforme with a combination of TCM and Western medicine. [6]

TCM prescription
DANG GUI SI NI TANG JIA JIAN
Chinese Angelica Root Counterflow Cold Decoction, with modifications

Dang Gui (Radix Angelicae Sinensis) 12g
Dan Shen (Radix Salviae Miltiorrhizae) 10g
Bai Shao (Radix Paeoniae Lactiflorae) 9g
Chi Shao (Radix Paeoniae Rubra) 9g
Tong Cao (Medulla Tetrapanacis Papyriferi) 6g
Fu Zi* (Radix Lateralis Aconiti Carmichaeli Praeparata) 6g
Xi Xin* (Herba cum Radice Asari) 3g
Zhi Gan Cao (Radix Glycyrrhizae, mix-fried with honey) 3g
Gan Jiang (Rhizoma Zingiberis Officinalis) 9g
Da Zao (Fructus Ziziphi Jujubae) 15g

One bag a day was used to prepare a decoction, taken twice a day.

Western medicine
Cinnarizine 25mg, vitamin E 100mg and anisodamine 10mg for oral administration three times a day. [i]

Results were seen after seven days.

Annular erythemas
环形红斑

Annular erythemas are a loose grouping of chronic, recurrent disorders characterized by circular or figurate lesions with a pale center and a raised erythematous margin.

In TCM, this condition is also known as *huo dan yin zhen* (Fire-cinnabar dormant papules) – in other words, a skin disease resembling a combination of erysipelas and urticaria – or *xue feng chuang* (Blood-Wind sore).

Clinical manifestations

- Annular erythemas generally appear in the middle-aged, without sex predilection. However, they may begin at any age.
- Eruptions usually involve the trunk, the limbs, the buttocks, and the medial aspect of the thighs, but rarely the face.
- Lesions manifest initially as one or several red papules, which gradually enlarge to form an annular or figurate shape with a raised margin and a flat center and a diameter that may extend to several centimeters. Confluent rings may appear as garlanded, arched, concentric, or fretted. New papules sometimes appear in the flattened center.

- Some papules may be active periodically over many years.
- In severe conditions, accompanying symptoms include slight fever and mild itching.

Differential diagnosis

Erythema multiforme
This disease is generally seen in early spring and late autumn with symmetrical involvement of the hands and feet and the extensor surfaces of the arm and leg. Eruptions typically manifest as "target" or "iris" lesions – erythema with raised purple borders surrounding a red patch, generally with a small vesicle in the center. In severe conditions, there may be erosion of the oral cavity and systemic symptoms such as high fever and painful joints.

Etiology and pathology

Wind-Heat, Summerheat or Summerheat-Damp can attack the skin and interstices (*cou li*) and obstruct the channels and network vessels, thereby spreading to affect the Xue level and leading to accumulation and

---

[i] Anisodamine is a drug structurally related to atropine, isolated from *Anisodus tanguticus*. It is available in China.

binding of pathogenic factors in the skin, thus causing the disease.

Pattern identification and treatment

INTERNAL TREATMENT

WIND-HEAT

Red skin eruptions spread relatively quickly, often with several rings coalescing into a garland-like shape. Slight itching is experienced. The tongue body is red with a thin white coating; the pulse is floating and rapid.

Treatment principle
Dredge Wind, clear Heat and cool the Blood.

Prescription
SI WU XIAO FENG SAN JIA JIAN
Four Agents Powder for Dispersing Wind, with modifications

Chao Niu Bang Zi (Fructus Arctii Lappae, stir-fried) 9g
Lian Qiao (Fructus Forsythiae Suspensae) 9g
Jin Yin Hua (Flos Lonicerae) 12g
Chi Shao (Radix Paeoniae Rubra) 9g
Zi Cao (Radix Arnebiae seu Lithospermi) 9g
Mu Dan Pi (Cortex Moutan Radicis) 9g
Bo He (Herba Menthae Haplocalycis) 4.5g
Jing Jie (Herba Schizonepetae Tenuifoliae) 4.5g
Fang Feng (Radix Ledebouriellae Divaricatae) 4.5g
Chan Tui‡ (Periostracum Cicadae) 3g
Sheng Di Huang (Radix Rehmanniae Glutinosae) 12g
Yu Quan San (Jade Spring Powder) 15g, wrapped

Explanation
- *Chao Niu Bang Zi* (Fructus Arctii Lappae, stir-fried), *Fang Feng* (Radix Ledebouriellae Divaricatae), *Jing Jie* (Herba Schizonepetae Tenuifoliae), *Lian Qiao* (Fructus Forsythiae Suspensae), *Chan Tui*‡ (Periostracum Cicadae), and *Bo He* (Herba Menthae Haplocalycis) dredge Wind and dissipate Heat, thrust pathogenic factors outward and alleviate itching.
- *Zi Cao* (Radix Arnebiae seu Lithospermi), *Mu Dan Pi* (Cortex Moutan Radicis), *Sheng Di Huang* (Radix Rehmanniae Glutinosae), and *Chi Shao* (Radix Paeoniae Rubra) cool the Blood and reduce erythema.
- *Yu Quan San* (Jade Spring Powder) clears Heat and drains Fire.

SUMMERHEAT-DAMP

Pale, hard and desquamative skin eruptions with a slightly raised rim are more pronounced in humid or muggy weather, similar to that encountered in summer in Southeast China. The tongue body is pale red with a thin, yellow and slightly greasy coating; the pulse is rapid.

Treatment principle
Transform Dampness and clear Heat, flush out Summerheat and free the network vessels.

Prescription
LIANG XUE WU GEN TANG JIA JIAN
Five Root Decoction for Cooling the Blood, with modifications

Zi Cao (Radix Arnebiae seu Lithospermi) 10g
Ban Lan Gen (Radix Isatidis seu Baphicacanthi) 10g
Qian Cao Gen (Radix Rubiae Cordifoliae) 10g
Ji Xue Teng (Caulis Spatholobi) 12g
Hai Feng Teng (Caulis Piperis Kadsurae) 12g
Ren Dong Teng (Caulis Lonicerae Japonicae) 12g
Ma Bian Cao (Herba cum Radice Verbenae) 12g
Hong Hua (Flos Carthami Tinctorii) 6g
Ling Xiao Hua (Flos Campsitis) 6g
Sheng Di Huang (Radix Rehmanniae Glutinosae) 6g
Mu Dan Pi (Cortex Moutan Radicis) 6g
Si Gua Luo (Fasciculus Vascularis Luffae) 6g
Huai Hua (Flos Sophorae Japonicae) 6g
Yi Yi Ren (Semen Coicis Lachryma-jobi) 30g
Chi Xiao Dou (Semen Phaseoli Calcarati) 30g
Xian Huo Xiang (Herba Agastaches seu Pogostemi Recens) 30g

Explanation
- *Zi Cao* (Radix Arnebiae seu Lithospermi), *Ban Lan Gen* (Radix Isatidis seu Baphicacanthi), *Qian Cao Gen* (Radix Rubiae Cordifoliae), *Ren Dong Teng* (Caulis Lonicerae Japonicae), and *Ma Bian Cao* (Herba cum Radice Verbenae) clear Heat and relieve Toxicity, free the network vessels and disperse eruptions.
- *Xian Huo Xiang* (Herba Agastaches seu Pogostemi Recens), *Yi Yi Ren* (Semen Coicis Lachryma-jobi) and *Chi Xiao Dou* (Semen Phaseoli Calcarati) clear Heat and flush out Summerheat.
- *Sheng Di Huang* (Radix Rehmanniae Glutinosae), *Mu Dan Pi* (Cortex Moutan Radicis), *Hong Hua* (Flos Carthami Tinctorii), *Ji Xue Teng* (Caulis Spatholobi), *Ling Xiao Hua* (Flos Campsitis), and *Huai Hua* (Flos Sophorae Japonicae) clear Heat from the Ying level and cool the Blood, relieve Toxicity and reduce erythema.
- *Si Gua Luo* (Fasciculus Vascularis Luffae) and *Hai Feng Teng* (Caulis Piperis Kadsurae) free the network vessels and transform Dampness.

General modifications
1. For fever, add *Shui Niu Jiao Fen*‡ (Cornu Bubali, powdered).
2. For pain in the limbs, add *Qin Jiao* (Radix Gentianae Macrophyllae), *Sang Zhi* (Ramulus Mori Albae) and *Mu Gua* (Fructus Chaenomelis).

3. For bright red eruptions and a dry mouth, add *Shi Gao* ‡ (Gypsum Fibrosum) and *Dan Zhu Ye* (Herba Lophatheri Gracilis).
4. For persistent, dull red eruptions, add *Tao Ren* (Semen Persicae) and *Su Mu* (Lignum Sappan).

PATENT HERBAL MEDICINES

For Deficiency-Excess complex patterns of long duration, take *Da Huang Zhe Chong Wan* (Rhubarb and Wingless Cockroach Pill) 3g, twice a day.

EXTERNAL TREATMENT

- For bright red, confluent, slightly itchy lesions, apply *Lu Hu Xi Ji* (Calamine and Giant Knotweed Wash Preparation) to the affected area once or twice a day.
- For pale red lesions with a little scaling, apply *Qing Liang Fen* (Cool Clearing Powder) one to three times a day.

ACUPUNCTURE

Points: GV-14 Dazhui, CV-12 Zhongwan, LI-11 Quchi, ST-36 Zusanli, and Ashi points (the area around the eruptions).
Technique: Apply the reducing method and retain the needles for 30 minutes after obtaining Qi. Treat once a day. A course consists of seven treatment sessions.

Explanation

- GV-14 Dazhui and LI-11 Quchi dissipate Wind and alleviate itching.
- CV-12 Zhongwan and ST-36 Zusanli fortify the Spleen and transform Dampness.

EAR ACUPUNCTURE

Points: Lung, Heart and Subcortex.
Technique: Retain the needles for 15 minutes. Treat once every other day. A course consists of five treatment sessions.

PRICKING TO BLEED METHOD

Points: BL-40 Weizhong and BL-57 Chengshan.

Technique: After sterilization, prick the points with a small three-edged needle and press the point slightly to squeeze some blood out. Treat once every five days. A course consists of three treatment sessions.

POINT LASER THERAPY

Points: BL-40 Weizhong and BL-57 Chengshan.
Technique: Apply laser therapy to each point for five minutes using a helium-neon laser apparatus. Treat once every other day. A course consists of ten treatment sessions.

Advice for the patient

- Pay attention to food hygiene.
- Do not eat raw ginger, garlic, chives, seafood, or spicy food (classified in Chinese medicine as stimulating food).
- Increase the intake of fresh fruit and vegetables.
- Take precautions to avoid insect bites.
- Build up the body's strength to prevent external contraction of Wind-Heat and Summerheat-Damp pathogenic factors.

Literature excerpt

In *Xu Lü He Wai Ke Yi An Yi Hua Ji* [A Collection of Xu Lühe's Medical Records on External Diseases], the author explains, "Erythema annulare centrifugum corresponds to *feng ban*, the Wind macules mentioned in *Yang Ke Xin De Ji: Sha Zhen Dan Ban Tong Yi Bian* [A Collection of Experiences in the Treatment of Sores: Differences and Similarities Between Patterns of Measles, Papules, Erysipelas, and Macules]. Red eruptions are usually caused by Fire in the Xue level. If itching is also felt, this means that Wind is involved. In this case, *Si Wu Xiao Feng San Jia Jian* (Four Agents Powder for Dispersing Wind, with modifications) [ii] is recommended."

Toxic erythema
中毒性红斑

Toxic erythema is an acute inflammatory skin disease characterized by generalized diffuse erythema. In Western medicine, the term toxic erythema is usually taken to mean an exanthematous, urticarial or erythema multiforme-type reaction to drugs. Chinese medicine adopts a slightly different approach to the cause of this disorder and the

---

[ii] Please refer to the Wind-Heat pattern in this section.

conditions described in this section, although often similar to those seen in drug eruptions, manifest as cutaneous reactions to spoiled or contaminated food or certain primary diseases.

In TCM, this disease is also known as *zhu wu zhong du* (poisoning due to various substances). Before an attack, there is often a history of consumption of food that has not been cleaned properly, especially fish and shellfish, or patients may have underlying diseases such as rheumatic diseases, pneumonia or malaria. In all of these instances, systemic erythema may result.

Clinical manifestations

- At the initial stage, the only skin lesions are small, isolated patches of erythema. As the disease develops, large patches of erythema spread throughout the body.
- In severe conditions, the buccal mucosa may be affected.
- Petechiae or hemorrhagic spots may be present in some cases.
- Significant desquamation, usually of bran-like scales, often occurs during the recovery phase.
- Itching of varying severity is likely.
- Systemic symptoms such as raging fever, loss of appetite, painful joints, constipation, and oliguria may accompany some cases.

Differential diagnosis

Exanthematous drug eruption
The patient has a history of drug allergy. Erythema, occasionally generalized, usually appears suddenly seven to ten days after starting the drug and reaches its peak in a few hours or two or three days. Eruptions may resemble those of scarlet fever (scarlatiniform) or measles (morbilliform) and present as symmetrically distributed, generalized, usually itchy red macules and papules. Identification of the factor triggering the eruption enables a differential diagnosis.

Etiology and pathology

Excessive consumption of spoiled or poorly-cleaned fish, seafood, meat, or poultry may stir Wind and induce the disease by damaging the Spleen and Stomach and generating Heat Toxins, both of which can lead to disharmony between the Spleen and Stomach and accumulation of Damp-Heat. Once Damp-Heat has been generated, it will burn the Ying and Xue levels. Heat Toxins spread outward to the skin and interstices (*cou li*), thus producing the erythema.

Pattern identification and treatment

INTERNAL TREATMENT

WIND-HEAT SPREADING TO THE SKIN
At the initial stage, a bright red morbilliform (measles-like) rash appears, which soon spreads throughout the body. The color blanches on pressure. Accompanying symptoms and signs include fever, aversion to cold, a sore and swollen throat, a preference for cold drinks, constipation, and short voidings of reddish urine. The tongue body is red with a thin yellow coating; the pulse is floating and rapid.

Treatment principle
Clear Heat and dispel Wind.

Prescription
YIN QIAO DA QING TANG JIA JIAN
Honeysuckle, Forsythia and Woad Leaf Decoction, with modifications

Jin Yin Hua (Flos Lonicerae) 12g
Lian Qiao (Fructus Forsythiae Suspensae) 12g
Da Qing Ye (Folium Isatidis seu Baphicacanthi) 9g
Chao Niu Bang Zi (Fructus Arctii Lappae, stir-fried) 9g
Jing Jie (Herba Schizonepetae Tenuifoliae) 3g
Bo He (Herba Menthae Haplocalycis) 3g, added 5 minutes before the end of the decoction process
Lü Dou Yi (Testa Phaseoli Radiati) 12g
Sheng Di Huang (Radix Rehmanniae Glutinosae) 12g
Mu Dan Pi (Cortex Moutan Radicis) 6g
Gan Cao (Radix Glycyrrhizae) 6g

Explanation
- *Jin Yin Hua* (Flos Lonicerae), *Lian Qiao* (Fructus Forsythiae Suspensae), *Da Qing Ye* (Folium Isatidis seu Baphicacanthi), *Gan Cao* (Radix Glycyrrhizae), and *Lü Dou Yi* (Testa Phaseoli Radiati) clear Heat from the Ying level and relieve Toxicity to protect the Heart.
- *Mu Dan Pi* (Cortex Moutan Radicis) and *Sheng Di Huang* (Radix Rehmanniae Glutinosae) cool the Blood and reduce erythema.
- *Chao Niu Bang Zi* (Fructus Arctii Lappae, stir-fried), *Jing Jie* (Herba Schizonepetae Tenuifoliae) and *Bo He* (Herba Menthae Haplocalycis) clear Heat and dredge Wind.

EXUBERANT TOXINS DUE TO BLOOD-HEAT
Lesions manifest as large patches of erythema, which may spread throughout the body. In some weight-bearing areas, such as the lumbosacral region and the

lower limbs, petechiae and ecchymoses that do not blanch on pressure are evident within the areas of erythema. Accompanying symptoms and signs include raging fever, a dry mouth, a sore and swollen throat, inhibited bending and stretching of the joints, and irregular urination and defecation. The tongue body is crimson or exhibits stasis marks and has a yellow and slightly dry coating; the pulse is rapid.

Treatment principle

Clear Heat and cool the Blood, relieve Toxicity and disperse erythema.

Prescription

XIAO BAN QING DAI SAN JIA JIAN

Indigo Powder for Dispersing Macules, with modifications

Qing Dai (Indigo Naturalis) 6g
Sheng Di Huang (Radix Rehmanniae Glutinosae) 30g
Mu Dan Pi (Cortex Moutan Radicis) 10g
Chi Shao (Radix Paeoniae Rubra) 10g
Da Huang (Radix et Rhizoma Rhei) 10g, added 10 minutes before the end of the decoction process
Zhi Mu (Rhizoma Anemarrhenae Asphodeloidis) 10g
Zhi Zi (Fructus Gardeniae Jasminoidis) 10g
Da Qing Ye (Folium Isatidis seu Baphicacanthi) 15g
Xuan Shen (Radix Scrophulariae Ningpoensis) 12g
Lü Dou Yi (Testa Phaseoli Radiati) 6g

Explanation

- *Qing Dai* (Indigo Naturalis), *Da Qing Ye* (Folium Isatidis seu Baphicacanthi), *Lü Dou Yi* (Testa Phaseoli Radiati), and *Zhi Zi* (Fructus Gardeniae Jasminoidis) clear Heat and relieve Toxicity.
- *Sheng Di Huang* (Radix Rehmanniae Glutinosae), *Mu Dan Pi* (Cortex Moutan Radicis) and *Chi Shao* (Radix Paeoniae Rubra) cool the Blood and reduce erythema.
- *Xuan Shen* (Radix Scrophulariae Ningpoensis) and *Zhi Mu* (Rhizoma Anemarrhenae Asphodeloidis) nourish Yin and clear Heat.
- *Da Huang* (Radix et Rhizoma Rhei) clears the Fu organs and drains Toxicity, frees the network vessels and reduces erythema.

General modifications

1. For Heat Toxins blocking the Wei and Qi levels, add *Shi Gao* ‡ (Gypsum Fibrosum), *Nan Sha Shen* (Radix Adenophorae), *Fu Ping* (Herba Spirodelae Polyrrhizae), and *Bai Mao Gen* (Rhizoma Imperatae Cylindricae).
2. For persistent high fever, add *Shui Niu Jiao* ‡ (Cornu Bubali), *Ling Yang Jiao** (Cornu Antelopis), *Sheng Di Huang Tan* (Radix Rehmanniae Glutinosae Carbonisata), and *Jin Yin Hua Tan* (Flos Lonicerae Carbonisata).
3. For sore and swollen throat, add *Shan Dou Gen* (Radix Sophorae Tonkinensis), *Ma Bo* (Sclerotium Lasiosphaerae seu Calvatiae), *She Gan* (Rhizoma Belamcandae Chinensis), and *Gua Jin Deng* (Calyx Physalis Alkekengi).
4. For abscesses and swellings, add *Ye Ju Hua* (Flos Chrysanthemi Indici), *Zi Hua Di Ding* (Herba Violae Yedoensitis), *Pu Gong Ying* (Herba Taraxaci cum Radice), and *Bai Hua She She Cao* (Herba Hedyotidis Diffusae).
5. For constipation, add *Chao Zhi Ke* (Fructus Citri Aurantii, stir-fried) and *Da Huang* (Radix et Rhizoma Rhei), the latter added 10 minutes before the end of the decoction process.
6. For poor appetite and nausea and vomiting, add *Zhu Ru* (Caulis Bambusae in Taeniis), *Huo Xiang* (Herba Agastaches seu Pogostemi), *Shen Qu* (Massa Fermentata), *Gu Ya* (Fructus Oryzae Sativae Germinatus), and *Mai Ya* (Fructus Hordei Vulgaris Germinatus).
7. For cough and hoarse voice, add *Jie Geng* (Radix Platycodi Grandiflori), *Mu Hu Die* (Semen Oroxyli Indici) and *Xuan Shen* (Radix Scrophulariae Ningpoensis).
8. For edema of the lips and eyelids, add *Fu Ping* (Herba Spirodelae Polyrrhizae), *Chan Tui* ‡ (Periostracum Cicadae), *Can Sha* ‡ (Excrementum Bombycis Mori), and *Bai Mao Gen* (Rhizoma Imperatae Cylindricae).
9. If erythema blanches under pressure, add *Zi Cao* (Radix Arnebiae seu Lithospermi) and *Huang Qin* (Radix Scutellariae Baicalensis).
10. If erythema does not blanch under pressure, add *Hong Hua* (Flos Carthami Tinctorii) and *Ling Xiao Hua* (Flos Campsitis).

EXTERNAL TREATMENT

- For bright red generalized erythema, apply *Qing Liang Fen* (Cool Clearing Powder) to the affected area.
- For sore and swollen throat, use *Xi Gua Shuang Pen Ji* (Watermelon Frost Spray Preparation) as an insufflation.

Clinical notes

Toxic erythema is an acute skin disease. The main treatment principle is to dredge Wind and relieve Toxicity, cool the Blood and reduce erythema.

- At the initial stage, *Yin Qiao San* (Honeysuckle and Forsythia Powder) can also be used to cool the Blood and relieve Toxicity; the prescription should be modified by removing *Dan Dou Chi* (Semen Sojae Praeparatum) and adding *Sheng Di Huang* (Radix

Rehmanniae Glutinosae), *Mu Dan Pi* (Cortex Moutan Radicis) and *Da Qing Ye* (Folium Isatidis seu Baphicacanthi) or similar ingredients.

- To nourish Yin and protect the Heart in patterns of exuberant Blood-Heat, *Xi Jiao Di Huang Tang* (Rhinoceros Horn and Rehmannia Decoction) with appropriate modifications can also be used.

Advice for the patient

- Avoid eating food that has not been cleaned properly or has started to go off.
- Use mild powders to alleviate itching such as *Qing Liang Fen* (Cool Clearing Powder) or *Fei Zi Fen* (Miliaria Powder).
- Do not wash with hot water.

Case history

Patient
Male, aged 40.

Clinical manifestations
The previous day, the patient had eaten some glutinous rice that had gone bad. Shortly afterwards, he started to suffer from abdominal discomfort and distension. During the night, the skin started to feel itchy all over the body and was red the following morning. In the afternoon, the patient's temperature reached 39.8°C. Accompanying symptoms and signs included mental exhaustion, stifling oppression in the chest, fever without sweating, constipation with no bowel movements for two days, and short voidings of reddish urine. Laboratory tests revealed a white blood cell count of 22.0×10^9/L.

By the time of the consultation, diffuse swollen erythema that blanched on pressure was evident on the face, trunk and limbs; petechial hemorrhage was noted in a few places on the legs. The tongue body was red with a white and greasy coating; the pulse was wiry, slippery and rapid.

Pattern identification
Damp-Heat caused by consumption of spoiled food binding with Toxins to scorch the Ying and Xue levels and surge to the exterior.

Treatment principle
Clear Heat and cool the Blood, relieve Toxicity and benefit the movement of Dampness.

Prescription ingredients
Xian Di Huang (Radix Rehmanniae Glutinosae Recens) 30g
Xian Lu Gen (Rhizoma Phragmitis Communis Recens) 30g
Da Qing Ye (Folium Isatidis seu Baphicacanthi) 30g
Ban Lan Gen (Radix Isatidis seu Baphicacanthi) 10g
Sang Ye (Folium Mori Albae) 10g
Chi Shao (Radix Paeoniae Rubra) 10g
Huang Qin (Radix Scutellariae Baicalensis) 10g

Hua Shi‡ (Talcum) 10g
Jin Yin Hua (Flos Lonicerae) 15g
Lian Qiao (Fructus Forsythiae Suspensae) 12g
Bai Xian Pi (Cortex Dictamni Dasycarpi Radicis) 15g
Zhi Zi (Fructus Gardeniae Jasminoidis) 6g
Gan Cao (Radix Glycyrrhizae) 3g

Second visit
The following day, after drinking two decoctions prepared from one bag of the prescription, the erythema was beginning to fade, bowel movements had begun again, the temperature had returned to normal, and the white blood cell count had dropped to 13.8×10^9/L. However, the itching had not improved and the patient still had a feeling of oppression in the chest. The tongue and pulse had not changed. *Zhi Ke* (Fructus Citri Aurantii) 4.5g was added to the prescription.

Third visit
After drinking another bag of the ingredients, 80 percent of the erythema had disappeared, but itching and slight desquamation were evident; the white blood cell count had fallen to 9.1×10^9/L. The patient's mood had improved and the oppression in the chest was much less pronounced. The tongue body was red with a white coating; the pulse was wiry and slippery.

Modified prescription ingredients
Jin Yin Hua (Flos Lonicerae) 12g
Bai Xian Pi (Cortex Dictamni Dasycarpi Radicis) 12g
Xian Di Huang (Radix Rehmanniae Glutinosae Recens) 15g
Xian Bai Mao Gen (Rhizoma Imperatae Cylindricae Recens) 15g
Chi Shao (Radix Paeoniae Rubra) 10g
Da Qing Ye (Folium Isatidis seu Baphicacanthi) 10g
Fu Ling (Sclerotium Poriae Cocos) 10g
Pu Gong Ying (Herba Taraxaci cum Radice) 10g
Dan Zhu Ye (Herba Lophatheri Gracilis) 10g
Liu Yi San (Six-To-One Powder) 18g

Fourth visit
After drinking one bag of this prescription, the redness and swelling had disappeared completely and the other symptoms had resolved. However, the patient had now lost his appetite. The tongue coating was slightly greasy; the pulse was deep and moderate. The prescription was therefore amended.

Treatment principle
Fortify the Spleen and harmonize the Stomach.

Prescription ingredients
Zhi Ke (Fructus Citri Aurantii) 4.5g
Chen Pi (Pericarpium Citri Reticulatae) 6g
Chao Gu Ya (Fructus Oryzae Sativae Germinatus, stir-fried) 10g
Zhu Ru (Caulis Bambusae in Taeniis) 6g
Jin Yin Hua (Flos Lonicerae) 10g
Bai Xian Pi (Cortex Dictamni Dasycarpi Radicis) 10g
Di Fu Zi (Fructus Kochiae Scopariae) 10g
Ju Hua (Flos Chrysanthemi Morifolii) 10g
Chi Shao (Radix Paeoniae Rubra) 10g

Discussion
In this case, consumption of spoiled food generated Damp-Heat, which bound with Toxins to scorch the Ying and Xue

levels and pour into the Lungs. The Lungs face the hundred vessels in the interior and govern the skin and hair in the exterior. Heat Toxins were therefore transported to the exterior to cause the disease.

The first prescription was designed to deal with Damp-Heat surging to the skin. *Jin Yin Hua* (Flos Lonicerae), *Lian Qiao* (Fructus Forsythiae Suspensae), *Da Qing Ye* (Folium Isatidis seu Baphicacanthi), *Ban Lan Gen* (Radix Isatidis seu Baphicacanthi), *Bai Xian Pi* (Cortex Dictamni Dasycarpi Radicis), and *Chi Shao* (Radix Paeoniae Rubra) clear Heat and relieve Toxicity; *Xian Di Huang* (Radix Rehmanniae Glutinosae Recens) and *Xian Lu Gen* (Rhizoma Phragmitis Communis Recens) clear Heat and cool the Blood; *Huang Qin* (Radix Scutellariae Baicalensis), *Zhi Zi* (Fructus Gardeniae Jasminoidis) and *Sang Ye* (Folium Mori Albae) clear Heat from the Heart and Lungs and drain Fire retained in the Triple Burner; and *Hua Shi*‡ (Talcum) and *Gan Cao* (Radix Glycyrrhizae) clear Heat and clear the orifices, benefit the movement of water and generate Body Fluids. After two bags of this prescription, the erythema was receding, the temperature had been reduced, urine and stool were regular, and the white blood cell count was within the normal range.

Since this disease was caused by the consumption of spoiled food, the Spleen and Stomach were damaged with the result that the patient lost his appetite once the erythema had disappeared. The greasy tongue coating signified that Damp-Heat in the Spleen and Stomach had not been completely dispersed. Although the combination of *Zhi Ke* (Fructus Citri Aurantii), *Chen Pi* (Pericarpium Citri Reticulatae), *Chao Gu Ya* (Fructus Oryzae Sativae Germinatus, stir-fried), and *Zhu Ru* (Caulis Bambusae in Taeniis) has a relatively bland Heat-clearing function, it was suitable in this case for fortifying the Spleen and harmonizing the Stomach. [7]

Modern clinical experience

Xu held that the pathology of toxic erythema due to administration of medical drugs was similar to that of eruptions due to Lung-Heat. His treatment principle therefore was to diffuse the Lungs and drain Heat, clear Heat from the Ying level and thrust eruptions outward and for this he used the formula listed on page 316. [8]

He treated ten patients (six male and four female, three under three years old, four between 8 and 18 years old and three between 41 and 47 years old). All ten had a history of antibiotic and antihistamine treatment; five had been treated with corticosteroids through intravenous drip. Lesions manifested as diffuse urticated erythematous plaques. All patients had temperatures between 38 and 40°C. Leucocytosis was present in all cases. Six patients had swollen tonsils.

Prescription
YIN QIAO DA QING TANG
Honeysuckle, Forsythia and Woad Leaf Decoction

Jin Yin Hua (Flos Lonicerae) 12g
Lian Qiao (Fructus Forsythiae Suspensae) 12g
Da Qing Ye (Folium Isatidis seu Baphicacanthi) 9g
Chao Niu Bang Zi (Fructus Arctii Lappae, stir-fried) 9g
Jing Jie (Herba Schizonepetae Tenuifoliae) 3g
Bo He (Herba Menthae Haplocalycis) 3g
Lü Dou Yi (Testa Phaseoli Radiati) 15g
Sheng Di Huang (Radix Rehmanniae Glutinosae) 15g
Mu Dan Pi (Cortex Moutan Radicis) 6g
Gan Cao (Radix Glycyrrhizae) 6g

Modifications
1. For large plaques of bright red wheals, *Huang Qin* (Radix Scutellariae Baicalensis), *Zi Cao* (Radix Arnebiae seu Lithospermi) and *Hong Hua* (Flos Carthami Tinctorii) were added.
2. For red, sore and swollen tonsils, *Xuan Shen* (Radix Scrophulariae Ningpoensis), *Shan Dou Gen* (Radix Sophorae Tonkinensis) and *Ma Bo* (Sclerotium Lasiosphaerae seu Calvatiae) were added.
3. For edema of the lips and face, *Chan Tui*‡ (Periostracum Cicadae), *Fu Ping* (Herba Spirodelae Polyrrhizae), *Che Qian Zi* (Semen Plantaginis), and *Dong Gua Pi* (Epicarpium Benincasae Hispidae) were added.
4. For cough and hoarse voice, *Jie Geng* (Radix Platycodi Grandiflori) and *Mu Hu Die* (Semen Oroxyli Indici) were added.
5. For swollen boils, *Ye Ju Hua* (Flos Chrysanthemi Indici) and *Zi Hua Di Ding* (Herba Violae Yedoensitis) were added.

The temperature returned to normal within two to three days of taking the decoction. The lesions resolved within seven to ten days.

Small vessel vasculitis
小血管血管炎

Vasculitis is inflammation of the blood vessel walls. It may be either a cutaneous phenomenon or part of a systemic disorder. Clinical manifestations depend on the size of the blood vessels affected and whether other organs are damaged. Small vessel vasculitis includes hypersensitivity vasculitis and anaphylactoid purpura (also known as Henoch-Schönlein purpura).

Hypersensitivity vasculitis is a serious condition with a high mortality. It shares various characteristics with polyarteritis nodosa, but presents with disseminated or diffuse vasculitis. Pathological changes mainly involve the small veins and arteries and the capillaries; this serves as a means for differentiating this type of vasculitis from polyarteritis nodosa, which involves medium muscular arteries, and from other types of vasculitis involving the large vessels. The clinical manifestations are caused by multiple-system pathological changes due to generalized microvessel infarction and hemorrhage. The renal, central nervous, pulmonary, musculoskeletal, and cardiac systems and the gastrointestinal tract may be involved.

Anaphylactoid purpura is a non-thrombocytopenic purpura occurring mainly in children under the age of 11, and is often preceded by a streptococcal or viral upper respiratory tract infection. It is a self-limiting and benign condition with an excellent long-term prognosis, although recurrences are possible. It is usually associated with other allergic manifestations such as urticaria, erythema, abdominal pain, hematuria, asthma, and acute arthralgia.

After consulting medical classics of past dynasties, Jiang Chunhua, a contemporary physician, put hypersensitivity vasculitis and anaphylactoid purpura into the category of *zi ban bing* (purple macule [purpura] disease) in TCM. However, other modern medical works also classify *pu tao yi* (grape epidemic, or hemorrhagic disease with purpura), recorded in *Wai Ke Qi Xuan* [Revelations of the Mystery of External Diseases], as anaphylactoid purpura.

The earliest description of a condition similar to *zi ban bing* (purple macule disease) has been found in *Jin Kui Yao Lue: Bai He Hu Huo Yin Yang Du Bing Mai Zheng Zhi* [Synopsis of Prescriptions from the Golden Cabinet: Pulse, Signs and Treatment of Lily Disease, Hu Huo Syndrome[iii] and Diseases Caused by Yin Yang Toxins[iv]].

Later medical classics such as *Zhu Bing Yuan Hou Lun* [A General Treatise on the Causes and Symptoms of Diseases], *Dan Xi Shou Jing* [Danxi's Handy Mirror] and *Yi Xue Ru Men* [Elementary Medicine] classified purple macular eruptions into different categories such as eruptions due to Warmth and Heat, internal injury, Toxins, Yang patterns, and Yin patterns; they also presented a detailed explanation of etiology and treatment, giving much useful clinical experience.

Clinical manifestations

Hypersensitivity vasculitis

- Fever and joint pain are the most common prodromal symptoms.

- Lesions usually manifest as painful, palpable purpura, but can also present as urticaria, papules, petechiae, nodules, or necrotic ulceration; they are generally pruritic.

- Skin eruptions usually appear at varying intervals as localized clusters of cutaneous hemorrhage on the lower limbs, or on the buttocks and flanks in bedridden patients. Individual lesions fade after one to four weeks, leaving pigmentation or atrophic scarring. Lesions vary in size from one millimeter to several centimeters and may resemble the annular lesions of erythema multiforme. Some lesions may enlarge to form painful nodules. Vesicles or bullae may be present in severe cases. Recurrence is possible.

- Abdominal pain is a common accompanying symptom. Nausea, vomiting, diarrhea, or melena (tarry stools) may also occur. Gastrointestinal hemorrhage is present in almost all patients; transfusion may be required if there is significant blood loss.

- Involvement of the kidneys may cause hypertension, acute glomerulonephritis, renal malfunction, and uremia. It is common to see microsopic hematuria and even macroscopic hematuria in cases of renal damage.

- Pulmonary involvement may exhibit no features other than radiological evidence of nodules or diffuse infiltrative lesions. In some cases, however, asthmatic symptoms, pleuritic pain or hemoptysis may occur.

[iii] A syndrome characterized by ulceration of the throat, anus and genitals, accompanied by mental confusion, uneasiness and restlessness.

[iv] The main manifestations of this condition include dark red macules on the face, generalized pain and sore throat.

- Arthralgia is a common symptom for most patients, but few suffer from obvious bursal synovitis. X-ray examination will not reveal any apparent bone erosion or joint deformity.
- Heart disorders such as pericarditis and myocarditis may be present; these may cause arrhythmias and may even be fatal in severe cases.
- Involvement of the central nervous system may lead to headache, diplopia, numbness, or hypoesthesia.
- *Serum sickness-like prodrome of acute infective hepatitis:* Some 10-20 percent of patients may develop acute viral hepatitis. Skin eruptions, urticaria and flitting polyarthritis occur during the incubation period one to six weeks prior to the appearance of jaundice. Acute arthritis is occasionally seen.

Anaphylactoid purpura

- Although this disease is seen most often in children, especially those in the 2-11 age range, it may occur in people of any age.
- Attacks usually follow viral or streptococcal upper respiratory tract infection in spring and may affect the skin, the joints, the kidneys, and the gastrointestinal tract.
- About 80 percent of patients exhibit the classic triad of palpable non-thrombocytopenic purpura, arthritis and abdominal pain.
- Skin eruptions usually occur on the buttocks and lower limbs, but may also spread to the arms. Lesions manifest as crops of 2-10 mm purpura which may coalesce.
- Ankles and knee joints are often involved with local swelling, a sensation of heat and tenderness. Arthritis is temporary in most cases.
- Gastrointestinal involvement may lead to severe cramping abdominal pain, intussusception, hemorrhage, protein-losing enteropathy, and occasionally perforation.
- About half of patients have renal problems manifesting as hematuria and proteinuria accompanied by swelling of the eyelids and lower limbs. Most renal involvement is mild, but may occasionally progress to renal failure.

Etiology and pathology

The external causes of this disease include Wind, Heat and Damp; the main internal factors relate to the Spleen. Both internal and external factors can result in the Blood not circulating in the vessels, but spilling into the external vessels, congealing in the skin and flesh and presenting as purpura. If the Zang-Fu organs are involved, there will be abdominal pain and blood in the stool and urine.

Exuberant Blood-Heat
External contraction of Wind-Heat or congenital sensitivity to drug Toxins damages the Ying and Xue levels, thus causing the frenetic movement of Blood-Heat. Exuberant Heat in the Xue level gives rise to purpura, with new lesions replacing old lesions as they fade. If Heat congests in the throat, this will result in sore throat.

Obstruction by Damp-Heat
When Damp-Heat invades the body, it usually fights with Qi and Blood, leading to Blood-Heat and damage to the Blood vessels. Consequently, the Blood spills outward to the skin and flesh, and Damp-Heat accumulates internally to obstruct the Stomach and Intestines.

Effulgent Yin Deficiency-Fire
Blood-Heat due to constitutional Yin Deficiency results in the internal stirring of Deficiency-Fire. Heat damages the Blood vessels and forces the Blood to leave the channels. As a result, Blood permeates into the skin and flesh and manifests as purpura.

Breakdown of the Spleen's control and containment function
The Spleen is the source of the transformation of Qi and Blood and functions to keep the Blood circulating inside the vessels. Underlying Deficiency of Spleen Qi, or excessive thought and preoccupation or improper diet damaging the Spleen means that the Spleen is Deficient and cannot control the Blood. Constitutional Deficiency or overwork or overstrain damaging Qi means that Qi is Deficient and cannot contain the Blood. When the control and containment function breaks down, the Blood does not remain in the channels and spills to the exterior, resulting in purpura.

Yang Deficiency of the Spleen and Kidneys
Fire cannot generate Earth with the result that the transportation and transformation function is impaired. Since Spleen Yang is Deficient, the Spleen cannot control the Blood, which overflows to produce purpura.

Pattern identification and treatment

INTERNAL TREATMENT

EXUBERANT BLOOD-HEAT
This pattern manifests as bright red lesions that subsequently gradually turn purple and do not blanch on pressure. Lesions are densely distributed, with crops appearing and disappearing regularly. Accompanying symptoms and signs include itching, or swollen and

painful joints. The tongue body is red with a thin yellow coating; the pulse is floating and rapid.

Treatment principle
Clear Heat, cool the Blood and dispel Wind, transform purpura and relieve Toxicity.

Prescription
XIAO BAN QING DAI SAN JIA JIAN
Indigo Powder for Dispersing Macules, with modifications

Qing Dai (Indigo Naturalis) 10g
Xuan Shen (Radix Scrophulariae Ningpoensis) 10g
Nan Sha Shen (Radix Adenophorae) 10g
Chai Hu (Radix Bupleuri) 10g
Zhi Mu (Rhizoma Anemarrhenae Asphodeloidis) 6g
Huang Lian (Rhizoma Coptidis) 6g
Gan Cao (Radix Glycyrrhizae) 6g
Lian Zi Xin (Plumula Nelumbinis Nuciferae) 6g
Shi Gao‡ (Gypsum Fibrosum) 15g
Sheng Di Huang (Radix Rehmanniae Glutinosae) 15g
Chao Niu Bang Zi (Fructus Arctii Lappae, stir-fried) 12g
Jing Jie (Herba Schizonepetae Tenuifoliae) 12g
Lü Dou Yi (Testa Phaseoli Radiati) 30g

Explanation
• *Qing Dai* (Indigo Naturalis), *Huang Lian* (Rhizoma Coptidis) and *Shi Gao*‡ (Gypsum Fibrosum) clear Heat from the Qi level and relieve Toxicity.
• *Xuan Shen* (Radix Scrophulariae Ningpoensis), *Nan Sha Shen* (Radix Adenophorae), *Sheng Di Huang* (Radix Rehmanniae Glutinosae), and *Zhi Mu* (Rhizoma Anemarrhenae Asphodeloidis) nourish Yin and clear Heat, cool the Ying level and protect Body Fluids.
• *Chai Hu* (Radix Bupleuri), *Chao Niu Bang Zi* (Fructus Arctii Lappae, stir-fried) and *Jing Jie* (Herba Schizonepetae Tenuifoliae) dissipate Wind and thrust pathogenic factors outward.
• *Lian Zi Xin* (Plumula Nelumbinis Nuciferae) and *Lü Dou Yi* (Testa Phaseoli Radiati) clear Heat from the Heart and relieve Toxicity, cool the Blood and reduce purpura.
• *Gan Cao* (Radix Glycyrrhizae) harmonizes the effects of the other ingredients.

OBSTRUCTION BY DAMP-HEAT
In this pattern, purpura is usually seen on the lower limbs, with dark purple hemorrhagic blisters and erosions often occurring in purpuric areas. Accompanying symptoms and signs include intense abdominal pain with bloody or black stool and swollen ankles in serious cases, or abdominal distension and slight pain with poor appetite and nausea and vomiting in mild cases. The tongue body is red or purple with a yellow and greasy coating; the pulse is soggy and rapid.

Treatment principle
Clear Heat and transform Dampness, invigorate the Blood and free the network vessels.

Prescription
SAN REN TANG, SHAO YAO GAN CAO TANG, SHI XIAO SAN HE FANG HUA CAI
Combined Formula of Three Kernels Decoction, Peony and Licorice Decoction and Sudden Smile Powder, with variations

Yi Yi Ren (Semen Coicis Lachryma-jobi) 15g
Hua Shi‡ (Talcum) 15g, wrapped
Chi Shao (Radix Paeoniae Rubra) 10g
Xing Ren (Semen Pruni Armeniacae) 10g
Pu Huang Tan (Pollen Typhae Carbonisatum) 10g
Gan Cao (Radix Glycyrrhizae) 10g
Tong Cao (Medulla Tetrapanacis Papyriferi) 6g
Dan Zhu Ye (Herba Lophatheri Gracilis) 6g
Bai Mao Gen (Rhizoma Imperatae Cylindricae) 30g
Chi Xiao Dou (Semen Phaseoli Calcarati) 30g
Mu Dan Pi (Cortex Moutan Radicis) 12g
Zi Cao (Radix Arnebiae seu Lithospermi) 12g

Explanation
• *Yi Yi Ren* (Semen Coicis Lachryma-jobi), *Hua Shi*‡ (Talcum), *Tong Cao* (Medulla Tetrapanacis Papyriferi), and *Dan Zhu Ye* (Herba Lophatheri Gracilis) clear Heat and transform Dampness.
• *Bai Mao Gen* (Rhizoma Imperatae Cylindricae), *Zi Cao* (Radix Arnebiae seu Lithospermi), *Mu Dan Pi* (Cortex Moutan Radicis), *Chi Shao* (Radix Paeoniae Rubra), and *Chi Xiao Dou* (Semen Phaseoli Calcarati) cool and invigorate the Blood, transform purpura and disperse swelling.
• *Gan Cao* (Radix Glycyrrhizae) and *Pu Huang Tan* (Pollen Typhae Carbonisatum) clear Heat and relieve Toxicity, transform Blood stasis and stop bleeding.
• *Xing Ren* (Semen Pruni Armeniacae) moistens the Intestines and frees the bowels.

EFFULGENT YIN DEFICIENCY-FIRE
Lesions manifest as constantly recurring dull purple patches with a scattered distribution. Accompanying symptoms and signs include irritability and restlessness due to Deficiency-Heat, reddening of the face, limpness and aching in the lower back and knees, hematuria, and proteinuria. The tongue body is red with a scant coating; the pulse is thready and rapid.

Treatment principle
Nourish Yin and clear Heat, bear Fire downward and stop bleeding.

Prescription
LIU WEI DI HUANG TANG JIA JIAN
Six-Ingredient Rehmannia Decoction, with modifications

Sheng Di Huang (Radix Rehmanniae Glutinosae) 12g
Chao Mu Dan Pi (Cortex Moutan Radicis, stir-fried) 12g
Xuan Shen (Radix Scrophulariae Ningpoensis) 12g
Da Ji (Herba seu Radix Cirsii Japonici) 12g
Xiao Ji (Herba Cephalanoploris seu Cirsii) 12g
Shan Yao (Radix Dioscoreae Oppositae) 30g
Bai Mao Gen (Rhizoma Imperatae Cylindricae) 30g
Fu Ling (Sclerotium Poriae Cocos) 15g
*Gui Ban** (Plastrum Testudinis) 15g, decocted for 30 minutes before adding the other ingredients
Gou Qi Zi (Fructus Lycii) 15g
Zi Cao (Radix Arnebiae seu Lithospermi) 15g
Ze Xie (Rhizoma Alismatis Orientalis) 15g

Explanation
- *Sheng Di Huang* (Radix Rehmanniae Glutinosae), *Chao Mu Dan Pi* (Cortex Moutan Radicis), *Shan Yao* (Radix Dioscoreae Oppositae), *Gou Qi Zi* (Fructus Lycii), and *Gui Ban** (Plastrum Testudinis) nourish Yin and clear Heat.
- *Da Ji* (Herba seu Radix Cirsii Japonici), *Xiao Ji* (Herba Cephalanoploris seu Cirsii), *Bai Mao Gen* (Rhizoma Imperatae Cylindricae), and *Zi Cao* (Radix Arnebiae seu Lithospermi) cool the Blood and stop bleeding.
- *Ze Xie* (Rhizoma Alismatis Orientalis) and *Xuan Shen* (Radix Scrophulariae Ningpoensis) enrich Yin and bear Fire downward; when Fire is eliminated, Blood will be calmed.
- *Fu Ling* (Sclerotium Poriae Cocos) quiets the Heart and Spirit.

BREAKDOWN OF THE SPLEEN'S CONTROL AND CONTAINMENT FUNCTION
In this pattern, the disease progresses slowly. Light or dark purpuric patches that do not blanch on pressure recur constantly over long periods. Accompanying symptoms and signs include abdominal distension, loose stools, nausea, poor appetite, a sallow yellow complexion or facial puffiness, spontaneous sweating, shortness of breath, listlessness, lassitude, palpitations, dizziness, blurred vision, and pale lips. The tongue body is pale with a scant coating; the pulse is deficient and thready.

Treatment principle
Fortify the Spleen and augment Qi to contain the Blood and stop bleeding.

Prescription
GUI PI TANG JIA JIAN
Decoction for Restoring the Spleen, with modifications

Dang Shen (Radix Codonopsitis Pilosulae) 15g

Zhi Huang Qi (Radix Astragali seu Hedysari, mix-fried with honey) 15g
Fu Shen (Sclerotium Poriae Cocos cum Ligno Hospite) 15g
Shu Di Huang (Radix Rehmanniae Glutinosae Conquita) 15g
Dang Gui (Radix Angelicae Sinensis) 10g
Chao Bai Shao (Radix Paeoniae Lactiflorae, stir-fried) 10g
Bai Zhu (Rhizoma Atractylodis Macrocephalae) 10g
Zhi Gan Cao (Radix Glycyrrhizae, mix-fried with honey) 10g
Long Yan Rou (Arillus Euphoriae Longanae) 12g
*Mu Xiang** (Radix Aucklandiae Lappae) 6g
E Jiao‡ (Gelatinum Corii Asini) 12g, dissolved in the prepared decoction

Explanation
- *Zhi Huang Qi* (Radix Astragali seu Hedysari, mix-fried with honey), *Dang Shen* (Radix Codonopsitis Pilosulae), *Dang Gui* (Radix Angelicae Sinensis), *Chao Bai Shao* (Radix Paeoniae Lactiflorae, stir-fried), *Bai Zhu* (Rhizoma Atractylodis Macrocephalae), *Shu Di Huang* (Radix Rehmanniae Glutinosae Conquita), *Zhi Gan Cao* (Radix Glycyrrhizae, mix-fried with honey), *Fu Shen* (Sclerotium Poriae Cocos cum Ligno Hospite), and *E Jiao* ‡ (Gelatinum Corii Asini) fortify the Spleen and augment Qi to contain the Blood and stop bleeding.
- *Long Yan Rou* (Arillus Euphoriae Longanae) strengthens the Heart with warmth and sweetness.
- *Mu Xiang** (Radix Aucklandiae Lappae) regulates Qi and prevents congestion caused by supplementing ingredients.

YANG DEFICIENCY OF THE SPLEEN AND KIDNEYS
This pattern has a slow onset and prolonged course. Lesions manifest as pale purple plaques that are cold to the touch and worsen on exposure to cold. Accompanying symptoms and signs include a pallid or dull purple complexion, dizziness, tinnitus, cold body and limbs, limpness and aching in the lower back and knees, poor appetite, loose stools, and abdominal pain that is relieved by pressure. The tongue body is pale or purplish with a scant coating; the pulse is thready and weak.

Treatment principle
Supplement the Kidneys and fortify the Spleen, warm Yang and contain the Blood.

Prescription
HUANG TU TANG JIA JIAN
Yellow Earth Decoction, with modifications

Zao Xin Tu (Terra Flava Usta) 45g, wrapped
Bai Zhu (Rhizoma Atractylodis Macrocephalae) 10g
Gan Cao (Radix Glycyrrhizae) 10g
E Jiao‡ (Gelatinum Corii Asini) 10g, dissolved in the prepared decoction

Fu Pen Zi (Fructus Rubi Chingii) 12g
Tu Si Zi (Semen Cuscutae) 12g
Xian He Cao (Herba Agrimoniae Pilosae) 12g
Huang Qin (Radix Scutellariae Baicalensis) 6g

Explanation

- *Fu Pen Zi* (Fructus Rubi Chingii), *Tu Si Zi* (Semen Cuscutae), *Zao Xin Tu* (Terra Flava Usta), and *Bai Zhu* (Rhizoma Atractylodis Macrocephalae) supplement the Kidneys and fortify the Spleen.
- *E Jiao* ‡ (Gelatinum Corii Asini), *Gan Cao* (Radix Glycyrrhizae) and *Xian He Cao* (Herba Agrimoniae Pilosae) warm Yang and contain the Blood.
- *Huang Qin* (Radix Scutellariae Baicalensis) clears Heat from the Lungs; once Heat is eliminated, purpura will be reduced.

General modifications

1. For high fever, add *Ling Yang Jiao** (Cornu Antelopis), *Shi Gao* ‡ (Gypsum Fibrosum), *Lü Dou Yi* (Testa Phaseoli Radiati), and *Gui Ban** (Plastrum Testudinis).
2. For swollen throat and nosebleed, add *Bei Dou Gen* (Rhizoma Menispermi), *Da Qing Ye* (Folium Isatidis seu Baphicacanthi), *Mai Men Dong* (Radix Ophiopogonis Japonici), *Nan Sha Shen* (Radix Adenophorae), and *Ma Bo* (Sclerotium Lasiosphaerae seu Calvatiae).
3. For red, swollen and painful joints, add *Gui Jian Yu* (Lignum Suberalatum Euonymi), *Qian Nian Jian* (Rhizoma Homalomenae), *Gou Ji* (Rhizoma Cibotii Barometz), *Hai Feng Teng* (Caulis Piperis Kadsurae), *Sang Zhi* (Ramulus Mori Albae), *Qin Jiao* (Radix Gentianae Macrophyllae), *Luo Shi Teng* (Caulis Trachelospermi Jasminoidis), and *Lao Guan Cao* (Herba Erodii seu Geranii).
4. For stubborn eruptions, add *Chi Xiao Dou* (Semen Phaseoli Calcarati), *Chun Pi* (Cortex Ailanthi Altissimae), *Zi Cao* (Radix Arnebiae seu Lithospermi), and *Zhi Mu* (Rhizoma Anemarrhenae Asphodeloidis).
5. For blood in the stool, add *Di Yu* (Radix Sanguisorbae Officinalis), *Huai Hua* (Flos Sophorae Japonicae) and *San Qi* (Radix Notoginseng).
6. For blood in the urine, add *Bai Mao Gen* (Rhizoma Imperatae Cylindricae), *Han Lian Cao* (Herba Ecliptae Prostratae) and *Xiao Ji* (Herba Cephalanoploris seu Cirsii).
7. For proteinuria, add *Yu Mi Xu* (Stylus Zeae Mays), *Lian Xu* (Stamen Nelumbinis Nuciferae), *Jin Ying Zi* (Fructus Rosae Laevigatae), *Qian Shi* (Semen Euryales Ferocis), and *Dong Gua Pi* (Epicarpium Benincasae Hispidae).
8. For abdominal pain, add *Yan Hu Suo* (Rhizoma Corydalis Yanhusuo), *Chuan Lian Zi* (Fructus Meliae Toosendan), *Mu Xiang** (Radix Aucklandiae Lappae), *Ru Xiang* (Gummi Olibanum), *Mo Yao* (Myrrha), *Chao Zhi Ke* (Fructus Citri Aurantii, stir-fried), and *Hou Po* (Cortex Magnoliae Officinalis).
9. For nausea and vomiting, add *Huang Lian* (Rhizoma Coptidis), *Jiang Ban Xia* (Rhizoma Pinelliae Ternatae, processed with ginger), *Zhu Ru* (Caulis Bambusae in Taeniis), and *Dao Dou Zi* (Semen Canavaliae).
10. For poor appetite, add *Sha Ren* (Fructus Amomi), *Ji Nei Jin* ‡ (Endothelium Corneum Gigeriae Galli) and *Jiao San Xian*, the scorch-fried combination of *Shan Zha* (Fructus Crataegi), *Shen Qu* (Massa Fermentata) and *Mai Ya* (Fructus Hordei Vulgaris Germinatus).
11. For Qi Deficiency, add *Huang Qi* (Radix Astragali seu Hedysari), *Dang Shen* (Radix Codonopsitis Pilosulae) and *Sheng Ma* (Rhizoma Cimicifugae).
12. For purple ecchymoses and a dull purple tongue, add powdered *San Qi* (Radix Notoginseng) or *Yun Nan Bai Yao* (Yunnan White).
13. For coma and delirium, add *Ling Yang Jiao Fen** (Cornu Antelopis, powdered) and *Shi Chang Pu* (Rhizoma Acori Graminei).

EMPIRICAL FORMULAE

- For Blood-Heat patterns, make a decoction with one of the following ingredients and take twice a day – *Da Zao* (Fructus Ziziphi Jujubae) 25g, *Lian Qiao* (Fructus Forsythiae Suspensae) 10g, *Gan Cao* (Radix Glycyrrhizae) 5g, or *Zi Zhu* (Folium Callicarpae) 5g.
- For frequent recurrence, use *Lei Gong Teng* (Radix Tripterygii Wilfordi) preparations:
  - Take 10ml three times a day of the syrup (each milliliter contains 1g of the crude herb).
  - Take 2-4 tablets three times a day (each tablet contains 3g of the crude herb).
  - **Caution:** Since *Lei Gong Teng* (Radix Tripterygii Wilfordi) is a toxic herb, it should not be taken if the white blood cell count is below 4.5×10^9/L.
- In the acute phase, take *Zi Cao* (Radix Arnebiae seu Lithospermi) extract in tablet form (equivalent to 4.5-6g a day of the crude herb) or decoct 24-30g of the crude herb and drink.

ACUPUNCTURE

Selection of points according to pattern identification

Points

- For Blood-Heat, select SP-10 Xuehai, SP-6 Sanyinjiao, LR-3 Taichong, and BL-40 Weizhong.
- For Spleen Deficiency, select BL-17 Geshu, BL-20 Pishu, SP-10 Xuehai, ST-36 Zusanli, and SP-6 Sanyinjiao.

Technique: Apply the reducing method for Excess patterns and the reinforcing method for Deficiency patterns.

After obtaining Qi, retain the needles for 5 minutes at BL-17 Geshu and BL-20 Pishu; then insert the needles perpendicularly at SP-10 Xuehai, ST-36 Zusanli, SP-6 Sanyinjiao, and LR-3 Taichong and retain for 30 minutes after obtaining Qi. BL-40 Weizhong is pricked to cause slight bleeding. Treat once every other day. A course consists of seven to ten treatment sessions.

Empirical points

Points: KI-1 Yongquan, EX-B-2 Jiaji T_7 and T_{11},[v] SP-6 Sanyinjiao, and SP-10 Xuehai.

Technique

- Needle KI-1 Yongquan with strong stimulation.
- Retain the needles in EX-B-2 Jiaji T_7 and T_{11} for five to eight minutes after obtaining Qi. After withdrawal, needle SP-6 Sanyinjiao and SP-10 Xuehai. Retain the needles for 30 minutes after obtaining Qi; manipulate them three times during this period. Apply the reinforcing method for Deficiency patterns and the reducing method for Excess patterns.
- Treat once a day for two weeks.

Explanation

- SP-10 Xuehai, LR-3 Taichong and BL-40 Weizhong cool the Blood and relieve Toxicity.
- BL-20 Pishu, ST-36 Zusanli and SP-6 Sanyinjiao supplement the Spleen to contain the Blood.
- BL-17 Geshu and EX-B-2 Jiaji T_7 and T_{11} transform Blood stasis and free the network vessels.

MOXIBUSTION

Points: BL-31 Shangliao, BL-32 Ciliao, BL-33 Zhongliao, BL-34 Xialiao, and GV-3 Yaoyangguan.

Technique: Place the patient in a prone position. To prevent scalds, apply some paraffin oil or Vaseline® to the points, cover with a piece of paper 7x7 cm square and place a slice of ginger about 0.25cm thick on the paper. Put a moxa cone 4cm in height and 6cm in diameter at the base on the ginger and ignite. The moxibustion points should feel warm throughout the 45-minute treatment session. Treat once a day. A course consists of seven treatment sessions.

EAR ACUPUNCTURE WITH SEEDS

Main points: Spleen, Liver and Stomach.

Auxiliary points: Lung, Mouth, Subcortex, and Triple Burner.

Technique: Attach *Wang Bu Liu Xing* (Semen Vaccariae Segetalis) seeds to the points with adhesive plaster. Ask the patient to press the points for one minute three to five times a day. Change the seeds every two days.

Clinical notes

- Blood-Heat patterns are commonly seen in the initial phase of this disease; the emphasis should therefore be placed on cooling the Blood and relieving Toxicity. However, for frequent recurrence, the treatment principle should focus on augmenting Qi and nourishing Yin, containing the Blood and reducing purpura. In the later stages, the Kidneys are often involved, and so stress should be placed on boosting the Kidneys and containing the Blood.
- As a general rule, recovery can be expected if attacks are triggered by external pathogenic factors, overeating of ginger and spicy food or drinking too much alcohol. In a minority of cases, the disease is prolonged, leading to effulgent Yin Deficiency-Fire or Qi failing to contain the Blood; in such cases, a cure will take much longer.

Advice for the patient

- Nourish Vital Qi (Zheng Qi), build up the body's strength and boost the body's defenses and immune levels by following a nutritious diet and exercising frequently.
- Take preventive measures to counteract invasion by the six pathogenic factors; avoid inducing factors such as drugs known to trigger the condition.
- Rest in bed or reduce physical activities in acute conditions or where bleeding is significant.
- Wear clothing appropriate to the weather conditions, follow a quieter lifestyle, avoid overwork and stress, and take precautions so as not to catch a cold.
- Avoid onions, ginger, garlic, chillis, mustard, and alcohol; reduce intake of fish, shellfish, milk and other food which may induce an attack or to which patients are hypersensitive.

Case history

Patient
Male, aged 24.

Clinical manifestations
One week previously, the patient had eaten too much stimulating food (prawns, shellfish and crabs) at a seaside picnic. Afterwards, he felt a slight swelling in the lower limbs accompanied by itching and found numerous small red papules on the legs. He then took chlorphenamine maleate for three days. However, the red papules did not disappear and the color

---

[v] M-BW-35 according to the system employed by the Shanghai College of Traditional Chinese Medicine.

gradually darkened. Accompanying symptoms and signs included a dry mouth, loose stools with three bowel movements a day, and irritability.

Examination revealed non-blanching purplish-red purpuric papules of varying sizes densely distributed bilaterally on the lower limbs from the feet to the thighs, being particularly obvious on the extensor surfaces. The lower limbs were slightly swollen. The tongue body was red with a thin yellow coating; the pulse was slippery and rapid. Routine blood and urine tests were normal.

Diagnosis

Anaphylactoid purpura (*pu tao yi*).

Pattern identification

Wind-Heat and Blood-Heat fighting, with Blood-Heat scorching the network vessels to cause the frenetic movement of Blood.

Treatment principle

Clear Heat and cool the Blood, invigorate the Blood to disperse purpura.

Prescription ingredients

Zi Cao (Radix Arnebiae seu Lithospermi) 15g
Qian Cao Gen (Radix Rubiae Cordifoliae) 15g
Bai Mao Gen (Rhizoma Imperatae Cylindricae) 30g
Ban Lan Gen (Radix Isatidis seu Baphicacanthi) 30g
Sheng Di Huang Tan (Radix Rehmanniae Glutinosae Carbonisata) 15g
Da Ji Tan (Herba seu Radix Cirsii Japonici Carbonisata) 15g
Xiao Ji Tan (Herba Cephalanoploris seu Cirsii Carbonisata) 15g
Jin Yin Hua Tan (Flos Lonicerae Carbonisata) 15g
Mu Dan Pi (Cortex Moutan Radicis) 15g
Che Qian Zi (Semen Plantaginis) 15g
Ze Xie (Rhizoma Alismatis Orientalis) 15g
Huai Niu Xi (Radix Achyranthis Bidentatae) 10g
Mu Gua (Fructus Chaenomelis) 10g
*Ling Yang Jiao Fen** (Cornu Antelopis, powdered) 0.6g, dissolved in the decoction

One bag a day was used to prepare a decoction, taken twice a day.

External application

Lu Hu Xi Ji (Calamine and Giant Knotweed Wash Preparation) was used to wash the affected area for 15 minutes once a day.

Second visit

After 14 bags of the decoction, the purplish-red color of the purpuric papules on the lower limbs had almost disappeared, and the swelling was significantly reduced. The stools were still loose and itching was slightly worse. The prescription was modified by adding *Bai Zhu* (Rhizoma Atractylodis Macrocephalae) 10g, *Fu Ling* (Sclerotium Poriae Cocos) 15g, *Bai Xian Pi* (Cortex Dictamni Dasycarpi Radicis) 30g, and *Ku Shen* (Radix Sophorae Flavescentis) 15g. The external wash continued as before.

Third visit

After 28 bags of the modified prescription, the lesions on the lower limbs had disappeared, as had the swelling. The stools

had returned to normal. Some pigmentation was left with slight itching. The tongue body was red with a white coating; the pulse was wiry and slippery. The patient was given a modified prescription.

Prescription ingredients

Zi Cao (Radix Arnebiae seu Lithospermi) 15g
Qian Cao Gen (Radix Rubiae Cordifoliae) 15g
Bai Mao Gen (Rhizoma Imperatae Cylindricae) 30g
Ban Lan Gen (Radix Isatidis seu Baphicacanthi) 30g
Xuan Shen (Radix Scrophulariae Ningpoensis) 15g
Chi Shao (Radix Paeoniae Rubra) 15g
Mu Dan Pi (Cortex Moutan Radicis) 15g
Bai Zhu (Rhizoma Atractylodis Macrocephalae) 10g
Fu Ling (Sclerotium Poriae Cocos) 15g
Bai Xian Pi (Cortex Dictamni Dasycarpi Radicis) 30g
Ku Shen (Radix Sophorae Flavescentis) 15g
Yi Yi Ren (Semen Coicis Lachryma-jobi) 30g
Huai Niu Xi (Radix Achyranthis Bidentatae) 10g
Mu Gua (Fructus Chaenomelis) 10g
San Qi Fen (Pulvis Radicis Notoginseng, powdered) 3g, dissolved in the prepared decoction
Dan Shen (Radix Salviae Miltiorrhizae) 15g

Fourteen bags were prescribed to consolidate the improvement. There was no external wash.

Discussion

This case had a rapid onset with symptoms such as red papules, irritability, dry mouth, a yellow tongue coating, and a slippery and rapid pulse. The pattern was therefore identified as Wind-Heat and Blood-Heat fighting. Blood-Heat exuberance causes the frenetic movement of Blood leading to Blood spilling out of the vessels and network vessels and then congealing, resulting in purpura.

The treatment principle of clearing Heat and cooling the Blood, and invigorating the Blood to disperse purpura was applied. In the prescription, *Sheng Di Huang Tan* (Radix Rehmanniae Glutinosae Carbonisata), *Da Ji Tan* (Herba seu Radix Cirsii Japonici Carbonisata), *Xiao Ji Tan* (Herba Cephalanoploris seu Cirsii Carbonisata), *Jin Yin Hua Tan* (Flos Lonicerae Carbonisata), and *Ban Lan Gen* (Radix Isatidis seu Baphicacanthi) clear Heat from the Blood, cool the Blood and stop bleeding; *Mu Dan Pi* (Cortex Moutan Radicis), *Zi Cao* (Radix Arnebiae seu Lithospermi), *Qian Cao Gen* (Radix Rubiae Cordifoliae), and *Bai Mao Gen* (Rhizoma Imperatae Cylindricae) cool and invigorate the Blood to stop bleeding, transform Blood stasis and disperse purpura; *Che Qian Zi* (Semen Plantaginis) and *Ze Xie* (Rhizoma Alismatis Orientalis) benefit the movement of water and disperse swelling; *Huai Niu Xi* (Radix Achyranthis Bidentatae) and *Mu Gua* (Fructus Chaenomelis) are channel conductors guiding the other materia medica downward; and *Ling Yang Jiao Fen** (Cornu Antelopis, powdered) strengthens the Heat-clearing effect.

The residual pigmentation resulted from Qi stagnation and Blood stasis, brought on by the length of the illness, which had weakened the patient's constitution. The addition of *Bai Zhu* (Rhizoma Atractylodis Macrocephalae), *Fu Ling* (Sclerotium Poriae Cocos), *Dan Shen* (Radix Salviae Miltiorrhizae), and *San Qi Fen* (Pulvis Radicis Notoginseng, powdered) therefore supplemented Qi in the Middle Burner, invigorated the Blood and transformed Blood stasis to disperse purpura. *Chi Shao* (Radix Paeoniae Rubra) and *Xuan Shen* (Radix Scrophulariae Ningpoensis) cooled the Blood, and *Bai Xian Pi* (Cortex Dictamni Dasycarpi Radicis), *Ku Shen* (Radix Sophorae Flavescentis) and *Yi Yi Ren* (Semen Coicis Lachryma-jobi) alleviated itching.

In treating this disease, it is important to remember that bleeding cannot be stopped without clearing Heat; the Blood will be calmed automatically if Heat is cleared. At same time, do not forget to regulate the Spleen to contain and control the Blood to treat the Root. [9]

Literature excerpts

Dan Xi Shou Jing [Danxi's Handy Mirror] states: "Purple macules are signs of intense Heat with a scorched black tongue and red face, and are caused by Yang Toxins. They are treated by *Yang Du Sheng Ma Tang* (Bugbane Decoction for Yang Toxins) and *Bai Hu Jia Ren Shen Tang* (White Tiger Decoction Plus Ginseng)."

In *Wai Ke Zheng Zong* [An Orthodox Manual of External Diseases], it says: "*Pu tao yi* (grape epidemic) is often seen in children if they are affected by untimely seasonal pathogenic factors, which are retained in the skin and form bluish-purple, grape-like macules on the body. Treatment at the initial stage should follow the principle of clearing Heat and cooling the Blood with *Ling Yang Jiao San* (Antelope Horn Powder); in the later stages, enrich and boost the interior with *Gui Pi Tang* (Decoction for Restoring the Spleen)."

Modern clinical experience

TREATMENT BASED ON PATTERN IDENTIFICATION
Li identified three patterns. [10]

- **Effulgent Yin Deficiency-Fire**

Prescription
LIU WEI DI HUANG TANG JIA JIAN
Six-Ingredient Rehmannia Decoction, with modifications

or

XI JIAO DI HUANG TANG HE DA BU YIN WAN JIA JIAN
Rhinoceros Horn and Rehmannia Decoction Combined With Major Yin Supplementation Pill, with modifications

Sheng Di Huang (Radix Rehmanniae Glutinosae) 15g
Shan Yao (Radix Dioscoreae Oppositae) 15g
Qian Cao Gen (Radix Rubiae Cordifoliae) 15g
Zi Cao (Radix Arnebiae seu Lithospermi) 15g

Xian He Cao (Herba Agrimoniae Pilosae) 6g
Huang Bai (Cortex Phellodendri) 10g
Zhi Mu (Rhizoma Anemarrhenae Asphodeloidis) 10g
Ce Bai Ye (Cacumen Biotae Orientalis) 10g
Mu Dan Pi (Cortex Moutan Radicis) 10g
Gui Ban* (Plastrum Testudinis) 15g

- **Heat forcing spillage of Blood**

Prescription
XI JIAO DI HUANG TANG
Rhinoceros Horn and Rehmannia Decoction, supported by *Yu Nü Jian* (Jade Lady Brew), *Qing Ying Tang* (Decoction for Clearing Heat from the Ying level) and *Da Bu Yin Wan* (Major Yin Supplementation Pill)

Shui Niu Jiao‡ (Cornu Bubali) 15g
Sheng Di Huang (Radix Rehmanniae Glutinosae) 10g
Mu Dan Pi (Cortex Moutan Radicis) 10g
Zi Cao (Radix Arnebiae seu Lithospermi) 15g
Xiao Ji (Herba Cephalanoploris seu Cirsii) 15g
Jin Yin Hua (Flos Lonicerae) 15g
Lian Qiao (Fructus Forsythiae Suspensae) 10g
Huai Hua (Flos Sophorae Japonicae) 15g
Chi Shao (Radix Paeoniae Rubra) 10g
Qian Cao Gen (Radix Rubiae Cordifoliae) 15g

- **Qi failing to contain the Blood**

Prescription
SI JUN ZI TANG JIA JIAN
Four Gentlemen Decoction, with modifications

Dang Shen (Radix Codonopsitis Pilosulae) 10g
Fu Ling (Sclerotium Poriae Cocos) 10g
Bai Zhu (Rhizoma Atractylodis Macrocephalae) 10g
Qu Mai (Herba Dianthi) 10g
Dang Gui (Radix Angelicae Sinensis) 10g
Chuan Xiong (Rhizoma Ligustici Chuanxiong) 10g
Bai Zhi (Radix Angelicae Dahuricae) 6g
Ting Li Zi (Semen Lepidii seu Descurainiae) 6g
Chen Pi (Pericarpium Citri Reticulatae) 6g
Da Fu Pi (Pericarpium Arecae Catechu) 6g

One bag a day was used to prepare a decoction, taken twice a day. Results were seen on average after 35 days (range: 11 to 86 days).

TREATMENT BASED ON DISEASE DIFFERENTIATION
Kong based his treatment on disease differentiation. [11]

Cutaneous purpura
Since, in the author's opinion, external Wind was another causative factor in addition to Heat Toxins, prescriptions for clearing Heat and cooling the Blood need to be modified by adding ingredients for dispelling

Wind such as *Fang Feng* (Radix Ledebouriellae Divaricatae), *Chan Tui*‡ (Periostracum Cicadae) and *Bai Ji Li* (Fructus Tribuli Terrestris).

Damage to the joints
In terms of pathology, damage to the joints in this disease is caused by Wind, Heat, Damp, or Blood stasis obstructing the channels and network vessels. Therefore, it is necessary to modify standard prescriptions such as those described in the treatment section above by adding ingredients such as *Qin Jiao* (Radix Gentianae Macrophyllae), *Wei Ling Xian* (Radix Clematidis) and *Ren Dong Teng* (Caulis Lonicerae Japonicae) to dispel Wind, clear Heat, overcome Dampness, and free the network vessels.

Digestive tract hemorrhage
This manifestation is generally associated with three factors: exuberant Fire causing the frenetic movement of Blood, Qi Deficiency leading to failure to store and control the Blood properly, and Blood stasis obstructing the vessels, thus causing the Blood to flow outside the channels. In this type of condition, the first step is to stop bleeding; the cause of the bleeding must then be established and appropriate treatment given. The prescription should include ingredients to cool the Blood, transform Blood stasis and stop bleeding such as *Sheng Di Huang* (Radix Rehmanniae Glutinosae), *Mu Dan Pi* (Cortex Moutan Radicis), *Chi Shao* (Radix Paeoniae Rubra), and *San Qi* (Radix Notoginseng).

Damage to the Kidneys
Kidney damage can be subdivided into four patterns:
* Wind-Heat complicated by Blood stasis, treated by dispelling Wind, cooling the Blood, transforming Blood stasis, and stopping bleeding.
* Wind-Damp-Heat complicated by Blood stasis, also treated by dispelling Wind, cooling the Blood, transforming Blood stasis, and stopping bleeding, but with the addition of some Heat-clearing ingredients such as *Huang Qin* (Radix Scutellariae Baicalensis) and *Huang Bai* (Cortex Phellodendri).
* Kidney Deficiency and Blood-Heat, treated by supplementing the Kidneys and cooling the Blood.
* Spleen and Kidney Deficiency, treated by supplementing the Kidneys and fortifying the Spleen.

SPECIAL PRESCRIPTIONS

1. **Zhang** formulated a basic prescription with modifications to treat anaphylactoid purpura. [12]

Treatment principle
Clear Heat and relieve Toxicity, cool the Blood and free the network vessels.

Prescription
HUA SHE XIAO DIAN TANG
Long-Noded Pit Viper Decoction for Dispersing Purpura

Qi She‡ (Agkistrodon) 5-10g
Chan Tui‡ (Periostracum Cicadae) 10g
Mu Dan Pi (Cortex Moutan Radicis) 10g
Fang Feng (Radix Ledebouriellae Divaricatae) 10g
Niu Xi (Radix Achyranthis Bidentatae) 10g
Sheng Di Huang (Radix Rehmanniae Glutinosae) 15g
Dan Shen (Radix Salviae Miltiorrhizae) 15g
Gan Cao (Radix Glycyrrhizae) 6g

Modifications
1. For severe abdominal pain, *Bai Shao* (Radix Paeoniae Lactiflorae) 10g and *Yan Hu Suo* (Rhizoma Corydalis Yanhusuo) 10g were added.
2. For blood in the urine, *Bai Mao Gen* (Rhizoma Imperatae Cylindricae) 30g, *Da Ji* (Herba seu Radix Cirsii Japonici) 15g and *Xiao Ji* (Herba Cephalanoploris seu Cirsii) 15g were added.
3. For blood in the stool, *Chao Huai Hua* (Flos Sophorae Japonicae, stir-fried) 30g and *Di Yu* (Radix Sanguisorbae Officinalis) 15g were added.
4. For swollen and painful joints, *Qin Jiao* (Radix Gentianae Macrophyllae) 15g and *Ren Dong Teng* (Caulis Lonicerae Japonicae) 30g were added.
5. For Qi and Blood Deficiency, *Huang Qi* (Radix Astragali seu Hedysari) 30g, *Dang Shen* (Radix Codonopsitis Pilosulae) 10g and *Da Zao* (Fructus Ziziphi Jujubae) 15g were added.
6. For effulgent Yin Deficiency-Fire, *Zhi Mu* (Rhizoma Anemarrhenae Asphodeloidis) 10g and *Huang Bai* (Cortex Phellodendri) 10g were added.
7. For exuberant Heat Toxins, *Jin Yin Hua* (Flos Lonicerae) 15g and *Shi Gao*‡ (Gypsum Fibrosum) 30g were added.

One bag a day was used to prepare a decoction, taken twice a day. A course of treatment lasted ten days. Results were generally seen after three courses.

2. **Zhu** treated this disease with a special formulation. [13]

Prescription
TUO MIN JIAN
Desensitization Brew

Yin Chai Hu (Radix Stellariae Dichotomae) 10-15g
Wu Mei (Fructus Pruni Mume) 10-15g
Wu Wei Zi (Fructus Schisandrae) 10-15g
Fang Feng (Radix Ledebouriellae Divaricatae) 6-10g

Modifications
1. Where the skin only was involved:
* For small, bright red, sparsely distributed eruptions accompanied by Wind-Heat exterior patterns, *Chan*

Tui ‡ (Periostracum Cicadae) 10g, *Jin Yin Hua* (Flos Lonicerae) 10g and *Lian Qiao* (Fructus Forsythiae Suspensae) 10g were added.

- For extensive eruptions in large patches accompanied by Blood-Heat patterns, *Sheng Di Huang* (Radix Rehmanniae Glutinosae) 15g, *Xuan Shen* (Radix Scrophulariae Ningpoensis) 15g, *Mu Dan Pi* (Cortex Moutan Radicis) 10g, *Chi Shao* (Radix Paeoniae Rubra) 12g, and *Zi Cao* (Radix Arnebiae seu Lithospermi) 30g were added.

2. For involvement of the joints, *Ren Dong Teng* (Caulis Lonicerae Japonicae) 15g, *Tong Cao* (Medulla Tetrapanacis Papyriferi) 15g and *Mu Gua* (Fructus Chaenomelis) 15g were added.

3. Abdominal patterns:

- For blood in the stool, *Xian He Cao* (Herba Agrimoniae Pilosae) 30g, *Di Yu* (Radix Sanguisorbae Officinalis) 15g and *Chao Huai Hua* (Flos Sophorae Japonicae, stir-fried) 15g were added.

- For abdominal pain, *Bai Shao* (Radix Paeoniae Lactiflorae) 30g and *Yan Hu Suo* (Rhizoma Corydalis Yanhusuo) 12g were added.

4. For involvement of the kidneys, where the patient was diagnosed with purpuric nephritis complicated by hematuria, *Da Ji* (Herba seu Radix Cirsii Japonici) 15g, *Xiao Ji* (Herba Cephalanoploris seu Cirsii) 15g, *Han Lian Cao* (Herba Ecliptae Prostratae) 15g, and *Bai Mao Gen* (Rhizoma Imperatae Cylindricae) 30g were added.

One bag a day was used to prepare a decoction, taken twice a day. Initial results were seen after two weeks.

3. **Zhang** followed the treatment principle of invigorating and cooling the Blood. [14]

Prescription ingredients

Qing Dai (Indigo Naturalis) 5g
Mu Dan Pi (Cortex Moutan Radicis) 10g
Chuan Xiong (Rhizoma Ligustici Chuanxiong) 10g
Zi Su Ye (Folium Perillae Frutescentis) 10g
Zi Cao (Radix Arnebiae seu Lithospermi) 10g
Dan Shen (Radix Salviae Miltiorrhizae) 20g
Sheng Di Huang (Radix Rehmanniae Glutinosae) 20g
Bai Mao Gen (Rhizoma Imperatae Cylindricae) 20g
Dang Gui (Radix Angelicae Sinensis) 15g
Chi Shao (Radix Paeoniae Rubra) 15g
Yi Mu Cao (Herba Leonuri Heterophylli) 15g
He Ye (Folium Nelumbinis Nuciferae) 6g

Modifications

1. For abdominal pain, *Bai Shao* (Radix Paeoniae Lactiflorae) 30g and *Gan Cao* (Radix Glycyrrhizae) 10g were added.
2. For painful joints, *Qin Jiao* (Radix Gentianae Macro-

phyllae) 12g and *Fang Feng* (Radix Ledebouriellae Divaricatae) 10g were added.

3. For Qi Deficiency, *Huang Qi* (Radix Astragali seu Hedysari) 20g and *Dang Shen* (Radix Codonopsitis Pilosulae) 20g were added.

One bag a day was used to prepare a decoction, taken twice a day. Results were seen after three weeks.

4. **Xu** modified *Xie Huang San* (Yellow-Draining Powder) to treat anaphylactoid purpura. [15]

Prescription
XIE HUANG SAN
Yellow-Draining Powder

Shi Gao ‡ (Gypsum Fibrosum) 10-15g
Zhi Zi (Fructus Gardeniae Jasminoidis) 10-15g
Huo Xiang (Herba Agastaches seu Pogostemi) 10-15g
Fang Feng (Radix Ledebouriellae Divaricatae) 10-15g
Zi Cao (Radix Arnebiae seu Lithospermi) 10-15g
Sheng Di Huang (Radix Rehmanniae Glutinosae) 20-25g
Da Huang (Radix et Rhizoma Rhei) 3-6g

Modifications

1. For exuberant Heat, *Da Huang* (Radix et Rhizoma Rhei) was added 10 minutes before the end of the decoction process.
2. For bright red purpura, accompanied by nosebleed or bleeding gums, *Da Huang Tan* (Radix et Rhizoma Rhei Carbonisatae) was used.
3. For dark purpura with frequent recurrence and long duration, *Jiu Zhi Da Huang* (Radix et Rhizoma Rhei, mix-fried with wine) was used.
4. For densely distributed, confluent purpura, *Mu Dan Pi* (Cortex Moutan Radicis) was added.
5. For raised, itchy purpura, *Qin Jiao* (Radix Gentianae Macrophyllae) and *Jing Jie* (Herba Schizonepetae Tenuifoliae) were added.
6. For swelling on the dorsum of the hands and feet, *Bai Mao Gen* (Rhizoma Imperatae Cylindricae) and *Che Qian Cao* (Herba Plantaginis) were added.
7. For swollen limb joints, *Chuan Niu Xi* (Radix Cyathulae Officinalis) and *Ji Xue Teng* (Caulis Spatholobi) were added.
8. For stabbing pain in the abdomen, *Shi Xiao San* (Sudden Smile Powder) was added.
9. For blood in the urine, *Bai Mao Gen* (Rhizoma Imperatae Cylindricae) and *Xian He Cao* (Herba Agrimoniae Pilosae) were added to the prescription; powdered *Hu Po* (Succinum) 0.5-1g and powdered *San Qi* (Radix Notoginseng) 1-3g were taken as an infusion.
10. For proteinuria, *Yi Mu Cao* (Herba Leonuri Heterophylli) and *Shi Gao* ‡ (Gypsum Fibrosum) were added.

One bag a day was used to prepare a decoction, taken twice a day. Results were seen within a range of 5 to 60 days.

5. **Wang** reported on the treatment of 120 cases of anaphylactoid purpura. [16]

Prescription
QING DAI YIN
Indigo Beverage

Qing Dai (Indigo Naturalis) 3g
Zi Cao (Radix Arnebiae seu Lithospermi) 9g
Bai Ji (Rhizoma Bletillae Striatae) 9g
Ru Xiang (Gummi Olibanum) 6g

Modifications
1. For mild purpura accompanied by an exterior pattern, *Jin Yin Hua* (Flos Lonicerae), *Ban Lan Gen* (Radix Isatidis seu Baphicacanthi), *Bai Zhi* (Radix Angelicae Dahuricae), and *Jiao Shan Zha* (Fructus Crataegi, scorch-fried) were added.
2. For Heat patterns in the Qi and Ying levels, *Ru Xiang* (Gummi Olibanum) was removed, and *Mu Dan Pi* (Cortex Moutan Radicis), *Xuan Shen* (Radix Scrophulariae Ningpoensis) and *Sheng Di Huang* (Radix Rehmanniae Glutinosae) were added.
3. For involvement of the joints, *Gou Teng* (Ramulus Uncariae cum Uncis), *Mu Gua* (Fructus Chaenomelis), *Wei Ling Xian* (Radix Clematidis), and *Ren Dong Teng* (Caulis Lonicerae Japonicae) were added.

One bag a day was added to 300ml of water, which was boiled down to 150ml, taken two or three times a day. Initial results were seen after two weeks.

TREATMENT WHEN THE KIDNEYS ARE INVOLVED
Anaphylactoid purpura may affect the kidneys and result in purpuric nephritis, in which case treatment can be difficult.

1. **Liu** treated 32 cases of infantile purpuric nephritis. [17]

Prescription
ZI SHEN TONG LUO TANG
Freeing the Network Vessels Decoction for Purpuric Nephritis

Zi Cao (Radix Arnebiae seu Lithospermi) 6-10g
Mu Dan Pi (Cortex Moutan Radicis) 6-10g
Chi Shao (Radix Paeoniae Rubra) 6-10g
Chuan Xiong (Rhizoma Ligustici Chuanxiong) 6-10g
Chan Tui‡ (Periostracum Cicadae) 6-10g
Dang Gui (Radix Angelicae Sinensis) 4-6g

Sheng Di Huang (Radix Rehmanniae Glutinosae) 10-15g
Yi Mu Cao (Herba Leonuri Heterophylli) 10-15g
Ji Xue Teng (Caulis Spatholobi) 10-15g
Zhu Ling (Sclerotium Polypori Umbellati) 10-15g
Fu Ling (Sclerotium Poriae Cocos) 10-15g
Bai Mao Gen (Rhizoma Imperatae Cylindricae) 10-15g

One bag a day was used to prepare a decoction, taken twice a day. A course of treatment lasted for one month. Results were usually seen after two courses.

2. **Chen** used a basic formula with modifications to treat this disease. [18]

Prescription
TUO MIN JIAN JIA WEI
Desensitization Brew, with additions

Yin Chai Hu (Radix Stellariae Dichotomae) 10-15g
Wu Mei (Fructus Pruni Mume) 10-15g
Wu Wei Zi (Fructus Schisandrae) 10-15g
Fang Feng (Radix Ledebouriellae Divaricatae) 3-10g

Modifications
1. For bright red purpura in Blood-Heat patterns, *Chan Tui*‡ (Periostracum Cicadae) 5g, *Zi Cao* (Radix Arnebiae seu Lithospermi) 15-30g, *Mu Dan Pi* (Cortex Moutan Radicis) 10g, *Chi Shao* (Radix Paeoniae Rubra) 9g, and *Sheng Di Huang* (Radix Rehmanniae Glutinosae) 12g were added.
2. For hematuria, *Xian He Cao* (Herba Agrimoniae Pilosae) 10-30g, *Bai Mao Gen* (Rhizoma Imperatae Cylindricae) 10-30g, *Qian Cao Gen* (Radix Rubiae Cordifoliae) 10-30g, and *Han Lian Cao* (Herba Ecliptae Prostratae) 10-30g were added.
3. For edema, *Ze Xie* (Rhizoma Alismatis Orientalis) 10g, *Yu Mi Xu* (Stylus Zeae Mays) 10-30g and *Che Qian Zi* (Semen Plantaginis) 10-30g were added.
4. For painful joints, *Tong Cao* (Medulla Tetrapanacis Papyriferi) 10g and *Mu Gua* (Fructus Chaenomelis) 6-15g were added.
5. For abdominal pain, *Bai Shao* (Radix Paeoniae Lactiflorae) 6-10g and *Yan Hu Suo* (Rhizoma Corydalis Yanhusuo) 6-10g were added.
6. For Qi Deficiency, *Huang Qi* (Radix Astragali seu Hedysari Praeparata) 10-15g and *Tai Zi Shen* (Radix Pseudostellariae Heterophyllae) 10-15g were added.

One bag a day was added to 300ml of water and used to prepare a decoction reduced to 100-150ml, taken two or three times a day. A course of treatment lasted for one month. Results were usually seen after two courses.

Erythromelalgia
红斑性肢痛症

Erythromelalgia is a rare episodic condition involving the extremities, with pronounced cutaneous vasodilatation when they are exposed to heat. It is usually bilateral and generally affects the feet more often than the hands. The condition produces a burning sensation, pain, mottled red skin, and a raised skin temperature.

Erythromelalgia may be idiopathic or occur in association with a myeloproliferative disorder (such as polycythemia rubra vera), lupus erythematosus, rheumatoid arthritis, gout, neurological diseases, or heavy metal poisoning.

In TCM, erythromelalgia is also known as *xue bi* (Blood Bi syndrome).

Clinical manifestations

- Erythromelalgia occurs most often in middle-aged men; women are seldom affected. Idiopathic erythromelalgia is commoner in younger individuals and is more frequently bilateral.
- The disease usually affects the feet bilaterally and is less likely to involve the hands; symptoms are most pronounced in the toes (occasionally in the fingers).
- The affected skin is rose-colored initially, subsequently turning dark red or purplish-red. The margins of the lesions are clearly demarcated.
- The temperature of the affected skin is 2-3°C higher than normal skin; accompanying symptoms and signs often include sweating, throbbing of the local arteries and dilatation of the veins.
- Burning, stabbing or distending pain often precedes erythema. Pain may be severe at night and may be precipitated by heat, exercise, standing for long periods, or dangling the feet.
- Attacks may last from a few minutes to several hours.
- Rest, soaking the feet in cold water, raising the affected limb, or baring the feet can bring about temporary alleviation. Small doses of acetylsalicylic acid (aspirin) may give symptomatic relief.
- This disease is usually chronic and exacerbates in summer. Persistent and repeated recurrences, often in secondary erythromelalgia, may trigger blood stasis, trophic skin changes and subcutaneous tissue damage; ulceration and gangrene or nail deformation may occur.

Differential diagnosis

Raynaud's disease
Although lesions may be similar to erythromelalgia, the skin is cold rather than hot. Raynaud's disease is more common in young women and involves the fingers more than the toes. During an attack, the extremities suddenly become cold and pale and then cyanotic; in the final stages, the affected area starts to feel warm and turns red. Those affected may only experience numbness followed by throbbing; intense pain is less common.

Etiology and pathology

Damp-Heat
Impairment of the Spleen's transportation function can result in internal generation of Damp-Heat, which pours downward to the feet and toes. When Damp-Heat enters the channels, Heat accumulates and obstructs the network vessels. Qi and Blood will then stagnate and cannot move freely, thus giving rise to the disease.

Retention of Fire
Excessive stimulation of the emotions can transform into Fire, impairing the functions of the Zang-Fu organs, damaging Yin and consuming Body Fluids. If this Fire binds in the toes, it will obstruct the vessels and inhibit the movement of Qi and Blood, thus causing the disease.

Pattern identification and treatment

INTERNAL TREATMENT

OBSTRUCTION BY DAMP-HEAT
This pattern manifests as swollen and intensely red skin, occasionally with edema. Burning or intense pain that worsens on exposure to heat may be felt. The tongue body is red with a yellow and thin or yellow and greasy coating; the pulse is slippery, rapid and soggy.

Treatment principle
Clear Heat and benefit the movement of Dampness, invigorate the Blood and free the network vessels.

Prescription
LONG DAN XIE GAN TANG JIA JIAN
Chinese Gentian Decoction for Draining the Liver, with modifications

Chao Long Dan Cao (Radix Gentianae Scabrae, stir-fried) 6g
Jiao Zhi Zi (Fructus Gardeniae Jasminoidis, scorch-fried) 6g
Chao Huang Bai (Cortex Phellodendri, stir-fried) 6g
Sheng Di Huang (Radix Rehmanniae Glutinosae) 15g
Chi Fu Ling (Sclerotium Poriae Cocos Rubrae) 15g
Ren Dong Teng (Caulis Lonicerae Japonicae) 15g
Si Gua Luo (Fasciculus Vascularis Luffae) 15g
Ji Xue Teng (Caulis Spatholobi) 15g
Niu Xi (Radix Achyranthis Bidentatae) 10g
Chi Xiao Dou (Semen Phaseoli Calcarati) 10g
Yi Yi Ren (Semen Coicis Lachryma-jobi) 10g
Qing Pi (Pericarpium Citri Reticulatae Viride) 10g

Explanation

- *Chao Long Dan Cao* (Radix Gentianae Scabrae, stir-fried), *Jiao Zhi Zi* (Fructus Gardeniae Jasminoidis, scorch-fried), *Chao Huang Bai* (Cortex Phellodendri, stir-fried), *Niu Xi* (Radix Achyranthis Bidentatae), and *Chi Fu Ling* (Sclerotium Poriae Cocos Rubrae) clear Heat and benefit the movement of Dampness.

- *Ren Dong Teng* (Caulis Lonicerae Japonicae), *Si Gua Luo* (Fasciculus Vascularis Luffae) and *Ji Xue Teng* (Caulis Spatholobi) free the network vessels and disperse swelling.

- *Sheng Di Huang* (Radix Rehmanniae Glutinosae), *Chi Xiao Dou* (Semen Phaseoli Calcarati), *Yi Yi Ren* (Semen Coicis Lachryma-jobi), and *Qing Pi* (Pericarpium Citri Reticulatae Viride) regulate Qi and invigorate the Blood, cool the Blood and alleviate pain.

ACCUMULATION OF RETAINED FIRE

This pattern manifests as red, swollen and painful toes. The scorching pain makes it feel as if the toes are being fried in oil. The patient is reluctant to put the feet on the ground. Some relief is obtained by soaking the feet in cold water, which reduces the pain and burning sensation slightly. The tongue body is red or crimson with a scant coating; the pulse is rapid and racing.

Treatment principle

Nourish Yin and clear Heat, dissipate Fire and alleviate pain.

Prescription
JIE DU YANG YIN TANG JIA JIAN
Decoction for Relieving Toxicity and Nourishing Yin, with modifications

Nan Sha Shen (Radix Adenophorae) 12g
Bei Sha Shen (Radix Glehniae Littoralis) 12g
*Shi Hu** (Herba Dendrobii) 12g
Xuan Shen (Radix Scrophulariae Ningpoensis) 12g
Gan Di Huang (Radix Rehmanniae Glutinosae Exsiccata) 12g
Tian Men Dong (Radix Asparagi Cochinchinensis) 12g
Mai Men Dong (Radix Ophiopogonis Japonici) 12g
Jin Yin Hua (Flos Lonicerae) 15g
Pu Gong Ying (Herba Taraxaci cum Radice) 15g
Dan Shen (Radix Salviae Miltiorrhizae) 15g
Huang Qi (Radix Astragali seu Hedysari) 15g
Si Gua Luo (Fasciculus Vascularis Luffae) 10g
Di Long‡ (Lumbricus) 10g
Gan Cao (Radix Glycyrrhizae) 10g

Explanation

- *Nan Sha Shen* (Radix Adenophorae), *Bei Sha Shen* (Radix Glehniae Littoralis), *Shi Hu** (Herba Dendrobii), *Xuan Shen* (Radix Scrophulariae Ningpoensis), *Gan Di Huang* (Radix Rehmanniae Glutinosae Exsiccata), *Tian Men Dong* (Radix Asparagi Cochinchinensis), and *Mai Men Dong* (Radix Ophiopogonis Japonici) nourish Yin and clear Heat.

- *Huang Qi* (Radix Astragali seu Hedysari), *Dan Shen* (Radix Salviae Miltiorrhizae) and *Gan Cao* (Radix Glycyrrhizae) augment Qi and invigorate the Blood, dissipate Fire and alleviate pain.

- *Jin Yin Hua* (Flos Lonicerae), *Pu Gong Ying* (Herba Taraxaci cum Radice), *Si Gua Luo* (Fasciculus Vascularis Luffae), and *Di Long‡* (Lumbricus) relieve Toxicity and free the network vessels, dissipate Blood stasis and alleviate pain.

PATENT HERBAL MEDICINES

- For accumulation of retained Fire, take *Pi Fu Bing Xue Du Wan* (Skin Disease Blood Toxicity Pill) 3g twice a day.

- To regulate and consolidate the effect of the treatment, take *Fu Fang Dan Shen Pian* (Compound Red Sage Root Tablet) 3g twice a day.

EXTERNAL TREATMENT

- For burning and distending pain, prepare a decoction with

  Dang Gui (Radix Angelicae Sinensis) 30g
  Ru Xiang (Gummi Olibanum) 30g
  Mo Yao (Myrrha) 30g
  Hong Hua (Flos Carthami Tinctorii) 15g

  Boil the ingredients twice in one liter of water to obtain a concentrated decoction of 300ml each time, allow to cool and use as a soak for the affected area twice a day.

- For inflamed skin and severe pain, mix *Yu Lu San* (Jade Dew Powder) to a paste with cold boiled water, or pound fresh *Ma Chi Xian* (Herba Portulacae Oleraceae) into a pulp; apply either of the preparations to the affected area once a day.

ACUPUNCTURE

Selection of points on the affected channels
Main points: SP-6 Sanyinjiao, KI-3 Taixi and LR-3 Taichong.

Auxiliary points

- For involvement of the feet, select ST-44 Neiting, LR-2 Xingjian, ST-41 Jiexi, GB-40 Qiuxu, and LR-4 Zhongfeng.
- For involvement of the hands, select LI-11 Quchi, LI-4 Hegu, LI-5 Yangxi, TB-5 Waiguan, and TB-4 Yangchi.

Selection of adjacent points
Main points: *Jing* (well) points on the affected toes.
Auxiliary point: ST-36 Zusanli.

Empirical points
LR-2 Xingjian (bilateral), GB-43 Xiaxi (bilateral) and GV-20 Baihui.

Technique
Apply the reinforcing method for Deficiency patterns and the reducing method for Excess patterns. Treat once every two days. A course consists of seven to ten treatment sessions.

Explanation

- ST-44 Neiting, LR-2 Xingjian, ST-41 Jiexi, and TB-5 Waiguan drain Heat and free the network vessels.
- SP-6 Sanyinjiao, GB-43 Xiaxi and KI-3 Taixi nourish Yin and alleviate pain.
- ST-36 Zusanli, LI-4 Hegu and LI-11 Quchi fortify the Spleen and transform Dampness.
- LR-3 Taichong, GB-40 Qiuxu and LR-4 Zhongfeng allow constrained Liver Qi to flow freely.
- LI-5 Yangxi and TB-4 Yangchi free Bi syndrome and alleviate pain.
- The *jing* (well) points on the toes clear Heat and relieve Toxicity, free the network vessels and alleviate pain.

EAR ACUPUNCTURE
Points: Liver, Subcortex and Endocrine.
Technique: Retain the needles for 15-20 minutes. Treat once every two days. A course consists of ten treatment sessions.

ELECTRO-ACUPUNCTURE AT EAR POINTS
Point prescription 1: Heart (bilateral) and Subcortex.
Point prescription 2: Sympathetic Nerve (bilateral) and Ear-Shenmen.

Point prescription 3: Heart (bilateral) and Ear-Shenmen.
Technique: Apply the three prescriptions alternately. Connect the needles to the apparatus and retain for 30 minutes. Treat once a day. A course consists of seven treatment sessions.

Clinical notes

- When treating this disease, consideration must be given to the duration of the burning sensation and the type of pain. A recently occurring burning sensation is generally attributable to Fire Toxins, while burning pain with a long history is more likely to be related to effulgent Yin Deficiency-Fire. Stabbing pain is a sign of involvement of the grandchild network vessels (*sun luo*), whereas distending pain is due to Spleen-Damp.
- Erythromelalgia will be alleviated if the primary disease (see the introduction to this section) is diagnosed and treated correctly.
- Some patients are likely to experience recurrence.

Advice for the patient

- Avoid long-term intake of warm or hot-natured foods, as these may damage Body Fluids, thus aggravating the condition.
- Try to remain optimistic and avoid getting depressed, worried, sad, or angry.

Literature excerpts

In *Zhu Bing Yuan Hou Lun* [A General Treatise on the Causes and Symptoms of Diseases], it states: "Heat diseases attack the hands and feet and enter the *jing* (well), *ying* (spring) and *shu* (transport) points of the Zang-Fu organs, which emerge on the hands and feet. Any Toxic pathogenic factors in the Zang-Fu organs pass along the channels and network vessels to attack the hands and feet, giving rise to redness, swelling and pain there."

In *Gu Jin Ming Yi Lin Zheng Jin Jian: Wai Ke Juan* [The Golden Mirror of Clinical Practice of Famous Doctors Ancient and Modern: External Diseases], Xi Jiuyi considered that erythromelalgia could be caused by pathogenic factors entering the Xue level and he obtained a satisfactory effect in treating the disease with TCM prescriptions for enriching Yin and cooling the network vessels. This corresponds to the theory of treating Yang hyperactivity by enriching Yin, as recorded in *Huang Di Nei Jing* [The Yellow Emperor's Classic of Internal Medicine], and to Wang Bing's commentary in *Huang Di Nei Jing Su Wen Zhu* [Notes on Simple Questions from the Yellow Emperor's Classic of Internal Medicine]: "To strengthen the governor of Water, restrict the brilliance of Yang." This treatment principle can regulate the functions of the vascular autonomic nerve system, which modern medicine considers to be responsible for erythromelalgia. For exuberant Heat, add a large dosage of *Shi Gao* ‡ (Gypsum Fibrosum) to clear Heat from the Qi level; and for flushing of the skin due to retained Heat, add *Shui Niu Jiao* ‡ (Cornu Bubali) and *Zi Cao* (Radix Arnebiae seu Lithospermi) to clear Heat from the Ying level.

Modern clinical experience

TREATMENT ACCORDING TO PATTERN IDENTIFICATION

Lan identified two patterns. [19]

• Blood-Dryness due to Spleen Deficiency

Treatment principle

Fortify the Spleen and nourish the Blood, cool the Blood and dispel Wind, free the network vessels and alleviate pain.

Prescription
REN DONG YI HAO FANG
Honeysuckle Stem No. 1 Formula

Huang Qi (Radix Astragali seu Hedysari) 30g
Ren Dong Teng (Caulis Lonicerae Japonicae) 30g
Dang Shen (Radix Codonopsitis Pilosulae) 20g
Gan Cao (Radix Glycyrrhizae) 5g
Dang Gui (Radix Angelicae Sinensis) 10g

Niu Xi (Radix Achyranthis Bidentatae) 10g
Qiang Huo (Rhizoma et Radix Notopterygii) 6g
Du Huo (Radix Angelicae Pubescentis) 6g
Chi Shao (Radix Paeoniae Rubra) 15g
Mu Dan Pi (Cortex Moutan Radicis) 15g
Bai Zhu (Rhizoma Atractylodis Macrocephalae) 15g
Fu Ling (Sclerotium Poriae Cocos) 15g
Xuan Shen (Radix Scrophulariae Ningpoensis) 15g

• Wind-Damp-Heat Toxins

Treatment principle

Clear Heat and relieve Toxicity, dispel Wind and eliminate Dampness, free the network vessels and alleviate pain.

Prescription
REN DONG ER HAO FANG
Honeysuckle Stem No. 2 Formula

Ren Dong Teng (Caulis Lonicerae Japonicae) 30g
Shi Gao ‡ (Gypsum Fibrosum) 30g
Zhi Mu (Rhizoma Anemarrhenae Asphodeloidis) 9g
Gui Zhi (Ramulus Cinnamomi Cassiae) 9g
Lian Qiao (Fructus Forsythiae Suspensae) 9g
Bai Shao (Radix Paeoniae Lactiflorae) 15g
Chi Shao (Radix Paeoniae Rubra) 15g
Sang Zhi (Ramulus Mori Albae) 15g
Wei Ling Xian (Radix Clematidis) 15g
Ban Zhi Lian (Herba Scutellariae Barbatae) 15g

One bag a day was used to prepare a decoction, taken twice a day. Three bags constituted a course of treatment. Results were seen after 20 courses.

Raynaud's disease
雷诺病

This is a paroxysmal disorder affecting the hands and feet due to episodic vasoconstriction of the arteries and arterioles, with sudden attacks of pallor and coldness in the fingers and toes lasting from a few minutes to longer than an hour.

Contraction of arteries near the skin surface is a natural response to cold, as restricting the flow of blood prevents loss of heat. These arteries also contract when blood is diverted to the muscles in response to emotional or physical stimuli. In Raynaud's disease, the response of the small arteries is exaggerated and slight cold or emotional stimulus may precipitate an attack. The disease may also be a symptom of a connective tissue disease, hyperviscosity of circulating blood, cryopathies, or repeated trauma ("vibration white finger" in pneumatic drill operators) and may resolve if an underlying cause is amenable to treatment.

Raynaud's disease is the name given to Raynaud's phenomenon when no cause is found. Causes of Raynaud's phenomenon include arterial occlusion, connective tissue disease, neurological disorders, and certain drugs such as beta-blockers.

Clinical manifestations

- Raynaud's disease is more common in women, with the age of onset usually under 40 years.
- The disease usually involves the extremities symmetrically, principally the fingers and less often the toes; occasionally the auricle, the tip of the nose or tongue, the cheeks, or the chin may also be involved.
- In the first stage of an attack, vasospasm results in ischemic manifestations, such as pale skin, cold fingers, stabbing pain, and perceptual abnormalities including numbness and rigidity of the fingers with difficulty in flexion and extension. This stage lasts a few minutes.
- In the second stage, relaxation of vasospasm results in skin swelling and cyanosis, with the skin turning dark blue or dark brown in serious cases, accompanied by stabbing pain and a throbbing sensation.
- In the third stage, the affected area starts to feel warm and turns red due to hyperemia. The throbbing sensation increases until normal color and function is restored.
- Attacks occur with increased frequency and severity in cold weather; ulceration may be present in severe cases, which may result in gangrene, although this is usually an indication of an underlying connective tissue disorder.
- Nails may be thinned or ridged.

Differential diagnosis

Thromboangiitis obliterans (Buerger's disease)
This condition usually involves the distal vessels of one lower limb and is predominantly seen in men under the age of 45 who are heavy smokers. Symptoms include intense pain on exertion, cold skin and a reduced or lost impulse of the dorsal artery of the foot. Gangrene may appear at the later stages.

Arteriosclerosis obliterans
This condition is a term describing chronic occlusive arterial disease affecting the aorta and its major branches, with ischemic symptoms such as intermittent claudication. Patients are mainly men aged over 50. The condition generally manifests on the lower limbs, and only occasionally on the upper limbs. Changing the position of the affected limb may induce variation in the skin color, with pallor on elevation and exacerbation of dusky cyanosis on dependence.

Etiology and pathology

- Internally, Yang Deficiency of the Spleen and Kidneys results in failure to warm the limbs properly.

- An invasion of pathogenic Cold results in Cold congealing and impeding the circulation of the Blood.
- Both internal and external factors can affect the circulation of the Blood, reducing or obstructing flow in the vessels and causing Qi stagnation and Blood stasis.

Pattern identification and treatment

INTERNAL TREATMENT

YANG DEFICIENCY OF THE SPLEEN AND KIDNEYS
This pattern manifests as persistent pallor and a freezing cold sensation in the limbs extending gradually, with numbness and pain in the extremities. In mild cases, the pallor may turn red and the extremities become swollen; in more severe cases, the skin remains pale or turns cyanotic. Accompanying symptoms and signs include cold and pain in the limbs, cyanosis of the lips and nails, lack of strength in the lower back and knees, a pale complexion, poor appetite, and loose stools. The tongue body is pale with a scant coating; the pulse is deep and thready.

Treatment principle
Warm and supplement the Spleen and Kidneys, expel Cold and free the network vessels.

Prescription
FU ZI LI ZHONG TANG JIA JIAN
Aconite Decoction for Regulating the Middle, with modifications

Fei Zi (Semen Torreyae Grandis) 10g
Gan Jiang (Rhizoma Zingiberis Officinalis) 10g
Bai Zhu (Rhizoma Atractylodis Macrocephalae) 10g
Zhi Gan Cao (Radix Glycyrrhizae, mix-fried with honey) 10g
Chuan Xiong (Rhizoma Ligustici Chuanxiong) 10g
Wang Bu Liu Xing (Semen Vaccariae Segetalis) 10g
Gui Zhi (Ramulus Cinnamomi Cassiae) 10g
Dang Shen (Radix Codonopsitis Pilosulae) 12g
Huang Qi (Radix Astragali seu Hedysari) 12g
Dan Shen (Radix Salviae Miltiorrhizae) 15g
Ji Xue Teng (Caulis Spatholobi) 15g
Lu Lu Tong (Fructus Liquidambaris) 6g

Explanation
- *Fei Zi* (Semen Torreyae Grandis), *Gan Jiang* (Rhizoma Zingiberis Officinalis), *Bai Zhu* (Rhizoma Atractylodis Macrocephalae), *Zhi Gan Cao* (Radix Glycyrrhizae, mix-fried with honey), *Dang Shen* (Radix Codonopsitis Pilosulae), and *Huang Qi* (Radix Astragali seu Hedysari) warm Yang and supplement the Kidneys, dissipate Cold and support the Spleen.

- *Wang Bu Liu Xing* (Semen Vaccariae Segetalis), *Gui Zhi* (Ramulus Cinnamomi Cassiae), *Chuan Xiong* (Rhizoma Ligustici Chuanxiong), *Dan Shen* (Radix Salviae Miltiorrhizae), and *Ji Xue Teng* (Caulis Spatholobi) invigorate the Blood and free the network vessels.

- *Lu Lu Tong* (Fructus Liquidambaris) frees the channels and invigorates the network vessels, expels Wind and dissipates Cold.

QI AND BLOOD DEFICIENCY

This pattern manifests as ice-cold extremities, with cyanosis in severe cases; the tips of the fingers become thinner and stiff due to lack of blood supply. Accompanying symptoms and signs include aversion to cold, lack of strength, shortness of breath, no desire to speak, a pale complexion, and occasional stabbing pain in the skin. The tongue body is pale red with a scant coating; the pulse is deep, thready and forceless.

Treatment principle
Augment Qi and warm Yang, nourish the Blood and free the network vessels.

Prescription
YI QI YANG XUE TANG JIA JIAN
Decoction for Augmenting Qi and Nourishing the Blood, with modifications

Huang Qi (Radix Astragali seu Hedysari) 30g
Dang Shen (Radix Codonopsitis Pilosulae) 15g
Dang Gui (Radix Angelicae Sinensis) 15g
Gui Zhi (Ramulus Cinnamomi Cassiae) 10g
Ji Xue Teng (Caulis Spatholobi) 10g
Shu Di Huang (Radix Rehmanniae Glutinosae Conquita) 10g
Yan Hu Suo (Rhizoma Corydalis Yanhusuo) 12g
Lu Lu Tong (Fructus Liquidambaris) 12g
Huo Xue Teng (Caulis seu Radix Schisandrae) 12g
Di Long‡ (Lumbricus) 6g
Shi Nan Teng (Caulis Photiniae) 12g
Dan Shen (Radix Salviae Miltiorrhizae) 6g
Su Mu (Lignum Sappan) 6g

Explanation

- *Huang Qi* (Radix Astragali seu Hedysari), *Dang Shen* (Radix Codonopsitis Pilosulae), *Dang Gui* (Radix Angelicae Sinensis), and *Gui Zhi* (Ramulus Cinnamomi Cassiae) augment Qi and warm Yang.

- *Ji Xue Teng* (Caulis Spatholobi), *Shu Di Huang* (Radix Rehmanniae Glutinosae Conquita) and *Huo Xue Teng* (Caulis seu Radix Schisandrae) nourish the Blood and free the network vessels.

- *Yan Hu Suo* (Rhizoma Corydalis Yanhusuo) and *Su Mu* (Lignum Sappan) free the network vessels and alleviate pain.

- *Di Long*‡ (Lumbricus), *Dan Shen* (Radix Salviae Miltiorrhizae), *Shi Nan Teng* (Caulis Photiniae), and *Lu Lu Tong* (Fructus Liquidambaris) dissipate Cold and dispel Bi syndrome, invigorate the Blood and free the network vessels.

INVASION BY EXTERNAL COLD

This pattern manifests as cold, numbness and pain in the extremities with a liking for warmth and a fear of cold. Warmth can alleviate the symptoms while exposure to cold results in pallor or cyanosis, followed by flushing. The tongue body is pale with a thin white coating; the pulse is thready and slow.

Treatment principle
Warm the channels and dissipate Cold, invigorate the Blood and free the network vessels.

Prescription
DANG GUI SI NI TANG JIA JIAN
Chinese Angelica Root Counterflow Cold Decoction, with modifications

Dang Gui (Radix Angelicae Sinensis) 30g
Huang Qi (Radix Astragali seu Hedysari) 30g
Gui Zhi (Ramulus Cinnamomi Cassiae) 15g
Hong Hua (Flos Carthami Tinctorii) 12g
Chuan Xiong (Rhizoma Ligustici Chuanxiong) 6g
Qiang Huo (Rhizoma et Radix Notopterygii) 6g
Xin Yi Hua (Flos Magnoliae) 6g
Gan Cao (Radix Glycyrrhizae) 6g
Qiang Huo (Rhizoma et Radix Notopterygii) 4.5g
Di Long‡ (Lumbricus) 4.5g
Dan Shen (Radix Salviae Miltiorrhizae) 4.5g
Ju Luo (Retinervus Fructus Citri Reticulatae) 4.5g

Explanation

- *Dang Gui* (Radix Angelicae Sinensis), *Huang Qi* (Radix Astragali seu Hedysari), *Gui Zhi* (Ramulus Cinnamomi Cassiae), *Xin Yi Hua* (Flos Magnoliae), and *Qiang Huo* (Rhizoma et Radix Notopterygii) warm Yang and dissipate Cold.

- *Chuan Xiong* (Rhizoma Ligustici Chuanxiong), *Hong Hua* (Flos Carthami Tinctorii), *Di Long*‡ (Lumbricus), *Dan Shen* (Radix Salviae Miltiorrhizae), and *Ju Luo* (Retinervus Fructus Citri Reticulatae) invigorate the Blood and free the network vessels.

- *Qiang Huo* (Rhizoma et Radix Notopterygii) dissipates Wind and dispels Cold, frees Bi syndrome and alleviates pain.

- *Gan Cao* (Radix Glycyrrhizae) augments Qi and regulates the Middle Burner, supports Vital Qi (Zheng Qi) and dispels pathogenic factors to treat the Root and the Manifestations simultaneously.

General modifications

1. For exclusive involvement of the hands, add *Jiang Huang* (Rhizoma Curcumae Longae) and *Sang Zhi* (Ramulus Mori Albae).

2. For exclusive involvement of the feet, add *Chuan Niu Xi* (Radix Cyathulae Officinalis) and *Mu Gua* (Fructus Chaenomelis).

3. For severe Cold, add *Pao Jiang* (Rhizoma Zingiberis Officinalis Praeparata), *Zhi Ma Huang** (Herba Ephedrae, mix-fried with honey) and *Fu Pen Zi* (Fructus Rubi Chingii).

4. For contracture of the extremities, add *Gou Teng* (Ramulus Uncariae cum Uncis), *Tian Ma** (Rhizoma Gastrodiae Elatae) and *Wu Gong* ‡ (Scolopendra Subspinipes).

5. For thinning or mild atrophy of the extremities in a prolonged disease, add *He Shou Wu* (Radix Polygoni Multiflori), *Tou Gu Cao* (Herba Speranskiae seu Impatientis), *Luo Shi Teng* (Caulis Trachelospermi Jasminoidis), and *Jiang Can* ‡ (Bombyx Batryticatus).

PATENT HERBAL MEDICINES

- Once the acute condition has been controlled, take three to five tablets of *Fu Fang Dan Shen Pian* (Compound Red Sage Root Tablet) two or three times a day.

- For pronounced Blood stasis, take *Tao Hong Si Wu Wan* (Peach Kernel and Safflower Four Agents Pill) 6g twice a day. These tablets may also be taken as an adjuvant to internal treatment.

EXTERNAL TREATMENT

- For local cyanosis, an ice-cold sensation and pallor and numbness of the skin, prepare a decoction with the following ingredients:

*Ma Huang** (Herba Ephedrae) 15g
Qiang Huo (Rhizoma et Radix Notopterygii) 15g
Xin Yi Hua (Flos Magnoliae) 15g
Cang Er Zi (Fructus Xanthii Sibirici) 30g
Xu Chang Qing (Radix Cynanchi Paniculati) 30g

Use the decoction to steam and then soak the affected area for 15-30 minutes twice a day.

- For a slightly reduced local temperature and mild cyanosis, apply *Hong Ling Jiu* (Red Spirit Wine) to the affected area two or three times a day. The effect is improved if gentle massage is given after application.

ACUPUNCTURE

Selection of points on the affected channels

Main points: HT-1 Jiquan, TB-4 Yangchi, SP-6 Sanyinjiao, and Bizhong (on the anterior side of the forearm between the radius and the ulna, at the midpoint of the line connecting the transverse wrist crease and the cubital crease).[vi]

Auxiliary points

- For a weak constitution, add CV-4 Guanyuan and ST-36 Zusanli.

- For depression, add LR-3 Taichong and LI-4 Hegu.

Selection of points according to disease differentiation

For involvement of the fingers of both hands
Main points: ST-12 Quepen and EX-UE-11 Shixuan.[vii]
Auxiliary points

- For involvement of the thumb and index finger, add LI-13 Shouwuli.

- For involvement of the middle finger, add PC-6 Neiguan.

- For involvement of the ring finger, add SI-8 Xiaohai.

For involvement of the toes
Main points: SP-6 Sanyinjiao and KI-6 Zhaohai.
Auxiliary points: EX-UE-11 Shixuan,[vii] GB-30 Huantiao and BL-54 Zhibian.

Empirical points

- For involvement of the upper limbs, select LI-4 Hegu, EX-UE-9 Baxie,[viii] LI-10 Shousanli, and TB-5 Waiguan.

- For involvement of the lower limbs, select EX-LE-10 Bafeng,[ix] SP-6 Sanyinjiao and ST-36 Zusanli.

Technique

Apply the even method to all the points with the exception of EX-UE-11 Shixuan, which are pricked to cause slight bleeding. Treat once a day. A course consists of fifteen treatment sessions.

Explanation

- TB-4 Yangchi, LI-10 Shousanli, ST-36 Zusanli, GB-30 Huantiao, CV-4 Guanyuan, and SP-6 Sanyinjiao warm Yang and dissipate Cold.

- HT-1 Jiquan, LI-4 Hegu, BL-54 Zhibian, LR-3 Taichong, KI-6 Zhaohai, TB-5 Waiguan, PC-6 Neiguan, LI-13 Shouwuli, and SI-8 Xiaohai free the channels and invigorate the network vessels.

[vi] M-UE-30 according to the system employed by the Shanghai College of Traditional Chinese Medicine.
[vii] M-UE-1 according to the system employed by the Shanghai College of Traditional Chinese Medicine.
[viii] M-UE-22 according to the system employed by the Shanghai College of Traditional Chinese Medicine.
[ix] M-LE-8 according to the system employed by the Shanghai College of Traditional Chinese Medicine.

- EX-UE-11 Shixuan, EX-LE-10 Bafeng, EX-UE-9 Baxie, ST-12 Quepen, and BL-54 Zhibian invigorate the Blood and dissipate Blood stasis.

MOXIBUSTION

Prescription 1: GV-14 Dazhui, GV-9 Zhiyang, GV-4 Mingmen, CV-13 Shangwan, and CV-12 Zhongwan.
Prescription 2: ST-36 Zusanli, BL-17 Geshu, BL-20 Pishu, BL-21 Weishu, and BL-23 Shenshu.
Technique: Choose two points from prescription 1 and one point from prescription 2 for each treatment session. Apply direct moxibustion to these points twice a day using seven to nine moxa cones per session. Treat for one month.

Clinical notes

- Treatment should concentrate on augmenting Qi, warming Yang, invigorating the Blood and transforming Blood stasis. The prescription is likely to be more effective with the addition of materia medica for freeing the grandchild network vessels (*sun luo*) such as *Xuan Fu Hua* (Flos Inulae) and *Si Gua Luo* (Fasciculus Vascularis Luffae).
- Acupuncture treatment benefits recovery, irrespective of whether the selection is based on empirical points or points along the affected channels.
- Treatment is most effective where the factors precipitating the attacks can be identified and avoided; otherwise, the disease tends to be chronic and treatment will take some time.
- Where the disease is a symptom of a primary focus (i.e. Raynaud's phenomenon), it will tend to clear up when that focus is treated.

Advice for the patient

- Do not expose the body to dampness or cold, keep warm, increase the amount of physical exercise, and try to avoid external trauma resulting in ulceration.
- Keep calm and try to reduce factors that may induce mental stress.
- Give up smoking and do not drink tea or coffee.
- Eat a well-balanced and nutritious diet.

Modern clinical experience

SPECIAL PRESCRIPTIONS

1. **Cao** formulated a basic prescription and modified it according to pattern identification. [20]

Prescription
ROU GAN JIE JING TANG
Decoction for Emolliating the Liver and Relieving Tetany

Bai Shao (Radix Paeoniae Lactiflorae) 30g
Gou Teng (Ramulus Uncariae cum Uncis) 30g
Zhi Gan Cao (Radix Glycyrrhizae, mix-fried with honey) 9g
Chai Hu (Radix Bupleuri) 9g
Mu Gua (Fructus Chaenomelis) 9g
Jiang Can‡ (Bombyx Batryticatus) 9g
Quan Xie‡ (Buthus Martensi) 6g, infused in the prepared decoction

Modifications according to pattern identification

1. For Cold congealing due to Yang Deficiency, *Dang Gui* (Radix Angelicae Sinensis), *Gui Zhi* (Ramulus Cinnamomi Cassiae), *Fu Zi** (Radix Lateralis Aconiti Carmichaeli Praeparata), *Ji Xue Teng* (Caulis Spatholobi), *Dang Shen* (Radix Codonopsitis Pilosulae), *Tong Cao* (Medulla Tetrapanacis Papyriferi), *Xi Xin** (Herba cum Radice Asari), and *Da Zao* (Fructus Ziziphi Jujubae) were added.

2. For Qi Deficiency and Blood stasis, *Dang Gui* (Radix Angelicae Sinensis), *Chuan Xiong* (Rhizoma Ligustici Chuanxiong), *Tao Ren* (Semen Persicae), *Hong Hua* (Flos Carthami Tinctorii), *Huang Qi* (Radix Astragali seu Hedysari), *Dang Shen* (Radix Codonopsitis Pilosulae), *Di Long*‡ (Lumbricus), *Ji Xue Teng* (Caulis Spatholobi), and *Gui Zhi* (Ramulus Cinnamomi Cassiae) were added.

3. For Liver Depression and Qi stagnation, *Zhi Shi* (Fructus Immaturus Citri Aurantii), *Chen Pi* (Pericarpium Citri Reticulatae), *Xiang Fu* (Rhizoma Cyperi Rotundi), *Dang Gui* (Radix Angelicae Sinensis), *Jiang Huang* (Rhizoma Curcumae Longae), and *Ji Xue Teng* (Caulis Spatholobi) were added.

One bag a day was used to prepare a decoction, taken twice a day. Results were seen after one month.

2. **Zhao** prepared a decoction for internal and external use. [21]

Prescription
WEN YANG TONG MAI YIN
Beverage for Warming Yang and Freeing the Blood Vessels

Dang Gui (Radix Angelicae Sinensis) 15g
Gui Zhi (Ramulus Cinnamomi Cassiae) 15g
Bai Shao (Radix Paeoniae Lactiflorae) 15g
Gan Cao (Radix Glycyrrhizae) 5g
Tong Cao (Medulla Tetrapanacis Papyriferi) 5g
Xi Xin* (Herba cum Radice Asari) 3g
Lu Jiao Jiao‡ (Gelatinum Cornu Cervi) 10g
Jiu Zhi Da Huang (Radix et Rhizoma Rhei, mix-fried with wine) 10g
Da Zao (Fructus Ziziphi Jujubae) 25g

Modifications

1. For persistent internal Cold, *Wu Zhu Yu* (Fructus Evodiae Rutaecarpae) 6g and *Sheng Jiang* (Rhizoma Zingiberis Officinalis Recens) 5g were added.
2. For excitability, *Long Gu* ‡ (Os Draconis) 30g and *Mu Li* ‡ (Concha Ostreae) 30g were added.
3. For intense pain, *Bai Zhi* (Radix Angelicae Dahuricae) 15g was added.
4. For severe cyanosis, *Shui Zhi* ‡ (Hirudo seu Whitmania) 5g and *Wu Ling Zhi* ‡ (Excrementum Trogopteri) 10g were added.

One bag a day was used to prepare a decoction, taken twice a day. The residue was boiled a third time and used to steam-wash the affected areas for 15-20 minutes, two or three times a day. Results were seen after one month.

3. **Liu** reported on the use of a modified classical formula. [22]

Prescription
FU ZI LI ZHONG TANG JIA WEI
Aconite Decoction for Regulating the Middle, with additions

Bai Zhu (Rhizoma Atractylodis Macrocephalae) 10-15g
Ru Xiang (Gummi Olibanum) 10-15g
Mo Yao (Myrrha) 10-15g
Dang Gui Wei (Extremitas Radicis Angelicae Sinensis) 10-15g
Di Long ‡ (Lumbricus) 10-15g
Chuan Xiong (Rhizoma Ligustici Chuanxiong) 10-15g
Dang Shen (Radix Codonopsitis Pilosulae) 20-30g
Shu Di Huang (Radix Rehmanniae Glutinosae Conquita) 20-30g
Huang Qi (Radix Astragali seu Hedysari) 20-30g
Rou Gui (Cortex Cinnamomi Cassiae) 15g
Gan Jiang (Rhizoma Zingiberis Officinalis) 5-15g
Zhi Gan Cao (Radix Glycyrrhizae, mix-fried with honey) 6-12g
Bai Shao (Radix Paeoniae Lactiflorae) 10-12g
Dan Shen (Radix Salviae Miltiorrhizae) 10-25g

One bag a day was used to prepare a decoction, taken three times a day. Results were seen after four to six weeks (34 days on average). Those treated successfully had experienced no recurrence after two years.

COMBINATION OF INTERNAL AND EXTERNAL TREATMENT
Bai treated Raynaud's disease with a combination of internal and external prescriptions. [23]

Internal prescription
WEN YANG QU YU TONG BI TANG
Decoction for Warming Yang, Dispelling Blood Stasis and Freeing Bi Syndrome

Lu Jiao Jiao ‡ (Gelatinum Cornu Cervi) 10g
Di Long ‡ (Lumbricus) 10g
Ru Xiang (Gummi Olibanum) 6g
Mo Yao (Myrrha) 6g
Dan Shen (Radix Salviae Miltiorrhizae) 30g
Huang Qi (Radix Astragali seu Hedysari) 30g
Gui Zhi (Ramulus Cinnamomi Cassiae) 10-20g
Dang Gui (Radix Angelicae Sinensis) 10-15g
Shen Jin Cao (Herba Lycopodii Japonici) 20g
Qiang Huo (Rhizoma et Radix Notopterygii) 6g
Xin Yi Hua (Flos Magnoliae) 6g
Sheng Jiang (Rhizoma Zingiberis Officinalis Recens) 12g

One bag a day was used to prepare a decoction, taken twice a day.

External prescription ingredients

Wu Jia Pi (Cortex Acanthopanacis Gracilistyli Radicis) 10g
Hai Tong Pi (Cortex Erythrinae) 10g
Sang Ji Sheng (Ramulus Loranthi) 10g
Ai Ye (Folium Artemisiae Argyi) 10g
Gui Zhi (Ramulus Cinnamomi Cassiae) 10g
Wei Ling Xian (Radix Clematidis) 20g
Shen Jin Cao (Herba Lycopodii Japonici) 20g
Lu Lu Tong (Fructus Liquidambaris) 15g

One bag a day was decocted to obtain 1500ml of liquid, which was cooled to around 55°C and then used several times a day as a soak for the extremities.

A course of treatment (internal and external) lasted for 15 days. Results were seen after two courses.

ACUPUNCTURE TREATMENT

1. **Xu** used the "setting the mountain on fire" method to treat this disease. [24]

Points
- LU-5 Chize and LI-4 Hegu were selected for involvement of the upper limb.
- ST-36 Zusanli and SP-6 Sanyinjiao were selected for involvement of the lower limb.
- If upper and lower limbs were both involved, all four points were needled.
- This treatment was combined with moxibustion with a moxa stick at CV-6 Qihai and CV-4 Guanyuan.

Technique
- LU-5 Chize and SP-6 Sanyinjiao were needled first

by applying the reducing method then the reinforcing method. The needles were not retained.

- LI-4 Hegu and ST-36 Zusanli were needled with 40-50mm filiform needles using the "setting the mountain on fire" method: With the left index finger pressing the point firmly, the right hand inserted and manipulated the needle. After obtaining Qi, the needle was thrust downward to the required depth and rotated by moving the thumb forward until there was a tight sensation around the tip of the needle. The needle was then lifted gently and thrust forcefully until there was a hot sensation; the needle was taken out and the hole pressed closed immediately. The needles were not retained.

- After the needles were withdrawn, moxibustion was applied to CV-6 Qihai and CV-4 Guanyuan with a moxa stick for 30 minutes.

The treatment was given once a day and ten treatment sessions made up a course. Results were seen after two courses.

2. **Wu** favored the warm needling method. [25]
Points: LI-4 Hegu, TB-5 Waiguan, LI-10 Shousanli, SP-6 Sanyinjiao, ST-36 Zusanli, and CV-4 Guanyuan.
Technique: The reinforcing method was applied after obtaining Qi. The needles were retained for 30 minutes. During this period, 5mm diameter moxa cones were attached to the needle handle and ignited. Three to five cones were used for each point.

The treatment was given once a day and ten treatment sessions made up a course. Results were seen after two courses.

COMBINATION OF TCM AND WESTERN MEDICINE

Hu combined TCM (internal and external treatment) and Western medicine to treat Raynaud's disease. [26]

Internal TCM prescription

*Ma Huang** (Herba Ephedrae) 15g
Dang Gui (Radix Angelicae Sinensis) 15g
Gui Zhi (Ramulus Cinnamomi Cassiae) 12g
Qiang Huo (Rhizoma et Radix Notopterygii) 12g
Du Huo (Radix Angelicae Pubescentis) 12g
Huang Qi (Radix Astragali seu Hedysari) 30g
Tao Ren (Semen Persicae) 10g

Di Long‡ (Lumbricus) 10g
Hong Hua (Flos Carthami Tinctorii) 10g

One bag a day was used to prepare a decoction, taken warm twice a day.

Modifications

1. For Kidney Yang Deficiency, *Rou Gui* (Cortex Cinnamomi Cassiae), *Yin Yang Huo* (Herba Epimedii) and *Rou Cong Rong* (Herba Cistanches Deserticolae) were added.
2. For severe Cold signs, *Wu Jia Pi* (Cortex Acanthopanacis Gracilistyli Radicis), *Hai Tong Pi* (Cortex Erythrinae), *Sang Ji Sheng* (Ramulus Loranthi), and *Gan Jiang* (Rhizoma Zingiberis Officinalis) were added.
3. For Qi stagnation, *Chen Pi* (Pericarpium Citri Reticulatae) and *Xiang Fu* (Rhizoma Cyperi Rotundi) were added.
4. For severe Blood stasis, *Ru Xiang* (Gummi Olibanum), *Mo Yao* (Myrrha), *San Leng* (Rhizoma Sparganii Stoloniferi), and *E Zhu* (Rhizoma Curcumae) were added.
5. For Qi Deficiency, *Xi Yang Shen* (Radix Panacis Quinquefolii) and *Huang Jing* (Rhizoma Polygonati) were added.

External TCM application

Wu Jia Pi (Cortex Acanthopanacis Gracilistyli Radicis) 30g
Hai Tong Pi (Cortex Erythrinae) 30g
Sang Ji Sheng (Ramulus Loranthi) 30g
Gui Zhi (Ramulus Cinnamomi Cassiae) 30g
Jiang Huang (Rhizoma Curcumae Longae) 30g
Bai Zhi (Radix Angelicae Dahuricae) 30g
Hai Feng Teng (Caulis Piperis Kadsurae) 30g
Tu Fu Ling (Rhizoma Smilacis Glabrae) 40g
*Xi Xin** (Herba cum Radice Asari) 15g
Gan Cao (Radix Glycyrrhizae) 10g

The decoction was used first to steam-wash the affected areas for 30 minutes and then as a soak for another 30 minutes, both three times a day. One bag was used every two days.

Western medicine

Intravenous infusion of 500ml of 5% glucose containing 90mg of papaverine administered once a day.

Results were seen after one month.

Chronic venous ulcer of the lower leg
慢性下肢溃疡

Chronic venous ulcer of the lower leg generally results from chronic venous insufficiency in the lower limb, often due to obesity. Such insufficiency results from valve incompetence in the deep and communicating veins in the leg, usually due to damage caused by thrombosis or infection. The condition is persistent, recurring and difficult to cure. Prolonged ulceration may result in the development of malignancy.

In TCM, chronic venous ulcer of the lower leg is also known as *qun bian chuang* (skirt hem sore).

Clinical manifestations

- Chronic venous ulcer of the lower leg occurs most frequently in the elderly and people who have to stand for lengthy periods.
- It can involve both the medial and lateral aspects of the lower third of the leg, but ulceration is most common in the region of the medial malleolus.
- In the initial stage, the condition appears subsequent to varicose veins or venous insufficiency. Heaviness of the legs and edema are often the first signs.
- Mild trauma results in superficial ulceration, gradually involving deeper layers of tissue.
- The lesion varies in size and may be round, oval or irregular in shape. Inflammatory pigmentation, scaling or crusting, and eczematoid changes may appear around the lesion. Allergic or irritant contact dermatitis may also develop after contact with Western medications or medicated bandages. Patients with psoriasis may develop scaling psoriatic changes around the ulcer (Koebner phenomenon).
- The lesion is purplish-red or dark red in color. Infection of the ulcer is common, resulting in the formation of colored slough and an unpleasant odor. Ulceration may persist for years without healing.
- If the ulcer remains indolent despite adequate treatment, or if the margin becomes raised, the possibility of malignant transformation should be suspected.

Differential diagnosis

Erythema induratum
Erythema appears on the lower limb in different sizes. Lesions manifest as subcutaneous nodules, which enlarge gradually to coalesce with the skin. The nodules are purplish-red, solid and slightly tender on pressure. They may disappear spontaneously, or heal with scarring after ulceration.

Other leg ulcers
Chronic leg ulcers also need to be differentiated from other types of leg ulcers. Arterial ulcers are generally deep, painful and gangrenous and are situated mostly on the foot or shin. Vasculitic ulcers develop from painful, palpable purpura into small "punched-out" ulcers; deep ulceration accompanying rheumatoid arthritis is usually due to vasculitis. The lower legs are also a common site for pyoderma gangrenosum, which evolves from a pustule or inflamed nodule into a painful, sharply demarcated ulcer that spreads rapidly over a purulent base.

Etiology and pathology

Wind-Heat-Damp Toxins
Overeating of spicy, dry, fatty, or sweet food will lead to impairment of the transportation function of the Spleen and Stomach. As a result, Damp-Heat will be generated internally. If this is complicated by an invasion of external Wind-Heat, the internal and external pathogenic factors will combine with each other; if retained in the interior for a long period, they will transform into Toxins. Damp-Heat affects the Yangming channel, which is abundant in Qi and Blood. Qi and Blood are steamed by the Wind-Heat-Damp Toxins, consuming the skin and flesh and leading to ulceration.

Stagnation of Cold-Damp
Cold pathogenic factors affecting the skin cause impairment of the movement of Qi and Blood in the channels and network vessels. Pathogenic Water and Dampness combine with Cold and are retained in the skin and flesh, eventually resulting in chronic ulcer of the lower leg.

Depletion of and damage to the Liver and Kidneys
If the disease persists, it will eventually involve the Kidneys. This will result in insufficiency of Essence and Blood; Toxins will stagnate and become even more difficult to transform. Since Qi and Blood are insufficiently nourished, movement in the network vessels and Blood vessels will be impeded. The lesions will therefore remain open for a lengthy period.

Trauma
The condition can be also triggered by cuts and other wounds, insect bites or breaking of the skin due to

scratching in skin diseases such as eczema.

Pattern identification and treatment

INTERNAL TREATMENT

WIND-HEAT-DAMP TOXINS

The lesions are mainly located on the medial aspect of the lower leg. The area around the ulcers is red, swollen and painful. Granulation is reddish-purple in color. The tongue body is red with a white or yellow coating; the pulse is deep and wiry, or rapid.

Treatment principle

Dispel Wind and percolate Dampness, relieve Toxicity and free the network vessels.

Prescription
SI SHENG WAN JIA JIAN
Four Fresh Agents Pill, with modifications

Di Long‡ (Lumbricus) 12g
Chao Jiang Can‡ (Bombyx Batryticatus, stir-fried) 12g
Bai Fu Zi (Rhizoma Typhonii Gigantei) 6g
Gui Zhi (Ramulus Cinnamomi Cassiae) 12g
Fu Ling Pi (Cortex Poriae Cocos) 15g
Mu Gua (Fructus Chaenomelis) 15g
Dan Shen (Radix Salviae Miltiorrhizae) 15g
Yi Yi Ren (Semen Coicis Lachryma-jobi) 30g
Ren Dong Teng (Caulis Lonicerae Japonicae) 30g
Chi Xiao Dou (Semen Phaseoli Calcarati) 30g

Explanation

- *Chao Jiang Can*‡ (Bombyx Batryticatus, stir-fried), *Bai Fu Zi* (Rhizoma Typhonii Gigantei) and *Gui Zhi* (Ramulus Cinnamomi Cassiae) dredge Wind and disperse swelling.
- *Fu Ling Pi* (Cortex Poriae Cocos), *Chi Xiao Dou* (Semen Phaseoli Calcarati), *Ren Dong Teng* (Caulis Lonicerae Japonicae), *Yi Yi Ren* (Semen Coicis Lachryma-jobi), and *Mu Gua* (Fructus Chaenomelis) transform Dampness and free the network vessels.
- *Di Long*‡ (Lumbricus) and *Dan Shen* (Radix Salviae Miltiorrhizae) invigorate the Blood and transform Blood stasis.
- When Wind is expelled and Blood stasis dissipated, the swelling will disappear and the pain will be alleviated.

STAGNATION OF COLD-DAMP

The affected leg is swollen and cold. Granulation and edema are present; the skin has a dull color. The pus is thin, clear and watery. The surface of the lesions is dark red or bluish-purple. The tongue body is pale red with a white coating; the pulse is deep, thready and forceless.

Treatment principle

Warm and transform Cold-Damp, invigorate the Blood and free the network vessels.

Prescription
GUI ZHI JIA DANG GUI TANG JIA JIAN
Cinnamon Twig Decoction plus Chinese Angelica Root, with modifications

Dang Gui (Radix Angelicae Sinensis) 15g
Huang Qi (Radix Astragali seu Hedysari) 20g
Dan Shen (Radix Salviae Miltiorrhizae) 20g
Chi Shao (Radix Paeoniae Rubra) 10g
Bi Xie (Rhizoma Dioscoreae Hypoglaucae seu Septemlobae) 10g
Tu Fu Ling (Rhizoma Smilacis Glabrae) 30g
Da Zao (Fructus Ziziphi Jujubae) 15g
Zhi Gan Cao (Radix Glycyrrhizae, mix-fried) 6g

Explanation

- *Dang Gui* (Radix Angelicae Sinensis), *Huang Qi* (Radix Astragali seu Hedysari), *Da Zao* (Fructus Ziziphi Jujubae), and *Gan Cao* (Radix Glycyrrhizae) augment Qi with warmth and sweetness.
- *Dan Shen* (Radix Salviae Miltiorrhizae) and *Chi Shao* (Radix Paeoniae Rubra) invigorate the Blood and transform Blood stasis.
- *Bi Xie* (Rhizoma Dioscoreae Hypoglaucae seu Septemlobae) and *Tu Fu Ling* (Rhizoma Smilacis Glabrae) transform Dampness and relieve Toxicity.

DEPLETION OF AND DAMAGE TO THE LIVER AND KIDNEYS

This pattern often occurs after febrile diseases or as a result of consumption of Kidney-Essence. The ulcers are mainly located on the medial aspect of the lower leg and the condition is likely to persist. The surface of the lesions is black and festering; the flesh is sunken. The pus is clear, thin and watery. Patients have a subjective feeling of persistent numbness. The tongue body is pale with a white coating; the pulse is thready.

Treatment principle

Nourish the Liver and supplement the Kidneys, free the network vessels and close sores.

Prescription
JIN KUI SHEN QI WAN JIA JIAN
Kidney Qi Pill from the Golden Cabinet, with modifications

Gan Di Huang (Radix Rehmanniae Glutinosae Exsiccata) 10g
Shan Zhu Yu (Fructus Corni Officinalis) 10g
Chao Mu Dan Pi (Cortex Moutan Radicis, stir-fried) 10g
Fu Ling (Sclerotium Poriae Cocos) 10g
Lu Jiao Pian‡ (Cornu Cervi, sliced) 12g

Huang Qi (Radix Astragali seu Hedysari) 12g
Shan Yao (Radix Dioscoreae Oppositae) 30g
Yi Yi Ren (Semen Coicis Lachryma-jobi) 30g
Chi Xiao Dou (Semen Phaseoli Calcarati) 30g
Chuan Niu Xi (Radix Cyathulae Officinalis) 6g
Qing Pi (Pericarpium Citri Reticulatae Viride) 6g
Si Gua Luo (Fasciculus Vascularis Luffae) 6g
Rou Gui (Cortex Cinnamomi Cassiae) 3g

Explanation

- *Gan Di Huang* (Radix Rehmanniae Glutinosae Exsiccata), *Shan Zhu Yu* (Fructus Corni Officinalis), *Lu Jiao Pian*‡ (Cornu Cervi, sliced), *Rou Gui* (Cortex Cinnamomi Cassiae), and *Huang Qi* (Radix Astragali seu Hedysari) augment Qi and warm Yang, based on the principle of the mutual rooting of Yin and Yang.

- *Fu Ling* (Sclerotium Poriae Cocos), *Shan Yao* (Radix Dioscoreae Oppositae), *Yi Yi Ren* (Semen Coicis Lachryma-jobi), and *Chi Xiao Dou* (Semen Phaseoli Calcarati) support the Spleen and transform Dampness.

- *Chuan Niu Xi* (Radix Cyathulae Officinalis) and *Mu Dan Pi* (Cortex Moutan Radicis) augment Qi and enrich Yin.

- *Qing Pi* (Pericarpium Citri Reticulatae Viride) and *Si Gua Luo* (Fasciculus Vascularis Luffae) regulate Qi and free the network vessels.

- The whole prescription has the effect of transforming Dampness without causing Dryness and supplementing Qi without causing stagnation.

General modifications

1. For lesions with blood oozing from the surface, add *Jiao Zhi Zi* (Fructus Gardeniae Jasminoidis, scorch-fried), *Ce Bai Tan* (Cacumen Biotae Orientalis Carbonisatum) and *Xian He Cao* (Herba Agrimoniae Pilosae).

2. For lesions with local inflammation and itching, add *Bai Xian Pi* (Cortex Dictamni Dasycarpi Radicis), *Di Fu Zi* (Fructus Kochiae Scopariae) and *Yi Mu Cao* (Herba Leonuri Heterophylli).

3. Where swelling is alleviated in the morning but aggravated in the evening, this is often associated with Qi Deficiency; *Dang Shen* (Radix Codonopsitis Pilosulae), *Bai Zhu* (Rhizoma Atractylodis Macrocephalae) and *Tai Zi Shen* (Radix Pseudostellariae Heterophyllae) should be added.

4. If the lesion appears black with no sign of regeneration of flesh, add *Rou Gui* (Cortex Cinnamomi Cassiae) and *Lu Jiao Jiao*‡ (Gelatinum Cornu Cervi).

5. If the lesion is very painful with no discharge of necrotic tissue, add *Zao Jiao Ci* (Spina Gleditsiae Sinensis), *Feng Fang*‡ (Nidus Vespae) and *Chuan Xiong* (Rhizoma Ligustici Chuanxiong).

6. For local varicose veins, add *Ze Lan* (Herba Lycopi Lucidi), *Dan Shen* (Radix Salviae Miltiorrhizae), *Ji Xue Teng* (Caulis Spatholobi), and *Huo Xue Teng* (Caulis seu Radix Schisandrae).

EXTERNAL TREATMENT

- At the initial stage with local inflammation, redness, swelling and pain, mix *Ru Yi Jin Huang San* (Agreeable Golden Yellow Powder) into a paste with honey and apply directly to the lesion.

- After the epidermis and dermis have been broken down and there is profuse exudation, make a decoction with *Ma Chi Xian* (Herba Portulacae Oleraceae) 60g, *Huang Bai* (Cortex Phellodendri) 20g and *Da Qing Ye* (Folium Isatidis seu Baphicacanthi) 30g; or *Bai Zhi* (Radix Angelicae Dahuricae) 15-30g, *Chuan Xiong* (Rhizoma Ligustici Chuanxiong) 15-30g and *Sang Piao Xiao*‡ (Oötheca Mantidis) 15-30g; or *Qian Li Guang* (Herba Senecionis Scandentis) 30g, *Ku Shen* (Radix Sophorae Flavescentis) 30g and *Wu Bei Zi*‡ (Galla Rhois Chinensis) 10g. Use the decoction as a wet compress for direct application to the affected area. This treatment is given two or three times a day.

- For exudation of thick pus, apply *Hua Du San* (Powder for Transforming Toxicity),ˣ the amount used depending on the extent of the lesions. Cover with *Fu Rong Gao* (Cotton Rose Flower Paste). Treat once a day. Classical formulae such as *San Xiang Gao* (Three Fragrances Paste) can also be used. When all the necrotic tissue has been eliminated and new tissue generated, use *Dong Fang Yi Hao Yao Gao* (Oriental Medicated Plaster No. 1) until the sores close.

- If there is any sign of malignancy, appropriate management should be implemented immediately (including referral to a doctor of Western medicine).

ACUPUNCTURE

Selection of points on the affected channels
Main points: SP-10 Xuehai, ST-36 Zusanli, SP-9 Yinlingquan, SP-6 Sanyinjiao, and SP-5 Shangqiu.
Auxiliary points: Three or four Ashi points 1cm from the border of the lesion on the affected channels. On each channel, insert two needles towards the center of the lesion, one following the course of the channel, the other against the course.

ˣ Alternatively, in those countries where this powder cannot be used, it can be replaced by *Jie Du Dan* (Special Pill for Relieving Toxicity) ground to a powder, although this preparation is not as effective.

Technique: The even method is applied to the main points. The Ashi points are needled with the needle directed toward the center of the lesion to a depth of 0.4-0.8 cun. After obtaining Qi, retain the needles for 15-30 minutes. Treat once a day.

Selection of points according to the location of the lesions

Points

- Where the lateral aspect of the lower leg is involved, select ST-36 Zusanli, GB-39 Xuanzhong and BL-57 Chengshan.
- Where the medial aspect of the lower leg is involved, select SP-10 Xuehai, LR-8 Ququan, SP-9 Yinlingquan, and KI-7 Fuliu.

Technique: Where the lateral aspect of the lower leg is involved, apply the reducing method; where the medial aspect of the lower leg is involved, apply the reinforcing method. For the peripheral area around the ulcerations, apply the leopard-spot needling technique to evacuate stagnant blood.[xi] Treat once a day.

Explanation

- SP-10 Xuehai and ST-36 Zusanli augment Qi and nourish the Blood.
- SP-9 Yinlingquan, SP-6 Sanyinjiao, SP-5 Shangqiu, and KI-7 Fuliu nourish Yin and clear Heat.
- GB-39 Xuanzhong, BL-57 Chengshan and LR-8 Ququan move Qi and free the network vessels.

MOXIBUSTION

Returning Yang moxibustion [xii]

Coarsely grind *Cao Wu** (Radix Aconiti Kusnezoffii) 100g, *Gan Jiang* (Rhizoma Zingiberis Officinalis) 100g, *Chi Shao* (Radix Paeoniae Rubra) 30g, *Bai Zhi* (Radix Angelicae Dahuricae) 30g, *Zhi Nan Xing* (Rhizoma Arisaematis Praeparata) 30g, *Rou Gui* (Cortex Cinnamomi Cassiae) 15g, *Dang Shen* (Radix Codonopsitis Pilosulae) 45g, and *Huang Qi* (Radix Astragali seu Hedysari) 45g. Wrap them in moxa roll paper to make a moxa stick for applying returning Yang moxibustion to the site of the lesions.

Direct moxibustion with a moxa stick

Clean the lesion first with physiological saline. Ignite a moxa stick and hold it over the affected area or apply "sparrow-pecking" moxibustion.

Warm moxibustion with a medicated moxa stick

Make a moxa stick by mixing 60g of moxa floss with a powder made by grinding *Liu Huang*‡ (Sulphur) 6g, *Song*

Xiang (Resina Pini) 6g, *Ru Xiang* (Gummi Olibanum) 6g, and *Mo Yao* (Myrrha) 6g. Ignite the moxa stick and hold it over the lesions for 10-15 minutes. Treat once a day.

POINT LASER THERAPY

Points: Ashi points (site of the lesions), ST-36 Zusanli and SP-6 Sanyinjiao.

Technique: Use a low-frequency helium-neon laser for 10-15 minutes at the Ashi points, and for two minutes at ST-36 Zusanli and SP-6 Sanyinjiao. Treat once a day.

Clinical notes

- Chronic ulcers on the lower leg are different in terms of Yin and Yang. Conditions involving the Yang channels on the lateral aspect of the leg are relatively straightforward to treat, whereas treatment of conditions involving the Yin channels on the medial aspect of the leg is much more difficult. This is due to the fact that the Yang channels are rich in Qi and Blood, whereas the Yin channels have a shortage of Qi and an excess of Blood or an excess of Qi and a shortage of Blood.
- Appropriate external treatment will relieve pain and aid healing of the lesions. If the condition is due to or accompanied by varicose veins, involvement of doctors of Western medicine for surgery is suggested as part of a combined treatment strategy.
- Acupuncture and moxibustion treatment help to limit ulceration in the local area, disperse swelling and alleviate pain with the result that these methods are often used in clinical practice.

Advice for the patient

- After the lesion heals, it is necessary to protect the local area by wearing an elastic bandage to prevent possible injury and recurrence.
- Where venous leg ulcers are linked to obesity, a diet aimed at weight loss is helpful.

Literature excerpts

According to *Wai Ke Shuo Yue* [Anthology of the Theory of External Diseases]: "Where chronic ulcer of the lower leg is accompanied by redness of the skin, this indicates that there is invasion by Heat; where the ulcer

---

[xi] One of the five ancient needling techniques whereby a three-edged needle is used to pierce small blood vessels around the affected area so as to evacuate stagnated blood and free the channels. The name is given because of the large number of hemorrhagic spots that appear during the process.

[xii] This moxibustion technique is so named because of the Yang-returning function of the ingredients used.

is accompanied by swelling, this indicates invasion by Damp; where it is accompanied by itching, this indicates invasion by Wind; where it is accompanied by pain, this indicates an Excess pattern; where the condition is alleviated in the morning and aggravated in the evening, this indicates sinking of Qi. In the initial stage, ulcers are generally caused by Wind, Heat and Damp Toxins; chronic conditions are often associated with sinking of Qi and Damp-Heat patterns."

In *Gu Jin Ming Yi Lin Zheng Jin Jian: Wai Ke Juan* [The Golden Mirror of Clinical Practice of Famous Doctors Ancient and Modern: External Diseases], Liu Jiren stated: "Patients suffering from this disease must not walk or stand for lengthy periods. Otherwise, Damp-Heat will pour down with Qi and Blood, which will make the condition even more difficult to cure. Although this disease is not fatal, it may linger for years.

"It is forbidden to scratch or burn the lesion or to make it drain by walking too much. Even though patients wish to recover rapidly, they should be careful not to break these rules. Patients have to put up with the pain and itching and abide strictly by the rules; the treatment will then work. If patients drink alcohol or have sex, their suffering will increase."

Modern clinical experience

SINGLE EMPIRICAL PRESCRIPTION

Xu treated this condition with an empirical prescription. [27]

Prescription ingredients

Ku Shen (Radix Sophorae Flavescentis) 30g
Bai Mao Gen (Rhizoma Imperatae Cylindricae) 30g
Bai Xian Pi (Cortex Dictamni Dasycarpi Radicis) 30g
Dan Shen (Radix Salviae Miltiorrhizae) 30g
Huang Qi (Radix Astragali seu Hedysari) 30g
She Chuang Zi (Fructus Cnidii Monnieri) 30g
Da Huang (Radix et Rhizoma Rhei) 6g, added 10 minutes before the end of the decoction process
Niu Xi (Radix Achyranthis Bidentatae) 12g
Huang Bai (Cortex Phellodendri) 10g
Gan Cao (Radix Glycyrrhizae) 10g

One bag a day was used to prepare a decoction, taken twice a day. The course of treatment ranged from two to eighteen months, averaging about four months. [27]

EXTERNAL TREATMENT

1. **Wu** applied *Fu Yang San* (Skin Ulcer Powder), manufactured by the Pharmaceutical Factory of Nanjing University, externally at a dosage modified according to the extent of the lesion. The dressing was changed once or twice a day if there was a large amount of exudate, but less frequently (once every other day or once every few days) once exudation diminished or stopped. The treatment continued until the lesion healed. One month constituted a course of treatment.

Results indicated that 573 out of 656 cases were treated successfully (87.4 percent), 77 showed various degrees of improvement (11.7 percent), and 6 had no effect (0.9 percent). Of those treated successfully, 197 needed one course of treatment, 213 two courses, 117 three courses and 46 four courses. No side-effects were noted. [28]

2. **Huang** combined *Zi Ding Gao* (Gromwell Root and Chinese Violet Paste) and *Sheng Ji San* (Flesh-Generating Powder) to treat chronic venous ulcer of the lower leg. [29]

Paste prescription
ZI DING GAO
Gromwell Root and Chinese Violet Paste

Zi Cao (Radix Arnebiae seu Lithospermi) 30g
Zi Hua Di Ding (Herba Violae Yedoensitis) 30g
Dang Gui (Radix Angelicae Sinensis) 20g
Fu Rong Ye (Folium Hibisci Mutabilis) 20g
Bai Ji (Rhizoma Bletillae Striatae) 20g
Ren Dong Teng (Caulis Lonicerae Japonicae) 15g
Bai Zhi (Radix Angelicae Dahuricae) 15g
Jin Yin Hua (Flos Lonicerae) 15g
Bing Pian (Borneolum) 3g

The ingredients were ground into a fine powder and passed through a 100-mesh sieve. The mixture was then combined with Vaseline® and sesame oil to make a paste, which was then sterilized in an autoclave before external application. The ointment was changed every other day.

For large, deep lesions with necrotic tissue and profuse exudation of pus, the lesion was excised, followed by repeated washing with hydrogen peroxide (H_2O_2). The second prescription, *Sheng Ji San* (Flesh-Generating Powder), was then spread over the surface of the lesion.

Powder prescription
SHENG JI SAN
Flesh-Generating Powder

Shu Shi Gao‡ (Gypsum Fibrosum Conquitum) 30g
Qian Dan‡ (Minium) 15g
Lu Gan Shi‡ (Calamina) 15g
Bing Pian (Borneolum) 3g

The lesion was then covered with a layer of Vaseline® and dressed with gauze. The dressing was changed every day. The treatment was continued until new tissue began to grow.

The treatment then switched back to external application of *Zi Ding Gao* (Gromwell Root and Chinese Violet

Paste) until crusts formed over the lesions, which healed after the crusts fell off. The course of treatment lasted 30 days.

INCREASED DOSE OF AN INDIVIDUAL INGREDIENT

Wang treated chronic venous ulcer of the lower leg by using a high dose of *Huang Qi* (Radix Astragali seu Hedysari). [30] He drew up the following prescription for internal treatment:

Huang Qi (Radix Astragali seu Hedysari) 80g
Dang Gui (Radix Angelicae Sinensis) 10g
Bai Mao Gen (Rhizoma Imperatae Cylindricae) 40g
Che Qian Cao (Herba Plantaginis) 12g

Modifications

- *Chuan Niu Xi* (Radix Cyathulae Officinalis) was added for pain at the mouth of the lesion.
- *Fu Ling* (Sclerotium Poriae Cocos) was added for puffy swelling of the face.
- *Ku Shen* (Radix Sophorae Flavescentis) was added for palpitations.

External treatment

Huang Lian Gan Ru Gao (Coptis, Calamine and Frankincense Paste) was applied once a day to the affected area.

In Dr. Wang's experience, chronic venous ulcer of the lower limb is mostly caused by Damp-Heat. Where pathogenic factors are exuberant, but Vital Qi (Zheng Qi) is not yet Deficient, the main treatment principle should be to clear Heat and eliminate Dampness. The ulcer will not heal unless Damp-Heat is eliminated. When the condition becomes chronic, Qi and Blood are likely to be Deficient, which will make it difficult for the lesion to heal.

Increasing the dosage of *Huang Qi* (Radix Astragali seu Hedysari) helps reinforce and supplement Vital Qi to increase the body's resistance. Under normal conditions, 30g of *Huang Qi* (Radix Astragali seu Hedysari) would be prescribed and the lesion would take about 30 days to heal. When the dosage is increased, the course of treatment can be shortened to 15-20 days and the result is more effective.

COMBINED TREATMENT WITH TCM AND LASER THERAPY

Guo treated this condition with a herbal soak. [31]

Prescription ingredients

Lian Qiao (Fructus Forsythiae Suspensae) 20g
Zi Hua Di Ding (Herba Violae Yedoensitis) 20g
Huang Bai (Cortex Phellodendri) 20g
Huang Qin (Radix Scutellariae Baicalensis) 20g
Pu Gong Ying (Herba Taraxaci cum Radice) 30g
Jin Yin Hua (Flos Lonicerae) 30g
Dang Gui (Radix Angelicae Sinensis) 15g
Chi Shao (Radix Paeoniae Rubra) 15g
Huang Qi (Radix Astragali seu Hedysari) 15g
Di Long ‡ (Lumbricus) 15g

Modifications

- For severe local pain, *Bai Jiang Cao* (Herba Patriniae cum Radice) 15g was added.
- For itching in the surrounding area, *Di Fu Zi* (Fructus Kochiae Scopariae) 15g, *Bai Xian Pi* (Cortex Dictamni Dasycarpi Radicis) 20g and *Tao Ren* (Semen Persicae) 15g were added.
- For varicose veins and hard, swollen nodules, *Hong Hua* (Flos Carthami Tinctorii) 10g was added.

The prescription was decocted and used warm to soak the affected area. The treatment was given twice daily with seven days making up a course. At the same time, treatment of the affected area with a helium-neon laser was also carried out twice a day for 10-15 minutes per session. Treatment ranged from 7 to 21 days (one to three courses).

References

1. Traditional Chinese Medicine Research Academy: Beijing Guang'anmen Hospital, *Zhu Ren Kang Lin Chuang Jing Yan Ji* [A Collection of Zhu Renkang's Clinical Experiences] (Beijing: People's Medical Publishing House, 1979), 160.

2. Shen Tongsheng, *Sheng Ma Lian Yi Tang Zhi Liao Duo Xing Hong Ban 82 Li Xiao Jie* [Summary of the Treatment of 82 Cases of Erythema Multiforme with *Sheng Ma Lian Yi Tang* (Bugbane, Forsythia and Coix Seed Decoction)], *Hu Nan Zhong Yi Za Zhi* [Hunan Journal of Traditional Chinese Medicine] 15, 1 (1999): 16.

3. Li Zhaoling, *Xiao Ban He Ji Zhi Liao Duo Xing Hong Ban 21 Li* [Treatment of 21 Cases of Erythema Multiforme with *Xiao Ban He Ji* (Dispersing Erythema Mixture)], *Hu Bei Zhong Yi Za Zhi* [Hubei Journal of Traditional Chinese Medicine] 18, 2 (1996): 6.

4. Lu Yan, *Gui Zhi Hong Hua Tang Zhi Liao Han Leng Xing Duo Xing Hong Ban* [Treatment of Cold-Type Erythema Multiforme with *Gui Zhi Hong Hua Tang* (Cinnamon Twig and Safflower Decoction)], *He Bei Zhong Yi* [Hebei Journal of Traditional Chinese Medicine] 18, 4 (1996): 10.

5. Zhong Dayuan, *Zhong Yao Zhi Liao Han Leng Xing Duo Xing Hong Ban 66 Li* [Chinese Materia Medica in the Treatment of 66 Cases of Cold-Type Erythema Multiforme], *Jiang Su Zhong Yi* [Jiangsu Journal of Traditional Chinese Medicine] 17, 7 (1996): 26.

6. Bao Zuoyi, *Zhong Xi Yi Jie He Zhi Liao Han Leng Xing Duo Xing Hong Ban 58 Li* [Treatment of 58 Cases of Cold-Type Erythema Multiforme with a Combination of TCM and Western Medicine], *Pi Fu Bing He Xing Bing* [Journal of Skin Diseases and Venereal Diseases] 20, 1 (1998): 30-31.

7. Beijing Hospital of Traditional Chinese Medicine, *Zhao Bing Nan Lin Chuan Jin Yan Ji* [A Collection of Zhao Bingnan's Clinical Experiences] (Beijing: People's Medical Publishing House, 1975), 169.

8. Xu Yihou, *Xu Yi Hou Pi Fu Bing Lin Chuang Jing Yan Ji Yao* [A Summary of Xu Yihou's Clinical Experiences in the Treatment of Skin Diseases] (Beijing: China Medical Science and Technology Publishing House, 1998), 202.

9. Zhang Zhili, *Zhang Zhi Li Pi Fu Bing Lin Chuang Jing Yan Ji Yao* [A Collection of Zhang Zhili's Clinical Experiences in the Treatment of Skin Diseases] (Beijing: China Medical Science and Technology Publishing House, 2001), 307.

10. Li Shaogui, *Bian Zheng Zhi Liao Guo Min Xing Zi Dian 56 Li* [Treatment of 56 Cases of Anaphylactoid Purpura Based on Pattern Identification], *Ji Lin Zhong Yi Yao* [Jilin Journal of Traditional Chinese Medicine] 6 (1996): 11.

11. Kong Zhaoxia, *Guo Min Xing Zi Dian 103 Li Bian Zhi Ti Hui* [Experience in Treating 103 Cases of Anaphylactoid Purpura Based on Pattern Identification], *Zhong Yi Za Zhi* [Journal of Traditional Chinese Medicine] 36, 1 (1995): 37-38.

12. Zhang Tingwei, *Hua She Xiao Dian Tang Zhi Liao Guo Min Xing Zi Dian 52 Li* [Treatment of 52 Cases of Anaphylactoid Purpura with *Hua She Xiao Dian Tang* (Long-Noded Pit Viper Decoction for Dispersing Purpura)], *Jiang Su Zhong Yi* [Jiangsu Journal of Traditional Chinese Medicine] 18, 10 (1997): 23.

13. Zhu Jichang, *Tuo Min Jian Jia Wei Zhi Liao Guo Min Xing Zi Dian 32 Li* [Treatment of 32 Cases of Anaphylactoid Purpura with Augmented *Tuo Min Jian* (Desensitization Brew)], *Zhe Jiang Zhong Yi Za Zhi* [Zhejiang Journal of Traditional Chinese Medicine] 31, 11 (1996): 501.

14. Zhang Mingya, *Huo Xue Liang Xue Fa Zhi Liao Guo Min Xing Zi Dian 22 Li* [Treatment of 22 Cases of Anaphylactoid Purpura with the Invigorating and Cooling the Blood Method], *Si Chuan Zhong* Yi [Sichuan Journal of Traditional Chinese Medicine] 8 (1996): 23.

15. Xu Dejun, *Xie Huang San Jia Jian Zhi Liao Guo Min Xing Zi Dian* [Treatment of Anaphylactoid Purpura with Modified *Xie Huang San* (Yellow-Draining Powder)], *Zhe Jiang Zhong Yi Za Zhi* [Zhejiang Journal of Traditional Chinese Medicine] 32, 6 (1997): 273.

16. Wang Zibin, *Qing Dai Yin Zhi Liao Guo Min Xing Zi Dian 120 Li* [Treatment of 120 Cases of Anaphylactoid Purpura with *Qing Dai Yin* (Indigo Beverage)], *Shan Dong Zhong Yi Za Zhi* [Shandong Journal of Traditional Chinese Medicine] 16, 6 (1997): 254.

17. Liu Jizhan, *Zi Shen Tong Luo Tang Zhi Liao Xiao Er Zi Dian Xing Shen Yan 32 Li* [Treatment of 32 Cases of Infantile Purpuric Nephritis with *Zi Shen Tong Luo Tang* (Freeing the Network Vessels Decoction for Purpuric Nephritis)], *Xin Zhong Yi* [New Journal of Traditional Chinese Medicine] 30, 3 (1998): 46.

18. Chen Changjiang, *Tuo Min Jian Jia Wei Zhi Liao Xiao Er Zi Dian Xing Shen Yan 23 Li* [Treatment of 23 Cases of Infantile Purpuric Nephritis with Augmented *Tuo Min Jian* (Desensitization Brew)], *Zhe Jiang Zhong Yi Za Zhi* [Zhejiang Journal of Traditional Chinese Medicine] 33, 9 (1998): 394.

19. Lan Qifang, *Bian Zheng Lun Zhi Hong Ban Xing Zhi Tong Zheng 36 Li Liao Xiao Guan Cha* [Observation of the Effectiveness of Treatment of 36 Cases of Erythromelalgia Based on Pattern Identification], *Xin Zhong Yi* [New Journal of Traditional Chinese Medicine] 29, 6 (1997): 21.

20. Cao Zhong, *Rou Gan Jie Jing Tang Wei Zhu Zhi Liao Lei Nuo Shi Bing* [Treatment of Raynaud's Disease Based on *Rou Gan Jie Jing Tang* (Decoction for Emolliating the Liver and Relieving Tetany)], *Zhong Yi Yao Xue Bao* [Journal of Traditional Chinese Medicine and Materia Medica] 2 (1994): 30-31.

21. Zhao Dianfa, *Wen Yang Tong Mai Yin Zhi Liao Lei Nuo Shi Bing 15 Li* [Treatment of 15 Cases of Raynaud's Disease with *Wen Yang Tong Mai Yin* (Beverage for Warming Yang and Freeing the Blood Vessels)], *Xin Jiang Zhong Yi Yao* [Xinjiang Journal of Traditional Chinese Medicine] 16, 2 (1998): 7-8.

22. Liu Jun, *Fu Zi Li Zhong Tang Jia Wei Zhi Liao Lei Nuo Shi Bing Liao Xiao Fen Xi* [Analysis of the Effectiveness of Treatment of Raynaud's Disease with Augmented *Fu Zi Li Zhong Tang* (Aconite Decoction for Regulating the Middle)], *He Bei Yi Xue* [Hebei Journal of Medicine] 4, 11 (1998): 89.

23. Bai Zhengping, *Zhong Yao Nei Wai Jie He Zhi Liao Lei Nuo Shi Bing 21 Li* [Treatment of 21 Cases of Raynaud's Disease with Combined Internal and External Application of Chinese Materia Medica], *He Nan Zhong Yi Xue Yuan Xue Bao* [Journal of Hunan College of Traditional Chinese Medicine] 19, 1 (1999): 44.

24. Xu Wenliang, *Shao Shan Huo Shou Fa Zhi Liao Lei Nuo Shi Bing 33 Li* [Treatment of 33 Cases of Raynaud's Disease with the Acupuncture Technique of Setting the Mountain on Fire], *Zhong Guo Zhen Jiu* [Chinese Journal of Acupuncture and Moxibustion] 17, 5 (1997): 285-6.

25. Wu Jie, *Wen Zhen Jiu Zhi Liao Lei Nuo Shi Bing 20 Li* [Treatment of 20 Cases of Raynaud's Disease with Warm Needling Moxibustion], *Shang Hai Zhen Jiu Za Zhi* [Shanghai Journal of Acupuncture and Moxibustion] 18, 1 (1999): 7.

26. Hu Guizhi, *Zhong Xi Yi Jie He Zhi Liao Lei Nuo Shi Bing* [Treatment of Raynaud's Disease with a Combination of TCM and Western Medicine], *Zhong Yuan Yi Kan* [Central Plains Medical Publications] 24, 10 (1997): 34-35.

27. Xu Huiyuan, *Zhong Yao Zhi Liao Xiao Tui Pi Fu Kui Yang De Guan Cha* [Survey of Chinese Herbal Treatments for Ulcers of the Lower Leg], *Shan Xi Zhong Yi* [Shanxi Journal of Traditional Chinese Medicine] 12, 2 (1996): 16-17.

28. Wu Yongjin, *Fu Yang San Zhi Liao Xia Zhi Kui Yang 656 Lin Chuang Bao Gao* [Clinical Report on the Treatment of 656 Cases of Ulcer of the Lower Limb with *Fu Yang San* (Skin Ulcer Powder)], *Lin Chuang Pi Fu Ke Za Zhi* [Journal of Clinical Dermatology] 27, 2 (1998): 104-105.

29. Huang Yadi, *Zi Ding Gao He Sheng Ji San Zhi Liao Xia Zhi Kui Yang 34 Li* [Treatment of 34 Cases of Ulcer of the Lower Limb with *Zi Ding Gao* (Gromwell Root and Chinese Violet Paste) and *Sheng Ji San* (Flesh-Generating Powder)], *Zhong Guo Zhong Xi Yi Jie He Za Zhi* [Chinese Journal of Integrated TCM and Western Medicine] 17, 11 (1997): 672.

30. Wang Junying, *Zhong Yong Sheng Huang Qi Zhi Liao Man Xing Xia Zhi Kui Yang De Ti Hui* [Experiences in Treating Chronic Ulcer of the Lower Leg with Increased Dosages of Raw *Huang Qi* (Radix Astragali seu Hedysari)], *Bei Jing Zhong Yi* [Beijing Journal of Traditional Chinese Medicine] 2 (1997): 18.

31. Guo Maoming, *Zhong Xi Yi Jie He Zhi Liao Xiao Tui Man Xing Kui Yang 34 Li Lin Chuang Guan Cha* [Clinical Observation of the Treatment of 34 Cases of Chronic Ulcer of the Lower Leg by Combining TCM and Western Medicine], *Shi Yong Zhong Xi Yi Jie He Za Zhi* [Practical Journal of Integrated TCM and Western Medicine] 11, 9 (1998): 778.

Bullous skin diseases

Bullous skin diseases cover a group of diseases with bullous lesions as their main feature. The causes of this group of diseases are not always clear, but most authorities believe that they fall within the scope of autoimmune and genetic diseases.

Blisters (vesicles and bullae) are accumulations of fluid within or under the epidermis. The type and appearance of a blister is determined by its location.

- Subcorneal blisters form beneath the stratum corneum, have a very thin roof and rupture easily; this type of blister occurs in bullous impetigo and pustular psoriasis.
- Intraepidermal blisters form within the epidermis (in the prickle cell layer); they also have a thin roof and rupture easily. This type of blister occurs in pemphigus, acute eczema and herpes.
- Subepidermal blisters form between the dermis and epidermis, have a much thicker roof and are therefore more tense; this type of blister occurs in bullous pemphigoid, dermatitis herpetiformis, bullous erythema multiforme, and cold or thermal injury.

Vesicles and bullae are found in numerous skin diseases such as bullous impetigo, erythema multiforme, pompholyx, acute eczema (particularly allergic contact dermatitis), and viral infections such as herpes simplex, herpes zoster and varicella (chickenpox), and may also occur after insect bites or in skin disorders due to physical agents.

The primary bullous diseases discussed in this chapter are serious but relatively uncommon diseases. In the treatment of these diseases, attention should be paid to the following aspects:

- careful nursing is needed to prevent secondary infection and complications;
- administration of various vitamins and compound proteins is required to rectify protein loss;
- early use of corticosteroids or immunosuppressive agents is advised in some intractable cases (in cooperation with Western medicine doctors).

Although there is no specific term in TCM covering this group of diseases, it is generally accepted that internal causes include accumulation of Heart-Fire and Spleen-Damp leading over a prolonged period to Spleen and Kidney Deficiency; and accumulation of Damp turbidity and fetal Toxins (Toxins inherited from the mother) wandering to the skin. Externally, this group of diseases is caused by Wind-Heat Toxins obstructing the skin and flesh.

Pemphigus
天疱疮

This is a relatively uncommon but potentially life-threatening autoimmune disease characterized mainly by flaccid superficial vesicles or bullae on the skin and oral mucosa.

It is divided clinically into four types – pemphigus vulgaris, pemphigus vegetans, pemphigus foliaceus, and pemphigus erythematosus – with pemphigus vulgaris being the most common.

In TCM, this disease is also known as *tian pao chuang* (heaven-borne blister sore).

Clinical manifestations

- Pemphigus is most commonly seen in the middle-aged and elderly.
- It usually involves the trunk, limb flexures, scalp, and oral mucosa.
- Lesions mainly manifest as intraepidermal blisters of varying size with flaccid walls and filled with clear fluid; the blisters break easily producing erosion and

exudate. Alternatively, vesicles and greasy yellow crusts appear on an erythematous patch.

- In some cases, papillomatous hyperplasia is noted on the erosive surface with foul-smelling, purulent secretion, followed by thick crusts. Sometimes large amounts of scale and crust form on the primary lesion.
- Nikolsky's sign is positive (separation of the stratum corneum from the underlying layers of the epidermis as a result of the application of slight shearing pressure).
- There is a strong association with underlying neoplasia.
- Different types of pemphigus have different characteristics:

Pemphigus vulgaris

This is the most common type of pemphigus and is seen most often in middle-aged people, presenting as extensive skin lesions and involvement of the oral mucosa (which usually precedes the skin manifestations). Nikolsky's sign is positive in areas subject to pressure or friction. Verrucous proliferation may occur on eroded surfaces after healing. The duration of the disease varies and few patients can be cured. Without treatment, most die of complications such as biochemical abnormalities and secondary infection; even with treatment, the mortality rate can be as high as 15 percent.

Pemphigus vegetans

This is a rare subtype of pemphigus vulgaris and is usually found in the groin, axillae or body folds. After the vesicular lesions rupture, granulomatous hyperplasia may gradually form on the erosive surface, with exudation of blood, serum and pus. Dry verrucous hyperkeratotic hyperplasia may develop in the final stage; this is a severe condition and is fatal for many patients.

Pemphigus foliaceus

Lesions initially involve the scalp, upper chest and back. Crusts form around the very superficial, easily ruptured blisters and moist peripheral areas as well as in areas without blisters or erosion, where exudation is also possible. The disease may persist for a lengthy period without healing, but it does not affect general health apart from some discomfort of the skin. However, when the whole body is involved, the disease may take on the appearance of exfoliative dermatitis with exfoliation, incomplete blisters, and serious erosion and exudation.

Pemphigus erythematosus

This may be a combination of localized pemphigus foliaceus and systemic lupus erythematosus (SLE) since the clinical and immunologic characteristics of SLE are present in addition to the features of pemphigus foliaceus. At the initial stage, this type resembles pemphigus foliaceus, with moist erythema, squamous keratotic lesions and crusts. Lesions involve the face, upper chest and back. Non-intact blisters are rare. Sunlight may aggravate the condition.

Table 8-1 Differentiation of pemphigus vulgaris against bullous pemphigoid and dermatitis herpetiformis

	Pemphigus vulgaris	Bullous pemphigoid	Dermatitis herpetiformis
Sex (male:female)	3:1	1:1	2:1
Age groups affected	Middle-aged and elderly	Mainly the elderly, but also young people and children sometimes	Mainly the young and middle-aged, rarely seen in children
Site of skin lesions	Trunk, limb flexures, scalp	Trunk, flexor aspects of limbs, body flexures	Elbows, knees, buttocks, upper back
Morphology of skin lesions	Flaccid intraepidermal vesicles extending peripherally to form shriveled bullae	Large, tense subepidermal blisters	Clustering, polymorphic lesions with small, tense blisters
Nikolsky's sign	Positive	Negative	Negative
Erosive surface	Mobile, large erosive surface, difficult to heal; heals without scarring	Non-mobile, small erosive surface, likely to heal rapidly	Small erosive surface, likely to heal
Oral lesions	May precede skin lesions; present in all cases in the final stage	Rare	Rare
Histopathology	Intraepidermal fissured blisters with acantholysis (separation of epidermal cells)	Subepidermal tension blisters without acantholysis	Subepidermal tension blisters without acantholysis
Immuno-fluorescence	Immunofluorescence in intercellular substance (antibodies binding to keratinocyte surface)	Sub-epidermal linear form, with circulating IgG antibodies binding to basement membrane zone	Fibrillar or granular IgA deposits in dermal papillae without circulating antibodies

Differential diagnosis

Differentiation is mainly made against bullous pemphigoid and dermatitis herpetiformis (see Table 8-1).

Etiology and pathology

- The main cause of this disease is the frenetic stirring of Heart-Fire complicated by Dampness resulting from dysfunction of the Spleen. Prolonged mental depression or other emotional disturbances cause Qi to stagnate, thus generating Heat. Heat retained in the Heart channel transforms into Fire. The Spleen governs the transformation and transportation of Water and Body Fluids. If this function is impaired, for example due to dietary irregularities, Dampness will form, eventually transforming into Heat and leading to Damp-Heat binding in the Spleen channel. Fire, Heat and Dampness accumulate internally, and Dampness follows Fire and Heat to the exterior to congest in the skin and flesh.
- If Damp-Heat accumulates in the skin over a long period, it will produce Toxins. If external pathogenic factors attack the body at the same time, they can combine with these internal Toxins to produce a pattern of exuberant Damp-Heat Toxins.
- Where Spleen-Damp predominates, the binding of Damp pathogenic factors in the skin and flesh leads to the appearance of multiple blisters, varying in size from one to several centimeters in diameter.
- Where Heart-Fire is predominant, the accumulation of Fire and Heat in the skin leads to patches of erythema and multiple blisters.
- Long-term accumulation of Damp-Heat transforms into Dryness, scorches the Body Fluids and consumes Qi. For this reason, both Qi and Yin will be damaged in the later stages of the disease.

Pattern identification and treatment

INTERNAL TREATMENT

EXUBERANT DAMP-HEAT TOXINS
This pattern is seen in pemphigus vulgaris and pemphigus foliaceus. Blisters appear first on the oral mucosa, rupturing to produce an erosive surface. They then occur all over the body, varying in size from 0.5cm to several centimeters in diameter. Blisters have flaccid walls, contain clear or bloody fluid and rupture easily, after which the eroded surface may be covered with purulent exudate. Accompanying symptoms and signs include pain in the mouth, shortness of breath, fever and chills, fatigue or irritability, a dry mouth, thirst with no desire for drinks, poor appetite, constipation, and reddish urine. The tongue body is red or dark red with a yellow and greasy coating; the pulse is wiry, slippery and rapid.

Treatment principle
Clear Heat and cool the Blood, eliminate Dampness and relieve Toxicity.

Prescription
QING WEN BAI DU YIN JIA JIAN
Beverage for Clearing Scourge and Vanquishing Toxicity, with modifications

Shui Niu Jiao‡ (Cornu Bubali) 15g
Sheng Di Huang (Radix Rehmanniae Glutinosae) 30g
Mu Dan Pi (Cortex Moutan Radicis) 10g
Chi Shao (Radix Paeoniae Rubra) 10g
Huang Qin (Radix Scutellariae Baicalensis) 10g
Huang Lian (Rhizoma Coptidis) 10g
Chao Zhi Mu (Rhizoma Anemarrhenae Asphodeloidis, stir-fried) 10g
Shi Gao‡ (Gypsum Fibrosum) 30g
Xuan Shen (Radix Scrophulariae Ningpoensis) 12g
Lian Qiao (Fructus Forsythiae Suspensae) 10g
Tong Cao (Medulla Tetrapanacis Papyriferi) 10g
Che Qian Zi (Semen Plantaginis) 10g, wrapped

Explanation
- *Shui Niu Jiao*‡ (Cornu Bubali), *Sheng Di Huang* (Radix Rehmanniae Glutinosae), *Xuan Shen* (Radix Scrophulariae Ningpoensis), *Chi Shao* (Radix Paeoniae Rubra), and *Mu Dan Pi* (Cortex Moutan Radicis) clear Heat and cool the Blood.
- *Chao Zhi Mu* (Rhizoma Anemarrhenae Asphodeloidis, stir-fried), *Lian Qiao* (Fructus Forsythiae Suspensae) and *Shi Gao*‡ (Gypsum Fibrosum) drain Fire with cold and bitterness, clear Heat from the Qi level and reduce fever.
- *Huang Qin* (Radix Scutellariae Baicalensis) and *Huang Lian* (Rhizoma Coptidis) clear Heat and dry Dampness, drain Fire and relieve Toxicity.
- *Tong Cao* (Medulla Tetrapanacis Papyriferi) and *Che Qian Zi* (Semen Plantaginis) eliminate Dampness and guide Heat downward.

ACCUMULATION OF SPLEEN-DAMP
This pattern is met in all types of pemphigus. Numerous blisters appear on the trunk, limbs and oral mucosa, varying in size from one to several centimeters in diameter. Blisters have flaccid walls and contain clear fluid. After rupture, an erosive surface forms with exudation and some crusting. Accompanying symptoms

and signs include fatigue, tired limbs, poor appetite, abdominal distension, and loose stools. The tongue body is pale with a white and greasy coating; the pulse is deep and soggy or slippery and thready.

Treatment principle
Clear Heat and transform Dampness.

Prescription
QING PI CHU SHI YIN JIA JIAN
Beverage for Clearing Heat from the Spleen and Eliminating Dampness, with modifications

Chi Fu Ling (Sclerotium Poriae Cocos Rubrae) 15g
Sheng Di Huang (Radix Rehmanniae Glutinosae) 15g
Lian Qiao (Fructus Forsythiae Suspensae) 15g
Yin Chen Hao (Herba Artemisiae Scopariae) 15g
Chao Cang Zhu (Rhizoma Atractylodis, stir-fried) 10g
Chao Bai Zhu (Rhizoma Atractylodis Macrocephalae, stir-fried) 10g
Mai Men Dong (Radix Ophiopogonis Japonici) 10g
Ze Xie (Rhizoma Alismatis Orientalis) 10g
Chao Zhi Ke (Fructus Citri Aurantii, stir-fried) 10g
Jiao Zhi Zi (Fructus Gardeniae Jasminoidis, scorch-fried) 6g
Huang Qin (Radix Scutellariae Baicalensis) 6g
Chi Xiao Dou (Semen Phaseoli Calcarati) 30g
Bai Hua She She Cao (Herba Hedyotidis Diffusae) 30g

Explanation
- *Chi Fu Ling* (Sclerotium Poriae Cocos Rubrae), *Yin Chen Hao* (Herba Artemisiae Scopariae), *Chao Zhi Ke* (Fructus Citri Aurantii, stir-fried), *Chao Cang Zhu* (Rhizoma Atractylodis, stir-fried), *Chao Bai Zhu* (Rhizoma Atractylodis Macrocephalae, stir-fried), *Ze Xie* (Rhizoma Alismatis Orientalis), and *Chi Xiao Dou* (Semen Phaseoli Calcarati) clear Heat and transform Dampness, fortify the Spleen and harmonize the Stomach.
- *Sheng Di Huang* (Radix Rehmanniae Glutinosae), *Mai Men Dong* (Radix Ophiopogonis Japonici), *Lian Qiao* (Fructus Forsythiae Suspensae), *Jiao Zhi Zi* (Fructus Gardeniae Jasminoidis, scorch-fried), *Huang Qin* (Radix Scutellariae Baicalensis), and *Bai Hua She She Cao* (Herba Hedyotidis Diffusae) cool the Blood and relieve Toxicity, enrich Yin and protect Body Fluids.

EXUBERANT HEAT AND DAMPNESS ACCUMULATION

This pattern is seen primarily in pemphigus erythematosus. Large patches of erythema and blisters of various sizes appear on the face, chest and back. Lesions are covered by oily scales and crusts; the scales peel off in layers. Accompanying symptoms and signs include irritability and restlessness, dry mouth, thirst with no desire for drinks, abdominal distension, and poor appetite. The tongue body is red with a yellow and greasy coating; the pulse is wiry and rapid, or slippery and rapid.

Treatment principle
Clear Heat, cool the Blood and eliminate Dampness.

Prescription
JIE DU XIE XIN TANG JIA JIAN
Decoction for Relieving Toxicity and Draining Fire from the Heart, with modifications

Huang Qin (Radix Scutellariae Baicalensis) 10g
Chao Niu Bang Zi (Fructus Arctii Lappae, stir-fried) 10g
Fang Feng (Radix Ledebouriellae Divaricatae) 10g
Hua Shi ‡ (Talcum) 10g, wrapped
Huang Lian (Rhizoma Coptidis) 6g
Chao Zhi Mu (Rhizoma Anemarrhenae Asphodeloidis, stir-fried) 6g
Zhi Zi (Fructus Gardeniae Jasminoidis) 6g
Jing Jie (Herba Schizonepetae Tenuifoliae) 6g
Shi Gao ‡ (Gypsum Fibrosum) 12g
Xuan Shen (Radix Scrophulariae Ningpoensis) 12g
Tong Cao (Medulla Tetrapanacis Papyriferi) 3g
Gan Cao (Radix Glycyrrhizae) 3g
Zi Cao (Radix Arnebiae seu Lithospermi) 15g

Explanation
- *Huang Qin* (Radix Scutellariae Baicalensis), *Zhi Zi* (Fructus Gardeniae Jasminoidis), *Chao Zhi Mu* (Rhizoma Anemarrhenae Asphodeloidis, stir-fried), *Huang Lian* (Rhizoma Coptidis), and *Shi Gao* ‡ (Gypsum Fibrosum) drain Fire with cold and bitterness, clear Heat from the Qi level and reduce fever.
- *Chao Niu Bang Zi* (Fructus Arctii Lappae, stir-fried), *Fang Feng* (Radix Ledebouriellae Divaricatae) and *Jing Jie* (Herba Schizonepetae Tenuifoliae) dissipate Wind and alleviate itching.
- *Zi Cao* (Radix Arnebiae seu Lithospermi) and *Xuan Shen* (Radix Scrophulariae Ningpoensis) cool the Blood and nourish Yin.
- *Hua Shi* ‡ (Talcum), *Tong Cao* (Medulla Tetrapanacis Papyriferi) and *Gan Cao* (Radix Glycyrrhizae) eliminate Dampness and guide Heat downward.

DAMAGE TO QI AND YIN

This pattern is seen in the later stages of all types of pemphigus. The condition tends to linger and responds slowly to treatment. Blisters appear intermittently. Dry crusts form and are difficult to shed. Accompanying symptoms and signs include listlessness, fatigue, tired limbs, shortness of breath, no desire to speak, spontaneous sweating or night sweating, thirst with a small fluid intake, irritability and restlessness, insomnia, abdominal distension, and poor appetite. The tongue body is pale with tooth marks and a thin white or peeling coating; the pulse is deep, thready and forceless.

Treatment principle
Augment Qi and nourish Yin, support Vital Qi (Zheng Qi) and consolidate the Root.

Prescription
SHEN QI ZHI MU TANG JIA JIAN
Ginseng, Astragalus and Anemarrhena Decoction, with modifications

Tian Men Dong (Radix Asparagi Cochinchinensis) 12g
Mai Men Dong (Radix Ophiopogonis Japonici) 12g
Huang Qi (Radix Astragali seu Hedysari) 12g
Dang Shen (Radix Codonopsitis Pilosulae) 12g
Bai Lian (Radix Ampelopsis Japonicae) 10g
Cang Zhu (Rhizoma Atractylodis) 10g
Bai Zhu (Rhizoma Atractylodis Macrocephalae) 10g
Chao Bai Shao (Radix Paeoniae Lactiflorae, stir-fried) 10g
Chi Fu Ling (Sclerotium Poriae Cocos Rubrae) 10g
Zhi Mu (Rhizoma Anemarrhenae Asphodeloidis) 15g
Jin Yin Hua (Flos Lonicerae) 15g
Shan Yao (Radix Dioscoreae Oppositae) 30g
Lü Dou Yi (Testa Phaseoli Radiati) 30g
Chi Xiao Dou (Semen Phaseoli Calcarati) 30g
Bai Hua She She Cao (Herba Hedyotidis Diffusae) 30g

Explanation
- *Huang Qi* (Radix Astragali seu Hedysari), *Dang Shen* (Radix Codonopsitis Pilosulae), *Cang Zhu* (Rhizoma Atractylodis), and *Bai Zhu* (Rhizoma Atractylodis Macrocephalae) augment Qi and support the Spleen, and consolidate the Root to ward off pathogenic factors.
- *Tian Men Dong* (Radix Asparagi Cochinchinensis), *Mai Men Dong* (Radix Ophiopogonis Japonici), *Chao Bai Shao* (Radix Paeoniae Lactiflorae, stir-fried), *Zhi Mu* (Rhizoma Anemarrhenae Asphodeloidis), and *Shan Yao* (Radix Dioscoreae Oppositae) nourish Yin and protect Body Fluids.
- *Chi Fu Ling* (Sclerotium Poriae Cocos Rubrae) and *Chi Xiao Dou* (Semen Phaseoli Calcarati) invigorate the Blood and transform Dampness.
- *Jin Yin Hua* (Flos Lonicerae), *Lü Dou Yi* (Testa Phaseoli Radiati), *Bai Hua She She Cao* (Herba Hedyotidis Diffusae), and *Bai Lian* (Radix Ampelopsis Japonicae) clear Heat and relieve Toxicity, close sores and absorb exudate.

General modifications
1. For raging fever and delirium, add *Lü Dou Yi* (Testa Phaseoli Radiati), *Gui Ban** (Plastrum Testudinis) and *Lian Zi* (Semen Nelumbinis Nuciferae).
2. For poor appetite or blisters in the oral mucosa, add *Bei Sha Shen* (Radix Glehniae Littoralis), *Bai Lian* (Radix Ampelopsis Japonicae), *Sha Ren* (Fructus Amomi), *Huo Xiang* (Herba Agastaches seu Pogostemi), and *Pei Lan* (Herba Eupatorii Fortunei).
3. For numerous, large blisters and severe erosion, add *Wu Jia Pi* (Cortex Acanthopanacis Gracilistyli Radicis), *Dong Gua Pi* (Epicarpium Benincasae Hispidae), *Zi Cao* (Radix Arnebiae seu Lithospermi), *Hong Hua* (Flos Carthami Tinctorii), *Fu Ling Pi* (Cortex Poriae Cocos), *Che Qian Zi* (Semen Plantaginis), and *Che Qian Cao* (Herba Plantaginis).
4. For profuse, foul-smelling exudate, add *Huo Xiang* (Herba Agastaches seu Pogostemi), *Pei Lan* (Herba Eupatorii Fortunei), *Yin Chen Hao* (Herba Artemisiae Scopariae), and *Yi Yi Ren* (Semen Coicis Lachryma-jobi).
5. For severe itching, add *Ku Shen* (Radix Sophorae Flavescentis), *Bai Xian Pi* (Cortex Dictamni Dasycarpi Radicis), *Di Fu Zi* (Fructus Kochiae Scopariae), and *Gou Teng* (Ramulus Uncariae cum Uncis).
6. For a sensation of burning heat and stabbing pain, add *Di Gu Pi* (Cortex Lycii Radicis), *Mu Dan Pi* (Cortex Moutan Radicis), *Chao Huang Lian* (Rhizoma Coptidis, stir-fried), and *Sang Bai Pi* (Cortex Mori Albae Radicis).
7. For mouth and tongue erosion, add *Jin Lian Hua* (Flos Trollii), *Jin Que Hua* (Flos Caraganae Sinicae), *Zang Qing Guo* (Fructus Immaturus Terminaliae Chebulae), and *Jin Guo Lan* (Tuber Tinosporae).
8. For weeping blisters after rupture, add *Huang Qi* (Radix Astragali seu Hedysari) and *Duan Mu Li*‡ (Concha Ostreae Calcinata).
9. For irritability, restlessness and insomnia, add *Lian Zi Xin* (Plumula Nelumbinis Nuciferae), *Lian Qiao Xin* (Semen Forsythiae Suspensae) and *Zhi Zi* (Fructus Gardeniae Jasminoidis).
10. For constipation, add *Xuan Ming Fen*‡ (Mirabilitum Depuratum), *Chao Zhi Ke* (Fructus Citri Aurantii, stir-fried) and *Da Huang* (Radix et Rhizoma Rhei).

PATENT HERBAL MEDICINES
- Take 0.5-1.0g twice a day of *Lei Gong Teng* (Radix Tripterygii Wilfordi) preparations, preferably in syrup or tablet form. These preparations are contraindicated for patients with a low white blood cell count because the herb has immunosuppressant properties.
- For erosion of the oral mucosa, take one or two tablets of *Jin Lian Hua Pian* (Globeflower Tablet) two or three times a day and allow to dissolve on the tongue.

EXTERNAL TREATMENT
- For small unruptured vesicles distributed over a large area, apply *Qing Dai San* (Indigo Powder) or *Qing Liang Gao* (Cool Clearing Paste) directly to the affected area; alternatively, the powder can be mixed into a paste with vegetable oil before application.
- For large vesicles or bullae with profuse watery exudate and obvious erosion after rupture, first prepare a

concentrated decoction with equal amounts of *Ma Chi Xian* (Herba Portulacae Oleraceae) and *Di Yu* (Radix Sanguisorbae Officinalis), or equal amounts of *Long Kui* (Herba Solani Nigri) and *Wu Bei Zi* ‡ (Galla Rhois Chinensis), or *Gan Cao* (Radix Glycyrrhizae) on its own, and use as a wet compress directly on the lesions. Then apply *Qing Dai San* (Indigo Powder) mixed to a paste with vegetable oil. If there are numerous thick crusts with scales, apply *Shi Du Gao* (Damp Toxin Paste).

- For ulceration and erosion of the oral mucosa, use *Xi Lei San* (Tin-Like Powder), *Xi Gua Shuang Pen Ji* (Watermelon Frost Spray Preparation) or *Zhu Huang San* (Pearl and Bezoar Powder) as an oral insufflation to the affected area three times a day.

Clinical notes

- Infections and complications may occur when treating this group of diseases, and therefore involvement of doctors of Western medicine is necessary. Pemphigus can be treated with a combination of TCM and Western medicine. However, complications related to the high doses of steroids or immunosuppressive drugs used to control the condition now cause more deaths than the disease itself.

- In the early stages of treatment with TCM, it is advisable to fortify the Spleen and transform Dampness, clear Heat and relieve Toxicity, with the emphasis being placed on the Spleen and Lungs. In the later stages, treat by augmenting Qi, nourishing Yin, supporting Vital Qi (Zheng Qi), and consolidating the Root, with the emphasis being placed on the Spleen and Kidneys.

- This disease is chronic and recurs frequently; the prognosis is poor.

Advice for the patient/carer

- Keep warm; do not scratch the skin to prevent secondary infection.
- Follow a high-protein, high-calorie and low-salt diet to increase the body's resistance to disease.
- Regular changes to the body position of patients confined to bed for long periods will help to prevent pressure sores.

Case histories

Case 1

Patient
Male, aged 42.

Clinical manifestations
Two years previously, blisters had begun to appear all over the patient's body, preceded by painful blisters in the mouth. The patient had attended the Western medicine department of the hospital and was treated with prednisone 15mg per day, which had prevented the condition from deteriorating. Two weeks ago, the patient had become very tired and the condition suddenly worsened with erosion in the mouth and generalized painful blisters.

Accompanying symptoms and signs included fever, irritability, thirst, constipation, and short voidings of reddish urine. Examination revealed numerous patches of moist erosion on the scalp, face, neck, chest, back, lower back, and groin. Numerous flaccid easily ruptured blisters were also to be found, some with bloody exudate after rupture. Nikolsky's sign was positive. Erosion was noted on the oral mucosa. The tongue body was red with a yellow and greasy coating; the pulse was wiry, slippery and slightly rapid.

Diagnosis
Pemphigus vulgaris (*tian pao chuang*).

Pattern identification
Exuberant Heart-Fire and accumulation of Spleen-Damp, with Heat accumulating in the Xue level.

Treatment principle
Drain Fire and cool the Blood, clear the Spleen and eliminate Dampness.

Prescription ingredients
Ling Yang Jiao Fen* (Cornu Antelopis, powdered) 0.6g
Zhi Zi (Fructus Gardeniae Jasminoidis) 10g
Huang Lian (Rhizoma Coptidis) 10g
Bai Zhu (Rhizoma Atractylodis Macrocephalae) 10g
Zhi Ke (Fructus Citri Aurantii) 10g
Yi Yi Ren (Semen Coicis Lachryma-jobi) 30g
Bi Xie (Rhizoma Dioscoreae Hypoglaucae seu Septemlobae) 10g
Fu Ling Pi (Cortex Poriae Cocos) 15g
Che Qian Cao (Herba Plantaginis) 15g
Che Qian Zi (Semen Plantaginis) 15g, wrapped
Ze Xie (Rhizoma Alismatis Orientalis) 15g
Chong Lou (Rhizoma Paridis) 15g
Bai Hua She She Cao (Herba Hedyotidis Diffusae) 30g

One bag a day was used to prepare a decoction, taken twice a day. The patient was also prescribed prednisone 40mg a day. [i]

Further visits
After seven bags of the decoction, the number of new blisters appearing had diminished and the patient's mood and appetite had improved. After another 14 bags, new blisters had stopped appearing, most of the erosion had dried, and the overall condition had stabilized.

The prescription was modified by removing *Gui Ban** (Plastrum Testudinis), *Zhi Zi* (Fructus Gardeniae Jasminoidis), *Huang Lian* (Rhizoma Coptidis), *Bi Xie* (Rhizoma Dioscoreae Hypoglaucae seu Septemlobae), *Che Qian Cao* (Herba Plantaginis), *Che Qian Zi* (Semen Plantaginis), and *Ze Xie* (Rhizoma Alismatis Orientalis), and adding *Huang Qi* (Radix Astragali seu Hedysari) 10g, *Dang Gui* (Radix Angelicae Sinensis) 10g,

Tai Zi Shen (Radix Pseudostellariae Heterophyllae) 15g, *Bai Bian Dou* (Semen Dolichoris Lablab) 10g, *Shan Yao* (Rhizoma Dioscoreae Oppositae) 10g, and *Dan Shen* (Radix Salviae Miltiorrhizae) 15g.

The patient took this prescription for a month with prednisone 15mg a day.[1] No new blisters had appeared during this period, indicating that this regime had brought the disease under control.

Discussion

In the first prescription, *Ling Yang Jiao Fen** (Cornu Antelopis, powdered) cools the Blood and relieves Toxicity, settles the Liver and quiets the Spirit; *Fu Ling Pi* (Cortex Poriae Cocos), *Bai Zhu* (Rhizoma Atractylodis Macrocephalae) and *Zhi Ke* (Fructus Citri Aurantii) fortify the Spleen, percolate Dampness and regulate Qi; *Huang Lian* (Rhizoma Coptidis) and *Zhi Zi* (Fructus Gardeniae Jasminoidis) drain Fire with cold and bitterness; *Ze Xie* (Rhizoma Alismatis Orientalis), *Che Qian Cao* (Herba Plantaginis), *Che Qian Zi* (Semen Plantaginis), *Yi Yi Ren* (Semen Coicis Lachryma-jobi), and *Bi Xie* (Rhizoma Dioscoreae Hypoglaucae seu Septemlobae) clear Heat and eliminate Dampness; and *Chong Lou* (Rhizoma Paridis) and *Bai Hua She She Cao* (Herba Hedyotidis Diffusae) clear Heat and relieve Toxicity.

In the modified prescription, *Huang Qi* (Radix Astragali seu Hedysari), *Tai Zi Shen* (Radix Pseudostellariae Heterophyllae), *Shan Yao* (Rhizoma Dioscoreae Oppositae), and *Bai Bian Dou* (Semen Dolichoris Lablab) were added to fortify the Spleen and eliminate Dampness, and *Dan Shen* (Radix Salviae Miltiorrhizae) and *Dang Gui* (Radix Angelicae Sinensis) were added to nourish and invigorate the Blood.[1]

Case 2

Patient
Female, aged 46.

Clinical manifestations
Erythema first started to appear on the patient's chest and back one year previously. Blisters subsequently appeared on the erythema. Crusts formed when the blisters burst. The number of blisters gradually increased, sometimes coalescing into patches. Accompanying symptoms and signs included distension and fullness in the stomach and abdomen, long voidings of clear urine and loose stools.

Examination revealed lesions on the chest, back, axillae, and umbilical region with an eroded surface and red areola; lesions were covered by oily crusts. New vesicles were widespread in these areas. The tongue body was pale and enlarged with a white coating; the pulse was deep, thready and moderate.

Diagnosis
Pemphigus erythematosus.

Pattern identification
Exuberant Dampness due to Spleen Deficiency complicated by external contraction of pathogenic Toxins.

Treatment principle
Fortify the Spleen and augment Qi, eliminate Dampness and relieve Toxicity.

Prescription ingredients
Huang Qi (Radix Astragali seu Hedysari) 15g
Tai Zi Shen (Radix Pseudostellariae Heterophyllae) 10g
Bai Zhu (Rhizoma Atractylodis Macrocephalae) 10g
Fu Ling (Sclerotium Poriae Cocos) 10g
Zhi Ke (Fructus Citri Aurantii) 10g
Yi Yi Ren (Semen Coicis Lachryma-jobi) 30g
Dong Gua Pi (Epicarpium Benincasae Hispidae) 30g
Da Fu Pi (Pericarpium Arecae Catechu) 15g
Bai Xian Pi (Cortex Dictamni Dasycarpi Radicis) 30g
Ku Shen (Radix Sophorae Flavescentis) 15g
Che Qian Zi (Semen Plantaginis) 15g
Ze Xie (Rhizoma Alismatis Orientalis) 15g
Chong Lou (Rhizoma Paridis) 15g
Bai Hua She She Cao (Herba Hedyotidis Diffusae) 30g
Sheng Di Huang (Radix Rehmanniae Glutinosae) 15g
Mu Dan Pi (Cortex Moutan Radicis) 15g

One bag a day was used to prepare a decoction, taken twice a day.

Second visit
After 14 bags of the ingredients, the condition had improved. The patient was told to continue with the same decoction with the addition of *Chen Pi* (Pericarpium Citri Reticulatae) 10g and *Bi Xie* (Rhizoma Dioscoreae Hypoglaucae seu Septemlobae) 15g to regulate Qi and fortify the Spleen.

Outcome
After another 30 bags of the decoction, no new blisters had appeared and the skin erosions had disappeared.

Discussion
This is a pattern of exuberant Dampness due to Spleen Deficiency complicated by external contraction of pathogenic Toxins so that the treatment principle of fortifying the Spleen and augmenting Qi, eliminating Dampness and relieving Toxicity was applied. In the prescription, *Huang Qi* (Radix Astragali seu Hedysari), *Tai Zi Shen* (Radix Pseudostellariae Heterophyllae), *Bai Zhu* (Rhizoma Atractylodis Macrocephalae), *Fu Ling* (Sclerotium Poriae Cocos) and *Zhi Ke* (Fructus Citri Aurantii) fortify the Spleen and augment Qi; *Yi Yi Ren* (Semen Coicis Lachryma-jobi), *Dong Gua Pi* (Epicarpium Benincasae Hispidae), *Da Fu Pi* (Pericarpium Arecae Catechu), *Bai Xian Pi* (Cortex Dictamni Dasycarpi Radicis), *Ku Shen* (Radix Sophorae Flavescentis), *Che Qian Zi* (Semen Plantaginis) and *Ze Xie* (Rhizoma Alismatis Orientalis) clear Heat and eliminate Dampness to guide out pathogenic factors; *Chong Lou* (Rhizoma Paridis) and *Bai Hua She She Cao* (Herba Hedyotidis Diffusae) clear Heat and relieve Toxicity; and *Sheng Di Huang* (Radix Rehmanniae Glutinosae) and *Mu Dan Pi* (Cortex Moutan Radicis) clear Heat and cool the Blood.[2]

---

[1] This will normally only be available on prescription from a registered doctor or registered pharmacist.

Literature excerpt

In *Wai Ke Zheng Zong* [An Orthodox Manual of External Diseases], it says: "Pemphigus is due to the frenetic stirring of Heart-Fire complicated by Spleen-Damp. The disease manifests differently depending on whether it occurs in the upper or lower body and whether the weather is hot or cold. When it occurs in the upper body, it is more likely to be due to Wind-Heat than Damp-Heat and the treatment principle should be to cool the Blood and dissipate Wind; when it occurs in the lower body, it is more likely to be due to Damp-Heat than Wind-Heat and the treatment principle should be to percolate Dampness. If the disease is not treated at an early stage, it may evolve into stubborn purpura, which is difficult to cure."

Modern clinical experience

PEMPHIGUS VULGARIS

1. **Zhang Zhili** treated pemphigus vulgaris with an empirical prescription. [3]

Pattern identification
Damp Toxins transforming into Heat which is retained in the Xue level.

Treatment principle
Clear Heat and eliminate Dampness, cool the Blood and relieve Toxicity.

Prescription
SHENG BAI QING HUANG TANG
Gypsum, Cogon Grass, Woad Leaf and Coptis Decoction

Bai Mao Gen (Rhizoma Imperatae Cylindricae) 30g
Shi Gao‡ (Gypsum Fibrosum) 30g
Da Qing Ye (Folium Isatidis seu Baphicacanthi) 30g
Ling Yang Jiao Fen* (Cornu Antelopis, powdered) 0.6g
Zi Hua Di Ding (Herba Violae Yedoensitis) 10g
Lian Zi Xin (Plumula Nelumbinis Nuciferae) 10g
Zhi Zi (Fructus Gardeniae Jasminoidis) 10g
Sheng Di Huang Tan (Radix Rehmanniae Glutinosae Carbonisata) 15g
Tian Hua Fen (Radix Trichosanthis) 15g
Huang Lian (Rhizoma Coptidis) 5g
Gan Cao (Radix Glycyrrhizae) 5g

Modifications
1. For severe pruritus, *Bai Xian Pi* (Cortex Dictamni Dasycarpi Radicis) 30g and *Ku Shen* (Radix Sophorae Flavescentis) 15g were added.
2. For generalized blisters with damp erosion, *Shan Yao* (Radix Dioscoreae Oppositae) 30g, *Bai Bian Dou* (Semen Dolichoris Lablab) 15g and *Yi Yi Ren* (Semen Coicis Lachryma-jobi) 30g were added.

3. For high fever, *Mu Dan Pi* (Cortex Moutan Radicis) 15g was added.
4. For oral erosion, *E Kou San* (Goose-Mouth Sore Powder) was used as an insufflation.

2. **Chen Tongyun** treated long-standing cases of pemphigus vulgaris. [4]

Pattern identification
Internal accumulation of Damp Toxins due to Spleen Deficiency.

Treatment principle
Fortify the Spleen and eliminate Dampness, clear Heat and transform Blood stasis.

Prescription ingredients
Cang Zhu (Rhizoma Atractylodis) 6g
Bai Zhu (Rhizoma Atractylodis Macrocephalae) 10g
Fu Ling (Sclerotium Poriae Cocos) 10g
Yi Yi Ren (Semen Coicis Lachryma-jobi) 15g
Bai Bian Dou (Semen Dolichoris Lablab) 10g
Long Dan Cao (Radix Gentianae Scabrae) 10g
Che Qian Zi (Semen Plantaginis) 15g
Ku Shen (Radix Sophorae Flavescentis) 15g
Di Fu Zi (Fructus Kochiae Scopariae) 10g
Bai Xian Pi (Cortex Dictamni Dasycarpi Radicis) 30g
Dan Shen (Radix Salviae Miltiorrhizae) 10g
Chi Shao (Radix Paeoniae Rubra) 10g
Ji Xue Teng (Caulis Spatholobi) 15g
Bai Ji Li (Fructus Tribuli Terrestris) 15g

One bag a day was used to prepare a decoction, taken twice a day. After 10 bags, acute inflammation was brought under control. *Long Dan Cao* (Radix Gentianae Scabrae), *Ku Shen* (Radix Sophorae Flavescentis) and *Bai Xian Pi* (Cortex Dictamni Dasycarpi Radicis) were removed from the prescription, and *Mu Dan Pi* (Cortex Moutan Radicis) 10g, *Fu Ling Pi* (Cortex Poriae Cocos) 10g, *Ren Dong Teng* (Caulis Lonicerae Japonicae) 15g, and *Ye Jiao Teng* (Caulis Polygoni Multiflori) 15g were added. The patients continued to take the modified prescription for two months.

PEMPHIGUS FOLIACEUS
Hu reported on Jiang Zezhong's empirical prescription for the treatment of pemphigus foliaceus. [5]

Prescription
SHI GAO SHENG DI TANG
Gypsum and Rehmannia Decoction

Shi Gao‡ (Gypsum Fibrosum) 30g
Sheng Di Huang (Radix Rehmanniae Glutinosae) 15g
Zhi Mu (Rhizoma Anemarrhenae Asphodeloidis) 15g
Xuan Shen (Radix Scrophulariae Ningpoensis) 15g
Jin Yin Hua (Flos Lonicerae) 15g

Da Huang (Radix et Rhizoma Rhei) 15g
Lian Qiao (Fructus Forsythiae Suspensae) 9g
Huang Lian (Rhizoma Coptidis) 9g
Mu Dan Pi (Cortex Moutan Radicis) 9g

Modifications
1. For loose stools, *Shan Yao* (Radix Dioscoreae Oppositae) was added.
2. For severe pruritus, *Huang Qi* (Radix Astragali seu Hedysari), *Dang Gui* (Radix Angelicae Sinensis), *Mai Men Dong* (Radix Ophiopogonis Japonici), and *Tu Fu Ling* (Rhizoma Smilacis Glabrae) were added.
3. For Qi and Blood Deficiency, *Huang Qi* (Radix Astragali seu Hedysari), *Bai Shao* (Radix Paeoniae Lactiflorae) and *Dang Gui* (Radix Angelicae Sinensis) were added.

Results were seen after 30 bags of the prescription. Another 20 bags were taken to consolidate the effect.

PEMPHIGUS AND BULLOUS PEMPHIGOID
Han used a combination of TCM and Western medicine to treat ten cases of pemphigus and six cases of bullous pemphigoid.[6] For the TCM treatment, he identified two patterns and treated accordingly.

- **Accumulation of Damp-Heat**

Prescription
YIN CHEN CHI XIAO DOU TANG JIA JIAN
Oriental Wormwood and Aduki Bean Decoction, with modifications

Yin Chen Hao (Herba Artemisiae Scopariae) 30g
Chi Xiao Dou (Semen Phaseoli Calcarati) 30g
Tu Fu Ling (Rhizoma Smilacis Glabrae) 30g
Ze Xie (Rhizoma Alismatis Orientalis) 10g
Chi Shao (Radix Paeoniae Rubra) 10g
*Fang Ji** (Radix Stephaniae Tetrandrae) 12g [ii]
Huang Bai (Cortex Phellodendri) 12g
Zhi Zi (Fructus Gardeniae Jasminoidis) 12g
Cang Zhu (Rhizoma Atractylodis) 12g
Fang Feng (Radix Ledebouriellae Divaricatae) 12g
Bai Zhu (Rhizoma Atractylodis Macrocephalae) 12g
Hei Zhi Ma (Semen Sesami Indici) 15g

Ku Shen (Radix Sophorae Flavescentis) 15g

- **Exuberant Heat Toxins**

Prescription
HUANG LIAN JIE DU TANG JIA JIAN
Coptis Decoction for Relieving Toxicity, with modifications

Huang Lian (Rhizoma Coptidis) 10g
Chan Tui‡ (Periostracum Cicadae) 12g
Zhi Zi (Fructus Gardeniae Jasminoidis) 12g
Huang Qin (Radix Scutellariae Baicalensis) 12g
Huang Bai (Cortex Phellodendri) 12g
Hong Teng (Caulis Sargentodoxae Cuneatae) 12g
Yi Yi Ren (Semen Coicis Lachryma-jobi) 20g
Cang Zhu (Rhizoma Atractylodis) 20g
Tu Fu Ling (Rhizoma Smilacis Glabrae) 15g

External treatment
For thick crusts that did not fall off, he prepared a decoction for use as an external wash once or twice a day.

Huang Bai (Cortex Phellodendri) 20g
Ai Ye (Folium Artemisiae Argyi) 20g
Da Huang (Radix et Rhizoma Rhei) 20g
Bai Xian Pi (Cortex Dictamni Dasycarpi Radicis) 20g
Jing Jie (Herba Schizonepetae Tenuifoliae) 15g
Fang Feng (Radix Ledebouriellae Divaricatae) 15g
Ku Shen (Radix Sophorae Flavescentis) 15g
Feng Fang‡ (Nidus Vespae) 30g
Di Fu Zi (Fructus Kochiae Scopariae) 30g
Ma Chi Xian (Herba Portulacae Oleraceae) 30g
Jin Yin Hua (Flos Lonicerae) 45g

Western medicine
Prednisone 10mg was prescribed for oral administration three times a day. For the ten most serious cases, an intravenous infusion with dexamethasone 10mg was administered once a day for one to two weeks. This medicine was then taken orally at a dosage of 10mg, three times a day. The dosage of dexamethasone was gradually reduced over a period of two to four months until it was discontinued, by which time most of the patients had recovered or shown a significant improvement.

[ii] In those countries where the use of *Fang Ji** (Radix Stephaniae Tetrandrae) is illegal, *Tong Cao* (Medulla Tetrapanacis Papyriferi) 10g can be substituted in this prescription.

Bullous pemphigoid
大疱性类天疱疮

Bullous pemphigoid is a rare, chronic, generalized, sub-epidermal blistering disease normally only seen in the elderly.

In TCM, this condition is also known as *huo chi chuang* (Fire-red sore).

Clinical manifestations

- Lesions usually occur on the trunk, axillae, inguinal groove, and the flexor surfaces of the limbs.
- Tense hemispherical vesicles and bullae appear on normal skin or on areas of erythema. The appearance of blisters may be preceded by urticarial eruptions. The blister wall is thick and blisters have good structural integrity. Firm pressure does not result in extension into normal skin (negative Nikolsky's sign).
- A minority (10-25 percent) of patients have oral lesions. Occasionally, the conjunctiva and vaginal mucosa are affected.
- Itching may be slight or severe. After rupture of the blisters, lesions form crusts and heal rapidly, leaving pigmented patches. Miliary papules are also sometimes seen.

Differential diagnosis

Pemphigus
Lesions mainly manifest as blisters of varying size with thin, flaccid walls, filled with clear fluid; the blisters break easily producing erosion and exudate. Scales and crusts may form on the primary lesion. Pemphigus can occur on any part of the body and may involve the oral mucosa (see also Table 8-1 in the Pemphigus section).

Dermatitis herpetiformis
Lesions manifest as symmetrically distributed, small, round vesicles on an erythematous base and generally involve the elbows, the knees, the extensor surfaces of the limbs, the base of the scalp, and the buttocks. This disease does not affect the oral mucosa. The initial eruption is itchy and progresses to form intensely burning lesions (see also Table 8-1 in the Pemphigus section).

Erythema multiforme
This disease has a rapid onset and is accompanied by systemic symptoms such as fever. It generally involves the dorsum of the hands and feet, the extensor surfaces of the arm and leg, and more rarely the face and neck. Lesions take a variety of forms, which may include vesicles or bullae. Bullae and erosions may also be present in the oral cavity. Each episode of erythema multiforme lasts approximately one month, and recurrences are fairly common. Erythema multiforme is likely to occur at a younger age than bullous pemphigoid.

Etiology and pathology

Bullous pemphigoid is caused by Heart-Fire due to accumulated Heat in the Heart channel and by Spleen-Damp due to Spleen Deficiency resulting in the Spleen failing to transport water and Dampness. Fire and Dampness then move outward to affect the skin. If the disease persists, Dampness and Fire transform into Dryness, which burns the Stomach and damages Body Fluids. By treating Heart-Fire and Spleen-Damp, Dryness is eliminated.

Pattern identification and treatment

INTERNAL TREATMENT

HEART-FIRE
Vesicles and bullae arise in erythematous skin. The eruption is often generalized, but the most common sites are the chest, abdomen and flexor surfaces of the limbs. Accompanying symptoms include fever, and aching and painful joints. The tongue body is red with a thin yellow coating; the pulse is rapid.

Treatment principle
Clear Heat from the Heart and relieve Toxicity.

Prescription
CHI DOU YIN JIA JIAN
Aduki Bean Beverage, with modifications

Chi Xiao Dou (Semen Phaseoli Calcarati) 15g
Zi Cao (Radix Arnebiae seu Lithospermi) 15g
Sheng Di Huang (Radix Rehmanniae Glutinosae) 10g
Mu Dan Pi (Cortex Moutan Radicis) 10g
Zhi Zi (Fructus Gardeniae Jasminoidis) 10g
Jin Yin Hua (Flos Lonicerae) 10g
Lian Qiao (Fructus Forsythiae Suspensae) 10g
Tong Cao (Medulla Tetrapanacis Papyriferi) 6g
Dan Zhu Ye (Herba Lophatheri Gracilis) 6g
Deng Xin Cao (Medulla Junci Effusi) 6g

Explanation
- *Sheng Di Huang* (Radix Rehmanniae Glutinosae), *Mu Dan Pi* (Cortex Moutan Radicis) and *Zi Cao* (Radix Arnebiae seu Lithospermi) clear Heat and cool the Blood.
- *Jin Yin Hua* (Flos Lonicerae), *Zhi Zi* (Fructus Gardeniae Jasminoidis) and *Lian Qiao* (Fructus Forsythiae Suspensae) clear Heat from the Heart and relieve Toxicity.
- *Chi Xiao Dou* (Semen Phaseoli Calcarati) invigorates the Blood and disperses swelling.
- *Tong Cao* (Medulla Tetrapanacis Papyriferi), *Dan Zhu Ye* (Herba Lophatheri Gracilis) and *Deng Xin Cao* (Medulla Junci Effusi) clear Heat from the Heart and guide out reddish urine to eliminate Heart-Fire Toxins from the body through urination.

SPLEEN-DAMP

This pattern manifests as a widespread distribution of tense-walled blisters. Exudation and erosion occur after rupture. Accompanying symptoms include poor appetite. The tongue body is enlarged and tender with a thin yellow coating; the pulse is slippery and rapid.

Treatment principle
Augment Qi and fortify the Spleen, transform Dampness and relieve Toxicity.

Prescription
WU LING SAN JIA JIAN
Poria Five Powder, with modifications

Dang Shen (Radix Codonopsitis Pilosulae) 10g
Bai Zhu (Rhizoma Atractylodis Macrocephalae) 10g
Huang Bai (Cortex Phellodendri) 10g
Fu Ling (Sclerotium Poriae Cocos) 10g
Cang Zhu (Rhizoma Atractylodis) 10g
Yi Yi Ren (Semen Coicis Lachryma-jobi) 15g
Yin Chen Hao (Herba Artemisiae Scopariae) 15g
Da Fu Pi (Pericarpium Arecae Catechu) 12g
Che Qian Zi (Semen Plantaginis) 12g
Di Fu Zi (Fructus Kochiae Scopariae) 12g
Bai Xian Pi (Cortex Dictamni Dasycarpi Radicis) 12g
Ku Shen (Radix Sophorae Flavescentis) 6g

Explanation
- *Dang Shen* (Radix Codonopsitis Pilosulae), *Fu Ling* (Sclerotium Poriae Cocos), *Bai Zhu* (Rhizoma Atractylodis Macrocephalae), *Cang Zhu* (Rhizoma Atractylodis), and *Yi Yi Ren* (Semen Coicis Lachryma-jobi) augment Qi and support the Spleen.
- *Huang Bai* (Cortex Phellodendri), *Yin Chen Hao* (Herba Artemisiae Scopariae), *Che Qian Zi* (Semen Plantaginis), and *Da Fu Pi* (Pericarpium Arecae Catechu) clear Heat and benefit the movement of Dampness, harmonize the Stomach and disperse swelling.
- *Bai Xian Pi* (Cortex Dictamni Dasycarpi Radicis), *Di Fu Zi* (Fructus Kochiae Scopariae) and *Ku Shen* (Radix Sophorae Flavescentis) relieve Toxicity and transform Dampness, expel pathogenic factors and alleviate itching.

General modifications
1. For fever, add *Jin Yin Hua* (Flos Lonicerae), *Huang Qin* (Radix Scutellariae Baicalensis) and *Ban Lan Gen* (Radix Isatidis seu Baphicacanthi).
2. For blood-filled blisters, add *Mu Dan Pi* (Cortex Moutan Radicis), *Xian He Cao* (Herba Agrimoniae Pilosae) and *Bai Mao Gen* (Rhizoma Imperatae Cylindricae).
3. For severe pruritus, add *Bai Xian Pi* (Cortex Dictamni Dasycarpi Radicis), *Chan Tui* ‡ (Periostracum Cicadae) and *Xu Chang Qing* (Radix Cynanchi Paniculati).

Clinical notes

- Since this disease is seen most frequently in the elderly, the addition of light supplementing materia medica to facilitate recovery is recommended (see Spleen-Damp pattern).
- In serious cases, treatment should be combined with administration of corticosteroids by a doctor of Western medicine.

Dermatitis herpetiformis
疱疹样皮炎

This chronic vesicular disease, which may last for decades, is seen most frequently in the young and middle-aged. The vesicles erupt in clusters, similar to herpes simplex, which gives the disease its name in English. Some authorities consider that it is related to the immune response of some individuals to gluten, which leads to gluten-sensitive enteropathy (celiac disease); dermatitis herpetiformis affects about 10% of celiac patients. However, although gluten-sensitive enteropathy is generally present, most patients with dermatitis herpetiformis are asymptomatic.

In TCM, dermatitis herpetiformis is also known as *zhi zhu huang* (spider sore) or *zi jie chuang* (purple scabies sore).

Clinical manifestations

- Most patients are in the 20-55 age range, with males twice as likely to be affected as females. It is rarely seen in patients of African or Asian origin.

- The disease generally involves the posterior axillary fold, the scapula, the base of the scalp, the sacrum, the buttocks, the knees, and the forearm, especially the extensor aspect near the elbow.

- At the initial stage, lesions manifest as symmetrical erythema, papules or urticarial wheals; clusters of small, round vesicles 3-4 mm in diameter appear on an erythematous base. The fluid in the vesicles is clear initially, but turns turbid later. Itching and burning are intense, with the result that vesicles are often broken by scratching to leave excoriations.

- Some patients have enteropathy as a complication, with diarrhea, abdominal pain and anemia. Some may also develop small bowel lymphoma.

- The disease tends to linger and recur, although this can be reduced by adherence to a gluten-free diet.

Differential diagnosis

Pemphigus
Lesions mainly manifest as blisters of varying size with thin, flaccid walls and filled with clear fluid; the blisters break easily producing erosion and exudate. Scales and crusts may form on the primary lesion. Pemphigus can occur on any part of the body and may involve the oral mucosa. Itching is not usually pronounced (see also Table 8-1 in the Pemphigus section).

Bullous pemphigoid
Lesions manifest as tense hemispherical vesicles and bullae on normal skin or on areas of erythema and usually involve the trunk, axillae, inguinal groove, and the flexor surfaces of the limbs. Itching may be slight or severe. After rupture of the blisters, lesions form crusts and heal rapidly, leaving pigmented patches. Some patients have oral lesions (see also Table 8-1 in the Pemphigus section).

Bullous impetigo
This is seen most frequently in children. Lesions manifest as thin-walled vesicles and bullae containing pus. They mainly involve the areas around the mouth and nose or on the limbs. The lesions rupture rapidly. The condition may become disseminated.

Scabies
Scabies is characterized by the development of vesicles and burrows in the skin at any site, characteristically at the wrist, the web of the fingers and the lower abdomen, with intense itching at night. Dermatitis herpetiformis lacks the grayish linear, curved or serpiginous burrows characteristic of scabies, but excoriations may make differentiation difficult.

Papular urticaria
Lesions, which usually involve the lumbosacral region, buttocks, trunk, and limbs, manifest initially as red, oval, infiltrative urticarial papules up to 5mm in diameter with papulovesicles or vesicles at the center. They may last for up to two weeks and recur in crops. Incidence is high among infants and young children, unlike dermatitis herpetiformis, which is rare in this age group.

Etiology and pathology

- If internal accumulation of Damp-Heat is complicated by externally-contracted Wind-Damp pathogenic factors, the three factors gather and fight in the skin and flesh to cause the disease. Fire and Heat spreading outward to the skin give rise to erythema, Dampness accumulating in the skin results in vesicles, and itching is due to Wind wandering through the skin and interstices (*cou li*).

- Retention of Fire Toxins in the Heart and Spleen channels leads to the formation of Blood-Heat, which generates Wind. This Wind then attacks the skin and interstices (*cou li*), gradually causing lesions to appear.

- Deficiency of the Spleen leads to impairment of its transformation and transportation function, causing internal accumulation of Damp-Heat. The condition is further complicated by invasion of Wind Toxins, which obstruct the channels and network vessels, resulting in undernourishment of the skin due to shortage of Blood.

- If the disease persists, Heat Toxins damage Body Fluids and consume the Blood, thus damaging Yin and depleting Blood; this in turn gives rise to Wind-Dryness and Blood-Dryness, depriving the skin of moisture.

Pattern identification and treatment

INTERNAL TREATMENT

FRENETIC STIRRING OF HEART-FIRE
Lesions manifest as papules, papulovesicles or vesicles on an erythematous base, either grouped in clusters or

becoming confluent to form large patches. The central part of the clusters or patches may resolve gradually with new lesions appearing at the periphery. Itching is intense, with obvious excoriation. A small amount of bloody exudate appears after scratching, followed by the formation of crusts. Accompanying symptoms include lassitude and poor appetite. The tongue body is red with a yellow coating; the pulse is rapid.

Treatment principle
Drain Fire and relieve Toxicity, dissipate Wind and alleviate itching.

Prescription
QIN LIAN JIE DU TANG JIA JIAN
Scutellaria and Coptis Decoction for Relieving Toxicity, with modifications

Huang Qin (Radix Scutellariae Baicalensis) 10g
Cang Zhu (Rhizoma Atractylodis) 10g
Bai Zhu (Rhizoma Atractylodis Macrocephalae) 10g
Ku Shen (Radix Sophorae Flavescentis) 10g
Fang Feng (Radix Ledebouriellae Divaricatae) 10g
Chao Huang Lian (Rhizoma Coptidis, stir-fried) 6g
Jiao Zhi Zi (Fructus Gardeniae Jasminoidis, scorch-fried) 6g
Chao Zhi Mu (Rhizoma Anemarrhenae Asphodeloidis, stir-fried) 4.5g
Chan Tui ‡ (Periostracum Cicadae) 4.5g
Huo Xiang (Herba Agastaches seu Pogostemi) 12g
Pei Lan (Herba Eupatorii Fortunei) 12g
Bai Xian Pi (Cortex Dictamni Dasycarpi Radicis) 12g
Di Fu Zi (Fructus Kochiae Scopariae) 12g
Liu Yi San (Six-To-One Powder) 30g, wrapped
Chi Xiao Dou (Semen Phaseoli Calcarati) 30g
Cang Er Zi (Fructus Xanthii Sibirici) 3g

Explanation
- *Chao Huang Lian* (Rhizoma Coptidis, stir-fried), *Huang Qin* (Radix Scutellariae Baicalensis) and *Jiao Zhi Zi* (Fructus Gardeniae Jasminoidis, scorch-fried) drain Fire and relieve Toxicity.
- *Huo Xiang* (Herba Agastaches seu Pogostemi), *Pei Lan* (Herba Eupatorii Fortunei) and *Liu Yi San* (Six-To-One Powder) aromatically transform turbidity and guide Heat downward.
- *Cang Zhu* (Rhizoma Atractylodis), *Bai Zhu* (Rhizoma Atractylodis Macrocephalae) and *Chi Xiao Dou* (Semen Phaseoli Calcarati) support the Spleen and dry Dampness.
- *Fang Feng* (Radix Ledebouriellae Divaricatae), *Ku Shen* (Radix Sophorae Flavescentis), *Chan Tui* ‡ (Periostracum Cicadae), and *Cang Er Zi* (Fructus Xanthii Sibirici) dredge Wind and alleviate itching.
- *Bai Xian Pi* (Cortex Dictamni Dasycarpi Radicis), *Di Fu Zi* (Fructus Kochiae Scopariae) and *Chao Zhi Mu*

(Rhizoma Anemarrhenae Asphodeloidis, stir-fried) relieve Toxicity and alleviate itching.

EXUBERANT DAMP ENCUMBERING THE SPLEEN
Lesions manifest mainly as clusters of itchy papulovesicles, vesicles and pustules. Exudation and maceration follow rupture of the lesions due to scratching. Accompanying symptoms and signs include diarrhea, abdominal pain and poor appetite. The tongue body is pale red with a thin white or thin, glossy and slightly greasy coating; the pulse is soggy and slippery.

Treatment principle
Fortify the Spleen and eliminate Dampness, dissipate Wind and alleviate itching.

Prescription
SHEN LING BAI ZHU SAN JIA JIAN
Ginseng, Poria and White Atractylodes Powder, with modifications

Jiao Bai Zhu (Rhizoma Atractylodis Macrocephalae, scorch-fried) 10g
Chao Bai Bian Dou (Semen Dolichoris Lablab, stir-fried) 10g
Fang Feng (Radix Ledebouriellae Divaricatae) 10g
Ze Xie (Rhizoma Alismatis Orientalis) 10g
Huo Xiang (Herba Agastaches seu Pogostemi) 12g
Shan Yao (Radix Dioscoreae Oppositae) 12g
Pei Lan (Herba Eupatorii Fortunei) 12g
Bai Xian Pi (Cortex Dictamni Dasycarpi Radicis) 12g
Di Fu Zi (Fructus Kochiae Scopariae) 12g
Huang Qin (Radix Scutellariae Baicalensis) 6g
Hu Huang Lian (Rhizoma Picrorhizae Scrophulariiflorae) 6g
Ku Shen (Radix Sophorae Flavescentis) 6g

Explanation
- *Huo Xiang* (Herba Agastaches seu Pogostemi), *Pei Lan* (Herba Eupatorii Fortunei), *Shan Yao* (Radix Dioscoreae Oppositae), *Chao Bai Bian Dou* (Semen Dolichoris Lablab, stir-fried), *Ze Xie* (Rhizoma Alismatis Orientalis), and *Jiao Bai Zhu* (Rhizoma Atractylodis Macrocephalae, scorch-fried) aromatically transform turbidity, augment Qi and support the Spleen.
- *Huang Qin* (Radix Scutellariae Baicalensis) and *Hu Huang Lian* (Rhizoma Picrorhizae Scrophulariiflorae) clear the Heart and drain Fire with cold and bitterness, and dry Dampness.
- *Fang Feng* (Radix Ledebouriellae Divaricatae) and *Ku Shen* (Radix Sophorae Flavescentis) dredge Wind and alleviate itching.
- *Di Fu Zi* (Fructus Kochiae Scopariae) and *Bai Xian Pi* (Cortex Dictamni Dasycarpi Radicis) relieve Toxicity and alleviate itching.

BLOOD-DRYNESS DUE TO YIN DEFICIENCY

This is a chronic and recurrent condition with erythematous and vesicular lesions. Excoriations, bloody crusts, and thickened and rough skin with pigmentation are also evident. Accompanying symptoms and signs include dizziness, lassitude, tired limbs, emaciation, and poor appetite. The tongue body is red with a scant coating; the pulse is thready and rapid.

Treatment principle

Nourish the Blood and moisten Dryness, enrich Yin and clear Heat.

Prescription

DANG GUI YIN ZI JIA JIAN

Chinese Angelica Root Drink, with modifications

Dang Gui (Radix Angelicae Sinensis) 10g
Chao Bai Shao (Radix Paeoniae Lactiflorae, stir-fried) 10g
Sheng Di Huang (Radix Rehmanniae Glutinosae) 10g
Shu Di Huang (Radix Rehmanniae Glutinosae Conquita) 10g
Xuan Shen (Radix Scrophulariae Ningpoensis) 10g
Mai Men Dong (Radix Ophiopogonis Japonici) 10g
Nan Sha Shen (Radix Adenophorae) 15g
He Shou Wu (Radix Polygoni Multiflori) 15g
Shan Yao (Radix Dioscoreae Oppositae) 15g
Bai Hua She She Cao (Herba Hedyotidis Diffusae) 15g
Bai Xian Pi (Cortex Dictamni Dasycarpi Radicis) 15g
Fang Feng (Radix Ledebouriellae Divaricatae) 12g
Gou Teng (Ramulus Uncariae cum Uncis) 12g
Tian Hua Fen (Radix Trichosanthis) 12g
Gan Cao (Radix Glycyrrhizae) 12g

Explanation

- *Dang Gui* (Radix Angelicae Sinensis), *Chao Bai Shao* (Radix Paeoniae Lactiflorae, stir-fried), *Sheng Di Huang* (Radix Rehmanniae Glutinosae), *Shu Di Huang* (Radix Rehmanniae Glutinosae Conquita), and *He Shou Wu* (Radix Polygoni Multiflori) nourish the Blood and moisten Dryness.

- *Nan Sha Shen* (Radix Adenophorae), *Tian Hua Fen* (Radix Trichosanthis), *Mai Men Dong* (Radix Ophiopogonis Japonici), *Xuan Shen* (Radix Scrophulariae Ningpoensis), *Shan Yao* (Radix Dioscoreae Oppositae), and *Gan Cao* (Radix Glycyrrhizae) enrich Yin and generate Body Fluids.

- *Bai Hua She She Cao* (Herba Hedyotidis Diffusae), *Bai Xian Pi* (Cortex Dictamni Dasycarpi Radicis), *Fang Feng* (Radix Ledebouriellae Divaricatae), and *Gou Teng* (Ramulus Uncariae cum Uncis) dissipate Wind and alleviate itching to aid healing of the excoriations.

General modifications

1. For irritability, restlessness and insomnia, add *He Huan Pi* (Cortex Albizziae Julibrissin), *Bai Zi Ren* (Semen Biotae Orientalis) and *Wu Wei Zi* (Fructus Schisandrae).

2. For poor appetite, add *Ji Nei Jin* ‡ (Endothelium Corneum Gigeriae Galli), *Shan Zha* (Fructus Crataegi), *Chao Gu Ya* (Fructus Setariae Italicae Germinatus, stir-fried), and *Chao Mai Ya* (Fructus Hordei Vulgaris Germinatus, stir-fried).

3. For weakness in the limbs and lassitude, add *Tu Si Zi* (Semen Cuscutae), *Gou Ji* (Rhizoma Cibotii Barometz) and *Xu Chang Qing* (Radix Cynanchi Paniculati).

4. For severe itching, add *Bai Ji Li* (Fructus Tribuli Terrestris), *Ku Shen* (Radix Sophorae Flavescentis), *Xi Xian Cao* (Herba Siegesbeckiae), and *Yi Mu Cao* (Herba Leonuri Heterophylli).

5. For lesions grouped on the back and lower back, add *Xi Xian Cao* (Herba Siegesbeckiae) and *Chao Du Zhong* (Cortex Eucommiae Ulmoidis, stir-fried).

6. For erosion and suppuration due to scratching, add *Pu Gong Ying* (Herba Taraxaci cum Radice), *Chong Lou* (Rhizoma Paridis) and *Ye Ju Hua* (Flos Chrysanthemi Indici).

EXTERNAL TREATMENT

- For lesions mainly characterized by papules and papulovesicles accompanied by intense itching, *Cang Fu Shui Xi Ji* (Atractylodes and Broom Cypress Wash Preparation) or *Lu Lu Tong Shui Xi Ji* (Sweetgum Fruit Wash Preparation) can be used as a wash for the affected area. Alternatively, the area can be washed with a decoction prepared from *Chu Tao Ye* (Folium Broussonetiae) 60g, *Xiang Fu* (Rhizoma Cyperi Rotundi) 60g and *Mu Zei* (Herba Equiseti Hiemalis) 30g.

- For relatively large amounts of exudate from vesicles and pustules, *Shi Liu Pi Shui Xi Ji* (Pomegranate Rind Wash Preparation) can be applied to the affected area as a wet compress. When the exudate has dried up, apply *Qing Dai San* (Indigo Powder) mixed to a paste with vegetable oil.

Clinical notes

- At the initial stage, follow the treatment principle of clearing Heat from the Heart, draining Fire, fortifying the Spleen, and transforming Dampness. In the later stages, treat by augmenting Qi and protecting Yin to reinforce Vital Qi (Zheng Qi) and consolidate the Root.

- External treatment is relatively effective in absorbing Dampness and closing sores, dissipating Wind and alleviating itching. Better results may be obtained if internal treatment is combined with external treatment.

- A wet compress should be applied promptly after blisters rupture with exudation and erosion, thus helping the area to dry as quickly as possible and preventing suppuration.

- The disease has a long duration with alternating periods of exacerbation and remission. It generally has a good prognosis and a low mortality rate. Where it is complicated by malignant tumors such as small bowel lymphoma, the prognosis is often poor. If the disease occurs in children, it will generally disappear during adolescence.

Advice for the patient

- Keep the affected area clean and dry. Avoid scratching and washing with hot water so as to prevent infection.

- Eat easily digestible and nutritious food. A gluten-free diet is recommended; it may be necessary to maintain this diet for several months. Rice can be eaten instead of other cereal products.

- In the rare cases where herpes or ulceration occurs in the mouth, attention should be paid to oral hygiene.

Case history

Patient
Male, aged 48.

Clinical manifestations
Erythema and recurrent crops of vesicles had occurred on the trunk and limbs for four years with intermittent exacerbation and remission. Pinhead to 0.5cm vesicles containing a clear fluid were seen around the mouth and on the trunk and limbs. Yellow crusts had formed in some places. Nikolsky's sign was negative. The tongue body was pale with a white and greasy coating; the pulse was wiry.

Pattern identification
Heat in the Heart channel and Dampness in the Spleen channel leading to the internal accumulation of Damp-Heat, which had spread outward to produce sores.

Treatment principle
Eliminate Dampness, clear Heat and relieve Toxicity.

Prescription ingredients
Huang Qin (Radix Scutellariae Baicalensis) 9g
Chi Fu Ling (Sclerotium Poriae Cocos Rubrae) 9g
Ze Xie (Rhizoma Alismatis Orientalis) 9g
Yi Yi Ren (Semen Coicis Lachryma-jobi) 9g
Chong Lou (Rhizoma Paridis) 9g

Lian Qiao (Fructus Forsythiae Suspensae) 9g
Bai Xian Pi (Cortex Dictamni Dasycarpi Radicis) 9g
Di Fu Zi (Fructus Kochiae Scopariae) 9g
Mu Dan Pi (Cortex Moutan Radicis) 9g
Chi Shao (Radix Paeoniae Rubra) 9g
Jin Yin Hua (Flos Lonicerae) 12g
Sheng Di Huang (Radix Rehmanniae Glutinosae) 30g

One bag a day was used to prepare a decoction, taken twice a day.

Second visit
After taking the decoction for one week, new vesicles had appeared and itching had intensified. The tongue body was pale with a thin white coating; the pulse was wiry, thready and slippery.

Revised treatment principle
The condition had lasted for a long time with damage to Yin and consumption of Blood; the treatment principle was therefore amended to nourishing Yin and eliminating Dampness.

Prescription ingredients
Sheng Di Huang (Radix Rehmanniae Glutinosae) 90g
Xuan Shen (Radix Scrophulariae Ningpoensis) 90g
Dan Shen (Radix Salviae Miltiorrhizae) 60g
Fu Ling (Sclerotium Poriae Cocos) 60g
Ze Xie (Rhizoma Alismatis Orientalis) 60g
She Chuang Zi (Fructus Cnidii Monnieri) 60g
Bai Xian Pi (Cortex Dictamni Dasycarpi Radicis) 60g
Gan Cao (Radix Glycyrrhizae) 30g

These ingredients were ground into a powder and made into 9g pills with honey. Two pills a day were taken. For external treatment, *Shi Zhen Fen* (Eczema Powder) was mixed with *Xiang You* (Oleum Sesami Seminis) and applied to the affected area.

Outcome
After three weeks, there were fewer blisters, but the itching still remained. The patient was told to continue taking the pills. After another two months, the number of blisters had been reduced further. Crusts had formed in a few places with dark pigmentation. The patient was told to continue with the pills for another month to consolidate the improvement. [7]

Literature excerpt

In *Wai Ke Bai Xiao Quan Shu* [A Compendium of the Effects of External Diseases], it says: "*Zi jie chuang* (purple scabies sore) is due to the accumulation of Toxins in the Zang-Fu organs. Pathogenic Qi steams in the Lungs, but since the Lungs govern the skin and hair, it moves along the channels and network vessels to the head and face, the skin on the body, and the hands and feet, producing purple, scabies-like sores that are painful and itchy. If the disease persists, accompanying symptoms can include vomiting and trance. The condition should be treated as quickly as possible."

Subcorneal pustulosis
角层下脓疱性皮肤病

This is a rare, chronic, benign, recurrent vesicopustular skin disease occurring most frequently in middle-aged women.

Clinical manifestations

- Subcorneal pustulosis occurs most frequently in middle-aged women with a female to male ratio of 4:1.
- The disease generally involves the inguinal groove, the axillae, the submammary region, the flexor aspect of the limbs, the dorsal aspect of the toes, and the web between the toes.
- At the initial stage, vesicles appear for a short time before changing into flaccid turbid pustules surrounded by a transient erythematous flare. Pustules may expand to form annular or gyrate shapes. After a few days, pustules dry up to form crusts or scales. Pale brown pigmentation is left after crusts or scales are shed.
- New pustules may appear on the original sites of the lesions several days, weeks or months after the old pustules heal.

Differential diagnosis

Impetigo
This is an infectious bacterial disease caused by staphylococci or streptococci. The skin reddens and small, fluid-filled, flaccid blisters appear. However, they quickly rupture to reveal an eroded base. A layer of thick, golden yellow crust forms after the fluid dries up. Impetigo mostly occurs in young people and is itchy.

Pemphigus
This disease usually affects the middle-aged and elderly. Lesions mainly involve the trunk and limbs and manifest as blisters of varying size with flaccid walls and filled with clear fluid; the blisters break easily producing erosion and exudate. Scale and crust may form on the primary lesion.

Etiology and pathology

- Fire resulting from emotional disturbances such as irascibility or impatience disturbs the Blood vessels causing Heat in the Blood to transform into Toxins, which move to the skin to cause the disease.
- Spleen Yang Deficiency or overintake of spicy food, fish or seafood can lead to Dampness encumbering the Middle Burner. If Dampness is retained for a long period, it transforms into Damp Toxins, which flow through the channels and network vessels to the skin and flesh, moving upward, downward or transversely to the limbs, gradually producing pustular eruptions.
- Since Dampness is sticky and clearing Heat Toxins is often difficult, the disease tends to recur.

Pattern identification and treatment

INTERNAL TREATMENT

HYPERACTIVITY OF HEART-FIRE
Eruptions are generalized, manifesting as disseminated blisters filled with turbid fluid and surrounded by areolae. Pustules may expand to form arcuate, annular or gyrate lesions. A sensation of mild itching may be experienced. The tongue body is red with a scant coating; the pulse is thready and rapid.

Treatment principle
Repress Fire with cold and bitterness.

Prescription
HUANG LIAN JIE DU TANG HE WU WEI XIAO DU YIN JIA JIAN
Coptis Decoction for Relieving Toxicity Combined With Five-Ingredient Beverage for Dispersing Toxicity, with modifications

Chao Huang Lian (Rhizoma Coptidis, stir-fried) 12g
Gan Cao (Radix Glycyrrhizae) 12g
Huang Qin (Radix Scutellariae Baicalensis) 10g
Huang Bai (Cortex Phellodendri) 10g
Jiao Zhi Zi (Fructus Gardeniae Jasminoidis, scorch-fried) 10g
Lian Qiao (Fructus Forsythiae Suspensae) 10g
Xuan Shen (Radix Scrophulariae Ningpoensis) 10g
Pu Gong Ying (Herba Taraxaci cum Radice) 12g
Chong Lou (Rhizoma Paridis) 12g
Ye Ju Hua (Flos Chrysanthemi Indici) 12g
Chi Shao (Radix Paeoniae Rubra) 12g
Bai Hua She She Cao (Herba Hedyotidis Diffusae) 15g
Yi Yi Ren (Semen Coicis Lachryma-jobi) 15g

Explanation
- *Chao Huang Lian* (Rhizoma Coptidis, stir-fried), *Huang Qin* (Radix Scutellariae Baicalensis), *Huang Bai* (Cortex Phellodendri), and *Jiao Zhi Zi* (Fructus Gardeniae

Jasminoidis, scorch-fried) repress Fire with cold and bitterness.

- *Pu Gong Ying* (Herba Taraxaci cum Radice), *Chong Lou* (Rhizoma Paridis), *Ye Ju Hua* (Flos Chrysanthemi Indici), and *Bai Hua She She Cao* (Herba Hedyotidis Diffusae) clear Heat and relieve Toxicity.
- *Xuan Shen* (Radix Scrophulariae Ningpoensis), *Lian Qiao* (Fructus Forsythiae Suspensae) and *Gan Cao* (Radix Glycyrrhizae) clear Heat from the Heart and protect Body Fluids.
- *Yi Yi Ren* (Semen Coicis Lachryma-jobi) and *Chi Shao* (Radix Paeoniae Rubra) invigorate the Blood and transform Dampness.

OBSTRUCTION OF DAMPNESS DUE TO SPLEEN DEFICIENCY

This pattern manifests as densely distributed pustules filled with a clear fluid at the top and turbid pus at the base. Pustules may coalesce and form eczematous plaques with crusting and scaling. The disease tends to recur with intervals of several days, weeks or months. The tongue body is pale red, enlarged and tender with a thin white coating; the pulse is soggy and thready.

Treatment principle
Clear Heat and transform Dampness, support the Spleen and consolidate the Root.

Prescription
XIE HUANG SAN JIA JIAN
Yellow-Draining Powder, with modifications

Huo Xiang (Herba Agastaches seu Pogostemi) 10g
Pei Lan (Herba Eupatorii Fortunei) 10g
Sheng Di Huang (Radix Rehmanniae Glutinosae) 10g
Shi Gao‡ (Gypsum Fibrosum) 15g, decocted for 30 minutes before adding the other ingredients
Che Qian Zi (Semen Plantaginis) 15g, wrapped
Shan Yao (Radix Dioscoreae Oppositae) 15g
Huang Qi (Radix Astragali seu Hedysari) 15g
Yi Yi Ren (Semen Coicis Lachryma-jobi) 30g
Chao Bai Bian Dou (Semen Dolichoris Lablab, stir-fried) 30g
Chi Xiao Dou (Semen Phaseoli Calcarati) 30g
Hei Da Dou (Semen Glycines Atrum) 30g
Dang Shen (Radix Codonopsitis Pilosulae) 12g
Bai Zhu (Rhizoma Atractylodis Macrocephalae) 12g
Sha Ren (Fructus Amomi) 8g, added 5 minutes before the end of the decoction process

Explanation
- *Huo Xiang* (Herba Agastaches seu Pogostemi), *Pei Lan* (Herba Eupatorii Fortunei), *Sha Ren* (Fructus Amomi), *Yi Yi Ren* (Semen Coicis Lachryma-jobi), *Chao Bai Bian Dou* (Semen Dolichoris Lablab, stir-fried), and *Shan Yao* (Radix Dioscoreae Oppositae) aromatically transform turbidity.
- *Dang Shen* (Radix Codonopsitis Pilosulae), *Bai Zhu* (Rhizoma Atractylodis Macrocephalae) and *Huang Qi* (Radix Astragali seu Hedysari) support the Spleen and consolidate the Root.
- *Shi Gao*‡ (Gypsum Fibrosum) clears Heat from the Qi level.
- *Che Qian Zi* (Semen Plantaginis) and *Chi Xiao Dou* (Semen Phaseoli Calcarati) invigorate the Blood and disperse swelling.
- *Hei Da Dou* (Semen Glycines Atrum) and *Sheng Di Huang* (Radix Rehmanniae Glutinosae) enrich Yin and moisten Dryness.

EXTERNAL TREATMENT
- For generalized lesions manifesting as blisters filled with a turbid liquid and slight exudation and erosion, apply *Di Hu Hu* (Sanguisorba and Giant Knotweed Paste) to the affected area twice a day.
- For lesions manifesting as pustules or eczematous eruptions, mix equal amounts of *Qu Shi San* (Powder for Dispelling Dampness) and *Qing Dai San* (Indigo Powder) into a paste with vegetable oil for external application to the affected area.

Clinical notes

- In treating this disease, it is important both to drain Heart-Fire, thus controlling the spread of the pustules, and to eliminate Dampness and fortify the Spleen, thus limiting the extent of erosive lesions.
- Since lesions occur most often in moist, covered areas, it is better to use mild external medications rather than strong and irritant preparations.
- This is a chronic, benign disease with frequent recurrence, but it does not generally affect the patient's general health.

References

1. Zhang Zhili, *Zhang Zhi Li Pi Fu Bing Lin Chuang Jing Yan Ji Yao* [A Collection of Zhang Zhili's Clinical Experiences in the Treatment of Skin Diseases] (Beijing: China Medical Science and Technology Publishing House, 2001), 295.
2. Zhang Zhili, *Zhang Zhi Li Pi Fu Bing Lin Chuang Jing Yan Ji Yao*, 292.

3. Hu Ximing (ed.), *Zhong Guo Zhong Yi Mi Fang Da Quan* [A Compendium of Secret Prescriptions of Traditional Chinese Medicine] (Shanghai: Wen Hui Publishing House, 1991), 434-6.

4. Lu Zhongxi, *Chen Tong Yun Zhi Liao Man Xing Jia Zu Xing Liang Xing Tian Pao Chuang De Jing Yan* [Chen Tongyun's Experiences in Treating Chronic Familial Benign Pemphigus], *Bei Jing Zhong Yi* [Beijing Journal of Traditional Chinese Medicine] 4 (1999): 3.

5. Hu Ximing (ed.), *Zhong Guo Zhong Yi Mi Fang Da Quan*, 436.

6. Han Lumin, *Zhong Xi Yi Jie He Zhi Liao Tian Pao Chuang Ji Lei Tian Pao Chuang* [Treatment of Pemphigus and Bullous Pemphigoid with a Combination of TCM and Western Medicine], *Zhong Guo Zhong Xi Yi Jie He Za Zhi* [Journal of Integrated TCM and Western Medicine] 18, 10 (1998): 632.

7. Traditional Chinese Medicine Research Academy: Beijing Guang'anmen Hospital, *Zhu Ren Kang Lin Chuang Jing Yan Ji* [A Collection of Zhu Renkang's Clinical Experiences] (Beijing: People's Medical Publishing House, 1979), 189.

Viral infections of the skin

Viruses are very small, simple microorganisms; they are intracellular parasites that multiply through replication. In the process of replication, viruses first attach themselves to specific receptors in the cell membrane. Through a process similar to phagocytosis, they enter the cytoplasm, where they synthesize capsid protein, the protective coat of the virus. The virus releases its own genetic material, which uses the synthetic machinery of the host cell in order to produce new viral nucleic acid and protein. Abundant new intact virus particles are later assembled inside the cell, and then released outside the cell to infect other cells.

This process causes the cessation of normal synthesis of protein or nucleic acid inside the cells, thus disrupting normal cellular metabolism. Disorder or death of cells will follow, which causes various symptoms and signs to occur.

The number of common viruses exceeds 500 and new viruses are still being discovered (the outbreak of the SARS virus in early 2003 being a good example). Viruses can be classified into the following categories according to their clinical manifestations:

- vesicular type, for example herpes simplex, herpes zoster, smallpox, and chickenpox viruses;
- eruptive type, for example measles and rubella viruses;
- neoplastic type, for example viruses causing various types of warts.

TCM attributes viral diseases to two causes:

- External Wind-Heat pathogenic factors settling in the Lungs and Stomach. The Lungs govern the skin and hair, and the Stomach takes in food and water. Where external pathogenic factors invade the Lungs and Stomach, it is extremely easy for them to be transformed into Damp-Heat Toxins, which then attack the skin and cause skin lesions such as papules and vesicles. These Toxins may move upward to attack the upper body, for example around the mouth, or downward to affect the lower body, manifesting for example as genital herpes or plantar warts; alternatively, they may reside in the Middle Jiao, manifesting for example as shingles. Where there is exuberance of Wind-Heat pathogenic factors, papular eruptions are likely to occur; where there is exuberance of Damp-Heat Toxins, the condition will manifest as a vesicular-type viral skin disease.

- Blood-Dryness due to Liver Deficiency impairs nourishment of Qi in the sinews and causes obstruction of the interstices (*cou li*) and the channels and network vessels. Warts may therefore occur.

Herpes simplex
单纯疱疹

Herpes simplex is caused by infection by the human herpes simplex virus (HSV) – HSV-1 is usually associated with oral infections and HSV-2 with genital infections. The herpes simplex virus is highly contagious and spreads through direct contact with infected individuals.

Infection takes place in two phases. The primary infection, which often occurs in childhood, causes skin or mucocutaneous infection which heals without scarring. During primary infection, the virus enters cutaneous nerve endings and is transmitted to dorsal root ganglia, where the non-replicating virus remains latent.

The secondary phase is caused by reactivation of the viral infection, with the virus travelling along the nerve fibers to cause recurrence of the herpes infection at the same anatomical location. Viral reactivation resulting in secondary phase herpes infection can be caused by local skin trauma (for example, abrasion, exposure to ultraviolet radiation or sunlight) or by systemic conditions (for example, febrile illness, respiratory tract infection, fatigue or stress, and menstruation).

In TCM, herpes simplex is also known as *re chuang* (Heat sore) or *re qi chuang* (Heat Qi sore). According to *Sheng Ji Zong Lu* [General Collection for Holy Relief], "*Re chuang* (Heat sore) is caused primarily by exuberant Heat with Wind Qi [pathogenic Wind] then taking advantage."

Clinical manifestations

- Any skin surface or mucous membrane may be affected by herpetic infection.
- In the initial stage, grouped papulovesicles and vesicles are seen on an erythematous base. The size of the vesicles is uniform, in contrast to the vesicles of herpes zoster. The clear fluid filling the vesicles subsequently becomes yellow and turbid. The vesicles finally burst, leaving an eroded base, which heals by drying up and forming a layer of crust. Slight pigmentation will be noticed after the crust peels off.
- The lesions of the primary infection normally last for around two weeks, but can persist for up to six weeks, whereas recurrent herpetic lesions usually heal within 10-14 days after onset.
- There may be feelings of itching, burning or tingling.

Differential diagnosis

Herpes zoster
The distribution of herpes zoster vesicles follows the dermatomal distribution of the involved peripheral nerve on one side of the body. The vesicles are of varying sizes, are grouped, and may extend to affect one or two adjacent dermatomes. Patients often complain of sharp pain, itching or burning in the prodromal phase before vesicles appear.

Impetigo
Impetigo commonly involves the face or the dorsum of the hand in children. It tends to occur in the spring or autumn. Thin-walled pustules form on the skin and break down with the formation of orange or golden yellow crusts. The pustules and crusts are infectious.

Etiology and pathology

- Pathogenic Wind-Heat can invade the body when it is weak due to Spleen-Stomach disharmony or menstruation. These pathogenic factors move along the channels and trigger an outbreak of herpes simplex around the mouth.

- Pathogenic Wind-Heat or Damp-Heat Toxins can also invade the body in persons of a weak or Deficient constitution; they can then move upward along the channels to produce herpes simplex around the mouth and nose or downward to trigger an outbreak in the genital region.
- Pathogenic Heat damages Body Fluids in an enduring illness, resulting in Yin Deficiency and internal Heat.

Pattern identification and treatment

INTERNAL TREATMENT

WIND-HEAT-DAMP TOXINS
This is an Excess-Heat pattern. It forms due to exuberant Heat Toxins scorching the Ying and Xue levels, resulting in pathogenic Wind-Heat overwhelming Deficiency to invade the body. This pattern is characterized by a relatively abrupt onset, short disease duration, skin lesions in the form of papulovesicles and vesicles, relatively severe erosions, subjective burning and tingling sensations, and occasional fever and coughing. The tongue body is red with a thin yellow coating; the pulse is floating and rapid.

Treatment principle
Dissipate Wind and clear Heat, transform Dampness and relieve Toxicity.

Prescription
XIN YI QING FEI YIN JIA JIAN
Magnolia Flower Beverage for Clearing the Lungs, with modifications

Huang Qin (Radix Scutellariae Baicalensis) 4.5g
Da Qing Ye (Folium Isatidis seu Baphicacanthi) 6g
Jiao Zhi Zi (Fructus Gardeniae Jasminoidis, scorch-fried) 6g
Pi Pa Ye (Folium Eriobotryae Japonicae) 6g
Sheng Ma (Rhizoma Cimicifugae) 6g
Yi Yi Ren (Semen Coicis Lachryma-jobi) 10g
Tian Men Dong (Radix Asparagi Cochinchinensis)10g
Mai Men Dong (Radix Ophiopogonis Japonici) 10g
Xuan Shen (Radix Scrophulariae Ningpoensis) 10g
Xin Yi Hua (Flos Magnoliae) 3g

Explanation
- *Da Qing Ye* (Folium Isatidis seu Baphicacanthi), *Huang Qin* (Radix Scutellariae Baicalensis), *Pi Pa Ye* (Folium Eriobotryae Japonicae), and *Xin Yi Hua* (Flos Magnoliae) clear Heat and diffuse the Lungs.
- *Jiao Zhi Zi* (Fructus Gardeniae Jasminoidis, scorch-fried) drains Excess-Fire from the Triple Burner, whereas *Xuan Shen* (Radix Scrophulariae Ningpoensis) treats Deficiency-Heat in the Liver and Kidneys. These two ingredients are used to support the first group of herbs.

- *Yi Yi Ren* (Semen Coicis Lachryma-jobi) and *Mai Men Dong* (Radix Ophiopogonis Japonici) transform Dampness and relieve Toxicity, nourish Yin and supplement the Lungs.
- *Sheng Ma* (Rhizoma Cimicifugae) relieves Toxicity and guides the action of the other ingredients up to the affected area, thus enhancing the effect in clearing and draining Heat from the Lungs and Stomach.

BINDING OF DAMP-HEAT

This pattern forms as a result of the presence of exuberant Fire in the Heart and Liver channels and Dampness being retained in the Spleen and Lung channels. Lesions occur primarily around the anogenital area, manifesting as vesicles on bright red erythema, with erosion and profuse exudation after the vesicles burst. Accompanying symptoms and signs include fatigue, lack of strength and yellow or reddish urine. The tongue body is red with a yellow and greasy coating; the pulse is slippery and rapid.

Treatment principle
Clear Heat and benefit the movement of Dampness, relieve Toxicity and dispel pathogenic factors.

Prescription
LONG DAN XIE GAN TANG JIA JIAN
Chinese Gentian Decoction for Draining the Liver, with modifications

Chao Long Dan Cao (Radix Gentianae Scabrae, stir-fried) 6g
Tong Cao (Medulla Tetrapanacis Papyriferi) 6g
Ze Xie (Rhizoma Alismatis Orientalis) 10g
Che Qian Zi (Semen Plantaginis) 10g, wrapped
Jiao Zhi Zi (Fructus Gardeniae Jasminoidis, scorch-fried) 10g
Gan Cao (Radix Glycyrrhizae) 10g
Huang Qin (Radix Scutellariae Baicalensis) 10g
Chai Hu (Radix Bupleuri) 3g
Da Qing Ye (Folium Isatidis seu Baphicacanthi) 10g
Yi Yi Ren (Semen Coicis Lachryma-jobi) 15g
Bai Mao Gen (Rhizoma Imperatae Cylindricae) 15g

Explanation
- Skin lesions in the lower part of the body are usually caused by Dampness and Heat binding. The prescription *Long Dan Xie Gan Tang* (Chinese Gentian Decoction for Draining the Liver), composed of the first eight ingredients, is used to treat the Root by clearing Heat, benefiting the movement of Dampness and expelling Damp-Heat from the Liver and Kidneys.
- As well as increasing the effect in relieving Toxicity, *Da Qing Ye* (Folium Isatidis seu Baphicacanthi), *Yi Yi Ren* (Semen Coicis Lachryma-jobi) and *Bai Mao Gen* (Rhizoma Imperatae Cylindricae) benefit the movement of Dampness and support the Spleen, and cool the Blood and reduce erythema. The effectiveness of this formula in clearing Heat and benefiting the movement of Dampness is greatly reinforced by the addition of these three ingredients.

QI AND YIN DEFICIENCY

The disease is persistent, with repeated eruptions of vesicles for prolonged periods. The tongue body is red with a scant coating; the pulse is thready and rapid.

Treatment principle
Augment Qi and nourish Yin, support Vital Qi (Zheng Qi) and consolidate the Root.

Prescription
REN SHEN GU BEN TANG JIA JIAN
Ginseng Decoction for Consolidating the Root, with modifications

Nan Sha Shen (Radix Adenophorae) 15g
Sheng Di Huang (Radix Rehmanniae Glutinosae) 15g
Huang Qi (Radix Astragali seu Hedysari) 10g
Bai Shao (Radix Paeoniae Lactiflorae) 10g
Gan Cao (Radix Glycyrrhizae) 10g
Mai Men Dong (Radix Ophiopogonis Japonici) 12g
Tian Men Dong (Radix Asparagi Cochinchinensis) 12g
Yi Yi Ren (Semen Coicis Lachryma-jobi) 12g
Shan Yao (Rhizoma Dioscoreae Oppositae) 12g
Sheng Ma (Rhizoma Cimicifugae) 6g
Ban Lan Gen (Radix Isatidis seu Baphicacanthi) 6g

Explanation
- *Nan Sha Shen* (Radix Adenophorae), *Huang Qi* (Radix Astragali seu Hedysari), *Bai Shao* (Radix Paeoniae Lactiflorae), *Sheng Di Huang* (Radix Rehmanniae Glutinosae), and *Gan Cao* (Radix Glycyrrhizae) augment Qi and nourish Yin to consolidate the Root.
- *Mai Men Dong* (Radix Ophiopogonis Japonici), *Tian Men Dong* (Radix Asparagi Cochinchinensis), *Yi Yi Ren* (Semen Coicis Lachryma-jobi), and *Shan Yao* (Rhizoma Dioscoreae Oppositae), with their sweet and moistening properties, nourish Lung and Spleen Yin.
- *Sheng Ma* (Rhizoma Cimicifugae) relieves Toxicity and bears Yang upward.
- *Ban Lan Gen* (Radix Isatidis seu Baphicacanthi) is an important herb for the treatment of viral diseases, being added to prescriptions to exercise a regulating function.

General modifications
1. For skin eruptions around the eyes, add *Qing Xiang Zi* (Semen Celosiae Argenteae), *Ju Hua* (Flos Chrysanthemi Morifolii) and *Sang Ye* (Folium Mori Albae).
2. For skin lesions that linger for years with repeated attacks, add *Xi Yang Shen** (Radix Panacis Quinquefolii), *Bai Wei* (Radix Cynanchi Atrati), *Bai Lian*

(Radix Ampelopsis Japonicae), and *Lü Dou Yi* (Testa Phaseoli Radiati).

3. For prickly itching and a pronounced sensation of burning pain, add *Gou Teng* (Ramulus Uncariae cum Uncis), *Shi Jue Ming*‡ (Concha Haliotidis), *Zi Cao* (Radix Arnebiae seu Lithospermi), and *Chan Tui* ‡ (Periostracum Cicadae).

PATENT HERBAL MEDICINES

* For Wind-Heat-Damp Toxin patterns, take *Huang Lian Shang Qing Wan* (Coptis Pill for Clearing the Upper Body) 3g twice a day.
* For patterns of Damp-Heat binding, take *Niu Huang Jie Du Wan* (Bovine Bezoar Pill for Relieving Toxicity) 1.5g twice a day.

EXTERNAL TREATMENT

* For severe erosion and exudation, apply *Ma Chi Xian Shui Xi Ji* (Purslane Wash Preparation) as a wet compress for 15 minutes once or twice a day.
* For small amounts of exudation, mix *Yu Lu San* (Jade Dew Powder) or *Qing Chui Kou San* (Indigo Mouth Insufflation Powder) into a paste with vegetable oil and apply to the affected areas.
* Apply *Huang Lian Ruan Gao* (Coptis Ointment) when crusts form with slight itching.

ACUPUNCTURE

Main points: BL-13 Feishu, GB-20 Fengchi and GV-23 Shangxing.

Auxiliary points

* For herpes in the facial region, add LI-4 Hegu and LU-10 Yuji.
* For herpes of the genital region, add BL-23 Shenshu, CV-4 Guanyuan and CV-6 Qihai.
* For recurrent herpes, add SP-6 Sanyinjiao and ST-36 Zusanli.

Technique: Use filiform needles and apply the even method. Retain the needles for 30 minutes after obtaining Qi. Moxibustion can be applied at ST-36 Zusanli. Treat once a day. A course consists of ten treatment sessions.

Explanation

* BL-13 Feishu, the back-*shu* point of the Lungs, diffuses Heat, dredges Wind and regulates Lung Qi.
* GB-20 Fengchi and GV-23 Shangxing dredge pathogenic factors, clear Heat, and regulate and harmonize the Qi and Xue levels.
* LI-4 Hegu and LU-10 Yuji clear Heat and diffuse the Lungs.
* BL-23 Shenshu, CV-4 Guanyuan and CV-6 Qihai regulate Original Qi (Yuan Qi) and dissipate pathogenic factors.
* ST-36 Zusanli and SP-6 Sanyinjiao support Vital Qi (Zheng Qi) and consolidate the Root.

EAR ACUPUNCTURE

Points: Lung, Stomach and Heart
Technique: Retain the needles for 30 minutes. Treat once every other day. A course consists of ten treatment sessions.

Clinical notes

* At the start of an attack of herpes simplex, the treatment principle should be to dredge Wind and clear Heat while supporting the Spleen and transforming Dampness. If it is impossible to prepare a herbal decoction, *Niu Huang Shang Qing Wan* (Bovine Bezoar Pill for Clearing the Upper Body) can be used as the main choice.
* For recurrent herpes simplex, especially if it occurs more frequently before menstruation or after stress, the treatment principle should be to augment Qi and nourish Yin. However, it is necessary to take the herbs for one to two months to reinforce the body's immunity and reduce the frequency of recurrence.
* A wet compress applied locally is useful when the skin lesions are characterized by inflammatory papulovesicles or exudation and erosion. External application of *Huang Lian Ruan Gao* (Coptis Ointment) to moisten the skin is recommended when crusts form or there is slight local itching.

Varicella (chickenpox)
水痘

Varicella (chickenpox) is an acute, highly infectious eruptive disease caused by the varicella zoster virus, transmitted by airborne droplets. It is characterized by maculopapular eruptions, blisters and crusting, which may be present simultaneously. It can occur all year round, but the majority of cases are seen in winter or spring.

The incidence of chickenpox is especially high among children aged one to six, although it can be contracted at any age. It can easily become epidemic in children's establishments (such as schools, kindergartens and nurseries).

The prognosis for chickenpox is generally good. Since an attack in childhood generally confers lifelong immunity, chickenpox is rare in adults, but the virus may reactivate in later life to cause herpes zoster (shingles).

In *Xiao Er Wei Sheng Zhong Wei Lun Fang: Pao Zhen Lun* [General Discussion on Children's Hygiene: Herpes], it says, "Eruptions with a thin skin like a water blister [vesicle] and drying easily after bursting are called chickenpox." Since the blisters are oval-shaped like a bean, are clear and contain a watery liquid, they are known in TCM as *shui dou* (water bean).[i]

Clinical manifestations

- There will be a history of contact with children suffering from chickenpox; the incubation period is 11-18 days.
- Skin eruptions begin on the trunk and spread to the face, scalp and limbs; the mucous membrane of the oral cavity and vagina may also be involved. Rarely in severe cases, necrosis occurs around the vesicles resulting in gangrenous ulceration.
- Eruptions occur in successive crops passing through the stages of macule, papule, vesicle, and pustule. The lesions finally dry out and form crusts which separate, usually without scarring unless there is superinfection.
- Patients are infectious from four days before the rash appears until all lesions have crusted; dry scabs are not infectious.
- Vesicles typically vary in size from 1mm to 5mm; they are surrounded by a red halo and are umbilicated.
- Moderate to intense itching is likely at the blister stage.

- Accompanying symptoms may include fever and general malaise.
- In adults, pneumonia may be a relatively common and serious complication; other possible complications include hepatitis and encephalitis.

Differential diagnosis

Impetigo
This disease is seen most often in young children and infants. Eruptions may grow to bullae 1-2 cm in diameter and contain a yellow turbid liquid or pus.

Herpes zoster (shingles)
The varicella zoster virus, responsible for chickenpox in children, may reactivate in adulthood to cause an attack of shingles. Lesions are generally unilaterally distributed along a single dermatome and rarely cross the midline. A severe burning pain is present.

Papular urticaria
Papular urticaria is a reaction to bites of insects such as fleas, mites or bedbugs where the actual source of the bite is unknown. Lesions initially manifest as red, oval, infiltrative wheals with papulovesicles or vesicles at the center and mainly involve the lumbosacral region, buttocks, trunk, and lower limbs. Incidence is high among infants and children. The lesions characteristically occur in irregular lines and clusters, may last for up to two weeks and recur in crops. Itching is likely.

Scabies
The main areas of involvement of scabies include the sides of the fingers, the webs between the fingers, the sides of the hands, the wrists, elbows, ankles and feet, and the genitals and buttocks. The characteristic scabies lesions – grayish linear, curved or serpiginous burrows – are generally intensely itchy.

Etiology and pathology

- Different generations of doctors have suggested different etiologies for this disease. Most of them consider the cause to be the result of an accumulation of Damp-Heat in children combined with externally-contracted seasonal pathogenic factors.

---

[i] In this instance, the character *dou* is the normal bean character with a sickness radical.

These factors fight the internal Damp-Heat and are retained in the Lung and Spleen channels.

- Since the Lungs of young children are relatively delicate, Wei Qi (Defensive Qi) may be insufficient to protect them against invasion by pathogenic factors. In winter and spring, they are vulnerable to attack by epidemic Wind-Heat and Damp-Heat.

- In mild cases, the Lungs are unable to diffuse and bear downwards, resulting in a series of symptoms relating to the Wei level. Since the pathogens are thrust outward through the exterior, the eruptions are red and moist and contain a transparent liquid.

- In severe cases, Dampness encumbers Spleen Yang, and the pathogenic factors will go deeper into the body resulting in symptoms relating to the Qi level. Since the pathogenic factors are unable to escape, lesions are dull purple and contain a dark, turbid liquid.

- Since seasonal pathogenic factors normally only damage the Wei and Qi levels and rarely involve the Ying level, it is relatively rare for symptoms to develop into a dangerous illness, especially in childhood.

Pattern identification and treatment

INTERNAL TREATMENT

WIND-HEAT WITH DAMPNESS (MILD PATTERN)

This pattern mainly involves the Wei level. The patient has a slight fever, nasal congestion and a runny nose, and starts to cough and sneeze. Chickenpox then develops after one to two days. The sparsely-distributed moist, oval red blisters show the characteristic "raindrop on a rose petal" appearance. They contain a transparent liquid, have a pale red halo and are itchy. Urine and stool are normal. The tongue coating is thin and white; the pulse is floating.

Treatment principle
Dredge Wind and clear Heat, relieve Toxicity and dispel Dampness.

Prescription
YIN QIAO SAN JIA JIAN
Honeysuckle and Forsythia Powder, with modifications

Jin Yin Hua (Flos Lonicerae) 10g
Lian Qiao (Fructus Forsythiae Suspensae) 6g
Dan Zhu Ye (Herba Lophatheri Gracilis) 6g
Jing Jie (Herba Schizonepetae Tenuifoliae) 6g
Lü Dou Yi (Testa Phaseoli Radiati) 12g
Jie Geng (Radix Platycodi Grandiflori) 4.5g
Chan Tui ‡ (Periostracum Cicadae) 4.5g
Da Qing Ye (Folium Isatidis seu Baphicacanthi) 4.5g
Zi Cao (Radix Arnebiae seu Lithospermi) 4.5g

Gan Cao (Radix Glycyrrhizae) 4.5g

Explanation
- *Jin Yin Hua* (Flos Lonicerae), *Lian Qiao* (Fructus Forsythiae Suspensae), *Da Qing Ye* (Folium Isatidis seu Baphicacanthi), *Zi Cao* (Radix Arnebiae seu Lithospermi), and *Gan Cao* (Radix Glycyrrhizae) clear and diffuse Wind-Heat, relieve Toxicity and reduce papules.

- *Jing Jie* (Herba Schizonepetae Tenuifoliae) and *Chan Tui* ‡ (Periostracum Cicadae) directly dissipate pathogenic Wind-Heat.

- *Lü Dou Yi* (Testa Phaseoli Radiati) relieves Toxicity to protect the Heart and prevent pathogenic factors from falling inward.

- *Dan Zhu Ye* (Herba Lophatheri Gracilis) guides Heat downward to dispel pathogenic Dampness from the urine.

- *Jie Geng* (Radix Platycodi Grandiflori) diffuses Lung Qi to reduce the degree of itching and achieve the effect of clearing Wind-Heat internally and dissipating it externally through the combination of herbs functioning on the upper and lower body.

EXUBERANT DAMP-HEAT (SEVERE PATTERN)
This pattern mainly involves the Qi and Ying levels. Skin lesions are large and densely distributed with a clearly-defined base surrounded by a bright red halo. Eruptions are dull purple and filled with a turbid liquid. Accompanying symptoms and signs include high fever, irritability, thirst, dry mouth and teeth, red lips and face, lassitude, mouth and tongue sores, and short voidings of reddish urine. The tongue coating is yellow, dry and thick; the pulse is slippery and rapid.

Treatment principle
Clear Heat, relieve Toxicity and cool the Blood.

Prescription
QING WEN BAI DU YIN JIA JIAN
Beverage for Clearing Scourge and Vanquishing Toxicity, with modifications

Lian Qiao (Fructus Forsythiae Suspensae) 10g
Huang Qin (Radix Scutellariae Baicalensis) 10g
Xuan Shen (Radix Scrophulariae Ningpoensis) 10g
Chi Shao (Radix Paeoniae Rubra) 10g
Jiao Zhi Zi (Fructus Gardeniae Jasminoidis, scorch-fried) 6g
Dan Zhu Ye (Herba Lophatheri Gracilis) 6g
Huang Lian (Rhizoma Coptidis) 6g
Zhi Mu (Rhizoma Anemarrhenae Asphodeloidis) 6g
Shi Gao ‡ (Gypsum Fibrosum) 12g
Da Qing Ye (Folium Isatidis seu Baphicacanthi) 12g
Zi Cao (Radix Arnebiae seu Lithospermi) 12g
Jin Yin Hua (Flos Lonicerae) 12g

Explanation

- *Shi Gao‡* (Gypsum Fibrosum), *Zhi Mu* (Rhizoma Anemarrhenae Asphodeloidis), *Dan Zhu Ye* (Herba Lophatheri Gracilis), *Xuan Shen* (Radix Scrophulariae Ningpoensis), and *Jiao Zhi Zi* (Fructus Gardeniae Jasminoidis, scorch-fried) clear and drain Heat Toxins from the Qi and Ying levels.

- *Huang Qin* (Radix Scutellariae Baicalensis) clears Heat from the Lungs.

- *Huang Lian* (Rhizoma Coptidis) and *Lian Qiao* (Fructus Forsythiae Suspensae) clear Heat from the Heart and combine with *Da Qing Ye* (Folium Isatidis seu Baphicacanthi), *Jin Yin Hua* (Flos Lonicerae), *Chi Shao* (Radix Paeoniae Rubra), and *Zi Cao* (Radix Arnebiae seu Lithospermi) to clear Heat Toxins from the skin and interstices (*cou li*).

- This combination clears Heat and relieves Toxicity in the Qi and Ying levels, the Zang-Fu organs, and the skin and interstices (*cou li*) to reduce fever and eliminate eruptions.

General modifications

1. For high fever, thirst, and irritability and restlessness, add *Han Shui Shi‡* (Calcitum), *Tian Hua Fen* (Radix Trichosanthis), *Gou Teng* (Ramulus Uncariae cum Uncis), *Bo He* (Herba Menthae Haplocalycis), added 5 minutes before the end of the decoction process, and *Niu Bang Zi* (Fructus Arctii Lappae).
2. For bullae, add *Yi Yi Ren* (Semen Coicis Lachryma-jobi) and *Dong Gua Pi* (Epicarpium Benincasae Hispidae).
3. For bleeding blisters, add *Da Ji* (Herba seu Radix Cirsii Japonici), *Xiao Ji* (Herba Cephalanoploris seu Cirsii) and *Pu Gong Ying* (Herba Taraxaci cum Radice).
4. For pustules, add *Ban Lan Gen* (Radix Isatidis seu Baphicacanthi), *Zi Hua Di Ding* (Herba Violae Yedoensitis) and *Chong Lou* (Rhizoma Paridis).
5. For necrosis, add *Bai Wei* (Radix Cynanchi Atrati), *Bai Hua She She Cao* (Herba Hedyotidis Diffusae) and *Bai Lian* (Radix Ampelopsis Japonicae).
6. For dull purple Toxic eruptions, add *Sheng Di Huang* (Radix Rehmanniae Glutinosae) and *Zi Cao* (Radix Arnebiae seu Lithospermi).
7. For mouth and tongue sores, add *Tong Cao* (Medulla Tetrapanacis Papyriferi), *Deng Xin Cao* (Medulla Junci Effusi) and *Sheng Di Huang* (Radix Rehmanniae Glutinosae).
8. For persistent itching, add *Jiang Can‡* (Bombyx Batryticatus) and *Tong Cao* (Medulla Tetrapanacis Papyriferi).
9. For dry stool or constipation, add *Da Huang* (Radix et Rhizoma Rhei) and *Gua Lou* (Fructus Trichosanthis).
10. For exudation after rupture of vesicle walls, add *Che Qian Zi* (Semen Plantaginis) and *Hua Shi‡* (Talcum).
11. For depletion of Body Fluids, add *Sha Shen* (Radix Glehniae seu Adenophorae), *Mai Men Dong* (Radix Ophiopogonis Japonici) and *Lu Gen* (Rhizoma Phragmitis Communis).
12. For residual Toxins, add *Huang Qin* (Radix Scutellariae Baicalensis) and *Lü Dou Yi* (Testa Phaseoli Radiati).
13. For confused Spirit and Mind, thirst with a desire to drink, or convulsions, add *Ling Yang Jiao Fen** (Cornu Antelopis, powdered).

EXTERNAL TREATMENT

- If the blisters are about to burst or exudation and erosion are relatively severe, use *Ma Chi Xian Shui Xi Ji* (Purslane Wash Preparation) as a wet compress on the affected skin three to five times a day.
- If erosion is complicated by suppuration, make *Qing Dai San* (Indigo Powder) into a paste with vegetable oil and apply to the affected area, or rub in *Qing Dai Gao* (Indigo Paste).
- For damage to the mucous membrane of the oral cavity, apply *Qing Chui Kou San* (Indigo Mouth Insufflation Powder) three or four times a day.

FOLK REMEDIES

- For mild cases, select one of the combinations below for a decoction and drink or use as a mouthwash:
  - *Jin Yin Hua* (Flos Lonicerae) 12g and *Gan Cao* (Radix Glycyrrhizae) 3g
  - *Xian Lu Gen* (Rhizoma Phragmitis Communis Recens) 60g and *Ye Ju Hua* (Flos Chrysanthemi Indici) 10g
  - *Ban Lan Gen* (Radix Isatidis seu Baphicacanthi) 30g and *Gan Cao* (Radix Glycyrrhizae) 4g
- Make a decoction with *Ye Ju Hua* (Flos Chrysanthemi Indici) 15g, *Lu Bian Ju* (Herba et Radix Kalimeridis) 15g and *Hai Jin Sha Teng* (Herba Lygodii Japonici) 30g and drink.
- Make a decoction with *Ku Shen* (Radix Sophorae Flavescentis) 30g, *Mang Xiao‡* (Mirabilitum) 30g and *Fu Ping* (Herba Spirodelae Polyrrhizae) 15g and use it as a wash or wet compress.
- Carrot and coriander soup: Boil 100g of carrots with 60g of coriander and drink as a tea. This soup is indicated for the initial stage of chickenpox as it will drive out the Toxins causing the eruption.

Clinical notes

- Make sure the bedroom is well-ventilated and has plenty of light. Ensure that the sick child is not in any direct draughts. Isolation until the last spot has crusted is necessary to prevent infection of others.

- During the eruptive stage, the child should be prevented from scratching the blisters in order to avoid scarring and infection. Nails should be cut and clothes changed frequently. It is advisable to refrain from having a bath in case this results in secondary infections.
- It is important to pay attention to oral hygiene. A mouthwash made from *Jin Yin Hua* (Flos Lonicerae) and *Gan Cao* (Radix Glycyrrhizae) can be used before meals to clean the oral cavity. If ulcers or erosions are present, apply *Lü Pao San* (Green Robe Powder) topically.
- Keep to a diet of light, easily digested food. Fatty and greasy food should be kept to a minimum. Fresh ginger, chilli and seafood should be avoided.

Literature excerpts

In *Jing Yue Quan Shu* [The Complete Works of Zhang Jingyue], it says: "Chickenpox usually starts with dozens of spots on the skin. Within a day, vesicles form on top of the spots. More spots and vesicles appear on the second and third days. Severe itching all over the body occurs on the fourth day when the tips of the vesicles burst; there may also be slight fever. Sweat-inducing food should be avoided. The disease has usually run its course after seven or eight days."

In *You You Ji Cheng* [A Complete Work on Pediatrics], it says: "Chickenpox is like smallpox with such symptoms as red face and lips, watery eyes, sneezing and coughing, or a runny nose with sticky discharge, and fever. Spots appear on the second or third day. Vesicles are pea-sized and transparent with a thin wall and crusting in the center; they appear and disappear quickly. If treated by warming methods, crusts will be slow to fall off and erosive eruptions will ensue. Ginger and chilli should be strictly avoided, as should bathing with cold water, otherwise sores and edema will result."

Herpes zoster (shingles)
带状疱疹

Herpes zoster (or shingles) is an acute infection of the nerves that supply certain areas of the skin. It is caused by reactivation of the varicella zoster virus that entered the cutaneous nerves in an earlier attack of chicken pox. The virus remains latent in the dorsal root ganglia for many years. It may be reactivated and migrate along the nerve to the skin to trigger an outbreak of herpes zoster when the immune system is depressed.

In TCM, herpes zoster is known as *chan yao huo dan* (girdling Fire cinnabar), *huo dai chuang* (Fire girdle sore) or *she chuan chuang* (snake string sore); herpes zoster of the head and neck is known as *huo zhu chuang* (Fire pearl sore); and herpes zoster complicated by infection is known as *she ke chuang* (snake nest sore).

Clinical manifestations

- Herpes zoster mainly affects people over 50 and the incidence rises with age. Younger people with weakened body conditions such as those with lymphoma and AIDS or those being treated with immunosuppressant drugs or chemotherapy may also be affected.
- Mild systemic symptoms are often observed prior to the development of the cutaneous lesions of herpes zoster, such as fatigue, poor appetite, headache, and fever. Pain, tingling and dysesthesia may precede the attack by days.
- Herpes zoster starts with inflammatory erythema and papules, which evolve into vesicles of varying sizes usually filled with clear transparent fluid and surrounded by areolae; vesicles may occasionally be filled with blood. The lesions are scattered in a dermatome distribution. However, the rash may also involve one or two adjacent dermatomes. In three or four days, the fluid inside the vesicles becomes turbid. Vesicles, which appear in successive crops, rupture and soon dry up leaving a crust. Crusts drop off in two to three weeks, leaving temporary pinkish marks or pigmentation locally, usually without scarring.
- Post-herpetic neuralgia is rare in patients under 40 years, but is more common in the elderly. Pain can persist for months after an attack, but in most cases subsides within 12 months.
- Although recurrence of the disease is not common, an attack of herpes zoster does not confer lifelong immunity and further episodes may take place.

Differential diagnosis

Pain preceding the attack may be mistaken for cardiac or pleural pain or for an acute abdominal emergency before typical herpetic eruptions appear.

Herpes simplex

Herpes simplex commonly occurs at mucocutaneous junctions, but may be present in any skin area. The vesicles are of uniform size, in contrast to the vesicles of herpes zoster. The condition may recur frequently, often after febrile diseases or skin trauma.

Etiology and pathology

- Failure of the transportation function of the Spleen results in Dampness. Internal Dampness moves outward to the skin and water accumulates in the flesh, forming a dense distribution of pearl-like vesicles.
- Qi Depression of the Liver and Heart leads to the generation of Heat; Heat retained over a prolonged period transforms into Fire. Heat and Fire congest in the skin and obstruct the channels and network vessels, resulting in such symptoms as erythema, papulovesicles and severe pain.
- Residual Toxins that become trapped in the channels and vessels impair the free circulation of Qi and result in Qi stagnation and Blood stasis. Qi cannot be diffused in the channels, often resulting in constant or stabbing pain.

Pattern identification and treatment

INTERNAL TREATMENT

DAMPNESS AND HEAT FIGHTING AND BINDING

The skin is slightly red in the diseased area and clusters of vesicles full of turbid fluid appear. Exudation or erosion may occur on rupture of the vesicles. Accompanying symptoms include pain, poor appetite and abdominal distension. The tongue body is pale red with a white or yellow greasy coating; the pulse is soggy and rapid, or slippery and rapid.

Treatment principle

Clear and transform Damp-Heat, cool the Blood and relieve Toxicity.

Prescription
YI REN CHI DOU TANG JIA JIAN
Coix Seed and Aduki Bean Decoction, with modifications

Yi Yi Ren (Semen Coicis Lachryma-jobi) 15g

Chi Xiao Dou (Semen Phaseoli Calcarati) 15g
Fu Ling Pi (Cortex Poriae Cocos) 12g
Jin Yin Hua (Flos Lonicerae) 12g
Di Fu Zi (Fructus Kochiae Scopariae) 12g
Sheng Di Huang (Radix Rehmanniae Glutinosae) 12g
Che Qian Zi (Semen Plantaginis) 10g
Che Qian Cao (Herba Plantaginis) 10g
Chi Shao (Radix Paeoniae Rubra) 10g
Ma Chi Xian (Herba Portulacae Oleraceae) 10g
Gan Cao (Radix Glycyrrhizae) 6g
Huo Xiang (Herba Agastaches seu Pogostemi) 9g
Pei Lan (Herba Eupatorii Fortunei) 9g

Explanation

- *Yi Yi Ren* (Semen Coicis Lachryma-jobi), *Chi Xiao Dou* (Semen Phaseoli Calcarati), *Fu Ling Pi* (Cortex Poriae Cocos), and *Di Fu Zi* (Fructus Kochiae Scopariae) clear Heat and transform Dampness.
- *Sheng Di Huang* (Radix Rehmanniae Glutinosae), *Chi Shao* (Radix Paeoniae Rubra), *Jin Yin Hua* (Flos Lonicerae), and *Gan Cao* (Radix Glycyrrhizae) support the first group of herbs by cooling the Blood and relieving Toxicity.
- *Huo Xiang* (Herba Agastaches seu Pogostemi) and *Pei Lan* (Herba Eupatorii Fortunei) aromatically transform turbid Dampness.
- *Che Qian Zi* (Semen Plantaginis) and *Che Qian Cao* (Herba Plantaginis) relieve Toxicity and clear Heat.
- *Ma Chi Xian* (Herba Portulacae Oleraceae) has a specific antiviral effect and is added to reinforce the actions of the original prescription.

EXUBERANT HEAT TOXINS

The skin in the affected areas appears bright red. Papules, papulovesicles and tensely distended vesicles, sometimes blood-filled, are present in clusters or strips. Patients have subjective sensations of burning or stabbing pain, which makes it difficult to sleep. Accompanying symptoms and signs include dry throat, a bitter taste in the mouth, yellow urine, and constipation. The tongue body is red with a yellow or dry and yellow coating; the pulse is wiry and rapid.

Treatment principle

Clear Heat and drain Fire, relieve Toxicity and alleviate pain.

Prescription
DA QING LIAN QIAO TANG JIA JIAN
Woad Leaf and Forsythia Decoction, with modifications

Da Qing Ye (Folium Isatidis seu Baphicacanthi) 9g
Xuan Shen (Radix Scrophulariae Ningpoensis) 9g
Ban Zhi Lian (Herba Scutellariae Barbatae) 9g
Huang Qin (Radix Scutellariae Baicalensis) 9g

Lian Qiao (Fructus Forsythiae Suspensae) 12g
Jin Yin Hua (Flos Lonicerae) 12g
Sheng Di Huang (Radix Rehmanniae Glutinosae) 12g
Ma Chi Xian (Herba Portulacae Oleraceae) 12-15g
Chao Mu Dan Pi (Cortex Moutan Radicis, stir-fried) 6g
Chi Shao (Radix Paeoniae Rubra) 6g
Lü Dou Yi (Testa Phaseoli Radiati) 15-30g

Explanation

- *Da Qing Ye* (Folium Isatidis seu Baphicacanthi), *Ban Zhi Lian* (Herba Scutellariae Barbatae), *Huang Qin* (Radix Scutellariae Baicalensis), *Jin Yin Hua* (Flos Lonicerae), and *Ma Chi Xian* (Herba Portulacae Oleraceae) clear Heat and relieve Toxicity.
- *Sheng Di Huang* (Radix Rehmanniae Glutinosae), *Chao Mu Dan Pi* (Cortex Moutan Radicis, stir-fried), *Chi Shao* (Radix Paeoniae Rubra), and *Lian Qiao* (Fructus Forsythiae Suspensae) support the first group of herbs by cooling the Blood and relieving Toxicity.
- *Lü Dou Yi* (Testa Phaseoli Radiati) was said in ancient times to have similar actions to *Xi Jiao** (Cornu Rhinoceri), in that it clears Heat from the Heart and relieves Toxicity; *Xuan Shen* (Radix Scrophulariae Ningpoensis) clears floating Fire due to Deficiency. These two ingredients work well in combination to relieve Toxicity and alleviate pain.

QI STAGNATION AND BLOOD STASIS

This syndrome is often found in the elderly; stagnation in the channels deprives the skin of normal nourishment so that symptoms such as constant or stabbing pain occur. There can be severe pain after all the eruptions have subsided, which makes sleep difficult. Other accompanying symptoms and signs include lack of appetite and irritability and restlessness The tongue body is red or dark red with a scant or thin white coating; the pulse is fine and rough.

Treatment principle

Regulate Liver Qi, free the network vessels and alleviate pain.

Prescription
JIN LING ZI SAN JIA JIAN

Sichuan Chinaberry Powder, with modifications

Chuan Lian Zi (Fructus Meliae Toosendan) 9g
Yu Jin (Radix Curcumae) 9g
Zi Cao (Radix Arnebiae seu Lithospermi) 9g
Yan Hu Suo (Rhizoma Corydalis Yanhusuo) 6-9g
Cu Chai Hu (Radix Bupleuri, processed with vinegar) 6g
Qing Pi (Pericarpium Citri Reticulatae Viride) 6g
Chao Bai Shao (Radix Paeoniae Lactiflorae, stir-fried) 12g
Dang Gui (Radix Angelicae Sinensis) 12g
Si Gua Luo (Fasciculus Vascularis Luffae) 10g

Explanation

- Since lingering pain is often associated with this pattern, *Chuan Lian Zi* (Fructus Meliae Toosendan), *Yu Jin* (Radix Curcumae), *Yan Hu Suo* (Rhizoma Corydalis Yanhusuo), *Cu Chai Hu* (Radix Bupleuri, processed with vinegar), and *Qing Pi* (Pericarpium Citri Reticulatae Viride) are used to regulate Qi and alleviate pain.
- *Bai Shao* (Radix Paeoniae Lactiflorae), *Dang Gui* (Radix Angelicae Sinensis), *Zi Cao* (Radix Arnebiae seu Lithospermi), and *Si Gua Luo* (Fasciculus Vascularis Luffae) support the first group of herbs by invigorating the Blood and freeing the network vessels, relieving Toxicity and reducing erythema.

General modifications

1. For persistent raging fever, add *Ling Yang Jiao** (Cornu Antelopis), *Lü Dou Yi* (Testa Phaseoli Radiati), *Jin Yin Hua Tan* (Flos Lonicerae Carbonisata), and *Sheng Di Huang Tan* (Radix Rehmanniae Glutinosae Carbonisata).
2. For a bitter taste in the mouth, dry throat and yellow urine, add *Jiao Zhi Zi* (Fructus Gardeniae Jasminoidis, scorch-fried), *Chao Long Dan Cao* (Radix Gentianae Scabrae, stir-fried), *Mai Men Dong* (Radix Ophiopogonis Japonici), and *Jie Geng* (Radix Platycodi Grandiflori).
3. For constipation, add *Jie Geng* (Radix Platycodi Grandiflori), and then *Chao Zhi Ke* (Fructus Citri Aurantii, stir-fried) and *Jiu Da Huang* (Radix et Rhizoma Rhei, processed with wine) for the final 10 minutes of decoction.
4. If erosion and exudation occur after eruptions break, add *Di Yu* (Radix Sanguisorbae Officinalis), *Cang Er Zi* (Fructus Xanthii Sibirici) and *Liu Yi San* (Six-to-One Powder), wrapped in *He Ye* (Folium Nelumbinis Nuciferae) or a clean cotton cloth.
5. For abdominal distension and loose stools, add *Da Fu Pi* (Pericarpium Arecae Catechu), *Chao Zhi Ke* (Fructus Citri Aurantii, stir-fried) and *Xiang Yuan* (Fructus Citri Medicae seu Wilsonii).
6. For poor appetite, add *Shen Qu* (Massa Fermentata) and *Chao Mai Ya* (Fructus Hordei Vulgaris Germinatus, stir-fried).
7. For dizziness and blurred vision, add *Chong Wei Zi* (Semen Leonuri Heterophylli), *Man Jing Zi* (Fructus Viticis) and *Chuan Xiong* (Rhizoma Ligustici Chuanxiong).
8. For persistent pain, add *Tian Ma** (Rhizoma Gastrodiae Elatae) and *Gou Teng* (Ramulus Uncariae cum Uncis).
9. For skin lesions on the lower limbs, add *Chuan Niu Xi* (Radix Cyathulae Officinalis) and *Mu Gua* (Fructus Chaenomelis).

10. For skin lesions in the lumbosacral region, add *Chao Du Zhong* (Cortex Eucommiae Ulmoidis, stir-fried) and *Xu Duan* (Radix Dipsaci).
11. For non-healing sores, add *Huang Qi* (Radix Astragali seu Hedysari), *Bai Lian* (Radix Ampelopsis Japonicae), *Dang Shen* (Radix Codonopsitis Pilosulae), and *Shan Yao* (Rhizoma Dioscoreae Oppositae).

PATENT HERBAL MEDICINES
- Take one 10ml phial of *Kang Bing Du Kou Fu Ye* (Antivirus Syrup) two or three times per day while the lesions are present.
- Take 3-5 tablets of *Nan Tong She Yao Pian* (Nantong Snake Tablet) two or three times a day. Alternatively, mix 10-15 tablets into a paste with 5-10 ml of vinegar and apply directly to the lesions once or twice a day. This is recommended in the initial stage of herpes zoster or for post-herpetic neuralgia.

EXTERNAL TREATMENT
- Before the vesicles burst, apply *Yu Lu Gao* (Jade Dew Ointment), or pound fresh *Lu Hui* (Herba Aloes) 10g to a pulp and mix with *Bing Pian* (Borneolum) 1g.
- When the vesicles have burst or if there is profuse exudation, prepare a decoction of *Ma Chi Xian* (Herba Portulacae Oleraceae) 30g, *Huang Lian* (Rhizoma Coptidis) 15g, *Huang Bai* (Cortex Phellodendri) 30g, and *Wu Bei Zi*‡ (Galla Rhois Chinensis) 15g and use as a wet compress.
- When the exudation decreases or the skin lesions have dried up, *Bing Shi San* (Borneol and Gypsum Powder) or *Huang Lian Ruan Gao* (Coptis Ointment) can be applied as a local dressing until crusts form.

ACUPUNCTURE
Selection of points on the affected channels
Main points: LI-11 Quchi, GV-12 Shenzhu, GB-34 Yanglingquan, and SP-6 Sanyinjiao.

Auxiliary points
- Add EX-HN-5 Taiyang,[ii] ST-8 Touwei and GB-14 Yangbai for involvement of the orbital region.
- Add ST-2 Sibai, BL-1 Jingming and ST-7 Xiaguan for involvement of the zygomatic region.
- Add ST-4 Dicang, ST-5 Daying and ST-6 Jiache for involvement of the lower jaw.
- Add SI-9 Jianzhen and HT-1 Jiquan if the axillary fossa is involved.
- Add LI-4 Hegu if the area above the umbilicus is affected.

- Add ST-36 Zusanli if the area below the umbilicus is affected.

Technique: Use the reducing method for young people, and the reinforcing method for older people and people with a weak constitution. Retain the needles for 30 minutes. Treat once a day. A course consists of ten treatment sessions.

Local points
Points: Ashi points (the site of the lesions).
Technique: Insert a no. 30-32 filiform needle obliquely underneath the skin lesion at an angle of 15-30° at points above, below, to the left, and to the right of the Ashi point. Retain the needles for 30 minutes after obtaining Qi; lightly rotate the needles three to five times during this period. Treat once a day. A course consists of ten treatment sessions.

Selection of points according to pattern identification
Main points: BL-18 Ganshu, LI-11 Quchi, TB-6 Zhigou, and Ashi points (the site of the lesions).

Auxiliary points
- For Dampness and Heat fighting and binding, add ST-44 Neiting, TB-5 Waiguan and GB-43 Xiaxi.
- For exuberant Heat Toxins, add LI-4 Hegu, GB-34 Yanglingquan and HT-7 Shenmen.

Technique: Apply the reducing method. Treat twice a day. A course consists of ten treatment sessions.

Acupuncture notes
- For extensive skin lesions, points are usually selected from the affected channels, whereas for circumscribed skin lesions, local points are normally employed.
- For obvious internal patterns, points should be selected according to pattern identification.
- Most points included in the prescriptions have the functions of alleviating pain by clearing Heat and transforming Dampness or relieving Toxicity and freeing the network vessels.
- These acupuncture points cannot be applied for the pattern of Qi stagnation and Blood stasis since the lesions will already have disappeared.

MOXIBUSTION
Encircling moxibustion
Points: Ashi points (the site of the lesions), BL-15 Xinshu and BL-18 Ganshu.
Technique: Perform direct moxibustion for 30-40 minutes until the skin reddens. Treat once a day.

---

ii M-HN-9 according to the system employed by the Shanghai College of Traditional Chinese Medicine.

Moxibustion at empirical points

Point: Spider Point.

Location: Ask the patient to sit upright. Measure the circumference of the patient's head with a length of thread. Place the thread around the neck from the front to the back and let the two ends dangle down so that they meet at a spot on the posterior midline at the thoracic level. This meeting point is known as the Spider Point.

Technique: Perform moxibustion with one to three moxa cones at this point. Treat once a day. A course consists of three treatment sessions.

EAR ACUPUNCTURE

Main points: Lung, Adrenal Gland and ear points corresponding to the areas of the body involved.

Auxiliary points: Ear-Shenmen, Endocrine, Sympathetic Nerve, Occiput, Liver, and Spleen.

Technique: Retain the needles in the ear points for 30 minutes. Treat once every other day. A course consists of seven treatment sessions.

PLUM-BLOSSOM NEEDLING

Points: Ashi points (the site of the lesions).

Technique: Ashi points in the area of the lesions can be strongly stimulated with a plum blossom needle until the herpes break and there is slight bleeding. The area is then cupped to suck out more exudate and blood. Finally, the local area is cleaned and *Bing Shi San* (Borneol and Gypsum Powder) applied externally; the area is then dressed with sterilized gauze. Treatment is given once every day. A course consists of three treatment sessions. The treatment procedure should be explained to patients before commencing.

Clinical notes

- In the initial stage of herpes zoster, herbal treatment and acupuncture treatment can be used alone or in combination to control pain as soon as possible. Acupuncture is particularly beneficial in alleviating pain. Herbal treatment works effectively in controlling the spread of skin lesions. The combination of a local wet compress with internal treatment helps to shorten the treatment period.

- Post-herpetic neuralgia, which may persist for many months, is a very troublesome problem, which acupuncture is relatively effective in treating. Combining acupuncture and internal treatment with *Huo Xue*

Xiao Yan Wan (Pill for Invigorating the Blood and Dispersing Inflammation) or *Nei Xiao Lian Qiao Wan* (Forsythia Internal Dispersion Pill) can help bring about better results.

- Herpes zoster usually heals without leaving any scar, but there may be residual depressed and depigmented scarring.

- The majority of patients with herpes zoster will not experience a recurrence of the disease. However, a small number of patients experience a second or third episode.

- For patients with severe and recurring herpes zoster, attention should be paid to the possibility of malignant tumors or chronic progressive immunologic disorders such as AIDS.

- Involvement of the ophthalmic division of the trigeminal nerve can result in corneal ulcers and scarring. Patients must be referred to a doctor of Western medicine immediately.

Modern clinical experience

SCALP ACUPUNCTURE FOR POST-HERPETIC NEURALGIA

Chen followed Jiao Shunfa's method for the classification of scalp areas. He selected the Sensory Area and the Foot Motor and Sensory Area contralateral to the skin lesions. No. 28 filiform needles 7 cm long were used. They were inserted quickly under the skin and advanced parallel to the scalp for about 5cm. The needles were rotated at a speed of 200 times per minute continuously for 1-2 minutes, once every 10-15 minutes. After three rotation sessions, the needles were retained for a further 30 minutes. Treatment was given once a day. Pain decreased after each treatment session. [1]

EXTERNAL TREATMENT

External treatments include the use of ointments, oils, lotions and powders. **Zhang** prepared a mixture of *Zi Cao* (Radix Arnebiae seu Lithospermi) and *Xiang You* (Oleum Sesami Seminis) in a ratio of 3:25; the mixture was then heated in a pot to 138°C. After 50 minutes, the oil was collected through a filter and cooled. It was then directly applied to the affected area 3-5 times a day. A course of treatment lasted seven days, with 20 out of 26 patients experiencing a significant improvement by the end of the course. [2]

Warts (verrucae)
疣

Warts are benign growths on the skin or mucous membranes that are caused by the human papillomavirus (HPV). Different types of HPV lead to different types of warts, for instance, HPV-1, 2 and 4 are found in common warts (verruca vulgaris) and plantar warts (verruca plantaris), whereas HPV-3 and 5 are found in plane or flat warts (verruca plana) and generalized verrucosis (epidermodysplasia verruciformis).

Trauma is an important factor in the spread of warts; infections occur when the wart virus in the scales of the skin comes into contact with breaches in the skin or mucous membranes. Cell-mediated immunity also plays a role in the occurrence of the disease; variations in immunity may explain differences in severity and duration.

In Chinese medicine, common patterns of warts can be classified as follows:

Patterns involving the Xue level

- Wind Dryness due to Blood Deficiency – this pattern develops due to Liver Deficiency and Blood Dryness with Qi in the sinews being deprived of nourishment. The treatment principle is to moisten Dryness and dissipate Wind.

- Qi stagnation and Blood congealing – this pattern is caused by exposure of the foot to water and Wind-Cold resulting in Qi stagnation and Blood congealing. The treatment principle is to enrich Kidney-Water and generate Liver-Blood.

Externally contracted Wind-Heat

- Pathogenic Wind accompanied by Heat – this pattern is characterized by skin lesions manifesting as slightly elevated, flat, smooth, and firm papules likely to occur on the face and the dorsum of the hand.

- Wind-Heat Toxins – the skin lesions in this pattern are characterized by solid, hemispherical, elevated papules with a shiny appearance and central umbilical-like depression. They may occur on any part of the body.

- For both these externally contracted Wind-Heat patterns, internal treatment should follow the principle of clearing Heat and relieving Toxicity, but external treatments differ. For pathogenic Wind accompanied by Heat, use *You Xi Fang* (Wart Wash Formula). For Wind-Heat Toxins, a three-edged needle is used after sterilization of the skin to prick the warts so that the white substance inside is squeezed out. This is followed by external application of *Niu Huang Jie Du Wan* (Bovine Bezoar Pill for Relieving Toxicity) ground into a powder and covered by gauze.

Common warts (verruca vulgaris)
寻常疣

Common warts usually appear on sites subject to minor injury, such as the hands, face, elbows, and knees, especially in young children. Spread is associated with trauma.

In TCM, common warts are also known as *qian ri chuang* (thousand-day sores).

Clinical manifestations

- Common warts commonly grow on the fingers, the dorsum of the hand, the edge of the foot, the face, or the genitals. They occasionally grow along the margin of nails in nail biters or in patients whose hands are frequently immersed in water.

- The warts start with pinpoint-like papules, which grow gradually to 0.5cm or even bigger. They are round or polygonal in shape with a rough surface and obvious hyperkeratosis. They are firm, elevated, and grayish-yellow, dirty yellow or dirty brown in color. Their surface breaks up skin lines. They assume a nipple-like shape as they proliferate, and are likely to bleed when rubbed or knocked. Thrombosed capillaries can occur in warts, manifesting as small black dots.

- Warts vary in number. They are usually multiple and can proliferate to many dozens. Single warts often remain unchanged for a long time.

Differential diagnosis

The diagnosis of common warts is usually obvious. However, where warts are present on the hand or foot, there may occasionally be confusion with corns (see plantar warts for a full differential diagnosis).

Etiology and pathology

- Wind-Heat in the Liver and Gallbladder, anger stirring Liver-Fire, or excessive pathogenic Qi settling in the Liver all lead to Blood-Dryness in the Liver Channel. The Blood therefore fails to nourish the sinews and sinew Qi cannot flourish. If there is then an external invasion of Wind, common warts develop.

- People in ancient times held the view that the Liver and Kidneys shared the same source. Hyperactive Liver-Fire gradually consumes Kidney-Water; Kidney Qi will therefore become undernourished and the sinews will lose moisture and nourishment, causing the development of common warts.

- As Gu Bohua has stressed in the modern era in *Shi Yong Zhong Yi Wai Ke Xue* [Practical Treatment of External Diseases with Traditional Chinese Medicine]: "Common warts grow because of external injury to the skin, infection by viruses or auto-inoculation after scratching."

Pattern identification and treatment

INTERNAL TREATMENT

WIND-HEAT IN THE LIVER AND GALLBLADDER

The duration of the disease is short. Skin lesions are generally numerous with a tendency to spread extensively. Patients may experience slight itching. The tongue body is red with a scant coating. The pulse is wiry and rapid.

Treatment principle

Clear the Liver and drain Fire, dredge Wind and flatten warts.

Prescription
QING GAN YI RONG TANG JIA JIAN
Decoction for Clearing the Liver and Boosting Nourishment, with modifications

Chai Hu (Radix Bupleuri) 6g
Chuan Xiong (Rhizoma Ligustici Chuanxiong) 6g
Jiao Zhi Zi (Fructus Gardeniae Jasminoidis, scorch-fried) 6g
Mu Gua (Fructus Chaenomelis) 6g
Fu Ling (Sclerotium Poriae Cocos) 10g
Shu Di Huang (Radix Rehmanniae Glutinosae Conquita) 10g
Bai Zhu (Rhizoma Atractylodis Macrocephalae) 10g
Chao Bai Shao (Radix Paeoniae Lactiflorae, stir-fried) 10g
Dang Gui (Radix Angelicae Sinensis) 10g
Jin Yin Hua (Flos Lonicerae) 15g
Ban Lan Gen (Radix Isatidis seu Baphicacanthi) 15g
Gou Teng (Ramulus Uncariae cum Uncis) 15g
Fang Feng (Radix Ledebouriellae Divaricatae) 15g
Yi Yi Ren (Semen Coicis Lachryma-jobi) 30g
Shi Jue Ming‡ (Concha Haliotidis) 30g
Shan Dou Gen (Radix Sophorae Tonkinensis) 15g

Explanation

- Where skin lesions are extensive, this is more likely to be caused by Blood-Dryness in the Liver channel and invasion of external Wind; *Chai Hu* (Radix Bupleuri), *Jiao Zhi Zi* (Fructus Gardeniae Jasminoidis, scorch-fried), *Gou Teng* (Ramulus Uncariae cum Uncis), *Fu Ling* (Sclerotium Poriae Cocos), *Shu Di Huang* (Radix Rehmanniae Glutinosae Conquita), *Bai Zhu* (Rhizoma Atractylodis Macrocephalae), *Chao Bai Shao* (Radix Paeoniae Lactiflorae, stir-fried), and *Dang Gui* (Radix Angelicae Sinensis) are therefore used to clear and emolliate the Liver in order to enrich and nourish sinew Qi.

- *Jin Yin Hua* (Flos Lonicerae), *Shan Dou Gen* (Radix Sophorae Tonkinensis) and *Ban Lan Gen* (Radix Isatidis seu Baphicacanthi) support the first group of herbs by clearing Heat and relieving Toxicity.

- *Mu Gua* (Fructus Chaenomelis), *Fang Feng* (Radix Ledebouriellae Divaricatae) and *Chuan Xiong* (Rhizoma Ligustici Chuanxiong) expel Wind and dissipate pathogenic factors.

- *Yi Yi Ren* (Semen Coicis Lachryma-jobi) and *Shi Jue Ming*‡ (Concha Haliotidis) soften hardness and eliminate warts.

LACK OF NOURISHMENT OF KIDNEY QI

The duration of the disease is long, during which time the warts appear and disappear without a complete cure. Alternatively, after treatment with corrosive substances (such as salicylic acid, formaldehyde or glutaraldehyde), the warts can blister with occasional exudation of blood. Other symptoms and signs include dizziness, tinnitus, weakness of the limbs, and lack of strength. The tongue body is pale red with a scant coating; the pulse is thready and rapid.

Treatment principle

Enrich Kidney-Water, calm the Liver and eradicate warts.

Prescription
GUI SHAO LIU WEI DI HUANG WAN JIA JIAN
Six-Ingredient Rehmannia Pill with Chinese Angelica
Root and Peony, with modifications

Shu Di Huang (Radix Rehmanniae Glutinosae Conquita) 10g
Fu Ling (Sclerotium Poriae Cocos) 10g
Dang Gui (Radix Angelicae Sinensis) 10g
Bai Shao (Radix Paeoniae Lactiflorae) 10g
Mu Dan Pi (Cortex Moutan Radicis) 10g
Shan Yao (Rhizoma Dioscoreae Oppositae) 15g
Shan Zhu Yu (Fructus Corni Officinalis) 15g
Sang Shen (Fructus Mori Albae) 15g
He Shou Wu (Radix Polygoni Multiflori) 15g
Ban Zhi Lian (Herba Scutellariae Barbatae) 6g
Chai Hu (Radix Bupleuri) 6g
Sang Zhi (Ramulus Mori Albae) 6g
Shi Jue Ming‡ (Concha Haliotidis) 30g
Yi Yi Ren (Semen Coicis Lachryma-jobi) 30g

Explanation
- The basic formula of *Shu Di Huang* (Radix Rehmanniae Glutinosae Conquita), *Fu Ling* (Sclerotium Poriae Cocos), *Dang Gui* (Radix Angelicae Sinensis), *Bai Shao* (Radix Paeoniae Lactiflorae), *Mu Dan Pi* (Cortex Moutan Radicis), *Shan Yao* (Rhizoma Dioscoreae Oppositae), and *Shan Zhu Yu* (Fructus Corni Officinalis) enriches the Kidneys and emolliates the Liver to nourish sinew Qi and prevent the growth of the warts.
- *He Shou Wu* (Radix Polygoni Multiflori) and *Sang Shen* (Fructus Mori Albae) support the first group of herbs by strengthening the Kidney-enriching effect.
- *Ban Zhi Lian* (Herba Scutellariae Barbatae), *Chai Hu* (Radix Bupleuri) and *Shi Jue Ming*‡ (Concha Haliotidis) relieve Toxicity and calm the Liver.
- *Yi Yi Ren* (Semen Coicis Lachryma-jobi) is effective at inhibiting the wart virus.
- *Sang Zhi* (Ramulus Mori Albae) works to guide the other ingredients along the channels to act directly on the affected area.

EXTERNAL TREATMENT
- For multiple, scattered warts, prepare a decoction with

  Ma Chi Xian (Herba Portulacae Oleraceae) 30g
  Cang Zhu (Rhizoma Atractylodis) 15g
  Feng Fang‡ (Nidus Vespae) 15g
  Bai Zhi (Radix Angelicae Dahuricae) 15g
  Chen Pi (Pericarpium Citri Reticulatae) 15g
  Xi Xin* (Herba cum Radice Asari) 10g
  She Chuang Zi (Fructus Cnidii Monnieri) 12g
  Ku Shen (Radix Sophorae Flavescentis) 12g

Use this decoction or *Xiang Mu Shui Xi Ji* (Cyperus and Scouring Rush Herb Wash Preparation) as an external wash or wet compress for 15-30 minutes once or twice a day.

- For single, large warts, apply oil made from *Ya Dan Zi* (Fructus Bruceae Javanicae) directly onto the warts without damaging the surrounding healthy skin. The treatment is applied once every two or three days until the wart drops off completely.

ACUPUNCTURE
Point: Ashi point (the mother wart).
Technique: Insert a filiform needle obliquely into the mother wart. Insert another four needles symmetrically around the wart. Retain the needles for 30 minutes. The treatment is repeated once every 2-3 days.

MOXIBUSTION
Direct moxibustion with a moxa stick
Point: Ashi point (the site of the wart).
Technique: Light one end of a moxa stick. Place the burning end directly on the top of the wart. If the patient cannot tolerate the burning pain, move the stick away slightly. Repeat the procedure until the wart looks scorched and dry. Crusts will normally fall off in 5-10 days and the wart will heal. If the first course of treatment does not work, repeat the procedure one week later.

EAR ACUPUNCTURE
Points: Lung, Subcortex, Endocrine, and points corresponding to the location of the lesions on the body.
Technique: Retain the needles for 15-30 minutes. Treat once a day. A course consists of ten treatment sessions.

FIRE NEEDLING
Point: Ashi point (the site of the wart).
Technique: After routine local disinfection, heat the needle in a flame, insert it quickly to a depth of about two-thirds of the body of the wart and withdraw it immediately. Insert the needle at three to five spots on the wart depending on its size. The wart will usually dry up and detach five to seven days after the treatment. The procedure must be explained to the patient before commencing the treatment.

RUBBING METHOD
Peel the skin from a fresh water chestnut (*Bi Qi*, Cormus Heliocharitis) and rub the white flesh against the body of the wart until the edge of the wart is softened with partial detachment and slight pinpoint bleeding. Treat three to four times a day. The wart will usually heal in a few days.

Clinical notes

- For patients with a strong constitution and large warts that are recent in onset, acupuncture, moxibustion and external treatment are recommended. For those with a weak constitution and multiple warts of long duration, internal herbal treatment should be given as the primary method, while acupuncture, moxibustion and external treatment should be used as secondary treatments.

- Some patients may experience redness, swelling and itching at sites of warts while taking herbs. These are signs indicating that treatment is effective and that the warts are going to shrivel and drop off. It is not advisable to discontinue the treatment upon such signs.

Advice for the patient

- Patients should be warned to avoid using topical preparations containing steroids, as these spread the infection.

- Try to avoid scratching the warts in order to prevent infection of new areas by autoinoculation.

Literature excerpt

According to *Yang Ke Xun Cui* [Essential Collection for the Treatment of Sores]: "If skin lesions on the hand are caused by malnourishment of the sinews because of Blood-Dryness due to Wind-Heat, follow the prescription of *Ba Wei Xiao Yao San* (Eight-Ingredient Free Wanderer Powder) plus *Huang Lian* (Rhizoma Coptidis). If the lesions are caused by Fire resulting from anger, follow the prescription of *Chai Hu Qing Gan Tang* (Bupleurum Decoction for Clearing the Liver). If they are caused by contraction of the sinews due to desiccation of the Kidneys and loss of Essence, follow the prescription of *Shen Qi Wan* (Kidney Qi Pill). Materia medica that are cold or cool in nature or have the function of bearing Fire downward must not be used. If these contraindications are ignored and such treatments are utilized, they may make the condition worse; in more serious cases, they may cause severe ulceration with swelling, pain and fever, possibly with bleeding, which may prove fatal."

Modern clinical experience

EMPIRICAL PRESCRIPTION

Guo prepared a formula called *Qu You Jian Ji* (Removing Warts Decoction) by boiling *Mu Zei* (Herba Equiseti Hiemalis) 30g and *Xiang Fu* (Rhizoma Cyperi Rotundi) 30g in water for 20 minutes in 800ml of water. The decoction was used once a day to soak the affected area for 30 minutes. Each wash was used three times. If the warts failed to come off in six months, *Ban Lan Gen* (Radix Isatidis seu Baphicacanthi) 30g and *Ku Shen* (Radix Sophorae Flavescentis) 30g were added to the original prescription for a second session of treatment. [3]

MOXIBUSTION

Qi reported on the technique of holding a burning moxa stick over each wart for 20 minutes at a time. The local temperature needed to be around 45°C to be effective. The treatment was carried out once a day. It was discontinued if there was no effect after two weeks. [4]

Plane warts (*verruca plana*)
扁平疣

Plane warts are flat-topped and slightly rough on the surface, which is often pigmented. They are usually around 2-3 mm in diameter and may need lighting in order to see their full extent. In TCM, plane warts are also known as *bian hou* (flat warts).

Clinical manifestations

- Plane warts are more commonly seen in children or young women.

- The most common sites of plane warts are on the face, especially the forehead and around the mouth and chin. Other common sites include the dorsum of the hands and the forearms. In a few cases, plane warts can be found on the nape, the scapular area and the legs.

- In the initial stage, plane warts are 1-3 mm in size. Smooth, flat-topped, and skin-colored or light brown, they can become prolific and widespread.

- Patients often complain of itching. Scratching can

make the warts spread in a line by autoinoculation of the virus.

- Although the duration may be lengthy and some lesions may last for years, spontaneous disappearance is possible. If the warts suddenly seem to increase in number, accompanied by symptoms such as itching, inflammation and elevation, this is usually an indication that they will resolve.

Etiology and pathology

Internal factors
Blood-Dryness due to Liver Deficiency results in the sinews and vessels being deprived of nourishment and the subsequent appearance of warts.

External factors
External Wind-Heat Toxins invade and fight in the skin and flesh, leading to Qi stagnation and Blood stasis

Pattern identification and treatment

INTERNAL TREATMENT

BLOOD-DRYNESS DUE TO LIVER DEFICIENCY
The skin lesions are disseminated and are a dark red color. Some may become confluent. Plaques may form due to proliferation. The tongue body is dark red with a scant coating. The pulse is wiry and rapid.

Treatment principle
Allow constrained Liver Qi to flow freely, quicken the Blood and dissipate warts.

Prescription
DAN ZHI XIAO YAO SAN JIA JIAN
Free Wanderer Powder with Tree Peony Root Bark and Gardenia, with modifications

Sheng Di Huang (Radix Rehmanniae Glutinosae) 12g
Dan Shen (Radix Salviae Miltiorrhizae) 12g
Fu Ling (Sclerotium Poriae Cocos) 12g
Yi Mu Cao (Herba Leonuri Heterophylli) 12g
Dang Gui (Radix Angelicae Sinensis) 10g
Bai Zhu (Rhizoma Atractylodis Macrocephalae) 10g
Chi Shao (Radix Paeoniae Rubra) 10g
Yi Yi Ren (Semen Coicis Lachryma-jobi) 15g
He Shou Wu (Radix Polygoni Multiflori) 15g
Zhi Zi (Fructus Gardeniae Jasminoidis) 6g
Mu Dan Pi (Cortex Moutan Radicis) 6g
*Chuan Shan Jia** (Squama Manitis Pentadactylae) 6g

Explanation
- *Sheng Di Huang* (Radix Rehmanniae Glutinosae), *Mu*

Dan Pi (Cortex Moutan Radicis), *Dan Shen* (Radix Salviae Miltiorrhizae), *Dang Gui* (Radix Angelicae Sinensis), *Chi Shao* (Radix Paeoniae Rubra), *Bai Zhu* (Rhizoma Atractylodis Macrocephalae), and *Fu Ling* (Sclerotium Poriae Cocos) support the Spleen, nourish the Blood and emolliate the Liver to treat the Root.
- *He Shou Wu* (Radix Polygoni Multiflori), *Yi Yi Ren* (Semen Coicis Lachryma-jobi), *Yi Mu Cao* (Herba Leonuri Heterophylli), *Chuan Shan Jia** (Squama Manitis Pentadactylae), and *Zhi Zi* (Fructus Gardeniae Jasminoidis) are used to support the first group of herbs by nourishing the Blood, eliminating warts, transforming Blood stasis, dissipating lumps, and clearing Heat. Therefore, any Fire resulting from Liver Depression and Qi stagnation can be cleared and sinew Qi can be enriched.

SPLEEN QI DEFICIENCY
The skin lesions are pale red in color and take a long time to disappear. Accompanying symptoms and signs include mental fatigue, lack of strength and poor appetite. The tongue body is pale red with a scant coating; the pulse is thready and weak.

Treatment principle
Augment Qi and support the Spleen, consolidate the Root and eliminate warts.

Prescription
GUI QI JIAN ZHONG TANG JIA JIAN
Chinese Angelica and Astragalus Decoction for Fortifying the Middle Burner, with modifications

Huang Qi (Radix Astragali seu Hedysari) 10g
Dang Gui (Radix Angelicae Sinensis) 10g
Bai Zhu (Rhizoma Atractylodis Macrocephalae) 10g
Bai Shao (Radix Paeoniae Lactiflorae) 10g
Gan Cao (Radix Glycyrrhizae) 10g
Yi Mu Cao (Herba Leonuri Heterophylli) 12g
Dan Shen (Radix Salviae Miltiorrhizae) 12g
Gan Di Huang (Radix Rehmanniae Glutinosae Exsiccata) 15g
*Chuan Shan Jia** (Squama Manitis Pentadactylae) 3g
Sheng Ma (Rhizoma Cimicifugae) 3g

Explanation
- The fact that the warts are difficult to get rid of indicates that Vital Qi (Zheng Qi) is too weak to ward off pathogenic factors. Therefore, *Dang Gui* (Radix Angelicae Sinensis), *Huang Qi* (Radix Astragali seu Hedysari), *Bai Zhu* (Rhizoma Atractylodis Macrocephalae), *Bai Shao* (Radix Paeoniae Lactiflorae), *Gan Di Huang* (Radix Rehmanniae Glutinosae Exsiccata), and *Gan Cao* (Radix Glycyrrhizae) are used to augment Qi with warmth and sweetness to support Spleen Yang.

- *Dan Shen* (Radix Salviae Miltiorrhizae), *Yi Mu Cao* (Herba Leonuri Heterophylli), *Chuan Shan Jia** (Squama Manitis Pentadactylae), and *Sheng Ma* (Rhizoma Cimicifugae) support the first group of herbs by invigorating the Blood, transforming Blood stasis and relieving Toxicity to flatten the warts.

EXTERNAL TREATMENT

- *You Xi Fang* (Wart Wash Formula) is recommended if there are multiple warts. Wash the affected area with the warm decoction for 15 minutes four or five times a day.
- For stubborn individual warts, wash the warts in warm water, then apply five pieces of mashed *Ya Dan Zi* (Fructus Bruceae Javanicae) directly onto the warts, avoiding the surrounding healthy skin. Cover the warts with a bandage. The warts usually come off in two to three days.

ACUPUNCTURE

Prescription 1
Points: LU-7 Lieque, LI-4 Hegu and ST-36 Zusanli.
Technique: Use filiform needles and apply the reducing method. Retain the needle for 30 minutes after obtaining Qi. Treat once a day. A course consists of ten treatment sessions.

Prescription 2
Point: EX-UE-5 Dagukong (located at the center of the dorsal transverse crease of the interphalangeal joint of the thumb).[iii]
Technique: Use filiform needles and apply the reducing method. Retain the needles for 30 minutes after obtaining Qi. Treat once a day. A course consists of ten treatment sessions.

Prescription 3
Main points: GB-20 Fengchi, LI-11 Quchi, LI-4 Hegu, EX-HN-5 Taiyang,[iv] GB-14 Yangbai, SP-10 Xuehai, and the Ashi point (the center of the mother wart).
Auxiliary points: One or two adjacent points from the channels in the local area of the lesions, for example, ST-6 Jiache and ST-7 Xiaguan.
Technique: Use filiform needles and apply subcutaneous needling on the facial points and the reducing method for the other points. Retain the needles for 30 minutes. The effect is improved if a no. 26-28 filiform needle is inserted perpendicularly to the base of the wart and one or two drops of blood are squeezed out. Treatment is given every other day. A course consists of seven treatment sessions.

Explanation
These prescriptions combine local and distal points:

- LI-4 Hegu, ST-36 Zusanli and SP-10 Xuehai support the Spleen and nourish the Blood to allow nourishment of the sinews.
- LU-7 Lieque, GB-20 Fengchi, LI-11 Quchi, EX-HN-5 Taiyang, and GB-14 Yangbai dredge Wind and dissipate Blood.

EAR ACUPUNCTURE

Ear needling
Points: Liver, Subcortex and Lung.
Technique: Retain the needles for 15 minutes. Treat every other day. A course consists of ten treatment sessions.

Embedding intradermal needles
Main points: Lung, Liver, Kidney, and Subcortex.
Auxiliary points: Ear points corresponding to the lesion areas on the body.
Technique: After routine disinfection, place the sterilized intradermal needles on the ear points without penetrating the skin. Attach them with adhesive plaster or tape. Repeat the treatment once every three days in summer, and once every seven days in winter. A course consists of five treatment sessions.

ELECTRO-ACUPUNCTURE
Point: EX-UE-5 Dagukong (empirical point).[iii]
Technique: After obtaining Qi, retain the needle for 25 minutes. Connect the needle to an electro-acupuncture stimulator at a frequency of 20 pulses per minute. Increase the frequency by one pulse per minute, thus gradually raising the intensity of stimulation until the patient's tolerance level is reached. Remove the needle after 25 minutes. Treat every other day. A course consists of seven treatment sessions.

PLUM-BLOSSOM NEEDLING
Location: The affected area on the first lateral line of the Bladder channel beside the bilateral cervical or thoracic vertebrae.
Technique: Tap three times up and down the first lateral line of the Bladder channel on the nape or back to produce moderate stimulation. Continue the treatment until the local skin becomes slightly red. The effect is improved by tapping the lesions with heavy stimulation until bleeding occurs. The treatment procedure should be explained to patients before commencing.

[iii] M-UE-15 according to the system employed by the Shanghai College of Traditional Chinese Medicine.
[iv] M-HN-9 according to the system employed by the Shanghai College of Traditional Chinese Medicine.

Clinical notes

- Plane warts mainly affect young men and women. If the skin lesions become inflamed or start to itch, patients should be told that there is no need to worry; this simply indicates that the medication is acting on the lesions, and is usually a sign that the warts are healing.

- Acupuncture and ear acupuncture are recommended for patients with a strong constitution; internal treatment for those with a weak constitution. Both internal and external treatments are needed for conditions of long duration.

- The prognosis for plane warts is good. But for patients with a weak constitution, the time needed for recovery will be relatively long.

Advice for the patient

Do not scratch the area containing warts, or wash the area with hot water.

Literature excerpt

Xu Yi Hou Pi Fu Bing Lin Chuang Jing Yan Ji Yao [A Summary of Xu Yihou's Clinical Experiences in the Treatment of Skin Diseases] states that the treatment for warts depends on which of the twelve channels are affected, as well as on the appearance, color and duration of the skin lesions.

Conditions that affect the Yang channels with surplus Qi settling in the Gallbladder channel are often associated with Blood-Dryness due to Wind-Heat. These conditions are usually Excess patterns.

Conditions involving the Yin channels are often the result of Water drying up due to Liver-Heat, which prevents Kidney Qi from flourishing and causes spasms due to lack of Essence. These conditions are usually Deficiency patterns and are of long duration.

The treatment principle for stubborn skin lesions should be to enrich the Kidneys, emolliate the Liver and support the Spleen. Although this is not a direct treatment for the warts, it can prove remarkably successful.

Modern clinical experience

EMPIRICAL PRESCRIPTIONS

1. **Cao** formulated an empirical prescription to treat plane warts. [5]

Prescription
QING YOU TANG
Decoction for Clearing Warts

Chai Hu (Radix Bupleuri) 6g
Ban Lan Gen (Radix Isatidis seu Baphicacanthi) 30g
Yi Yi Ren (Semen Coicis Lachryma-jobi) 30g
Zhen Zhu Mu‡ (Concha Margaritifera) 30g
Ci Shi‡ (Magnetitum) 30g
Da Qing Ye (Folium Isatidis seu Baphicacanthi) 20g

The ingredients were decocted three times, with the first and second decoctions taken internally in the morning and evening, and the third preparation used as an external wash. Ten days constituted a course of treatment; on average, treatment lasted for two courses.

2. **Wu** treated 113 cases of plane warts with *Fu Fang Ma Chi Xian Chong Ji* (Purslane Compound Soluble Granules). [6]

Prescription ingredients

Ma Chi Xian (Herba Portulacae Oleraceae)
Zi Cao (Radix Arnebiae seu Lithospermi)
Ban Lan Gen (Radix Isatidis seu Baphicacanthi)
Jin Yin Hua (Flos Lonicerae)
Yi Yi Ren (Semen Coicis Lachryma-jobi)
Chi Shao (Radix Paeoniae Rubra)
Dan Shen (Radix Salviae Miltiorrhizae)
Xiang Fu (Rhizoma Cyperi Rotundi)
Mu Zei (Herba Equiseti Hiemalis)
Bai Ji Li (Fructus Tribuli Terrestris)
Chan Tui‡ (Periostracum Cicadae)

Fifteen grams of the granules were taken orally three times a day. The dosage was halved for children under 8 years old. Results were seen after a course of treatment lasting for one month.

3. **Qin** treated plane warts with *Qu You Fang* (Formula for Eliminating Warts). [7]

Prescription ingredients

Hu Zhang (Radix et Rhizoma Polygoni Cuspidati) 15g
Da Qing Ye (Folium Isatidis seu Baphicacanthi) 15g
Zi Cao (Radix Arnebiae seu Lithospermi) 9g
E Zhu (Rhizoma Curcumae) 9g
Mu Dan Pi (Cortex Moutan Radicis) 9g
Gan Cao (Radix Glycyrrhizae) 5g
Dang Gui (Radix Angelicae Sinensis) 10g
Zhen Zhu Mu‡ (Concha Margaritifera) 30g
Ci Shi‡ (Magnetitum) 30g

One bag was used to prepare a decoction, taken twice a day. Ten days constituted a course and results were seen after three continuous courses.

4. **Hong** treated plane warts with *Yin Lan Tao You Tang* (Honeysuckle, Isatis Root and Peach Kernel Decoction for Treating Warts) used internally and externally. [8]

Prescription ingredients

Jin Yin Hua (Flos Lonicerae) 30g
Ban Lan Gen (Radix Isatidis seu Baphicacanthi) 30g
Pu Gong Ying (Herba Taraxaci cum Radice) 30g
Yi Yi Ren (Semen Coicis Lachryma-jobi) 30g
Xia Ku Cao (Spica Prunellae Vulgaris) 30g
Wa Leng Zi‡ (Concha Arcae) 30g
Chi Shao (Radix Paeoniae Rubra) 10g
Mu Dan Pi (Cortex Moutan Radicis) 10g
Tao Ren (Semen Persicae) 10g
*Chuan Shan Jia** (Squama Manitis Pentadactylae) 10g
Mu Zei (Herba Equiseti Hiemalis) 10g
Gan Cao (Radix Glycyrrhizae) 10g
Zhi Zi (Fructus Gardeniae Jasminoidis) 15g
Huang Qin (Radix Scutellariae Baicalensis) 15g

The dosage was halved for children under 10 years old. One bag of the ingredients was used per day, decocted three times for internal use. It was then decocted for a fourth time with the addition of *Ya Dan Zi* (Fructus Bruceae Javanicae) 7-10g and *E Zhu* (Rhizoma Curcumae) 20-30g. The decoction was strained and the residue discarded. A piece of gauze was soaked in the herbal decoction and rubbed against warts while still warm for at least 15 minutes three times a day. Results were seen after a course of treatment lasting for four weeks.

5. **Chen** treated 153 cases of plane warts with *Huo Xue Jie Du Tang* (Decoction for Invigorating the Blood and Relieving Toxicity) used internally and externally. [9]

Prescription ingredients

Hong Hua (Flos Carthami Tinctorii) 10g
Zi Cao (Radix Arnebiae seu Lithospermi) 10g
*Chuan Shan Jia** (Squama Manitis Pentadactylae) 15g
Ma Chi Xian (Herba Portulacae Oleraceae) 15g
Mu Zei (Herba Equiseti Hiemalis) 15g
Yi Mu Cao (Herba Leonuri Heterophylli) 15g
Dan Shen (Radix Salviae Miltiorrhizae) 15g
Xia Ku Cao (Spica Prunellae Vulgaris) 15g
Bai Jiang Cao (Herba Patriniae cum Radice) 30g
Yi Yi Ren (Semen Coicis Lachryma-jobi) 30g

One bag a day was used to prepare a decoction, taken in the morning and evening. The ingredients were boiled for a third time, with 50-100ml of vinegar being added to the decoction at the end. This was applied directly to the skin lesions once a day, with the affected area being rubbed until the skin became red or hot. Results indicated that 95 patients were cured, 32 experienced a significant effect, 21 some effect, and 5 no effect.

TREATMENT ACCORDING TO PATTERN IDENTIFICATION

1. **Meng** identified three different patterns for plane warts: [10]

- **Wind-Heat settling in the exterior**
Treatment principle: Dredge Wind, release the exterior and clear Heat.
Prescription: *Yin Qiao San Jia Jian* (Honeysuckle and Forsythia Powder, with modifications according to the patient's condition).

- **Qi stagnation and Blood stasis**
Treatment principle: Soothe the Liver, regulate Qi and transform Blood stasis.
Prescription: *Xiao Yao San* (Free Wanderer Powder) or *Tao Hong Si Wu Tang* (Peach Kernel and Safflower Four Agents Decoction).

- **Blood-Dryness due to hyperactivity of the Liver**
Treatment principle: Calm the Liver, nourish the Blood and moisten Dryness.
Prescription: *Tian Ma Gou Teng Yin Jia Jian* (Gastrodia and Uncaria Beverage, with modifications according to the patient's condition).

2. **Zhang** classified plane warts into two types with a different treatment for each type. [11]

- **Wind-Heat restricting the exterior**

Prescription
BIAN PING YOU YI HAO
Plane Warts Prescription No. 1

Sang Ye (Folium Mori Albae) 15g
Ju Hua (Flos Chrysanthemi Morifolii) 10g
Jin Yin Hua (Flos Lonicerae) 10g
Huang Qin (Radix Scutellariae Baicalensis) 6g
Zi Cao (Radix Arnebiae seu Lithospermi) 15g
Ban Lan Gen (Radix Isatidis seu Baphicacanthi) 15g
Ma Chi Xian (Herba Portulacae Oleraceae) 15g
Zhe Bei Mu (Bulbus Fritillariae Thunbergii) 6g
Bo He (Herba Menthae Haplocalycis) 6g
Chi Shao (Radix Paeoniae Rubra) 10g
Mu Dan Pi (Cortex Moutan Radicis) 10g
Gan Cao (Radix Glycyrrhizae) 6g

- **Phlegm and Blood stasis retained in the exterior**

Prescription
BIAN PING YOU ER HAO
Plane Warts Prescription No. 2

Tu Bei Mu (Tuber Bolbostemmatis) 15g
Yi Yi Ren (Semen Coicis Lachryma-jobi) 30g
Ban Lan Gen (Radix Isatidis seu Baphicacanthi) 15g

Feng Fang‡ (Nidus Vespae) 10g
Zi Cao (Radix Arnebiae seu Lithospermi) 10g
Bai Zhi (Radix Angelicae Dahuricae) 6g
Dan Shen (Radix Salviae Miltiorrhizae) 15g
Chi Shao (Radix Paeoniae Rubra) 10g
Zhen Zhu Mu‡ (Concha Margaritifera) 15g
Tao Ren (Semen Persicae) 10g
Hu Zhang (Radix et Rhizoma Polygoni Cuspidati) 10g

LOCAL TREATMENT

In recent years, ingredients used in formulae for the external treatment of plane warts fall into three major categories:

- dispelling Wind and clearing Heat
- transforming Blood stasis and dissipating lumps
- eliminating Dampness and relieving Toxicity

Ingredients that occur in more than ten prescriptions include *Ban Lan Gen* (Radix Isatidis seu Baphicacanthi), *Xiang Fu* (Rhizoma Cyperi Rotundi) and *Mu Zei* (Herba Equiseti Hiemalis); and those that occur in more than three prescriptions include *Tao Ren* (Semen Persicae), *Chai Hu* (Radix Bupleuri), *Zi Cao* (Radix Arnebiae seu Lithospermi), *Ku Shen* (Radix Sophorae Flavescentis), *Yi Yi Ren* (Semen Coicis Lachryma-jobi), *Bai Xian Pi* (Cortex Dictamni Dasycarpi Radicis), *Ma Chi Xian* (Herba Portulacae Oleraceae), and *Di Fu Zi* (Fructus Kochiae Scopariae). External treatments are mainly in the form of washes, tinctures and pastes. [12]

Plantar warts (verruca plantaris)
跖疣

These lesions are often solitary and are distributed over pressure areas of the sole. When they overlie a bony prominence and are associated with marked hyperkeratosis, pain and tenderness may be severe.

In TCM, plantar warts are also known as *zu hou* (foot warts).

Clinical manifestations

- Plantar warts occur on the sole of the foot or in the web between the toes.
- Individual plantar warts present as keratinized, firm, callus-like maculopapules, up to 1cm or more in diameter. Pricking or rubbing the lesion may cause slight bleeding. Dark punctate spots (thrombosed capillaries) are revealed on paring.
- The number of plantar warts varies. Multiple plantar warts may coalesce into plaques known as mosaic warts. In such cases, tenderness is obvious.

Differential diagnosis

Callus

A callus is a diffuse thickening of the horny layers of the skin as a result of frequent pressure or friction, which is often profession-related. They are usually painless. The thickening is greatest in the center, and grows thinner towards the edge of the area. Skin lines remain apparent in calluses, unlike in plantar warts.

Corn (clavus)

A corn typically occurs on an area of intense local pressure. It is commonly caused by the pressure of tight-fitting shoes. So-called soft corns occur in the web space between the toes, related to ill-fitting shoes which squeeze the toes together. Soft corns are often macerated. Corns consist of a central hard core of keratin which disturbs the skin lines. Applying pressure to corns often results in pain. Paring the surface keratin reveals a shiny central area, in contrast to the dark vessels of a pared wart.

Etiology and pathology

- Damp-Heat accumulating internally leads to the obstruction and stagnation of Qi and Blood. As a result, Qi in the sinews is deprived of nourishment and warts gradually appear.
- Plantar warts may also grow due to viral infection following skin trauma or autoinoculation after scratching.

Pattern identification and treatment

INTERNAL TREATMENT

DAMP-HEAT ACCUMULATING INTERNALLY

In the initial stage, a slightly raised wart is noticed on the sole of the foot or between the toes. There is slight bleeding when knocked. Tenderness is obvious. The tongue body is red with a scant coating; the pulse is wiry and rapid.

Treatment principle
Dispel Dampness and clear Heat, soften hardness and eradicate warts.

Prescription
CHAN YOU RUAN JIAN TANG JIA JIAN
Decoction for Eradicating Warts and Softening Hardness, with modifications

Ci Shi ‡ (Magnetitum) 30g
Dai Zhe Shi ‡ (Haematitum) 30g
Mu Li ‡ (Concha Ostreae) 30g
Zhen Zhu Mu ‡ (Concha Margaritifera) 30g
Di Gu Pi (Cortex Lycii Radicis) 15g
Yi Yi Ren (Semen Coicis Lachryma-jobi) 15g
Fu Ling Pi (Cortex Poriae Cocos) 15g
Hong Hua (Flos Carthami Tinctorii) 6g
Tao Ren (Semen Persicae) 6g
Shan Ci Gu (Pseudobulbus Shancigu) 6g
Chai Hu (Radix Bupleuri) 6g
Chuan Niu Xi (Radix Cyathulae Officinalis) 10g

Explanation
- Ci Shi ‡ (Magnetitum), Dai Zhe Shi ‡ (Haematitum), Mu Li ‡ (Concha Ostreae), and Zhen Zhu Mu ‡ (Concha Margaritifera) calm the Liver and soften hardness.
- Hong Hua (Flos Carthami Tinctorii), Tao Ren (Semen Persicae), Chuan Niu Xi (Radix Cyathulae Officinalis), and Shan Ci Gu (Pseudobulbus Shancigu) invigorate the Blood and soften hardness.
- Yi Yi Ren (Semen Coicis Lachryma-jobi) and Fu Ling Pi (Cortex Poriae Cocos) dispel Dampness.
- Di Gu Pi (Cortex Lycii Radicis) and Chai Hu (Radix Bupleuri) clear Heat.
- The prescription contains more ingredients to soften hardness than to eliminate Dampness; this is due to the fact that lesions on the foot are subjected to pressure and therefore become harder.

HEAT TOXINS ATTACKING THE SKIN
Skin lesions may be extensive, especially over the heads of the metatarsals and between the toes. Slight pain is experienced. The pulse is rapid and the tongue body is red with a scant coating.

Treatment principle
Clear Heat and relieve Toxicity, invigorate the Blood and dissipate lumps.

Prescription
GONG YING TAO REN TANG
Dandelion and Peach Kernel Decoction

Da Qing Ye (Folium Isatidis seu Baphicacanthi) 15g
Ban Lan Gen (Radix Isatidis seu Baphicacanthi) 15g
Pu Gong Ying (Herba Taraxaci cum Radice) 30g
Sheng Di Huang (Radix Rehmanniae Glutinosae) 9g
San Leng (Rhizoma Sparganii Stoloniferi) 9g
E Zhu (Rhizoma Curcumae) 9g
Tao Ren (Semen Persicae) 9g
Jiang Can ‡ (Bombyx Batryticatus) 9g
Bai Bu (Radix Stemonae) 9g
Feng Fang ‡ (Nidus Vespae) 9g
Gan Cao (Radix Glycyrrhizae) 4g

Explanation
- Da Qing Ye (Folium Isatidis seu Baphicacanthi), Ban Lan Gen (Radix Isatidis seu Baphicacanthi), Bai Bu (Radix Stemonae), Gan Cao (Radix Glycyrrhizae), Pu Gong Ying (Herba Taraxaci cum Radice), and Feng Fang ‡ (Nidus Vespae) clear Heat and relieve Toxicity.
- Sheng Di Huang (Radix Rehmanniae Glutinosae), San Leng (Rhizoma Sparganii Stoloniferi), E Zhu (Rhizoma Curcumae), Tao Ren (Semen Persicae), and Jiang Can ‡ (Bombyx Batryticatus) invigorate the Blood and soften hardness.
- The location of the skin lesions and the difficulty in removing them are taken into consideration in this formula. In addition to taking the decoction internally, the prescription can also be used as a soak for the affected area of the foot, thus increasing effectiveness.

General modifications
1. For very firm lesions with thick skin, add Chuan Shan Jia* (Squama Manitis Pentadactylae Praeparata), Dan Shen (Radix Salviae Miltiorrhizae) and Wu Mei (Fructus Pruni Mume).
2. If there is severe pain in the affected area, add Shi Jue Ming ‡ (Concha Haliotidis) and Wu Gong ‡ (Scolopendra Subspinipes).

EXTERNAL TREATMENT
- For isolated lesions, apply Shui Jing Gao (Crystal Paste) or oil made from Ya Dan Zi (Fructus Bruceae Javanicae) directly onto the warts without damaging the surrounding healthy skin. The treatment is applied once every two or three days until the warts are destroyed.
- For numerous lesions, use Xiang Mu Shui Xi Ji (Cyperus and Scouring Rush Herb Wash Preparation) or Gou Ji Shui Xi Ji (Cibot Wash Preparation) as concentrated preparations for soaking the foot.

ACUPUNCTURE
Points: KI-3 Taixi, BL-60 Kunlun and ST-36 Zusanli.
Technique: Apply the reducing method. Retain the needles for 30 minutes after obtaining Qi. Treat once

every other day. A course consists of ten treatment sessions.

Explanation: KI-3 Taixi, BL-60 Kunlun and ST-36 Zusanli augment Qi, support the Spleen and enrich Kidney Yin. Both Earlier Heaven and Later Heaven Qi are supported so that Yin and Blood are nourished and sinew Qi augmented, with the result that the warts are flattened.

MOXIBUSTION

Point: Ashi point (the site of the warts).
Technique: Light a moxa cone on the top of the wart; the base of the cone should cover about four-fifths of the surface of the wart. Use three to five cones in each treatment session. Treat once a day. A course consists of ten treatment sessions.

EAR ACUPUNCTURE

Points: Liver, Subcortex, Endocrine, and ear points corresponding to the locations of the skin lesions on the feet.
Technique: Retain the needles for 30 minutes. Treat once every other day. A course consists of ten treatment sessions.

Clinical notes

- Plantar warts often occur in individuals whose feet are prone to hyperhidrosis. External treatment by soaking the foot in herbal preparations combined with internal administration of Chinese materia medica or acupuncture and moxibustion treatment yields the best results.
- Since the lesions are thick and firm, patients should be encouraged to persist with the treatment for at least four to six weeks. At the end of the healing process, the skin will be smooth without scarring.

Advice for the patient

- Take measures to prevent hyperhidrosis of the foot, such as wearing socks and shoes of natural materials like cotton and leather.
- Avoid putting pressure on the plantar warts.

Case history

Patient
Female, aged 22.

Clinical manifestations
The patient had been suffering from plantar warts for two weeks; the warts affected her normal gait when walking.

Physical examination showed 12 warts, 2-3mm in size, on the sole of her left foot. The lesions were slightly raised and very painful.

Treatment principle
Soften hardness and dissipate lumps, invigorate the Blood and alleviate pain.

Prescription
CI BEI HE JI
Magnetite and Cowrie Shell Compound Preparation

Ci Shi‡ (Magnetitum) 30g
Zi Bei Chi‡ (Concha Mauritiae) 30g
Dai Zhe Shi‡ (Haematitum) 30g
Mu Li‡ (Concha Ostreae) 30g
Di Gu Pi (Cortex Lycii Radicis) 30g
Hong Hua (Flos Carthami Tinctorii) 6g
Tao Ren (Semen Persicae) 9g
Huai Niu Xi (Radix Achyranthis Bidentatae) 9g
Bai Shao (Radix Paeoniae Lactiflorae) 9g
Huang Bai (Cortex Phellodendri) 4g
Shan Ci Gu (Pseudobulbus Shancigu) 4g
Shi Jue Ming‡ (Concha Haliotidis) 15g
Chuan Shan Jia* (Squama Manitis Pentadactylae) 9g

Shi Jue Ming‡ (Concha Haliotidis) was added to treat the severe pain, *Chuan Shan Jia** (Squama Manitis Pentadactylae) to treat the hardness and thickness of the lesions. One bag a day was used to prepare a decoction, taken twice a day.

Outcome
After the patient finished two bags of the medication, the warts softened. After six bags, they came off and healed. [13]

Literature excerpt

In *Wai Ke Shu Yao* [Essentials of External Diseases], it says: "This disease is similar to the formation of nodules due to Blood-Dryness. External treatment with corrosive medications and internal treatment with ingredients that relieve Toxicity but also dry the Blood will result in the Essence and Blood becoming even more Deficient. At the same time, these ingredients may injure the sinews, which are governed by the Liver. As a result, the sores will rupture and the condition will deteriorate."

Modern clinical experience

INTERNAL TREATMENT
Guan adopted the treatment principle of invigorating the Blood and softening hardness. [14]

Prescription ingredients

Hong Hua (Flos Carthami Tinctorii) 9g
Tao Ren (Semen Persicae) 9g
Yu Jin (Radix Curcumae) 9g
Niu Xi (Radix Achyranthis Bidentatae) 9g

Chuan Shan Jia* (Squama Manitis Pentadactylae) 9g
Tou Gu Cao (Herba Speranskiae seu Impatientis) 12g
Zhen Zhu Mu‡ (Concha Margaritifera) 30g
Mu Li‡ (Concha Ostreae) 30g
Hai Ge Ke‡ (Concha Meretricis seu Cyclinae) 30g

One bag a day was used to prepare a decoction, taken twice a day. Results were seen after 10-14 days.

EXTERNAL TREATMENT

1. **Zhang et al** used a decoction as an external soak. [15]

Prescription ingredients

Xiang Fu (Rhizoma Cyperi Rotundi) 60g
Mu Zei (Herba Equiseti Hiemalis) 60g
Ban Lan Gen (Radix Isatidis seu Baphicacanthi) 30g
Wu Mei (Fructus Pruni Mume) 30g
Xi Xian Cao (Herba Siegesbeckiae) 30g

The ingredients were decocted and used to soak the affected area for 10-15 minutes two or three times a day.

2. **Cheng et al** also adopted external treatment with a soak. [16]

Prescription
RE JIN TUO YOU TANG
Warm Soak Decoction for Shedding Warts

Mu Zei (Herba Equiseti Hiemalis) 30g
Dan Shen (Radix Salviae Miltiorrhizae) 30g
Yi Yi Ren (Semen Coicis Lachryma-jobi) 30g
Ban Lan Gen (Radix Isatidis seu Baphicacanthi) 30g
Xiang Fu (Rhizoma Cyperi Rotundi) 20g
Chuan Xiong (Rhizoma Ligustici Chuanxiong) 20g
Hong Hua (Flos Carthami Tinctorii) 12g
Zi Cao (Radix Arnebiae seu Lithospermi) 15g

The ingredients were decocted and used to soak the affected area for 20-30 minutes twice a day.

Measles
麻疹

Measles is one of the four main children's exanthematous diseases; in Western countries, immunization programs have largely restricted outbreaks to isolated cases and epidemics are rare.

Measles is an acute infectious disease caused by the RNA virus passing through the respiratory tract. Symptoms include fever, coughing, nasal congestion or runny nose, aversion to light, watery eyes, macules on the mucous membranes inside the mouth (Koplik's spots), and red papules 1-2 mm in diameter on the face and spreading all over the body. Scaling and pigmentation may occur following disappearance of the eruption.

The incidence of measles is highest among children aged between six months and five years. Since measles antibodies can be transferred from the pregnant mother to the fetus, the newborn baby acquires passive immunity from its mother for the first three to four months after birth.

As the baby grows older, the level of measles antibodies in its body decreases gradually, disappearing at the age of six to eight months. Once exposed to infection, the child is susceptible to catching the disease.

Complete recovery is the normal outcome in rich countries but measles is a serious and often fatal disease in many poor countries.

Recurrence is very rare since lifelong immunity normally develops after the first infection.

Clinical manifestations

- Measles mostly occurs in children under the age of five years. It can be seen all year around, but it tends to be epidemic in winter and spring (in those instances where immunization does not reach required numbers in a population).
- The average incubation period is nine to eleven days.
- The prodromal phase generally lasts for four days and symptoms may include high fever, conjunctival congestion, aversion to light, increased discharge from the eyes, a runny nose with sticky and purulent discharge, coughing, and occasionally nausea, vomiting and diarrhea. Koplik's spots (small red spots with white centers, located on the inside of the mouth) may appear two to three days after onset of the disease; they begin to disappear as the maculopapular rash appears.
- Eruptive phase: Eruptions first appear behind the ears, along the hairline and on the face, and then spread rapidly to the neck, upper limbs, trunk, and

lower limbs. Eruptions are rose-colored maculo-papular lesions with blanching on pressure. The rash develops completely within two to five days. During the eruptive stage, the temperature can rise to 41°C and systemic symptoms can worsen. Lymph nodes in the neck, liver and spleen are enlarged.

- Recovery phase: Five to seven days after eruption of the measles rash, the temperature drops and eruptions gradually disappear, followed by dark brown pigmentation and scaling. The whole course of the disease lasts about two weeks.

- Although measles is not usually associated with complications in otherwise healthy children, morbidity and mortality rates in undernourished children or those already suffering from other diseases can be relatively high. The most common complications are febrile fits, chest infection, otitis media, meningitis, diarrhea and vomiting, and keratoconjunctivitis. In the immunosuppressed, there may be fatal giant cell pneumonitis. Intrauterine infection may cause spontaneous abortion or premature delivery. The most serious complication is the rare subacute sclerosing panencephalitis (headache, lassitude, fits, and cerebral damage) from which 15 percent die and 25 percent develop deafness or permanent brain damage.

Differential diagnosis

Table 9-1 details the main points of differential diagnosis between measles and other childhood diseases.

Etiology and pathology

Measles is a highly infectious febrile disease caused by seasonal epidemic Toxins and is Yang in nature. The Qi of the Zang organs in young children is not very strong, and their defense system is weak. A child's body is full of Yang Qi, which makes it susceptible to this kind of epidemic Toxin. After the onset of the disease, these two Yangs (the Yang nature of the disease and the Yang Qi of the child) will combine to affect the body; Heat ferments and transforms into Fire, leading to a range of warm-febrile disease symptoms.

Table 9-1 Differential diagnosis between measles and other childhood diseases

	Measles	Scarlet fever	Rubella	Roseola infantum
General symptoms	Prodromal phase generally lasts for four days with high fever, watery eyes, nasal discharge, and Koplik's spots; symptoms are relatively severe	Prodromal phase generally lasts for four days with severe general symptoms, swollen and enlarged tonsils, a red, sore and swollen throat, and a strawberry-colored tongue	Mild general symptoms, slightly red and swollen eyes, slight temperature and headache, sore and enlarged lymph nodes behind the ears	Sudden onset of high fever, but the temperature subsides after two to three days; general symptoms are mild
Sequence of skin eruptions	Eruptions first appear behind the ears, along the hairline and on the face, and then spread rapidly to the neck, upper limbs, trunk, and lower limbs within two to five days	Eruption is completely expressed within one day, spreading over the neck, trunk and limbs	Eruption is completely expressed within one day, spreading from the head and face to the trunk and limbs	Sequential distribution is from the neck to the face, trunk and limbs within 24 hours
Features of eruptions	Small or large rose-colored maculopapular eruptions, which may become confluent; scaling and pigmentation after disappearance of eruptions	Diffuse reddening of the skin, tiny raised papules in the skin creases, reddening blanches on pressure, extensive desquamation after disappearance of the eruption	Light red or pink macules or papules	Macular eruptions begin as the fever subsides; the small, pink macules remain discrete or become confluent without itching, scaling or pigmentation

Pattern identification and treatment

INTERNAL TREATMENT

FAVORABLE PATTERNS

INITIAL FEVER PHASE

This phase lasts from the onset of fever to the first appearance of skin eruptions, usually three to four days. Symptoms and signs include fever, aversion to wind, coughing, a runny nose, swollen throat and hoarse voice, red and swollen eyes, lacrimation, fatigue and generalized heaviness, reduced appetite, or nausea and vomiting and diarrhea. The tongue coating is thin and white or slightly yellow; the pulse is rapid and floating. The fever lasts for two to three days; Koplik's spots can be seen on the mucosa of the mouth.

Treatment principle

Release the exterior with coolness and acridity.

Prescription

SHENG MA GE GEN TANG HE YIN QIAO SAN JIA JIAN

Bugbane and Kudzu Vine Decoction Combined With Honeysuckle and Forsythia Powder, with modifications

Sheng Ma (Rhizoma Cimicifugae) 6g
Ge Gen (Radix Puerariae) 6g
Jing Jie Sui (Spica Schizonepetae Tenuifoliae) 6g
Dan Dou Chi (Semen Sojae Praeparatum) 6g
Chao Niu Bang Zi (Fructus Arctii Lappae, stir-fried) 10g
Lian Qiao (Fructus Forsythiae Suspensae) 10g
Dan Zhu Ye (Herba Lophatheri Gracilis) 10g
Jin Yin Hua (Flos Lonicerae) 15g
Lu Gen (Rhizoma Phragmitis Communis) 15g

Explanation

- *Sheng Ma* (Rhizoma Cimicifugae), *Ge Gen* (Radix Puerariae) and *Jing Jie Sui* (Spica Schizonepetae Tenuifoliae) release the exterior and vent papules.
- *Dan Dou Chi* (Semen Sojae Praeparatum), *Chao Niu Bang Zi* (Fructus Arctii Lappae, stir-fried), *Lian Qiao* (Fructus Forsythiae Suspensae), *Dan Zhu Ye* (Herba Lophatheri Gracilis), *Jin Yin Hua* (Flos Lonicerae), and *Lu Gen* (Rhizoma Phragmitis Communis) clear Heat and relieve Toxicity.

ERUPTIVE PHASE

This phase lasts from the first appearance of skin eruptions until they are fully expressed, usually three to four days. Symptoms include an increase in temperature, thirst with an increased intake of fluids, increased coughing, lassitude, sore limbs, red and slightly swollen eyes with profuse discharge and aversion to light, irritability and restlessness, somnolence, or possibly mental confusion and convulsions. Tiny, 1-2 mm diameter, rose-colored maculopapular eruptions that feel rough to the touch start to appear behind the ear, then gradually spread over the body. Initially, the eruptions are discrete and bright red, gradually becoming confluent, with the color changing to dark red. The tongue body is red with a yellow coating; the pulse is rapid and surging.

Treatment principle

Relieve Toxicity and vent papules, while clearing Heat from the Qi level.

Prescription

QING JIE TOU BIAO TANG JIA JIAN

Decoction for Clearing Heat, Relieving Toxicity and Venting the Exterior, with modifications

Xi He Liu (Cacumen Tamaricis) 6g
Chan Tui ‡ (Periostracum Cicadae) 6g
Sheng Ma (Rhizoma Cimicifugae) 6g
Ge Gen (Radix Puerariae) 6g
Chao Niu Bang Zi (Fructus Arctii Lappae, stir-fried) 6g
Jin Yin Hua (Flos Lonicerae) 15g
Zi Cao (Radix Arnebiae seu Lithospermi) 15g
Shi Gao ‡ (Gypsum Fibrosum) 15g, decocted for
  30 minutes before adding the other ingredients
Lian Qiao (Fructus Forsythiae Suspensae) 10g
Zhi Mu (Rhizoma Anemarrhenae Asphodeloidis) 10g
Gan Cao (Radix Glycyrrhizae) 10g

Explanation

- *Xi He Liu* (Cacumen Tamaricis), *Sheng Ma* (Rhizoma Cimicifugae), *Chan Tui* ‡ (Periostracum Cicadae), and *Ge Gen* (Radix Puerariae) release the exterior and vent papules.
- *Chao Niu Bang Zi* (Fructus Arctii Lappae, stir-fried) vents papules and relieves Toxicity.
- *Shi Gao* ‡ (Gypsum Fibrosum) and *Zhi Mu* (Rhizoma Anemarrhenae Asphodeloidis) clear Heat from the Qi level.
- *Jin Yin Hua* (Flos Lonicerae) and *Lian Qiao* (Fructus Forsythiae Suspensae) clear Heat, relieve Toxicity and cool the Blood.
- *Zi Cao* (Radix Arnebiae seu Lithospermi) and *Gan Cao* (Radix Glycyrrhizae) clear Heat and relieve Toxicity.

RECOVERY PHASE

This phase lasts from the full expression of the eruptions to their disappearance, usually three to four days. Eruptions start to disappear in order of their appearance. The temperature drops, coughing is reduced, the mind becomes clear and the appetite improves, although a slight thirst remains. The tongue body is red with a scant coating; the pulse is thready, rapid and forceless.

Treatment principle
Nourish Yin and clear Heat.

Prescription
ZHU YE SHI GAO TANG JIA JIAN
Lophatherum and Gypsum Decoction, with modifications

Dan Zhu Ye (Herba Lophatheri Gracilis) 6g
Gan Cao (Radix Glycyrrhizae) 6g
Shi Gao ‡ (Gypsum Fibrosum) 30g, decocted for
  30 minutes before adding the other ingredients
Tai Zi Shen (Radix Pseudostellariae Heterophyllae) 12g
Mai Men Dong (Radix Ophiopogonis Japonici) 12g
Jing Mi (Semen Oryzae) 12g
Tian Hua Fen (Radix Trichosanthis) 10g
Shan Yao (Rhizoma Dioscoreae Oppositae) 10g
Bai Wei (Radix Cynanchi Atrati) 10g

Explanation
- *Dan Zhu Ye* (Herba Lophatheri Gracilis), *Gan Cao* (Radix Glycyrrhizae), *Shi Gao* ‡ (Gypsum Fibrosum), *Bai Wei* (Radix Cynanchi Atrati), and *Tian Hua Fen* (Radix Trichosanthis) clear Heat.
- *Tai Zi Shen* (Radix Pseudostellariae Heterophyllae), *Mai Men Dong* (Radix Ophiopogonis Japonici), *Jing Mi* (Semen Oryzae), and *Shan Yao* (Rhizoma Dioscoreae Oppositae) supplement Qi and nourish Yin.

UNFAVORABLE PATTERNS

MEASLES TOXINS BLOCKING THE LUNGS

Symptoms and signs include persistent high fever, irritability and restlessness, wheezing and oppression in the chest, coughing and Phlegm rale, and incomplete eruption of dull-colored papules. The tongue body is crimson with a yellow and greasy coating; the pulse is rapid, floating, agitated, and racing.

Treatment principle
Clear Heat and relieve Toxicity, diffuse the Lungs and open blockage.

Prescription
MA XING SHI GAN TANG JIA JIAN
Ephedra, Apricot Kernel, Gypsum, and Licorice Decoction, with modifications

*Ma Huang** (Herba Ephedrae) 6g
Tao Ren (Semen Persicae) 6g
Zhi Ke (Fructus Citri Aurantii) 6g
Si Gua Luo (Fasciculus Vascularis Luffae) 6g
Xing Ren (Semen Pruni Armeniacae) 10g
Gan Cao (Radix Glycyrrhizae) 10g
Lian Qiao (Fructus Forsythiae Suspensae) 10g
Qian Hu (Radix Peucedani) 10g

Shi Gao ‡ (Gypsum Fibrosum) 30g, decocted for
  30 minutes before adding the other ingredients
Jin Yin Hua (Flos Lonicerae) 15g
Yu Xing Cao (Herba Houttuyniae Cordatae) 15g
Xian Lu Gen (Rhizoma Phragmitis Communis Recens) 20g

Explanation
- *Ma Huang** (Herba Ephedrae) and *Xing Ren* (Semen Pruni Armeniacae) diffuse the Lungs.
- *Lian Qiao* (Fructus Forsythiae Suspensae), *Jin Yin Hua* (Flos Lonicerae), *Shi Gao* ‡ (Gypsum Fibrosum), *Yu Xing Cao* (Herba Houttuyniae Cordatae), and *Xian Lu Gen* (Rhizoma Phragmitis Communis Recens) clear Heat and relieve Toxicity.
- *Tao Ren* (Semen Persicae) cools and invigorates the Blood.
- *Zhi Ke* (Fructus Citri Aurantii), *Si Gua Luo* (Fasciculus Vascularis Luffae) and *Qian Hu* (Radix Peucedani) transform Phlegm.
- *Gan Cao* (Radix Glycyrrhizae) harmonizes the effects of the other ingredients in the prescription.

MEASLES TOXINS ATTACKING THE HEART

Symptoms and signs include high fever, mental confusion, restlessness, nausea and vomiting, convulsions, and fainting due to emotional upsets. Lesions quickly disappear after erupting or fuse into dark purple patches. The lips and tongue are purple or crimson and the tongue has a dry, yellow coating; the pulse is thready and rapid.

Treatment principle
Clear Heat and relieve Toxicity, open the orifices and extinguish Wind.

Prescription
QING YING TANG JIA JIAN
Decoction for Clearing Heat from the Ying Level, with modifications

Shui Niu Jiao ‡ (Cornu Bubali) 30g
Sheng Di Huang (Radix Rehmanniae Glutinosae) 12g
Xuan Shen (Radix Scrophulariae Ningpoensis) 12g
Jin Yin Hua (Flos Lonicerae) 12g
Lian Qiao (Fructus Forsythiae Suspensae) 12g
Mai Men Dong (Radix Ophiopogonis Japonici) 10g
Dan Shen (Radix Salviae Miltiorrhizae) 10g
Huang Lian (Rhizoma Coptidis) 6g
Dan Zhu Ye (Herba Lophatheri Gracilis) 6g

Explanation
- *Shui Niu Jiao* ‡ (Cornu Bubali) cools the Blood and clears Heat.
- *Jin Yin Hua* (Flos Lonicerae), *Lian Qiao* (Fructus Forsythiae Suspensae), *Huang Lian* (Rhizoma Coptidis),

and *Dan Zhu Ye* (Herba Lophatheri Gracilis) clear Heat and relieve Toxicity.

- *Sheng Di Huang* (Radix Rehmanniae Glutinosae), *Xuan Shen* (Radix Scrophulariae Ningpoensis) and *Mai Men Dong* (Radix Ophiopogonis Japonici) enrich Yin and clear Heat.

- *Dan Shen* (Radix Salviae Miltiorrhizae) invigorates the Blood.

MEASLES TOXINS ATTACKING THE THROAT

Symptoms and signs include a sore and swollen throat, difficulty in swallowing, a hoarse voice, possibly with breathing difficulties, wheezing and Phlegm rale, hic-coughing after drinking, a grayish-green facial complexion, irritability, restlessness and disquiet, dull purple lips and tongue, a yellow tongue coating, and a rapid pulse.

Treatment principle
Clear Heat and relieve Toxicity, benefit the throat and disperse swelling.

Prescription
QING YAN XIA TAN TANG JIA JIAN
Decoction for Clearing the Throat and Causing Phlegm to Descend, with modifications

Xuan Shen (Radix Scrophulariae Ningpoensis) 10-12g
Jie Geng (Radix Platycodi Grandiflori) 10-12g
Chao Niu Bang Zi (Fructus Arctii Lappae, stir-fried) 10-12g
Zhe Bei Mu (Bulbus Fritillariae Thunbergii) 10-12g
Gua Lou (Fructus Trichosanthis) 10-12g
She Gan (Rhizoma Belamcandae Chinensis) 6g
Jing Jie (Herba Schizonepetae Tenuifoliae) 6g
Shan Dou Gen (Radix Sophorae Tonkinensis) 10g
Lian Qiao (Fructus Forsythiae Suspensae) 10g

Explanation
- *Xuan Shen* (Radix Scrophulariae Ningpoensis) clears Heat and cools the Blood.
- *Jie Geng* (Radix Platycodi Grandiflori), *Chao Niu Bang Zi* (Fructus Arctii Lappae, stir-fried), *She Gan* (Rhizoma Belamcandae Chinensis), *Shan Dou Gen* (Radix Sophorae Tonkinensis), and *Lian Qiao* (Fructus Forsythiae Suspensae) clear Heat, relieve Toxicity and benefit the throat.
- *Jing Jie* (Herba Schizonepetae Tenuifoliae) vents papules.
- *Zhe Bei Mu* (Bulbus Fritillariae Thunbergii) and *Gua Lou* (Fructus Trichosanthis) clear Heat and transform Phlegm.

COMPLICATIONS FOLLOWING MEASLES

TIDAL FEVER
Symptoms and signs include continuous low-grade fever that worsens in the evening, emaciation, dry mouth and throat, night sweating, and palpitations. The tongue body is red with a scant coating; the pulse is thready and rapid.

Treatment principle
Nourish Yin and vent Heat.

Prescription
QING HAO BIE JIA TANG JIA JIAN
Sweet Wormwood and Turtle Shell Decoction, with modifications

*Bie Jia** (Carapax Amydae Sinensis) 12g, decocted for 30 minutes before adding the other ingredients
Qing Hao (Herba Artemisiae Chinghao) 6g
Yin Chai Hu (Radix Stellariae Dichotomae) 6g
Bai Wei (Radix Cynanchi Atrati) 10g
Zhi Mu (Rhizoma Anemarrhenae Asphodeloidis) 10g
Huang Bai (Cortex Phellodendri) 10g
Chi Shao (Radix Paeoniae Rubra) 10g
Sheng Di Huang (Radix Rehmanniae Glutinosae) 10g
Mu Dan Pi (Cortex Moutan Radicis) 10g

Explanation
- *Bie Jia** (Carapax Amydae Sinensis), *Zhi Mu* (Rhizoma Anemarrhenae Asphodeloidis) and *Sheng Di Huang* (Radix Rehmanniae Glutinosae) nourish Yin and clear Heat.
- *Qing Hao* (Herba Artemisiae Chinghao), *Yin Chai Hu* (Radix Stellariae Dichotomae), *Bai Wei* (Radix Cynanchi Atrati), *Chi Shao* (Radix Paeoniae Rubra), *Huang Bai* (Cortex Phellodendri), and *Mu Dan Pi* (Cortex Moutan Radicis) clear Deficiency-Heat.

Note: Where *Bie Jia** (Carapax Amydae Sinensis) is not available as a result of its endangered species status, it can be replaced in this prescription by *Hu Huang Lian* (Rhizoma Picrorhizae Scrophulariiflorae)

DIARRHEA OR DYSENTERY
Symptoms and signs include intermittent abdominal pain, diarrhea with pus and blood, and abdominal urgency and tenesmus. The tongue body is red with a yellow and greasy coating; the pulse is rapid and soggy.

Treatment principle
Harmonize the Middle Burner, relieve Toxicity, clear the Intestines, and stop diarrhea.

Prescription
GE GEN QIN LIAN TANG HE MU XIANG BING LANG WAN JIA JIAN
Kudzu, Scutellaria and Coptis Decoction Combined With Aucklandia and Areca Pill, with modifications

Ge Gen (Radix Puerariae) 10g
Huang Qin (Radix Scutellariae Baicalensis) 10g
Huang Lian (Rhizoma Coptidis) 10g
Bai Shao (Radix Paeoniae Lactiflorae) 10g
Bai Tou Weng (Radix Pulsatillae Chinensis) 10g
Mu Xiang* (Radix Aucklandiae Lappae) 6g
Bing Lang* (Semen Arecae Catechu) 6g
Chen Pi (Pericarpium Citri Reticulatae) 3g
Gan Cao (Radix Glycyrrhizae) 3g

Explanation
- *Ge Gen* (Radix Puerariae), the sovereign herb of the prescription, releases flesh, vents eruptions and reduces fever, thus releasing the exterior, and bears clear Yang upward to stop diarrhea, thus harmonizing the interior.
- *Huang Qin* (Radix Scutellariae Baicalensis), *Huang Lian* (Rhizoma Coptidis) and *Bai Tou Weng* (Radix Pulsatillae Chinensis) clear Heat and dry Dampness in the Stomach and Large Intestine with cold and bitterness.
- *Mu Xiang** (Radix Aucklandiae Lappae), *Bing Lang** (Semen Arecae Catechu) and *Bai Shao* (Radix Paeoniae Lactiflorae) regulate Qi and move the Blood, and guide out stagnation to alleviate pain.
- *Chen Pi* (Pericarpium Citri Reticulatae) regulates Qi and loosens the Intestines.
- *Gan Cao* (Radix Glycyrrhizae) harmonizes the Middle Burner, and regulates and harmonizes the actions of the other herbs in the prescription.

SUPPURATIVE INFLAMMATION OF THE CHEEK
Symptoms and signs include severe swelling of the cheeks with scorching heat and pain on contact, and difficulty in opening the mouth and chewing, possibly accompanied by purulent discharge. The tongue body is red with a yellow coating; the pulse is rapid.

Treatment principle
Clear Heat and relieve Toxicity, reduce swelling and alleviate pain.

Prescription
PU JI XIAO DU YIN JIA JIAN
Universal Salvation Beverage for Dispersing Toxicity, with modifications

Huang Qin (Radix Scutellariae Baicalensis) 9g
Huang Lian (Rhizoma Coptidis) 9g
Xuan Shen (Radix Scrophulariae Ningpoensis) 9g
Jin Yin Hua (Flos Lonicerae) 9g
Lian Qiao (Fructus Forsythiae Suspensae) 9g
Ma Bo (Sclerotium Lasiosphaerae seu Calvatiae) 9g
Niu Bang Zi (Fructus Arctii Lappae) 9g
Ban Lan Gen (Radix Isatidis seu Baphicacanthi) 15g
Chai Hu (Radix Bupleuri) 6g
Gan Cao (Radix Glycyrrhizae) 3g

Explanation
- *Huang Qin* (Radix Scutellariae Baicalensis), *Huang Lian* (Rhizoma Coptidis), *Xuan Shen* (Radix Scrophulariae Ningpoensis), *Jin Yin Hua* (Flos Lonicerae), *Lian Qiao* (Fructus Forsythiae Suspensae), *Ban Lan Gen* (Radix Isatidis seu Baphicacanthi), *Gan Cao* (Radix Glycyrrhizae), and *Ma Bo* (Sclerotium Lasiosphaerae seu Calvatiae) clear Heat and relieve Toxicity.
- *Gan Cao* (Radix Glycyrrhizae) and *Ma Bo* (Sclerotium Lasiosphaerae seu Calvatiae) also alleviate pain.
- *Niu Bang Zi* (Fructus Arctii Lappae) reduces swelling.
- *Chai Hu* (Radix Bupleuri) abates fever.

MOUTH GAN
Symptoms and signs include mouth sores, erosion of the mucous membrane of the mouth, swollen and bleeding gums, bad breath, and constipation. The tongue body is red with a yellow and greasy coating; the pulse is slippery and rapid.

Treatment principle
Clear Heat and relieve Toxicity, harmonize the Blood and reduce swelling.

Prescription
QING WEN BAI DU YIN JIA JIAN
Beverage for Clearing Scourge and Vanquishing Toxicity, with modifications

Shi Gao‡ (Gypsum Fibrosum) 20g, decocted for 30 minutes before adding the other ingredients
Sheng Di Huang (Radix Rehmanniae Glutinosae) 9g
Zhi Zi (Fructus Gardeniae Jasminoidis) 9g
Huang Qin (Radix Scutellariae Baicalensis) 9g
Mu Dan Pi (Cortex Moutan Radicis) 9g
Xuan Shen (Radix Scrophulariae Ningpoensis) 9g
Lian Qiao (Fructus Forsythiae Suspensae) 9g
Dan Zhu Ye (Herba Lophatheri Gracilis) 6g
Da Huang (Radix et Rhizoma Rhei) 6g, added 10 minutes before the end of the decoction process

In addition, apply *Bing Huang San* (Borneol, Cat-Tail Pollen and Phellodendron Powder) to the affected area as an insufflation.

Explanation
- *Huang Qin* (Radix Scutellariae Baicalensis), *Xuan Shen*

(Radix Scrophulariae Ningpoensis), *Lian Qiao* (Fructus Forsythiae Suspensae), and *Dan Zhu Ye* (Herba Lophatheri Gracilis) clear Heat and relieve Toxicity.

- *Shi Gao*‡ (Gypsum Fibrosum) clears Heat and reduces swelling.

- *Sheng Di Huang* (Radix Rehmanniae Glutinosae) and *Mu Dan Pi* (Cortex Moutan Radicis) clear Heat and harmonize the Blood.

- *Zhi Zi* (Fructus Gardeniae Jasminoidis), *Xuan Shen* (Radix Scrophulariae Ningpoensis) and *Da Huang* (Radix et Rhizoma Rhei) harmonize the Blood and reduce swelling.

General modifications

1. For persistent high fever, add *Chan Tui*‡ (Periostracum Cicadae), *Jiang Can*‡ (Bombyx Batryticatus) and *Lu Gen* (Rhizoma Phragmitis Communis).
2. For high fever with convulsions, add *Gou Teng* (Ramulus Uncariae cum Uncis), *Ling Yang Jiao** (Cornu Antelopis), *Di Long*‡ (Lumbricus), and *Quan Xie*‡ (Buthus Martensi).
3. For a red, sore and swollen throat, add *She Gan* (Rhizoma Belamcandae Chinensis) and *Ban Lan Gen* (Radix Isatidis seu Baphicacanthi).
4. For nausea and vomiting, add *Zi Su Ye* (Folium Perillae Frutescentis), *Zhu Ru* (Caulis Bambusae in Taeniis) and *Fa Ban Xia* (Rhizoma Pinelliae Ternatae Praeparata).
5. For severe cough, add *Qian Hu* (Radix Peucedani) and *Xing Ren* (Semen Pruni Armeniacae).
6. For cough with sticky phlegm, add *Chuan Bei Mu* (Bulbus Fritillariae Cirrhosae) and *Sang Bai Pi* (Cortex Mori Albae Radicis).
7. For cough with scant phlegm, add *Sha Shen* (Radix Glehniae seu Adenophorae) and *Ju Luo* (Retinervus Fructus Citri Reticulatae).
8. For dull purple eruptions, add *Dan Shen* (Radix Salviae Miltiorrhizae) and *Hong Hua* (Flos Carthami Tinctorii).
9. For eruptions forming dull purple patches, add *Sheng Di Huang* (Radix Rehmanniae Glutinosae), *Mu Dan Pi* (Cortex Moutan Radicis), *Chi Shao* (Radix Paeoniae Rubra), and *Zi Cao* (Radix Arnebiae seu Lithospermi).
10. For persistent low-grade fever, add *Di Gu Pi* (Cortex Lycii Radicis) and *Yin Chai Hu* (Radix Stellariae Dichotomae).
11. For reduced appetite, add *Huo Xiang* (Herba Agastaches seu Pogostemi), *Mai Ya* (Fructus Hordei Vulgaris Germinatus) and *Shen Qu* (Massa Fermentata).
12. For constipation, add *Da Huang* (Radix et Rhizoma Rhei).
13. For wheezing with profuse phlegm, add *Tian Zhu Huang* (Concretio Silicea Bambusae) and *Xian Zhu Li* (Succus Bambusae Recens).
14. For non-eruption of papules, add *Fu Ping* (Herba Spirodelae Polyrrhizae) and *Chan Tui*‡ (Periostracum Cicadae).
15. For mental confusion and restlessness, add *Shui Niu Jiao*‡ (Cornu Bubali), *Mu Dan Pi* (Cortex Moutan Radicis) and *Sheng Di Huang* (Radix Rehmanniae Glutinosae).

EXTERNAL TREATMENT

Initial fever phase

- Decoct *Zi Su Ye* (Folium Perillae Frutescentis) 30g, *Fu Ping* (Herba Spirodelae Polyrrhizae) 30g and *Xi He Liu* (Cacumen Tamaricis) 15g in 600ml of water. Use the medicated liquid to steam-wash the body for 15-20 minutes, two or three times a day for one or two days.

- Add 15-30g of one or two of the following herbs – *Ma Huang** (Herba Ephedrae), *Fu Ping* (Herba Spirodelae Polyrrhizae), *Xi He Liu* (Cacumen Tamaricis), or *Xiang Cai* (Herba cum Radice Coriandri) – to 60ml of *Huang Jiu* (Vinum Aureum). Decoct in 300ml of water and use for fuming and steaming; alternatively, dip a towel in the liquid and rub the face, trunk and limbs.

Eruptive phase

- Decoct 90-150g of fresh *Zhu Ma Gen* (Radix Boehmeriae Niveae) in water and use warm to wash the body. Rub the skin dry and cover with a quilt, allowing the patient to sweat slightly. This method can also help to vent papules.

- Add *Nen Liu Zhi* (Ramulus Tener Salicis) 250g, *Xing Xing Cao* (Herba Eragrosti) 120g and *Chan Tui*‡ (Periostracum Cicadae) 60g to 6 liters of water and boil for 15 minutes. Cool to a comfortable temperature and use it to wash the body until slight sweating is induced. Treat once a day for two or three days. Keep the patient out of draughts at all times. This treatment is indicated for severe cases of measles in children where eruptions are dense, dark red and incompletely expressed.

ACUPUNCTURE

Main points: BL-13 Feishu, DU-14 Dazhui and LI-11 Quchi.

Auxiliary points

- In the initial fever stage, add LU-7 Lieque and LI-4 Hegu.

- In the eruptive phase, add LI-4 Hegu, LU-5 Chize and ST-36 Zusanli.

Technique: Insert obliquely downward to a depth of 0.3-0.5 cun at BL-13 Feishu; insert obliquely against the channel to a depth of 0.5-0.8 cun at LU-7 Lieque; perpendicular insertion at the other points. Apply the reducing method and retain the needles for 15-20 minutes; manipulate the needles every five minutes.

Explanation

- BL-13 Feishu, DU-14 Dazhui and LI-11 Quchi clear Heat from the Lungs and dredge Wind.
- LU-7 Lieque and LI-4 Hegu clear Heat and expel Wind.
- LI-4 Hegu, LU-5 Chize and ST-36 Zusanli fortify the Spleen, nourish the Blood and dredge Wind.

FOLK REMEDIES

- *Xiao Du San* (Powder for Dispersing Toxicity): Grind 30g each of *Di Long* ‡ (Lumbricus) and *Fang Feng* (Radix Ledebouriellae Divaricatae) into a fine powder and take 10g orally with 15ml each of rice wine and water (the proportion of water can be increased for young children). This treatment is indicated for non-eruption of measles.
- *Chan Tui Yi Wu San* (Cicada Slough Powder): Grind 30g of *Chan Tui* ‡ (Periostracum Cicadae) into a powder. Decoct 10g in water over a low heat, drain and drink warm. This decoction is indicated in the initial fever and eruptive phases to clear Heat and vent papules.
- Boil 30-60g of fresh pomelo leaves and use as a wash to facilitate eruption of the rash.
- Decoct *Xi He Liu* (Cacumen Tamaricis) 15g and *Fu Ping* (Herba Spirodelae Polyrrhizae) 10g and drink. This remedy is indicated for the initial fever stage, as it can facilitate eruption of the rash.
- Decoct *Zi Cao* (Radix Arnebiae seu Lithospermi) 10g, *Jin Yin Hua* (Flos Lonicerae) 15g and *Gan Cao* (Radix Glycyrrhizae) 6g and drink. This remedy has a preventive function for the disease and also reduces Toxicity.

Clinical notes

- During outbreaks of measles, children who have not previously contracted the disease or been vaccinated against it are at risk from infection. A child who has contracted measles should be isolated until no longer contagious.
- Make sure the bedroom is quiet, warm, well ventilated, and not too bright. The sick child should be kept out of draughts and direct sunlight, and fluctuations in temperature should be avoided.
- The child should be fed on a nourishing and light fluid or semi-fluid diet. Pungent, spicy, fatty, and greasy foods should be completely avoided.
- In addition, particular attention should be paid to oral, nasal and eye hygiene in order to prevent secondary infections.
- The seriousness of the possible complications of measles should not be minimized. In children who develop unfavorable patterns, TCM treatment should be combined with Western medicine to avoid fatal complications.

Literature excerpts

In *Ma Zhen Ji Cheng* [Collected Abstracts on Measles], it says: "Papules are caused by Heat accumulating in the Lungs and Stomach. Treatment should concentrate on clearing pathogenic Heat from these two channels. Once Heat has been cleared, the symptoms will disappear."

In *Dou Zhen Xin Fa* [Experiences in Treating Pox and Papules], it says: "Since measles involves Fire, its treatment is different from that of chickenpox in that herbs for chickenpox can be warm or cool, whereas only herbs for clearing Heat and relieving Toxicity are used in the treatment of measles.

"*Jing Fang Bai Du San* (Schizonepeta and Ledebouriella Powder for Vanquishing Toxicity), *Hua Ban Tang* (Decoction for Transforming Macules) and *Liang Ge San* (Powder for Cooling the Diaphragm) are three treasured formulae for measles.

"If papules are still not visible after six or seven days of fever, this indicates latent measles due to a thick skin and blocked interstices (*cou li*), or to attack by Wind-Cold, or to a history of vomiting and diarrhea. It should be treated urgently with formulae for drawing Toxins from the interior and releasing the exterior. Use *Ma Huang Tang* (Ephedra Decoction); remove *Xing Ren* (Semen Pruni Armeniacae), and add *Chan Tui* ‡ (Periostracum Cicadae) and *Sheng Ma* (Rhizoma Cimicifugae)."

References

1. Chen Xiuqian, *Tou Zhen Zhi Liao Dai Zhuang Pao Zhen Hou Yi Liu Shen Jing Tong 37 Li* [Scalp Acupuncture in the Treatment of 37 Cases of Post-Herpetic Neuralgia], *Zhong Guo Pi Fu Xing Bing Xue Za Zhi* [Chinese Journal of Dermatology and Venereology] 10, 1 (1996): 50.
2. Zhang Hao, *Zi Cao You Wai Tu Zhi Liao Dai Zhuang Pao*

Zhen 26 Li [External Application of *Zi Cao You* (Gromwell Root Oil) in the Treatment of 26 Cases of Herpes Zoster], *Zhong Yi Wai Zhi Za Zhi* [Journal of Traditional Chinese Medicine External Treatments] 5, 2 (1996): 18.

3. Guo Gang, *Liu Shen Wan Zhi Liao Xun Chang You He Bian Ping You* [*Liu Shen Wan* (Six Spirits Pill) in the Treatment of Common Warts and Plane Warts], *Bei Jing Zhong Yi Yao Da Xue Xue Bao* [Journal of Beijing University of Traditional Chinese Medicine] 18, 4 (1995): 48.

4. Qi Ying, *Ai Tiao Yan Xun Fa Zhi Liao Xun Chang You* [Treatment of Common Warts by Fumigation with a Moxa Stick], *He Nan Zhong Yi* [Henan Journal of Traditional Chinese Medicine] 19, 4 (1999): 59.

5. Cao Shanbin, *Zi Ni Qing You Tang Zhi Liao Bian Ping You 32 Li Liao Xiao Guan Cha* [Observation of the Effectiveness of the Empirical Prescription *Qing You Tang* (Decoction for Clearing Warts) in the Treatment of 32 Cases of Plane Warts], *Pi Fu Xing Bing Xue Za Zhi* [Journal of Dermatology and Venereology] 4, 2 (1998): 32.

6. Wu Ziqin, *Fu Fang Ma Chi Xian Chong Ji Zhi Liao Bian Ping You 113 Li Lin Chuang Guan Cha* [Clinical Observation of *Fu Fang Ma Chi Xian Chong Ji* (Purslane Compound Soluble Granules) in the Treatment of 113 Cases of Plane Warts], *Xin Zhong Yi* [New Journal of Traditional Chinese Medicine] 31, 5 (1999): 46.

7. Qin Xiaojuan, *Qu You Fang Zhi Liao Bian Ping You 65 Li* [Treatment of 65 Cases of Plane Warts with *Qu You Fang* (Formula for Eliminating Warts)], *Hei Long Jiang Zhong Yi Yao* [Heilongjiang Journal of Traditional Chinese Medicine and Materia Medica] 3 (1996): 16.

8. Hong Shide, *Yin Lan Tao You Tang Zhi Liao Bian Ping You 68 Li* [Treatment of 68 Cases of Plane Warts with *Yin Lan Tao You Tang* (Honeysuckle, Isatis Root and Peach Kernel Decoction for Treating Warts)], *Yun Nan Zhong Yi Xue Yuan Xue Bao* [Journal of Yunnan College of Traditional Chinese Medicine] 21, 1 (1998): 51.

9. Chen Guoqin, *Huo Xue Jie Du Tang Zhi Liao Bian Ping You 153 Li* [Treatment of 153 Cases of Plane Warts with *Huo Xue Jie Du Tang* (Decoction for Invigorating the Blood and Relieving Toxicity)], *Hu Bei Zhong Yi Za Zhi* [Hubei Journal of Traditional Chinese Medicine] 21, 3 (1999): 104.

10. Meng Li, *Bian Ping You De Fen Xing Lun Zhi* [Treatments for Plane Warts Classified According to Patterns], *He Nan Zhong Yi* [Henan Journal of Traditional Chinese Medicine] 18, 2 (1998): 40.

11. Zhang Yuankui, *Zhong Yi Yao Zhi Liao Bian Ping You 60 Li* [Treatment of 60 Cases of Plane Warts with Traditional Chinese Medicine], *Shi Yong Zhong Xi Yi Jie He Za Zhi* [Practical Journal of Integrated TCM and Western Medicine] 11, 5 (1998): 434.

12. Tian Qingle, *Bian Ping You De Zhong Yao Wai Zhi Jin Kuang* [Recent External Treatments for Plane Warts Using Chinese Materia Medica], *Zhong Yi Wai Zhi Za Zhi* [Journal of Traditional Chinese Medicine External Treatments] 7, 4 (1998): 22-23.

13. Cheng Yunqian, *Zhong Yi Pi Fu Bing Xue Jian Bian* [Dermatology in Traditional Chinese Medicine: Concise Edition] (Xi'an: Shaanxi People's Publishing House, 1979), 85.

14. Guan Fen, *Shi Yong Zhong Yi Pi Fu Bing Xue* [Practical Dermatology in Traditional Chinese Medicine] (Lanzhou: Gansu People's Publishing House, 1981), 71.

15. Zhang Manhua et al., *Zhong Yi Pi Fu Bing Xue Jing Hua* [Essentials of Dermatology in Traditional Chinese Medicine] (Guangzhou: Guangdong Higher Education Publishing House, 1988), 125.

16. Cheng Qiusheng et al, *Pi Fu Bing Zhong Yi Jin Zi Liao Fa* [Soaks in the Treatment of Skin Diseases with Traditional Chinese Medicine] (Xi'an: Northwest University Publishing House, 1993), 95.

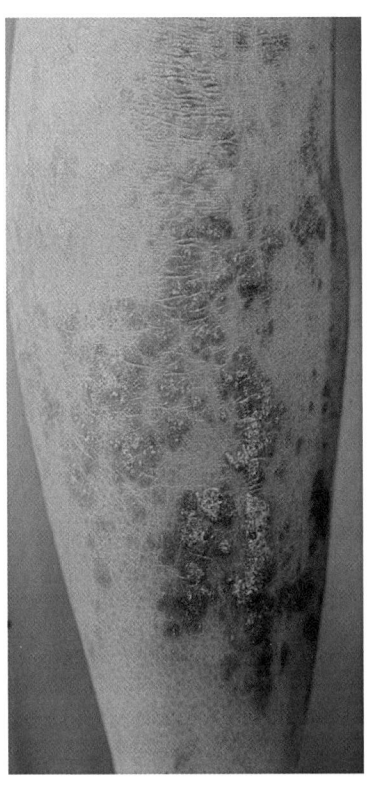

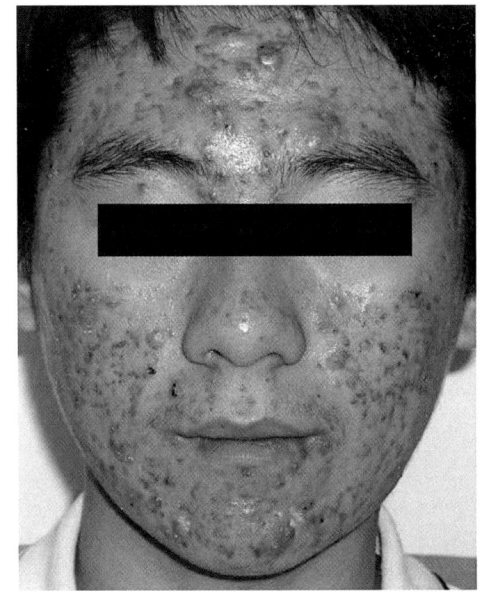

Figure 11 Erythema multiforme
Bullous and target lesions involving the hands. The scattered or clustered lesions are usually numerous.

Figure 10 Lichen planus
Intensely pruritic flat-topped shiny papules with an irregular, sharply-defined angulated border have evolved from their initial pink color to purplish-red. Lesions that persist may develop into confluent hypertrophic plaques. Mucous membranes are involved in many cases.

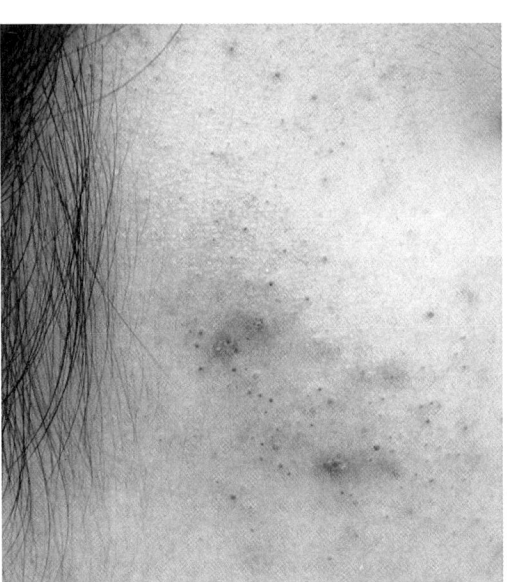

Figures 12, 13 Acne
Acne is common among adolescents and young adults, with lesions generally appearing on the face, chest and back. At the initial stage, lesions may manifest as open comedones or blackheads (left), caused by keratin and sebum plugging the pilosebaceous orifice, or closed comedones or whiteheads, small white or grayish papules caused by occlusion of the follicle opening. As the disease develops, lesions may evolve into inflammatory papules or pustules (right).

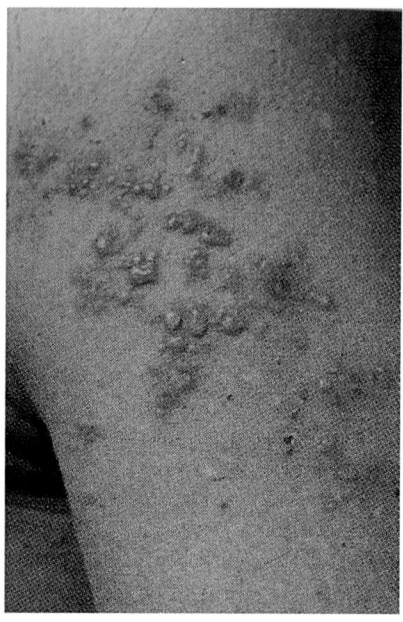

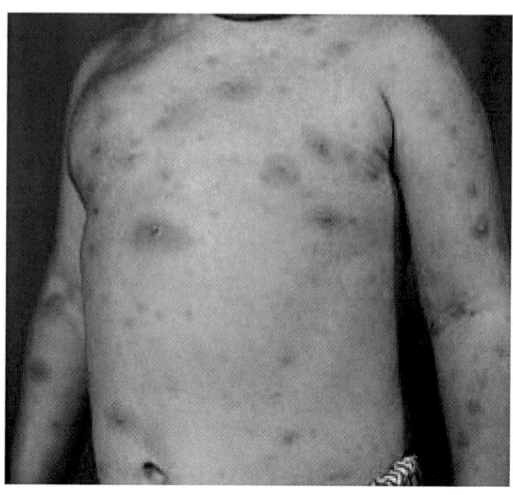

Figure 15 Varicella (chickenpox)
Skin eruptions begin on the trunk and spread to the face, scalp and limbs. Eruptions occur in successive crops passing through the stages of macule, papule, vesicle, and pustule. Vesicles typically vary in size from 1mm to 5mm and are surrounded by a red halo.

Figure 14 Dermatitis herpetiformis
Clusters of small, round, tense vesicles appear on an erythematous base. The fluid in the vesicles is clear initially, but turns turbid later. Itching and burning are intense, with the result that vesicles are often broken by scratching to leave excoriations.

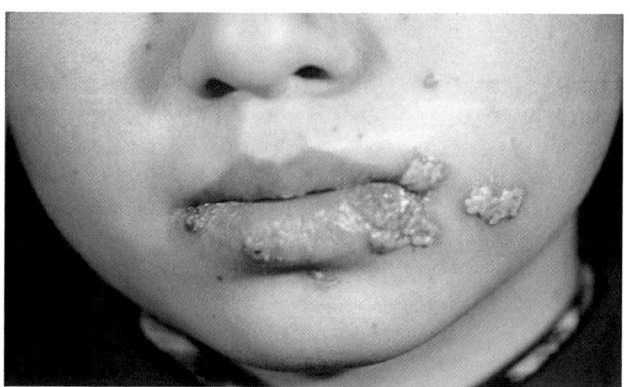

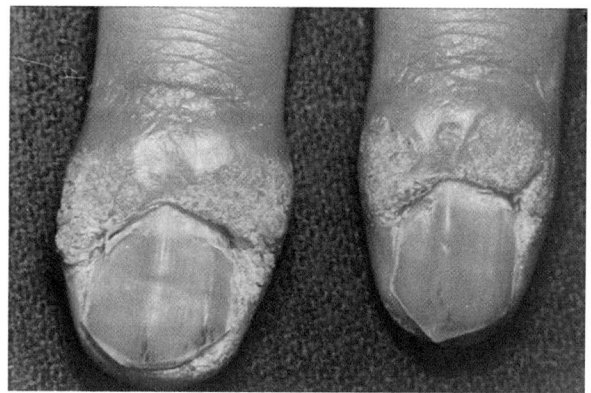

Figure 16 Herpes simplex
Grouped papulovesicles and vesicles have arisen on an erythematous base; some of the fluid filling the vesicles has become yellow and turbid.

Figure 17 Common warts (verruca vulgaris)
Common warts growing in a typical location, on the fingers and periungual region. Warts are likely to bleed when rubbed or knocked.

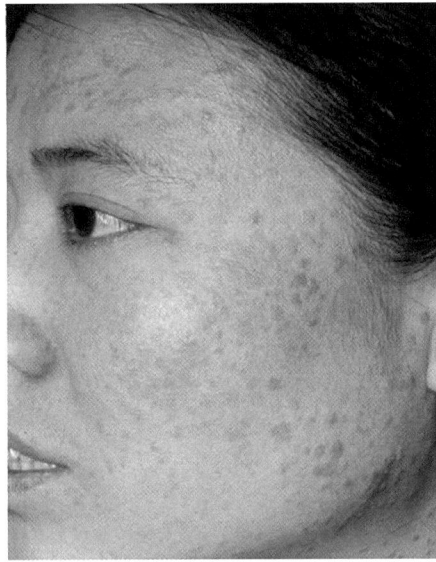

Figure 18 Plane warts (verruca plana)
Plane warts often involve the face; smooth, flat-topped and skin-colored or light brown, they can become prolific and widespread. Although some warts may last for years, spontaneous disappearance is possible.

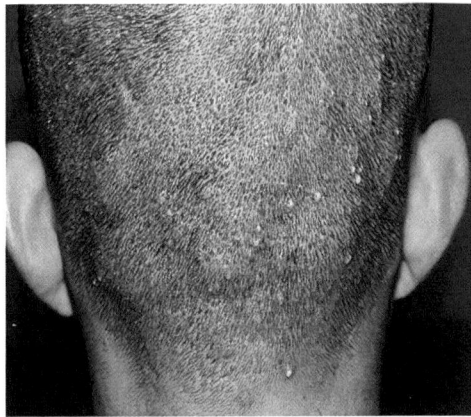

Figure 19 Folliculitis
Multiple papules and pustules manifesting on the scalp; folliculitis can affect any hair-bearing area of the body.

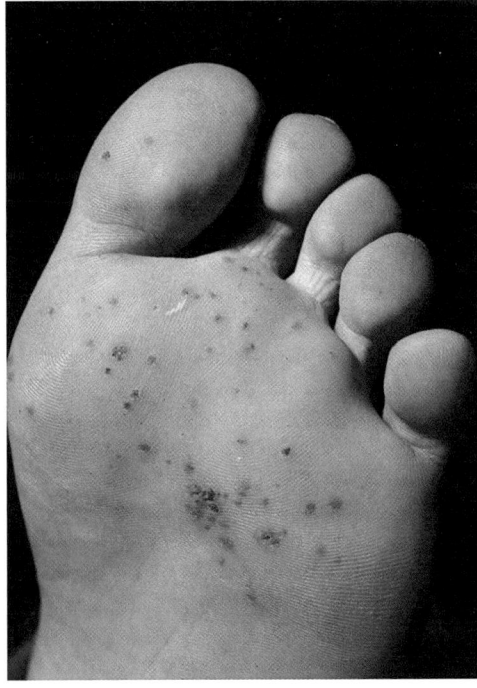

Figure 20 Plantar warts (verruca plantaris)
Often distributed over pressure areas of the sole, plantar warts present as keratinized, firm, callus-like maculopapules, sometimes up to 1 cm in diameter.

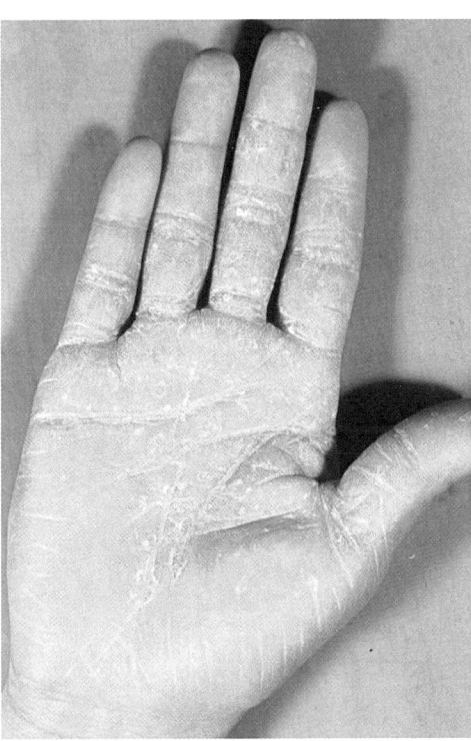

Figure 21 Tinea manuum
Small transparent pinpoint vesicles have dried up to be covered with layers of white scale. The skin on the palm has become dry, rough and thick with fissuring along creases. Tinea manuum is usually asymmetrical and is frequently seen in association with tinea pedis.

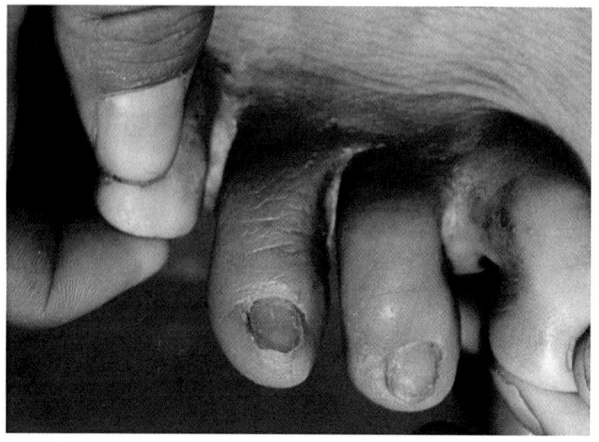

Figure 22 Tinea pedis
In interdigital tinea pedis, small vesicles appear between the toes. Repeated rubbing causes white, macerated skin. Pruritus is likely.

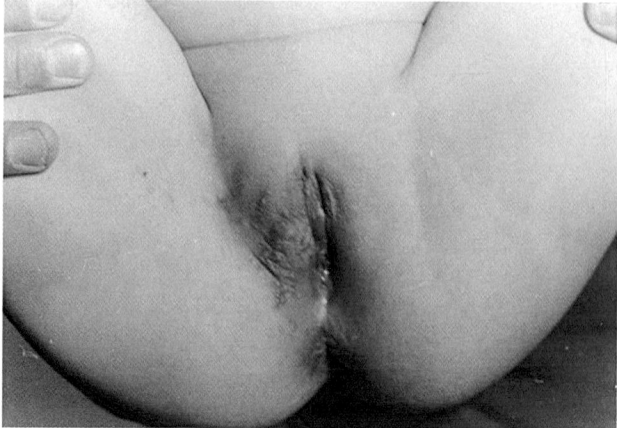

Figure 23 Vulval pruritus
A dry, thickened vulva due to repeated scratching is usually found on examination.

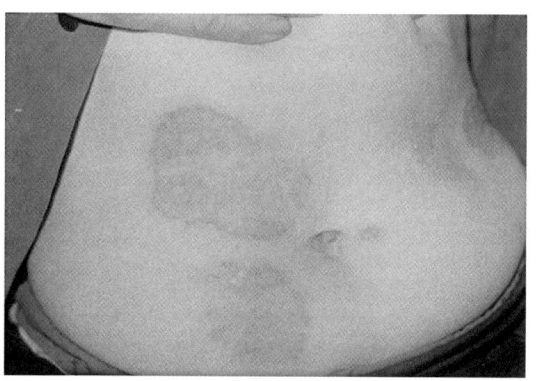

Figure 24 Tinea corporis (ringworm of the body)
Classic tinea lesions on the lower abdomen, forming sharply circumscribed circular patches. Central healing and elevated borders are also typical of ringworm.

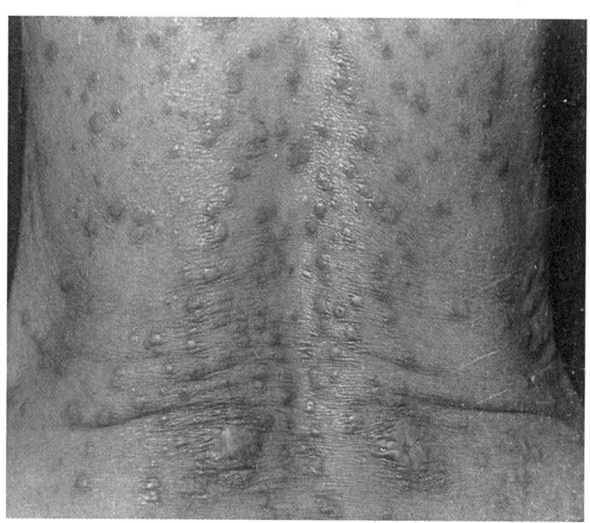

Figure 25 Nodular prurigo
Sites of predilection for this chronic condition include the upper and lower limbs and the back. The rough hemispherical nodules, produced by repeated scratching or rubbing, are firm on palpation.

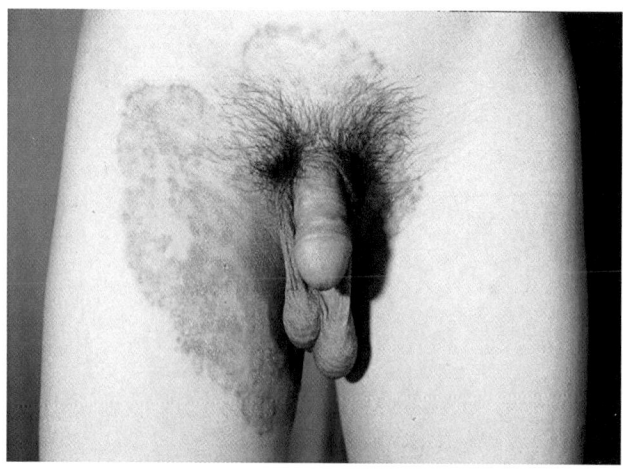

Figure 26 Tinea cruris (jock itch)
The lesion initially appears as a red scaly patch with a narrow, elevated, well-defined border; the patch spreads gradually from the crural fold to the thigh and buttocks. Later, small vesicles or pustules may form at the border of the lesion, while the center heals, sometimes with temporary pigmentation. There is often intolerable local itching.

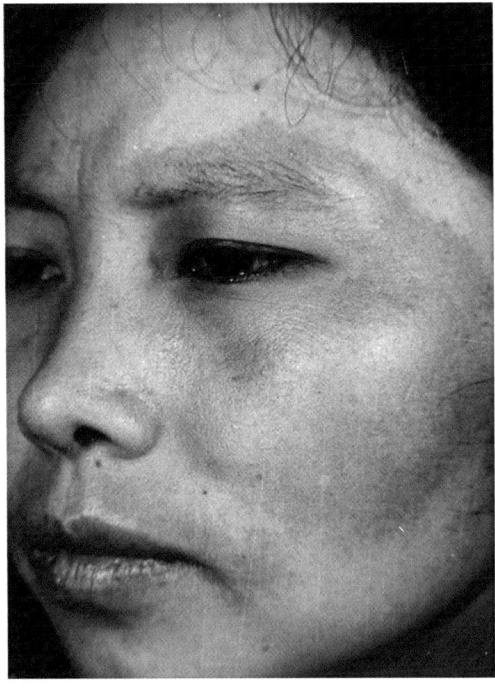

Figure 27 Melasma (chloasma)
Dark brown hyperpigmented patches mainly involve the forehead, the cheeks, the perioral and perinasal areas, and the chin. Pregnant women in the second and third trimesters and women taking oral contraceptives are most likely to be affected.

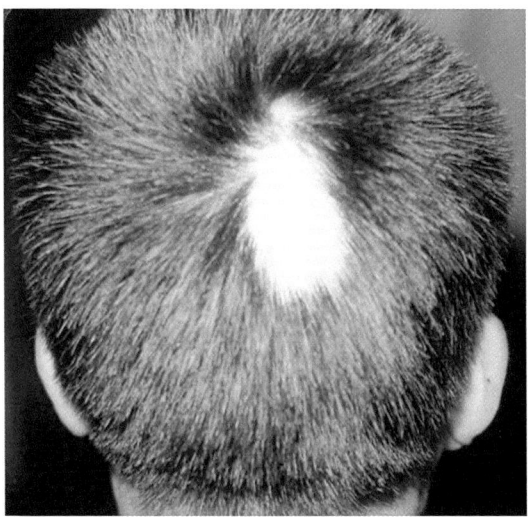

Figure 28 Alopecia areata
Hair loss was sudden in this clearly-defined oval area of the scalp.

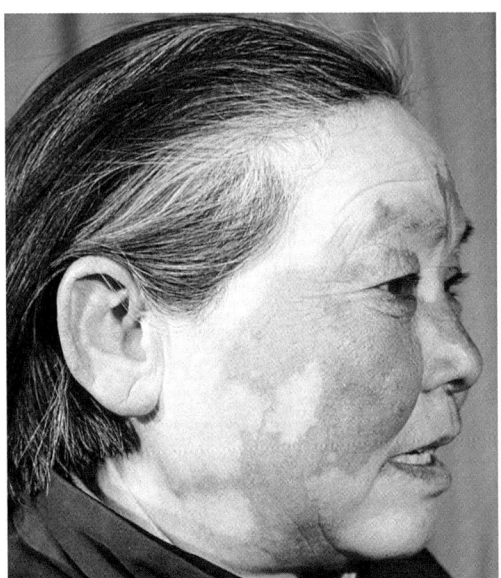

Figure 29 Vitiligo
Circumscribed symmetrically-distributed depigmented patches with sharply demarcated borders are especially striking in darker-skinned individuals.

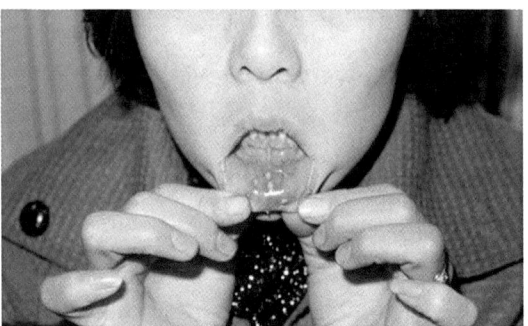

Figure 30 Recurrent aphthous stomatitis
These mouth ulcers appear individually, unlike the clusters of herpetic stomatitis. Small papules on the labial mucosa rupture to form superficial, oval, yellowish-white ulcers with a red areola.

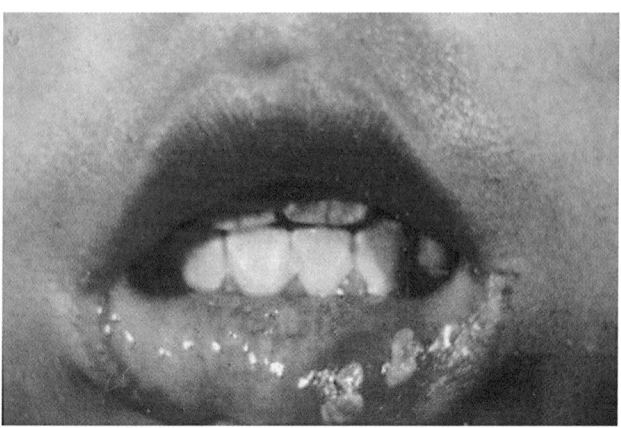

Figure 31 Herpetic stomatitis
Lesions manifest as small clusters of tiny vesicles; they may break after several hours and become ulcerative. A sensation of burning heat and stabbing pain is felt.

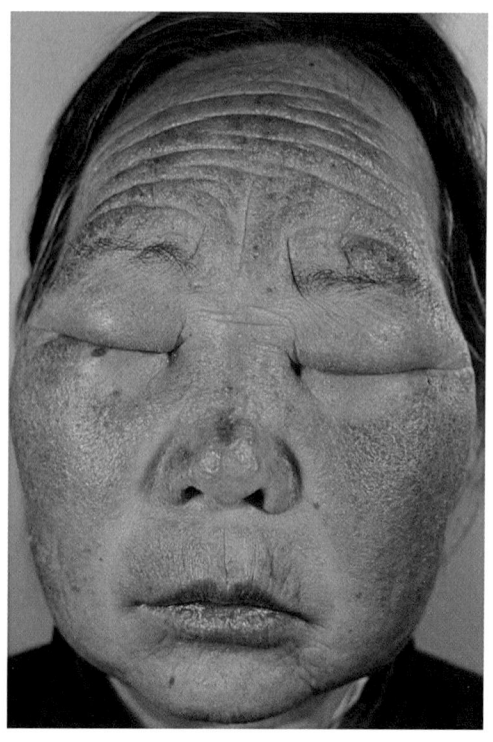

Figure 32 Phytophotodermatitis
After consumption of three-colored amaranth and sun exposure, this patient suffered an acute phototoxic reaction. Skin folds around wrinkles have been spared from the eruption.

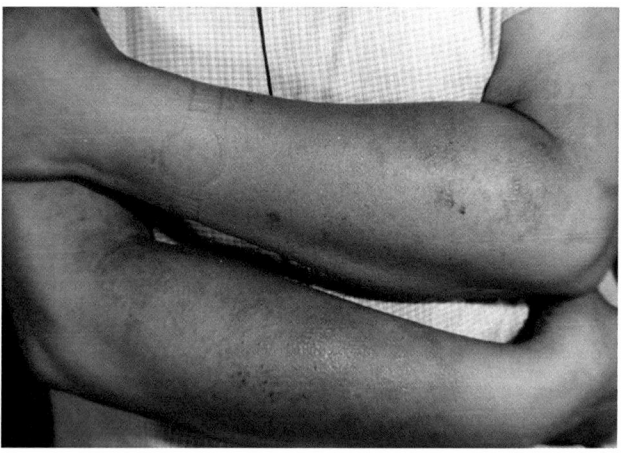

Figure 33 Polymorphic light eruption
Flushed red skin at the sites of exposure to strong sunlight have developed into slightly raised itchy erythema with well-defined margins; small red papules subsequently appeared on the erythema.

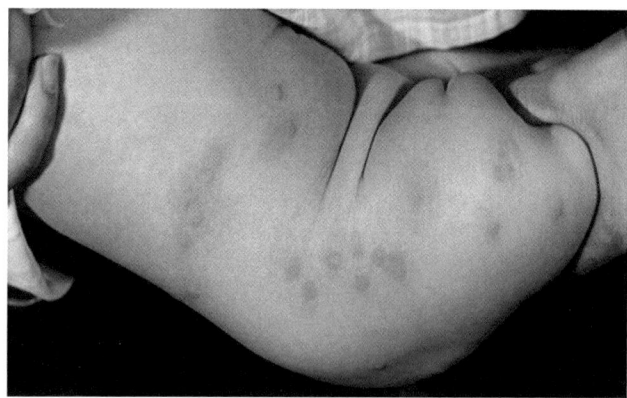

Figure 34 Papular urticaria (insect bites)
Incidence is high among infants and young children, usually involving the lumbosacral region, buttocks and limbs. Lesions manifest initially as red, oval, infiltrative urticarial papules with papulovesicles or vesicles at the center, characteristically occurring in irregular lines and clusters.

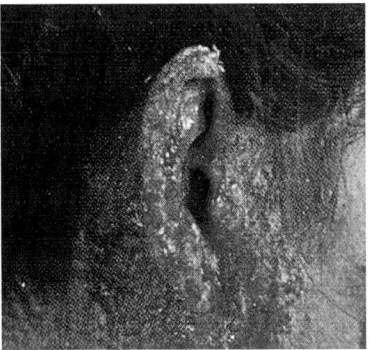

Figure 1 Infectious eczematoid dermatitis
Purulent discharge from a primary focus (in this case, otitis media) has given rise to eczematoid lesions such as papules, papulovesicles, vesicles, erosion, and purulent crusts around the focus.

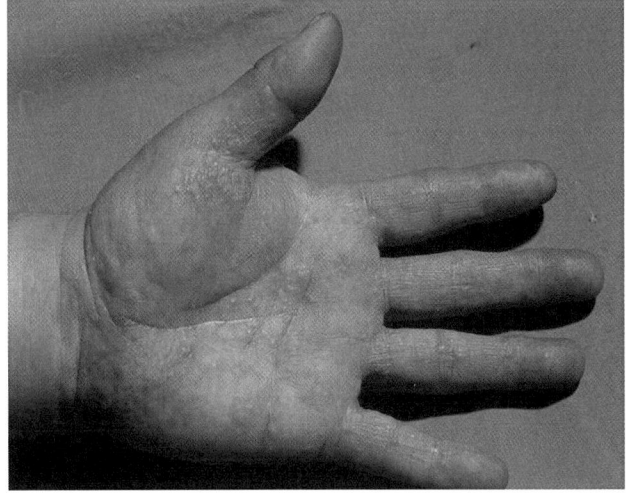

Figure 2 Pompholyx
Lesions manifest as deep-seated domed vesicles filled with a clear and glistening fluid, which may occasionally turn turbid. There is usually symmetrical involvement of the palms and sides of the fingers, and less frequently the soles of the feet. Scaling and peeling follow drying of the vesicles.

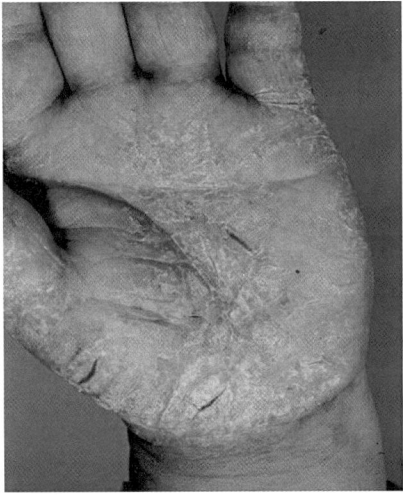

Figure 3 Hand eczema
In this chronic condition, the skin on the palm has become dry and rough with painful fissuring.

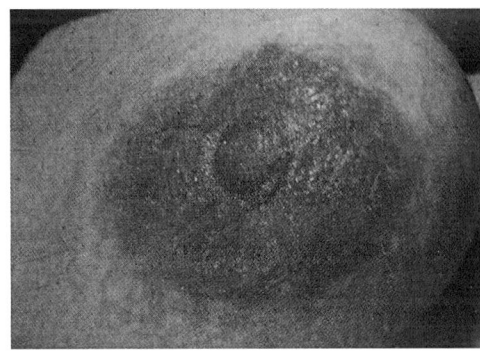

Figure 4 Nipple eczema
Dark red maculopapules appear on the nipples and areolae with slight exudation and erosion or dryness and desquamation. Lesions may be painful and itchy.

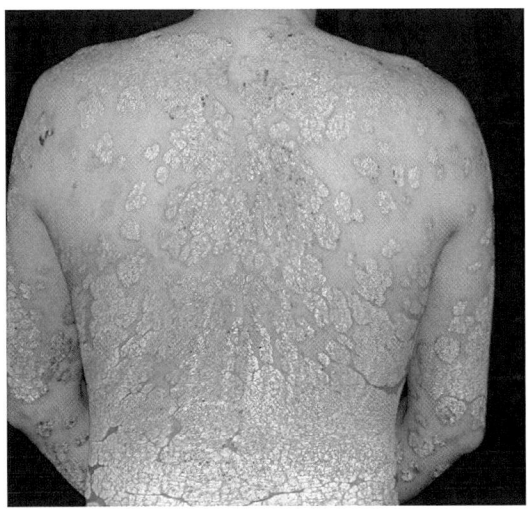

Figure 5 Psoriasis
Extensive plaque psoriasis on the back. These thick red plaques have sharply defined borders and are covered by large dry silvery-white scales.

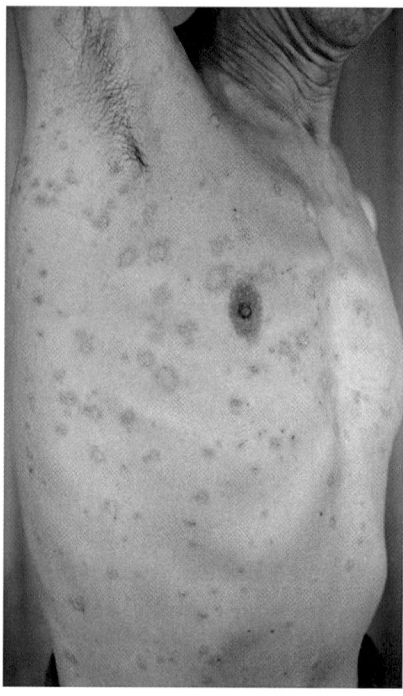

Figure 6 Pityriasis rosea
Reddish-brown oval plaques on the trunk are covered by a thin layer of bran-like scales; the longitudinal axis of the plaques is oriented along the lines of the ribs.

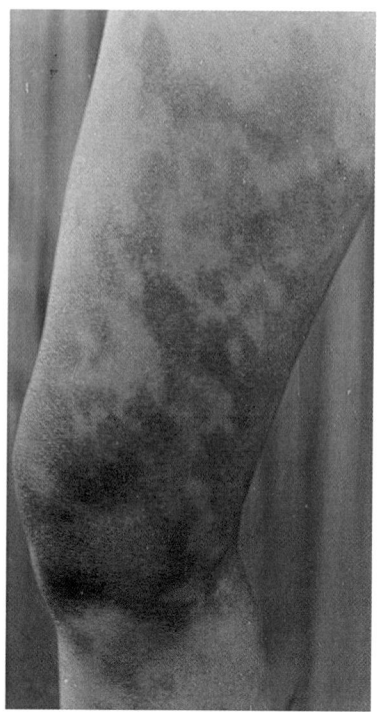

Figure 7 Parapsoriasis (chronic superficial dermatitis)
Round, oval or irregularly-shaped pale red and dull red patches with clearly-defined margins covered by a small amount of scale on the inner thigh. This disease may develop into cutaneous T-cell lymphoma.

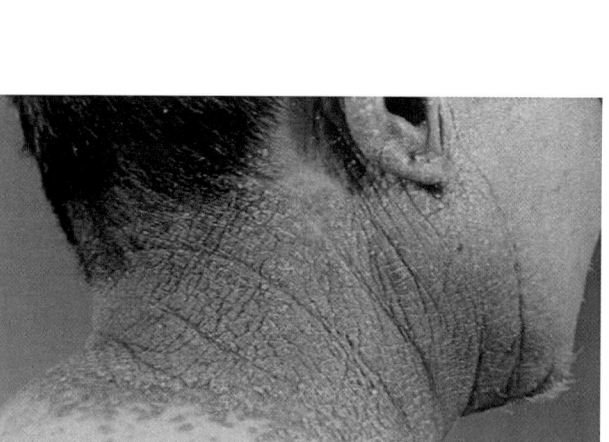

Figure 8 Pityriasis rubra pilaris
Redness and bran-like scaling of the neck have extended to the lower jaw. The original papules have merged into large red plaques covered by grayish-white scale.

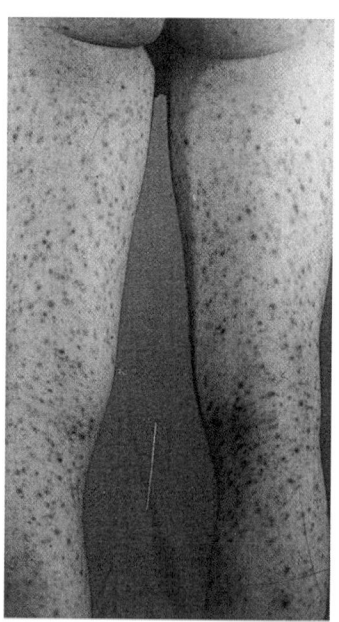

Figure 9 Pityriasis lichenoides (acute varioliform type)
Pale red papules are densely distributed on the flexor aspects of the legs of a teenage boy. The recurrence of crops of lesions means that the simultaneous presence of lesions at different stages is characteristic of this disease.

Bacterial infections of the skin

Normal skin usually provides an excellent barrier against infection. However, where the skin's defenses are breached or otherwise broken down, bacteria and other microorganisms can penetrate the skin to reproduce and cause disease.

The following situations cause a greater risk for infection:

- Various types of eczema (including atopic eczema and contact dermatitis), certain fungal infections and many other skin conditions are characterized by pruritus, with the result that patients may scratch repeatedly. The first barrier of the skin, the stratum corneum or horny layer, will be damaged or removed, allowing the invasion of bacteria.
- Diabetic patients are more likely to have skin infections due to poor blood flow to the skin.
- Small children tend to be infected by bacteria because their skin is thin and delicate, and their body resistance is weak.
- Several immunodeficiency conditions such as steroid therapy, AIDS, Chediak-Higashi syndrome, and Wiskott-Aldrich syndrome predispose to bacterial skin infections.
- Primary viral disease such as herpes simplex can lead to impetigo.
- Other organisms such as fleas or lice break the skin and with repeated scratching may lead to bacterial infection.

The resident flora of normal skin are usually harmless microorganisms, chiefly bacteria, mites and yeasts, which cluster in irregularities in the stratum corneum and in hair follicles. The most common bacteria causing skin infections include *Staphylococcus aureus* or *Streptococcus pyogenes*, which are both Gram-positive bacteria.

Bacterial infections of the skin can be classified into the following categories according to the pathogenesis and clinical manifestations of skin lesions:

- Primary infections of the skin, which are caused by the direct invasion of pathogens into the skin.
- Secondary infections of the skin, which develop as a complication of primary skin diseases.
- Systemic infections: For skin lesions in systemic bacterial infections such as bacteremia and scarlet fever, the multiplying bacteria release a large number of toxic substances such as collagenase, proteases and hyaluronidase, which help to disseminate the pathogens. Leucocidin destroys the white blood cells, erythrogenic toxin results in erythema, and endotoxin leads to elevated body temperature and lesions in some internal organs.

In TCM, the etiology of bacterial infections can be summarized as follows:

- External pathogenic factors – external contraction of Summerheat Toxins or retention of Fire Toxins in the skin and interstices (*cou li*).
- Diet – a diet rich in spicy and greasy foods creates internal Heat Toxins, which can obstruct the channels and network vessels.
- Weak constitution – a weak constitution means that the body fails to eliminate Toxins, with Heat Toxins consequently spreading out to the skin.
- Invasion of Toxic pathogenic factors – skin infections can also develop due to physical destruction of the skin and mucous membranes resulting from insect bites or scratching, which allows the invasion of Toxic pathogenic factors.

Impetigo
脓疱病

Impetigo is a suppurative skin disease caused by coagulase-positive staphylococci, streptococci or a combination of both organisms. It is highly contagious and spreads through autoinoculation or contact with infected people. In TCM, impetigo is also known as *huang shui chuang* (yellow water sore).

Clinical manifestations

- Impetigo is seen most often in children, and is usually more frequent in the summer and autumn.
- It normally occurs around the nose and mouth or on the limbs and usually follows a break in the skin from a cut, a cold sore or eczema.
- Pustules are the major skin lesions of impetigo. The condition may start with vesicles, which soon grow to bullae 1-2 cm in diameter and filled with a clear fluid. Gradually the fluid will become turbid. There may be indistinct surrounding erythema.
- In some cases, vesicles develop over an area of erythema and soon progress to form pustules full of sticky fluid surrounded by an erythematous margin.
- In both conditions, the walls of the pustules are thin and flaccid, breaking easily to reveal an eroded base. Spread of the infected fluid results in new lesions of impetigo at the edge of existing patches or in new patches developing nearby. A layer of thick, golden yellow crust forms after the fluid dries up.
- Impetigo is itchy.
- There may be regional lymphadenopathy, accompanied by fever in severe cases. Rarely, complications such as septicemia or glomerulonephritis may develop.

Differential diagnosis

Varicella (chickenpox)

Two to three weeks after exposure to the varicella virus, there is a brief prodromal illness of fever, headache and malaise. This is followed by the quick progression of macules to papules to vesicles to pustules in a matter of hours. Skin eruptions begin on the trunk and spread to the face, scalp and limbs. The fever subsides as soon as new spots stop occurring. The spots crust over and usually heal without scarring. Varicella is most commonly seen in the winter and spring.

Papular urticaria

Papular urticaria is a reaction to bites of insects such as fleas, mites or bedbugs where the actual source of the bite is unknown. Lesions initially manifest as red, oval, infiltrative wheals with papulovesicles or vesicles at the center and mainly involve the lumbosacral region, buttocks, trunk, and lower limbs. Incidence is high among infants and children. The lesions characteristically occur in irregular lines and clusters, may last for up to two weeks and recur in crops. This condition is very itchy but not infectious.

Pemphigus

Pemphigus is an autoimmune condition usually affecting adults after the age of 40. Thin-walled vesicles of various sizes are seen on the trunk, limb flexures and scalp, often preceded by lesions on the oral mucosa. The vesicles break easily leaving moist eroded areas. Nikolsky's sign is positive (separation of the stratum corneum from the underlying layers of the epidermis as a result of the application of slight shearing pressure).

Etiology and pathology

Accumulation of Spleen-Damp

Dietary irregularities such as overeating of greasy food or seafood or irregular mealtimes will impair the Spleen's transformation and transportation function resulting in Spleen-Damp accumulating internally and spreading to the skin and flesh on the limbs. In cases of recurrent impetigo, pathogenic Toxins damage Vital Qi (Zheng Qi), thus causing Deficiency of Spleen Qi.

Weakness of the interstices (*cou li*)

In the heat of summer, it is easy for Summerheat-Damp pathogenic factors to invade, impairing the functional activities of Qi and inhibiting the smooth flow of Qi. Children's skin is especially tender and delicate and can easily be invaded by Summerheat-Damp and Wind pathogenic factors, particularly where children have a weak constitution. When Heat in the flesh combines with Dampness in the Spleen, impetigo occurs.

Heat Toxins invading the exterior

In summer, when it is hot and humid, Heat Toxins will predominate and attack the skin surface to cause impetigo. If children play outdoors when the wind is blowing or the sun is strong, Summerheat can allow Heat Toxins or Wind-Heat to attack the skin and bring on impetigo.

Pattern identification and treatment

INTERNAL TREATMENT

WIND-DAMP-HEAT

This pattern is usually seen in the initial stage of impetigo. Yellow 1-2 mm papules appear suddenly in various locations, subsequently developing into bullae, accompanied by local itching. The tongue body is red with a thin yellow coating; the pulse is floating and rapid.

Treatment principle

Dredge Wind and clear Heat, transform Dampness and relieve Toxicity.

Prescription
SHENG MA XIAO DU YIN JIA JIAN
Bugbane Beverage for Relieving Toxicity, with modifications

Dang Gui Wei (Extremitas Radicis Angelicae Sinensis) 10g
Chi Shao (Radix Paeoniae Rubra) 10g
Jiao Zhi Zi (Fructus Gardeniae Jasminoidis, scorch-fried) 10g
Lian Qiao (Fructus Forsythiae Suspensae) 10g
Jin Yin Hua (Flos Lonicerae) 15g
Ye Ju Hua (Flos Chrysanthemi Indici) 15g
Pu Gong Ying (Herba Taraxaci cum Radice) 15g
Sheng Ma (Rhizoma Cimicifugae) 6g
Jie Geng (Radix Platycodi Grandiflori) 6g
Chao Huang Qin (Radix Scutellariae Baicalensis, stir-fried) 3g
Chao Huang Lian (Rhizoma Coptidis, stir-fried) 3g
Gan Cao (Radix Glycyrrhizae) 4.5g

Explanation
- *Dang Gui Wei* (Extremitas Radicis Angelicae Sinensis) is predominantly warm and combines with *Chi Shao* (Radix Paeoniae Rubra) to invigorate the Blood so as to expel Wind and clear Heat.
- *Lian Qiao* (Fructus Forsythiae Suspensae), *Jin Yin Hua* (Flos Lonicerae) and *Jie Geng* (Radix Platycodi Grandiflori) dissipate Wind and clear Heat.
- *Ye Ju Hua* (Flos Chrysanthemi Indici), *Sheng Ma* (Rhizoma Cimicifugae), *Pu Gong Ying* (Herba Taraxaci cum Radice), and *Gan Cao* (Radix Glycyrrhizae) clear Heat and relieve Toxicity, eliminate swelling and treat sores.
- *Jiao Zhi Zi* (Fructus Gardeniae Jasminoidis, scorch-fried), *Chao Huang Qin* (Radix Scutellariae Baicalensis, stir-fried) and *Chao Huang Lian* (Rhizoma Coptidis, stir-fried) clear Heat, transform Dampness and relieve Toxicity.
- In the initial stage of impetigo, the main factor is binding of pathogenic Wind-Damp. When Wind is expelled and Dampness transformed, Heat can be cleared.

DAMP-HEAT
This pattern is marked by numerous bullae surrounded by areolae, or ruptured bullae with exudation of turbid fluid, inflammatory infiltration involving the surrounding areas, and local pain and itching. Accompanying symptoms and signs include generalized fever and regional lymph node enlargement. The tongue body is red with a yellow and greasy coating; the pulse is slippery and rapid.

Treatment principle
Clear Heat and transform Dampness, relieve Toxicity and flush out Summerheat.

Prescription
QIN LIAN PING WEI SAN JIA JIAN
Scutellaria and Coptis Powder for Calming the Stomach, with modifications

Jin Yin Hua (Flos Lonicerae) 15g
Di Fu Zi (Fructus Kochiae Scopariae) 15g
Ye Ju Hua (Flos Chrysanthemi Indici) 15g
Huo Xiang (Herba Agastaches seu Pogostemi) 10g
Pei Lan (Herba Eupatorii Fortunei) 10g
Ze Xie (Rhizoma Alismatis Orientalis) 10g
Jiao Zhi Zi (Fructus Gardeniae Jasminoidis, scorch-fried) 10g
Pu Gong Ying (Herba Taraxaci cum Radice) 10g
Chao Huang Qin (Radix Scutellariae Baicalensis, stir-fried) 6g
Ku Shen (Radix Sophorae Flavescentis) 6g
Tong Cao (Medulla Tetrapanacis Papyriferi) 6g
Bai Mao Gen (Rhizoma Imperatae Cylindricae) 30g
Chi Xiao Dou (Semen Phaseoli Calcarati) 30g

Explanation
- *Huo Xiang* (Herba Agastaches seu Pogostemi), *Pei Lan* (Herba Eupatorii Fortunei), *Ze Xie* (Rhizoma Alismatis Orientalis), *Bai Mao Gen* (Rhizoma Imperatae Cylindricae), *Chi Xiao Dou* (Semen Phaseoli Calcarati), *Huang Qin* (Radix Scutellariae Baicalensis), *Ku Shen* (Radix Sophorae Flavescentis), and *Di Fu Zi* (Fructus Kochiae Scopariae) transform Dampness and clear Summerheat.
- *Jin Yin Hua* (Flos Lonicerae), *Ye Ju Hua* (Flos Chrysanthemi Indici), *Pu Gong Ying* (Herba Taraxaci cum Radice), *Jiao Zhi Zi* (Fructus Gardeniae Jasminoidis, scorch-fried), *Chao Huang Qin* (Radix Scutellariae Baicalensis, stir-fried), and *Tong Cao* (Medulla Tetrapanacis Papyriferi) clear Heat and relieve Toxicity.
- The first group of herbs focuses on treating pathogenic Dampness, the second group on treating Heat. When pathogenic Damp-Heat is cleared, the disease can be controlled.

FINAL STAGE AFTER ELIMINATION OF DAMP-HEAT
The main manifestations of this pattern include the drying up of oozing skin lesions with yellow or yellowish-black crusts forming over the lesions, sometimes accompanied by itching. The lesions heal after the crusts fall off. The tongue body is normal with a thin yellow coating; the pulse is thready and rapid.

Treatment principle
Relieve residual Toxicity, augment Qi and protect Yin.

Prescription
SI MIAO TANG JIA JIAN
Mysterious Four Decoction, with modifications

Huang Qi (Radix Astragali seu Hedysari) 10g

Jin Yin Hua (Flos Lonicerae) 10g
Lian Qiao (Fructus Forsythiae Suspensae) 10g
Xuan Shen (Radix Scrophulariae Ningpoensis) 10g
Fu Ling Pi (Cortex Poriae Cocos) 10g
Chi Xiao Dou (Semen Phaseoli Calcarati) 15g
Lü Dou Yi (Testa Phaseoli Radiati) 12g
Nan Sha Shen (Radix Adenophorae) 12g
Yi Yi Ren (Semen Coicis Lachryma-jobi) 12g
Bai Mao Gen (Rhizoma Imperatae Cylindricae) 30g

Explanation

- In the final stage of impetigo, Heat has been cleared and Toxicity relieved. The main symptom remaining is itching.
- *Huang Qi* (Radix Astragali seu Hedysari) and *Nan Sha Shen* (Radix Adenophorae) augment Qi and protect Yin to support Vital Qi (Zheng Qi) and alleviate itching.
- *Yi Yi Ren* (Semen Coicis Lachryma-jobi), *Chi Xiao Dou* (Semen Phaseoli Calcarati) and *Fu Ling Pi* (Cortex Poriae Cocos) clear residual Damp pathogenic factors to alleviate itching.
- *Jin Yin Hua* (Flos Lonicerae), *Xuan Shen* (Radix Scrophulariae Ningpoensis), *Lian Qiao* (Fructus Forsythiae Suspensae), *Bai Mao Gen* (Rhizoma Imperatae Cylindricae), and *Lü Dou Yi* (Testa Phaseoli Radiati) clear Heat and relieve Toxicity to alleviate itching.

General modifications

1. For oppression in the chest and poor appetite, add *Bai Bian Dou* (Semen Dolichoris Lablab) and *Sha Ren* (Fructus Amomi).
2. For exuberant Heart-Fire, add *Lian Zi Xin* (Plumula Nelumbinis Nuciferae) and *Zhi Zi* (Fructus Gardeniae Jasminoidis).
3. For hyperactive Wind-Heat with signs such as itching due to pathogenic Wind settling in the skin, add *Chan Tui*‡ (Periostracum Cicadae) and *Bo He* (Herba Menthae Haplocalycis).
4. For pronounced Wind-Damp signs such as itchy skin, add *Bai Xian Pi* (Cortex Dictamni Dasycarpi Radicis) and *Qian Cao Gen* (Radix Rubiae Cordifoliae).
5. For short voidings of yellow urine, add *Che Qian Zi* (Semen Plantaginis), *Chong Lou* (Rhizoma Paridis) and *Deng Xin Cao* (Medulla Junci Effusi).
6. For blood in the urine, add *Da Ji* (Herba seu Radix Cirsii Japonici), *Xiao Ji* (Herba Cephalanoploris seu Cirsii) and *Xian He Cao* (Herba Agrimoniae Pilosae).
7. For puffy swelling of the legs, add *Zhu Ling* (Sclerotium Polypori Umbellati), *Che Qian Zi* (Semen Plantaginis) and *Ze Xie* (Rhizoma Alismatis Orientalis).

EXTERNAL TREATMENT

- For lesions manifesting mainly as vesicles and pustules, use *Qing Dai San* (Indigo Powder) or *Er Bai San* (Two Whites Powder). Mix to a paste with an appropriate quantity of vegetable oil or *Hua Jiao You* (Chinese Prickly Ash Oil) for application to the affected areas.
- For erosion and infiltration after the blisters have burst, make a decoction with *Pu Gong Ying* (Herba Taraxaci cum Radice) 20g and *Zi Hua Di Ding* (Herba Violae Yedoensitis) 20g, or prepare *Ma Chi Xian Shui Xi Ji* (Purslane Wash Preparation) or *Shi Liu Pi Shui Xi Ji* (Pomegranate Rind Wash Preparation); use as an external wash or wet compress. Then mix *Qing Dai San* (Indigo Powder) and *Qu Shi San* (Powder for Dispelling Dampness) with vegetable oil for application to the lesions.
- For any remaining crusts, apply *Si Huang Gao* (Four Yellows Paste).

Clinical notes

- In the initial stages of impetigo, it is important to focus on relieving Toxicity rather than on supporting Vital Qi (Zheng Qi). Formulae such as *Wu Wei Xiao Du Yin* (Five-Ingredient Beverage for Dispersing Toxicity) can be used as alternatives to those listed above.
- In the later stages of impetigo, concentrate on supporting Vital Qi (Zheng Qi) rather than on relieving Toxicity. Use formulae such as *Si Miao Tang* (Mysterious Four Decoction).
- *Chi Xiao Dou* (Semen Phaseoli Calcarati), *Fu Ling* (Sclerotium Poriae Cocos), *Yi Yi Ren* (Semen Coicis Lachryma-jobi), *Zhe Bei Mu* (Bulbus Fritillariae Thunbergii), and other materia medica for transforming Dampness and dissipating lumps can be included at any stage.
- External treatment is also important. Application of *Qing Dai San* (Indigo Powder) at the initial stage can often prevent further development of the disease.
- Acute glomerulonephritis may follow streptococcal (crusted) impetigo, especially in very young children. In such cases, patients should be referred immediately to a doctor of Western medicine for treatment with antibiotics.

Advice for the patient

- To prevent transmission of the disease, pillowcases, towels and flannels should not be shared and should be boiled after use. Clothes should be changed regularly.
- Patients should avoid skin-to-skin contact with others.

Literature excerpt

In *Wai Ke Zheng Zong* [An Orthodox Manual of External Diseases], it says: "Yellow blisters suddenly appear on the face, ears and neck. They soon break, followed by exudation of thick, turbid fluid. The surrounding areas are soon involved. The outbreak is usually accompanied by pain and itching. The disease is caused by exposure to sun and wind and sudden contraction of Damp-Heat, or by internal Wind stirring Fire as a result of an improper diet producing Damp-Heat internally."

Modern clinical experience

EXTERNAL TREATMENT

1. **Wang** treated 200 cases of impetigo with his own empirical powder preparation prescription. [1]

Prescription
KU LU HUANG SAN
Prepared Alum, Calamine and Phellodendron Bark Powder

Ku Fan ‡ (Alumen Praeparatum) 60g
Lu Gan Shi ‡ (Calamina) 60g
Huang Bai (Cortex Phellodendri) 60g
Huang Lian (Rhizoma Coptidis) 10g
Bing Pian (Borneolum) 6g

The ingredients were ground to a fine powder and sieved. The powder was either applied directly to the lesions, with the amount depending on the size of the lesions, or mixed to a paste with *Xiang You* (Oleum Sesami Seminis) or boiled water and then applied. Treatment was given once or twice a day. Results were seen after two to ten days.

2. **Cao** prepared a decoction for use as an external wash to treat 98 impetigo patients. [2]

Prescription ingredients

Ku Shen (Radix Sophorae Flavescentis) 30g
Bai Bu (Radix Stemonae) 30g
She Chuang Zi (Fructus Cnidii Monnieri) 30g
He Shi (Fructus Carpesii) 30g

Tu Jin Pi (Cortex Pseudolaricis) 30g
Tu Fu Ling (Rhizoma Smilacis Glabrae) 30g
Yu Xing Cao (Herba Houttuyniae Cordatae) 30g
Bai Xian Pi (Cortex Dictamni Dasycarpi Radicis) 20g
Di Fu Zi (Fructus Kochiae Scopariae) 20g
Xu Chang Qing (Radix Cynanchi Paniculati) 20g
Bai Zhi (Radix Angelicae Dahuricae) 10g
Chan Tui ‡ (Periostracum Cicadae) 10g

The prescription was decocted in 7.5 liters of water and used as an external wash. Treatment was given for 5-10 minutes twice a day. Results were seen after one course of treatment lasting five days; 77 patients recovered completely, 9 improved and 12 showed no effect.

3. **Bao** prepared a paste to treat 43 cases of impetigo. [3]

Prescription
FU FANG BEI FAN SHI HU JI
Compound Chinese Gall, Prepared Alum and Talcum Paste Preparation

Wu Bei Zi ‡ (Galla Rhois Chinensis) 10g
Ku Fan ‡ (Alumen Praeparatum) 5g
Hua Shi ‡ (Talcum) 5g
Qing Dai (Indigo Naturalis) 5g
Bing Pian (Borneolum) 2g

The ingredients were ground into a fine powder and mixed to a paste with 100ml of 75% ethanol before being stored in a sealed bottle. After removing the crusts from the lesions, the paste was applied directly. Treatment was given three times a day. Results were seen after five to eight days.

4. **Zhao** prepared a rub by mixing 2.4g of *Zhu Huang San* (Pearl and Bezoar Powder) with 100ml of gentian violet solution. The lesions were first cleaned with physiological saline or 3% hydrogen peroxide and the lotion applied directly to the lesions with cotton wool. Treatment was administered three to four times a day until the lesions healed. Results were generally seen after four or five days; some patients responded more quickly, and a few cases took more than six days before any improvement was seen. [4]

Ethyma
臁疮

Ecthyma is an ulcerative pyoderma of the skin caused by group A beta-hemolytic streptococci (GABHS). Since ecthyma extends into the dermis, it is often referred to as a deeper form of impetigo. GABHS may cause a primary infection or may secondarily infect pre-existing wounds. Tissue damage from skin conditions such as excoriations, insect bites and inflammation or other conditions such as diabetes predispose patients to ecthyma, as does overcrowding and poor hygiene.

In TCM, ecthyma is also known as *nong ke chuang* (purulent nest sore).

Clinical manifestations

- Ecthyma is most common in children or elderly adults.
- The condition occurs mainly on the lower limbs.
- Lesions begin as a vesicle or pustule overlying an inflamed area of skin. This deepens into a dermal ulceration covered with a hard crust. Removal of the crust discloses an ulcer which is deepest in the center. A deep ulcer will have a raised and indurated margin.
- Ecthyma heals with scarring.
- There are often accompanying symptoms such as pain, itching, fever, and enlargement of local lymph nodes.

Differential diagnosis

Impetigo
The lesions of impetigo are normally shallow and occur around the nose and mouth as well as on the limbs. In impetigo, the walls of the pustules are thin and flaccid, breaking easily to reveal an eroded base in contrast to the ulcers formed in ecthyma.

Furuncles
Furuncles commonly occur on the head, face, neck, and buttocks. The lesion has an indurated swollen base and a tense, shining surface. Pus appears on the top of the lesion. Severe pain is diminished after removal of the purulent core.

Etiology and pathology

- Heat in the Lung channel and Dampness in the Spleen channel combine to form Damp-Heat, which accumulates internally and steams outward to the skin and interstices (*cou li*), transforming into Toxins and generating Worms, which ferment to produce abscesses.
- If the body is constitutionally weak, there is disharmony between Qi and Blood and external Heat Toxins may be contracted; exuberant Heat putrefies the flesh, giving rise to ecthyma.
- Ecthyma can be a secondary problem of other con-

ditions such as scabies, insect bites, varicella (chickenpox), neglected external injury, or wasting and thirsting disease. The patient suffers from severe itching, which if satiated, can allow external Heat Toxins to penetrate the broken skin.

Pattern identification and treatment

INTERNAL TREATMENT

DAMP-HEAT
This pattern is characterized by relatively few, circumscribed, discretely distributed pustules developing on the lower limbs, surrounded by an erythematous margin. The lesion may discharge thick pus or may be covered by a thick yellow purulent crust. There may be pain; itching is very frequent. The tongue body is red with a thin yellow coating; the pulse is soggy and rapid.

Treatment principle
Clear Heat and relieve Toxicity, and benefit the movement of Dampness by bland percolation.

Prescription
HUANG LIAN JIE DU TANG JIA JIAN
Coptis Decoction for Relieving Toxicity, with modifications

Chao Huang Lian (Rhizoma Coptidis, stir-fried) 6g
Lian Zi Xin (Plumula Nelumbinis Nuciferae) 6g
Huang Bai (Cortex Phellodendri) 10g
Huang Qin (Radix Scutellariae Baicalensis) 10g
Cang Zhu (Rhizoma Atractylodis) 10g
Chi Fu Ling (Sclerotium Poriae Cocos Rubrae) 10g
Chuan Niu Xi (Radix Cyathulae Officinalis) 10g
Pu Gong Ying (Herba Taraxaci cum Radice) 15g
Ren Dong Teng (Caulis Lonicerae Japonicae) 15g
Zi Hua Di Ding (Herba Violae Yedoensitis) 15g
Yi Yi Ren (Semen Coicis Lachryma-jobi) 15g
Che Qian Zi (Semen Plantaginis) 30g, wrapped
Chi Xiao Dou (Semen Phaseoli Calcarati) 30g

Explanation
- *Chao Huang Lian* (Rhizoma Coptidis, stir-fried), *Huang Qin* (Radix Scutellariae Baicalensis), *Huang Bai* (Cortex Phellodendri), and *Lian Zi Xin* (Plumula Nelumbinis Nuciferae) drain Fire with cold and bitterness to clear Heat Toxins.
- *Pu Gong Ying* (Herba Taraxaci cum Radice), *Ren Dong Teng* (Caulis Lonicerae Japonicae), *Zi Hua Di Ding* (Herba Violae Yedoensitis), and *Chi Xiao Dou* (Semen Phaseoli Calcarati) clear Heat and relieve Toxicity.
- *Chi Fu Ling* (Sclerotium Poriae Cocos Rubrae), *Yi Yi Ren* (Semen Coicis Lachryma-jobi) and *Che Qian Zi*

(Semen Plantaginis) percolate Dampness and clear Heat.

- *Cang Zhu* (Rhizoma Atractylodis) and *Chuan Niu Xi* (Radix Cyathulae Officinalis) transform Dampness and act as channel conductors to guide the other ingredients to the affected areas.

DISHARMONY BETWEEN QI AND BLOOD
This pattern presents with numerous pustules or vesicles containing thin clear fluid, but without any distinct areola. Slight itching is experienced. Accompanying symptoms and signs include emaciation, a white facial complexion, poor appetite, or slight fever. The tongue body is pale red with a white coating; the pulse is deep, thready and rapid.

Treatment principle
Augment Qi, supplement the Blood and relieve Toxicity.

Prescription
SI WU TANG JIA WEI
Four Agents Decoction, with additions

Dang Gui (Radix Angelicae Sinensis) 10g
Bai Shao (Radix Paeoniae Lactiflorae) 10g
Tian Men Dong (Radix Asparagi Cochinchinensis) 10g
Mai Men Dong (Radix Ophiopogonis Japonici) 10g
Dang Shen (Radix Codonopsitis Pilosulae) 10g
Huang Qi (Radix Astragali seu Hedysari) 12g
Sheng Di Huang (Radix Rehmanniae Glutinosae) 12g
Yi Yi Ren (Semen Coicis Lachryma-jobi) 12g
Chao Bai Zhu (Rhizoma Atractylodis Macrocephalae, stir-fried) 12g
Chuan Xiong (Rhizoma Ligustici Chuanxiong) 6g
Gan Cao (Radix Glycyrrhizae) 6g
Chai Hu (Radix Bupleuri) 6g
Jin Yin Hua (Flos Lonicerae) 15g
Bai Hua She She Cao (Herba Hedyotidis Diffusae) 15g

Explanation
- *Dang Shen* (Radix Codonopsitis Pilosulae), *Chao Bai Zhu* (Rhizoma Atractylodis Macrocephalae, stir-fried), *Huang Qi* (Radix Astragali seu Hedysari), and *Gan Cao* (Radix Glycyrrhizae) augment Qi.
- *Dang Gui* (Radix Angelicae Sinensis), *Chuan Xiong* (Rhizoma Ligustici Chuanxiong), *Bai Shao* (Radix Paeoniae Lactiflorae), and *Sheng Di Huang* (Radix Rehmanniae Glutinosae) nourish the Blood.
- *Tian Men Dong* (Radix Asparagi Cochinchinensis), *Mai Men Dong* (Radix Ophiopogonis Japonici) and *Yi Yi Ren* (Semen Coicis Lachryma-jobi) nourish Yin and support the Spleen.
- *Jin Yin Hua* (Flos Lonicerae), *Bai Hua She She Cao* (Herba Hedyotidis Diffusae) and *Chai Hu* (Radix Bupleuri) relieve Toxicity and reduce fever.

SECONDARY INFECTION BY HEAT TOXINS
Scratch marks and excoriations are often present on the skin. Ulcers form under surface crusts. Lesions are surrounded by a bright red areola. Pain and itching are experienced. The tongue body is red with a scant coating; the pulse is rapid.

Treatment principle
Clear Heat, relieve Toxicity and alleviate itching.

Prescription
WU WEI XIAO DU YIN JIA JIAN
Five-Ingredient Beverage for Dispersing Toxicity, with modifications

Jin Yin Hua (Flos Lonicerae) 15g
Pu Gong Ying (Herba Taraxaci cum Radice) 15g
Zi Hua Di Ding (Herba Violae Yedoensitis) 15g
Dang Gui (Radix Angelicae Sinensis) 10g
Chi Shao (Radix Paeoniae Rubra) 10g
Chen Pi (Pericarpium Citri Reticulatae) 10g
Qiang Huo (Rhizoma et Radix Notopterygii) 10g
Fang Feng (Radix Ledebouriellae Divaricatae) 10g
Bai Ji Li (Fructus Tribuli Terrestris) 10g
Bai Hua She She Cao (Herba Hedyotidis Diffusae) 12g
Tian Hua Fen (Radix Trichosanthis) 12g

Explanation
- *Jin Yin Hua* (Flos Lonicerae), *Zi Hua Di Ding* (Herba Violae Yedoensitis), *Pu Gong Ying* (Herba Taraxaci cum Radice), and *Bai Hua She She Cao* (Herba Hedyotidis Diffusae) relieve Toxicity.
- *Qiang Huo* (Rhizoma et Radix Notopterygii), *Fang Feng* (Radix Ledebouriellae Divaricatae) and *Bai Ji Li* (Fructus Tribuli Terrestris) alleviate itching.
- *Dang Gui* (Radix Angelicae Sinensis), *Chi Shao* (Radix Paeoniae Rubra), *Chen Pi* (Pericarpium Citri Reticulatae), and *Tian Hua Fen* (Radix Trichosanthis) invigorate the Blood and reduce erythema.

EXTERNAL TREATMENT
- At the initial stage before the vesicles or pustules have ulcerated, mix *Qing Dai San* (Indigo Powder) or *Qing Bai San* (Green-White Powder) into a paste with vegetable oil for external application.
- For profuse pus, prepare a decoction with equal portions of *Pu Gong Ying* (Herba Taraxaci cum Radice), *Ye Ju Hua* (Flos Chrysanthemi Indici) and *Ma Chi Xian* (Herba Portulacae Oleraceae). Soak several layers of gauze in the medicated lotion and apply to the affected area as a wet compress for 15 minutes.
- For smaller amounts of pus, make a decoction with *Pu Gong Ying* (Herba Taraxaci cum Radice) 20g and

Zi Hua Di Ding (Herba Violae Yedoensitis) 20g and apply to the affected area three or four times a day.

- Ruptured lesions can be treated by a decoction prepared with

Qing Hao (Herba Artemisiae Chinghao) 30g
Yu Xing Cao (Herba Houttuyniae Cordatae) 30g
Huang Bai (Cortex Phellodendri) 20g
Da Huang (Radix et Rhizoma Rhei) 10g
Jin Yin Hua (Flos Lonicerae) 30g
Tu Fu Ling (Rhizoma Smilacis Glabrae) 20g
Bing Pian (Borneolum) 2g

Use to wash the affected area for 15 minutes once or twice a day.

Clinical notes

- At the initial stage, treatment focuses on clearing Heat and transforming Dampness, while relieving Toxicity and freeing the network vessels; in the later stages, it focuses on warming Yang and augmenting Qi, while relieving Toxicity and closing sores.
- The lesions may take a long time to heal, anywhere from weeks to months. In such cases, scars remain after the lesions heal.

Advice for the patient

- Hygiene is important: use bactericidal soap and change bed sheets, towels and clothing frequently.
- Patients should avoid skin-to-skin contact.
- Cut the fingernails to prevent spread of infection through scratching.

Case history

Patient
Male, aged 6.

Clinical manifestations
Five days previously, the patient had developed vesicles 0.5-1.5 cm in diameter on the head and face; these vesicles subsequently spread to the limbs and trunk, gradually filling with pus to form superficial abscesses, especially on the legs. At the time of the consultation, the pustules had ruptured and become very painful. The inguinal lymph nodes were enlarged and painful. The patient had a temperature of 39.5°C, which was even higher at night. Accompanying symptoms included poor appetite, dry mouth and yellow urine. The tongue body was red with a yellow coating; the pulse was rapid and racing.

Pattern identification
As the disease occurred in summer, the pattern was identified

as pathogenic Summerheat and Dampness settling in the skin; these pathogenic factors could not be drained externally and finally involved the Xue level.

Treatment principle
Clear Heat.

Prescription ingredients
Jin Yin Hua (Flos Lonicerae) 15g
Ren Dong Teng (Caulis Lonicerae Japonicae) 15g
Lian Qiao (Fructus Forsythiae Suspensae) 9g
Chi Fu Ling (Sclerotium Poriae Cocos Rubrae) 9g
Che Qian Zi (Semen Plantaginis) 9g, wrapped
Jiao Zhi Zi (Fructus Gardeniae Jasminoidis, scorch-fried) 9g
Lü Dou Yi (Testa Phaseoli Radiati) 9g
Huang Lian (Rhizoma Coptidis) 2g
Huang Qin (Radix Scutellariae Baicalensis) 4.5g
Liu Yi San (Six-To-One Powder) 12g, wrapped
Mu Dan Pi (Cortex Moutan Radicis) 6g
Dan Zhu Ye (Herba Lophatheri Gracilis) 10g

External application
Huang Ling Dan (Yellow Spirit Special Pill) was mixed to a paste with sesame oil and applied externally to the lesions, twice a day. *Fu Rong Gao* (Cotton Rose Flower Paste) was applied twice a day to the inguinal lymph nodes.

Outcome
After following the treatment for two days, local and systemic symptoms started to diminish gradually. After another four days, the patient recovered.[5]

Literature excerpt

In *Wai Ke Tu Shuo* [Illustrated Explanations of External Diseases], it says: "*Nong ke chuang* (purulent nest sores) are as big as soybeans and contain yellow pus. They are very painful. They usually result from Damp-Heat due to Spleen Deficiency. Treat internally with *Shen Xiao Tuo Li San* (Wondrous Effect Powder for Drawing Out Toxins from the Interior) plus *Cang Zhu* (Rhizoma Atractylodis) and *Fang Feng* (Radix Ledebouriellae Divaricatae), and apply *Pu Ji Dan* (Universal Salvation Special Pill) externally."

Modern clinical experience

TREATMENT ACCORDING TO PATTERN IDENTIFICATION

1. **Zhu** identified three patterns for the treatment of ecthyma.[6]

- **Initial stage**

Treatment principle
Clear Heat, benefit the movement of Dampness and relieve Toxicity.

Prescription

Er Miao Wan (Mysterious Two Pill) combined with *Wu Shen Tang* (Five Spirits Decoction)

- **Later stages (with Qi and Blood Deficiency)**

Treatment principle

Supplement Qi and Blood.

Prescription

Shi Quan Da Bu Wan (Perfect Major Supplementation Pill) combined with *Si Miao Tang* (Mysterious Four Decoction)

- **Qi fall due to Spleen Qi Deficiency**

Treatment principle

Augment Qi, bear Yang upward and relieve Toxicity.

Prescription

Bu Zhong Yi Qi Tang (Decoction for Supplementing the Middle and Augmenting Qi) plus *Ren Dong Teng* (Caulis Lonicerae Japonicae) and *Tu Fu Ling* (Rhizoma Smilacis Glabrae)

2. **Gu** identified two patterns for the treatment of ecthyma. [7]

- **Damp-Heat**

Treatment principle

Clear Heat and transform Dampness.

Prescription ingredients

Huang Lian (Rhizoma Coptidis) 10g
Huang Qin (Radix Scutellariae Baicalensis) 10g
Jin Yin Hua (Flos Lonicerae) 15g
Lian Qiao (Fructus Forsythiae Suspensae) 15g
Chi Shao (Radix Paeoniae Rubra) 10g
Mu Dan Pi (Cortex Moutan Radicis) 10g
Chi Fu Ling (Sclerotium Poriae Cocos Rubrae) 10g
Yi Yi Ren (Semen Coicis Lachryma-jobi) 15g
Gan Cao (Radix Glycyrrhizae) 6g
Bi Xie (Rhizoma Dioscoreae Hypoglaucae seu Septemlobae) 10g

- **Exuberant Toxins due to Deficiency of Vital Qi (Zheng Qi)**

Treatment principle

Augment Qi, supplement the Blood and relieve Toxicity.

Prescription ingredients

Huang Qi (Radix Astragali seu Hedysari) 15g
Jiao Bai Zhu (Rhizoma Atractylodis Macrocephalae, scorch-fried) 10g
Dang Gui (Radix Angelicae Sinensis) 10g
Jin Yin Hua (Flos Lonicerae) 15g
Pu Gong Ying (Herba Taraxaci cum Radice) 10g

Chen Pi (Pericarpium Citri Reticulatac) 10g
Zao Jiao Ci (Spina Gleditsiae Sinensis) 6g
Gan Cao (Radix Glycyrrhizae) 6g
Fu Ling (Sclerotium Poriae Cocos) 10g
Yi Yi Ren (Semen Coicis Lachryma-jobi) 15g

3. **Deng** combined treatment based on pattern identification with an external application. [8]

- **Stagnation of Damp-Heat**

This pattern is present at the initial stage of ulceration with exuberant pathogenic factors and strong Vital Qi (Zheng Qi).

Treatment principle

Clear Heat and benefit the movement of Dampness, transform stagnation and free the network vessels.

Prescription ingredients

Huang Bai (Cortex Phellodendri) 10g
Cang Zhu (Rhizoma Atractylodis) 10g
Yi Yi Ren (Semen Coicis Lachryma-jobi) 15g
Bi Xie (Rhizoma Dioscoreae Hypoglaucae seu Septemlobae) 10g
Fu Ling (Sclerotium Poriae Cocos) 10g
Ze Xie (Rhizoma Alismatis Orientalis) 15g
Chi Xiao Dou (Semen Phaseoli Calcarati) 15g
Che Qian Zi (Semen Plantaginis) 15g
Pu Gong Ying (Herba Taraxaci cum Radice) 10g
Ban Zhi Lian (Herba Scutellariae Barbatae) 15g
Bai Hua She She Cao (Herba Hedyotidis Diffusae) 30g
Mu Dan Pi (Cortex Moutan Radicis) 10g
Niu Xi (Radix Achyranthis Bidentatae) 10g
Ze Lan (Herba Lycopi Lucidi) 10g
Dan Shen (Radix Salviae Miltiorrhizae) 10g

- **Qi Deficiency and Blood stasis**

This pattern is present in the later stages of ulceration, with persistent non-healing sores.

Treatment principle

Augment Qi and fortify the Spleen, nourish Ying Qi (Nutritive Qi) and harmonize the Blood.

Prescription ingredients

Dang Shen (Radix Codonopsitis Pilosulae) 10g
Bai Zhu (Rhizoma Atractylodis Macrocephalae) 10g
Fu Ling (Sclerotium Poriae Cocos) 10g
Huang Qi (Radix Astragali seu Hedysari) 15g
Shan Yao (Radix Dioscoreae Oppositae) 10g
Bai Bian Dou (Semen Dolichoris Lablab) 10g
Yi Yi Ren (Semen Coicis Lachryma-jobi) 15g
Chen Pi (Pericarpium Citri Reticulatae) 10g
Dang Gui (Radix Angelicae Sinensis) 10g
Dan Shen (Radix Salviae Miltiorrhizae) 10g
Hong Hua (Flos Carthami Tinctorii) 10g

Ji Xue Teng (Caulis Spatholobi) 15g
Chuan Xiong (Rhizoma Ligustici Chuanxiong) 10g
Ze Lan (Herba Lycopi Lucidi) 10g

External application

Da Huang (Radix et Rhizoma Rhei) 50g
Bai Lian (Radix Ampelopsis Japonicae) 30g
Di Yu (Radix Sanguisorbae Officinalis) 30g
Bai Zhi (Radix Angelicae Dahuricae) 30g
Er Cha (Pasta Acaciae seu Uncariae) 30g
Qing Dai (Indigo Naturalis) 20g
Xue Jie (Resina Draconis) 20g
Bing Pian (Borneolum) 10g

The ingredients were ground into a fine powder and applied to the lesions, which were then dressed with gauze prepared with *Tie Gu San Gao* (Iron Hoop Powder Paste). *Bai Ji* (Rhizoma Bletillae Striatae) 50g and *Zhen Zhu Fen*‡ (Pearl Powder) 30g were added for non-healing ulcers. The powder was applied once a day until the lesions healed.

SINGLE EMPIRICAL PRESCRIPTION

Li treated ecthyma with *Shen Miao Tang* (Mysterious Spirit Decoction). [9]

Prescription ingredients

Jin Yin Hua (Flos Lonicerae) 30g
Yi Yi Ren (Semen Coicis Lachryma-jobi) 30g
Lian Qiao (Fructus Forsythiae Suspensae) 12g
Fu Ling (Sclerotium Poriae Cocos) 12g
Ze Xie (Rhizoma Alismatis Orientalis) 9g
Chao Cang Zhu (Rhizoma Atractylodis, stir-fried) 9g
Chao Huang Bai (Cortex Phellodendri, stir-fried) 9g
Niu Xi (Radix Achyranthis Bidentatae) 9g
Fang Ji* (Radix Stephaniae Tetrandrae) 9g
Qin Jiao (Radix Gentianae Macrophyllae) 9g
Dang Gui (Radix Angelicae Sinensis) 9g
Chi Shao (Radix Paeoniae Rubra) 9g

Modifications

1. For severe itching, *Fang Feng* (Radix Ledebouriellae Divaricatae) was added.
2. For non-healing of sores after discharge of pus, *Ze Xie* (Rhizoma Alismatis Orientalis) was removed and *Huang Qi* (Radix Astragali seu Hedysari) added.

One bag was used to prepare a decoction, taken twice a day. Results were seen after 5-70 bags.

Folliculitis
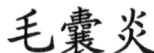

Folliculitis is an inflammation of the hair follicles caused by infection (coagulase-positive staphylococci) or physical or chemical irritation. The most common form of superficial folliculitis is idiopathic. More serious forms of folliculitis involve the deep portion of the hair follicle, are usually more symptomatic, and may cause scarring.

In TCM, folliculitis is also known as *fa ji chuang* (hairline sore).

Clinical manifestations

- The primary lesion in folliculitis is a papule or pustule with a central hair, which may not always be seen.
- A gridlike pattern of multiple red papules and/or pustules on hair-bearing areas of the body may occur.
- Typical body sites affected are the face, scalp, thighs, axillae, and inguinal area.
- Patients experience burning pain or itching in the affected area.

- Folliculitis involving an eyelash is called a hordeolum or stye.
- Deep folliculitis inflames the entire follicular structure and tends to be more symptomatic.
- Healing may result in formation of keloids, or in atrophic scars with alopecia.

Differential diagnosis

Folliculitis decalvans

Folliculitis decalvans on the hairline is very similar to *fa ji chuang* (hairline sore); however, it heals to leave patchy alopecia where the hair never regrows.

Furuncles (boils)

Furuncles form in adjacent hair follicles and are more deeply located than the lesions of folliculitis. Furuncles are usually relatively large, firm and swollen. They have a shiny, tight surface, and are red, hot and painful. When mature, there is a necrotic core in the center. Upon rupture and discharge of the abscess, they have a crater-like appearance.

Etiology and pathology

Retention of Damp-Heat internally

This pattern is often seen in people with an improper diet such as overintake of greasy or sweet food, which impairs the functions of the Spleen, or in people who are overweight and therefore have profuse Dampness and Phlegm. Pathogenic Dampness combines with Heat in the flesh, and when this is complicated by an invasion of external Wind, exuberant Wind-Heat or Damp-Heat moves upward or outward to cause the disease.

Hyperactivity of Fire due to Blood Deficiency

Constitutional Deficiency results in hyperactivity of Fire in the Heart channel due to Blood Deficiency. Vital Qi (Zheng Qi) is too weak to defeat pathogenic factors, giving rise to repeated attacks of folliculitis that may persist for years without healing. Where Vital Qi (Zheng Qi) cannot ward off pathogenic factors, Damp-Heat Toxins may also attack and obstruct the channels and network vessels, leading to a proliferation of sores and boils that are hard to treat.

Pattern identification and treatment

INTERNAL TREATMENT

EXUBERANT WIND-HEAT TOXINS

This pattern has an acute onset. Numerous red papules with pustular or papulopustular heads appear on the posterior hairline or other hair-bearing areas of the body. Areolae surround the lesions. A local burning sensation or pain and itching may occur. Accompanying symptoms and signs include dry throat, thirst, constipation, and short voidings of yellow urine. The tongue body is red with a thin, yellow coating; the pulse is rapid, or slippery and rapid.

Treatment principle

Dredge Wind, clear Heat and relieve Toxicity.

Prescription
SHENG MA XIAO DU YIN JIA JIAN

Bugbane Beverage for Relieving Toxicity, with modifications

Sheng Ma (Rhizoma Cimicifugae) 6g
Qiang Huo (Rhizoma et Radix Notopterygii) 6g
Fang Feng (Radix Ledebouriellae Divaricatae) 6g
Bai Zhi (Radix Angelicae Dahuricae) 6g
Jie Geng (Radix Platycodi Grandiflori) 6g
Gan Cao (Radix Glycyrrhizae) 6g
Jin Yin Hua (Flos Lonicerae) 10g
Lian Qiao (Fructus Forsythiae Suspensae) 10g
Chi Shao (Radix Paeoniae Rubra) 10g

Dang Gui (Radix Angelicae Sinensis) 10g
Chao Niu Bang Zi (Fructus Arctii Lappae, stir-fried) 10g
Tian Hua Fen (Radix Trichosanthis) 10g
Ye Ju Hua (Flos Chrysanthemi Indici) 12g
Chong Lou (Rhizoma Paridis) 12g

Explanation

- *Sheng Ma* (Rhizoma Cimicifugae), *Qiang Huo* (Rhizoma et Radix Notopterygii), *Fang Feng* (Radix Ledebouriellae Divaricatae), and *Chao Niu Bang Zi* (Fructus Arctii Lappae, stir-fried) dredge Wind and clear Heat.
- *Jin Yin Hua* (Flos Lonicerae), *Lian Qiao* (Fructus Forsythiae Suspensae), *Ye Ju Hua* (Flos Chrysanthemi Indici), and *Chong Lou* (Rhizoma Paridis) relieve Toxicity and dissipate lumps.
- *Gan Cao* (Radix Glycyrrhizae) clears Heat and relieves Toxicity.
- *Bai Zhi* (Radix Angelicae Dahuricae), *Jie Geng* (Radix Platycodi Grandiflori), *Dang Gui* (Radix Angelicae Sinensis), and *Tian Hua Fen* (Radix Trichosanthis) eliminate pathogenic factors from the interior, expel pus, dissipate lumps, and alleviate pain.
- *Chi Shao* (Radix Paeoniae Rubra) dissipates Blood stasis and disperses swelling to alleviate pain.

DAMP-HEAT BINDING TO PRODUCE TOXINS

Successive crops of lesions (pustules or occasionally papulopustules) develop, often located on the posterior hairline. Crusts form after the pus drains. The tongue body is red with a yellow and greasy coating; the pulse is slippery, or slippery and rapid.

Treatment principle

Clear Heat and eliminate Dampness, dissipate Wind and relieve Toxicity.

Prescription
FENG FANG SAN JIA JIAN

Hornet Nest Powder, with modifications

Feng Fang‡ (Nidus Vespae) 6g
Ze Xie (Rhizoma Alismatis Orientalis) 12g
Zi Hua Di Ding (Herba Violae Yedoensitis) 12g
Chi Fu Ling (Sclerotium Poriae Cocos Rubrae) 12g
Chi Shao (Radix Paeoniae Rubra) 12g
Jin Yin Hua (Flos Lonicerae) 15g
Pu Gong Ying (Herba Taraxaci cum Radice) 15g
Qiang Huo (Rhizoma et Radix Notopterygii) 4.5g
Tu Bei Mu (Tuber Bolbostemmatis) 10g
Sheng Ma (Rhizoma Cimicifugae) 10g

Explanation

- *Zi Hua Di Ding* (Herba Violae Yedoensitis), *Chi Fu Ling* (Sclerotium Poriae Cocos Rubrae), *Ze Xie*

416 DERMATOLOGY IN TRADITIONAL CHINESE MEDICINE

(Rhizoma Alismatis Orientalis), *Qiang Huo* (Rhizoma et Radix Notopterygii), and *Sheng Ma* (Rhizoma Cimicifugae) dissipate Wind, transform Blood stasis and disperse swelling to treat Heat Toxins.

- *Feng Fang* ‡ (Nidus Vespae), *Jin Yin Hua* (Flos Lonicerae), *Pu Gong Ying* (Herba Taraxaci cum Radice), *Chi Shao* (Radix Paeoniae Rubra), and *Tu Bei Mu* (Rhizoma Bolbostemmatis) relieve Toxicity, expel pus and dissipate lumps.

- *Feng Fang* ‡ (Nidus Vespae) is especially recommended for persistent folliculitis that is difficult to heal because of its effectiveness in dissipating Wind and relieving Toxicity.

RETENTION OF PATHOGENIC FACTORS DUE TO DEFICIENCY OF VITAL QI (ZHENG QI)

This pattern occurs in cases of depletion and damage to Qi and Blood due to constitutional Deficiency, and manifests as a pallid complexion, pale lesions capped by pustules and slight pain. Lesions usually involve the head, are often recurrent and may persist for years. Accompanying symptoms and signs include difficulty in getting to sleep and palpitations. The tongue body is pale red, possibly with stasis marks; the pulse is thready and rapid.

Treatment principle
Augment Qi and draw out Toxins.

Prescription
TUO LI XIAO DU SAN JIA JIAN
Powder for Drawing Out Toxins from the Interior, with modifications

Huang Qi (Radix Astragali seu Hedysari) 12g
Dang Shen (Radix Codonopsitis Pilosulae) 12g
Mai Men Dong (Radix Ophiopogonis Japonici) 12g
*Shi Hu** (Herba Dendrobii) 12g
Chong Lou (Rhizoma Paridis) 12g
Dang Gui (Radix Angelicae Sinensis) 12g
Zi Hua Di Ding (Herba Violae Yedoensitis) 15g
Pu Gong Ying (Herba Taraxaci cum Radice) 15g
Jin Yin Hua (Flos Lonicerae) 15g
Bai Hua She She Cao (Herba Hedyotidis Diffusae) 15g
Sheng Di Huang (Radix Rehmanniae Glutinosae) 10g
Zhe Bei Mu (Bulbus Fritillariae Thunbergii) 10g
Chen Pi (Pericarpium Citri Reticulatae) 10g
Tian Men Dong (Radix Asparagi Cochinchinensis) 10g

Explanation
- *Dang Shen* (Radix Codonopsitis Pilosulae), *Huang Qi* (Radix Astragali seu Hedysari) and *Dang Gui* (Radix Angelicae Sinensis) augment Qi.
- *Tian Men Dong* (Radix Asparagi Cochinchinensis),

Mai Men Dong (Radix Ophiopogonis Japonici), *Shi Hu** (Herba Dendrobii), and *Sheng Di Huang* (Radix Rehmanniae Glutinosae) enrich Yin.

- *Chong Lou* (Rhizoma Paridis), *Zi Hua Di Ding* (Herba Violae Yedoensitis), *Pu Gong Ying* (Herba Taraxaci cum Radice), *Jin Yin Hua* (Flos Lonicerae), and *Bai Hua She She Cao* (Herba Hedyotidis Diffusae) clear Heat and relieve Toxicity.

- *Zhe Bei Mu* (Bulbus Fritillariae Thunbergii) and *Chen Pi* (Pericarpium Citri Reticulatae) expel pus and dissipate lumps.

EXTERNAL TREATMENT

- At the initial stage, with local redness, swelling and pain, apply *Yuan Hua Shui Xi Ji* (Genkwa Wash Preparation) or *Cang Fu Shui Xi Ji* (Atractylodes and Broom Cypress Wash Preparation) externally once a day.

- For red and swollen lesions before rupture, use one of the following as an external application once a day – *Leng Shui Dan* (Cold Water Special Pill), *Fu Rong Gao* (Cotton Rose Flower Paste), *Tie Gu San Gao* (Iron Hoop Powder Paste), or *Xiao Yan Gao* (Paste for Dispersing Inflammation).

- Medicated powders such as *Er Bai San* (Two Whites Powder), *Ru Yi Jin Huang San* (Agreeable Golden Yellow Powder) or *Yu Lu San* (Jade Dew Powder) can be used for all types of folliculitis. Mix into a paste with an appropriate quantity of vegetable oil, *Dan Huang You* (Egg Yolk Oil) or vinegar and apply directly to the affected area two or three times a day.

ACUPUNCTURE
Main points: GV-14 Dazhui, GV-13 Taodao, GB-20 Fengchi, BL-10 Tianzhu, GB-12 Wangu, and Xinjian (located 1.5 cun lateral to the space between C₄ and C₅).
Auxiliary points: BL-65 Shugu, GB-43 Xiaxi, BL-67 Zhiyin, BL-64 Jinggu, GB-40 Qiuxu, GB-44 Zuqiaoyin, GB-41 Zulinqi, and BL-66 Zutonggu.
Technique: Apply the reducing method to the points. Retain the needles for 30 minutes after obtaining Qi. Treat once every one or two days. A course consists of seven treatment sessions.

Explanation
- The main points dredge Wind and clear Heat, relieve Toxicity and dissipate lumps.
- The auxiliary points, all located on the foot, dissipate Heat, relieve Toxicity and disperse swelling.

MOXIBUSTION
Points: Ashi points (the site of the lesions).
Technique: Cover the Ashi point with 0.2 cm thick slices of garlic and place a moxa cone on top of each

garlic slice. Burn ten moxa cones each time at each Ashi point. Treat once a day. A course consists of ten treatment sessions.

Indications: This treatment is recommended for chronic folliculitis.

COMBINED ACUPUNCTURE AND MOXIBUSTION

Points: GB-20 Fengchi, LI-11 Quchi and BL-40 Weizhong.

Technique: Apply the reducing method to the points. After withdrawing the needles, heat the affected area with a moxa stick for 15-20 minutes. Treat once a day. A course consists of ten treatment sessions.

EAR ACUPUNCTURE

Points: Occiput, Ear-Shenmen, Adrenal Gland, and Heart.

Technique: Retain needles in the ear points for 30-60 minutes each time. Treat once a day.

COMBINED BLEEDING AND FIRE-CUPPING TREATMENT

Point: BL-40 Weizhong.

Technique: Use a filiform needle to prick BL-40 Weizhong to cause bleeding. Then apply fire-cupping to the point, leaving the cup in place for 10 minutes. Alternatively, prick some points around ruptured pustules, and apply the same cupping method. Treat once every two or three days.

Clinical notes

- If folliculitis involves the back of the neck in overweight patients, it is generally due to Damp-Heat binding to produce Toxins. Treatment with *Feng Fang San* (Hornet Nest Powder) is recommended (see above).

- For stubborn or recurrent folliculitis or folliculitis characterized by severe pain, moxibustion treatment or combined bleeding and fire-cupping treatment are recommended. Both methods help to relieve symptoms and shorten the time required for treatment.

- Combining external with internal treatment can help to reduce pain and accelerate the healing process, regardless of whether there is only local redness and pain or whether pustules have already formed.

- In some cases, individual lesions of folliculitis may coalesce into plaques; small patches of alopecia may be left when the lesions heal.

- The possibility of latent diabetes should be considered for patients with persistent folliculitis.

Case history

Patient
Male, aged 33.

Clinical manifestations
The patient had suffered from folliculitis on the back of the neck for 10 years. He had tried several types of treatment, and although each one worked temporarily, the folliculitis would recur the following year, being particularly bad in the summer and autumn.

Physical examination indicated that the posterior hairline on the neck was red and swollen. There were several discrete red or dark red follicular papules 2-3 mm in diameter with a central hair. Some had already become pustules.

Diagnosis
Chronic folliculitis.

Treatment
Moxibustion on garlic at Ashi points (the lesions). Three to five cones were burnt at each point. For the first six days of treatment, the patient felt no pain when the moxa cones were burnt. From the seventh day of treatment onward, the patient felt pain after two-thirds of each moxa cone was burnt.

Outcome
After one course of ten sessions, the inflammation was relieved. The pustules ruptured, but the necrotic core was difficult to drain. After a second course of ten treatment sessions, the 0.5 cm deep necrotic core was finally drained, after which the patient did not feel any pain locally. Following a third course of treatment, the lesions dried up and were covered by a crust. Follow-up visits over the next five years indicated no recurrence of the disease. [10]

Literature excerpt

In *Liu Juan Zi Gui Yi Fang* [Liu Juanzi's Remedies Left Behind by Ghosts], it says: "Millet-like sores, white at the top and red at the base, grow along the hairline. There is severe stabbing pain. For folliculitis with sudden onset, small lesions, abscesses, pain, and itching, treatment is relatively straightforward; folliculitis with repeated onset and long duration tends to be chronic and treatment is difficult."

Modern clinical experience

INTERNAL TREATMENT

1. **Zhu** differentiated folliculitis into Excess or Deficiency patterns. [11]

- **Excess patterns**

Treatment principle
Dissipate Blood stasis and relieve Toxicity.

Prescription
XIAO YAN FANG
Formula for Dispersing Inflammation

Huang Lian (Rhizoma Coptidis) 6g
Gan Cao (Radix Glycyrrhizae) 6g
Huang Qin (Radix Scutellariae Baicalensis) 10g
Mu Dan Pi (Cortex Moutan Radicis) 10g
Chi Shao (Radix Paeoniae Rubra) 10g
Jin Yin Hua (Flos Lonicerae) 10g
Chong Lou (Rhizoma Paridis) 10g
Lian Qiao (Fructus Forsythiae Suspensae) 10g
Xiao Bo (Radix seu Caulis Berberidis) 9g

• **Deficiency patterns**

Treatment principle
Support Vital Qi (Zheng Qi) and draw out Toxins.

Prescription
TUO LI XIAO DU SAN
Powder for Drawing Out Toxins from the Interior

Huang Qi (Radix Astragali seu Hedysari) 10g
Dang Shen (Radix Codonopsitis Pilosulae) 10g
Tian Men Dong (Radix Asparagi Cochinchinensis) 10g
Mai Men Dong (Radix Ophiopogonis Japonici) 10g
*Shi Hu** (Herba Dendrobii) 10g
Zi Hua Di Ding (Herba Violae Yedoensitis) 10g
Ye Ju Hua (Flos Chrysanthemi Indici) 10g
Xiao Bo (Radix seu Caulis Berberidis) 10g
Sheng Di Huang (Radix Rehmanniae Glutinosae) 30g

For both patterns, one bag a day was used to prepare a decoction, taken twice a day for 14 days.

2. **Qian** held that folliculitis was caused by Damp-Heat together with an external invasion of Wind-Fire. [12]

Prescription
YUE BI TANG JIA WEI
Maidservant from Yue Decoction, with additions

*Ma Huang** (Herba Ephedrae) 6g
Shi Gao ‡ (Gypsum Fibrosum) 20g
Gan Cao (Radix Glycyrrhizae) 10g
Da Zao (Fructus Ziziphi Jujubae) 10g
Sheng Jiang (Rhizoma Zingiberis Officinalis Recens) 6g
Zi Hua Di Ding (Herba Violae Yedoensitis) 15g
Chong Lou (Rhizoma Paridis) 10g

One bag a day was used to prepare a decoction, taken twice a day. Improvement was usually seen within one week of treatment.

EXTERNAL TREATMENT

1. **Xu Lühe** used *Huang Xiang Bing* (Phellodendron Bark and Frankincense Cake), made by mixing powdered *Huang Bai* (Cortex Phellodendri) 30g and *Ru Xiang* (Gummi Olibanum) 9g into a paste with a decoction prepared with *Huai Hua* (Flos Sophorae Japonicae) 3g. The paste was applied externally once or twice a day. [13]

2. **Shi Hanzhang** recommended *Feng Fang You Gao* (Hornet Nest Oil Paste). [14]

Prescription ingredients
Feng Fang ‡ (Nidus Vespae) 20g
Xue Yu ‡ (Crinis Hominis) 15g
Xiang You (Oleum Sesami Seminis) 50g
Mi La ‡ (Cera) 10g

Method
Feng Fang ‡ (Nidus Vespae) and *Xue Yu* ‡ (Crinis Hominis) were calcined and ground into a fine powder. *Xiang You* (Oleum Sesami Seminis) was then brought to the boil, *Mi La* ‡ (Cera) melted in it, and the powdered ingredients added. The paste was applied to the lesions as a compress. The dressing was changed every day. The author of the report has used this paste in his practice for many years and has found it to be effective.

3. **Xiang** treated folliculitis with a rub preparation. [15]

Prescription
SAN HUANG CHA JI
Three Yellows Rub Preparation

Huang Lian (Rhizoma Coptidis) 15g
Huang Bai (Cortex Phellodendri) 12g
Da Huang (Radix et Rhizoma Rhei) 30g
Jin Yin Hua (Flos Lonicerae) 30g

The ingredients were ground to a powder, added to 500ml of water and cooked over a mild heat to obtain 100-150ml of a decoction, which was rubbed over the affected area. The treatment was given three to five times per day.

Folliculitis decalvans
脱发性毛囊炎

Folliculitis decalvans is a destructive type of folliculitis, which results in permanent hair loss on healing. Most patients have seborrhea or have a long history of seborrheic eczema.

Clinical manifestations

- Folliculitis decalvans usually occurs in young people.
- The condition predominantly affects the hair-bearing scalp, but may also involve places where beard, pubic and axillary hair grows.
- The lesion starts with follicular erythema or a papule and later becomes a pustule. A round or elliptical scar is left on healing of the lesion. Discrete erythema, pustules or cicatricial baldness may develop around the scar.
- Patients experience local itching. The disease is prolonged, persisting for years or even decades.

Differential diagnosis

Folliculitis decalvans must be distinguished from scarring baldness resulting from other diseases such as favus, lichen planus, cutaneous lupus erythematosus, and lupus vulgaris barbae. Identification of the fungi causing favus will identify baldness resulting from this disease, and biopsy will distinguish baldness resulting from the other conditions.

Etiology and pathology

Damp-Heat brewing to produce Toxins
Overeating of fatty, greasy, sweet, or spicy foods or excessive alcohol consumption will lead to Dampness accumulating internally. If Dampness is retained in the body for a long period, it will transform into Heat. When the pathogenic factors move up to the head, folliculitis decalvans occurs.

Heat accumulating in the Heart and Liver channels
Internal damage due to the seven emotions can lead to hyperactivity of Liver-Fire, eventually resulting in exuberant Heat accumulating in the Heart and Liver channels. When Heat scorches upward to the head, it can cause folliculitis decalvans.

Pattern identification and treatment

INTERNAL TREATMENT

DAMP-HEAT BREWING TO PRODUCE TOXINS
At the initial stage, miliaria-like papules appear on the scalp with a central hair, a surrounding red erythematous halo and a pustular head. Accompanying symptoms and signs include local itching and pain, a feeling of oppression in the chest, poor appetite, irregular bowel movements, and yellow or reddish urine. The tongue body is red with a thin, yellow and greasy coating; the pulse is slippery and rapid.

Treatment principle
Clear Heat and benefit the movement of Dampness, relieve Toxicity and dispel pathogenic factors.

Prescription
CHU SHI JIE DU TANG JIA JIAN
Decoction for Eliminating Dampness and Relieving Toxicity, with modifications

Huang Qin (Radix Scutellariae Baicalensis) 10g
Niu Bang Zi (Fructus Arctii Lappae) 10g
Lian Qiao (Fructus Forsythiae Suspensae) 10g
Liu Yi San (Six-To-One Powder) 10g, wrapped
Long Dan Cao (Radix Gentianae Scabrae) 10g
Ze Xie (Rhizoma Alismatis Orientalis) 12g
Jin Yin Hua (Flos Lonicerae) 15g
Chi Fu Ling (Sclerotium Poriae Cocos Rubrae) 15g
Bai Zhi (Radix Angelicae Dahuricae) 6g
Qiang Huo (Rhizoma et Radix Notopterygii) 6g

Explanation
- *Huang Qin* (Radix Scutellariae Baicalensis), *Lian Qiao* (Fructus Forsythiae Suspensae) and *Jin Yin Hua* (Flos Lonicerae) drain Fire and relieve Toxicity with cold and bitterness.
- *Long Dan Cao* (Radix Gentianae Scabrae), *Chi Fu Ling* (Sclerotium Poriae Cocos Rubrae), *Ze Xie* (Rhizoma Alismatis Orientalis), and *Liu Yi San* (Six-To-One Powder) benefit the movement of Dampness, clear Heat and relieve Toxicity.
- *Niu Bang Zi* (Fructus Arctii Lappae), *Bai Zhi* (Radix Angelicae Dahuricae) and *Qiang Huo* (Rhizoma et Radix Notopterygii) dredge Wind, disperse swelling and alleviate pain.

HEAT ACCUMULATING IN THE HEART AND LIVER CHANNELS

The 5-10 mm lesions have an inflammatory halo and ooze pus and blood. Accompanying symptoms and signs include irritability, dry mouth with a desire for cold drinks, constipation, and reddish urine. The tongue body is deep red with a scant coating; the pulse is wiry and rapid.

Treatment principle
Cool the Blood and relieve Toxicity

Prescription
LIANG XUE JIE DU TANG JIA JIAN
Decoction for Cooling the Blood and Relieving Toxicity, with modifications

Chao Zhi Zi (Fructus Gardeniae Jasminoidis, stir-fried) 10g
Chao Long Dan Cao (Radix Gentianae Scabrae, stir-fried) 10g
Chao Mu Dan Pi (Cortex Moutan Radicis, stir-fried) 10g
Chi Shao (Radix Paeoniae Rubra) 10g
Pu Gong Ying (Herba Taraxaci cum Radice) 12g
Ye Ju Hua (Flos Chrysanthemi Indici) 12g
Jin Yin Hua (Flos Lonicerae) 12g
Zhe Bei Mu (Bulbus Fritillariae Thunbergii) 12g
Lian Qiao (Fructus Forsythiae Suspensae) 12g
Sheng Di Huang (Radix Rehmanniae Glutinosae) 30g
Zi Hua Di Ding (Herba Violae Yedoensitis) 15g

Explanation

- *Chao Zhi Zi* (Fructus Gardeniae Jasminoidis, stir-fried), *Chao Long Dan Cao* (Radix Gentianae Scabrae, stir-fried), *Chao Mu Dan Pi* (Cortex Moutan Radicis, stir-fried), *Chi Shao* (Radix Paeoniae Rubra), and *Sheng Di Huang* (Radix Rehmanniae Glutinosae) cool the Blood and relieve Toxicity to disperse swelling and reduce inflammation.

- *Pu Gong Ying* (Herba Taraxaci cum Radice), *Jin Yin Hua* (Flos Lonicerae), *Lian Qiao* (Fructus Forsythiae Suspensae), *Ye Ju Hua* (Flos Chrysanthemi Indici), *Zhe Bei Mu* (Bulbus Fritillariae Thunbergii), and *Zi Hua Di Ding* (Herba Violae Yedoensitis) relieve Toxicity, disperse swelling and dissipate lumps.

EXTERNAL TREATMENT

Apply *Yuan Hua Shui Xi Ji* (Genkwa Wash Preparation) to the affected area or prepare a decoction with the following ingredients for use a wash or wet compress:

Cang Er Zi (Fructus Xanthii Sibirici) 60g
Ku Shen (Radix Sophorae Flavescentis) 10g
Lu Lu Tong (Fructus Liquidambaris) 10g

Ming Fan‡ (Alumen) 10g
Huang Bai (Cortex Phellodendri) 15g

ACUPUNCTURE

Main points: GV-14 Dazhui, LI-11 Quchi, LI-4 Hegu, and TB-5 Waiguan.
Auxiliary points: ST-36 Zusanli, GB-20 Fengchi, BL-40 Weizhong, GB-41 Zulinqi, GB-40 Qiuxu, and BL-60 Kunlun.
Technique: Apply the reducing method. Retain the needles for 15-30 minutes after obtaining Qi. Treat once a day. A course consists of seven treatment sessions.

Explanation

- GV-14 Dazhui, GB-20 Fengchi, LI-4 Hegu, and TB-5 Waiguan dissipate Wind and disperse swelling.
- BL-40 Weizhong, LI-11 Quchi and BL-60 Kunlun clear Fire and drain Toxicity.
- ST-36 Zusanli, GB-41 Zulinqi and GB-40 Qiuxu relieve Toxicity to alleviate pain.

MOXIBUSTION

Points: GV-14 Dazhui or over the lesions.
Technique: Cover the points with 0.2 cm thick slices of garlic and place a moxa cone on top of each garlic slice. Burn ten moxa cones each time at each point. Treat once a day. A course consists of ten treatment sessions.

Clinical notes

- Treatment should start immediately symptoms appear in order to prevent permanent baldness. Internal administration of Chinese materia medica combined with moxibustion increases the effectiveness of the treatment.
- Treat pustules as soon as possible to prevent the formation of scars; this is crucial to preventing permanent baldness.
- Wet compresses with a decoction of *Yuan Hua Shui Xi Ji* (Genkwa Wash Preparation) disperse swelling and alleviate pain.

Advice for the patient

- Hygiene of the scalp is important. Wash the hair regularly.
- Avoid spicy, rich, greasy, and sweet foods, and do not drink alcohol.

Sycosis barbae
须疮

Sycosis barbae is a suppurative folliculitis that often affects the beard and moustache areas. In TCM, it is also known as *yang hu chuang* (beard sore).

Clinical manifestations

- Sycosis most commonly affects men aged 30 to 40.
- Lesions start with an edematous erythema, progressing to papule or pustule formation around a hair follicle. After the pustule ruptures, it will dry to form a crust.
- The lesions often go through a chronic cyclical process, during which old lesions heal while new ones grow.
- Patients experience a local sensation of burning or itching.

Differential diagnosis

Tinea barbae

Tinea develops slowly in contrast to folliculitis. Follicular fungal infection is usually limited to one area of the beard. The main manifestations include grouped pustules, edema, infiltration, and obvious inflammation. Although this resembles sycosis barbae, microscopy will show fungi.

Etiology and pathology

Damp and Heat Toxins

Frequent overindulgence in rich, greasy and spicy foods, and excessive alcohol consumption leads to impairment of the Spleen's transformation and transportation function. This causes Dampness and Heat to accumulate and bind, and when they spread outward to the skin and flesh, moist lesions result. In more severe cases, retained Dampness may be transformed into Heat; exuberant Heat putrefies the flesh, leading to the formation of pustules.

Phlegm and Blood stasis binding

Exuberant Dampness accumulates in the Middle Burner and impairs the Spleen's transformation and transportation function, leading to the collection of water and Dampness and the formation of Phlegm, which binds with Blood stasis caused by the persistence of the condition.

Pattern identification and treatment

INTERNAL TREATMENT

EXUBERANT HEAT TOXINS

This pattern manifests as patches of inflamed red skin on the lower jaw with groups of pustules. Local pain and itching are experienced. The tongue body is red with a thin yellow coating; the pulse is wiry and rapid.

Treatment principle

Clear Heat and relieve Toxicity, fortify the Spleen and dry Dampness.

Prescription

QIN ZHI PING WEI SAN JIA JIAN
Scutellaria and Gardenia Powder for Calming the Stomach, with modifications

Huang Qin (Radix Scutellariae Baicalensis) 10g
Chao Mu Dan Pi (Cortex Moutan Radicis, stir-fried) 10g
Chi Fu Ling (Sclerotium Poriae Cocos Rubrae) 10g
Jiao Zhi Zi (Fructus Gardeniae Jasminoidis, scorch-fried) 10g
Sheng Di Huang (Radix Rehmanniae Glutinosae) 15g
Chao Zhi Ke (Fructus Citri Aurantii, stir-fried) 6g
Hou Po (Cortex Magnoliae Officinalis) 6g
Cang Zhu (Rhizoma Atractylodis) 6g
Chen Pi (Pericarpium Citri Reticulatae) 6g
Sheng Ma (Rhizoma Cimicifugae) 4.5g
Bai Hua She She Cao (Herba Hedyotidis Diffusae) 30g
Yin Chen Hao (Herba Artemisiae Scopariae) 30g

Explanation

- *Huang Qin* (Radix Scutellariae Baicalensis), *Jiao Zhi Zi* (Fructus Gardeniae Jasminoidis, scorch-fried), *Chi Fu Ling* (Sclerotium Poriae Cocos Rubrae), and *Yin Chen Hao* (Herba Artemisiae Scopariae) clear Heat and transform Dampness.
- *Cang Zhu* (Rhizoma Atractylodis), *Hou Po* (Cortex Magnoliae Officinalis), *Chao Zhi Ke* (Fructus Citri Aurantii, stir-fried), and *Chen Pi* (Pericarpium Citri Reticulatae) dry Dampness with warmth and acridity.
- *Bai Hua She She Cao* (Herba Hedyotidis Diffusae) relieves Toxicity.
- *Sheng Ma* (Rhizoma Cimicifugae) alleviates itching.
- *Sheng Di Huang* (Radix Rehmanniae Glutinosae) and *Chao Mu Dan Pi* (Cortex Moutan Radicis, stir-fried) cool the Blood and reduce inflammation.

EXUBERANT DAMP TOXINS

This pattern is characterized by a discrete distribution of pustules on inflamed red skin with erosion and exudation. The tongue body is red with a yellow and greasy coating; the pulse is soggy and rapid.

Treatment principle

Benefit the movement of Dampness by bland percolation, clear Heat and relieve Toxicity.

Prescription
DAO CHI SAN JIA JIAN
Powder for Guiding Out Reddish Urine, with modifications

Sheng Di Huang (Radix Rehmanniae Glutinosae) 12-15g
Hua Shi‡ (Talcum) 12-15g, wrapped in He Ye (Folium Nelumbinis Nuciferae) for decoction
Chi Fu Ling (Sclerotium Poriae Cocos Rubrae) 12-15g
Tong Cao (Medulla Tetrapanacis Papyriferi) 6g
Dan Zhu Ye (Herba Lophatheri Gracilis) 6g
Che Qian Cao (Herba Plantaginis) 10g
Che Qian Zi (Semen Plantaginis) 10g
Yin Chen Hao (Herba Artemisiae Scopariae) 30g
Bai Xian Pi (Cortex Dictamni Dasycarpi Radicis) 10g

Explanation

- Hua Shi‡ (Talcum), Chi Fu Ling (Sclerotium Poriae Cocos Rubrae), Tong Cao (Medulla Tetrapanacis Papyriferi), Yin Chen Hao (Herba Artemisiae Scopariae), Che Qian Cao (Herba Plantaginis), Che Qian Zi (Semen Plantaginis), and Dan Zhu Ye (Herba Lophatheri Gracilis) clear Heat and benefit the movement of Dampness.
- Sheng Di Huang (Radix Rehmanniae Glutinosae) and Bai Xian Pi (Cortex Dictamni Dasycarpi Radicis) cool the Blood and relieve Toxicity.

PHLEGM AND BLOOD STASIS BINDING

This condition is chronic with repeated attacks. Papular or pustular lesions come and go. Local stabbing pain is experienced. The tongue body is dark with stasis marks; the pulse is rough.

Treatment principle

Clear Heat and transform Phlegm, invigorate the Blood and dissipate lumps.

Prescription
CHU SHI SAN YU TANG JIA JIAN
Decoction for Eliminating Dampness and Dissipating Blood Stasis, with modifications

Tao Ren (Semen Persicae) 10g
Cang Zhu (Rhizoma Atractylodis) 10g
Chi Shao (Radix Paeoniae Rubra) 10g
Chen Pi (Pericarpium Citri Reticulatae) 10g
Chuan Niu Xi (Radix Cyathulae Officinalis) 10g

Fa Ban Xia (Rhizoma Pinelliae Ternatae Praeparata) 10g
Zhe Bei Mu (Bulbus Fritillariae Thunbergii) 12g
Huang Qi (Radix Astragali seu Hedysari) 12g
Ze Lan (Herba Lycopi Lucidi) 12g
Huang Bai (Cortex Phellodendri) 12g
Dang Gui (Radix Angelicae Sinensis) 6g
Shan Ci Gu (Pseudobulbus Shancigu) 6g

Explanation

- Huang Qi (Radix Astragali seu Hedysari) and Dang Gui (Radix Angelicae Sinensis) augment Qi and invigorate the Blood.
- Tao Ren (Semen Persicae) and Chi Shao (Radix Paeoniae Rubra) transform Blood stasis and dissipate lumps.
- Chuan Niu Xi (Radix Cyathulae Officinalis) and Ze Lan (Herba Lycopi Lucidi) invigorate the Blood and dispel Blood stasis.
- Chen Pi (Pericarpium Citri Reticulatae), Cang Zhu (Rhizoma Atractylodis) and Fa Ban Xia (Rhizoma Pinelliae Ternatae Praeparata) regulate Qi and transform Phlegm.
- Zhe Bei Mu (Bulbus Fritillariae Thunbergii) and Shan Ci Gu (Pseudobulbus Shancigu) dissipate lumps and eliminate scars.
- Huang Bai (Cortex Phellodendri) drains Ministerial Fire.
- As this condition is persistent, the treatment combines supplementing and offensive ingredients.

EXTERNAL TREATMENT

- For pustules or oozing lesions, apply Cang Fu Shui Xi Ji (Atractylodes and Broom Cypress Wash Preparation) as a wet compress once or twice a day.
- If pustules are the main manifestation, mix Qing Bai San (Green-White Powder) to a paste with Xiang You (Oleum Sesami Seminis) and apply externally to the affected area twice a day.

ACUPUNCTURE AND MOXIBUSTION
Points: GB-20 Fengchi, LI-11 Quchi and BL-40 Weizhong
Technique: Apply the reducing method and retain the needles for 30 minutes after obtaining Qi. At the same time, a lit moxa stick can be used over the affected areas on the lower jaw for 10-30 minutes.
Indications: This treatment is particularly recommended for chronic conditions with repeated attacks without obvious erythema.

Explanation

- GB-20 Fengchi and LI-11 Quchi dissipate Wind and eliminate Dampness to alleviate itching.
- BL-40 Weizhong drains Heat and relieves Toxicity to eliminate pain.

- Once itching and pain are alleviated, the lesions will subside.

Clinical notes

- It is important to determine whether Dampness is more predominant than Heat or vice versa and then treat as described above.
- Acupuncture and moxibustion therapy are recommended for chronic, persistent conditions. Treat once every other day. Changes can be expected after three to five treatment sessions.
- Sycosis barbae is often a stubborn condition. Starting treatment at an early stage improves the chances of complete recovery.

Advice for the patient

- Keep the lesion area clean. Avoid touching the beard.

- Avoid sweet, rich, greasy, and spicy foods, and alcohol.

Literature excerpt

In *Wai Ke Yi An Hui Bian* [A Collection of Case Histories Relating to External Diseases], it says: "In the prescription *Qin Lian Ping Wei San* (Scutellaria and Coptis Powder for Calming the Stomach) used to treat *yang hu chuang* (beard sore), ...*Huang Qin* (Radix Scutellariae Baicalensis) and *Huang Lian* (Rhizoma Coptidis) transform Damp-Heat with cold and bitterness. When added to *Ping Wei San* (Calming the Stomach Powder), they act with *Hou Po* (Cortex Magnoliae Officinalis) and *Cang Zhu* (Rhizoma Atractylodis) to dry Dampness, and with *Chen Pi* (Pericarpium Citri Reticulatae) to fortify the Spleen. If the Spleen is strong, Dampness will be expelled; if Heat is cleared, itching will stop. Exudation from the lesions will stop when Dampness is eliminated."

Furuncles (boils) and carbuncles
疖与痈

Furuncles, or boils, are painful, erythematous, papular lesions that are related to a deep infection of the hair follicle. The infecting agent is usually *Staphylococcus aureus*. The condition may evolve from superficial folliculitis. If several adjacent follicles are deeply infected with these bacteria, the lesion becomes a carbuncle. Furuncles and carbuncles are often related to impaired immunity, diabetes, frequent scratching, and friction.

Clinical manifestations

- Furuncles can affect any hair-bearing site, particularly those subject to friction or sweating. They are most common on the neck, axillae, buttocks, groin, anterior thighs, and waist.
- Lesions manifest initially as papules, later growing larger and firmer and becoming red. Tenderness and pain are noted. In two to three days, an abscess will form with a central necrotic core. It crusts and heals within one to two weeks.
- Some cases tend to be chronic with old furuncles healing and new ones growing continuously (furunculosis).

- Where several furuncles join together to form a carbuncle, a swollen, painful, suppurating area will be formed with discharge of pus from different points.
- Common sites for carbuncles include the back of the neck, the upper and lower back, the buttocks, and the lateral thighs.
- Systemic symptoms such as fever and chills may occur when the carbuncle is inflamed.

Differential diagnosis

Cystic acne
This often involves the facial area and the back and chest. The lesion starts with a white or grayish papule (closed comedone) containing white or turbid material, which can be released when the lesion is squeezed. Some patients have multiple lesions, where the papules develop into red or dark red nodules or cysts, located deeper in the skin. The surface of large cysts is fluctuant when palpated.

Hidradenitis suppurativa
Hidradenitis suppurativa is more common in young or middle-aged women, with lesions usually occurring in

the axillae, the groin, the area under the female breast, and the anogenital region. The lesion starts with a tender red subcutaneous nodule, which gradually enlarges; further lesions develop. The overlying skin finally ruptures and a small amount of purulent fluid is discharged. Fistulae may form.

Etiology and pathology

FURUNCLES
Accumulation and binding of Dampness and Fire
Excessive intake of sweet food, which can cause a feeling of fullness in the Middle Burner, and fatty food, which can generate internal Heat, impairs the Spleen's normal transportation function. As a result, Dampness and Fire bind together, accumulating to produce Toxins in the skin.

Blood-Heat due to Yin Deficiency
Patients with wasting and thirsting disease often develop Dryness and Heat of the Zang-Fu organs as well as effulgent Yin Deficiency-Fire. Fire scorches Stomach Yin and the Body Fluids are unable to nourish the skin and flesh properly; the circulation of Ying Qi (Nutritive Qi) and Wei Qi (Defensive Qi) is also impaired. Externally contracted pathogenic Wind-Heat can then invade. The internal and external factors combine and are retained in the skin layer, causing the formation of furuncles.

CARBUNCLES
Carbuncles on the neck are usually due to pathogenic Wind, those on the lower back and hypochondrium to stagnation, and those on the lower limbs to Damp Toxins.

Fire Toxins
Stagnation of Fire Toxins results in binding of Qi and Blood, causing obstruction of the channels and network vessels in the skin and flesh, thus leading to the formation of carbuncles.

Binding Depression of the seven emotions
Binding depression of the emotions results in internal generation of Yin-Fire, which obstructs the channels and network vessels to result in carbuncles.

Pattern identification and treatment

INTERNAL TREATMENT

ACCUMULATION AND BINDING OF DAMPNESS AND FIRE
Sites commonly involved include the neck, back, axillae, and buttocks. Furuncles appear as round, firm nodules, which are initially red, swollen, hot and painful, and later soften with the formation of abscesses with yellow heads; yellow pus exudes on rupture. Accompanying symptoms and signs include fever, thirst, headache, and generalized pain. The tongue body is red with a thin, yellow coating; the pulse is floating and rapid, or soggy and rapid.

Treatment principle
Clear Heat and transform Dampness, relieve Toxicity and dissipate lumps.

Prescription
WU WEI XIAO DU YIN JIA JIAN
Five-Ingredient Beverage for Dispersing Toxicity, with modifications

Ye Ju Hua (Flos Chrysanthemi Indici) 12g
Pu Gong Ying (Herba Taraxaci cum Radice) 12g
Tian Kui Zi (Tuber Semiaquilegiae) 12g
Chi Shao (Radix Paeoniae Rubra) 12g
Jin Yin Hua (Flos Lonicerae) 15g
Dang Gui (Radix Angelicae Sinensis) 10g
Zi Hua Di Ding (Herba Violae Yedoensitis) 10g
Gan Cao (Radix Glycyrrhizae) 10g
Zhe Bei Mu (Bulbus Fritillariae Thunbergii) 6g
Tian Hua Fen (Radix Trichosanthis) 6g

Explanation
- *Ye Ju Hua* (Flos Chrysanthemi Indici), *Pu Gong Ying* (Herba Taraxaci cum Radice), *Jin Yin Hua* (Flos Lonicerae), *Zi Hua Di Ding* (Herba Violae Yedoensitis), and *Tian Kui Zi* (Tuber Semiaquilegiae) clear Heat and relieve Toxicity, transform Dampness and disperse swelling.
- *Gan Cao* (Radix Glycyrrhizae) clears Heat and relieves Toxicity.
- *Chi Shao* (Radix Paeoniae Rubra) and *Dang Gui* (Radix Angelicae Sinensis) invigorate the Blood, alleviate pain and disperse swelling.
- *Zhe Bei Mu* (Bulbus Fritillariae Thunbergii) relieves Toxicity and dissipates lumps.
- *Tian Hua Fen* (Radix Trichosanthis) relieves Toxicity and expels pus.
- This prescription can be used at the initial stage when pathogenic factors are exuberant.

BLOOD-HEAT DUE TO YIN DEFICIENCY
Single swollen boils appear at various body sites, or are confined to one location. Lesions appear successively and tend to persist. Dull red abscesses form slowly. Accompanying symptoms and signs include dry mouth, swift digestion with rapid hungering, irritability, insomnia, and yellow or reddish urine. The tongue body is red with a scant coating; the pulse is deficient and rapid.

Treatment principle

Enrich Yin and clear Heat, support Vital Qi (Zheng Qi) and draw out Toxins.

Prescription

ZI CUI TANG JIA WEI

Enriching the Pancreas Decoction, with additions

Sheng Di Huang (Radix Rehmanniae Glutinosae) 15g
Huang Qi (Radix Astragali seu Hedysari) 15g
Nan Sha Shen (Radix Adenophorae) 15g
Bei Sha Shen (Radix Glehniae Littoralis) 15g
Pu Gong Ying (Herba Taraxaci cum Radice) 15g
Jin Yin Hua (Flos Lonicerae) 15g
Shan Yao (Radix Dioscoreae Oppositae) 30g
Shan Zhu Yu (Fructus Corni Officinalis) 12g
Xuan Shen (Radix Scrophulariae Ningpoensis) 12g
Shi Hu* (Herba Dendrobii) 12g
Tian Men Dong (Radix Asparagi Cochinchinensis) 12g
Mai Men Dong (Radix Ophiopogonis Japonici) 12g
Deng Xin Cao (Medulla Junci Effusi) 6g
Dan Zhu Ye (Herba Lophatheri Gracilis) 6g
Lian Zi Xin (Plumula Nelumbinis Nuciferae) 6g

Explanation

- *Huang Qi* (Radix Astragali seu Hedysari), *Nan Sha Shen* (Radix Adenophorae), *Bei Sha Shen* (Radix Glehniae Littoralis), *Shan Yao* (Radix Dioscoreae Oppositae), *Shan Zhu Yu* (Fructus Corni Officinalis), *Tian Men Dong* (Radix Asparagi Cochinchinensis), *Mai Men Dong* (Radix Ophiopogonis Japonici), *Shi Hu** (Herba Dendrobii), and *Sheng Di Huang* (Radix Rehmanniae Glutinosae) augment Qi and nourish Yin.

- *Pu Gong Ying* (Herba Taraxaci cum Radice), *Jin Yin Hua* (Flos Lonicerae), *Xuan Shen* (Radix Scrophulariae Ningpoensis), *Dan Zhu Ye* (Herba Lophatheri Gracilis), *Deng Xin Cao* (Medulla Junci Effusi), and *Lian Zi Xin* (Plumula Nelumbinis Nuciferae) clear Heat, relieve Toxicity and dissipate lumps.

- This prescription can be used in the later stages of the condition when Vital Qi (Zheng Qi) is Deficient.

WIND-WARMTH FIRE TOXINS

With this pattern, carbuncles appear most often on the neck. Lesions are red, swollen and painful with hard, protruding surfaces. Accompanying symptoms and signs include fever, aversion to cold, headache, reddish urine, and constipation. The tongue body is red with a thin yellow coating; the pulse is floating and rapid.

Treatment principle

Arrest Wind and clear Heat, relieve Toxicity and dissipate lumps.

Prescription

YE JU BAI DU TANG JIA JIAN

Wild Chrysanthemum Decoction for Vanquishing Toxicity, with modifications

Ye Ju Hua (Flos Chrysanthemi Indici) 12g
Pu Gong Ying (Herba Taraxaci cum Radice) 12g
Zi Hua Di Ding (Herba Violae Yedoensitis) 12g
Zhe Bei Mu (Bulbus Fritillariae Thunbergii) 10g
Xuan Shen (Radix Scrophulariae Ningpoensis) 10g
Jie Geng (Radix Platycodi Grandiflori) 10g
Lian Qiao (Fructus Forsythiae Suspensae) 10g
Chi Shao (Radix Paeoniae Rubra) 10g
Gan Cao (Radix Glycyrrhizae) 6g

Explanation

- *Ye Ju Hua* (Flos Chrysanthemi Indici), *Pu Gong Ying* (Herba Taraxaci cum Radice), *Zi Hua Di Ding* (Herba Violae Yedoensitis), *Xuan Shen* (Radix Scrophulariae Ningpoensis), and *Chi Shao* (Radix Paeoniae Rubra) clear Heat, relieve Toxicity and disperse swelling.

- *Zhe Bei Mu* (Bulbus Fritillariae Thunbergii) and *Jie Geng* (Radix Platycodi Grandiflori) dispel Wind and dissipate lumps.

- *Lian Qiao* (Fructus Forsythiae Suspensae) dissipates Wind-Heat and relieves Toxicity.

- *Gan Cao* (Radix Glycyrrhizae) harmonizes the properties of the other ingredients.

QI DEPRESSION TRANSFORMING INTO TOXINS

With this pattern, carbuncles appear most often on the lower back and hypochondrium and only evolve slowly. Lesions are swollen, often with a dull pain in the affected area. Pus is discharged if the skin becomes inflamed. The tongue body is red with a thin white coating; the pulse is wiry and rapid.

Treatment principle

Dredge Qi and relieve Depression, soften hardness and disperse swelling.

Prescription

CHAI HU QING GAN YIN JIA JIAN

Bupleurum Beverage for Clearing the Liver, with modifications

Chai Hu (Radix Bupleuri) 6g
Huang Qin (Radix Scutellariae Baicalensis) 6g
Yu Jin (Radix Curcumae) 6g
Chuan Xiong (Rhizoma Ligustici Chuanxiong) 6g
Jin Yin Hua (Flos Lonicerae) 12g
Pu Gong Ying (Herba Taraxaci cum Radice) 12g
Fu Ling (Sclerotium Poriae Cocos) 12g
Zhe Bei Mu (Bulbus Fritillariae Thunbergii) 12g

Jiang Can‡ (Bombyx Batryticatus) 12g
Chi Shao (Radix Paeoniae Rubra) 10g
Dang Gui (Radix Angelicae Sinensis) 10g
Zi Hua Di Ding (Herba Violae Yedoensitis) 10g
Chuan Lian Zi (Fructus Meliae Toosendan) 10g

Explanation

- *Chai Hu* (Radix Bupleuri), *Yu Jin* (Radix Curcumae), *Chuan Xiong* (Rhizoma Ligustici Chuanxiong), and *Chuan Lian Zi* (Fructus Meliae Toosendan) move Qi and relieve Depression.
- *Huang Qin* (Radix Scutellariae Baicalensis), *Jin Yin Hua* (Flos Lonicerae), *Pu Gong Ying* (Herba Taraxaci cum Radice), and *Zi Hua Di Ding* (Herba Violae Yedoensitis) clear Heat, relieve Toxicity and disperse swelling.
- *Jiang Can* ‡ (Bombyx Batryticatus), *Fu Ling* (Sclerotium Poriae Cocos), *Zhe Bei Mu* (Bulbus Fritillariae Thunbergii), and *Dang Gui* (Radix Angelicae Sinensis) soften hardness and dissipate lumps.
- *Chi Shao* (Radix Paeoniae Rubra) disperses swelling to alleviate pain.

General modifications

1. For dry, bound stool, add *Da Huang* (Radix et Rhizoma Rhei) and *Gua Lou Ren* (Semen Trichosanthis).
2. Where pus has formed, add *Zao Jiao Ci* (Spina Gleditsiae Sinensis) and *Chuan Shan Jia*** (Squama Manitis Pentadactylae).

EXTERNAL TREATMENT

Initial stage

- To disperse swelling and alleviate pain, choose one of the following and apply externally to the lesions:

  Yu Lu San (Jade Dew Powder)
  Ru Yi Jin Huang San (Agreeable Golden Yellow Powder)
  Tie Gu San Gao (Iron Hoop Powder Paste)
  Qing Dai San (Indigo Powder)

- One or two of the following materia medica can also be pounded to a pulp and applied to the affected area:

  Pu Gong Ying (Herba Taraxaci cum Radice)
  Ye Ju Hua (Flos Chrysanthemi Indici)
  Bai Jiang Cao (Herba Patriniae cum Radice)
  Lu Bian Ju (Herba et Radix Kalimeridis)

- If the redness, swelling and pain are severe, apply *Fu Rong Gao* (Cotton Rose Flower Paste) to the boils.
- At the initial stage of carbuncles, apply *Jin Huang Gao* (Golden Yellow Paste) or *Yu Lu Gao* (Jade Dew Ointment) to the affected area.

Later stages

To generate flesh and close the lesion after it has burst, apply a small amount of *Qing Dai San* (Indigo Powder) or *Bing Shi San* (Borneol and Gypsum Powder) to the opening of the wound and dress the lesion with *Huang Lian Ruan Gao* (Coptis Ointment) or *Huang Lian Gan Ru Gao* (Coptis, Calamine and Frankincense Paste). Change the dressing every day.

ACUPUNCTURE

Main points: GV-14 Dazhui, LI-11 Quchi, LI-4 Hegu, and TB-5 Waiguan.

Auxiliary points: ST-36 Zusanli, GB-20 Fengchi, BL-40 Weizhong, GB-41 Zulinqi, GB-40 Qiuxu, and BL-60 Kunlun.

Technique: Apply the reducing method and retain the needles for 30 minutes after obtaining Qi. Treat once a day. A course consists of seven treatment sessions.

Explanation

- GV-14 Dazhui, LI-11 Quchi and LI-4 Hegu clear Heat and relieve Toxicity.
- GB-41 Zulinqi, GB-20 Fengchi and TB-5 Waiguan regulate Qi and disperse swelling.
- ST-36 Zusanli, BL-40 Weizhong, GB-40 Qiuxu, and BL-60 Kunlun augment Qi and nourish Yin.

MOXIBUSTION

Direct moxibustion with a moxa stick

Give moxibustion by keeping an ignited moxa stick directly over the lesion until a local sensation of mild heat is felt. Treat once a day.

Indirect moxibustion with a moxa stick

Cover the lesion with a piece of *Feng Fang* ‡ (Nidus Vespae). Then give moxibustion by keeping an ignited moxa stick over the skin. Continue until it is too hot for the patient. After moxibustion, use sterilized gauze to dress lesions where abscesses have not yet formed.

Moxibustion with *Deng Xin Cao* (Medulla Junci Effusi)

Main point: Guqizhuma (located 0.5 cun lateral to the midline, level with T$_{10}$, bilateral).

Auxiliary points

- For boils on the head, add TB-20 Jiaosun and TB-18 Chimai.
- For lesions above the waist, add GB-21 Jianjing, SI-15 Jianzhongshu and SI-14 Jianwaishu.
- For lesions below the waist, add BL-31 Shangliao, BL-32 Ciliao, BL-33 Zhongliao, and BL-34 Xialiao.

Technique: Dip one end of *Deng Xin Cao* (Medulla Junci Effusi) into *Xiang You* (Oleum Sesami Seminis) or vegetable oil. After igniting the end, scorch the points briefly until a popping sound is heard as the rush burns the skin. Keep the points clean and dry after treatment. Crusts will form at the points and drop off after a few days. Treat once a week. Three treatment sessions make up a course. Practitioners should exercise great caution with this method; the patient's consent must be obtained before treatment.

EAR ACUPUNCTURE
Points: Occiput, Ear-Shenmen, Adrenal Gland, and points corresponding to the sites of the skin lesions.
Technique: Retain the needles for 30 minutes. Treat once a day. A course consists of seven treatment sessions.

SEVEN-STAR NEEDLING
After routine disinfection of the area around a boil, tap gently from the periphery to the center three to five times. Afterwards, give moxibustion if the patient is willing to accept it. Treat once a day. A course consists of seven treatment sessions. If the patient has a weak constitution or the lesion has persisted for a long time, performing moxibustion at LI-4 Hegu and ST-36 Zusanli improves the effectiveness of the treatment.

Clinical notes

- Correct pattern identification is very important for the effective treatment of furuncles. This is particularly so for Blood-Heat due to Yin Deficiency, which can be misdiagnosed as a Heat Toxin pattern because of the recurrence and persistence of the lesions. If treatment is given with ingredients that relieve Toxicity with cold and bitterness, this may damage Yin, create Dryness and promote hyperactivity of Fire.
- In the early stages of furuncles, treatment should focus on clearing Heat, relieving Toxicity, drawing out Toxins and dissipating lumps. Restrict to a minimum the use of ingredients for subduing Fire with cold and bitterness.
- Treatment of carbuncles should focus on dispersing swelling, drawing out Toxins and supplementing Qi. Commonly used materia medica include *Huang Qi* (Radix Astragali seu Hedysari), *Dang Gui* (Radix Angelicae Sinensis), *Dang Shen* (Radix Codonopsitis Pilosulae), *Xuan Shen* (Radix Scrophulariae Ningpoensis), *Chuan Xiong* (Rhizoma Ligustici Chuanxiong), and *Zao Jiao Ci* (Spina Gleditsiae Sinensis).
- Where carbuncles are very painful, add *Nei Xiao Lian Qiao Wan* (Forsythia Internal Dispersion Pill), which is very effective at transforming Toxicity and alleviating pain.

Advice for the patient

- Avoid rich and greasy foods.
- Keep the skin and fingernails clean.

Literature excerpt

In *Tai Ping Sheng Hui Fang* [Peaceful Holy Benevolent Prescriptions], it says: "Furuncles are caused by Wind, Cold and Damp pathogenic factors fighting with the Blood to bind and accumulate. In addition, when people exert themselves, Yang Qi floats outward and sweating occurs. If sweat meets Cold and Dampness fighting in the channels and network vessels, Cold will obstruct the Blood, which cannot circulate properly, thus causing furuncles."

Modern clinical experience

INTERNAL TREATMENT
Zhou used *Yi Shen Gong Du Tang* (Decoction for Boosting the Kidneys and Attacking Toxicity) to treat 95 cases of persistent furuncles. [16]

Prescription ingredients

Shu Di Huang (Radix Rehmanniae Glutinosae Conquita) 5-30g
Shan Zhu Yu (Fructus Corni Officinalis) 5-30g
Shan Yao (Rhizoma Dioscoreae Oppositae) 5-30g
Rou Cong Rong (Herba Cistanches Deserticolae) 5-30g
Tu Bie Chong‡ (Eupolyphaga seu Steleophaga) 0.5-10g
Shui Zhi‡ (Hirudo seu Whitmania) 0.5-10g
Quan Xie‡ (Buthus Martensi) 0.5-10g
*Tian Ma** (Rhizoma Gastrodiae Elatae) 5-10g
Gou Teng (Ramulus Uncariae cum Uncis) 5-10g

Modifications
1. For Kidney Yang Deficiency, *Gui Zhi* (Ramulus Cinnamomi Cassiae) 2-10g, *Bu Gu Zhi* (Fructus Psoraleae Corylifoliae) 5-30g and *Jiang Can*‡ (Bombyx Batryticatus) 3-30g were added.
2. For Kidney Yin Deficiency, *Sang Shen* (Fructus Mori Albae) 3-30g, *Xuan Shen* (Radix Scrophulariae Ningpoensis) 3-30g and *Di Long*‡ (Lumbricus) 3-30g were added.
3. For Qi Deficiency, *Huang Qi* (Radix Astragali seu Hedysari) 5-30g and *Dang Shen* (Radix Codonopsitis Pilosulae) 5-30g were added.
4. For lesions on the face, head or arms, *Fang Feng* (Radix Ledebouriellae Divaricatae) 5-30g and *Man Jing Zi* (Fructus Viticis) 5-30g were added.
5. For lesions around the waist or on the legs, *Du Zhong* (Cortex Eucommiae Ulmoidis) 5-15g and *Chuan Niu Xi* (Radix Cyathulae Officinalis) 5-15g were added.
6. For lesions that often occur in spring and autumn, *Han Shui Shi*‡ (Calcitum) 3-25g and *Yi Yi Ren* (Semen Coicis Lachryma-jobi) 3-25g were added.

One bag was used to prepare a decoction, taken twice a day. A course of treatment lasted for 40-60 days. After six months, 51 cases had recovered completely, 35 had experienced some improvement and 9 had seen no effect.

EXTERNAL TREATMENT

Cai combined two external applications.[17] He first ground the following ingredients into a fine powder:

Tian Xian Zi (Semen Hyoscyami) 50g
Teng Huang (Resina Garciniae) 10g
Zhe Bei Mu (Bulbus Fritillariae Thunbergii) 10g
Chong Lou (Rhizoma Paridis) 10g
Chi Shao (Radix Paeoniae Rubra) 15g
Ru Xiang (Gummi Olibanum) 6g
Mo Yao (Myrrha) 6g
Bing Pian (Borneolum) 3g

Then he prepared a decoction of the following herbs in 500ml of water:

Da Huang (Radix et Rhizoma Rhei) 30g
Huang Qin (Radix Scutellariae Baicalensis) 30g
Huang Bai (Cortex Phellodendri) 15g
Huang Lian (Rhizoma Coptidis) 5g

The powder was mixed into a paste with cold boiled water. A 1-2 cm layer of paste was placed on a piece of gauze slightly larger than the affected area and then applied to the lesions. Other pieces of gauze were soaked in the decoction and then applied on the top of the first piece of gauze. This procedure was carried out three times a day until the lesions subsided.

Pyogenic paronychia (whitlow)
化脓性甲沟炎

Pyogenic paronychia is inflammation of the skin around the edge of a fingernail or toenail. A break in the skin or cuticle due to minor trauma, hangnail or excessive manicuring allows bacteria to enter and cause infection.

In TCM, this condition is also known as *dai zhi* (substitute finger).

Clinical manifestations

- The tissue around the nail appears swollen and inflamed. The swelling then spreads and abscesses form around the fingernail or toenail. The end of the finger or toe turns red and can swell up to a considerable size.
- In some cases, abscesses form along the edge of the nail, which may then eventually come off.
- Severe pain occurs locally since there is little room for swelling in the nail area.
- Some patients also have other symptoms such as fever, headache and poor appetite.

Etiology and pathology

- The lesion develops because exuberant Blood-Heat accumulates in the fingers to generate Heat Toxins, which flow along the channels impairing the normal circulation of Qi; an abscess finally forms.
- In addition, contact with dirty objects or puncture wounds caused by splinters or fish bones allow

infection by Toxins and pathogenic factors, which can result in paronychia if they settle in the skin and flesh or in the channels and network vessels.

Pattern identification and treatment

INTERNAL TREATMENT

ACCUMULATION OF HEAT TOXINS

Inflammation, redness and swelling at the side of the nail are characteristic of the initial stage of the condition; the swelling can expand to a considerable size. Persistent local burning pain is likely. Accompanying symptoms and signs include headache, fever, constipation, and short voidings of reddish urine. The tongue body is red with a thin yellow coating; the pulse is slippery and rapid.

Treatment principle
Clear Heat and relieve Toxicity, invigorate the Blood and alleviate pain.

Prescription
QING RE JIE DU YIN JIA JIAN
Beverage for Clearing Heat and Relieving Toxicity, with modifications

Jin Yin Hua (Flos Lonicerae) 10g
Pu Gong Ying (Herba Taraxaci cum Radice) 10g
Mu Dan Pi (Cortex Moutan Radicis) 10g
Chi Shao (Radix Paeoniae Rubra) 10g
Gan Cao (Radix Glycyrrhizae) 10g

Da Huang (Radix et Rhizoma Rhei) 10g, added 10 minutes before the end of the decoction process

Zhi Zi (Fructus Gardeniae Jasminoidis) 10g

Lian Qiao (Fructus Forsythiae Suspensae) 12g

Zhe Bei Mu (Bulbus Fritillariae Thunbergii) 12g

Chi Xiao Dou (Semen Phaseoli Calcarati) 12g

Chao Zhi Ke (Fructus Citri Aurantii, stir-fried) 6g

Explanation

- *Jin Yin Hua* (Flos Lonicerae), *Pu Gong Ying* (Herba Taraxaci cum Radice) and *Gan Cao* (Radix Glycyrrhizae) clear Heat and relieve Toxicity.

- *Mu Dan Pi* (Cortex Moutan Radicis) and *Chi Shao* (Radix Paeoniae Rubra) cool the Blood and relieve Toxicity.

- *Zhi Zi* (Fructus Gardeniae Jasminoidis) and *Lian Qiao* (Fructus Forsythiae Suspensae) clear Heat in the Heart and relieve Toxicity.

- *Chao Zhi Ke* (Fructus Citri Aurantii, stir-fried) and *Da Huang* (Radix et Rhizoma Rhei) free the Fu organs and relieve Toxicity.

- *Zhe Bei Mu* (Bulbus Fritillariae Thunbergii) and *Chi Xiao Dou* (Semen Phaseoli Calcarati) transform Dampness and expel pus.

- The prescription focuses on relieving Toxicity and dispersing swelling to alleviate pain. Toxicity is relieved in four ways – by clearing Heat, by cooling the Blood, by clearing Heart-Heat, and by freeing the Fu organs. Once pus and Toxins disappear, swelling is dispersed and pain alleviated.

EXUBERANT HEAT TOXINS

Yellowish-green abscesses form under or beside the nail. There is persistent local throbbing pain. Discharge of pus is difficult as the skin does not rupture. Accompanying symptoms and signs include high fever, thirst, difficulty in getting to sleep because of the pain, dry stools, and short voidings of reddish urine. The tongue body is red with a thin yellow coating; the pulse is surging and rapid.

Treatment principle

Clear Heat and relieve Toxicity to diffuse and drain Toxic pathogenic factors.

Prescription

JIE DU PAI NONG TANG JIA JIAN

Decoction for Relieving Toxicity and Expelling Pus, with modifications

Zi Hua Di Ding (Herba Violae Yedoensitis) 12g

Pu Gong Ying (Herba Taraxaci cum Radice) 12g

Ye Ju Hua (Flos Chrysanthemi Indici) 12g

Chi Shao (Radix Paeoniae Rubra) 10g

Zhe Bei Mu (Bulbus Fritillariae Thunbergii) 10g

Jie Geng (Radix Platycodi Grandiflori) 10g

Zao Jiao Ci (Spina Gleditsiae Sinensis) 10g

Chi Xiao Dou (Semen Phaseoli Calcarati) 30g

Sang Zhi (Ramulus Mori Albae) 6g

Gan Cao (Radix Glycyrrhizae) 6g

Ling Yang Jiao Fen* (Cornu Antelopis, powdered) 0.6g, infused in the prepared decoction

Explanation

- *Zi Hua Di Ding* (Herba Violae Yedoensitis), *Pu Gong Ying* (Herba Taraxaci cum Radice), *Ye Ju Hua* (Flos Chrysanthemi Indici), and *Gan Cao* (Radix Glycyrrhizae) clear Heat and relieve Toxicity to disperse swelling.

- *Chi Shao* (Radix Paeoniae Rubra), *Zhe Bei Mu* (Bulbus Fritillariae Thunbergii), *Jie Geng* (Radix Platycodi Grandiflori), *Zao Jiao Ci* (Spina Gleditsiae Sinensis), and *Chi Xiao Dou* (Semen Phaseoli Calcarati) expel pus and draw out Toxins to alleviate pain.

- *Sang Zhi* (Ramulus Mori Albae) is a channel conductor herb.

- *Ling Yang Jiao Fen** (Cornu Antelopis, powdered) strengthens the effect in clearing Heat and relieving Toxicity to alleviate pain.

EXTERNAL TREATMENT

- For non-ruptured lesions characterized by local redness and swelling, apply *Yu Lu Gao* (Jade Dew Ointment) or *Xiao Yan Gao* (Paste for Dispersing Inflammation) twice a day.

- For abscesses that are under the nail with difficult discharge of pus, use fire needling to burst the abscess.[i] Then apply *Ba Jia Gao* (Nail-Removing Plaster) to the affected nail. Renew the plaster once every other day. After two to three plasters, the nail will soften and come off. Continue the treatment with materia medica for generating flesh.

- If lesions have already ruptured, apply *Shou Gan Sheng Ji Yao Fen* (Medicated Powder for Promoting Contraction and Generating Flesh) or *Bing Shi San* (Borneol and Gypsum Powder) and cover with *Fu Rong Gao* (Cotton Rose Flower Paste). Treat once a day.

ACUPUNCTURE

Points

- For lesions on the hand, use GV-10 Lingtai as the main point in combination with LI-4 Hegu.

---

[i] Fire needling is a needling method using specially made thick needles. The needle is normally 2-3 cun in length and 0.5-1 mm in diameter. The needle is heated in a flame until red, then inserted into the lesion to treat swelling and pain.

- For lesions on the foot, use LR-2 Xingjian as the main point in combination with LR-3 Taichong and SP-6 Sanyinjiao.

Technique: The reducing method is applied. Stimulate the points without retaining the needles. The treatment is given daily. For abscesses that have not ruptured, prick with a needle to drain the pus.

Explanation

- GV-10 Lingtai clears Heat and relieves Toxicity.
- LI-4 Hegu dissipates Wind-Heat.
- LR-2 Xingjian, LR-3 Taichong and SP-6 Sanyinjiao clear and drain Heat Toxins in the Liver and Spleen channels.

MOXIBUSTION

Point: Ashi point (the site of ulcerated abscesses).
Technique: Clean the affected area with physiological saline. Then apply moxibustion with a moxa stick for 20-30 minutes, once a day.

Clinical notes

- When an abscess forms, the lesion should be pricked immediately with a needle to release the pus; alternatively, Western medical techniques can be used to incise the lesion to drain the pus. The aim is to prevent pus Toxins from further affecting the tendons (septic tendonitis) and bones (osteomyelitis).
- Internal treatment should focus on clearing Heat, relieving Toxicity, transforming Dampness, and expelling pus. A good effect can be achieved by

using assistants like *Sang Zhi* (Ramulus Mori Albae) as channel conductors.

- When the pain is severe, take *Huo Xue Zhi Tong San* (Powder for Invigorating the Blood and Alleviating Pain) 1.5g twice a day with warm boiled water. This powder is very effective for freeing the network vessels, dispersing swelling and alleviating pain.
- If treatment starts immediately at the initial stage, and pus is drained when the abscess forms, the prognosis for the condition is good. Otherwise, there is a risk of infection penetrating to the bone, resulting in osteomyelitis.

Advice for the patient

- Avoid damaging or injuring the nails.
- Keep the hands dry and clean.

Literature excerpt

In *Zheng Zhi Zhun Sheng* [Standards of Diagnosis and Treatment], it says: "The nails are the extension of the sinews. The sinews depend on the Blood for nourishment. When there is Blood-Heat, it will move to the ends of the fingers resulting in the fingers becoming swollen and hot and abscesses forming. In severe cases, the nails will come off. This is very similar to *ju* abscess of the fingers, but, as there is no accumulation of Toxins, the skin does not turn dark. Although the disease may persist, it will not be fatal."

Erysipelas
丹毒

Erysipelas is an acute inflammatory skin disorder caused by streptococcal infection, generally *Streptococcus pyogenes*. Streptococci usually enter the skin through a split or break in the surface, often located behind the ear or between the toes, in the latter case associated with tinea pedis. Repeated infection can lead to persistent lymphedema.

In TCM, this condition is known as *dan du* (cinnabar Toxin) as a result of the bright red color of the lesions. Facial erysipelas is also known as *bao tou huo dan* (head Fire cinnabar), or as *da tou wen* (massive head scourge) in severe cases; erysipelas on the leg is also called *liu huo*

(flowing Fire); and erysipelas in children is known as *chi you dan* (red wandering cinnabar).

Clinical manifestations

- Erysipelas usually involves the lower leg or face and ears, but may also appear on the buttocks, hands and feet. In children, lesions are often situated on the abdomen.
- The appearance of skin lesions is preceded by a prodromal phase of fever, chills and malaise, sometimes

accompanied by loss of appetite and vomiting; this phase usually lasts between 4 and 48 hours.

- At the initial stage, lesions manifest as localized bright red or purplish-red edematous erythema with irregular, sharply demarcated and rapidly expanding borders. The surface of the lesions is tense, shiny and hot. Some vesicles or bloody blisters may appear on the plaques.

- The condition is usually accompanied by sensations of moderate to severe itching, burning, tenderness, and pain.

- The eruption reaches a peak in 5-7 days and then subsides gradually over the following one to two weeks.

- Raging fever and headache or delirium and loss of consciousness may occur in severe cases.

- Repeated attacks can occur in the same area leading to lymphedema since lymphatic drainage is impaired. This is most likely in patients with venous stasis or venous ulcers of the lower limbs.

- Guttate psoriasis may follow a streptococcal infection (see Chapter 4).

Differential diagnosis

Stasis eczema
Erysipelas on the leg should be differentiated from stasis eczema, which manifests at the acute stage with eczematoid lesions (papules, vesicles, erosion, exudation, and crusts) and lacks the advancing red plaques and systemic symptoms of erysipelas.

Allergic contact dermatitis
Facial erysipelas should be differentiated from allergic contact dermatitis, which may also present with itching and burning sensations, but which lacks the prodromal symptoms and tenderness of erysipelas.

Angioedema
Facial erysipelas should also be differentiated from angioedema on the face. In angioedema, lesions generally manifest as circumscribed edema with ill-defined borders and a tight, shiny, uniform pink or flesh-colored surface. There may be a sensation of burning pain, but itching is not pronounced. Prodromal symptoms are absent.

Etiology and pathology

Intense Fire due to Wind-Heat
When the Heart is harassed over a long period by irritability, intense Heart-Fire will accumulate internally. Since the Heart pertains to Fire and the Heart governs the Blood, this will result in Heat in the Xue level. When this is complicated by repeated external contraction of Wind-Heat, the internal and external factors will combine. Wind and Fire will fan one another to produce Fire Toxins. Lesions are located on the face because pathogenic Wind and Fire tend to ascend.

Retention of Fire in the Liver channel
A rash and impatient nature, sudden anger or emotional depression will result in Qi Depression generating Fire. Hyperactivity of Fire in the Liver channel forces Blood to spill outward to the thoracic and lumbar regions making the skin as red as cinnabar with a sensation of burning heat and stabbing pain.

Exuberant Fire due to Damp-Heat
Dietary irregularities with excessive consumption of bitter, spicy, aromatic, or fried foods or alcohol will damage the Spleen and Stomach and impair their transportation and transformation function. Damp-Heat will be generated internally, eventually transforming into Fire Toxins, which rush to the skin to appear as intense inflammation. Damp-Heat generated internally may also pour down to the lower limbs, manifesting as vesicles.

Fetal Heat
During pregnancy, the mother's preference for fatty, sweet, spicy, or fried food or overindulgence in fish and seafood can result in impairment of the Spleen's transportation function and the generation of Damp-Heat in the interior, which can be passed on to the fetus. If this is subsequently complicated by external pathogenic Heat attacking the baby's delicate skin and flesh, erysipelas can result.

Toxic pathogenic factors attacking the interior
Scratching, picking the nose or ear, insect bites, or trauma allow Toxic pathogenic factors to enter the body.

Pattern identification and treatment

INTERNAL TREATMENT

WIND-HEAT
This pattern mainly involves the face or the upper part of the body. Lesions are inflamed and swollen with sharply demarcated borders and a tense, shiny surface. Sensations of burning heat and pain are usual. Prodromal symptoms include fever, chills, headache, and nausea and vomiting. The tongue body is bright red with a thin yellow coating; the pulse is floating and rapid or slippery and rapid.

Treatment principle
Clear Heat and relieve Toxicity, extinguish Wind and disperse swelling.

Prescription
PU JI XIAO DU YIN JIA JIAN
Universal Salvation Beverage for Dispersing Toxicity, with modifications

Chao Niu Bang Zi (Fructus Arctii Lappae, stir-fried) 10g
Chi Shao (Radix Paeoniae Rubra) 10g
Sang Ye (Folium Mori Albae) 10g
Chao Huang Qin (Radix Scutellariae Baicalensis, stir-fried) 10g
Chao Huang Lian (Rhizoma Coptidis, stir-fried) 3g
Jiao Zhi Zi (Fructus Gardeniae Jasminoidis, scorch-fried) 3g
Jin Yin Hua (Flos Lonicerae) 12g
Ye Ju Hua (Flos Chrysanthemi Indici) 12g
Lian Qiao (Fructus Forsythiae Suspensae) 12g
Ban Lan Gen (Radix Isatidis seu Baphicacanthi) 12g
Chao Mu Dan Pi (Cortex Moutan Radicis, stir-fried) 6g
Chan Tui ‡ (Periostracum Cicadae) 6g

Explanation

- *Chao Niu Bang Zi* (Fructus Arctii Lappae, stir-fried), *Sang Ye* (Folium Mori Albae), *Jin Yin Hua* (Flos Lonicerae), *Chan Tui* ‡ (Periostracum Cicadae), and *Ye Ju Hua* (Flos Chrysanthemi Indici) dissipate Wind and disperse swelling.
- *Chi Shao* (Radix Paeoniae Rubra), *Chao Mu Dan Pi* (Cortex Moutan Radicis, stir-fried), *Lian Qiao* (Fructus Forsythiae Suspensae), and *Jiao Zhi Zi* (Fructus Gardeniae Jasminoidis, scorch-fried) cool the Blood and relieve Toxicity.
- *Ban Lan Gen* (Radix Isatidis seu Baphicacanthi), *Chao Huang Lian* (Rhizoma Coptidis, stir-fried) and *Chao Huang Qin* (Radix Scutellariae Baicalensis, stir-fried) drain Fire and relieve Toxicity.

LIVER-FIRE

The swollen and red lesions characteristic of this pattern usually involve the chest, abdomen, back, lower back, and hip regions. Stabbing pain and a sensation of burning heat are normally felt. Accompanying symptoms and signs include dry mouth with a bitter taste and short voidings of yellow urine. The tongue body is red with a scant or thin yellow coating; the pulse is wiry and rapid.

Treatment principle
Clear Heat from the Liver and drain Fire, cool the Blood and reduce erythema.

Prescription
CHAI HU QING GAN YIN JIA JIAN
Bupleurum Beverage for Clearing the Liver, with modifications

Chai Hu (Radix Bupleuri) 4.5g
Chao Mu Dan Pi (Cortex Moutan Radicis, stir-fried) 4.5g
Chao Long Dan Cao (Radix Gentianae Scabrae, stir-fried) 4.5g
Chao Huang Lian (Rhizoma Coptidis, stir-fried) 4.5g

Chao Huang Qin (Radix Scutellariae Baicalensis, stir-fried) 6g
Jiao Zhi Zi (Fructus Gardeniae Jasminoidis, scorch-fried) 6g
Lian Qiao (Fructus Forsythiae Suspensae) 6g
Chao Zhi Mu (Rhizoma Anemarrhenae Asphodeloidis, stir-fried) 6g
Jin Yin Hua (Flos Lonicerae) 15g
Lü Dou Yi (Testa Phaseoli Radiati) 15g
Sheng Di Huang (Radix Rehmanniae Glutinosae) 12g
Shi Gao ‡ (Gypsum Fibrosum) 12g
Yi Yi Ren (Semen Coicis Lachryma-jobi) 30g
Chi Xiao Dou (Semen Phaseoli Calcarati) 30g

Explanation

- *Chao Mu Dan Pi* (Cortex Moutan Radicis, stir-fried), *Chao Huang Lian* (Rhizoma Coptidis, stir-fried), *Chao Huang Qin* (Radix Scutellariae Baicalensis, stir-fried), *Jiao Zhi Zi* (Fructus Gardeniae Jasminoidis, scorch-fried), and *Lian Qiao* (Fructus Forsythiae Suspensae) drain Fire and relieve Toxicity.
- *Shi Gao* ‡ (Gypsum Fibrosum), *Chao Zhi Mu* (Rhizoma Anemarrhenae Asphodeloidis, stir-fried), *Sheng Di Huang* (Radix Rehmanniae Glutinosae), *Yi Yi Ren* (Semen Coicis Lachryma-jobi), and *Chi Xiao Dou* (Semen Phaseoli Calcarati) cool the Blood and clear Heat from the Qi level.
- *Lü Dou Yi* (Testa Phaseoli Radiati) and *Jin Yin Hua* (Flos Lonicerae) relieve Toxicity and reduce erythema.
- *Chai Hu* (Radix Bupleuri) and *Chao Long Dan Cao* (Radix Gentianae Scabrae, stir-fried) clear and drain Excess-Fire from the Liver and Gallbladder.

DAMP-HEAT

Lesions usually involve the lower leg and ankle and manifest as shiny tense patches of circumscribed edematous erythema. Vesicles, blood-filled blisters or necrosis may occasionally be seen. Lesions may recur in places or may be exacerbated by overstrain or high temperatures. Accompanying symptoms and signs include fatigue in the legs and poor appetite. The tongue body is red with a thin, yellow and slightly greasy coating; the pulse is thready and slippery, or deep and soggy.

Treatment principle
Clear Heat and transform Dampness, harmonize the Blood and free the network vessels.

Prescription
BI XIE SHEN SHI TANG JIA JIAN
Yam Rhizome Decoction for Percolating Dampness, with modifications

Bi Xie (Rhizoma Dioscoreae Hypoglaucae seu Septemlobae) 10g
Lian Qiao (Fructus Forsythiae Suspensae) 10g

Dang Gui (Radix Angelicae Sinensis) 10g
Ma Bian Cao (Herba cum Radice Verbenae) 10g
Chi Shao (Radix Paeoniae Rubra) 10g
Chao Mu Dan Pi (Cortex Moutan Radicis, stir-fried) 4.5g
Chao Huang Bai (Cortex Phellodendri, stir-fried) 6g
Cang Zhu (Rhizoma Atractylodis) 6g
Chuan Niu Xi (Radix Cyathulae Officinalis) 6g
Qing Pi (Pericarpium Citri Reticulatae Viride) 6g
Chi Xiao Dou (Semen Phaseoli Calcarati) 15g
Ren Dong Teng (Caulis Lonicerae Japonicae) 15g
Yi Yi Ren (Semen Coicis Lachryma-jobi) 30g

Explanation

- *Bi Xie* (Rhizoma Dioscoreae Hypoglaucae seu Septemlobae), *Yi Yi Ren* (Semen Coicis Lachryma-jobi), *Chao Huang Bai* (Cortex Phellodendri, stir-fried), *Cang Zhu* (Rhizoma Atractylodis), *Chuan Niu Xi* (Radix Cyathulae Officinalis), and *Qing Pi* (Pericarpium Citri Reticulatae Viride) clear Heat, percolate Dampness and benefit the movement of water.
- *Ma Bian Cao* (Herba cum Radice Verbenae), *Ren Dong Teng* (Caulis Lonicerae Japonicae), *Lian Qiao* (Fructus Forsythiae Suspensae), and *Chi Xiao Dou* (Semen Phaseoli Calcarati) relieve Toxicity and free the network vessels.
- *Chao Mu Dan Pi* (Cortex Moutan Radicis, stir-fried), *Chi Shao* (Radix Paeoniae Rubra) and *Dang Gui* (Radix Angelicae Sinensis) invigorate and cool the Blood and reduce erythema.

FETAL HEAT

This pattern occurs in infants. The skin in the abdomen becomes inflamed and swollen and feels burning hot when touched. In severe cases, the erythema advances in all directions. Accompanying symptoms and signs include fever, irritability and restlessness, persistent crying, and, in serious cases, convulsions or loss of consciousness. The tongue body is red with a scant coating; the pulse is rapid and the finger vein is purple.

Treatment principle

Clear Fire and relieve Toxicity, cool the Blood and reduce erythema.

Prescription
QING HUO XIAO DAN TANG JIA JIAN
Decoction for Clearing Fire and Dispersing Erysipelas, with modifications

Sheng Di Huang (Radix Rehmanniae Glutinosae) 10g
Chao Mu Dan Pi (Cortex Moutan Radicis, stir-fried) 6g
Xuan Shen (Radix Scrophulariae Ningpoensis) 6g
Chi Shao (Radix Paeoniae Rubra) 6g
Lü Dou Yi (Testa Phaseoli Radiati) 15g
Lian Qiao (Fructus Forsythiae Suspensae) 4.5g

Gan Cao (Radix Glycyrrhizae) 4.5g
Tian Hua Fen (Radix Trichosanthis) 4.5g
Chuan Niu Xi (Radix Cyathulae Officinalis) 4.5g

Explanation

- *Sheng Di Huang* (Radix Rehmanniae Glutinosae), *Chao Mu Dan Pi* (Cortex Moutan Radicis, stir-fried), *Xuan Shen* (Radix Scrophulariae Ningpoensis), *Chi Shao* (Radix Paeoniae Rubra), *Lü Dou Yi* (Testa Phaseoli Radiati), *Lian Qiao* (Fructus Forsythiae Suspensae), and *Tian Hua Fen* (Radix Trichosanthis) clear Heat from the Heart and drain Fire to reduce erythema.
- *Chuan Niu Xi* (Radix Cyathulae Officinalis) acts as a channel conductor to guide the other ingredients to the affected area.
- *Gan Cao* (Radix Glycyrrhizae) harmonizes the properties of the other ingredients and relieves Toxicity.

ATTACK BY TOXINS

Inadequate or delayed treatment at the initial stage of the disease may cause a rapid deterioration. The swollen red lesions extend rapidly and neighboring lymph nodes may enlarge. Accompanying symptoms and signs include raging fever, irritability and restlessness, headache, vomiting, and delirium. The tongue body is crimson with a thin yellow coating; the pulse is surging, large and forceless.

Treatment principle

Clear Heat from the Ying level and cool the Blood, protect the Heart and quiet the Spirit.

Prescription
XI JIAO DI HUANG TANG JIA JIAN
Rhinoceros Horn and Rehmannia Decoction

Sheng Di Huang Tan (Radix Rehmanniae Glutinosae Carbonisata) 30g
Jin Yin Hua Tan (Flos Lonicerae Carbonisatus) 30g
Lü Dou Yi (Testa Phaseoli Radiati) 30g
Chao Mu Dan Pi (Cortex Moutan Radicis, stir-fried) 6g
Zi Cao (Radix Arnebiae seu Lithospermi) 6g
Chao Huang Lian (Rhizoma Coptidis, stir-fried) 6g
Lian Qiao (Fructus Forsythiae Suspensae) 6g
Chi Shao (Radix Paeoniae Rubra) 6g
Gan Cao (Radix Glycyrrhizae) 6g
Dan Zhu Ye (Herba Lophatheri Gracilis) 10g
Shui Niu Jiao ‡ (Cornu Bubali) 15g, decocted for 30 minutes before adding the other ingredients

Explanation

- *Sheng Di Huang Tan* (Radix Rehmanniae Glutinosae Carbonisata), *Jin Yin Hua Tan* (Flos Lonicerae Carbonisatus), *Lü Dou Yi* (Testa Phaseoli Radiati), *Lian Qiao* (Fructus Forsythiae Suspensae), and *Chao Huang Lian* (Rhizoma Coptidis, stir-fried) clear Heat from the Ying level and relieve Toxicity to protect the Heart.

- *Dan Zhu Ye* (Herba Lophatheri Gracilis) clears Heat through urination.
- *Shui Niu Jiao*‡ (Cornu Bubali) cools the Blood and quiets the Spirit.
- *Chi Shao* (Radix Paeoniae Rubra), *Chao Mu Dan Pi* (Cortex Moutan Radicis, stir-fried) and *Zi Cao* (Radix Arnebiae seu Lithospermi) cool the Blood, relieve Toxicity and reduce erythema.
- *Gan Cao* (Radix Glycyrrhizae) harmonizes the properties of the other ingredients and relieves Toxicity.

EXTERNAL TREATMENT

- For bright red and swollen lesions, apply *Si Huang Gao* (Four Yellows Paste) to the affected area twice a day or mix *Da Huang San* (Rhubarb Powder) or *Yu Lu San* (Jade Dew Powder) to a paste with vegetable oil, cooled boiled water or syrup and apply twice a day.
- Where the redness and swelling gradually subsides, but does not disappear, rub in *Chong He San* (Harmonious Flow Powder) with *Xiao Yan Gao* (Paste for Dispersing Inflammation) twice a day.
- For lesions on the leg, prepare a decoction with
  - *Zi Su Ye* (Folium Perillae Frutescentis) 15g and *Shi Chang Pu* (Rhizoma Acori Graminei) 15g;
  - or *Hai Tong Pi* (Cortex Erythrinae) 12g, *Jiang Huang* (Rhizoma Curcumae Longae) 12g and *Cang Zhu* (Rhizoma Atractylodis) 12g;
  - or *Yin Chen Hao* (Herba Artemisiae Scopariae) 10g, *Sheng Jiang* (Rhizoma Zingiberis Officinalis Recens) 10g and *Can Sha*‡ (Excrementum Bombycis Mori) 10g;
  - or *Gui Zhi* (Ramulus Cinnamomi Cassiae) 6g and *Bai Zhu* (Rhizoma Atractylodis Macrocephalae) 6g.

Use the decoction when hot to steam the affected area, then allow it to cool to lukewarm before using it as a soak. Treat two or three times a day.

ACUPUNCTURE

Selection of points according to pattern identification
Main points: SP-8 Diji, SP-10 Xuehai, SP-6 Sanyinjiao, ST-40 Fenglong, and LR-3 Taichong.
Auxiliary points: SP-9 Yinlingquan, SP-5 Shangqiu, ST-36 Zusanli, and LR-5 Ligou.

Empirical points
Main points: GV-14 Dazhui, LI-11 Quchi, ST-43 Xiangu, and BL-40 Weizhong.
Auxiliary points: EX-HN-5 Taiyang,ⁱⁱ LI-4 Hegu and ST-36 Zusanli.

General modifications
1. For headache, add EX-HN-5 Taiyang and GB-20 Fengchi.
2. For nausea and vomiting, add PC-6 Neiguan.
3. For constipation, add ST-40 Fenglong and ST-37 Shangjuxu.
4. For lesions on the face, add ST-8 Touwei, ST-2 Sibai and TB-17 Yifeng.
5. For lesions on the legs, add GB-39 Xuanzhong and BL-60 Kunlun.

Technique
Apply the reducing method and retain the needles for 30 minutes after obtaining Qi. Treat once a day. A course of treatment consists of seven sessions.

Explanation
- SP-8 Diji, SP-10 Xuehai, SP-6 Sanyinjiao, ST-40 Fenglong, and SP-9 Yinlingquan clear and drain Damp-Heat from the Spleen and Stomach, relieve Toxicity and alleviate itching.
- SP-5 Shangqiu, ST-36 Zusanli, and LR-5 Ligou support Vital Qi (Zheng Qi) and expel pathogenic factors.
- LR-3 Taichong dissipates Wind.
- EX-HN-5 Taiyang and GB-20 Fengchi dissipate Wind to treat headache.
- PC-6 Neiguan bears counterflow Qi downward to treat nausea and vomiting.
- ST-40 Fenglong and ST-37 Shangjuxu free the Fu organs to treat constipation.
- ST-8 Touwei, ST-2 Sibai, TB-17 Yifeng, GB-39 Xuanzhong, and BL-60 Kunlun perform a similar function to materia media channel conductors.

MOXIBUSTION
Point: Ashi point (induration at the center of the line joining LI-15 Jianyu and LI-11 Quchi).
Technique: Position a slice of garlic on the point and place a moxa cone on top. Burn 5-7 cones per session. Treat once a day. A course of treatment consists of five sessions.

EAR ACUPUNCTURE
Points: Ear-Shenmen, Adrenal Gland, Subcortex, and Occiput.
Technique: Retain the needles for 30 minutes. Treat once a day. A course of treatment consists of seven sessions.

SEVEN-STAR NEEDLING
Points: Ashi points (red and swollen areas).

ⁱⁱ M-HN-9 according to the system employed by the Shanghai College of Traditional Chinese Medicine.

Technique: After routine sterilization, tap the areas gently until a small amount of blood appears. Treat once every two days.
Indication: Recurrent erysipelas.

Clinical notes

- Treatment of erysipelas depends on whether the upper, central or lower parts of the body are affected:
1. Lesions on the head and face are generally caused by Wind-Heat Toxins and can be treated with *Qing Wen Bai Du Yin* (Beverage for Clearing Scourge and Vanquishing Toxicity) in addition to the prescription detailed above.
2. Lesions on the trunk are generally caused by Heat Toxins attacking the interior and can be treated by *Huang Lian Jie Du Tang* (Coptis Decoction for Relieving Toxicity) in addition to the prescription detailed above.
3. Lesions on the legs and feet are generally caused by Damp Toxins and can be treated by *San Miao Wan* (Mysterious Three Pill) in addition to the prescription detailed above.
- The use of acupuncture for dredging Wind, draining Fire, dispersing swelling, and alleviating itching increases the effectiveness of the treatment.
- Where the cause of the original infection that allowed *Streptococci* to penetrate can be identified, for example tinea pedis, it should also be treated.
- Where the disease recurs repeatedly, the possibility of a chronic infectious focus should be investigated.

Case histories

Case 1

Patient
Male, aged 64.

Clinical manifestations
Ten days previously, the patient had begun to suffer from fever and chills, followed by the appearance of painful red and swollen lesions on the forehead, the cheeks and the bridge of the nose. Accompanying symptoms and signs included oppression in the chest, irritability, nausea, poor appetite, constipation, and short voidings of reddish urine.

Examination revealed a temperature of 38°C and sharply demarcated bright red swollen lesions with a sensation of burning pain. Numerous small vesicles had appeared on the bridge of the nose, some of which had ruptured with erosion or scabs. The tongue body was crimson with a yellow and greasy coating; the pulse was surging, rapid and forceful. Tests indicated a higher-than-normal white blood cell count.

Diagnosis
Facial erysipelas (*bao tou huo dan*).

Pattern identification
Exuberant Heat Toxins, Blood-Heat due to Yin Deficiency.

Treatment principle
Clear Heat and relieve Toxicity, cool the Blood and protect Yin.

Prescription ingredients
Jin Yin Hua (Flos Lonicerae) 24g
Pu Gong Ying (Herba Taraxaci cum Radice) 15g
Zi Hua Di Ding (Herba Violae Yedoensitis) 15g
Da Qing Ye (Folium Isatidis seu Baphicacanthi) 12g
Ban Lan Gen (Radix Isatidis seu Baphicacanthi) 18g
Chi Shao (Radix Paeoniae Rubra) 10g
Bai Mao Gen (Rhizoma Imperatae Cylindricae) 30g
Jiao Zhi Zi (Fructus Gardeniae Jasminoidis, scorch-fried) 10g
Jie Geng (Radix Platycodi Grandiflori) 5g
Da Huang (Radix et Rhizoma Rhei) 10g, added 10 minutes before the end of the decoction process
Huang Qin (Radix Scutellariae Baicalensis) 10g
Zhu Ru (Caulis Bambusae in Taeniis) 10g
Hua Shi‡ (Talcum) 10g

One bag a day was used to prepare a decoction, taken twice a day.

External treatment
Qu Du Yao Fen (Medicated Powder for Eliminating Toxins) 60g and powdered *Bing Pian* (Borneolum) 3g were mixed to a paste with warm water for application twice a day to the affected area. iii

Second visit
After one bag of the internal treatment, the constipation and the feeling of oppression in the chest had been relieved, but the patient's temperature had risen to 38.8°C. *Da Huang* (Radix et Rhizoma Rhei) and *Hua Shi*‡ (Talcum) were removed from the prescription and *Xuan Shen* (Radix Scrophulariae Ningpoensis) 18g and *Huang Lian* (Rhizoma Coptidis) 6g added.

Third visit
After one bag of the ingredients, the temperature fell to 37.7°C, the irritability and nausea had ceased and the patient was beginning to get his appetite back. The redness and swelling on the face was improving and the vesicles had dried and crusted. After another three bags, the redness and swelling had disappeared, but there were two painful areas behind the ears. The patient was very thirsty. The tongue body was red with a whitish-yellow coating; the pulse was wiry and slippery.

Treatment principle
Clear Heat, relieve Toxicity and nourish Yin.

---

iii In those countries where certain ingredients of *Qu Du Yao Fen* (Medicated Powder for Eliminating Toxins) mean that its use is not permitted, *Qing Dai San* (Indigo Powder) may be applied instead.

Prescription ingredients

Jin Yin Hua (Flos Lonicerae) 10g
Lian Qiao (Fructus Forsythiae Suspensae) 10g
Ju Hua (Flos Chrysanthemi Morifolii) 10g
Pu Gong Ying (Herba Taraxaci cum Radice) 10g
Jiao Zhi Zi (Fructus Gardeniae Jasminoidis, scorch-fried) 10g
Long Dan Cao (Radix Gentianae Scabrae) 5g
Zi Cao (Radix Arnebiae seu Lithospermi) 10g
Sheng Di Huang (Radix Rehmanniae Glutinosae) 30g
Mu Dan Pi (Cortex Moutan Radicis) 10g
Zi Hua Di Ding (Herba Violae Yedoensitis) 10g
Huang Qin (Radix Scutellariae Baicalensis) 6g
Chi Shao (Radix Paeoniae Rubra) 10g

Outcome

After three bags of the new prescription, all the symptoms had disappeared and the white blood cell count had returned to normal. [18]

Case 2

Patient

Woman, aged 67.

Clinical manifestations

Two years previously, red, swollen and painful lesions had appeared on the anterior aspect of the patient's lower left leg, accompanied by fever, chills and generalized malaise. The patient was treated by her local hospital clinic for erysipelas and the symptoms were relieved. However, the condition recurred four times with the same manifestations and could only be kept under control by strong doses of antibiotics. Four days previously, the symptoms had recurred once again.

Examination revealed a temperature of 39.5°C, which made the patient irritable. A red and swollen lesion 8 x 15 cm with a sharply demarcated border was noted on the anterior aspect of the lower left leg. The lymph node in the left inguinal groove was enlarged and tender. The area between the toes on the left foot was red and swollen with maceration, erosion and a small amount of exudation. The tongue body was red with a thin white coating; the pulse was deep, thready and slightly rapid. Tests indicated a higher-than-normal white blood cell count.

Diagnosis

Acute flare-up of recurrent erysipelas on the leg (*liu huo*).

Pattern identification

Damp Toxins and pathogenic Heat obstructing the channels and network vessels.

Treatment principle

Clear Heat, cool the Blood and relieve Toxicity, invigorate the Blood and free the network vessels.

Prescription ingredients

Ren Dong Teng (Caulis Lonicerae Japonicae) 30g

Lian Qiao (Fructus Forsythiae Suspensae) 15g
Ban Lan Gen (Radix Isatidis seu Baphicacanthi) 30g
Huang Qin (Radix Scutellariae Baicalensis) 10g
Huang Lian (Rhizoma Coptidis) 10g
Huang Bai (Cortex Phellodendri) 10g
Zhi Zi (Fructus Gardeniae Jasminoidis) 10g
Zi Hua Di Ding (Herba Violae Yedoensitis) 15g
Sheng Di Huang (Radix Rehmanniae Glutinosae) 15g
Mu Dan Pi (Cortex Moutan Radicis) 15g
Chi Shao (Radix Paeoniae Rubra) 15g
Ze Lan (Herba Lycopi Lucidi) 15g
Dan Shen (Radix Salviae Miltiorrhizae) 15g
Ji Xue Teng (Caulis Spatholobi) 30g
Niu Xi (Radix Achyranthis Bidentatae) 10g
Shi Gao ‡ (Gypsum Fibrosum) 30g, decocted for 30 minutes before adding the other ingredients

External treatment

Hua Du San Gao (Powder Paste for Transforming Toxicity)[iv] was applied to lesions on the lower leg. A 2% gentian violet solution was applied between the toes and allowed to dry before application of 1% *Lü Yang You* (Chloramphenicol and Zinc Oxide Oil).[v] Small balls of tissue were then placed between the toes to keep the area dry.

Outcome

After seven bags of the decoction, the patient's temperature had returned to normal and the redness and swelling were gradually subsiding. After another seven bags, the redness and swelling had completely disappeared, as had all other symptoms. The patient was then prescribed *Huo Xue Xiao Yan Wan* (Pill for Invigorating the Blood and Dispersing Inflammation) and *Da Huang Zhe Chong Wan* (Rhubarb and Wingless Cockroach Pill), both 6g twice a day, for one month to consolidate the treatment. A follow-up visit one year later indicated no recurrence of the disease. [19]

Literature excerpt

In *Yang Ke Xin De Ji* [A Collection of Experiences in the Treatment of Sores], it says: "*Da tou wen* [severe facial erysipelas] is caused by seasonal or epidemic pathogenic Heat Toxins infecting the body. Pulse diagnosis is an important part of the treatment. The pulse may be slippery and rapid, floating and surging, deep and tight, or wiry and rough. A floating and rapid pulse indicates that pathogenic factors are still in the exterior and the condition can be treated with *Xi Jiao Sheng Ma Tang* (Rhinoceros and Bugbane Decoction). A deep and rough pulse indicates that pathogenic factors have penetrated deep inside the body and Toxins are exuberant; *Hua Du Wan* (Pill for Transforming Toxicity) should be used to attack the Toxins immediately. Patients with constipation due to Excess-Heat should be prescribed *Da Huang Wan* (Rhubarb Pill) to free the bowels."

---

iv In those countries where certain ingredients of this paste mean that its use is not permitted, *Fu Rong Gao* (Cotton Rose Flower Paste) may be applied instead.
v Usually only available on prescription.

Modern clinical experience

INTERNAL TREATMENT

1. **Bai** formulated an empirical prescription to treat 50 cases of recurrent erysipelas. [20]

Prescription
YIN HUA JIE DU TANG
Honeysuckle Decoction for Relieving Toxicity

Jin Yin Hua (Flos Lonicerae) 30g
Yi Yi Ren (Semen Coicis Lachryma-jobi) 30g
Mu Dan Pi (Cortex Moutan Radicis) 20g
Ye Ju Hua (Flos Chrysanthemi Indici) 20g
Dan Shen (Radix Salviae Miltiorrhizae) 20g
Huang Bai (Cortex Phellodendri) 12g
Tian Hua Fen (Radix Trichosanthis) 12g
Cang Zhu (Rhizoma Atractylodis) 5g
Gan Cao (Radix Glycyrrhizae) 6g

Modifications
1. For exuberant Damp-Heat, *Sheng Di Huang* (Radix Rehmanniae Glutinosae) 15g, *Niu Bang Zi* (Fructus Arctii Lappae) 10g and *Jiang Can* ‡ (Bombyx Batryticatus) 10g were added.
2. For Damp-Heat pouring down, *Dan Shen* (Radix Salviae Miltiorrhizae) was removed and *Bi Xie* (Rhizoma Dioscoreae Hypoglaucae seu Septemlobae) 10g and

Che Qian Zi (Semen Plantaginis) 15g were added.
3. For fever, *Shi Gao* ‡ (Gypsum Fibrosum) 30g and *Zhi Mu* (Rhizoma Anemarrhenae Asphodeloidis) 15g were added.

One bag a day was used to prepare a decoction, taken twice a day for 15 days. Follow-up visits after six months suggested the treatment had been successful in 45 cases.

2. **Wang** also treated erysipelas internally. [21]

Prescription
YIN HUANG JIE DU TANG
Honeysuckle and Scutellaria Decoction for Relieving Toxicity

Jin Yin Hua (Flos Lonicerae) 30g
Zi Hua Di Ding (Herba Violae Yedoensitis) 20g
Che Qian Zi (Semen Plantaginis) 10g
Niu Xi (Radix Achyranthis Bidentatae) 10g
Mu Dan Pi (Cortex Moutan Radicis) 15g
Huang Qin (Radix Scutellariae Baicalensis) 12g
Yi Yi Ren (Semen Coicis Lachryma-jobi) 12g
Bi Xie (Rhizoma Dioscoreae Hypoglaucae seu Septemlobae) 12g

One bag a day was used to prepare a decoction, taken twice a day. Earliest results were seen after four days, but in some stubborn cases up to 32 days were needed.

Erythema induratum (Bazin's disease)
硬结性红斑

Erythema induratum, a mycobacterial infection, is also known as Bazin's disease or tuberculosis indurativa subcutanea. It is characterized by subcutaneous nodular lesions on the flexor aspect of the lower leg in young women. The nodules may break down to form necrotic ulcers that leave scars after healing. The disease is almost invariably preceded by tuberculosis (however the etiological relationship to that disease is debated).

Erythema induratum is known in TCM as *fei fa* or *fei chuai fa* (deep-rooted calf sore).

Clinical manifestations

- Erythema induratum is usually seen in young women, often as a complication of tuberculosis of the internal organs.

- The disease is likely to occur on the flexor aspect of the lower leg with symmetrical distribution but relatively few lesions.
- Lesions manifest as subcutaneous nodules, which enlarge gradually to coalesce with the skin. The nodules are purplish-red, solid and slightly tender on pressure but do not protrude above the skin surface. They may disappear spontaneously, or may ulcerate and leave scars after healing.

Differential diagnosis

Erythema nodosum
An acute vasculitis that affects dermis and fat, erythema nodosum causes multiple tender red nodules that are usually most prominent on the shin. The nodules never

break down to form ulcers and generally start to resolve gradually within a few weeks.

Polyarteritis nodosa

A vasculitic disorder of the medium and small arteries, polyarteritis nodosa manifests as segmental inflammatory infiltration and fibrinoid necrosis of the vessel walls leading to diminished blood flow. Tender subcutaneous nodules appear along the lines of the arteries. Overlying skin may ulcerate or develop individual or multiple purpuric nodules that are small and hard, often accompanied by intolerable pain. Apart from causing skin lesions, the disease may also involve internal organs such as the kidneys or heart.

Etiology and pathology

Yin Deficiency of the Lungs and Kidneys

Persistent coughing, as in tuberculosis, damages Lung Yin to result in Lung Qi Deficiency, which affects the Kidneys. An enduring illness causes Kidney Yin Deficiency, which affects the Lungs. Yin and Blood Deficiency lead to obstruction of Qi in the channels and impairment of the movement of Blood, finally resulting in Qi stagnation and Blood stasis. Plaques and nodules appear in the skin and flesh. If there is a concurrent Deficiency-Cold pattern, the surface color of the plaques or nodules will remain unchanged; occasionally, the temperature may rise slightly in the affected areas.

Cold-Damp restraining the exterior

Cold-Damp invading the fleshy exterior will cause Qi stagnation and Blood stasis. As a result, hard, dark-red or purplish-red nodules will form with a diffuse swelling.

Qi stagnation and Blood stasis

In *Xue Zheng Lun* [A Treatise on Blood Patterns], it says: "The Blood that leaves the channels is already separated from the Blood that is nourishing the body. They are already apart and no longer in harmony." Once Blood stasis forms, no matter whether it is caused by Cold-Damp, Damp-Heat, or Qi and Blood Deficiency, it may lead to stagnation of the channels and network vessels or stasis and obstruction in the Zang-Fu organs. Nodules and plaques are dark red or purplish-red. Accompanying symptoms and signs include obvious pain, irritability and restlessness with a sensation of heat, and profuse sweating.

Pattern identification and treatment

INTERNAL TREATMENT

YIN DEFICIENCY OF THE LUNGS AND KIDNEYS

Plaques and hard nodules appear in the skin and flesh;

the skin does not change color. The lesions subsequently ulcerate, discharging a thin, clear fluid; at this stage, lesions will persist and are difficult to cure. Accompanying symptoms and signs include tidal fever, night sweating, dry cough, and a feverish sensation in the center of the palms and soles accompanied by irritability and restlessness. The tongue body is red with a scant coating; the pulse is thready and rapid.

Treatment principle

Supplement the Lungs and boost the Kidneys, invigorate the Blood and soften hardness.

Prescription

NEI XIAO LUO LI WAN JIA JIAN
Scrofula Internal Dispersion Pill, with modifications

Sheng Di Huang (Radix Rehmanniae Glutinosae) 15g
Xuan Shen (Radix Scrophulariae Ningpoensis) 10g
Mai Men Dong (Radix Ophiopogonis Japonici) 10g
*Bie Jia** (Carapax Amydae Sinensis) 10g
Tu Si Zi (Semen Cuscutae) 10g
Xu Duan (Radix Dipsaci) 10g
Nü Zhen Zi (Fructus Ligustri Lucidi) 10g
Huang Qin (Radix Scutellariae Baicalensis) 10g
Bai Bu (Radix Stemonae) 10g
Yu Xing Cao (Herba Houttuyniae Cordatae) 10g
Dan Shen (Radix Salviae Miltiorrhizae) 10g
Ji Xue Teng (Caulis Spatholobi) 10g
Xia Ku Cao (Spica Prunellae Vulgaris) 30g
Mu Li‡ (Concha Ostreae) 30g
Zhe Bei Mu (Bulbus Fritillariae Thunbergii) 6g
Shan Ci Gu (Pseudobulbus Shancigu) 6g

Explanation

- *Sheng Di Huang* (Radix Rehmanniae Glutinosae), *Xuan Shen* (Radix Scrophulariae Ningpoensis), *Mai Men Dong* (Radix Ophiopogonis Japonici), *Xu Duan* (Radix Dipsaci), *Nü Zhen Zi* (Fructus Ligustri Lucidi), *Huang Qin* (Radix Scutellariae Baicalensis), and *Tu Si Zi* (Semen Cuscutae) enrich Yin and clear Heat to supplement the Lungs and Kidneys.
- *Bie Jia** (Carapax Amydae Sinensis), *Dan Shen* (Radix Salviae Miltiorrhizae) and *Ji Xue Teng* (Caulis Spatholobi) nourish Yin and invigorate the Blood.
- *Bai Bu* (Radix Stemonae), *Xia Ku Cao* (Spica Prunellae Vulgaris), *Zhe Bei Mu* (Bulbus Fritillariae Thunbergii), *Mu Li‡* (Concha Ostreae), *Shan Ci Gu* (Pseudobulbus Shancigu), and *Yu Xing Cao* (Herba Houttuyniae Cordatae) transform Phlegm, dissipate nodules, soften hardness, and free the network vessels.

QI STAGNATION AND COLD CONGEALING

A number of firm, purplish-red or dark red nodules and

lumps appear on the flexor aspect of the lower leg; the swelling is elevated or protruding with distending pain. The patient's limbs are cold. This pattern often occurs in winter when it is cold. The tongue body is pale red with a thin white coating; the pulse is deep, thready and rough.

Treatment principle
Warm Yang and dissipate Cold, free stagnation and soften hardness.

Prescription
YANG HE TANG JIA JIAN
Harmonious Yang Decoction, with modifications

*Zhi Ma Huang** (Herba Ephedrae, mix-fried with honey) 6g
Pao Jiang (Rhizoma Zingiberis Officinalis Praeparata) 6g
Chao Bai Jie Zi (Semen Sinapis Albae, stir-fried) 6g
Shu Di Huang (Radix Rehmanniae Glutinosae Conquita) 30g
Zhe Bei Mu (Bulbus Fritillariae Thunbergii) 10g
Ju Hong (Pars Rubra Epicarpii Citri Erythrocarpae) 10g
Hai Zao (Herba Sargassi) 10g
Kun Bu (Thallus Laminariae seu Eckloniae) 10g
Huang Yao Zi (Rhizoma Dioscoreae Bulbiferae) 6g
Bai Yao Zi (Tuber Stephaniae Cepharanthae) 6g
Feng Fang‡ (Nidus Vespae) 6g
Chuan Xiong (Rhizoma Ligustici Chuanxiong) 12g
Dang Gui (Radix Angelicae Sinensis) 12g
Dan Shen (Radix Salviae Miltiorrhizae) 12g
Jiang Can‡ (Bombyx Batryticatus) 4.5g
Quan Xie‡ (Buthus Martensi) 3g

Explanation
- *Zhi Ma Huang** (Herba Ephedrae, mix-fried with honey), *Pao Jiang* (Rhizoma Zingiberis Officinalis Praeparata) and *Chao Bai Jie Zi* (Semen Sinapis Albae, stir-fried) warm Yang and dissipate Cold.
- *Zhe Bei Mu* (Bulbus Fritillariae Thunbergii), *Ju Hong* (Pars Rubra Epicarpii Citri Erythrocarpae), *Hai Zao* (Herba Sargassi), *Kun Bu* (Thallus Laminariae seu Eckloniae), *Jiang Can*‡ (Bombyx Batryticatus), *Huang Yao Zi* (Rhizoma Dioscoreae Bulbiferae), and *Bai Yao Zi* (Tuber Stephaniae Cepharanthae) regulate Qi and transform Phlegm, dissipate nodules and disperse swelling.
- *Chuan Xiong* (Rhizoma Ligustici Chuanxiong), *Feng Fang*‡ (Nidus Vespae) and *Quan Xie*‡ (Buthus Martensi) free stagnation and soften hardness.
- *Shu Di Huang* (Radix Rehmanniae Glutinosae Conquita), *Dan Shen* (Radix Salviae Miltiorrhizae) and *Dang Gui* (Radix Angelicae Sinensis) nourish and invigorate the Blood.

QI STAGNATION AND BLOOD STASIS
Plaques and hard nodules are relatively large; the skin is purplish-red or dark red. There is severe distending pain in the lower leg, worse when walking. The tongue body is dull purple, possibly with stasis spots; the pulse is thready and rough.

Treatment principle
Regulate Qi and invigorate the Blood, free the network vessels and dissipate nodules.

Prescription
TONG LUO FANG JIA JIAN
Formula for Freeing the Network Vessels, with modifications

Dang Gui (Radix Angelicae Sinensis) 10g
Chi Shao (Radix Paeoniae Rubra) 10g
Ze Lan (Herba Lycopi Lucidi) 10g
Qian Cao Gen (Radix Rubiae Cordifoliae) 10g
Tao Ren (Semen Persicae) 10g
Qing Pi (Pericarpium Citri Reticulatae Viride) 6g
Xiang Fu (Rhizoma Cyperi Rotundi) 6g
Wang Bu Liu Xing (Semen Vaccariae Segetalis) 6g
Hong Hua (Flos Carthami Tinctorii) 6g
Chuan Niu Xi (Radix Cyathulae Officinalis) 12g
Tu Bei Mu (Tuber Bolbostemmatis) 12g

Explanation
- *Dang Gui* (Radix Angelicae Sinensis), *Chi Shao* (Radix Paeoniae Rubra), *Ze Lan* (Herba Lycopi Lucidi), *Qian Cao Gen* (Radix Rubiae Cordifoliae), *Tao Ren* (Semen Persicae), and *Hong Hua* (Flos Carthami Tinctorii) invigorate and cool the Blood to free the network vessels.
- *Qing Pi* (Pericarpium Citri Reticulatae Viride), *Xiang Fu* (Rhizoma Cyperi Rotundi) and *Wang Bu Liu Xing* (Semen Vaccariae Segetalis) regulate Qi and free the network vessels.
- *Chuan Niu Xi* (Radix Cyathulae Officinalis) and *Tu Bei Mu* (Tuber Bolbostemmatis) relieve Toxicity and transform Phlegm.

General modifications
1. For persistent hard nodules, add *Ju He* (Semen Citri Reticulatae), *Tian Hua Fen* (Radix Trichosanthis) and *Ji Nei Jin*‡ (Endothelium Corneum Gigeriae Galli).
2. For persistent low-grade fever, add *Yin Chai Hu* (Radix Stellariae Dichotomae) and *Di Gu Pi* (Cortex Lycii Radicis).
3. For ruptured lesions that are difficult to close, add *Dang Shen* (Radix Codonopsitis Pilosulae), *Huang Qi* (Radix Astragali seu Hedysari), *Lu Jiao Pian*‡ (Cornu Cervi, sliced), *Shan Yao* (Radix Dioscoreae Oppositae), and *Bai Lian* (Radix Ampelopsis Japonicae).
4. For persistent puffy swelling around the ankles, add *Bi Xie* (Rhizoma Dioscoreae Hypoglaucae seu Septemlobae), *Chen Pi* (Pericarpium Citri Reticulatae) and a large dose of *Huang Qi* (Radix Astragali seu Hedysari).

EXTERNAL TREATMENT

- If hard nodules do not dissipate, mix *Zi Se Xiao Zhong Fen* (Purple Powder for Dispersing Swelling) with *Hei Bu Yao Gao* (Black Cloth Medicated Paste) for external application to the affected area.
- If hard nodules are about to break down, apply *Lü Yun Gao* (Green Cloud Paste) to the affected area.
- For non-healing lesions, apply *Mao Yan Cao Gao* (Crescent Euphorbia Paste) or *Feng Fang Gao* (Hornet Nest Paste) to the affected area.
- If granulation in the lesion appears red and active, apply *Bing Shi San* (Borneol and Gypsum Powder) and cover with *Gan Cao You* (Licorice Oil) or *Dan Huang You* (Egg Yolk Oil).

MOXIBUSTION

Point: Ashi points (the site of the lesions).
Technique: Cut a garlic clove into slices and use to cover the lesions. Place a moxa cone on each garlic slice and light. Retain until it is too hot for the patient. Repeat for a further three cones. This treatment is given once a day. Seven treatments make up a course.
Indications: This type of moxibustion therapy helps to disperse nodules that have not ruptured, and to reduce exudate and promote granulation if the lesion has already ruptured.

Clinical notes

- Moxibustion is recommended for the treatment of erythema induratum with or without breakdown of nodules and ulceration. For nodules that have not broken down, it has the functions of dispersing swelling and alleviating pain; for lesions that have already ulcerated, it helps to close the lesion and generate flesh.
- Nodules that break down to form necrotic ulcers are often associated with Yin Deficiency and a weak constitution. During treatment, attention should therefore be paid to nourishing Yin, augmenting Qi, supporting Vital Qi (Zheng Qi), and drawing out Toxicity. In such cases, *Bai He Gu Jin Tang* (Lily Bulb Decoction for Consolidating Metal) combined with *Tao Hong Si Wu Tang* (Peach Kernel and Safflower Four Agents Decoction) is recommended.
- If tuberculosis is diagnosed and active, usual isolation procedures and precautions should be carried out.

Case history

Patient
Adult female, age unspecified.

Clinical manifestations
The patient had consulted two years previously for erythema on the medial aspect of the right thigh. The erythema later turned purple and firm nodules developed. One year later, similar lesions appeared on the medial aspect of the left thigh. Hospital biopsy confirmed the condition as erythema induratum.

Examination revealed hard, dull purple nodules on the right thigh forming a plaque measuring 4 x 6 cm; the nodules were slightly tender on pressure. Other symptoms included dizziness and blurred vision, which sometimes caused the patient to faint, flushed face, restless sleep, irritability, palpitations, and a dry mouth. The tongue body was red with a white coating; the pulse was wiry and forceful.

Pattern identification
Hyperactivity of Liver-Fire, disharmony of the network vessels, Qi stagnation and Blood stasis, and accumulation of Phlegm-turbidity.

Treatment principle
Invigorate the Blood and transform stasis, clear Fire and transform Phlegm.

Prescription ingredients
Dang Gui (Radix Angelicae Sinensis) 6g
Hong Hua (Flos Carthami Tinctorii) 6g
Chi Shao (Radix Paeoniae Rubra) 6g
Mu Dan Pi (Cortex Moutan Radicis) 6g
Niu Xi (Radix Achyranthis Bidentatae) 6g
Kun Bu (Thallus Laminariae seu Eckloniae) 9g
Hai Zao (Herba Sargassi) 9g
Xia Ku Cao (Spica Prunellae Vulgaris) 9g
Mu Li‡ (Concha Ostreae) 15g
Zhi Bi Hu‡ (Gekko Swinhoana, mix-fried) 9g
Shan Ci Gu (Pseudobulbus Shancigu) 2g

After seven bags of this prescription taken twice a day, the nodules were subsiding and the skin was beginning to return to a normal color. However, the patient still complained of dizziness and a distending pain in the head.

Further treatment
The treatment was continued with additional attention being paid to calming the Liver and extinguishing Wind. *Ju Hua* (Flos Chrysanthemi Morifolii) 6g, *Zhen Zhu Mu*‡ (Concha Margaritifera) 30g and *Gou Teng* (Ramulus Uncariae cum Uncis) 10g were added to the prescription.

Outcome
After two months' treatment with the modified prescription, the hard, swollen nodules had disappeared completely. Dizziness, palpitations and the flushing on the face all showed considerable improvement. The patient was told to follow the modified prescription for another ten days to consolidate the improvement and to take one tablet of *Fu Fang Dan Shen Pian* (Compound Red Sage Root Tablet) once a day. [22]

Literature excerpts

According to *Yi Zong Jin Jian: Wai Ke Xin Fa Yao Jue* [Golden Mirror of Medicine: Important Decisions in

Treating External Diseases]: *"Fei chuai fa* occurs in the calf. … If the lesion is red and inflamed, with an elevated swelling, and painful with exudation of pus mixed with blood, the prognosis is good. The condition complies with the normal course of the disease. If the lesion is dark purple with a diffuse swelling, which flattens or sinks, produces thin clear discharge, and there is pain in the lymph node, the prognosis is poor. The condition does not comply with the normal course of the disease."

In *Yang Ke Xun Cui* [Essential Collection for the Treatment of Sores], it says: "How can we interpret the disease characterized by deep-rooted sores in the calf (*fei chuai fa*), accompanied by fever and chills, irritability and restlessness? It is associated with the Kidney channel and occurs because of insufficiency of Kidney-Water resulting in the accumulation of Heat.

"The ancient classics indicate that the disease is difficult to cure. Treatment can be given by using *Huo Ming Yin* (Life-Giving Beverage) plus *Niu Xi* (Radix Achyranthis Bidentatae), *Mu Gua* (Fructus Chaenomelis) and *Huang Bai* (Cortex Phellodendri); for the elderly and people with a weak constitution, use *Ba Zhen Tang* (Eight Treasure Decoction) plus *Niu Xi* (Radix Achyranthis Bidentatae). Patients with Deficiency patterns are difficult to treat; in such cases, use *Shen Qi Wan* (Kidney Qi Pill) or *Shi Quan Da Bu Tang* (Perfect Major Supplementation Decoction). If there is exudation of pus and blood on breakdown of the nodules, the prognosis is good; if thin watery fluid is exuded, the prognosis is poor."

Modern clinical experience

Zhu emphasized that the selection of ingredients for this treatment should take the involvement of the Xue level into account. He alluded to Tang Rongchuan in *Xue Zheng Lun* [A Treatise on Blood Patterns]: "Once there is Blood stasis, irrespective of whether it has formed recently or has been present for some time, it must be dispersed. Once it has been eliminated, Cold, Heat, Wind or Dampness cannot linger in the body." [23]

Treatment principle
Free the network vessels and dispel Blood stasis, move Qi and invigorate the Blood.

Prescription
TONG LUO HUO XUE FANG JIA JIAN
Formula for Freeing the Network Vessels and Invigorating the Blood, with modifications

Dang Gui Wei (Extremitas Radicis Angelicae Sinensis) 9g
Chi Shao (Radix Paeoniae Rubra) 9g
Tao Ren (Semen Persicae) 9g
Hong Hua (Flos Carthami Tinctorii) 9g
Ze Lan (Herba Lycopi Lucidi) 9g
Qian Cao Gen (Radix Rubiae Cordifoliae) 9g
Qing Pi (Pericarpium Citri Reticulatae Viride) 9g
Xiang Fu (Rhizoma Cyperi Rotundi) 9g
Wang Bu Liu Xing (Semen Vaccariae Segetalis) 9g
Di Long‡ (Lumbricus) 9g
Niu Xi (Radix Achyranthis Bidentatae) 9g

Modifications
1. For inflamed, red and swollen nodules at the initial stage, accompanied by yellow urine, constipation, a red tongue body, and a slippery and rapid pulse, add *Sheng Di Huang* (Radix Rehmanniae Glutinosae), *Mu Dan Pi* (Cortex Moutan Radicis), *Da Qing Ye* (Folium Isatidis seu Baphicacanthi), and *Jin Yin Hua* (Flos Lonicerae) to cool the Blood and clear Heat.
2. For larger, dull purple plaques, with a pale tongue body and a thready, slippery pulse, add *Ma Huang** (Herba Ephedrae) and *Gui Zhi* (Ramulus Cinnamomi Cassiae) to warm the channels and free the network vessels.
3. For persistent erythema, add *Zhi Chuan Shan Jia** (Squama Manitis Pentadactylae, mix-fried), *Hai Zao* (Herba Sargassi) and *Shan Ci Gu* (Pseudobulbus Shancigu) to soften hardness and dissipate nodules.
4. For persistent non-healing ulcers, add *Dang Shen* (Radix Codonopsitis Pilosulae), *Zhi Huang Qi* (Radix Astragali seu Hedysari, mix-fried with honey) and *Shu Di Huang* (Radix Rehmanniae Glutinosae Conquita) to augment Qi and supplement the Blood.
5. For persistent puffy swelling around the ankle, add *Bi Xie* (Rhizoma Dioscoreae Hypoglaucae seu Septemlobae), *Chen Pi* (Pericarpium Citri Reticulatae) and a high dose of *Huang Qi* (Radix Astragali seu Hedysari) to move Qi and benefit the movement of water.
6. For pain and soreness in the joints, add *Xi Xian Cao* (Herba Siegesbeckiae), *Qin Jiao* (Radix Gentianae Macrophyllae) and *Mu Gua* (Fructus Chaenomelis) to dispel Wind and overcome Dampness.

Erythrasma
红癣

Erythrasma is a condition marked by superficial infection of areas prone to friction and is caused by *Corynebacterium minutissimum*. It is known as *dan xuan* (cinnabar tinea) in TCM. This name was actually given in the modern era in reference to the lesion characterized by reddish-brown tinea-like patches.

Clinical manifestations

- Erythrasma occurs more commonly in young men in a body flexure where the thin skin is easily traumatized, such as the genitals, groin, axillae, and toes.
- The pale brown or pinkish non-inflamed lesion is round or irregular in shape; some fine scaling may be observed on the surface.

Differential diagnosis

Erythrasma should be differentiated from tinea corporis, tinea cruris, tinea pedis, and pityriasis versicolor. Fungus examination and culture, and examination with Wood's light – a long-wave ultraviolet light – will help to establish the diagnosis; erythrasma fluoresces coral pink due to the presence of porphyrins.

Etiology and pathology

- The condition frequently develops because of Wind, Dampness or Worms being retained in the interstices after they have attacked the warm body.

- It may also occur because of stagnation of Damp-Heat in the pores as a result of wearing clothes soaked in sweat.
- Erythrasma may also be passed on by infection.

Treatment

EXTERNAL TREATMENT
Since the lesion often involves areas where the skin is tender, strongly-irritant external medications should not be used. *Tu Jin Pi Ding* (Golden Larch Bark Tincture), *Dian Dao San Xi Ji* (Reversal Powder Wash Preparation) or *Yang Ti Gen Jiu* (Curled Dock Root Wine) can be selected as appropriate depending on the state of the lesions.

Clinical notes

External treatment only is recommended for erythrasma. In the initial stage, apply *Tu Jin Pi Ding* (Golden Larch Bark Tincture) or *Dian Dao San Xi Ji* (Reversal Powder Wash Preparation) to the affected area. Where there is a small amount of desquamation, apply *Yang Ti Gen Jiu* (Curled Dock Root Wine).

Advice for the patient

- Continue the external medication for an additional one to two weeks after the lesion heals in order to prevent recurrence.
- Sterilize underwear frequently by boiling in water and drying in the sun.

References

1. Wang Xinmin, *Zi Ni Ku Lu Huang San Zhi Liao Nong Pao Chuang 200 Li* [Treatment of 200 Cases of Impetigo with the Empirical Prescription *Ku Lu Huang San* (Prepared Alum, Calamine and Phellodendron Bark Powder)], *Zhong Yi Wai Zhi Za Zhi* [Journal of Traditional Chinese Medicine External Treatments] 6, 5 (1997): 43.
2. Cao Zhigang, *Zhong Yao Xi Fang Zhi Liao Nong Pao Chuang* [Treatment of Impetigo with a Chinese Materia Medica Wash Formula], *Jiang Su Zhong Yi* [Jiangsu Journal of Traditional Chinese Medicine] 19, 5 (1998): 28-29.
3. Bao Zuoyi, *Fu Fang Bei Fan Shi Hu Ji Zhi Liao Nong Pao Chuang 43 Li* [Treatment of 43 Cases of Impetigo with *Fu Fang Bei Fan Shi Hu Ji* (Compound Chinese Gall, Prepared Alum and Talcum Paste Preparation)], *Xin Yi Xue* [New Journal of Medicine] 27, 11 (1996): 565.
4. Zhao Mingnan, *Zhu Zi He Ji Zhi Liao Nong Pao Chuang 103 Li Liao Xiao Guan Cha* [Clinical Observation of the Effectiveness of Treating 103 Cases of Impetigo with a Combination of *Zhu Huang San* (Pearl and Bezoar Powder) and Gentian Violet Solution], *Xin Yi Xue* [New Journal of Medicine] 27, 10 (1996): 514.

5. Xu Fusong, *Xu Lü He Wai Ke Yi An Yi Hua Ji* [A Collection of Xu Lühe's Medical Records and Notes on External Diseases] (Beijing: China Science and Technology Publishing House, 1986), 421-2.

6. Zhu Renkang, *Zhong Yi Wai Ke Xue* [External Diseases in Traditional Chinese Medicine] (Beijing: People's Medical Publishing House, 1987), 358.

7. Gu Bohua, *Shi Yong Zhong Yi Wai Ke Xue* [Practical Treatment of External Diseases with Traditional Chinese Medicine] (Shanghai: Shanghai Science and Technology Publishing House, 1985), 423.

8. Deng Xiaoyuan, *Fen Xing Zhi Liao Lian Chuang 38 Li Lin Chuang Guan Cha* [Clinical Observation of the Treatment of 38 Cases of Ecthyma Based on Pattern Identification], *Si Chuan Zhong Yi* [Sichuan Journal of Traditional Chinese Medicine] 7 (1996): 44.

9. Li Weili, *Shen Miao Tang Zhi Liao Lian Chuang 83 Li* [Treatment of 83 Cases of Ecthyma with *Shen Miao Tang* (Mysterious Spirit Decoction)], *Shan Xi Zhong Yi* [Shanxi Journal of Traditional Chinese Medicine] 12, 4 (1996): 6-7.

10. Tian Conghuo, *Zhen Jiu Yi Xue Yan Ji* [Collected Experiences in Acupuncture and Moxibustion] (Beijing: Science and Technology Documents Publishing House, 2000), 761.

11. Zhu Renkang, *Zhong Yi Wai Ke Xue*, 571.

12. Qian Weishan, *Yue Bi Tang Jia Wei Zhi Liao Fa Ji Chuang* [Treatment of Folliculitis with Augmented *Yue Bi Tang* (Maidservant from Yue Decoction)], *Jiang Su Yi Yao* [Jiangsu Journal of Medicine] 1 (1973): 30.

13. Du Huaitang (ed.), *Zhong Guo Dang Dai Ming Yi Yan Fang Da Quan* [A Compendium of Empirical Prescriptions Made by Famous Contemporary Chinese Doctors] (Shijiazhuang: Hebei Science and Technology Publishing House, 1990), 405.

14. Ibid., 404.

15. Xiang Junting, *San Huang Cha Ji Zhi Liao Fei Chuang (Mao Nang Yan)* [Treatment of Folliculitis with *San Huang Cha Ji* (Three Yellows Rub Preparation)], *Hu Bei Zhong Yi Za Zhi* [Hubei Journal of Traditional Chinese Medicine] 20, 3 (1998): 62.

16. Zhou Yuzhu, *Yi Shen Gong Du Tang Zhi Liao Jie Bing 95 Li* [Treatment of 95 Cases of Furuncles with *Yi Shen Gong Du Tang* (Decoction for Boosting the Kidneys and Attacking Toxicity)], *An Hui Zhong Yi Xue Yuan Xue Bao* [Journal of Anhui College of Traditional Chinese Medicine] 12, 4 (1992): 14.

17. Cai Wenmo, *Tian Xian Xiao Du Gao Zhi Liao Jie Zhong 46 Li Liao Xiao Guan Cha* [Observation of the Effectiveness of Treatment of 46 Cases of Furuncles with *Tian Xian Xiao Du Gao* (Henbane Seed Paste for Dispersing Swelling)], *Xin Jiang Zhong Yi Yao* [Xinjiang Journal of Traditional Chinese Medicine and Materia Medica] 2 (1995): 19.

18. Beijing Hospital of Traditional Chinese Medicine, *Zhao Bing Nan Lin Chuang Jing Yan Ji* [A Collection of Zhao Bingnan's Clinical Experiences] (Beijing: People's Medical Publishing House, 1975), 52.

19. An Jiafeng and Zhang Fan, *Zhang Zhi Li Pi Fu Bing Yi An Xuan Cui* [A Collection of Zhang Zhili's Skin Disease Cases] (Beijing: People's Medical Publishing House, 1994), 214.

20. Bai Landi, *Zi Ni Yin Hua Jie Du Tang Zhi Liao Dan Du 50 Li* [Treatment of 50 Cases of Erysipelas with the Empirical Prescription *Yin Hua Jie Du Tang* (Honeysuckle Decoction for Relieving Toxicity)], *Zhong Guo Zhong Xi Yi Jie He Za Zhi* [Journal of Integrated TCM and Western Medicine] 16, 2 (1996): 108.

21. Wang Longchuan, *Yin Huang Jie Du Tang Zhi Liao Dan Du De Liao Xiao Guan Cha* [Observation of the Effectiveness of *Yin Huang Jie Du Tang* (Honeysuckle and Scutellaria Decoction for Relieving Toxicity) in the Treatment of Erysipelas], *Xin Jiang Zhong Yi Yao* [Xinjiang Journal of Traditional Chinese Medicine and Materia Medica] 16, 3 (1998): 20-21.

22. Xu Fusong, *Xu Lü He Wai Ke Yi An Yi Hua Ji*, 422.

23. Zhu Renkang, *Zhu Ren Kang Lin Chuang Jing Yan Ji* [A Collection of Zhu Renkang's Clinical Experiences] (Beijing: People's Medical Publishing House, 1979), 165-166.

Fungal infections of the skin

Fungi are a very simple kind of plant that lack the chlorophyll that enables other plants to form carbohydrates from the carbon dioxide in the air. They are widespread in nature, but relatively few are pathogenic to humans. Fungal infection in humans is mainly caused by two groups of fungi – dermatophytes, whose usual method of reproduction is by forming spores, which grow to produce a mycelium (a mass of filaments, or hyphae), and yeasts, which reproduce by budding.

Dermatophytes are responsible for most human fungal infections. Dermatophytes survive on dead keratin found in the stratum corneum, the hair and the nails. Immunosuppression may allow dermatophyte infections to infect deeper layers of skin and in severe cases to disseminate systemically.

Three genera are recognized:
- *Trichophyton*, which infect the skin, nails and hair
- *Microsporum*, which infect the skin and hair
- *Epidermophyton*, which infect the skin and nails

The inflammation caused by dermatophytes is due to delayed hypersensitivity or the metabolic products of the fungi. Zoophilic species of fungi (those transmitted from animals to humans) generally cause more severe inflammation than anthropophilic species (transmitted from person to person).

The main skin diseases caused by yeasts include pityriasis versicolor and candidiasis. Candidal balanitis is considered in this chapter, a discussion of oral candidiasis (thrush) can be found in Chapter 15 (Regional disorders), and the role of *Candida albicans* in diaper dermatitis (nappy rash) and intertrigo is described in Chapters 3 and 17 respectively.

In TCM, fungal infections of the skin are mainly attributed to *chong* (Worms). The Western terminology of ringworm, or tinea (Latin for worm), historically reflects a similar understanding. In TCM these infections are also related to invasion by Wind, Heat and Damp pathogenic factors. After pathogenic Worms and external pathogenic factors invade the body, they fight with Wei Qi (Defensive Qi) and bind with Body Fluids. If they accumulate and are not dissipated, tinea will occur.

If the condition persists, the Ying and Xue levels will lose moisture, and the skin and hair will become dry since they will be deprived of adequate nourishment. If there is also retention of Dampness, exudation will occur. Where the condition is persistent, both Qi and Blood will be damaged and the disease will be difficult to cure.

Tinea capitis (ringworm of the scalp)
头癣

Tinea capitis is caused by dermatophyte infection of the scalp and hair. It occurs most often in prepubertal children. The responsible organism varies in different countries. Tinea capitis is infectious, spreading by direct contact, clothing, hairdressing implements, or contact with infected animals. Fungi of animal origin result in more intensely inflamed lesions than those caused by fungi transmitted from person to person.

In TCM, tinea capitis is known as *tu chuang* (bald scalp sore); it can also be referred to according to the various characteristic skin lesions – "gray patch ringworm" is known as *bai tu chuang* (bald white scalp sore), kerion as *chi tu* (red baldness), and favus as *fei chuang* (fat sore).

Clinical manifestations

Although there are many ways of classifying tinea capitis, the most useful method for the practitioner is based on the clinical manifestations. Most cases of tinea capitis begin with one or several patches of scaling or alopecia.

Three basic clinical patterns of infection are recognized:

- "Gray patch ringworm" – this pattern is characterized by round or irregular scaly lesions of grayish-white patches. Hairs usually break off 3-4 mm above the skin surface with white sheaths left at the root of the affected hairs. The scalp is not inflamed and healing occurs without scarring. This type is commonly caused by *Microsporum audouinii*.

- Kerion – a severe inflammatory reaction with boggy induration and multiple, dark red, round or oval discharging abscesses is known as a kerion. It frequently causes scarring alopecia. Any species of fungus may cause this, but it is particularly associated with infection by zoophilic fungi such as *Microsporum canis*, *Trichophyton mentagrophytes* or *Trichophyton verrucosum*.

- Favus is a rare cause of tinea capitis in Western countries. The causative organism is *Trichophyton schoenleinii*. Skin lesions are typically saucer-shaped and lusterless, with foul-smelling yellow crusts of varying size. A single hair may appear through the center of the crust. Healing results in atrophic areas with scarring alopecia.

Differential diagnosis

Alopecia areata
The gray patch ringworm pattern of tinea capitis should be differentiated from alopecia areata, which is characterized by the sudden appearance of one or several clearly defined round or oval patches of hair loss, generally 1-4 cm in size. The skin is smooth and white or may have short stubs of hair at the margins of lesions (so-called "exclamation mark hairs", about 4mm in length and tapering toward the scalp). Inflammation and scaling are absent.

Psoriasis of the scalp
The scalp is bright red or dark red and is covered by layers of silvery-white scale. The hair may form matted bundles in the area of the skin lesions, which often spread beyond the hairline. Areas of scaling may be interspersed with normal skin. Similar lesions may also be present on other parts of the body. Lesions are frequently exacerbated in winter and alleviated in summer.

Seborrheic eczema
Seborrheic eczema is a chronic inflammatory condition mainly affecting hair-bearing areas of the head and body. An itchy red or yellowish-red scaly or exudative erythematous eruption affects the scalp and scalp margins, the sides of the nose, the eyebrows, and the ears.

The presternal and interscapular areas and body flexures may also be involved. On the scalp, the condition may be accompanied by marked dandruff.

Etiology and pathology

- When the Zang-Fu organs are in disharmony and the exterior is weak, Wind-Damp or Wind-Heat Toxins can attack the scalp to cause the disease.

- Damp-Heat steams in the Spleen and Stomach and rises; if retained internally over a long period, Damp-Heat weakens Wei Qi (Defensive Qi), thus allowing invasion by Worms, which destroy the hair root and cause tinea capitis.

- Tinea capitis may also result from infection by Toxins through contact with hairdressing equipment or dirty clothes, hats or pillowcases.

Pattern identification and treatment

INTERNAL TREATMENT

DAMP-HEAT TRANSFORMING INTO TOXINS (KERION)
Follicles are raised and the affected area is inflamed and swollen with surface pustules. Pressure on the lesion will cause exudation of pus and provoke pain and itching. Other symptoms include dry mouth and enlargement of the lymph nodes in the neck. The tongue body is red with a thin yellow coating; the pulse is thready and rapid.

Treatment principle
Clear Heat and transform Dampness, relieve Toxicity and dissipate nodules.

Prescription
QU DU TANG JIA JIAN
Decoction for Expelling Toxicity, with modifications

Jin Yin Hua (Flos Lonicerae) 10g
Fang Feng (Radix Ledebouriellae Divaricatae) 10g
Zi Hua Di Ding (Herba Violae Yedoensitis) 10g
Huang Qin (Radix Scutellariae Baicalensis) 10g
Niu Bang Zi (Fructus Arctii Lappae) 10g
Chi Shao (Radix Paeoniae Rubra) 10g
Gan Cao (Radix Glycyrrhizae) 10g
Lian Qiao (Fructus Forsythiae Suspensae) 12g
Pu Gong Ying (Herba Taraxaci cum Radice) 12g
Bai Hua She She Cao (Herba Hedyotidis Diffusae) 15g
Yin Chen Hao (Herba Artemisiae Scopariae) 15g
Yi Yi Ren (Semen Coicis Lachryma-jobi) 15g
Chi Fu Ling (Sclerotium Poriae Cocos Rubrae) 15g

Explanation
- *Yi Yi Ren* (Semen Coicis Lachryma-jobi), *Chi Fu Ling* (Sclerotium Poriae Cocos Rubrae) and *Yin Chen Hao* (Herba Artemisiae Scopariae) clear Heat and transform Dampness.
- *Fang Feng* (Radix Ledebouriellae Divaricatae) and *Niu Bang Zi* (Fructus Arctii Lappae) dredge Wind and alleviate itching.
- *Jin Yin Hua* (Flos Lonicerae), *Zi Hua Di Ding* (Herba Violae Yedoensitis), *Lian Qiao* (Fructus Forsythiae Suspensae), *Pu Gong Ying* (Herba Taraxaci cum Radice), and *Bai Hua She She Cao* (Herba Hedyotidis Diffusae) relieve Toxicity and disperse swelling.
- *Chi Shao* (Radix Paeoniae Rubra) and *Huang Qin* (Radix Scutellariae Baicalensis) cool the Blood and reduce erythema.
- *Gan Cao* (Radix Glycyrrhizae) clears Heat and relieves Toxicity.

BINDING OF WIND-DAMP (FAVUS)
Lesions manifest as red papules and pustules with erosion and exudation accompanied by a fetid odor. The hair is dry and withered with hair loss in severe cases. The tongue body is red with a scant coating; the pulse is rapid.

Treatment principle
Dissipate Wind and eliminate Dampness, cool the Blood and relieve Toxicity. [i]

Prescription
JING FANG SAN JIA JIAN
Schizonepeta and Ledebouriella Powder, with modifications

Jing Jie (Herba Schizonepetae Tenuifoliae) 6g
Fang Feng (Radix Ledebouriellae Divaricatae) 6g
Chao Niu Bang Zi (Fructus Arctii Lappae, stir-fried) 6g
Lian Qiao (Fructus Forsythiae Suspensae) 6g
Xuan Shen (Radix Scrophulariae Ningpoensis) 10g
Tian Hua Fen (Radix Trichosanthis) 10g
Zhe Bei Mu (Bulbus Fritillariae Thunbergii) 10g
Chi Shao (Radix Paeoniae Rubra) 10g
Sheng Di Huang (Radix Rehmanniae Glutinosae) 12g
Jin Yin Hua (Flos Lonicerae) 12g
He Shou Wu (Radix Polygoni Multiflori) 12g

Explanation
- *Jing Jie* (Herba Schizonepetae Tenuifoliae), *Fang Feng* (Radix Ledebouriellae Divaricatae) and *Niu Bang Zi* (Fructus Arctii Lappae) dredge Wind and alleviate itching.

- *Tian Hua Fen* (Radix Trichosanthis), *Xuan Shen* (Radix Scrophulariae Ningpoensis), *Sheng Di Huang* (Radix Rehmanniae Glutinosae), and *He Shou Wu* (Radix Polygoni Multiflori) enrich Yin and eliminate Dampness.
- *Jin Yin Hua* (Flos Lonicerae), *Lian Qiao* (Fructus Forsythiae Suspensae), *Chi Shao* (Radix Paeoniae Rubra), and *Zhe Bei Mu* (Bulbus Fritillariae Thunbergii) relieve Toxicity and invigorate the Blood, dissipate nodules and eliminate sores.

PATENT HERBAL MEDICINES
For gray patch ringworm, take *Fang Feng Tong Sheng San* (Ledebouriella Powder that Sagely Unblocks) 6g three times a day with warm boiled water.

EXTERNAL TREATMENT
External treatment for tinea capitis should focus on killing Worms and alleviating itching while ensuring that the infected hairs are plucked out. *Tu Chuang Gao* (Bald Scalp Sore Paste) can be applied directly to the lesions. Alternatively, *Fei Chuang Gao* (Fat Sore Paste) can be used to treat favus; in those countries where the use of certain ingredients contained in this paste are not permitted, *Tu Jin Pi Ding* (Golden Larch Bark Tincture) can be applied instead.

Alternatives for treatment of gray patch ringworm include:
- *Ku Lian You* (Chinaberry Oil): Put 30g of crushed fresh *Chuan Lian Zi* (Fructus Meliae Toosendan) into cottonseed oil and cook until the herb turns dry. Filter off the oil and apply it externally to the lesions two or three times a day.
- *Bai Cao Shuang You* (Weed Soot Oil): Grind *Bai Cao Shuang* (Fuligo Herbarum Ustarum) to a powder and mix with sesame oil. Apply the oil externally to the lesions two or three times a day.

ACUPUNCTURE
Points: LI-11 Quchi and KI-2 Rangu.
Technique: Apply the reducing method and retain the needles for 30 minutes. Treat once a day. A course consists of seven treatment sessions.

Explanation
LI-11 Quchi and KI-2 Rangu dredge Wind and expel pathogenic factors, nourish Yin and moisten the skin. Combining the two points can help to alleviate itching and heal the lesion.

---

[i] In Chinese medicine, lesions characterized by red papules and pustules are considered to be related to Blood-Heat, hence the treatment principle of cooling the Blood and relieving Toxicity.

MOXIBUSTION

Direct moxibustion with a moxa stick

After cleaning the affected area, move a lit moxa stick over the lesion for 5-10 minutes using the sparrow-pecking method. The treatment is given once every other day. A course consists of five treatment sessions.

Indirect moxibustion with moxa cones

Points: KI-2 Rangu and ST-36 Zusanli
Technique: Place a slice of clean, fresh ginger on the points. Burn five to seven moxa cones on the ginger slice at each point. The treatment is given once a day. A course consists of ten treatment sessions.

Clinical notes

- Treatment of tinea capitis generally focuses on external application. Local treatment of these conditions usually includes ingredients for killing Worms and alleviating itching such as *Chuan Lian Zi* (Fructus Meliae Toosendan), *Liu Huang*‡ (Sulphur), *Mu Jin Pi* (Cortex Hibisci Syriaci Radicis) and *Ku Shen* (Radix Sophorae Flavescentis). In classical formulae, heavy metals such as *Qing Fen*‡ (Calomelas), *Mi Tuo Seng*‡ (Lithargyrum) and *Zhu Sha*‡ (Cinnabaris) are often recommended. Due to their toxicity, such treatments are generally no longer permitted in Western countries.
- The addition of internal treatment, acupuncture and moxibustion aids the healing process where there is exudation and erosion of lesions.
- If favus is not treated in time, permanent alopecia may result.

Advice for the patient

- All hairdressing equipment must be properly sterilized to prevent the disease from spreading.
- All pillowcases, clothes, hats, and combs used by patients with tinea capitis should be thoroughly sterilized. Hair or scale shed by patients should be destroyed.

Modern clinical experience

Zhang Zanchen formulated a soak to treat tinea capitis.[1]

Prescription

XUAN YAO JIN YE
Medicated Soak for Tinea

Bai Bu (Radix Stemonae) 9g
Bing Lang* (Semen Arecae Catechu) 9g
Bai Ji (Rhizoma Bletillae Striatae) 9g
Mu Bie Zi (Semen Momordicae Cochinchinensis) 9g
Tu Jin Pi (Cortex Pseudolaricis) 9g
Bai Zhi (Radix Angelicae Dahuricae) 9g
Ban Mao‡ (Mylabris) 4.5g, remove head and feet and stir-fry with rice
Zhang Nao (Camphora) 4.5g
Tu Da Huang (Radix Rumicis Madaio) 15g

These ingredients were soaked in 250 ml of sorghum liquor for a week. The medicated liquor was then applied externally once or twice a day. This formula should not be used for lesions with erosion.

Tinea manuum (ringworm of the hands)
手癣

Tinea manuum is a chronic dermatophytosis of the hand caused by *Trichophyton rubrum*. It mainly involves the palm and the webs between the fingers but may extend to the dorsum of the hand. It may also be accompanied by tinea pedis on the sole of the foot, manifesting as fine white scales and bleeding on rupture of the skin. Local itching or pain are also possible.

In TCM, the type of tinea manuum occurring on the palm of the hand is also known as *e zhang feng* (goose-foot Wind).

Clinical manifestations

- Tinea manuum is usually asymmetrical and is frequently seen in association with tinea pedis.
- Lesions mainly involve the center of the palm and the palmar aspect of the fingers.
- In the initial stage, small transparent pinpoint vesicles appear, which quickly rupture with a small amount of exudate. They soon dry up and are

covered with layers of white scale. Later, the affected skin becomes dry, rough and thick, and may crack or fissure, resulting in pain and difficulty in bending and stretching the hand and fingers.

- The condition is aggravated in summer and alleviated in winter. If not treated, the symptoms can persist for years.
- Local blistering provokes intolerable itching.
- Where tinea manuum involves the dorsum of the hand, lesions resemble those of tinea corporis. The nails are also frequently affected.

Differential diagnosis

Contact dermatitis

Tinea manuum of the palm may be difficult to differentiate from irritant or allergic contact dermatitis, especially at the chronic stage. Identification of possible causes is usually the best guide to differentiation and treatment. Individuals with a history of atopic eczema are often more susceptible to irritants causing contact dermatitis. In addition, the association with the lesions of tinea pedis is absent.

Recurrent focal palmar peeling (keratolysis exfoliativa)

This condition tends to occur at the end of spring or autumn and involves the bilateral palms. At the initial stage, lesions appear as pinpoint white spots containing no fluid. The lesions gradually extend and eventually produce scaling and peeling. The center of the scaly area may turn red and tender. After desquamation of the horny layer, the skin underneath returns to normal. The condition resolves spontaneously, but may recur once or more a year.

Etiology and pathology

Pathogenic Worms can take advantage of Qi and Blood Deficiency to invade. If Wind and Damp pathogenic factors have accumulated in the skin and flesh, Qi and Blood cannot perform their moistening and nourishing functions, thus depriving the skin of proper nourishment.

Pattern identification and treatment

INTERNAL TREATMENT

BINDING OF WIND-DAMP

At the initial stage, pinpoint vesicles appear on the palm and the palmar aspect of the fingers; these vesicles burst on scratching, producing a small amount of exudate. The skin peels off after the lesions dry up, leaving annular scaling. The skin is dry and patients frequently experience intolerable itching. The tongue body is pale red with a scant coating; the pulse is floating and rapid.

Treatment principle
Dispel Wind and benefit the movement of Dampness, boost the Kidneys and relieve Toxicity.

Prescription
LIU WEI DI HUANG TANG JIA JIAN
Six-Ingredient Rehmannia Decoction

Sheng Di Huang (Radix Rehmanniae Glutinosae) 12g
Fu Ling (Sclerotium Poriae Cocos) 12g
Shan Zhu Yu (Fructus Corni Officinalis) 12g
Chao Bai Shao (Radix Paeoniae Lactiflorae, stir-fried) 12g
Mai Men Dong (Radix Ophiopogonis Japonici) 12g
Chao Mu Dan Pi (Cortex Moutan Radicis, stir-fried) 10g
Ze Xie (Rhizoma Alismatis Orientalis) 10g
Shan Yao (Rhizoma Dioscoreae Oppositae) 30g
Chai Hu (Radix Bupleuri) 6g
Shi Chang Pu (Rhizoma Acori Graminei) 6g

Explanation
- *Sheng Di Huang* (Radix Rehmanniae Glutinosae), *Mai Men Dong* (Radix Ophiopogonis Japonici), *Ze Xie* (Rhizoma Alismatis Orientalis), and *Fu Ling* (Sclerotium Poriae Cocos) enrich Yin and transform Dampness.
- *Chao Bai Shao* (Radix Paeoniae Lactiflorae, stir-fried), *Chao Mu Dan Pi* (Cortex Moutan Radicis, stir-fried), *Shan Yao* (Rhizoma Dioscoreae Oppositae), and *Shan Zhu Yu* (Fructus Corni Officinalis) boost the Kidneys and consolidate the Root.
- *Chai Hu* (Radix Bupleuri) and *Shi Chang Pu* (Rhizoma Acori Graminei) dredge Wind and dissipate Heat to alleviate itching.
- Herbs for boosting the Kidneys are included because dry skin or skin peeling off after the lesions dry up is related to insufficiency of Kidney Yin resulting in lack of nourishment of the skin. Herbs for dissipating Heat are included because there is always an indication of Heat or Fire in itchiness (whether accompanied by Wind, Dampness or Dryness); *Huang Di Nei Jing: Su Wen* [The Yellow Emperor's Classic of Internal Medicine: Simple Questions] says that "all painful and itching sores are ascribed to the Heart [Fire]."

BLOOD-DRYNESS DUE TO SPLEEN DEFICIENCY

The skin in the affected area is thick and rough with deep and wide fissures due to a persistent condition or unsuccessful treatment. Pain and itching occur following fissuring. The palm resembles the webbed foot of a goose. Dryness and pain in the palm result in impaired manual dexterity. The tongue body is dry and lacking in moisture; the pulse is deficient, thready and rapid.

Treatment principle
Nourish the Blood and moisten Dryness, support the Spleen and secure the Root.

Prescription
DANG GUI YIN ZI JIA JIAN
Chinese Angelica Root Drink, with modifications

Dang Gui (Radix Angelicae Sinensis) 6g
Chuan Xiong (Rhizoma Ligustici Chuanxiong) 6g
Gui Zhi (Ramulus Cinnamomi Cassiae) 6g
Gan Cao (Radix Glycyrrhizae) 6g
He Shou Wu (Radix Polygoni Multiflori) 15g
Huang Jing (Rhizoma Polygonati) 15g
Sheng Di Huang (Radix Rehmanniae Glutinosae) 15g
Shu Di Huang (Radix Rehmanniae Glutinosae Conquita) 15g
Chao Bai Shao (Radix Paeoniae Lactiflorae, stir-fried) 15g
Shan Yao (Rhizoma Dioscoreae Oppositae) 12g
Tian Men Dong (Radix Asparagi Cochinchinensis) 12g
Mai Men Dong (Radix Ophiopogonis Japonici) 12g
*Shi Hu** (Herba Dendrobii) 12g
Chao Bai Bian Dou (Semen Dolichoris Lablab, stir-fried) 12g
Yu Zhu (Rhizoma Polygonati Odorati) 12g

Explanation
- *He Shou Wu* (Radix Polygoni Multiflori), *Huang Jing* (Rhizoma Polygonati), *Tian Men Dong* (Radix Asparagi Cochinchinensis), *Mai Men Dong* (Radix Ophiopogonis Japonici), *Shi Hu** (Herba Dendrobii), and *Yu Zhu* (Rhizoma Polygonati Odorati) enrich Yin and moisten Dryness.
- *Dang Gui* (Radix Angelicae Sinensis), *Chuan Xiong* (Rhizoma Ligustici Chuanxiong), *Chao Bai Shao* (Radix Paeoniae Lactiflorae, stir-fried), *Sheng Di Huang* (Radix Rehmanniae Glutinosae), and *Shu Di Huang* (Radix Rehmanniae Glutinosae Conquita) nourish the Blood and moisten the skin.
- *Gui Zhi* (Ramulus Cinnamomi Cassiae) warms the channels and harmonizes the Blood.
- *Chao Bai Bian Dou* (Semen Dolichoris Lablab, stir-fried), *Shan Yao* (Rhizoma Dioscoreae Oppositae) and *Gan Cao* (Radix Glycyrrhizae) support the Spleen and consolidate the Root.

EXTERNAL TREATMENT
- For papulovesicular and scaly lesions, use *Fu Ping Cu* (Duckweed Vinegar Preparation), *Huo Xiang Jin Pao Ji* (Agastache/Patchouli Soak Preparation), *E Zhang Feng Jin Pao Ji* (Soak Preparation for Goose-Foot Wind), or *Cu Pao Fang* (Vinegar Soak Formula) to soak the affected area for 20 minutes two or three times a day; alternatively, *E Zhang Feng Xuan Yao Shui* (Goose-Foot Wind Tinea Lotion), *Tu Jin Pi Bai Bu Ding* (Golden Larch Bark and Stemona Root Tincture) or *Fu Fang Tu Jin Pi Ding* (Compound Golden Larch Bark Tincture) can be used as a wash.
- For lesions with slight exudation and erosion or with vesicles, prepare a decoction with *Huang Ding Shui Xi Ji* (Siberian Solomonseal and Cloves Wash Preparation) or *Huang Jing Shui Xi Ji* (Siberian Solomonseal Wash Preparation) and use as a wet compress on the lesions. Then apply *Mie Xuan Zhi Shi Fen* (Powder for Eliminating Tinea and Alleviating Dampness) or *Yang Ti Gen San* (Curled Dock Root Powder).
- For dry skin or painful, cracked skin, first use *Er Fan San* (Alum and Melanterite Powder) to prepare a steam-wash, then apply *Run Ji Gao* (Flesh-Moistening Paste), *Gan Cao You* (Licorice Oil), *Tu Da Huang Gao* (Madaio Dock Root Paste), or *Dong Fan San* (Minium and Alum Powder) mixed to a paste with vegetable oil.

ACUPUNCTURE

Selection of points on the affected channels
PC-6 Neiguan, LI-4 Hegu, PC-8 Laogong, SP-6 Sanyinjiao, ST-36 Zusanli, KI-3 Taixi, BL-60 Kunlun, and BL-9 Yuzhen.

Selection of points according to clinical manifestations
- For vesicles, select LI-4 Hegu, PC-6 Neiguan and ST-40 Fenglong.
- For cracking of the skin, select PC-6 Neiguan, SP-6 Sanyinjiao and ST-36 Zusanli.

Technique
Apply the reducing method. Use lifting and thrusting needle manipulation without retaining the needles. Treat once a day. A course consists of ten treatment sessions.

Explanation
- PC-6 Neiguan, LI-4 Hegu and PC 8 Laogong clear the Heart and drain Fire.
- BL-9 Yuzhen arrests Wind and clears Heat.
- SP-6 Sanyinjiao, ST-36 Zusanli, BL-60 Kunlun, KI-3 Taixi, and ST-40 Fenglong enrich Yin and eliminate Dampness.

MOXIBUSTION
Points: Ashi points (the site of the lesions).
Technique: Give moxibustion by burning 5-10 moxa cones on top of slices of *Sheng Fu Zi** (Radix Lateralis Aconiti Carmichaeli Cruda) placed on the Ashi points.

OTHER TREATMENT METHODS
Soaking with soya milk
Place *Hua Jiao* (Pericarpium Zanthoxyli) 15g and *Tou*

Gu Cao (Herba Speranskiae seu Impatientis) 15g in a pot, add two large bowls of soya milk and bring to the boil. Allow the liquid to cool to lukewarm and soak the hand in it for two hours a day for three or four days. This treatment is suitable when vesicles are present.

Baking method

First apply *Gan Cao You* (Licorice Oil) mixed with *Yang Ti Gen San* (Curled Dock Root Powder) to the lesions. Then heat the affected area with an electric hair-drier for 20-30 minutes once or twice a day. This treatment is suitable once layers of white scale appear.

Clinical notes

- For cases of recurrent tinea manuum, an effective result can be achieved by treating the disease in summer when it is aggravated; use *Fu Ping Cu* (Duckweed Vinegar Preparation), *Huo Xiang Jin Pao Ji* (Agastache/Patchouli Soak Preparation) or *E Zhang Feng Jin Pao Ji* (Soak Preparation for Goose-Foot Wind).
- For painful tinea manuum with dry and cracked skin, or papulovesicles with severe itching, combining internal treatment, external soaks and direct application of *Gan Cao You* (Licorice Oil) mixed with *Yang Ti Gen San* (Curled Dock Root Powder) for two to three weeks will prove effective.
- Patients with tinea pedis should be treated as early as possible to prevent occurrence or aggravation of tinea manuum.
- Although tinea manuum is a stubborn condition to treat, a cure can be effected by focusing on removal of the causative factors through regular and persevering treatment.

Case history

Patient

Female, aged 34.

Clinical manifestations

The patient had been suffering from *e zhang feng* (goose-foot Wind, tinea manuum) for 12 years. In the previous summer, 1-2 mm vesicles had appeared in the center of the palms, followed by scaling of the skin and dryness resulting in intolerable itching. In the winter, the skin on the palms was rough and the fingertips were chapped and painful with bleeding.

Pattern identification

Externally contracted Damp, Heat and Wind Toxins. These Toxins had accumulated in the skin, obstructing Qi and Blood and depriving the skin of nourishment.

Treatment principle

Dredge Wind and dispel Dampness, kill Worms and alleviate itching.

Prescription

FU PING SAN

Duckweed Powder

Fu Ping (Herba Spirodelae Polyrrhizae) 12g
Jiang Can‡ (Bombyx Batryticatus) 12g
Bai Xian Pi (Cortex Dictamni Dasycarpi Radicis) 12g
Jing Jie (Herba Schizonepetae Tenuifoliae) 10g
Fang Feng (Radix Ledebouriellae Divaricatae) 10g
Du Huo (Radix Angelicae Pubescentis) 10g
Qiang Huo (Rhizoma et Radix Notopterygii) 10g
Zao Jiao (Fructus Gleditsiae Sinensis) 10g
*Chuan Wu** (Radix Aconiti Carmichaeli) 10g
*Cao Wu** (Radix Aconiti Kusnezoffii) 10g
Wei Ling Xian (Radix Clematidis) 10g
Xian Feng Xian Hua (Flos Impatientis Balsaminae Recens) one stalk, without the root

Method

The powder was steeped in one liter of mature vinegar for 24 hours, then simmered over a low heat for 30 minutes. The residues were filtered out and the hand soaked in the medicated vinegar for 10-20 minutes, three times a day.

Outcome

The condition resolved at the end of three preparations. [2]

Modern clinical experience

See under tinea pedis (athlete's foot).

Tinea pedis (athlete's foot)
足癣

Tinea pedis is a dermatophyte infection of the skin most commonly caused by *Trichophyton rubrum*; other causative organisms are *Trichophyton mentagrophytes* var. *interdigitale* and *Epidermophyton floccosum*. It mainly affects

the webs between the toes and the plantar surface or dorsum of the foot, occasionally extending to the ankle.

In TCM, tinea pedis is also known as *jiao qi chuang* (foot Qi sore) or *jiao shi qi* (foot damp Qi).

Clinical manifestations

- Tinea pedis is common in adults, especially young males. The sharing of communal washing facilities (for example, changing room showers) or swimming pools can result in infection (arthrospores can survive in human scale for 12 months).
- Fungal infection may be aggravated by tight-fitting shoes, which promote sweating.
- Although this disease may present with the classic ringworm pattern, most infections occur between the toes or on the sole.

Interdigital tinea pedis

- Lesions commonly involve the toes and the plantar border.
- Small vesicles appear between the toes, particularly in the fourth and fifth interspace, or along the plantar border. There is frequently superinfection with other organisms. The vesicles rupture when rubbed; fluid oozes out, giving off a fishy smell. Repeated rubbing between the toes will cause white, macerated skin. When the macerated skin comes off, a bright red erosive base is visible. Some vesicles may turn purple, white or yellow.
- Some cases are characterized by dryness and itching between the toes with rough skin and desquamation; there may be pain due to the formation of fissures.
- Pruritus is likely.
- The disease is aggravated in winter and alleviated in summer. It often persists for a long period and can be difficult to cure.

"Moccasin-type" tinea pedis

- The entire sole is usually infected and covered by fine, diffuse dry white scale.
- Pruritus is likely.
- Infection is likely to be associated with tinea manuum, with one foot and both hands or both feet and one hand being involved.
- This type of tinea pedis is particularly resistant to treatment.

Vesicular tinea pedis

- Vesicles evolve rapidly on the sole or the dorsum of the foot, either merging into bullae or collecting under the thick surface of the sole.
- Recurrent crops of vesicles may occur at the same sites or at distant locations. These itchy vesicles are an id (dermatophytid) reaction, representing an allergic response to the fungus.

Differential diagnosis

INTERDIGITAL TINEA PEDIS

Erythrasma

Erythrasma occurs more commonly in young men in a body flexure where the thin skin is easily traumatized, such as the area between the toes. The pale brown or pinkish non-inflamed lesion is round or irregular in shape; some fine scaling may be observed on the surface. Fungus examination and culture, and examination with Wood's light – a long-wave ultraviolet light – will help to establish the diagnosis; erythrasma fluoresces coral pink due to the presence of porphyrins.

"MOCCASIN-TYPE" TINEA PEDIS

Chronic eczema

This condition often evolves from recurring acute or subacute eczema or may be a manifestation of contact dermatitis. Characteristic lesions manifest as dry, rough, thickened, and scaling skin, deepening and widening of the cleavage lines of the skin, and hyperpigmentation or hypopigmentation. Itching may be moderate or intense. Parallel involvement of one or both hands is more likely with tinea pedis.

Recurrent focal palmar peeling (keratolysis exfoliativa)

This condition tends to occur at the end of spring or autumn and involves the bilateral soles. At the initial stage, lesions appear as pinpoint white spots containing no fluid. The lesions gradually extend and eventually produce scaling and peeling. The center of the scaly area may turn red and tender. After desquamation of the horny layer, the skin underneath returns to normal. The condition resolves spontaneously, but may recur once or more a year.

VESICULAR TINEA PEDIS

Pompholyx

Vesicular tinea pedis should be differentiated from pompholyx, which usually has symmetrical involvement of the soles. At the initial stage, lesions manifest as a sudden eruption of deep-seated domed vesicles. Vesicles are filled with a clear and glistening fluid. Scaling and peeling follow drying of the vesicles. Itching varies from moderate to severe.

Palmoplantar pustulosis (pustular psoriasis)

The disease mainly occurs on the palms and soles, in a symmetrical distribution, with the soles being affected more often, especially in the plantar arch. At the initial stage, small vesicles appear on an erythematous base, rapidly evolving into sterile 3-10 mm pustules of varying colors, usually yellow or brown. After five to seven days, the fluid in the pustules is absorbed, the pustules dry up and desquamation follows. After a certain time, crops of pustules will reappear.

Etiology and pathology

Damp-Heat pouring down

Soaking by water or dampness, sitting or lying in a damp environment, or living in a humid place will allow invasion of the body by Damp Toxins, which pour down along the channels to the foot. When Damp Toxins accumulate and bind in the foot, tinea pedis occurs with maceration and erosion.

Invasion of pathogenic factors due to Deficiency of Vital Qi (Zheng Qi)

Enduring diseases will inevitably result in Deficiency and the Kidneys will finally be involved. The Kidneys dominate the Lower Burner. Kidney Deficiency leads to Emptiness and Deficiency in the channels and network vessels. Wind-Damp and Damp-Heat pathogenic factors take advantage of this Deficiency to invade the skin and fight with Vital Qi (Zheng Qi) in the skin and flesh, thus causing tinea pedis with itching and desquamation.

Other factors

Contact with shoes and socks used by an infected person, or walking on contaminated floors can also cause invasion by Toxic pathogenic factors.

Pattern identification and treatment

INTERNAL TREATMENT

DAMP-HEAT POURING DOWN

The skin between the toes is macerated; there is erosion and exudation accompanied by a fishy smell. Rubbing will cause the macerated skin to peel off and reveal a moist erosive base; the exudate is thick and sticky. Infection by pathogenic factors after the macerated skin has been rubbed off will result in erosion with severe pain, local inflammation and swelling; walking may be difficult. The tongue body is red with a scant coating or a thin yellow coating; the pulse is soggy and rapid.

Treatment principle

Clear Heat and benefit the movement of Dampness, relieve Toxicity and disperse swelling.

Prescription
WU SHEN TANG JIA JIAN
Five Spirits Decoction, with modifications

Jin Yin Hua (Flos Lonicerae) 15g

Zi Hua Di Ding (Herba Violae Yedoensitis) 15g
Yi Yi Ren (Semen Coicis Lachryma-jobi) 15g
Chi Fu Ling (Sclerotium Poriae Cocos Rubrae) 15g
Huang Bai (Cortex Phellodendri) 10g
Chuan Niu Xi (Radix Cyathulae Officinalis) 10g
Ze Xie (Rhizoma Alismatis Orientalis) 10g
Chao Mu Dan Pi (Cortex Moutan Radicis, stir-fried) 10g
Che Qian Zi (Semen Plantaginis) 10g, wrapped
Qing Pi (Pericarpium Citri Reticulatae Viride) 6g

Explanation

- *Yi Yi Ren* (Semen Coicis Lachryma-jobi), *Chi Fu Ling* (Sclerotium Poriae Cocos Rubrae), *Che Qian Zi* (Semen Plantaginis), *Ze Xie* (Rhizoma Alismatis Orientalis), *Huang Bai* (Cortex Phellodendri), and *Chuan Niu Xi* (Radix Cyathulae Officinalis) clear Heat and benefit the movement of Dampness.
- *Jin Yin Hua* (Flos Lonicerae), *Zi Hua Di Ding* (Herba Violae Yedoensitis) and *Chao Mu Dan Pi* (Cortex Moutan Radicis, stir-fried) relieve Toxicity and disperse swelling.
- *Qing Pi* (Pericarpium Citri Reticulatae Viride) regulates Qi and alleviates pain.

INVASION OF WIND DUE TO KIDNEY DEFICIENCY

This condition is persistent and difficult to cure. There is often unbearable itching between the toes, or puffy swelling or exudation, or dry itching with desquamation; the skin between the toes may also fissure. Pain will be provoked on exposure to heat or water. The tongue body is pale red with a scant coating; the pulse is deficient and thready.

Treatment principle

Supplement Kidney Qi, dissipate Wind and benefit the movement of Dampness.

Prescription
XI JIAO SAN JIA JIAN
Rhinoceros Horn Powder, with modifications

Gan Di Huang (Radix Rehmanniae Glutinosae Exsiccata) 12g
Shan Zhu Yu (Fructus Corni Officinalis) 12g
Huang Qi (Radix Astragali seu Hedysari) 12g
*Tian Ma** (Rhizoma Gastrodiae Elatae) 10g
Qiang Huo (Rhizoma et Radix Notopterygii) 10g
Fang Feng (Radix Ledebouriellae Divaricatae) 10g
Chao Huang Qin (Radix Scutellariae Baicalensis, stir-fried) 10g
Da Fu Pi (Pericarpium Arecae Catechu) 6g
Chao Zhi Ke (Fructus Citri Aurantii, stir-fried) 6g
Wu Shao She ‡ (Zaocys Dhumnades) 6g
Bai Xian Pi (Cortex Dictamni Dasycarpi Radicis) 15g
Shan Yao (Rhizoma Dioscoreae Oppositae) 15g
Ze Xie (Rhizoma Alismatis Orientalis) 15g

Explanation

- *Sheng Di Huang* (Radix Rehmanniae Glutinosae), *Shan Zhu Yu* (Fructus Corni Officinalis) and *Shan Yao* (Rhizoma Dioscoreae Oppositae) enrich and supplement the Liver and Kidneys.
- *Chao Zhi Ke* (Fructus Citri Aurantii, stir-fried), *Qiang Huo* (Rhizoma et Radix Notopterygii) and *Fang Feng* (Radix Ledebouriellae Divaricatae) dissipate external Wind to alleviate itching.
- *Tian Ma** (Rhizoma Gastrodiae Elatae) and *Wu Shao She‡* (Zaocys Dhumnades) extinguish internal Wind.
- *Huang Qi* (Radix Astragali seu Hedysari) augments Qi and consolidates the exterior.
- *Bai Xian Pi* (Cortex Dictamni Dasycarpi Radicis), *Huang Qin* (Radix Scutellariae Baicalensis), *Da Fu Pi* (Pericarpium Arecae Catechu), and *Ze Xie* (Rhizoma Alismatis Orientalis) eliminate Dampness and relieve Toxicity to alleviate pain.

EXTERNAL TREATMENT

- Where lesions are primarily white and macerated, first soak the foot in *Shi Liu Pi Shui Xi Ji* (Pomegranate Rind Wash Preparation). Then apply *Hua Rui Shi San* (Ophicalcite Powder) or *Qu Shi San* (Powder for Dispelling Dampness) to the lesions.
- For red and swollen lesions with erosion and exudation accompanied by infection by Toxins, use *Huang Ding Shui Xi Ji* (Siberian Solomonseal and Cloves Wash Preparation) as a soak for the foot. Then mix *Qing Dai San* (Indigo Powder) and *Zhen Jun Miao Tie San* (True Gentleman's Wondrous Powder for External Application) to a paste with vegetable oil and apply to the affected area.
- Where the skin is dry, scaly and fissured ("moccasin type" tinea pedis), apply *Run Ji Gao* (Flesh-Moistening Paste) to the lesions once or twice a day.
- Where lesions are primarily vesicular, use *Gan Ge Shui Xi Ji* (Kudzu Vine Root Wash Preparation) or *Lou Lu Tang* (Globethistle Root Decoction), or prepare a decoction with *Yi Zhi Huang Hua* (Herba Solidaginis) 15g, or *Wang Bu Liu Xing* (Semen Vaccariae Segetalis) 30g and *Ming Fan‡* (Alumen) 9g. Use as a soak or wet compress for the foot; apply twice a day.

ACUPUNCTURE

Selection of points on the affected channels
Main points: LI-4 Hegu, SI-3 Houxi, TB-3 Zhongzhu, and EX-UE-9 Baxie. [ii]

Auxiliary points: PC-7 Daling, SP-6 Sanyinjiao and KI-3 Taixi.

Selection of points according to the type of disease

- For the macerating type of tinea pedis, select BL-9 Yuzhen (bilateral).
- For the vesicular type, select BL-57 Chengshan itself or a point 0.5 cun below it.

Technique
Apply the reducing method and retain the needles for 30 minutes. Treat once every one or two days. A course consists of ten treatment sessions.

Explanation

- Distal points such as LI-4 Hegu, TB-3 Zhongzhu, SI-3 Houxi, SP-6 Sanyinjiao, KI-3 Taixi, and PC-7 Daling enrich Yin and drain Fire to eliminate itching.
- EX-UE-9 Baxie disperses swelling and relieves Toxicity.
- BL-57 Chengshan and BL-9 Yuzhen eliminate Dampness and dissipate Wind to relieve Toxicity.

Clinical notes

- Lesions on the foot are usually associated with Dampness. In the course of pattern differentiation, it is important to distinguish between Damp-Heat and Cold-Damp (white macerated lesions between the toes are related to Cold-Damp). If Damp-Heat predominates, the treatment should focus on clearing Heat and benefiting the movement of Dampness; if Cold-Damp predominates, concentrate on dissipating Cold and dispelling Dampness.
- Where the condition is characterized by exudation, maceration and erosion, the main external treatments are washes and soaks for the foot, with *Gan Ge Shui Xi Ji* (Kudzu Vine Root Wash Preparation) and *Shi Liu Pi Shui Xi Ji* (Pomegranate Rind Wash Preparation) being especially effective. Once the condition has reached the stage of cracked and scaly skin, pastes or ointments are more appropriate (see external treatment above).
- Patients should be encouraged to persist with the treatment until a complete cure is obtained in order to prevent infection of the hand and avoid the occurrence of tinea manuum or tinea unguium. The length of treatment will vary depending on the patient's condition.

[ii] M-UE-22 according to the system employed by the Shanghai College of Traditional Chinese Medicine.

Advice for the patient

- Pay attention to personal hygiene and do not wear other people's shoes or socks.
- Wash the feet with warm water every evening before going to bed.
- Use shower shoes when bathing at home or in public places.

Case history

Patient
Female, aged 34.

Clinical manifestations
When the patient came for her first visit, she had not been able to walk for the previous two weeks due to a painful and swollen left foot. This was accompanied by pain and swelling in the left groin. Physical examination showed that the dorsum of the left foot was red and swollen with pitting edema. Crusting, erosion, and exudation of clear fluid and pus was noted between the toes. Tenderness was still evident in the left inguinal groove.

Pattern identification
Damp-Heat pouring down, transforming into Fire Toxins.

Treatment principle
Clear Heat and relieve Toxicity, benefit the movement of Dampness and disperse swelling.

Internal prescription ingredients
Chi Fu Ling (Sclerotium Poriae Cocos Rubrae) 9g
Huang Qin (Radix Scutellariae Baicalensis) 9g
Ze Xie (Rhizoma Alismatis Orientalis) 9g
Mu Dan Pi (Cortex Moutan Radicis) 9g
Chong Lou (Rhizoma Paridis) 9g
Lian Qiao (Fructus Forsythiae Suspensae) 9g
Che Qian Zi (Semen Plantaginis) 9g, wrapped
Liu Yi San (Six-To-One Powder) 9g, wrapped
Pu Gong Ying (Herba Taraxaci cum Radice) 15g

One bag a day was used to prepare a decoction, taken twice a day.

External prescription ingredients
Di Yu (Radix Sanguisorbae Officinalis) 60g
Ma Chi Xian (Herba Portulacae Oleraceae) 60g
Huang Bai (Cortex Phellodendri) 60g

One bag a day was used to prepare a decoction for use as a wet compress.

Further treatment
After three days, the swelling and inflammation were subsiding and the erosion and exudation were diminishing. Pyogenic secretion had ceased, pain was alleviated and the lump and tenderness in the inguinal groove had disappeared. The same internal treatment was followed with the addition of *Er*

Miao Wan (Mysterious Two Pill) 9g twice a day. The wet compress was the same as before.

Outcome
After another three days of treatment, the swelling and redness had disappeared completely. The webs between the toes were dry and slightly itchy. The patient was told to apply a mixture of *Liu Yi San* (Six-To-One Powder) 9g and *Ku Fan* ‡ (Alumen Praeparatum) 3g between the toes. After five days, the condition was cured, but treatment was continued by soaking the foot in *Cu Pao Fang* (Vinegar Soak Formula) for half an hour every evening to prevent recurrence. [3]

Modern clinical experience

TREATMENTS USING VINEGAR-BASED SOLUTIONS

1. **Yang** treated tinea manuum with a wash formula. [4]

Prescription
FU FANG ER FAN XI JI
Compound Alum and Melanterite Wash Preparation

Ku Fan ‡ (Alumen Praeparatum) 15g
Huang Jing (Rhizoma Polygonati) 15g
Duan Lü Fan ‡ (Melanteritum Rubrum) 15g
Er Cha (Pasta Acaciae seu Uncariae) 10g
Ce Bai Ye (Cacumen Biotae Orientalis) 10g
Tu Jin Pi (Cortex Pseudolaricis) 10g
Ding Xiang (Flos Caryophylli) 3g
Xue Jie (Resina Draconis) 2g

The ingredients were ground into a fine powder and soaked in 500 ml of vinegar for a week. They were then filtered through two layers of gauze and the liquid was stored. The residue was soaked for another week in a further 500 ml of vinegar. The medicated vinegar was again filtered through two layers of gauze. A 10 percent concentration of the wash preparation results from mixing the two medicated vinegar liquids together.

A total of 139 patients were treated with the wash formula, while 77 patients in a comparison group were treated with a 10 percent concentration of *E Zhang Feng Yao Ye* (Medicated Lotion for Goose-Foot Wind) prepared by diluting *E Zhang Feng Zhi Yang Fen* (Powder for Alleviating Goose-Foot Wind Itching), made by the Shanghai Huangpu Pharmaceutical Factory, in vinegar. Patients in both groups soaked the affected hand in the medicated preparations for 15-20 minutes twice a day. Seven treatments made up a course. Most patients followed two treatment courses.

Fu Fang Er Fan Xi Ji (Compound Alum and Melanterite Wash Formula) was found to be clinically more effective than the comparison formula. In the wash formula group, 104 patients (74.8 percent) recovered completely, another

31 (22.3 percent) showed varying degrees of improvement and 4 (2.9 percent) experienced no effect; in the comparison group, 47 patients (61.0 percent) recovered completely, 25 (32.5 percent) showed varying degrees of improvement and 5 (6.5 percent) experienced no effect.

Adverse effects manifested as a mild or moderate burning sensation in the local area during days 1-3 of treatment in the wash formula group and during days 1-5 of treatment in the comparison group. This had no influence on the therapeutic result.

2. **Lu** prepared a soak to treat both tinea manuum and tinea pedis. [5]

Prescription
KE XUAN TANG
Restraining Tinea Decoction

Da Feng Zi (Semen Hydnocarpi) 20g
Wu Jia Pi (Cortex Acanthopanacis Gracilistyli Radicis) 18g
She Tui ‡ (Exuviae Serpentis) 12g
Shi Hua (Parmelia) 12g
Teng Huang (Resina Garciniae) 12g
Hai Tong Pi (Cortex Erythrinae) 12g
She Chuang Zi (Fructus Cnidii Monnieri) 12g
Tu Jin Pi (Cortex Pseudolaricis) 15g
Jin Gu Cao (Herba Ajugae Decumbentis) 15g
Ji Xue Teng (Caulis Spatholobi) 15g
Ku Shen (Radix Sophorae Flavescentis) 30g

The ingredients were soaked in 1000 ml of vinegar for three hours and then brought to the boil over a mild heat. The medicated vinegar was collected through a gauze filter. Patients were treated by placing the affected hand or foot in a bowl, covering with the medicated vinegar and soaking for 40 minutes twice a day.

3. **Chen** treated tinea pedis with an empirical prescription for a soak. [6]

Prescription
KE XUAN JIN PAO JI
Soak Preparation for Restraining Tinea

Huang Bai (Cortex Phellodendri) 15g
Zao Jiao (Fructus Gleditsiae Sinensis) 15g
Ming Fan ‡ (Alumen) 10g

The ingredients were soaked in 500ml of vinegar for two hours and then filtered through gauze. The medicated vinegar was heated to an appropriate temperature (around 35°C for normal skin, lower for cracked skin or skin that is more sensitive to heat) before soaking the affected foot for 20 minutes twice a day. One medicated vinegar soak can be used for ten days. Thirty days made up a course.

TREATMENTS USING WATER-BASED SOLUTIONS

1. **Ruan** prepared a decoction to treat tinea pedis. [7]

Prescription
KU SHEN TANG
Flavescent Sophora Root Decoction

Ku Shen (Radix Sophorae Flavescentis) 30g
Bai Xian Pi (Cortex Dictamni Dasycarpi Radicis) 30g
She Chuang Zi (Fructus Cnidii Monnieri) 30g
Di Fu Zi (Fructus Kochiae Scopariae) 30g
Da Feng Zi (Semen Hydnocarpi) 30g
Huang Bai (Cortex Phellodendri) 20g
Hua Jiao (Pericarpium Zanthoxyli) 20g
Fang Feng (Radix Ledebouriellae Divaricatae) 20g
Ming Fan ‡ (Alumen) 20g
Wu Mei (Fructus Pruni Mume) 20g

The ingredients were boiled in 3 liters of water for 20 minutes and the liquid was then poured off and retained. The residue was boiled again in 2 liters of water for 15-20 minutes and the liquid poured off and retained. The two decoctions were mixed together and divided into two portions for soaking and washing the affected foot for 30-40 minutes twice a day. Five days made up a course of treatment. If the disease was not cured after the first course, a second course was followed.

The wash can be used for different manifestations of tinea pedis – erosion, desquamation and cornification, vesicles, and combined erosion and vesicles.

2. **Li** adopted a combined steaming and soaking method to treat tinea pedis. [8]

Prescription ingredients

Huang Jing (Rhizoma Polygonati) 30g
Fang Feng (Radix Ledebouriellae Divaricatae) 30g
Da Huang (Radix et Rhizoma Rhei) 30g
Ku Shen (Radix Sophorae Flavescentis) 30g
Bai Bu (Radix Stemonae) 30g
Huang Qin (Radix Scutellariae Baicalensis) 30g
Huang Bai (Cortex Phellodendri) 30g
Huang Lian (Rhizoma Coptidis) 15g

The ingredients were decocted in 3 liters of water. The affected foot was steamed with the boiling decoction until the skin was moist and then soaked in the warmest-bearable decoction for 30 minutes once every evening for four to six consecutive evenings. The results were even better when the insole of the shoe was soaked in the medicated preparation and then dried before use. This treatment was effective for tinea pedis with maceration, vesicles, scaling, and cornification.

3. Cui prepared a water-based soak for tinea pedis. [9]

Prescription
SI YE TANG
Four-Leaf Decoction

Liu Ye (Folium Salicis) 25g
Qing Yang Shu Ye (Folium Populi) 25g
Yu Shu Ye (Folium Ulmi) 25g
Pu Gong Ying (Herba Taraxaci cum Radice) 25g

The ingredients were covered with a double depth of water and decocted for 15-20 minutes. The decoction was then used to soak the affected foot for 10 minutes, several times a day.

Modifications

- For patients with a foul smell from the feet, *Huo Xiang* (Herba Agastaches seu Pogostemi) 15g, *Pei Lan* (Herba Eupatorii Fortunei) 15g, *He Ye* (Folium Nelumbinis Nuciferae) 15g, *Jin Yin Hua* (Flos Lonicerae) 30g, and *Zi Hua Di Ding* (Herba Violae Yedoensitis) 30g were added.
- For patients with sweaty feet, *Huang Bai* (Cortex Phellodendri) 15g, *Cang Zhu* (Rhizoma Atractylodis) 30g, *Cang Er Cao* (Caulis et Folium Xanthii Sibirici) 50g, and *Bai Ji Li* (Fructus Tribuli Terrestris) 30g were added.

Tinea unguium (ringworm of the nail)
甲癣

Tinea unguium is caused by infection of the finger or toe nail plate by dermatophytes (principally *Trichophyton mentagrophytes* or *Trichophyton rubrum*). It may occur due to direct infection by fungi as a result of external injury to the nail, or may develop simultaneously with tinea manuum and/or tinea pedis. A complete cure for the condition is difficult to achieve because the thickness of the nails prevents medications from reaching the diseased area.

In TCM, tinea unguium is also known as *hui zhi jia* (ashen nail), *you hui zhi jia* (oily ashen nail) or *e zhao feng* (goose claw wind).

Clinical manifestations

- Fungal infection of the nails increases with age.
- Toenails, especially the nail of the big toe, are usually more affected than fingernails. It is rare for all nails to be affected.
- At the initial stage, the distal part of the finger or toe nail becomes lusterless with gradual thickening and atrophy, finally separating from the nail bed.
- In severe cases, fungal infection leads to the nail becoming decayed, fragmented or deformed. The nail plate becomes brittle and easily broken with an uneven surface.
- Where the nail plate is infected by *Candida albicans*, paronychia (whitlow) is possible. The nail groove is red and swollen, but seldom suppurative.

Differential diagnosis

Psoriasis
In up to 50 percent of psoriasis cases, pathological changes to the finger and toe nails (pitting, distal separation from the nail bed, discoloration, and subungual hyperkeratosis) occur. The most common manifestation of psoriasis, pitting of the nail, does not occur with fungal infection. Tinea unguium may also develop simultaneously with tinea manuum and/or tinea pedis.

Brittleness of the nails (onychorrhexis)
The nail is fragile and breaks easily. This condition is often associated with hands being frequently immersed in alkaline water.

Thickening of the nail
The nail thickens as a result of complications following trauma of the nail or another skin disease such as psoriasis.

Discoloration of the nail
The nail is discolored in spots or bands; sometimes the entire nail is affected. This condition may be associated with the use of certain medications such as antimalarial drugs, cancer chemotherapeutic agents, and minocycline.

Etiology and pathology

- *Huang Di Nei Jing: Su Wen* [The Yellow Emperor's Classic of Internal Medicine: Simple Questions] says: "The

Liver governs the sinews and its bloom is in the nails." Deficiency of Liver-Blood will lead to malnutrition of the nails, which may then become diseased.

- This disease has an external origin in pathogenic Worms and an internal origin in Liver Deficiency, which allows invasion of pathogenic factors.

- For patients with tinea manuum or tinea pedis scratching the affected hand or foot with the fingers may result in the nails becoming infected and tinea unguium developing.

Pattern identification and treatment

INTERNAL TREATMENT

DEFICIENCY OF LIVER-BLOOD

Deficiency of Liver-Blood results in the Blood being unable to nourish the nails properly, with the disease becoming chronic. The nail begins to decay and turns grayish-white. It then becomes fragmented or separates from the nail bed.

Treatment principle

Nourish Liver-Blood.

Prescription

BU GAN TANG JIA JIAN

Supplementing the Liver Decoction, with modifications

Dang Gui (Radix Angelicae Sinensis) 10g
Bai Shao (Radix Paeoniae Lactiflorae) 10g
Mai Men Dong (Radix Ophiopogonis Japonici) 10g
Shan Zhu Yu (Fructus Corni Officinalis) 10g
Mu Gua (Fructus Chaenomelis) 10g
Shu Di Huang (Radix Rehmanniae Glutinosae Conquita) 15g
Chuan Xiong (Rhizoma Ligustici Chuanxiong) 6g
Gan Cao (Radix Glycyrrhizae) 6g
Bu Gu Zhi (Fructus Psoraleae Corylifoliae) 6g
He Shou Wu (Radix Polygoni Multiflori) 12g
Sang Shen (Fructus Mori Albae) 12g
Gou Qi Zi (Fructus Lycii) 12g

Explanation

- *Dang Gui* (Radix Angelicae Sinensis), *Bai Shao* (Radix Paeoniae Lactiflorae), *Shu Di Huang* (Radix Rehmanniae Glutinosae Conquita), *Chuan Xiong* (Rhizoma Ligustici Chuanxiong), *He Shou Wu* (Radix Polygoni Multiflori), *Shan Zhu Yu* (Fructus Corni Officinalis), *Sang Shen* (Fructus Mori Albae), *Mai Men Dong* (Radix Ophiopogonis Japonici), and *Gou Qi Zi* (Fructus Lycii) enrich and moisten the Liver and Kidneys.

- *Mu Gua* (Fructus Chaenomelis) and *Bu Gu Zhi* (Fructus Psoraleae Corylifoliae) strengthen the bones and act as channel conductors; they can help the new nail to grow.

- *Gan Cao* (Radix Glycyrrhizae) harmonizes the properties of the other ingredients.

Modifications

1. If the disease involves the fingernails, add *Gui Zhi* (Ramulus Cinnamomi Cassiae), *Sang Zhi* (Ramulus Mori Albae) and *Jiang Huang* (Rhizoma Curcumae Longae).

2. If the disease involves the toenails, add *Niu Xi* (Radix Achyranthis Bidentatae), *Qing Pi* (Pericarpium Citri Reticulatae Viride) and *Chai Hu* (Radix Bupleuri). [iii]

EXTERNAL TREATMENT

Direct application of medication

Lightly scrape the affected nail with a sharp blade. Then apply *Tu Jin Pi Ding* (Golden Larch Bark Tincture) directly to the nail two or three times a day. Continue the treatment until the new nail grows.

Soaking

Soak the nail in *Cu Pao Fang* (Vinegar Soak Formula) or *E Zhang Feng Jin Pao Ji* (Soak Preparation for Goose-Foot Wind) for 30 minutes a day. When the surface of the nail softens, scrape off the residue with a sharp blade.

Cloth-wrap

Take *Feng Xian Hua* (Flos Impatientis Balsaminae) 30g and *Ming Fan* ‡ (Alumen) 9g; or *Tu Da Huang* (Radix Rumicis Madaio) 3g, *Feng Xian Hua Geng* (Caulis Impatientis Balsaminae) one stalk and *Ku Fan* ‡ (Alumen Praeparatum) 6g, and pound to a pulp. Apply to the affected nail and wrap in a piece of cloth. Change the dressing daily.

Medicated plaster

Heat *Hei Se Ba Gao Gun* (Black Medicated Plaster Stick) and apply to the affected nail. Change the plaster every three to five days. [iv]

Application of plaster and lotion

Apply *Ba Jia Gao* (Nail-Removing Plaster) to the

[iii] This is an instance of the use of herbs of opposing properties to induce a desired effect; in this case *Chai Hu* (Radix Bupleuri) is used to facilitate the ability of *Niu Xi* (Radix Achyranthis Bidentatae) to go downward. The dosage of *Chai Hu* (Radix Bupleuri) should be much smaller than that of *Niu Xi* (Radix Achyranthis Bidentatae), for example in a 1:4 ratio, so that *Niu Xi* (Radix Achyranthis Bidentatae) is stronger and leads the herbs down to the feet.

[iv] This treatment has proven very effective clinically, but some ingredients may not be permitted in certain countries.

affected nail. Change the dressing every three to five days until the nail is removed. Then apply *Tu Jin Pi Ding* (Golden Larch Bark Tincture) until the new nail grows.

MOXIBUSTION

Direct moxibustion
Place 3mm moxa cones near the edge and in the center of the affected nail. Burn for 10-15 minutes, two or three times a day.

Indirect moxibustion
Peel a head of garlic. Pound the cloves to a pulp or cut them into slices. Place a thin layer of cloth over the affected nail, and put the mashed or sliced garlic on top. Ignite the moxa cone and place it on top of the garlic. If the patient feels a burning pain, pause for a moment before continuing. Treat for 10 minutes once every three days until the condition is cleared.

Clinical notes

- Particular attention should be paid to means of preventing and treating tinea manuum and tinea pedis in order to prevent them spreading and causing tinea unguium.
- For patients with a weak constitution, combining external treatment with internal use of herbal decoctions or patent herbal remedies for enriching the Liver and supplementing the Kidneys will help to increase the effectiveness of the treatment.

Advice for the patient

- Tinea unguium is a stubborn disease. Patients must be prepared to persevere when following external treatment for the condition as they will usually need to continue for about six months.
- When treating with soak preparations, first soak the affected nail for at least 10-15 minutes. Then scrape the affected nail with a sharp blade. Finally, apply external medication to the lesion.

Literature excerpt

In *Wai Ke Zheng Zhi Quan Sheng Ji* [A Life-Saving Manual of the Diagnosis and Treatment of External Diseases], it says: "To treat *you hui zhi jia* (oily ashen nail), pound white *Feng Xian Hua* (Flos Impatientis Balsaminae) to a pulp and wrap round the affected nail. Change the dressing daily. Continue the treatment until the new nail grows."

Tinea corporis (ringworm of the body)
体癣

Tinea corporis is a superficial dermatophyte infection of the smooth skin – the skin of the trunk and limbs (excluding the feet, hands and groin) and the facial skin (excluding the beard area in men). The main pathogenic fungi involved include *Microsporum* and *Trichophyton*.

In TCM, tinea corporis is also known as *yuan xuan* (coin tinea).

Clinical manifestations

- Lesions usually involve the trunk, limbs, face (excluding the beard area in men), or neck.
- Lesions start with grouped red papules or papulovesicles, which gradually increase in number and size and spread outward to form single or multiple sharply circumscribed circular, semicircular or concentric erythema. Lesions gradually heal in the center but are elevated at the borders (known as an "active edge") with clusters of red papules or papulovesicles. Thin, fine scaling may sometimes be noted.
- Patients may experience mild to severe itching.
- The condition is often aggravated in summer but alleviated or absent in winter. However, it may recur the following summer.

Differential diagnosis

Nummular eczema (discoid eczema)
Although nummular eczema mainly involves the limbs, it may also occur on the buttocks and the trunk. Lesions manifest as very itchy, sharply demarcated, coin-shaped plaques 1-5 cm in diameter formed from

the confluence of densely distributed red papules or vesicles. Lesions may be acute with clear or bloody exudate and crusting, or chronic with erythema and scaling. The central healing and peripheral scaling of tinea corporis usually permit differentiation.

Psoriasis

Psoriasis usually involves the extensor aspect of the limbs, especially the extensor aspect of the elbows and knees, but sometimes spreads to affect the whole body. The nails and scalp may also be involved. Lesions manifest as erythematous papules covered by silvery-white scales as opposed to the fine scaling of tinea corporis. If the scales of psoriasis are removed, bleeding points appear (Auspitz's sign).

Pityriasis rosea

Lesions manifest as multiple pale red, yellowish-brown or reddish-brown oval plaques, gradually turning rosy. The plaques have a discrete distribution, with the long axes of the lesions following the lines of cleavage of the skin. A fine scale often remains within the border of the plaque, resulting in a characteristic "collarette" ring of scale. Pityriasis rosea is often preceded by a herald patch. The disease is self-limited and usually clears spontaneously within one or two months.

Etiology and pathology

- Tinea corporis mainly occurs as a result of Wind, Damp, Heat, and Worms invading the skin. In summer especially, Damp-Heat pathogenic factors are likely to attack the skin and flesh. Heat in the skin combined with profuse sweating or moist skin can trigger or aggravate the disease.
- Infection caused by contact with clothes used by a patient with tinea corporis can also lead to the disease.
- Contact with cats, dogs or other pets infected by tinea is an additional causative factor.

Treatment

EXTERNAL TREATMENT

- For lesions marked by papules and papulovesicles, use *Xuan Jiu* (Wine Preparation for Tinea), *Xi Xuan Fang* (Tinea Wash Formula), *Xuan Yao Shui Er Hao* (No. 2 Medicated Lotion for Tinea), or *Xuan Yao Shui San Hao* (No. 3 Medicated Lotion for Tinea).
- For lesions with erosion and exudation, use *Qing Dai San* (Indigo Powder), *Yang Ti Gen San* (Curled Dock Root Powder) or *Hua Rui Shi San* (Ophicalcite Powder). Once the lesions are dry, apply *Xuan Yao Shui Er Hao* (No. 2 Medicated Lotion for Tinea) or *Xuan Yao*

Shui San Hao (No. 3 Medicated Lotion for Tinea).
- For lesions with dryness, desquamation or fissuring of the skin, use *Tu Jin Pi Ding* (Golden Larch Bark Tincture).

ACUPUNCTURE
Points

- For lesions on the upper half of the body, select PC-3 Quze, LI-11 Quchi, LI-4 Hegu, and LI-15 Jianyu.
- For lesions on the lower half of the body, select GB-30 Huantiao, GB-31 Fengshi, GB-38 Yangfu, SP-10 Xuehai, SP-6 Sanyinjiao, BL-40 Weizhong, and BL-60 Kunlun.

Technique: Apply the reducing method and retain the needles for 30 minutes. Treat once a day. A course consists of ten treatment sessions.

Explanation

- LI-11 Quchi, LI-4 Hegu, PC-3 Quze, and LI-15 Jianyu dredge Wind and clear Heat to alleviate itching.
- GB-30 Huantiao, GB-31 Fengshi, GB-38 Yangfu, SP-10 Xuehai, SP-6 Sanyinjiao, BL-40 Weizhong, and BL-60 Kunlun enrich Yin, moisten Dryness, invigorate the Blood, and alleviate itching.

PLUM-BLOSSOM NEEDLING (WITH MOXIBUSTION)

Points: Affected areas (the site of the lesions).
Technique: Tap heavily to produce strong stimulation or use moxibustion after needling. This treatment is effective in alleviating itching and reducing papules.

Clinical notes

- Internal treatment is not generally required for this condition.
- The best procedure for the treatment of tinea corporis is as follows: First wash the lesions with lukewarm water. Where lesions are characterized by dryness, itching and papules, or desquamation, apply liquid medications before using medications in powder form. If lesions are present in folds of the skin or are marked by slight erosion, apply medications in powder form immediately after washing the affected area. Use of ointments should be kept to the minimum, and avoided entirely if possible.
- Acupuncture treatment cannot directly inhibit the growth of fungi. However, it helps to alleviate itching and prevent patients from scratching and is therefore beneficial in aiding recovery.
- Particular attention should be paid to the means of preventing and treating tinea manuum, tinea pedis,

tinea unguium, and tinea capitis to prevent spread of the infection to other areas.

Advice for the patient

- Avoid contact with towels or public baths used by patients with tinea.
- Do not touch cats, dogs or other pets with tinea.
- Continue the medications for one week after the lesions disappear to ensure a complete cure.

Literature excerpt

In *Wai Tai Mi Yao* [Secrets of a Frontier Official], it says: "In this type of tinea, the coin-shaped papules lie dormant in the skin and flesh, then enlarge gradually in round or oval patches. Local pain and itching occur. Worms grow at the site of the lesions. Scratching the lesions leads to exudation."

Tinea cruris (jock itch)
股癣

Tinea cruris is a superficial dermatophyte infection of the inguinal groove, almost exclusively in adult males and can be considered as a special manifestation of tinea corporis affecting the groin.

The disease occurs in the summer after sweating and in the winter when additional layers of clothing are worn. The moist environment of the groin allows the infection to spread. Infection may also occur through contact, particularly sexual contact.

In TCM, tinea cruris is also known as *yin xuan* (genital region tinea).

Clinical manifestations

- The main sites for tinea cruris include the medial aspect of the thigh and the genital region; the disease may spread to the anus and perianal area.
- The main symptom is pruritus. Skin lesions manifest as papules, vesicles or papulovesicles depending on the pathogenic fungi involved. However, even if one type only of pathogenic fungus is the cause of the infection, lesions may vary in shape or form, being bead-like, papulovesicular, round, annular, or granular.
- In the early stage, the lesion appears as a red scaly patch that spreads gradually from the crural fold to the thigh and the buttocks. The patch has a narrow, elevated, well-defined border that is often inflamed. Later, small vesicles or pustules may form at the border of the lesion, while the center heals, sometimes with temporary pigmentation. The lesion spreads evenly from the center to the peripheral area in single or multiple annular shapes, a classic ringworm pattern.

- In a few cases, tinea cruris may spread to involve the scrotum. The deep color and folds of the scrotum make it difficult to distinguish inflammation and scaling. There is often intolerable local itching.
- Skin lesions typically have a quick onset where *Epidermophyton floccosum* is the main pathogenic fungus. Where *Trichophyton rubrum* is the cause, the onset is slow and the lesion may spread from the buttocks to the lower back and abdomen, occasionally accompanied by pain. In severe cases, there may be secondary bacterial infection.

Differential diagnosis

Erythrasma
With erythrasma, the slightly scaly lesions appear pale brown or pinkish. There is no inflammatory ring around the edge of the lesion and itching is absent.

Candidiasis
Candidiasis in the genital region occurs more often in women. The lesion has no well-defined border. It often involves the mucous membranes and skin folds with a sticky, white secretion. Where men are affected, the infection is more likely to spread to the scrotum than is the case with tinea cruris.

Genital eczema
This eczema occurs initially in the scrotum or vulva before spreading to the crural region and perineum. Lesions start with papules and erythema, which may later form thick crusts.

Intertrigo

This condition may involve the axillae and submammary folds as well as the crural region. Lesions manifest as pink, moist, glistening plaques, often accompanied by painful fissuring in the skin creases.

Other

Tinea cruris should also be differentiated from other conditions such as annular erythema, psoriasis, pityriasis rosea, and lichen simplex chronicus (neurodermatitis). Microscopic examination for fungus may be necessary.

Etiology and pathology

- In the heat of summer, there tends to be profuse sweating and moisture in the groin. As this moisture is slow to evaporate, the area is damp most of the time. Damp-Heat accumulates gradually and after a certain period, this will result in Worm Toxins invading the skin and flesh to cause the disease.

- Poor personal hygiene, such as wearing dirty underwear or infrequent bathing or showering, will allow Damp Toxins to invade the groin and genital area.

- Patients with tinea manuum or tinea pedis may infect other parts of the body through contact with the hand after scratching the lesions.

Pattern identification and treatment

INTERNAL TREATMENT

ACCUMULATION OF DAMP-HEAT

Manifestations of this pattern include moisture and profuse sweating in the crural region. Intertrigo and exudation occur with local pain and itching. Accompanying symptoms and signs include a dry mouth with a bitter taste and short voidings of reddish urine. The tongue body is red with a yellow coating; the pulse is wiry and rapid.

Treatment principle

Clear Heat and dry Dampness, kill Worms and alleviate itching.

Prescription

ER MIAO WAN JIA JIAN

Mysterious Two Pill, with modifications

Chao Huang Bai (Cortex Phellodendri, stir-fried) 10g
Chao Long Dan Cao (Radix Gentianae Scabrae, stir-fried) 10g
Jiao Zhi Zi (Fructus Gardeniae Jasminoidis, scorch-fried) 10g
Chi Fu Ling (Sclerotium Poriae Cocos Rubrae) 10g
Cang Zhu (Rhizoma Atractylodis) 15g
Sheng Di Huang (Radix Rehmanniae Glutinosae) 12g

Che Qian Zi (Semen Plantaginis) 12g, wrapped
Bi Xie (Rhizoma Dioscoreae Hypoglaucae seu Septemlobae) 12g
Bai Mao Gen (Rhizoma Imperatae Cylindricae) 30g
Bai Xian Pi (Cortex Dictamni Dasycarpi Radicis) 6g
Ku Shen (Radix Sophorae Flavescentis) 6g
Wei Ling Xian (Radix Clematidis) 6g

Explanation

- *Chao Huang Bai* (Cortex Phellodendri, stir-fried), *Chao Long Dan Cao* (Radix Gentianae Scabrae, stir-fried), *Jiao Zhi Zi* (Fructus Gardeniae Jasminoidis, scorch-fried), *Bai Xian Pi* (Cortex Dictamni Dasycarpi Radicis), *Ku Shen* (Radix Sophorae Flavescentis), and *Wei Ling Xian* (Radix Clematidis) clear Heat and relieve Toxicity, kill Worms and alleviate itching.

- *Chi Fu Ling* (Sclerotium Poriae Cocos Rubrae), *Cang Zhu* (Rhizoma Atractylodis), *Bi Xie* (Rhizoma Dioscoreae Hypoglaucae seu Septemlobae), and *Che Qian Zi* (Semen Plantaginis) benefit the movement of Dampness and transform Toxicity.

- *Sheng Di Huang* (Radix Rehmanniae Glutinosae) and *Bai Mao Gen* (Rhizoma Imperatae Cylindricae) cool the Blood and relieve Toxicity to reduce erythema.

EXTERNAL TREATMENT

- The skin of the folds in the crural area is thin and tender; strong, irritant medications should be avoided, or adverse effects such as redness and swelling are likely to occur. At the initial stage of the condition, medicated vinegar can be used externally; this is prepared by soaking an appropriate amount of *Shi Da Gong Lao Ye* (Folium Mahoniae) in vinegar for five days and removing the residue. Alternative liquid treatments for external use include *Yin Xuan You* (Genital Region Tinea Oil), or *Yin Xuan Yao Shui Yi Hao* (No. 1 Medicated Lotion for Genital Region Tinea).

- To reduce sweating and moisture in the crural region, apply *Yang Ti Gen San* (Curled Dock Root Powder) or *Hua Rui Shi San* (Ophicalcite Powder) to the lesions.

- For thick, dry and itchy lesions, use *Yang Ti Gen San* (Curled Dock Root Powder) or *Zhi Yang Gao* (Paste for Alleviating Itching).

- For moderate to severe itching and slight exudation, grind equal amounts of *Liu Huang* ‡ (Sulphur) and *Wu Zhu Yu* (Fructus Evodiae Rutaecarpae) into a fine powder and then mix them into a paste with vegetable oil for application to the affected area twice a day until the condition is cured.

- Prepare a wash with the following ingredients:

Huo Xiang (Herba Agastaches seu Pogostemi) 20g

Hu Zhang (Radix et Rhizoma Polygoni Cuspidati) 20g
Da Huang (Radix et Rhizoma Rhei) 20g
Ku Shen (Radix Sophorae Flavescentis) 20g
She Chuang Zi (Fructus Cnidii Monnieri) 20g
Bai Bu (Radix Stemonae) 20g

Decoct the herbs in one liter of cold water and boil down to 700ml of liquid, which is used to wash the affected area twice a day until the condition is cured. This wash can be used at all stages of the disease.

ACUPUNCTURE
Points: CV-3 Zhongji, SP-6 Sanyinjiao and KI-3 Taixi.
Technique: Apply the reinforcing method and retain the needles for 30 minutes. Treat once a day. A course consists of ten treatment sessions.

Explanation
CV-3 Zhongji, SP-6 Sanyinjiao and KI-3 Taixi are used to regulate the Chong and Ren vessels, and enrich the Liver and supplement the Kidneys to consolidate the Root. Although not a direct treatment for tinea, it will help the healing process.

SEVEN-STAR NEEDLING
Follow routine procedures for disinfecting the site of the lesions. Tap gently with a seven-star needle until the skin becomes slightly red or there is slight bleeding with a burning sensation. If the skin in the lesion area is thick, tapping can be stronger. Treat once every one or two days. A course consists of five treatment sessions. After the itching disappears, continue the treatment for another three to five sessions to consolidate the therapeutic effect.

Clinical notes

- Since tinea cruris involves the medial aspect of the thigh and the genital region, medication used externally should be strong enough to kill Worms without injuring or irritating the skin and exacerbating the condition. Therefore, the concentration of the medications used is of great importance.
- Particular attention should be paid to tinea manuum, tinea pedis, tinea unguium, and tinea corporis to avoid tinea cruris infection through contact.
- External medication containing steroids is contraindicated for local use. Strongly-alkaline soap should not be used for washing the affected area.
- Where elderly patients have persistent tinea cruris, consideration should be given to the possibility of an association with diabetes.
- The prognosis for tinea cruris is good if patients

correctly follow the treatment and pay particular attention to personal hygiene, otherwise recurrence is possible.

Advice for the patient

- Wear shower shoes when using a public or family bathing facility, and wear clean underclothing, thus preventing reinfection.
- Keep the genital region clean and dry.
- Take a shower or bath daily.

Case history

Patient
Male, aged 15.

Clinical manifestations
The patient developed redness, swelling and itching in the inguinal grooves after swimming. He was diagnosed with tinea corporis affecting the groin by the dermatology department of the local clinic and given Undecylenate Tinea Lotion for external usage. The lesions worsened after use of the medication, turning purplish-brown with sharply circumscribed borders. He was then prescribed *Huo Huang Jin Ji Tang* (Agastache/Patchouli and Siberian Solomonseal Soak Preparation) for a sitz bath and *Xiao Feng San* (Powder for Dispersing Wind) for internal administration. The condition continued to worsen. Eruptions spread extensively in the groin and scrotum with itching and exudation. The urine was deep yellow in color and the tongue was red at the tip.

Pattern identification
Damp-Heat accumulating in the lower body with the excess spilling to the skin.

Treatment principle
Clear and drain Damp-Heat.

Treatment regime
1. *Pi Yan Xi Ji* (Dermatitis Wash Preparation) for washing the lesions twice a day.
2. *Qing Dai San* (Indigo Powder) mixed with *Cha You* (Oleum Camelliae Oleiferae Seminis, tea oil) for external application to the lesions twice a day.
3. Decoction for internal administration

Internal prescription ingredients
Long Dan Cao (Radix Gentianae Scabrae) 3g
Sheng Gan Cao (Radix Glycyrrhizae Cruda) 3g
Jiao Zhi Zi (Fructus Gardeniae Jasminoidis, scorch-fried) 9g
Ze Xie (Rhizoma Alismatis Orientalis) 9g
Che Qian Zi (Semen Plantaginis) 9g
Chai Hu (Radix Bupleuri) 2g
Huang Qin (Radix Scutellariae Baicalensis) 6g
Tong Cao (Medulla Tetrapanacis Papyriferi) 6g
Huang Bai (Cortex Phellodendri) 6g

Sheng Di Huang (Radix Rehmanniae Glutinosae) 12g
Di Fu Zi (Fructus Kochiae Scopariae) 10g

One bag a day was used to prepare the decoction, taken twice a day.

Outcome
After five days, the red eruptions were clearly fading. Itching was reduced and exudation had ceased. The urine had turned clear and the tongue body was paler. The patient was cured after another five days of this treatment. [10]

Candidal balanitis
念珠菌龟头炎

The yeast *Candida albicans* is a normal inhabitant of the mouth, gut and vaginal tract, and may become pathogenic as a result of certain predisposing factors such as diabetes, obesity, skin maceration, pregnancy, the use of oral contraceptives, or treatment with antibiotics or topical steroids. The yeast usually only infects the outer layers of the epidermis, spreading under the stratum corneum and peeling it away, leading to the characteristic red, bare, glistening surface with a scaling, advancing border. Rarely it can become systematized, especially in the immunosuppressed.

In TCM, candidal balanitis is also known as *xiu kou gan* (cuff canker sore), first referred to in *Yi Zong Jin Jian* [The Golden Mirror of Medicine].

Clinical manifestations

- The uncircumcised penis offers an ideal warm and moist environment for infection by *Candida albicans* under the foreskin, but circumcised patients may also be infected.
- Infection in men generally occurs after sexual intercourse with an infected partner, but can also arise in the absence of sexual contact. (Genital candidiasis in women commonly manifests as a sore itchy vulvovaginitis, with white plaques adhering to inflamed mucous membranes and a whitish discharge.)
- Lesions are characterized by a glistening surface with red pinpoint papules and pustules and a slightly scaling margin. White exudate may be present. Where inflammation is intense, erosion and ulceration may result.
- The infection may spread to the groin area.

Differential diagnosis

Psoriasis
A red plaque on the glans penis with a well-defined border is a possible presentation of plaque psoriasis.

Plaques may persist for months or years. There is no discharge.

Etiology and pathology

Damp-Heat pouring down
Damp-Heat pouring down in the Liver channel causes the disease since the Liver channel passes around the genitals. The uncircumcised foreskin and infrequent washing increase the possibility of the condition arising since foul turbidity and moisture can accumulate beneath the foreskin.

Damp-Heat accumulating to form Toxins
A preference for sweet or fatty food and alcohol results in accumulation of Damp-Heat in the Spleen, subsequently descending toward the penis to collect and bind there to cause the disease.

Pattern identification and treatment

INTERNAL TREATMENT

DAMP-HEAT POURING DOWN
This pattern is characterized by sudden onset with a red and swollen glans penis and sharp or stabbing pain on urination that worsens with friction. Accompanying symptoms and signs include fever, aversion to cold, irritability and restlessness, dry mouth, and lassitude. The tongue body is red with a thin, yellow and slightly greasy coating; the pulse is slippery and rapid.

Treatment principle
Clear Heat and transform Dampness, relieve Toxicity and expel pathogenic factors.

Prescription
LONG DAN XIE GAN TANG JIA JIAN
Chinese Gentian Decoction for Draining the Liver, with modifications

Chao Long Dan Cao (Radix Gentianae Scabrae, stir-fried) 6g

Jiao Zhi Zi (Fructus Gardeniae Jasminoidis, scorch-fried) 6g
Chao Huang Qin (Cortex Scutellariae Baicalensis, stir-fried) 6g
Tong Cao (Medulla Tetrapanacis Papyriferi) 6g
Chai Hu (Radix Bupleuri) 6g
Chi Fu Ling (Sclerotium Poriae Cocos Rubrae) 15g
Ma Bian Cao (Herba cum Radice Verbenae) 15g
Ren Dong Teng (Caulis Lonicerae Japonicae) 15g
Bai Jiang Cao (Herba Patriniae cum Radice) 15g
Yu Xing Cao (Herba Houttuyniae Cordatae) 15g
Che Qian Cao (Herba Plantaginis) 30g
Sheng Di Huang (Radix Rehmanniae Glutinosae) 10g

Explanation

- *Chao Long Dan Cao* (Radix Gentianae Scabrae, stir-fried), *Jiao Zhi Zi* (Fructus Gardeniae Jasminoidis, scorch-fried), *Chao Huang Qin* (Cortex Scutellariae Baicalensis, stir-fried), and *Chi Fu Ling* (Sclerotium Poriae Cocos Rubrae) clear Heat and dry Dampness.
- *Ren Dong Teng* (Caulis Lonicerae Japonicae) and *Tong Cao* (Medulla Tetrapanacis Papyriferi) free the network vessels and disperse swelling.
- *Yu Xing Cao* (Herba Houttuyniae Cordatae), *Bai Jiang Cao* (Herba Patriniae cum Radice), *Ma Bian Cao* (Herba cum Radice Verbenae), and *Che Qian Cao* (Herba Plantaginis) clear Heat, relieve Toxicity and dispel Dampness.
- *Chai Hu* (Radix Bupleuri) dredges the Liver and relieves Depression.
- *Sheng Di Huang* (Radix Rehmanniae Glutinosae) regulates Qi and nourishes the Blood, cools the Blood and alleviates pain.

DAMP-HEAT ACCUMULATING TO FORM TOXINS

Ulcerating sores gradually develop on the penis with exudation, a foul smell, and local swelling with burning pain. Adjacent lymph nodes are swollen and walking is affected. Accompanying symptoms and signs include dribbling urination or inhibited urination. The tongue body is red with a thin yellow coating; the pulse is wiry and rapid.

Treatment principle

Clear Heat and benefit the movement of Dampness, relieve Toxicity and cool the Blood.

Prescription
YIN HUA JIE DU TANG JIA JIAN

Honeysuckle Flower Decoction for Relieving Toxicity, with modifications

Jin Yin Hua (Flos Lonicerae) 30g
Bai Mao Gen (Rhizoma Imperatae Cylindricae) 30g
Lian Qiao (Fructus Forsythiae Suspensae) 10g
Mu Dan Pi (Cortex Moutan Radicis) 10g

Jiao Zhi Zi (Fructus Gardeniae Jasminoidis, scorch-fried) 10g
Huang Bai (Cortex Phellodendri) 10g
Che Qian Zi (Semen Plantaginis) 10g, wrapped
Chi Shao (Radix Paeoniae Rubra) 12g
Zi Hua Di Ding (Herba Violae Yedoensitis) 12g
Gan Cao (Radix Glycyrrhizae) 15g
Bai Hua She She Cao (Herba Hedyotidis Diffusae) 15g

Explanation

- *Jin Yin Hua* (Flos Lonicerae), *Bai Hua She She Cao* (Herba Hedyotidis Diffusae), *Lian Qiao* (Fructus Forsythiae Suspensae), *Zi Hua Di Ding* (Herba Violae Yedoensitis), and *Gan Cao* (Radix Glycyrrhizae) clear Heat and relieve Toxicity.
- *Huang Bai* (Cortex Phellodendri), *Jiao Zhi Zi* (Fructus Gardeniae Jasminoidis, scorch-fried), *Mu Dan Pi* (Cortex Moutan Radicis), and *Che Qian Zi* (Semen Plantaginis) clear Heat and benefit the movement of Dampness.
- *Chi Shao* (Radix Paeoniae Rubra) and *Bai Mao Gen* (Rhizoma Imperatae Cylindricae) clear Heat and cool the Blood to eliminate local swelling with burning pain.

EXTERNAL TREATMENT

- For a red and swollen penis with significant exudation, use *Ma Chi Xian Shui Xi Ji* (Purslane Wash Preparation) or *Long Dan Cao Shui Xi Ji* (Chinese Gentian Wash Preparation) to wash the affected area for 15 minutes once a day.
- Prepare a decoction with *Huang Bai* (Cortex Phellodendri) 30g and *Gan Cao* (Radix Glycyrrhizae) 15g; or *Huang Bai* (Cortex Phellodendri) 15g, *Jin Yin Hua* (Flos Lonicerae) 12g and *Zi Hua Di Ding* (Herba Violae Yedoensitis) 12g. Allow to cool and apply as a cold compress on the affected area or use to wash away any purulent discharge. Then apply one of *Yang Ti Gen San* (Curled Dock Root Powder), *Qing Chui Kou San* (Indigo Mouth Insufflation Powder) or *Qing Dai San* (Indigo Powder) directly or mixed into a paste with sunflower oil. Treat once or twice a day.

Clinical notes

- For internal treatment, the principles of clearing Heat and benefiting the movement of Dampness, cooling the Blood and relieving Toxicity are of particular importance. *Long Dan Cao* (Radix Gentianae Scabrae), *Chi Fu Ling* (Sclerotium Poriae Cocos Rubrae), *Ma Bian Cao* (Herba cum Radice Verbenae) and *Bai Jiang Cao* (Herba Patriniae cum Radice) are commonly used for this purpose.

- It is better to apply wash preparations for external treatment; do not use pastes because they will make erosion worse.

Advice for the patient

Wash the penis frequently, particularly the area under the foreskin.

Pityriasis versicolor (tinea versicolor)
花斑癣

Pityriasis versicolor is a superficial chronic fungal infection of the skin caused by *Malassezia furfur*, the pathogenic form of *Pityrosporum orbiculare*, a normal inhabitant of the scalp. It mainly occurs in summer, involving areas with a dense distribution of sweat glands. This is the reason why it is also known in TCM as *han ban* (sweat macules).

Clinical manifestations

- Pityriasis versicolor mainly occurs on the chest and back, but may also spread to the upper arms, neck and abdomen.
- It occurs mainly in adults (generally young adults), especially in summer or in hot and humid climates; those people with a tendency to sweat profusely are more likely to be affected.
- Lesions start with multiple small macules, which soon enlarge to round or oval macular nail-sized patches covered by a layer of fine scaling. Lesions may be pale white, pale red, yellowish-brown, or dark brown, tending to be paler in dark or tanned skin and darker in untanned skin. Lesions may not be noticeable in fair-skinned persons in winter.
- Patients may experience slight itching, but their main concern is normally the appearance of the skin.
- Pityriasis versicolor is contagious and recurrent.

Differential diagnosis

Vitiligo
White macules without scaling appear in a discrete, vaguely symmetrical distribution on normal-colored skin. Lesions vary in size and have well-defined borders. The hairs growing inside the white macules also turn white. There is no pain or itching.

Pityriasis rosea
This condition starts with a herald patch. Smaller patches then appear on the trunk. Lesions manifest as oval or round erythema, the long axes of which follow the lines of cleavage of the skin. Fine, bran-like scaling is noted.

Pityriasis alba
Pityriasis alba generally involves the face, particularly the area around the mouth, and the chin, cheeks and forehead; involvement of other locations is less common. Lesions usually manifest as white or pale pink patches of varying size and indistinct borders. Their surface is usually covered by fine dry scales. Slight itching may occur with very dry lesions.

Seborrheic eczema of the trunk
This condition is usually limited to the presternal and interscapular regions. Lesions present as scaly, erythematous patches. The scalp and face are also likely to be affected.

Etiology and pathology

- Pityriasis versicolor often develops due to a combination of internal Heat and an invasion of Wind-Damp. These pathogenic factors are retained in the skin and interstices (*cou li*), thus causing the disease.
- Wearing sweat-drenched clothes followed by exposure to the sun leads to Summerheat-Damp invading and stagnating in the pores.

Treatment

PATENT HERBAL MEDICINES
Treat with *Fang Feng Tong Sheng Wan* (Ledebouriella Pill that Sagely Unblocks) to dispel Wind and transform Dampness, and kill Worms to alleviate itching. Take 3g, twice a day with warm boiled water. This treatment is recommended for persistent cases.

EXTERNAL TREATMENT
- Wash the affected area with soap. Mix *Yang Ti Gen San* (Curled Dock Root Powder) with vinegar and

apply externally if the lesion is red or brown; if the lesion is white, rub the powder in with a slice of fresh ginger. Treat once a day. Do not wash the affected area immediately after application of the medication.

- Apply *Tu Jin Pi Ding* (Golden Larch Bark Tincture) or *Pu Xuan Shui* (Universal Tinea Lotion) to the lesions two or three times a day until the condition is cured.
- For stubborn lesions, grind equal amounts of *Zhe Bei Mu* (Bulbus Fritillariae Thunbergii) and *Tian Nan Xing* (Rhizoma Arisaematis) to a fine powder and apply with a slice of fresh ginger once or twice a day.
- For significant scaling, decoct *Xia Ku Cao* (Spica Prunellae Vulgaris) 30g in 500ml of water and wash the lesions daily for seven days, after which the scaling should decrease.

Clinical notes

- Treatment of pityriasis versicolor should focus on external application of medication to the affected area. Start the treatment with a low concentration of one of the external treatment medications, then gradually increase the concentration.
- Pityriasis versicolor can be cured, but it may recur in some cases in the heat of summer.

Advice for the patient

- Avoid contact with clothes worn by patients with pityriasis versicolor.
- It is also important to keep the skin clean and to disinfect underwear by boiling.

Literature excerpt

In *Wai Ke Da Cheng* [A Compendium of External Diseases], it says: "This disease is commonly known as *han ban* (sweat macules). Lesions are dark as a result of Blood stasis or white as a result of Qi stagnation. In both conditions, Wind-Damp invades the body while it is hot. These pathogenic factors are then retained in the skin and interstices (*cou li*). Scratching may lead to scaling without provoking pain."

Modern clinical experience

In the literature, reports on treatment of pityriasis versicolor refer mainly to external application, sometimes accompanied by internal treatment.

EXTERNAL TREATMENT
Liang reported on the external application of a rub. [11]

Prescription
WU BEI ZI SAN
Chinese Gall Powder

Wu Bei Zi‡ (Galla Rhois Chinensis) 30g
Liu Huang‡ (Sulphur) 20g
Bai Fu Zi (Rhizoma Typhonii Gigantei) 10g
Ku Fan‡ (Alumen Praeparatum) 15g

The ingredients were ground into a fine powder and mixed into a paste with vinegar. The medicated paste was applied by rubbing it into the affected area with a cucumber stalk. Treatment took place twice a day for the first ten days, and then continued once a day for a further two weeks. Results were seen at the end of this course.

COMBINED INTERNAL AND EXTERNAL TREATMENT
Li combined a decoction with external treatment. [12]

Prescription ingredients

Fang Feng (Radix Ledebouriellae Divaricatae) 18g
Chuan Xiong (Rhizoma Ligustici Chuanxiong) 10g
Ju Hua (Flos Chrysanthemi Morifolii) 15g
Mu Dan Pi (Cortex Moutan Radicis) 15g
Bai Xian Pi (Cortex Dictamni Dasycarpi Radicis) 15g
Cang Er Zi (Fructus Xanthii Sibirici) 12g
Di Fu Zi (Fructus Kochiae Scopariae) 12g

One bag a day was used to prepare a decoction, taken twice a day. For simultaneous external treatment, he used *Fu Fang Shui Yang Suan Ruan Gao* (Compound Salicylic Ointment) prepared by grinding *Mu Dan Pi* (Cortex Moutan Radicis) 30g and mixing it with 350g of Vaseline® and 120g of powdered salicylic acid. Patients were also advised to avoid spicy food, fish and seafood during the treatment. Results were seen after a ten-day course of treatment.

References

1. Wang Yuxi (ed.), *Shi Yong Zhong Yi Wai Ke Fang Ji Da Ci Dian* [Dictionary of Practical TCM Formulae for External Treatment] (Beijing: Traditional Chinese Medicine Publishing House, 1993), 936.

2. Xu Yihou, *Shan Cang Gui Wai Ke Jing Yan Ji* [A Collection of Shan Canggui's Experiences in Treating External Diseases] (Wuhan: Hubei Science and Technology Publishing House, 1984), 58.

3. Traditional Chinese Medicine Research Academy: Beijing Guang'anmen Hospital, *Zhu Ren Kang Lin Chuang Jing Yan Ji* [A Collection of Zhu Renkang's Clinical Experiences] (Beijing: People's Medical Publishing House, 1979), 79.

4. Yang Zhibo, *Fu Fang Er Fan Xi Ji Zhi Liao Shou Xuan De Lin Chuang Yu Shi Yan Yan Jiu* [Clinical and Experimental Study on the Treatment of Tinea Manuum with *Fu Fang Er Fan Xi Ji* (Compound Alum and Melanterite Wash Preparation)], *Zhong Guo Zhong Xi Yi Jie He Za Zhi* [Journal of Integrated TCM and Western Medicine] 17, 3 (1997): 150.

5. Lu Mingren, *Zhong Yao Ke Xuan Tang Wai Xi Zhi Liao E Zhang Feng 100 Li* [Treatment of 100 Cases of *E Zhang Feng* (Goose-Foot Wind) by an External Wash with the Chinese Herbal Preparation *Ke Xuan Tang* (Restraining Tinea Decoction)], *Liao Ning Zhong Yi Za Zhi* [Liaoning Journal of Traditional Chinese Medicine] 23, 3 (1996): 119.

6. Chen Wangen, *Zi Ni Ke Xuan Jin Pao Ji Zhi Liao Jiao Xuan Lin Chuang Liao Xiao Guan Cha* [Observation of the Clinical Effectiveness of Treating Tinea Pedis with the Empirical Prescription *Ke Xuan Jin Pao Ji* (Soak Preparation for Restraining Tinea)], *Zhong Guo Nong Cun Yi Xue* [Chinese Rural Medicine] 24, 3 (1996): 54.

7. Ruan Maorong, *Ku Shen Tang Zhi Liao Jiao Xuan 216 Li* [Treatment of 216 Cases of Tinea Pedis with *Ku Shen Tang* (Flavescent Sophora Root and Cnidium Fruit Decoction)], *Ren Min Jun Yi* [Medical Journal of the People's Army] 41, 5 (1998): 366-7.

8. Li Jianguo, *Yan Fang Zhi Liao Shou Zu Xuan 50 Li* [Treatment of 50 Cases of Tinea Manuum and Tinea Pedis with Empirical Prescriptions], *Ren Min Jun Yi* [Medical Journal of the People's Army] 41, 2 (1998): 114.

9. Cui Yinchun, *Si Ye Tang Jian Xi Zhi Liao Jiao Xuan Gan Ran* [Treatment of Tinea Pedis Infection with *Si Ye Tang* (Four-Leaf Decoction)], *Zhong Yi Za Zhi* [Journal of Traditional Chinese Medicine] 37, 7 (1996): 423.

10. Xu Fusong, *Xu Lü He Wai Ke Yi An Yi Hua Ji* [A Collection of Xu Lühe's Medical Records and Notes on External Diseases] (Nanjing: Jiangsu Science and Technology Publishing House, 1980), 309.

11. Liang Baohui, *Wu Bei Zi San Wai Ca Zhi Liao Hua Ban Xuan 21 Li* [External Treatment of 21 Cases of Pityriasis Versicolor Using *Wu Bei Zi San* (Chinese Gall Powder) as a Rub], *Zhong Yi Wai Zhi Za Zhi* [Journal of Traditional Chinese Medicine External Treatments] 8, 2 (1999): 14.

12. Li Chenggong, *Zhong Yi Yao Zhi Liao Hua Ban Xuan 85 Li* [Treatment of 85 Cases of Pityriasis Versicolor with Chinese Materia Medica], *Guang Xi Zhong Yi Za Zhi* [Guangxi Journal of Traditional Chinese Medicine] 21, 1 (1998): 33.

Pruritus and prurigo

Although the etiology of the diseases discussed in this chapter is often unknown or unclear, emotional factors frequently appear to play a role in their occurrence. The skin is richly supplied with nerves, with the greatest density occurring in the hands, face and genital region. Most free sensory nerve endings are found in the dermis, but some encroach into the epidermis. Free nerve endings detect stimuli such as heat, itching and pain. Itching is characteristic of many skin diseases and occurs as the result of stimulation of free nerve endings lying near the junction of the dermis and epidermis.

Skin diseases which may have functional or organic disorders of the nervous system as a possible cause include pruritus, prurigo and lichen simplex chronicus (or neurodermatitis, see Chapter 3); these diseases can be triggered or aggravated by factors such as depression, stress or anxiety. This chapter focuses on pruritus and prurigo, where itching is the main manifestation of the condition; itching present as a symptom of a skin disorder is discussed under the relevant disorder.

In general terms, TCM considers that there are three main etiologies for these conditions:

- Pathogenic Wind, Dampness and Heat settle in the skin, obstructing the channels and network vessels and inhibiting the movement of Qi, thus causing itching.
- Emotional factors such as depression or anxiety lead to disharmony of Qi and Blood, resulting in stagnation of Liver Qi.
- Dietary irregularities such as excessive intake of spicy or rich food damage and deplete Yin and Blood. Consequently, the skin is deprived of nourishment or will be affected by Blood-Heat.

Pruritus
皮肤瘙痒症

Pruritus may be generalized or localized. The term generalized pruritus is normally used for patients with itching but with no detectable primary disorder of the skin. Some patients have marked secondary features of excoriation that affect all sites except the mid-back that cannot be reached by the patient (the "butterfly" sign). Many patients with idiopathic pruritus appear to have generally fine scaly skin and itching responds to emollients. Some may have an underlying systemic disease, but 50% have no obvious underlying abnormality.

Systemic conditions clearly associated with generalized pruritus include obstructive biliary disease, uremia, lymphomas, leukemias, thyrotoxicosis, polycythemia rubra vera, iron deficiency, and pregnancy. Other causes are drugs, parasitic infestations and psychogenic; dry skin in the elderly may also cause itching.

Localized pruritus is caused by localized friction, trichomoniasis, pinworm, or leukorrhea.

In TCM, this condition is also known as *feng sao yang* (Wind itch).

Clinical manifestations

- Pruritus is usually generalized or affects large areas of the body.
- It is more common in adults, particularly in the elderly.
- In cases of generalized pruritus, complete sparing of areas that are not accessible suggests that any rash is secondary to scratching.
- Most widespread pruritus is due to skin disease rather than systemic causes.
- There are no primary rashes associated with pruritus, which is paroxysmal and worse at night.
- Secondary lesions such as scratch marks, crusts or eczematoid lesions, or lichenification may occur as a

result of scratching.
• Systemic symptoms vary from case to case.

Differential diagnosis

Urticaria, scabies, insect bites, and drug eruptions present with itching; however, these conditions are associated with primary rashes. Pruritus is differentiated by intense itching without any primary rash.

Etiology and pathology

Internal and external Wind play a major role in the etiology of this disease, either alone or in combination.

External factors
The six external pathogenic factors – Wind, Dryness, Summerheat, Fire, Dampness and Cold – can attack the skin and interstices (*cou li*) and fight with Blood and Qi. These pathogenic factors move around in the skin, obstructing Qi in the channels and leading to pruritus. Pathogenic Wind is the most important of these factors, since it can combine with other factors and wander through the skin to cause itching. In addition, friction or contact with fur, feathers or artificial fabrics may also induce pruritus.

Blood-Heat generating Wind
Young or middle-aged people are full of Qi and Blood. In many instances, Blood-Heat brews internally due to external invasion of pathogenic factors. Blood-Heat generates Wind; exuberant Wind then results in itching.

Qi and Blood Deficiency
In the elderly and infirm or those with a weak constitution due to chronic illnesses, Qi Deficiency often leads to Wei Qi (Defensive Qi) being unable to consolidate the exterior, allowing pathogenic Wind to attack. Blood Deficiency results in the skin being deprived of moisture and nourishment. In the long term, this can lead to obstruction of Qi and Blood and stagnation in the channels and vessels. If Qi cannot flow freely in the channels, pruritus may result.

Dietary irregularities
Excessive consumption of fish, seafood, spicy, and greasy food, or alcohol may damage the transformation and transportation function of the Spleen and Stomach resulting in Damp-Heat being generated internally. The two pathogens bind together to transform into Heat and generate Wind, which cannot be drained internally or thrust outward externally, but is retained in the skin, hair and interstices (*cou li*), resulting in pruritus. In addition, food substances stirring internal Wind often produce severe Heart-Fire, causing Blood-Heat to attack the skin, again giving rise to pruritus.

Emotional factors
Depression, irritability, anxiety, stress, and other emotional factors may impair the functional activities of Qi in the Zang-Fu organs. This results in the five emotions transforming into Fire and Blood-Heat brewing internally. When Heat is transformed, it stirs Wind, thus leading to pruritus.

Depletion of Essence and Blood
Qi and Blood will be Deficient in patients with chronic or recurrent diseases; in the elderly and infirm, depletion of the Essence and Blood is to be expected. Blood Deficiency generates internal Wind. The skin is deprived of moisture and nourishment, resulting in pruritus.

Pattern identification and treatment

INTERNAL TREATMENT

BLOOD-HEAT GENERATING WIND
This pattern is encountered more commonly in the young and middle-aged with exuberant Qi and Blood; it occurs more often in summer. Internal factors such as irritability and restlessness or overindulgence in spicy, aromatic or roast food may lead to Blood-Heat generating Wind, resulting in pruritus. Scratch marks and crusts may cover the whole body. Itching is likely to be severe in summer, when Yang Qi is predominant in nature, as external Heat mixes with internal Heat. Itching is alleviated by cold. The tongue body is red with a thin yellow coating; the pulse is wiry and rapid.

Treatment principle
Cool the Blood and clear Heat, dissipate Wind and alleviate itching.

Prescription
ZHI YANG XI FENG TANG JIA JIAN
Decoction for Alleviating Itching and Extinguishing Wind, with modifications

Sheng Di Huang (Radix Rehmanniae Glutinosae) 15g
Long Gu ‡ (Os Draconis) 15g
Mu Li ‡ (Concha Ostreae) 15g
Xuan Shen (Radix Scrophulariae Ningpoensis) 10g
Dang Gui (Radix Angelicae Sinensis) 10g
Bai Ji Li (Fructus Tribuli Terrestris) 10g
Dan Shen (Radix Salviae Miltiorrhizae) 10g
Fang Feng (Radix Ledebouriellae Divaricatae) 6g
Gan Cao (Radix Glycyrrhizae) 6g
Chan Tui ‡ (Periostracum Cicadae) 6g
Huang Qin (Radix Scutellariae Baicalensis) 6g

Explanation
• *Sheng Di Huang* (Radix Rehmanniae Glutinosae), *Xuan Shen* (Radix Scrophulariae Ningpoensis) and

Huang Qin (Radix Scutellariae Baicalensis) clear Heat and cool the Blood.

- *Fang Feng* (Radix Ledebouriellae Divaricatae), *Bai Ji Li* (Fructus Tribuli Terrestris) and *Chan Tui* ‡ (Periostracum Cicadae) dissipate Wind and alleviate itching.
- *Dang Gui* (Radix Angelicae Sinensis) and *Dan Shen* (Radix Salviae Miltiorrhizae) invigorate the Blood and free the network vessels to assist *Fang Feng* (Radix Ledebouriellae Divaricatae) and the other ingredients in alleviating itching.
- *Long Gu* ‡ (Os Draconis), *Mu Li* ‡ (Concha Ostreae) and *Gan Cao* (Radix Glycyrrhizae) extinguish Wind and alleviate itching.

EXUBERANT WIND
This pattern is often encountered in spring, when Wood dominates. Looseness of the flesh and interstices (*cou li*) allows external Wind to invade. If this Wind is retained over a long period, it eventually transforms into Heat, resulting in itching. Typical signs are generalized itching not restricted to a fixed location and bleeding on scratching, which stops very quickly. Lesions are dry with crusts, and infection and suppuration are rare. Lichenification occurs if the disease lasts for a long time. The tongue body is red with a thin yellow coating; the pulse is wiry and rapid.

Treatment principle
Arrest Wind and clear Heat, vanquish Toxicity and alleviate itching.

Prescription
WU SHE QU FENG TANG JIA JIAN
Black-Tail Snake Decoction for Expelling Wind, with modifications

Xu Chang Qing (Radix Cynanchi Paniculati) 6g
Qiang Huo (Rhizoma et Radix Notopterygii) 6g
Chan Tui ‡ (Periostracum Cicadae) 6g
Jing Jie (Herba Schizonepetae Tenuifoliae) 6g
Huang Qin (Radix Scutellariae Baicalensis) 6g
Fang Feng (Radix Ledebouriellae Divaricatae) 10g
Lian Qiao (Fructus Forsythiae Suspensae) 10g
Jin Yin Hua (Flos Lonicerae) 10g
Chi Xiao Dou (Semen Phaseoli Radiati) 15g
Gou Teng (Ramulus Uncariae cum Uncis) 15g
Bai Ji Li (Fructus Tribuli Terrestris) 15g

Explanation
- *Xu Chang Qing* (Radix Cynanchi Paniculati), *Chan Tui* ‡ (Periostracum Cicadae) and *Gou Teng* (Ramulus Uncariae cum Uncis) arrest Wind and alleviate itching.
- *Qiang Huo* (Rhizoma et Radix Notopterygii), *Jing Jie* (Herba Schizonepetae Tenuifoliae), *Fang Feng* (Radix Ledebouriellae Divaricatae), and *Bai Ji Li* (Fructus

Tribuli Terrestris) dissipate Wind and alleviate itching.
- Both of these groups of materia medica alleviate itching, but the first group is more effective for expelling Toxicity, whereas the second group is better for dissipating Wind.
- *Huang Qin* (Radix Scutellariae Baicalensis), *Lian Qiao* (Fructus Forsythiae Suspensae), *Jin Yin Hua* (Flos Lonicerae), and *Chi Xiao Dou* (Semen Phaseoli Radiati) clear Heat and vanquish Toxicity.

WIND-DAMP-HEAT SETTLING IN THE SKIN
This pattern is encountered more often in summer and is more likely to affect young and middle-aged people as well as those who overindulge in greasy, sweet or rich food, resulting in Dampness accumulating in the body. After external contraction of pathogenic Wind, Wind and Dampness contend, resulting in pruritus.

Where there is exuberance of Wind, the main symptom is intense itching. In *Wai Ke Qi Xuan* [Revelations of the Mystery of External Diseases], it says: "The pattern often occurs on the inner and outer shanks, extending up to the knees and down to the ankles, with the itching being generated by pathogenic Wind invading the Blood." Constant scratching or washing in very hot water will result in the local area becoming eczematoid. The tongue body is pale red with a white and greasy coating; the pulse is wiry and slippery.

Treatment principle
Dispel Wind and overcome Dampness, clear Heat and alleviate itching.

Prescription
QUAN CHONG FANG JIA JIAN
Scorpion Formula, with modifications

Gou Teng (Ramulus Uncariae cum Uncis) 6g
Zao Jiao Ci (Spina Gleditsiae Sinensis) 6g
Ku Shen (Radix Sophorae Flavescentis) 6g
Bai Ji Li (Fructus Tribuli Terrestris) 12g
Xi Xian Cao (Herba Siegesbeckiae) 12g
Bai Xian Pi (Cortex Dictamni Dasycarpi Radicis) 12g
Huang Bai (Cortex Phellodendri) 12g
Yi Yi Ren (Semen Coicis Lachryma-jobi) 15g
Chi Xiao Dou (Semen Phaseoli Radiati) 15g
Mu Dan Pi (Cortex Moutan Radicis) 10g
Fang Feng (Radix Ledebouriellae Divaricatae) 10g

Explanation
- *Gou Teng* (Ramulus Uncariae cum Uncis), *Zao Jiao Ci* (Spina Gleditsiae Sinensis), *Ku Shen* (Radix Sophorae Flavescentis), *Fang Feng* (Radix Ledebouriellae Divaricatae), *Bai Xian Pi* (Cortex Dictamni Dasycarpi Radicis), *Xi Xian Cao* (Herba Siegesbeckiae), and *Bai Ji Li*

(Fructus Tribuli Terrestris) dissipate Wind and dispel Dampness, expel pathogenic factors and alleviate itching.

- *Huang Bai* (Cortex Phellodendri), *Yi Yi Ren* (Semen Coicis Lachryma-jobi), *Chi Xiao Dou* (Semen Phaseoli Radiati), and *Mu Dan Pi* (Cortex Moutan Radicis) clear Heat, transform Dampness, and relieve Toxicity.

WIND-COLD FETTERING THE EXTERIOR

This pattern occurs more often in winter, with generalized itching mostly affecting exposed areas such as the head, face, neck, and hands. Although considered as a Yin pattern, the root of the disease is an insufficiency of Yang Qi, which means that the body cannot ward off external Cold, leading to external contraction of Wind-Cold. Pruritus will be induced or aggravated by cold or by sudden changes of temperature such as when entering a warm room from the cold. Itching will ease while sweating or when in a warm environment. The skin is usually dry with tiny bran-like scales. The tongue body is pale red with a thin white coating; the pulse is floating and tight or floating and moderate.

Treatment principle

Dissipate Cold and dispel Wind, release the exterior and alleviate itching.

Prescription
GUI ZHI MA HUANG GE BAN TANG JIA JIAN

Cinnamon Twig and Ephedra Half-and-Half Decoction, with modifications

Ma Huang* (Herba Ephedrae) 1.5g
Gui Zhi (Ramulus Cinnamomi Cassiae) 1.5g
Chao Bai Shao (Radix Paeoniae Lactiflorae, stir-fried) 6g
Jie Geng (Radix Platycodi Grandiflori) 6g
Jing Jie (Herba Schizonepetae Tenuifoliae) 6g
Fang Feng (Radix Ledebouriellae Divaricatae) 6g
Gan Jiang (Rhizoma Zingiberis Officinalis) 6g
Qiang Huo (Rhizoma et Radix Notopterygii) 4.5g
Du Huo (Radix Angelicae Pubescentis) 4.5g
Gan Cao (Radix Glycyrrhizae) 4.5g
Da Zao (Fructus Ziziphi Jujubae) 15g

Explanation

- *Ma Huang** (Herba Ephedrae), *Gui Zhi* (Ramulus Cinnamomi Cassiae), *Chao Bai Shao* (Radix Paeoniae Lactiflorae, stir-fried), *Gan Cao* (Radix Glycyrrhizae), *Da Zao* (Fructus Ziziphi Jujubae), and *Gan Jiang* (Rhizoma Zingiberis Officinalis) harmonize the Ying and Wei levels to expel Cold from the skin and interstices (*cou li*).
- *Jing Jie* (Herba Schizonepetae Tenuifoliae), *Fang Feng* (Radix Ledebouriellae Divaricatae), *Qiang Huo* (Rhizoma et Radix Notopterygii), *Jie Geng* (Radix Platycodi Grandiflori), and *Du Huo* (Radix Angelicae Pubescentis), dredge Wind and dissipate Cold, disperse Wind and alleviate itching.

BLOOD DEFICIENCY GENERATING WIND

This pattern is encountered more commonly in the elderly or in people with a weak constitution and occurs more frequently in autumn and winter. Deficiency of Qi and Blood generates internal Wind and the skin is deprived of nourishment, resulting in dry skin and bran-like scales. Itching is worse at night; scratching leads to crusts and scratch marks all over the body. After a certain time, the skin may become lichenified. Accompanying symptoms and signs include fatigue, a pale facial complexion, lack of energy during the day and difficulty in sleeping at night, palpitations, and poor appetite. The tongue body is pale red with a scant or thin white coating; the pulse is deficient, thready and rapid.

Treatment principle

Nourish the Blood and disperse Wind, moisten Dryness and alleviate itching.

Prescription
YANG XUE RUN FU YIN JIA JIAN

Decoction for Nourishing the Blood and Moistening the Skin, with modifications

Dang Gui (Radix Angelicae Sinensis) 10g
Tian Men Dong (Radix Asparagi Cochinchinensis) 10g
Mai Men Dong (Radix Ophiopogonis Japonici) 10g
Tian Hua Fen (Radix Trichosanthis) 10g
Huang Qi (Radix Astragali seu Hedysari) 10g
Sheng Di Huang (Radix Rehmanniae Glutinosae) 15g
Shu Di Huang (Radix Rehmanniae Glutinosae Conquita) 15g
He Shou Wu (Radix Polygoni Multiflori) 15g
Gou Teng (Ramulus Uncariae cum Uncis) 15g
Huang Qin (Radix Scutellariae Baicalensis) 6g
Hong Hua (Flos Carthami Tinctorii) 6g
Tao Ren (Semen Persicae) 6g
Zao Jiao Ci (Spina Gleditsiae Sinensis) 4.5g
Sheng Ma (Rhizoma Cimicifugae) 4.5g

Explanation

- *Dang Gui* (Radix Angelicae Sinensis), *Sheng Di Huang* (Radix Rehmanniae Glutinosae), *Shu Di Huang* (Radix Rehmanniae Glutinosae Conquita), *Tao Ren* (Semen Persicae), and *Hong Hua* (Flos Carthami Tinctorii) nourish the Blood to disperse Wind.
- *Tian Men Dong* (Radix Asparagi Cochinchinensis), *Mai Men Dong* (Radix Ophiopogonis Japonici), *Tian Hua Fen* (Radix Trichosanthis), and *He Shou Wu* (Radix Polygoni Multiflori) emolliate the Liver, boost the Kidneys, nourish Yin, and moisten Dryness.

- *Gou Teng* (Ramulus Uncariae cum Uncis), *Zao Jiao Ci* (Spina Gleditsiae Sinensis), *Huang Qin* (Radix Scutellariae Baicalensis), and *Sheng Ma* (Rhizoma Cimicifugae) disperse Wind and alleviate itching.
- *Huang Qi* (Radix Astragali seu Hedysari) consolidates the exterior and supports Vital Qi (Zheng Qi) to prevent the invasion of external pathogenic factors.
- Itching will disappear once internal Wind is dispelled.

BLOOD STASIS

This pattern may happen at any age and in any season. Usually, itching occurs most frequently at areas subject to constant pressure or friction such as the waist, the lumbosacral region, the dorsum of the foot, and the wrist. Clusters of scratch marks can be seen; sometimes scratching breaks the skin and blood seeps to the exterior. Purple striae may also be visible. Accompanying symptoms and signs include a dark facial complexion and purple lips. The tongue body is dark, possibly with stasis marks, and has a scant coating; the pulse is thready and rough.

Treatment principle

Invigorate the Blood and transform Blood stasis, disperse Wind and alleviate itching.

Prescription
HUO XUE QU FENG TANG JIA JIAN

Decoction for Invigorating the Blood and Dispelling Wind, with modifications

Dang Gui (Radix Angelicae Sinensis) 10g
Tao Ren (Semen Persicae) 10g
Yi Mu Cao (Herba Leonuri Heterophylli) 10g
Fang Feng (Radix Ledebouriellae Divaricatae) 10g
Jing Jie (Herba Schizonepetae Tenuifoliae) 6g
Hong Hua (Flos Carthami Tinctorii) 6g
Gan Cao (Radix Glycyrrhizae) 6g
Chan Tui‡ (Periostracum Cicadae) 6g
Chi Shao (Radix Paeoniae Rubra) 6g
Bai Ji Li (Fructus Tribuli Terrestris) 12g
Gou Teng (Ramulus Uncariae cum Uncis) 12g

Explanation
- *Dang Gui* (Radix Angelicae Sinensis), *Tao Ren* (Semen Persicae), *Hong Hua* (Flos Carthami Tinctorii), *Chi Shao* (Radix Paeoniae Rubra), and *Yi Mu Cao* (Herba Leonuri Heterophylli) invigorate the Blood and transform Blood stasis, free the network vessels and alleviate itching.
- *Jing Jie* (Herba Schizonepetae Tenuifoliae), *Chan Tui*‡ (Periostracum Cicadae) and *Fang Feng* (Radix Ledebouriellae Divaricatae) disperse Wind and alleviate itching.
- *Bai Ji Li* (Fructus Tribuli Terrestris) and *Gou Teng* (Ramulus Uncariae cum Uncis) extinguish Wind and

alleviate itching.
- *Jing Jie* (Herba Schizonepetae Tenuifoliae), *Chan Tui*‡ (Periostracum Cicadae) and *Fang Feng* (Radix Ledebouriellae Divaricatae) disperse external Wind, whereas *Bai Ji Li* (Fructus Tribuli Terrestris) and *Gou Teng* (Ramulus Uncariae cum Uncis) extinguish internal Wind. The effect in alleviating itching is much more evident when herbs from both groups are used.
- *Gan Cao* (Radix Glycyrrhizae) harmonizes the properties of the other ingredients.

WEAKNESS OF WEI QI DUE TO SPLEEN DEFICIENCY

This pattern is usually caused by overindulgence in fish and seafood, or through contact with fur and feathers. Intensity of itching varies over time. Scratch marks with tiny crusts are often found on the skin. Accompanying symptoms and signs include shortness of breath, lack of strength, no desire to speak, tiredness, and dry or loose stools. The tongue body is pale red with a scant or thin coating; the pulse is deficient, thready and weak.

Treatment principle

Fortify the Spleen and augment Qi to assist in consolidating the exterior.

Prescription
REN SHEN JIAN PI TANG JIA JIAN

Ginseng Decoction for Fortifying the Spleen, with modifications

Dang Shen (Radix Codonopsitis Pilosulae) 10-12g
Huang Qi (Radix Astragali seu Hedysari) 10-12g
Tu Chao Bai Zhu (Rhizoma Atractylodis Macrocephalae, stir-fried with earth) 10g
Chen Pi (Pericarpium Citri Reticulatae) 10g
Fang Feng (Radix Ledebouriellae Divaricatae) 10g
Fu Ling Pi (Cortex Poriae Cocos) 12-15g
Jing Jie (Herba Schizonepetae Tenuifoliae) 6g
Sha Ren (Fructus Amomi) 6g, added 5 minutes before the end of the decoction process
Zhi Ke (Fructus Citri Aurantii) 6g
Mei Gui Hua (Flos Rosae Rugosae) 6g
Gan Cao (Radix Glycyrrhizae) 6g
Huang Lian (Rhizoma Coptidis) 1.5g
*Mu Xiang** (Radix Aucklandiae Lappae) 3-6g

Explanation
- *Dang Shen* (Radix Codonopsitis Pilosulae), *Huang Qi* (Radix Astragali seu Hedysari), *Bai Zhu* (Rhizoma Atractylodis Macrocephalae), *Chen Pi* (Pericarpium Citri Reticulatae), *Fu Ling Pi* (Cortex Poriae Cocos), *Mu Xiang** (Radix Aucklandiae Lappae), and *Sha Ren* (Fructus Amomi) augment Qi and fortify the Spleen to consolidate the Root.

- *Fang Feng* (Radix Ledebouriellae Divaricatae), *Jing Jie* (Herba Schizonepetae Tenuifoliae) and *Zhi Ke* (Fructus Citri Aurantii) dissipate Wind and alleviate itching to treat the Manifestations.
- *Huang Lian* (Rhizoma Coptidis) clears Heart-Fire.
- *Mei Gui Hua* (Flos Rosae Rugosae) soothes the Liver and regulates Qi. Not only does it assist *Dang Shen* (Radix Codonopsitis Pilosulae) and *Huang Qi* (Radix Astragali seu Hedysari) to augment Qi and fortify the Spleen, it also helps *Fang Feng* (Radix Ledebouriellae Divaricatae) and *Jing Jie* (Herba Schizonepetae Tenuifoliae) to dissipate Wind and alleviate itching.

General modifications

1. For pruritus in the upper part of the body, add *Fu Pen Zi* (Fructus Rubi Chingii), *Sang Ye* (Folium Mori Albae) and *Ju Hua* (Flos Chrysanthemi Morifolii).
2. For pruritus in the lower part of the body, add *Chao Du Zhong* (Cortex Eucommiae Ulmoidis, stir-fried), *Sang Ji Sheng* (Ramulus Loranthi) and *Niu Xi* (Radix Achyranthis Bidentatae).
3. For generalized pruritus, add *Fu Ping* (Herba Spirodelae Polyrrhizae), *Bai Ji Li* (Fructus Tribuli Terrestris), *Ku Shen* (Radix Sophorae Flavescentis), *Bai Xian Pi* (Cortex Dictamni Dasycarpi Radicis), and *Di Fu Zi* (Fructus Kochiae Scopariae).
4. For stubborn pruritus, add *Chuan Xiong* (Rhizoma Ligustici Chuanxiong), *Wu Shao She*‡ (Zaocys Dhumnades), *Quan Xie*‡ (Buthus Martensi), and *Wei Ling Xian* (Radix Clematidis).
5. For oozing and exudation, add *Jiang Can*‡ (Bombyx Batryticatus), *Fu Ling Pi* (Cortex Poriae Cocos), *Yin Chen Hao* (Herba Artemisiae Scopariae), and *Chi Xiao Dou* (Semen Phaseoli Radiati).
6. To prevent infection of excoriations, add *Jiao Zhi Zi* (Fructus Gardeniae Jasminoidis, scorch-fried), *Huang Bai* (Cortex Phellodendri), *Bai Hua She She Cao* (Herba Hedyotidis Diffusae), *Pu Gong Ying* (Herba Taraxaci cum Radice), and *Ye Ju Hua* (Flos Chrysanthemi Indici).
7. For severe Blood-Heat, add *Di Yu* (Radix Sanguisorbae Officinalis) and *Zi Cao* (Radix Arnebiae seu Lithospermi).
8. For severe Wind, add *Fang Feng* (Radix Ledebouriellae Divaricatae) and *Quan Xie*‡ (Buthus Martensi).
9. For lichenification, add *Jiang Huang* (Rhizoma Curcumae Longae), *E Zhu* (Rhizoma Curcumae), *Mu Dan Pi* (Cortex Moutan Radicis), *Dan Shen* (Radix Salviae Miltiorrhizae), and *E Jiao*‡ (Gelatinum Corii Asini).
10. For thirst and constipation, add *Da Huang* (Radix et Rhizoma Rhei) 10 minutes before the end of the decoction process, and *Zhi Mu* (Rhizoma Anemarrhenae Asphodeloidis).
11. For palpitations and insomnia, add *Suan Zao Ren* (Semen Ziziphi Spinosae), *Bai Zi Ren* (Semen Biotae Orientalis) and *Ye Jiao Teng* (Caulis Polygoni Multiflori).
12. For mental and physical fatigue, add *He Shou Wu* (Radix Polygoni Multiflori) and *Ren Shen* (Radix Ginseng).
13. For aversion to cold and cold limbs, add *Fu Pen Zi* (Fructus Rubi Chingii).
14. For Blood Deficiency, add *Dang Gui* (Radix Angelicae Sinensis) and *Sang Shen* (Fructus Mori Albae).

PATENT HERBAL MEDICINES

- For exuberant Wind patterns, take *Wu She Zhi Yang Wan* (Black-Tail Snake Pill for Alleviating Itching) 3g twice a day.
- For Wind-Damp-Heat settling in the skin, take *Er Miao Wan* (Mysterious Two Pill) 1g and *Fang Feng Tong Sheng Wan* (Ledebouriella Pill that Sagely Unblocks) 1g twice a day.
- For Blood Deficiency generating Wind, take *Liu Wei Di Huang Wan* (Six-Ingredient Rehmannia Pill) 1.5g and *Fang Feng Tong Sheng Wan* (Ledebouriella Pill that Sagely Unblocks) 1.5g twice a day.
- For Blood stasis, take *Fu Fang Dan Shen Pian* (Compound Red Sage Root Tablet) 1.5g and *Wu She Zhi Yang Wan* (Black-Tail Snake Pill for Alleviating Itching) 1.5g twice a day.

EXTERNAL TREATMENT

- For **generalized pruritus**, select three or four of the materia medica listed below and use 30-60g of each in a decoction used warm as a general body wash.

  Di Fu Zi (Fructus Kochiae Scopariae)
  Fu Ping (Herba Spirodelae Polyrrhizae)
  Yi Mu Cao (Herba Leonuri Heterophylli)
  Si Gua Luo (Fasciculus Vascularis Luffae)
  Mu Zei (Herba Equiseti Hiemalis)
  Xiang Fu (Rhizoma Cyperi Rotundi)
  Can Sha‡ (Excrementum Bombycis Mori)
  Jin Qian Cao (Herba Lysimachiae)
  Wu Zhu Yu (Fructus Evodiae Rutaecarpae)
  Hou Po (Cortex Magnoliae Officinalis)
  She Chuang Zi (Fructus Cnidii Monnieri)

- For **localized pruritus**, rub the affected area with an appropriate amount of one of the following:

  Ku Shen Jiu (Flavescent Sophora Root Wine)
  San Shi Shui (Three Stones Lotion)
  Bai Bu Ding (Stemona Root Tincture)

  Then apply *Qing Liang Fen* (Cool Clearing Powder) or *Gan Shi San* (Calamine Powder).

- For dry, itchy and lichenified skin, apply *Huang Lian Ruan Gao* (Coptis Ointment) or *Run Ji Gao* (Flesh-Moistening Paste) to the affected area.

ACUPUNCTURE

Selection of points according to pattern identification

Blood-Heat generating Wind
Main points: GB-20 Fengchi, GV-14 Dazhui and SP-10 Xuehai.
Auxiliary points: GV-16 Fengfu, LI-11 Quchi and ST-36 Zusanli.

Exuberant Wind
Main points: GB-20 Fengchi, GV-16 Fengfu, GV-20 Baihui, and SP-10 Xuehai.
Auxiliary points: LR-3 Taichong, GV-14 Dazhui and GB-34 Yanglingquan.

Wind-Damp-Heat settling in the skin
Main points: ST-38 Tiaokou, ST-40 Fenglong, CV-12 Zhongwan, and LI-11 Quchi.
Auxiliary points: GB-20 Fengchi, CV-10 Xiawan and ST-36 Zusanli.

Wind-Cold fettering the exterior
Main points: CV-6 Qihai, CV-4 Guanyuan, ST-36 Zusanli, GV-20 Baihui, and GB-20 Fengchi.
Auxiliary points: BL-23 Shenshu, CV-12 Zhongwan and SP-6 Sanyinjiao.

Blood Deficiency generating Wind
Main points: SP-10 Xuehai, BL-17 Geshu, ST-36 Zusanli, and SP-6 Sanyinjiao.
Auxiliary points: GV-20 Baihui, ST-40 Fenglong and LR-2 Xingjian.

Blood stasis
Main points: SP-10 Xuehai, BL-17 Geshu, ST-36 Zusanli, and SP-6 Sanyinjiao.
Auxiliary points: GV-20 Baihui, ST-40 Fenglong and LR-2 Xingjian.

Weakness of Wei Qi due to Spleen Deficiency
Main points: SP-6 Sanyinjiao, SP-10 Xuehai, SP-8 Diji, CV-12 Zhongwan, and LI-11 Quchi.
Auxiliary points: ST-36 Zusanli, ST-25 Tianshu and ST-40 Fenglong.

Technique
Apply the reinforcing method for Deficiency patterns and the reducing method for Excess patterns. Retain the needles for 30 minutes after obtaining Qi. Treat once a day. A course consists of ten treatment sessions.

Selection of points according to disease
Generalized pruritus
Main points: LI-11 Quchi and SP-10 Xuehai.
Auxiliary points: LI-4 Hegu, ST-36 Zusanli and BL-13 Feishu.

Localized pruritus
Main points: LR-11 Yinlian and CV-2 Qugu.
Auxiliary points: SP-9 Yinlingquan and SP-6 Sanyinjiao.

Technique
Apply the reducing method for Excess patterns and the reinforcing method for Deficiency patterns. Retain the needles for 30 minutes after obtaining Qi. Treat once a day. A course consists of ten treatment sessions.

Explanation
- GB-20 Fengchi, GV-16 Fengfu and BL-13 Feishu dissipate Wind and alleviate itching.
- SP-10 Xuehai, BL-17 Geshu, LR-11 Yinlian, and CV-2 Qugu invigorate the Blood and alleviate itching.
- ST-40 Fenglong, ST-38 Tiaokou, CV-6 Qihai, SP-8 Diji, ST-25 Tianshu, and CV-12 Zhongwan transform Dampness and alleviate itching.
- GV-20 Baihui, CV-10 Xiawan and GV-14 Dazhui dissipate Cold and alleviate itching.
- BL-23 Shenshu and CV-4 Guanyuan warm the Kidneys and alleviate itching.
- LR-3 Taichong, GB-34 Yanglingquan and LR-2 Xingjian regulate Qi and alleviate itching.
- In *Su Wen* [Simple Questions], it says that all painful and itching sores are ascribed to the Heart. SP-10 Xuehai, ST-36 Zusanli, LI-4 Hegu, LI-11 Quchi, SP-9 Yinlingquan, and SP-6 Sanyinjiao are used to fortify the Spleen and generate Blood to nourish the Heart.

MOXIBUSTION
Points: BL-17 Geshu, SP-10 Xuehai, BL-18 Ganshu, and SP-6 Sanyinjiao.
Technique: Apply direct moxibustion to the points for 5-10 minutes. Treat once a day. A course consists of seven treatment sessions.

Explanation
These points nourish the Blood, emolliate the Liver and alleviate itching

EAR ACUPUNCTURE
Prescription 1: Ear-Shenmen, Sympathetic Nerve, Adrenal Gland, Endocrine, Lung, and itching points (the location of lesions on the body).
Prescription 2: Ear-Shenmen, Lung, Allergy, and Endocrine.
Technique: Retain the needles for 30 minutes. Treat once or twice a day for two weeks, alternating the prescriptions.

SCALP ACUPUNCTURE

Points: Upper 2/5 of bilateral Sensory Areas and bilateral Foot Motor Areas.

Technique: Insert the needles horizontally and rotate with small amplitude for about one minute. Retain the needles for 30 minutes. Treat once a day. A course consists of seven treatment sessions.

Explanation

Needling these areas not only supports Vital Qi (Zheng Qi) and consolidates the Root, it also expels pathogenic factors to alleviate itching.

ELECTRO-ACUPUNCTURE

Prescription 1: SP-6 Sanyinjiao, ST-36 Zusanli, SP-10 Xuehai, and LI-11 Quchi.

Prescription 2: CV-4 Guanyuan, CV-2 Qugu, SP-6 Sanyinjiao, BL-32 Ciliao, LR-11 Yinlian, and Zhuogushang (slightly lateral to the point 2 cun above the midpoint of the line between the greater trochanter and the tip of the coccyx).

Technique: Alternate between prescriptions. Retain the needles for 30 minutes after obtaining Qi. Treat once every two days. A course consists of ten treatment sessions.

WRIST AND ANKLE THERAPY

Points

- For generalized pruritus, select Upper Region I (on the flexor side of the forearm, two finger-widths above the wrist crease, at the radial side of the ulna where thumb pressure creates the greatest concavity).
- For localized pruritus, select Lower Region I (three finger-widths above the highest point of the medial malleolus, at the medial border of the Achilles tendon).

Technique: Using a 3 cun filiform needle, make an oblique insertion proximally to a depth of 1.5-2.0 cm. Retain the needle for 15-30 minutes. Treat once a day or every two days. A course consists of ten treatment sessions.

Clinical notes

- Pruritus is one of the most frequently encountered symptoms in skin diseases and may in itself be a symptom of a disease process. In treatment, it is important to clarify whether a Deficiency or an Excess pattern is involved.
- For Excess patterns, attention should be paid to dredging Wind to alleviate itching and freeing the network vessels to alleviate itching.

- For Deficiency patterns, it is important to regulate the functions of the Liver and Kidneys.
- Acupuncture is very effective in alleviating itching and quieting the Spirit.
- Examine the skin carefully for skin dryness (xerosis), dermographism or subtle signs of scabies before investigating possible systemic causes.
- The primary disease should be treated first if the pruritus is caused by internal disorders.
- Where an underlying disease process is suspected, Western medical tests are recommended (in particular tests relating to the liver, gallbladder, kidney, endocrine function, and blood sugar levels).

Advice for the patient

- Avoid scratching to prevent secondary infection.
- Avoid frequent washing with soap or with very hot water.
- Soft, non-irritating clothing should be used in contact with the skin.
- Avoid alcohol and spicy food, restrict intake of fish or seafood and try to increase consumption of vegetables and fruit. It is important to keep bowel movements regular.

Case history

Patient
Male, aged 54.

Clinical manifestations
Eight months previously, the patient had an allergic reaction after dyeing his hair. The swelling subsided after treatment but episodes of pruritus on the scalp and face recurred frequently, exacerbated after drinking alcohol. The itching made the patient irritable and he only found relief by scratching so hard that the skin was broken and bleeding occurred. The condition worsened in the summer with sweating. The pruritus had recently spread to become generalized, affecting sleep so much that the patient felt dizzy and weak; other symptoms included a bitter taste in the mouth and severe indigestion.

On examination, the skin was rough with linear excoriations, some of which had formed bloody crusts; some lichenification was evident. Follicular papules had appeared at a few sites. The tongue was red at the tip with a white and greasy coating; the pulse was slippery and slightly rapid.

Pattern identification
Accumulation and obstruction of Wind-Damp, depriving the skin and flesh of nourishment.

Treatment principle
Dispel Wind and eliminate Dampness, nourish the Blood and moisten the skin.

Prescription
QUAN CHONG FANG HE QING PI CHU SHI YIN JIA JIAN
Scorpion Formula Combined With Beverage for Clearing Heat from the Spleen and Eliminating Dampness, with modifications

Quan Xie ‡ (Buthus Martensi) 6g
Zao Jiao Ci (Spina Gleditsiae Sinensis) 6g
Bai Ji Li (Fructus Tribuli Terrestris) 30g
Bai Xian Pi (Cortex Dictamni Dasycarpi Radicis) 30g
Ku Shen (Radix Sophorae Flavescentis) 15g
Che Qian Zi (Semen Plantaginis) 15g
Che Qian Cao (Herba Plantaginis) 15g
Ze Xie (Rhizoma Alismatis Orientalis) 10g
Bai Zhu (Rhizoma Atractylodis Macrocephalae) 10g
Zhi Ke (Fructus Citri Aurantii) 10g
Sheng Di Huang (Radix Rehmanniae Glutinosae) 15g
Huai Hua (Flos Sophorae Japonicae) 30g
Dang Gui (Radix Angelicae Sinensis) 10g
Ye Jiao Teng (Caulis Polygoni Multiflori) 30g
Di Fu Zi (Fructus Kochiae Scopariae) 15g
Fang Feng (Radix Ledebouriellae Divaricatae) 10g

One bag a day was used to prepare a decoction, taken twice a day.

External treatment
A decoction was prepared with *Ma Chi Xian* (Herba Portulacae Oleraceae) 30g, allowed to cool and then used to wash the affected area once a day. This was followed by rubbing in a mixture of *Xiong Huang Jie Du San* (Realgar Powder for Relieving Toxicity) [i] 15g and *Bai Bu Ding* (Stemona Root Tincture) 60ml.

Second visit
After 14 bags of the decoction, the itching had improved significantly. The patient could sleep six hours at night, his appetite had improved and he felt much better. The prescription was amended by removing *Quan Xie* ‡ (Buthus Martensi), *Che Qian Cao* (Herba Plantaginis) and *Huai Hua* (Flos Sophorae Japonicae) and adding *Dan Shen* (Radix Salviae Miltiorrhizae) 15g, *Ji Xue Teng* (Caulis Spatholobi) 30g, *Chi Shao* (Radix Paeoniae Rubra) 15g, and *Chan Tui* (Periostracum Cicadae) 10g. External treatment remained the same.

Outcome
After another 14 bags of the decoction, the itching had stopped and all the symptoms had vanished. Examination of the skin surface indicated no trace of the excoriations or bloody crusts, although some lichenification remained. The patient was told to continue taking the internal prescription for another four weeks to consolidate the treatment and to use 5% *Hei Dou Liu You Ruan Gao* (Black Soybean and Vaseline® Ointment) twice a day for external application.

Discussion
Pruritus is an itchy skin condition without primary skin lesions but with such secondary lesions as excoriation, bloody crusts, pigmentation, and lichenification. It is relatively diffi-

cult to treat due to the variety of causes leading to the itching. Therefore, it is important to search for the real cause of the disease and identify patterns carefully.

This case is one of pruritus caused by accumulation and obstruction of Wind-Damp, depriving the skin and flesh of nourishment. Exuberant Wind scurries from place to place with no fixed location to cause generalized itching, whereas exuberant Dampness makes the skin thicker and prevents the sensation of itching from being dissipated. The most appropriate treatment principle is to dispel Wind and eliminate Dampness, nourish the Blood and moisten the skin.

In the prescription, *Quan Xie* ‡ (Buthus Martensi), *Zao Jiao Ci* (Spina Gleditsiae Sinensis), *Fang Feng* (Radix Ledebouriellae Divaricatae) and *Bai Ji Li* (Fructus Tribuli Terrestris) expel Wind and alleviate itching; *Ku Shen* (Radix Sophorae Flavescentis), *Bai Xian Pi* (Cortex Dictamni Dasycarpi Radicis), *Che Qian Zi* (Semen Plantaginis), *Che Qian Cao* (Herba Plantaginis), *Ze Xie* (Rhizoma Alismatis Orientalis) and *Di Fu Zi* (Fructus Kochiae Scopariae) dispel Dampness and alleviate itching; *Bai Zhu* (Rhizoma Atractylodis Macrocephalae) and *Zhi Ke* (Fructus Citri Aurantii) clear Heat from the Spleen and eliminate Dampness; *Sheng Di Huang* (Radix Rehmanniae Glutinosae) and *Huai Hua* (Flos Sophorae Japonicae) clear Heat and cool the Blood; and Dang Gui (Radix Angelicae Sinensis) and *Ye Jiao Teng* (Caulis Polygoni Multiflori) nourish the Blood and moisten the skin. In the amended prescription, *Dan Shen* (Radix Salviae Miltiorrhizae), *Ji Xue Teng* (Caulis Spatholobi), *Chi Shao* (Radix Paeoniae Rubra), and *Chan Tui* ‡ (Periostracum Cicadae) were added to invigorate the Blood and dissipate Wind and strengthen the general effect.

This type of pruritus is usually caused by improper diet and pathogenic Wind after drinking alcohol. Therefore, anything that stirs Wind such as smoking, alcohol, strong tea, or any spicy food or seafood is likely to be an important internal factor in this type of skin problem.

External treatment for pruritus should also be applied flexibly depending on the type of illness and pattern identification:

- In cases with internal accumulation of Damp-Heat with infection due to scratching accompanied by red and swollen skin lesions, *Ma Chi Xian Shui Xi Ji* (Purslane Wash Preparation) can be used to wash the affected area.
- For severe itching, *She Chuang Zi* (Fructus Cnidii Monnieri), *Ku Shen* (Radix Sophorae Flavescentis) and *Di Fu Zi* (Fructus Kochiae Scopariae) can be used to prepare a decoction for use as an external wash.
- For genital or anal itching, *She Chuang Zi Xi Ji* (Cnidium Fruit Wash Preparation) can be used for a sitz bath.
- For vulval pruritus, *Qu Shi San* (Powder for Dispelling Dampness) or *Xin San Miao San* (New Mysterious Three Powder) mixed with *Gan Cao You* (Licorice Oil) or vegetable oil can be applied.
- For chronic skin lesions, 5% *Hei Dou Liu You Ruan Gao* (Black Soybean and Vaseline® Ointment) or *Zhi Yang Gao* (Paste for Alleviating Itching) can be used.

[i] In those countries where the use of certain ingredients contained in this powder is not permitted, *Qing Dai San* (Indigo Powder) can be applied instead.

It is also very important that patients co-operate in the treatment. Elderly patients with pruritus should not take frequent baths, and when they do have a bath, the water should be warm rather than hot and the soap neutral (neither acid nor alkali). A light diet is recommended and spicy food avoided. Clothing (especially underwear) should be soft and loose and made of cotton rather than artificial fabrics. Wool or feather material should not touch the skin directly. [1]

Literature excerpt

In *Wai Ke Da Cheng* [A Compendium of External Diseases], it says: "Sores, pain and itching are all caused by Fire." It also says: "Exuberant Wind may cause itching, because Wind is the manifestation of Fire. For itching due to Wind-Heat settling in the skin, it is important to dredge Wind. *Qu Feng Huan Ji Wan* (Pill for Dispelling Wind and Regenerating the Flesh) and *Ku Shen Wan* (Flavescent Sophora Root Pill) are recommended. For itching due to internal Wind-Heat and Blood Deficiency, it is important to cool the Blood and moisten Dryness."

Modern clinical experience

INTERNAL TREATMENT

1. **Gao** reported on the treatment of stubborn pruritus.[2]

Prescription
XIAO FENG SAN JIA WEI
Powder for Dispersing Wind, with additions

Dang Gui (Radix Angelicae Sinensis) 10g
Zhi Mu (Rhizoma Anemarrhenae Asphodeloidis) 10g
Ku Shen (Radix Sophorae Flavescentis) 10g
Hei Zhi Ma (Semen Sesami Indici) 10g
Jing Jie (Herba Schizonepetae Tenuifoliae) 10g
Niu Bang Zi (Fructus Arctii Lappae) 10g
Sheng Di Huang (Radix Rehmanniae Glutinosae) 25g
Fang Feng (Radix Ledebouriellae Divaricatae) 15g
Cang Zhu (Rhizoma Atractylodis) 15g
Shi Gao‡ (Gypsum Fibrosum) 15g
Chan Tui‡ (Periostracum Cicadae) 6g
Tong Cao (Medulla Tetrapanacis Papyriferi) 6g
Gan Cao (Radix Glycyrrhizae) 5g

One bag a day was used to prepare a decoction, taken twice a day for two weeks.

2. **Wu** recommended *Si Wu Tang Jia Wei* (Four Agents Decoction, with additions).[3]

Prescription ingredients

Dang Gui (Radix Angelicae Sinensis) 15g
Sheng Di Huang (Radix Rehmanniae Glutinosae) 15g
He Shou Wu (Radix Polygoni Multiflori) 15g

Huang Qi (Radix Astragali seu Hedysari) 15g
Bai Shao (Radix Paeoniae Lactiflorae) 10g
Chuan Xiong (Rhizoma Ligustici Chuanxiong) 10g

Modifications
1. For exuberant Wind, *Jing Jie* (Herba Schizonepetae Tenuifoliae) 10g, *Fang Feng* (Radix Ledebouriellae Divaricatae) 10g and *Bai Ji Li* (Fructus Tribuli Terrestris) 15g were added.
2. For exuberant Damp, *Huang Bai* (Cortex Phellodendri) 15g, *Cang Zhu* (Rhizoma Atractylodis) 15g and *Ku Shen* (Radix Sophorae Flavescentis) 15g were added.
3. For hyperactivity of Liver Yang, *Sang Ye* (Folium Mori Albae) 15g, *Ju Hua* (Flos Chrysanthemi Morifolii) 15g and *Gou Qi Zi* (Fructus Lycii) 15g were added.
4. For insomnia, *Wu Wei Zi* (Fructus Schisandrae Chinensis) 10g, *Mu Li*‡ (Concha Ostreae) 30g, and *Zhen Zhu Mu*‡ (Concha Margaritifera) 30g were added.

One bag a day was used to prepare a decoction, taken twice a day for 20 days.

3. **Li** reported on the use of *Di Fu Yin* (Broom Cypress Fruit Beverage).[4]

Prescription ingredients

Di Fu Zi (Fructus Kochiae Scopariae) 15g
Dan Shen (Radix Salviae Miltiorrhizae) 15g
Sheng Di Huang (Radix Rehmanniae Glutinosae) 15g
Bai Xian Pi (Cortex Dictamni Dasycarpi Radicis) 15g
She Chuang Zi (Fructus Cnidii Monnieri) 9g
Ku Shen (Radix Sophorae Flavescentis) 9g
Xuan Shen (Radix Scrophulariae Ningpoensis) 6g
Di Long‡ (Lumbricus) 6g
Chan Tui‡ (Periostracum Cicadae) 3g
Can Sha‡ (Excrementum Bombycis Mori) 3g

One bag a day was used to prepare a decoction, taken twice a day. Six days made up a course of treatment. Results were seen after two to three courses.

4. **Wu** treated pruritus with *Zhi Yang Tang* (Decoction for Alleviating Itching).[5]

Prescription ingredients

Fang Feng (Radix Ledebouriellae Divaricatae) 10g
Chan Tui‡ (Periostracum Cicadae) 10g
Wei Ling Xian (Radix Clematidis) 10g
Dang Gui (Radix Angelicae Sinensis) 10g
Cang Zhu (Rhizoma Atractylodis) 10g
Sheng Di Huang (Radix Rehmanniae Glutinosae) 15g
Huang Bai (Cortex Phellodendri) 15g
Bai Xian Pi (Cortex Dictamni Dasycarpi Radicis) 15g
Ku Shen (Radix Sophorae Flavescentis) 15g

Di Fu Zi (Fructus Kochiae Scopariae) 15g
Gan Cao (Radix Glycyrrhizae) 6g

One bag a day was used to prepare a decoction, taken twice a day. Results were seen after two to three weeks.

EXTERNAL TREATMENT

1. **Liu** treated pruritus with an external wash. [6]

Prescription ingredients

She Chuang Zi (Fructus Cnidii Monnieri) 30g
Ku Shen (Radix Sophorae Flavescentis) 30g
Di Fu Zi (Fructus Kochiae Scopariae) 20g
Hua Jiao (Pericarpium Zanthoxyli) 15g
Cang Er Zi (Fructus Xanthii Sibirici) 15g
Bai Xian Pi (Cortex Dictamni Dasycarpi Radicis) 15g
Huang Bai (Cortex Phellodendri) 15g
Bai Ji Li (Fructus Tribuli Terrestris) 12g
Shi Chang Pu (Rhizoma Acori Graminei) 12g
Jing Jie (Herba Schizonepetae Tenuifoliae) 12g
Fang Feng (Radix Ledebouriellae Divaricatae) 12g
Gan Cao (Radix Glycyrrhizae) 6g

The ingredients were decocted in 3 liters of water and used to wash the affected area for 15-30 minutes twice a day. Results were seen within two weeks.

2. **Duan** also used an external wash to treat pruritus. [7]

Prescription ingredients

Fang Feng (Radix Ledebouriellae Divaricatae) 20g
Huang Qi (Radix Astragali seu Hedysari) 20g
Dang Gui (Radix Angelicae Sinensis) 15g

Huang Bai (Cortex Phellodendri) 10g
Hong Hua (Flos Carthami Tinctorii) 10g
Chuan Xiong (Rhizoma Ligustici Chuanxiong) 10g
Liu Huang‡ (Sulphur) 10g
Ku Shen (Radix Sophorae Flavescentis) 10g

The ingredients were decocted in 3 liters of water and used to wash the affected area for 15 minutes once or twice a day. Improvements were seen within three to six days.

ACUPUNCTURE

Zhang designed the following acupuncture treatment. [8]
Points: GB-20 Fengchi, BL-15 Xinshu, BL-17 Geshu, and PC-6 Neiguan.
Technique

- At GB-20 Fengchi, a 2 cun filiform needle was inserted obliquely toward the tip of the nose to a depth of 1.0-1.5 cun, with the needle being manipulated to allow the sensation to radiate to the forehead.
- At BL-15 Xinshu and BL-17 Geshu, 1.5 cun filiform needles were inserted at an angle of 30° toward the spinal column to a depth of 0.5-0.8 cun.
- At PC-6 Neiguan, a 1.5 cun filiform needle was inserted toward the elbow to a depth of 1.0-1.2 cun, with the needle being manipulated to allow a numbing and distending sensation to radiate to the elbow.
- The needles were retained for 30 minutes. Treatment was given once a day, with ten treatment sessions making up a course. There was an interval of three days between courses.

Results were seen after two courses.

Vulval and scrotal pruritus
女阴及阴囊瘙痒

Itching of the skin in the genital region may be associated with friction, sweating or irritation and often accompanies genital skin diseases; sometimes, no obvious cause is found. Persistence of itching and scratching often leads to lichenification.

In TCM, vulval pruritus is known as *yin yang* (pudendal itch), scrotal pruritus as *yin nang sao yang* (scrotal itch).

Clinical manifestations

- In vulval pruritus, pronounced excoriations in the greater lips of the vulva (labia majora) and mons

pubis, or a dry, thickened vulva are usually found on examination.
- Vulval pruritus is often associated with irregular menstruation or increased intensity of itching prior to menstruation. Breast distension, abdominal pain and menstrual clots may accompany menstruation.
- In scrotal pruritus, itching of the scrotum may spread to involve the penis in severe cases. Excoriation, bloody scabs or lichenification may be seen locally.
- In both conditions, itching may occur during the day, but more often appears or worsens at night. The itch-scratch cycle is commonly self-perpetuating.

Differential diagnosis

The genital region is a common site for skin diseases with itching as one of their symptoms. Candidal infection, intertrigo, erythrasma, psoriasis, contact dermatitis, lichen simplex chronicus (neurodermatitis), and pubic lice infection should be excluded on the basis of their primary lesions.

Etiology and pathology

- The Liver and Kidney channels pass through the genital region. When turbid Dampness forms due to Spleen Deficiency and accumulates to transform into Heat, Damp-Heat can flow along the Liver channel to the genitals, spreading moisture and itching. In addition, Kidney Yang Deficiency will impair transportation of Spleen Yang, leading to Dampness pouring down to the genital region; again, accumulation of Dampness will result in Heat.

- Depletion and Deficiency in the Kidney channel may allow external Wind-Heat to invade, leading to the dryness, itching and possibly fissuring in the genital region.

- Excessive sexual activity damages the Liver and Kidneys, resulting in internal generation of Deficiency-Heat due to Yin Deficiency of the Liver and Kidneys. Since the local area is then deprived of moisture and nourishment, pruritus occurs.

Pattern identification and treatment

INTERNAL TREATMENT

DAMP-HEAT
This pattern is seen in vulval and scrotal pruritus. Itching fluctuates in intensity. There is erosion and slight exudation following excoriation. The tongue body is red with a thin yellow coating; the pulse is wiry and rapid.

Treatment principle
Clear the Liver and transform Dampness.

Prescription
ZHI BAI DI HUANG WAN JIA JIAN
Anemarrhena, Phellodendron and Rehmannia Pill, with modifications

Yan Shui Chao Huang Bai (Cortex Phellodendri, stir-fried with brine) 6g
Chao Zhi Mu (Rhizoma Anemarrhenae Asphodeloidis, stir-fried) 6g
Chao Mu Dan Pi (Cortex Moutan Radicis, stir-fried) 6g
Sheng Di Huang (Radix Rehmanniae Glutinosae) 12g

Shan Zhu Yu (Fructus Corni Officinalis) 12g
Che Qian Zi (Semen Plantaginis) 12g, wrapped
Ze Xie (Rhizoma Alismatis Orientalis) 12g
Fu Ling (Sclerotium Poriae Cocos) 12g
Gou Teng (Ramulus Uncariae cum Uncis) 15g
Xiao Hui Xiang (Fructus Foeniculi Vulgaris) 3g
Chai Hu (Radix Bupleuri) 3g

Explanation
- *Yan Shui Chao Huang Bai* (Cortex Phellodendri, stir-fried with brine), *Chao Zhi Mu* (Rhizoma Anemarrhenae Asphodeloidis, stir-fried), *Chao Mu Dan Pi* (Cortex Moutan Radicis, stir-fried), *Sheng Di Huang* (Radix Rehmanniae Glutinosae), and *Chai Hu* (Radix Bupleuri) clear Heat retained in the Liver and Kidney channels.
- *Che Qian Zi* (Semen Plantaginis), *Ze Xie* (Rhizoma Alismatis Orientalis) and *Fu Ling* (Sclerotium Poriae Cocos) percolate Dampness and transform turbidity.
- *Shan Zhu Yu* (Fructus Corni Officinalis), *Gou Teng* (Ramulus Uncariae cum Uncis) and *Xiao Hui Xiang* (Fructus Foeniculi Vulgaris) transform Dampness and regulate Qi, extinguish Wind and alleviate itching.

KIDNEY DEFICIENCY
This pattern is seen in vulval pruritus. When the condition persists for a long period, the local area becomes dry with fissuring. The tongue body is red with a scant coating; the pulse is thready and weak.

Treatment principle
Warm the Kidneys and invigorate the Blood.

Prescription
CHEN XIANG WAN JIA JIAN
Eaglewood Pill, with modifications

Sheng Di Huang (Radix Rehmanniae Glutinosae) 12g
Shu Di Huang (Radix Rehmanniae Glutinosae Conquita) 12g
Shan Yao (Radix Dioscoreae Oppositae) 12g
Hu Lu Ba (Semen Trigonellae Foeni-graeci) 12g
Li Zhi He (Semen Litchi Chinensis) 12g
Chen Xiang (Lignum Aquilariae Resinatum) 3g
Chai Hu (Radix Bupleuri) 3g
Chao Du Zhong (Cortex Eucommiae Ulmoidis, stir-fried) 10g
She Chuang Zi (Fructus Cnidii Monnieri) 10g

Explanation
- *Sheng Di Huang* (Radix Rehmanniae Glutinosae), *Shu Di Huang* (Radix Rehmanniae Glutinosae Conquita), *Shan Yao* (Radix Dioscoreae Oppositae), *Hu Lu Ba* (Semen Trigonellae Foeni-graeci), and *Chao Du Zhong* (Cortex Eucommiae Ulmoidis, stir-fried) warm the Kidneys to secure the Root.

- *Chai Hu* (Radix Bupleuri) and *She Chuang Zi* (Fructus Cnidii Monnieri) dispel Dampness and alleviate itching.
- *Li Zhi He* (Semen Litchi Chinensis) and *Chen Xiang* (Lignum Aquilariae Resinatum) warm and moisten the Liver and Kidneys.

LIVER AND KIDNEY DEFICIENCY

This pattern is seen in scrotal pruritus. Itching varies from mild to severe. Accompanying symptoms and signs include dizziness, lack of strength in the limbs, and insomnia. The tongue body is pale red with a scant coating; the pulse is deep and thready.

Treatment principle

Enrich the Liver and supplement the Kidneys.

Prescription

MAI WEI DI HUANG TANG JIA JIAN

Ophiopogon and Rehmannia Decoction, with modifications

Mai Men Dong (Radix Ophiopogonis Japonici) 12g
Gan Di Huang (Radix Rehmanniae Glutinosae Exsiccata) 12g
Fu Shen (Sclerotium Poriae Cocos cum Ligno Hospite) 12g
Bai Shao (Radix Paeoniae Lactiflorae) 12g
Suan Zao Ren (Semen Ziziphi Spinosae) 12g
Chao Du Zhong (Cortex Eucommiae Ulmoidis, stir-fried) 10g
Gou Teng (Ramulus Uncariae cum Uncis) 10g
Xu Chang Qing (Radix Cynanchi Paniculati) 10g
Wu Wei Zi (Fructus Schisandrae) 6g

Explanation

- *Mai Men Dong* (Radix Ophiopogonis Japonici), *Wu Wei Zi* (Fructus Schisandrae) and *Suan Zao Ren* (Semen Ziziphi Spinosae) nourish Liver and Kidney Yin with sweetness and sourness.
- *Xu Chang Qing* (Radix Cynanchi Paniculati), *Bai Shao* (Radix Paeoniae Lactiflorae) and *Gan Di Huang* (Radix Rehmanniae Glutinosae Exsiccata) nourish and invigorate the Blood to alleviate itching.
- *Fu Shen* (Sclerotium Poriae Cocos cum Ligno Hospite), *Chao Du Zhong* (Cortex Eucommiae Ulmoidis, stir-fried) and *Gou Teng* (Ramulus Uncariae cum Uncis) nourish the Liver, boost the Kidneys and quiet the Spirit.

EXTERNAL TREATMENT

- If pruritus is accompanied by mild exudation, use *Lu Lu Tong Shui Xi Ji* (Sweetgum Fruit Wash Preparation) to wash the area once a day.
- If pruritus is accompanied by lichenification or slight fissuring, apply *Huang Lian Ruan Gao* (Coptis Ointment) or *Run Ji Gao* (Flesh-Moistening Paste) to the affected area once a day.

ACUPUNCTURE AND MOXIBUSTION

Vulval pruritus

Main point: CV-3 Zhongji.
Auxiliary points: ST-30 Qichong, SP-9 Yinlingquan, SP-6 Sanyinjiao, KI-6 Zhaohai, and LR-3 Taichong.

Scrotal pruritus

Main points: BL-40 Weizhong and BL-23 Shenshu.
Auxiliary points: GB-30 Huantiao and SP-10 Xuehai. Moxibustion at LR-1 Dadun should also be given for this condition.

Technique

Apply the reducing method for Excess patterns and the reinforcing method for Deficiency patterns. Retain the needles for 30 minutes after obtaining Qi. Treat once a day. A course consists of ten treatment sessions.

Explanation

- CV-3 Zhongji, ST-30 Qichong and LR-3 Taichong regulate Qi and alleviate itching.
- SP-9 Yinlingquan, SP-6 Sanyinjiao and KI-6 Zhaohai fortify the Spleen and eliminate Dampness to alleviate itching.
- BL-40 Weizhong and SP-10 Xuehai nourish and invigorate the Blood.
- BL-23 Shenshu, GB-30 Huantiao and LR-1 Dadun warm the Kidneys and dissipate Cold.

Case history

Patient

Female, aged 40.

Clinical manifestations

The patient had suffered from itching in the pudenda for the previous six months. Itching was intense before and after menstruation. Vaginal discharge was profuse, clear and thin. The patient had attended the gynecology department of a local hospital, where "no mycotic or trichomonal infection was found."

The skin on the labia majora and minora, the vaginal orifice and the medial aspect of the thighs was swollen with some lichenification. Persistent scratching and rubbing had caused some of the pubic hair to fall out. The tongue body was pale, enlarged and tender with tooth marks; the tongue coating was white and greasy with a yellowish center. The pulse was wiry and slippery.

Pattern identification

Exuberant Dampness due to Spleen Deficiency, with the skin and flesh being deprived of nourishment.

Treatment principle

Fortify the Spleen and eliminate Dampness, nourish the Blood and moisten the skin.

Prescription
BI XIE SHEN SHI TANG HE YANG XUE RUN FU TANG JIA JIAN
Yan Rhizome Decoction for Percolating Dampness Combined With Decoction for Nourishing the Blood and Moistening the Skin, with modifications

Bai Zhu (Rhizoma Atractylodis Macrocephalae) 10g
Yi Yi Ren (Semen Coicis Lachryma-jobi) 30g
Zhi Ke (Fructus Citri Aurantii) 10g
Bi Xie (Rhizoma Dioscoreae Hypoglaucae seu Septemlobae) 10g
Long Dan Cao (Radix Gentianae Scabrae) 10g
Sheng Di Huang (Radix Rehmanniae Glutinosae) 15g
Huang Bai (Cortex Phellodendri) 15g
*Fang Ji** (Radix Stephaniae Tetrandrae) 10g[ii]
Ku Shen (Radix Sophorae Flavescentis) 15g
Bai Xian Pi (Cortex Dictamni Dasycarpi Radicis) 30g
Che Qian Zi (Semen Plantaginis) 15g
Che Qian Cao (Herba Plantaginis) 15g
Ze Xie (Rhizoma Alismatis Orientalis) 10g
Dang Gui (Radix Angelicae Sinensis) 10g
Ye Jiao Teng (Caulis Polygoni Multiflori) 30g

One bag a day was used to prepare a decoction, taken twice a day.

Prescription for external application

She Chuang Zi (Fructus Cnidii Monnieri) 10g
Bai Xian Pi (Cortex Dictamni Dasycarpi Radicis) 15g
Di Fu Zi (Fructus Kochiae Scopariae) 15g
Ma Chi Xian (Herba Portulacae Oleraceae) 15g
Huang Bai (Cortex Phellodendri) 10g
Ku Shen (Radix Sophorae Flavescentis) 15g
Bai Bu (Radix Stemonae) 10g

A decoction prepared with these ingredients was used lukewarm for a sitz bath, once a day. Then 5% *Hei Dou Liu You Ruan Gao* (Black Soybean and Vaseline® Ointment) was applied to the affected area, followed by *Zhi Yang Fen* (Powder for Alleviating Itching).

Second visit
After 14 bags of the decoction, the pruritus was significantly alleviated, vaginal discharge had lessened and the swelling was gradually subsiding. The tongue body was pale with a white coating. The prescription was amended by removing *Che Qian Cao* (Herba Plantaginis) and *Long Dan Cao* (Radix Gentianae Scabrae) and adding *Dan Shen* (Radix Salviae Miltiorrhizae) 15g and *Ji Xue Teng* (Caulis Spatholobi) 15g.

Outcome
The treatment continued for a further 14 bags. The pruritus stopped, systemic symptoms were relieved, and local swelling and excoriations disappeared, although slight lichenification remained.

Discussion
Vulval pruritus is often associated with profuse vaginal discharge. In this case, there is genital itching and profuse leukorrhea. The tongue body is pale with a white coating, and the pulse is wiry and slippery. The pattern can therefore be identified as exuberant Dampness due to Spleen Deficiency, with the skin and flesh being deprived of nourishment. In the prescription, *Bai Zhu* (Rhizoma Atractylodis Macrocephalae), *Yi Yi Ren* (Semen Coicis Lachryma-jobi), *Zhi Ke* (Fructus Citri Aurantii), and *Bi Xie* (Rhizoma Dioscoreae Hypoglaucae seu Septemlobae) clear Heat from the Spleen and eliminate Dampness; *Long Dan Cao* (Radix Gentianae Scabrae), *Sheng Di Huang* (Radix Rehmanniae Glutinosae), *Huang Bai* (Cortex Phellodendri), and *Fang Ji** (Radix Stephaniae Tetrandrae) clear Heat and benefit the movement of Dampness; *Ku Shen* (Radix Sophorae Flavescentis) and *Bai Xian Pi* (Cortex Dictamni Dasycarpi Radicis) dredge Wind and alleviate itching; *Che Qian Cao* (Herba Plantaginis), *Che Qian Zi* (Semen Plantaginis) and *Ze Xie* (Rhizoma Alismatis Orientalis) eliminate Dampness and benefit the movement of water; and *Dang Gui* (Radix Angelicae Sinensis) and *Ye Jiao Teng* (Caulis Polygoni Multiflori) nourish the Blood and moisten the skin.[9]

Literature excerpt

In *Yi Xue Liu Yao* [Six Essentials of Medical Criteria], it says: "Vulval pruritus is caused by Damp-Heat in the Liver, which is treated with *Xie Gan Tang* (Decoction for Draining the Liver). If this condition occurs in a thin person, it is Yin Deficiency; the main formula will be *Kan Li Sha* (Fire and Water Hexagram Granules) for oral administration and a decoction of *She Chuang Zi* (Fructus Cnidii Monnieri) as an external wash."

Modern clinical experience

COMBINED INTERNAL AND EXTERNAL TREATMENT

1. **Ling** treated vulval pruritus with a basic prescription and modified it according to pattern differentiation.[10]

Treatment principle
Supplement Qi and invigorate the Blood, dry Dampness, clear Heat and relieve Toxicity.

Basic prescription for internal treatment
DANG GUI NIAN TONG TANG JIA WEI
Chinese Angelica Root Decoction for Assuaging Pain, with additions

Qiang Huo (Rhizoma et Radix Notopterygii) 6g
Fang Feng (Radix Ledebouriellae Divaricatae) 10g
Sheng Ma (Rhizoma Cimicifugae) 6g
Ge Gen (Radix Puerariae) 10g
Dang Shen (Radix Codonopsitis Pilosulae) 10g

[ii] In those countries where the use of *Fang Ji** (Radix Stephaniae Tetrandrae) is illegal, *Tong Cao* (Medulla Tetrapanacis Papyriferi) 10g can be substituted in this prescription.

Ku Shen (Radix Sophorae Flavescentis) 6g
Cang Zhu (Rhizoma Atractylodis) 10g
Bai Zhu (Rhizoma Atractylodis Macrocephalae) 10g
Zhu Ling (Sclerotium Polypori Umbellati) 12g
Ze Xie (Rhizoma Alismatis Orientalis) 12g
Huang Qin (Radix Scutellariae Baicalensis) 10g
Zhi Mu (Rhizoma Anemarrhenae Asphodeloidis) 10g
Dang Gui (Radix Angelicae Sinensis) 10g
Yin Chen Hao (Herba Artemisiae Scopariae) 12g
Gan Cao (Radix Glycyrrhizae) 3g
Huang Bai (Cortex Phellodendri) 10g
Chuan Xin Lian (Herba Andrographitis Paniculatae) 10g
Shui Qin Cai (Herba et Radix Oenanthes Benghalensis) 10g
Xian Ren Zhang (Radix et Caulis Opuntiae Dillenii) 20g

Modifications

1. For Damp Toxins pouring down, remove *Ge Gen* (Radix Puerariae), *Qiang Huo* (Rhizoma et Radix Notopterygii) and *Bai Zhu* (Rhizoma Atractylodis Macrocephalae) and add *Jin Qian Cao* (Herba Lysimachiae) 30g, *Tu Fu Ling* (Rhizoma Smilacis Glabrae) 30g and *Wu Gong*‡ (Scolopendra Subspinipes) 6g.

2. For Damp-Heat in the Liver and Gallbladder, remove *Ge Gen* (Radix Puerariae) and *Qiang Huo* (Rhizoma et Radix Notopterygii) and add *Yu Jin* (Radix Curcumae) 10g and *Yan Hu Suo* (Rhizoma Corydalis Yanhusuo) 10g.

3. For Blood Deficiency with Damp-Heat, remove *Ge Gen* (Radix Puerariae), *Qiang Huo* (Rhizoma et Radix Notopterygii) and *Fang Feng* (Radix Ledebouriellae Divaricatae) and add *Sheng Di Huang* (Radix Rehmanniae Glutinosae) 15g and *Bai Shao* (Radix Paeoniae Lactiflorae) 10g.

4. For Yin Deficiency with Damp-Heat, remove *Ge Gen* (Radix Puerariae), *Qiang Huo* (Rhizoma et Radix Notopterygii), *Fang Feng* (Radix Ledebouriellae Divaricatae), *Cang Zhu* (Rhizoma Atractylodis), and *Zhu Ling* (Sclerotium Polypori Umbellati) and add *Sheng Di Huang* (Radix Rehmanniae Glutinosae) 15g, *Mu Dan Pi* (Cortex Moutan Radicis) 15g, *Shan Yao* (Radix Dioscoreae Oppositae) 30g, *Shan Zhu Yu* (Fructus Corni Officinalis) 10g, *Gou Qi Zi* (Fructus Lycii) 15g, and *Bai Shao* (Radix Paeoniae Lactiflorae) 10g.

External application prescription
KU SHEN ER HUANG TANG
Two Yellows Decoction with Flavescent Sophora Root

Ku Shen (Radix Sophorae Flavescentis) 20g
Da Huang (Radix et Rhizoma Rhei) 20g
Bai Zhi (Radix Angelicae Dahuricae) 20g
Qing Hao (Herba Artemisiae Chinghao) 20g
Ai Ye (Folium Artemisiae Argyi) 20g
Huang Lian (Rhizoma Coptidis) 10g
Da Ye An Ye (Folium Eucalypti Globuli) 30g

The ingredients were decocted in one liter of water and used to steam-wash the area twice a day. This external treatment could be used with any of the above patterns. Results were assessed after two weeks.

EXTERNAL TREATMENT

1. **Sun** treated vulval pruritus with a steam-wash. [11]

Prescription
BAI SHE TANG
Dittany and Cnidium Decoction

She Chuang Zi (Fructus Cnidii Monnieri) 50g
Bai Xian Pi (Cortex Dictamni Dasycarpi Radicis) 50g
Huang Bai (Cortex Phellodendri) 50g
Jing Jie (Herba Schizonepetae Tenuifoliae) 15g
Fang Feng (Radix Ledebouriellae Divaricatae) 15g
Ku Shen (Radix Sophorae Flavescentis) 15g
Long Dan Cao (Radix Gentianae Scabrae) 15g
Bo He (Herba Menthae Haplocalycis) 10g, added
   5 minutes before the end of the decoction process

The ingredients were used to prepare a decoction for steam-washing the area twice a day for 15 minutes. A course of treatment lasted 10-15 days.

2. **Zhang** also prepared a steam-wash to treat vulval pruritus. [12]

Prescription
LANG DU TANG
Chinese Wolfsbane Decoction

Lang Du (Radix Euphorbiae Fischerianae) 12g
Ku Shen (Radix Sophorae Flavescentis) 12g
Bai Tou Weng (Radix Pulsatillae Chinensis) 12g
She Chuang Zi (Fructus Cnidii Monnieri) 12g
Di Fu Zi (Fructus Kochiae Scopariae) 12g
Cang Zhu (Rhizoma Atractylodis) 12g
Ku Fan‡ (Alumen Praeparatum) 12g
Lian Qiao (Fructus Forsythiae Suspensae) 20g

The ingredients were decocted in 1500 ml of water for 30 minutes and then used to steam and wash the area twice a day for ten days. This prescription has been used to treat vulval pruritus, trichomonas vaginitis and vulvar eczema.

3. **Wu** prepared a decoction for use as a sitz bath to treat vulval pruritus. [13]

Prescription
HU ZHANG KU MU TANG
Giant Knotweed, Flavescent Sophora Root and Rose-of-Sharon Root Bark Decoction

Hu Zhang (Radix et Rhizoma Polygoni Cuspidati) 100g
Ku Shen (Radix Sophorae Flavescentis) 50g
Mu Jin Pi (Cortex Hibisci Syriaci Radicis) 50g

The ingredients were decocted in 4500 ml of water, which was reduced to 4000 ml; 200 ml of the decoction was used for a sitz bath for 10-15 minutes twice a day. A course of treatment lasted 7-14 days.

ACUPUNCTURE

Liu treated vulval pruritus with ear and body points.[14]

- **Damp-Heat pouring down**
Ear points: Shenmen, Triple Burner and Liver.
Body point: LR-3 Taichong (bilateral).

- **Yin Deficiency and Blood-Dryness**
Ear points: Kidney, Ovary and Endocrine.

Body point: SP-10 Xuehai (bilateral).

Technique

- The ear points were needled with 0.5 cun filiform needles inserted to a depth of 0.2-0.3 cun and rotated continuously for 5-10 minutes before being removed. One ear was needled for each treatment alternately.
- The body points were needled with the even method, with the needles retained for 30 minutes.
- The treatment was given once every two days. A course consisted of ten treatment sessions. Results were seen within three courses of treatment.

Nodular prurigo
结节性痒疹

Prurigo is a loosely applied term used to describe a range of unconnected itchy skin diseases. It is generally applied when excoriations, thickening or nodules develop as a result of scratching. TCM refers to prurigo as *yang zhen* (itchy papules).

Nodular prurigo is a chronic idiopathic itchy condition usually seen in middle-aged women who develop discrete nodules 5-30 mm in diameter, most commonly on the extensor aspects of the limbs, as a result of scratching. The original cause of the scratching is usually obscure, although some patients have a background of atopic diseases. Emotional stress may play a part. Similar nodular lesions can be seen in patients with a long-standing systemic cause of pruritus. Some authorities consider nodular prurigo to be a nodular form of lichen simplex chronicus (neurodermatitis).

In TCM, this condition is also known as *ma jie* (horse scabies).

Clinical manifestations

- Onset is gradual, mainly involving the upper and lower limbs and occasionally the back.
- Initially the skin lesions are pale red papules. These develop into hemispherical nodules up to 30mm in diameter. They have a rough surface area and are reddish-brown or grayish-brown in color. The nodules are firm on palpation. Excoriated bloody crusting is present.
- Nodules may be few and widely spaced in some individuals; in others, they are numerous and may

appear in a linear arrangement. Lesions are produced by repeated scratching or rubbing.
- The disease is a chronic condition.

Differential diagnosis

Common warts (verruca vulgaris)

Common warts appear most frequently on sites subject to trauma (fingers, elbows, knees, face, and scalp), but may spread elsewhere. Round or polygonal in shape with a rough surface and obvious hyperkeratosis, they are firm, elevated and grayish-yellow, dirty yellow or dirty brown in color. Their surface breaks up skin lines. In most cases, verrucae are not itchy and there are no accompanying symptoms.

Papular urticaria

This condition represents a reaction to insect bites and incidence is highest among infants and young children. The lumbosacral region, buttocks and trunk may be involved as well as the limbs. Lesions, which recur in crops, manifest initially as red urticarial papules up to 5 mm in diameter with papulovesicles or vesicles at the center. Distribution is uneven in number and configuration.

Hypertrophic lichen planus

Eruptions in lichen planus usually involve the flexor surfaces of the wrists and forearms, and the lower legs around and above the ankles. Lesions manifest as intensely pruritic dull red flat-topped shiny papules with an irregular, sharply defined angulated border. The surface of the lesions exhibits a lacy white pattern of lines

(Wickham's striae). Lesions that persist, most frequently on the shins, may develop into confluent hypertrophic plaques. These lesions can become hyperkeratotic with a coarse surface covered by scales.

Etiology and pathology

- Nodular prurigo develops when an improper diet and Spleen-Stomach disharmony result in Damp-Heat brewing internally. When combined with invasion by external Wind, pathogenic Wind, Dampness and Heat fight each other, accumulating and binding in the skin and flesh. Where pathogenic Wind is virulent, itching can be intense.

- Where Toxic fluids from the bite or sting of a poisonous insect invade the interior, they can combine with external pathogenic Wind and internal accumulation of Dampness to block the channels and network vessels, causing stagnation of Qi and Blood and resulting in itching. Nodules gradually form due to scratching rather than from the bite or sting itself.

- Dampness is characterized by heaviness and turbidity. When it pours down along the channels, it tends to sink to the lower leg. Since Dampness is sticky and slimy by nature, the disease tends to linger for a long time.

Pattern identification and treatment

INTERNAL TREATMENT

DAMP, HEAT AND WIND TOXINS
The condition is of short duration, manifesting with rough reddish-brown nodules, intense itching and turbid bloody exudate with crusting. Accompanying symptoms and signs include irritability, thirst, irregular bowel movements, and yellow or reddish urine. The tongue body is red with a greasy coating; the pulse is slippery and rapid.

Treatment principle
Eliminate Dampness and clear Heat, dredge Wind and alleviate itching.

Prescription
QUAN CHONG FANG
Scorpion Formula

Jing Jie (Herba Schizonepetae Tenuifoliae) 10g
Fang Feng (Radix Ledebouriellae Divaricatae) 10g
Dang Gui (Radix Angelicae Sinensis) 10g
Chi Shao (Radix Paeoniae Rubra) 10g
Bai Shao (Radix Paeoniae Lactiflorae) 10g

Ze Xie (Rhizoma Alismatis Orientalis) 10g
Zao Jiao Ci (Spina Gleditsiae Sinensis) 6g
Quan Xie‡ (Buthus Martensi) 6g
Ku Shen (Radix Sophorae Flavescentis) 10-15g
Bai Xian Pi (Cortex Dictamni Dasycarpi Radicis) 10-15g
Bi Xie (Rhizoma Dioscoreae Hypoglaucae seu Septem-lobae) 10-15g
Che Qian Zi (Semen Plantaginis) 10-15g, wrapped

Explanation
- *Jing Jie* (Herba Schizonepetae Tenuifoliae), *Fang Feng* (Radix Ledebouriellae Divaricatae) and *Ku Shen* (Radix Sophorae Flavescentis) dissipate Wind and alleviate itching.
- *Dang Gui* (Radix Angelicae Sinensis), *Chi Shao* (Radix Paeoniae Rubra), *Bai Shao* (Radix Paeoniae Lactiflorae), and *Zao Jiao Ci* (Spina Gleditsiae Sinensis) invigorate the Blood and dissipate nodules.
- *Ze Xie* (Rhizoma Alismatis Orientalis), *Bi Xie* (Rhizoma Dioscoreae Hypoglaucae seu Septemlobae) and *Che Qian Zi* (Semen Plantaginis) clear Heat and dry Dampness.
- *Quan Xie*‡ (Buthus Martensi) and *Bai Xian Pi* (Cortex Dictamni Dasycarpi Radicis) relieve Toxicity and alleviate itching.

BLOOD STASIS OBSTRUCTING THE SKIN AND FLESH
The condition is of long duration, manifesting with large and hard verruca-like nodules with a rough surface and grayish-brown color. Itching is intense. Accompanying symptoms and signs include a dark complexion, sleeplessness and listlessness. The tongue body is dark red with stasis marks and a scant coating; the pulse is rough.

Treatment principle
Invigorate the Blood, soften hardness, free the network vessels, and alleviate itching.

Prescription
DA HUANG ZHE CHONG WAN
Rhubarb and Wingless Cockroach Pill

Jiu Zhi Da Huang (Radix et Rhizoma Rhei, processed with wine) 10g
Tao Ren (Semen Persicae) 10g
Chi Shao (Radix Paeoniae Rubra) 10g
Qing Pi (Pericarpium Citri Reticulatae Viride) 10g
Sheng Di Huang (Radix Rehmanniae Glutinosae) 15g
Chao Huang Qin (Radix Scutellariae Baicalensis, stir-fried) 15g
Dan Shen (Radix Salviae Miltiorrhizae) 15g
Xi Xian Cao (Herba Siegesbeckiae) 12g
Chao Zhi Ke (Fructus Citri Aurantii, stir-fried) 12g
Chen Pi (Pericarpium Citri Reticulatae) 12g
Chuan Xiong (Rhizoma Ligustici Chuanxiong) 6g

Explanation

- *Jiu Zhi Da Huang* (Radix et Rhizoma Rhei, processed with wine), *Tao Ren* (Semen Persicae), *Chi Shao* (Radix Paeoniae Rubra), *Dan Shen* (Radix Salviae Miltiorrhizae), and *Chuan Xiong* (Rhizoma Ligustici Chuanxiong) transform Blood stasis and dissipate nodules.
- *Qing Pi* (Pericarpium Citri Reticulatae Viride), *Chen Pi* (Pericarpium Citri Reticulatae), *Xi Xian Cao* (Herba Siegesbeckiae) and *Chao Zhi Ke* (Fructus Citri Aurantii, stir-fried) dissipate Wind and alleviate itching.
- *Sheng Di Huang* (Radix Rehmanniae Glutinosae) and *Chao Huang Qin* (Radix Scutellariae Baicalensis, stir-fried) cool and nourish the Blood.

PATENT HERBAL MEDICINES

- For Damp, Heat and Wind Toxin patterns, take *Wu She Zhi Yang Wan* (Black-Tail Snake Pill for Alleviating Itching) 3g twice a day with warm boiled water for one month.
- For patterns of Blood stasis obstructing the skin and flesh, take *San Jie Ling* (Efficacious Remedy for Dissipating Nodules) 3g twice a day or *Huo Xue Xiao Yan Wan* (Pill for Invigorating the Blood and Dispersing Inflammation) 3g twice a day with warm boiled water for one month. Alternatively, *Nei Xiao Lian Qiao Wan* (Forsythia Internal Dispersion Pill) 6g twice a day may be taken.

EXTERNAL TREATMENT

- If the nodules are small without deep infiltration, dip a broken leaf of fresh *Lu Hui* (Herba Aloes) in *Qing Dai San* (Indigo Powder) and spread the powder over the affected areas. Alternatively, apply fresh cucumber or water chestnut dipped in *Xin San Miao San* (New Mysterious Three Powder) to the lesions.
- If the nodules become more extensive, prepare a condensed decoction of *Lu Lu Tong Shui Xi Ji* (Sweetgum Fruit Wash Preparation) or *Cang Fu Shui Xi Ji* (Atractylodes and Broom Cypress Wash Preparation) and apply to the nodules as a wet compress or wash.
- If the nodules are large with deep infiltration, heat *Hei Se Ba Gao Gun* (Black Medicated Plaster Stick) and apply it to the nodules; alternatively, *Kang Fu Ying Gao* (Healthy Skin Plaster) can be used.

Clinical notes

- Internal treatment of all types of prurigo use the methods of dissipating nodules and transforming

stasis in addition to dissipating Wind and dispelling Dampness. These methods result in freeing the channels and network vessels and relieving stasis and stagnation, thus treating itching.
- External treatments, either washes or other external applications, are effective for local lesions.
- Nodular prurigo is a stubborn disease and usually responds slowly to the treatment; treatment for extensive periods (one to six months) will therefore be required.

Advice for the patient

- Avoid breaking the skin by scratching, as secondary infection may occur.
- Avoid fish, seafood, spicy food, and fried food.

Case history

Patient
Female, 20 years old.

Clinical manifestations
The patient had suffered from lumps on the upper limbs with intense itching for over two months. On examination, about 50 grayish-brown, firm, coniform or hemispherical nodules 0.5-2 cm in diameter were found on the extensor aspects of the upper limbs. Their surface was rough and covered with crusts. The tongue body was pale red with a thin white coating; the pulse was slippery and moderate.

Pattern identification
Accumulation of stubborn Dampness due to congealing of Damp Toxins, which resulted in obstruction of Qi and Blood.

Treatment principle
Soothe the Liver and regulate Qi, invigorate the Blood and transform Blood stasis, eliminate Dampness and alleviate itching.

Prescription
Internal treatment: *Xiao Yao Wan* (Free Wanderer Pill) 6g in the morning and *Da Huang Zhe Chong Wan* (Rhubarb and Wingless Cockroach Pill) 5g in the evening.
External treatment: *Hei Se Ba Gao Gun* (Black Medicated Plaster Stick) for application to the lesions. [iii]

Second visit
After one month's treatment, the patient's condition was only slightly improved, so the treatment principle was changed.

Treatment principle
Eliminate Dampness and relieve Toxicity, dredge Wind, invigorate the Blood and transform Blood stasis.

[iii] In those countries where the use of certain ingredients contained in this plaster is not permitted, *Hei Dou Liu You Ruan Gao* (Black Soybean and Vaseline® Ointment) can be applied instead.

Prescription ingredients

Ku Shen (Radix Sophorae Flavescentis) 15g

Chi Shao (Radix Paeoniae Rubra) 15g

Dang Gui (Radix Angelicae Sinensis) 15g

Dan Shen (Radix Salviae Miltiorrhizae) 15g

Bai Ji Li (Fructus Tribuli Terrestris) 30g

Bai Xian Pi (Cortex Dictamni Dasycarpi Radicis) 30g

Fang Feng (Radix Ledebouriellae Divaricatae) 10g

Quan Xie‡ (Buthus Martensi) 6g

One bag a day was used to prepare a decoction, taken twice a day. Meanwhile, the patient continued to take one 5g pill of *Da Huang Zhe Chong Wan* (Rhubarb and Wingless Cockroach Pill) a day and to use the same external application over the lesion.

Outcome

After one month, itching had been alleviated, small nodules had flattened and turned dull brown in color, and large nodules had shrunk and softened.

Treatment continued with *Qin Jiao Wan* (Large-Leaf Gentian Pill) 6g and *Da Huang Zhe Chong Wan* (Rhubarb and Wingless Cockroach Pill) 6g, both twice a day, for one more month.

After three months' treatment, all the nodules had flattened and the itching had disappeared; some patches of hyperpigmentation remained. [15]

Literature excerpt

Zhao Bing Nan Lin Chuang Jing Yan Ji [A Collection of Zhao Bingnan's Clinical Experiences] records that in the treatment of nodular prurigo in its initial stage, the principle is to dredge Wind, alleviate itching, eliminate Dampness, and relieve Toxicity with large doses of *Jing Jie* (Herba Schizonepetae Tenuifoliae), *Fang Feng* (Radix Ledebouriellae Divaricatae), *Ku Shen* (Radix Sophorae Flavescentis), *Bai Ji Li* (Fructus Tribuli Terrestris), *Bai Xian Pi* (Cortex Dictamni Dasycarpi Radicis), and *Quan Xie*‡ (Buthus Martensi).

At a later period when the nodules grow larger and firmer, in addition to the previous principles treat them with herbs for invigorating the Blood and softening hardness such as *Chi Shao* (Radix Paeoniae Rubra), *Dang Gui* (Radix Angelicae Sinensis), *Dan Shen* (Radix Salviae Miltiorrhizae), *Xi Xian Cao* (Herba Siegesbeckiae), and *Da Huang* (Radix et Rhizoma Rhei) in moderate or heavy doses. Alternatively, treat them with patent herbal medicines such as *Da Huang Zhe Chong Wan* (Rhubarb and Wingless Cockroach Pill) or *San Jie Ling* (Efficacious Remedy for Dissipating Nodules).

Where there are signs of Spleen-Stomach disharmony, resulting in failure of the transformation and transportation function, add *Zhi Ke* (Fructus Citri Aurantii), *Hou Po* (Cortex Magnoliae Officinalis) and *Chen Pi* (Pericarpium Citri Reticulatae) to the prescription.

Modern clinical experience

INTERNAL TREATMENT

Mu treated nodular prurigo with *Chai Hu Jia Long Gu Mu Li Tang Jia Jian* (Bupleurum Decoction Plus Dragon Bone and Oyster Shell, with modifications). [16]

Prescription ingredients

Chai Hu (Radix Bupleuri) 6g

Huang Qin (Radix Scutellariae Baicalensis) 6g

Fa Ban Xia (Rhizoma Pinelliae Ternatae Praeparata) 10g

Fu Ling (Sclerotium Poriae Cocos) 10g

Long Gu‡ (Os Draconis) 3g

Mu Li‡ (Concha Ostreae) 3g

Chan Tui‡ (Periostracum Cicadae) 6g

He Huan Pi (Cortex Albizziae Julibrissin) 10g

Da Zao (Fructus Ziziphi Jujubae) 15g

Gan Cao (Radix Glycyrrhizae) 6g

Sheng Jiang (Rhizoma Zingiberis Officinalis Recens) 10g

Most patients responded within a month of using this treatment, although some cases required two months.

COMBINATION OF EXTERNAL AND INTERNAL TREATMENT

Xu combined internal treatment with an external steam-wash. [17]

Internal treatment prescription

Fang Feng (Radix Ledebouriellae Divaricatae) 10g

Bai Ji Li (Fructus Tribuli Terrestris) 10g

Dan Shen (Radix Salviae Miltiorrhizae) 10g

Di Fu Zi (Fructus Kochiae Scopariae) 10g

Xu Chang Qing (Radix Cynanchi Paniculati) 10g

Dang Gui (Radix Angelicae Sinensis) 10g

Chi Shao (Radix Paeoniae Rubra) 10g

Kun Bu (Thallus Laminariae seu Eckloniae) 10g

Xia Ku Cao (Spica Prunellae Vulgaris) 10g

Ku Shen (Radix Sophorae Flavescentis) 10g

Zao Jiao Ci (Spina Gleditsiae Sinensis) 10g

Bai Xian Pi (Cortex Dictamni Dasycarpi Radicis) 15g

Ji Xue Teng (Caulis Spatholobi) 15g

One bag a day was used to prepare a decoction, taken twice a day.

External treatment prescription

Ye Ju Hua (Flos Chrysanthemi Indici) 15g

Jin Yin Hua (Flos Lonicerae) 15g

Da Ye An Ye (Folium Eucalypti Globuli) 15g

Huang Bai (Cortex Phellodendri) 10g

Wu Bei Zi‡ (Galla Rhois Chinensis) 10g

Cang Zhu (Rhizoma Atractylodis) 10g

Chi Shi Zhi‡ (Halloysitum Rubrum) 10g

Chi Shao (Radix Paeoniae Rubra) 10g
Chuan Xiong (Rhizoma Ligustici Chuanxiong) 10g
Sang Zhi (Ramulus Mori Albae) 10g
Ming Fan‡ (Alumen) 30g
Hong Hua (Flos Carthami Tinctorii) 5g

The ingredients were used to prepare a decoction for steaming then washing the affected area for 30 minutes a day. Most patients responded to the combined treatment after 10 to 60 days.

Prurigo of pregnancy
妊娠痒疹

Prurigo of pregnancy refers to a kind of pruritic eruption which begins during the mid-trimester of pregnancy. It may disappear spontaneously before term or rapidly after delivery.

Clinical manifestations

- The onset of the condition is generally three to four months after conception and it usually disappears at the latest within three months of delivery. The condition rarely occurs in subsequent pregnancies.
- Skin lesions usually occur on the upper part of the trunk and the proximal portion of the limbs.
- Lesions usually manifest as papules, papulovesicles and wheals up to 5mm in diameter, symmetrically distributed on both sides of the body, but occasionally randomly over the whole body.
- Intense itching may disturb sleep. Lichenification results from scratching.

Etiology and pathology

This condition is caused by Blood stasis obstructing the skin and interstices (*cou li*).

Treatment

EXTERNAL TREATMENT
A decoction of the following ingredients can be used to wash the affected area once or twice a day.

Jin Qian Cao (Herba Lysimachiae) 30g
Xiang Fu (Rhizoma Cyperi Rotundi) 15g
Wu Zhu Yu (Fructus Evodiae Rutaecarpae) 15g
Ku Shen (Radix Sophorae Flavescentis) 15g

Clinical notes

- Prurigo of pregnancy is primarily treated externally.
- If the skin condition is severe, the patient should be referred to a practitioner of Western medicine for administration of oral antihistamines to reduce symptoms.

References

1. An Jiafeng and Zhang Peng, *Zhang Zhi Li Pi Fu Bing Yi An Xuan Cui* [A Collection of Zhang Zhili's Skin Disease Cases] (Beijing: People's Medical Publishing House, 1994), 155.
2. Gao Ruihong, *Xiao Feng San Jia Wei Zhi Liao Wan Gu Xing Sao Yang 120 Li Lin Chuang Guan Cha* [Clinical Observation of the Treatment of 120 Cases of Stubborn Pruritus with Augmented *Xiao Feng San* (Powder for Dispersing Wind)], *Hei Long Jiang Zhong Yi Yao* [Heilongjiang Journal of Traditional Chinese Medicine and Materia Medica] 6 (1997): 33-34.
3. Wu Yanhua, *Si Wu Tang Jia Wei Zhi Liao Pi Fu Sao Yang Zheng 38 Li* [Treatment of 38 Cases of Pruritus with Augmented *Si Wu Tang* (Four Agents Decoction)] *Ling Nan Pi Fu Xing Bing Ke Za Zhi* [Lingnan Journal of Dermatology and Venereology] 4, 1 (1997): 28-29.
4. Li Xiufang, *Ding Lu Sheng Yun Yong Di Fu Yin Zhi Liao Sao Yang Bing De Jing Yan* [Ding Lusheng's Experiences in Treating Pruritus with *Di Fu Yin* (Broom Cypress Fruit Beverage)] *Xin Jiang Zhong Yi Yao* [Xinjiang Journal of Traditional Chinese Medicine and Materia Medica] 16, 1

(1998): 56-57.

5. Wu Meirong, *Zhi Yang Tang Zhi Liao Pi Fu Sao Yang Zheng* [Treatment of Pruritus with *Zhi Yang Tang* (Decoction for Alleviating Itching)], *He Bei Yi Xue Yuan Xue Bao* [Journal of Hebei Medical College] 15, 2 (1994): cover 3.

6. Liu Jinfeng, *Zhong Yao Wai Yong Zhi Liao Pi Fu Sao Yang Zheng 56 Li* [External Application of Chinese Materia Medica in the Treatment of 56 Cases of Pruritus] *Zhong Yi Wai Zhi Za Zhi* [Journal of Traditional Chinese Medicine External Treatments] 8, 3 (1999): 43.

7. Duan Xiang'ai, *Zhong Yao Xun Xi Zhi Liao Pi Fu Sao Yang Zheng 25 Li* [Treatment of 25 Cases of Pruritus by Steam-Washing with Chinese Materia Medica], *Zhong Yi Wai Zhi Za Zhi* [Journal of Traditional Chinese Medicine External Treatments] 5, 3 (1996): 34.

8. Zhang Liansheng, *Zhen Ci Zhi Liao Pi Fu Sao Yang Zheng 65 Li* [Acupuncture Treatment of 65 Pruritus Cases] *Zhong Guo Zhen Jiu* [Chinese Acupuncture and Moxibustion] 18, 2 (1998): 74.

9. An Jiafeng and Zhang Peng, *Zhang Zhi Li Pi Fu Bing Yi An Xuan Cui*, 156.

10. Ling Suibai, *Bian Zheng Zhi Liao Yin Yang 520 Li* [Treatment of 520 Cases of Vulval Pruritus Based on Pattern Identification], *Zhe Jiang Zhong Yi Za Zhi* [Zhejiang Journal of Traditional Chinese Medicine] 21, 7 (1986): 303.

11. Sun Fengzhi, *Bai She Tang Zhi Liao Nü Yin Sao Yang 400 Li* [Treatment of 400 Cases of Vulval Pruritus with *Bai She Tang* (Dittany and Cnidium Decoction)], *Zhong Yi Yao Xin Xi* [Traditional Chinese Medicine and Materia Medica News] 13, 1 (1996): 38.

12. Zhang Xuelu, *Lang Du Tang Xun Xi Zhi Liao Yin Yang 30 Li* [Treatment of 30 Cases of Vulval Pruritus by Steam-Washing with *Lang Du Tang* (Chinese Wolfsbane Decoction)], *Zhong Yi Wai Zhi Za Zhi* [Journal of Traditional Chinese Medicine External Treatments] 7, 2 (1998): 44.

13. Wu Riliang, *Hu Zhang Ku Mu Tang Zuo Yu Zhi Liao Yin Yang 100 Li* [Treatment of 100 Cases of Vulval Pruritus with a Sitz Bath Prepared with *Hu Zhang Ku Mu Tang* (Giant Knotweed, Flavescent Sophora Root and Rose-of-Sharon Root Bark Decoction)], *Zhe Jiang Zhong Yi Za Zhi* [Zhejiang Journal of Traditional Chinese Medicine] 26, 8 (1991): 352.

14. Liu Min, *Er Zhen Wei Zhu Bian Zheng Zhi Liao Yin Yang 80 Li* [Ear Acupuncture in the Treatment of 80 Cases of Vulval Pruritus Based on Pattern Identification], *Xin Zhong Yi* [New Journal of Traditional Chinese Medicine] 29, 11 (1997): 23.

15. Beijing Hospital of Traditional Chinese Medicine, *Zhao Bing Nan Lin Chuang Jing Yan Ji* [A Collection of Zhao Bingnan's Clinical Experiences] (Beijing: People's Medical Publishing House, 1975), 196.

16. Mu Xiangqin, *Chai Hu Jia Long Gu Mu Li Tang Zhi Liao Jie Jie Xing Yang Zhen 28 Li* [Treatment of 28 Cases of Nodular Prurigo with *Chai Hu Jia Long Gu Mu Li Tang* (Bupleurum Decoction plus Dragon Bone and Oyster Shell)], *Tian Jin Zhong Yi* [Tianjin Journal of Traditional Chinese Medicine] 16, 2 (1999): 39-40.

17. Xu Chuanlian, *Zhong Yao Nei Fu Xun Xi Zhi Liao Jie Jie Xing Yang Zhen 16 Li* [Treatment of 16 Cases of Nodular Prurigo with Chinese Materia Medica for Internal Administration and External Steam-Washing], *He Nan Zhong Yi* [Henan Journal of Traditional Chinese Medicine] 19, 2 (1999): 37-38.

Disorders of pigmentation

Normal skin color is related to two factors:
- Pigments in the skin and subcutaneous tissues – melanin (produced by melanocytes in the basal layer of the epidermis), carotene (found in the stratum corneum and subcutaneous fat) and oxyhemoglobin (present in the blood).
- Differences in skin anatomy, mainly involving the thickness of the skin, especially the stratum corneum and the stratum granulosum – where the epidermis is thin, the skin takes on the color of the blood in the dermopapillary vessels; where the stratum granulosum is thick, the skin lacks transparency and appears darker.

Apart from abnormal increase or decrease in pigmentation, morbid skin color changes can also be related to other factors such as drugs (amiodarone, clofazimine, mepacrine, and phenothiazines), metals (gold, silver, bismuth), foreign bodies (tattoos, application of cosmetic powders), deposition of metabolic pigments (jaundice), and pathological changes to the skin (thickening, thinning, edema, inflammation, infiltration, and necrosis).

Skin diseases related to abnormality of melanocytes and melanogenesis may be due to genetic and environmental factors. Some pigmentation disorders result from variations in the number of melanocytes or melanocyte dysfunction:
- Melanocyte hyperactivity can lead to melasma (chloasma) due to endocrine changes.
- An increase in the number of melanocytes can lead to melanocytic nevi, café au lait spots and nevus spilus.
- Melanocyte underactivity can occur in atopic eczema, pityriasis alba, psoriasis, and post-inflammatory hypopigmentation.
- A reduction in the number of melanocytes leads to depigmentation in such disorders as vitiligo and halo nevus.
- Abnormality of tyrosine metabolism results in little or no melanin being made in the skin; this occurs in albinism, an autosomal recessive disorder.

In TCM, the etiology of pigmentation disorders is related to external factors, especially invasion by Wind pathogenic factors, which may disturb Qi and Blood and cause pigment dysfunction, and to internal factors, essentially disharmony of the Zang-Fu organs, particularly the Liver, Spleen and Kidneys.

Melasma (chloasma)
黄褐斑

Melasma is yellow or brown pigmentary discoloration of the skin, manifesting as macules on the face of genetically predisposed women. It is related to numerous factors, such as pregnancy, oral contraceptives and sex hormone dysfunction. Exposure to sunlight and nervous disorders may also be responsible.

In TCM, melasma is known as *mian chen* (dusty complexion).

Clinical manifestations

- Melasma mainly affects pregnant women in the second and third trimesters and women taking oral contraceptives.
- Pigmentation is symmetrical and mainly involves the forehead, cheeks, perioral and perinasal areas, and chin.

- Lesions manifest as light to dark brown hyperpigmented macules or patches of varying size and shape. They may become darker and larger during pregnancy and aggravation of hepatic diseases, but turn lighter or disappear postpartum, after stopping contraceptives or in the recovery phase of hepatic diseases.
- Pigmentation evolves slowly and is more evident after exposure to sunlight.

Etiology and pathology

- The face depends on nourishment by the Zang organs to maintain its color and bloom. Any disturbance of the functions of the Zang organs can result in the facial skin being deprived of nourishment and patches appearing.
- Emotional disturbances can injure the Zang-Fu organs and impair the functional activities of Qi; for example, sudden anger damages the Liver, excessive thought and preoccupation damages the Spleen, and fear and shock damage the Kidneys.
- Emotional depression affects the function of the Liver in governing the normal movement of Qi. Therefore, Qi stagnates and transforms into Fire, which in turn prevents Qi and Blood from ascending to nourish the face; brown macules will eventually appear.
- Dietary irregularities, predilection for one of the five flavors, or excessive fatigue impair the Spleen and Stomach in their transportation and transformation function and lead to the formation of Damp-Heat in the Middle Burner. In addition, the Spleen cannot generate enough Qi and Blood to moisten the face. If Dampness and Heat bind and steam upward to the head and face, melasma will gradually spread from the area around the eyes to the area around the mouth and nose, and possibly to the forehead, deepening in color.
- Excessive sexual activity damages the Essence and Heart and Kidney Yin in the long term, depleting Water, which therefore fails to control Fire. Deficiency-Fire flames upward preventing the face from being moistened or nourished and resulting in brown macules.

Pattern identification and treatment

INTERNAL TREATMENT

LIVER DEPRESSION AND QI STAGNATION

This pattern mainly affects women with infertility or irregular menstruation. Since the Liver opens into the eyes, melasma therefore frequently occurs in the area around the eyes. Lesions manifest as clearly defined pale brown to dark brown macules or patches of varying size distributed symmetrically in a butterfly shape on both cheeks and around the eyes. Accompanying symptoms and signs include distension and fullness in the chest and hypochondrium, irritability, restlessness and irascibility, and poor appetite. Patients also suffer from deeper pigmentation and pain or distension in the breasts prior to periods. The tongue body is red with a thin white coating; the pulse is wiry and slippery.

Treatment principle
Dredge the Liver and regulate Qi, invigorate the Blood and reduce macules.

Prescription
XIAO YAO SAN JIA JIAN
Free Wanderer Powder, with modifications

Chai Hu (Radix Bupleuri) 10g
Qing Pi (Pericarpium Citri Reticulatae Viride) 10g
Chen Pi (Pericarpium Citri Reticulatae) 10g
Chuan Lian Zi (Fructus Meliae Toosendan) 10g
Dang Gui (Radix Angelicae Sinensis) 10g
Fu Ling (Sclerotium Poriae Cocos) 12g
Chao Bai Shao (Radix Paeoniae Lactiflorae, stir-fried) 12g
Bai Zhu (Rhizoma Atractylodis Macrocephalae) 12g
Hong Hua (Flos Carthami Tinctorii) 6g
Ling Xiao Hua (Flos Campsitis) 6g
Sheng Di Huang (Radix Rehmanniae Glutinosae) 15g

Explanation

- *Chai Hu* (Radix Bupleuri), *Qing Pi* (Pericarpium Citri Reticulatae Viride), *Chen Pi* (Pericarpium Citri Reticulatae), and *Chuan Lian Zi* (Fructus Meliae Toosendan) soothe the Liver and regulate Qi.
- *Dang Gui* (Radix Angelicae Sinensis), *Chao Bai Shao* (Radix Paeoniae Lactiflorae, stir-fried), *Hong Hua* (Flos Carthami Tinctorii), *Ling Xiao Hua* (Flos Campsitis), and *Sheng Di Huang* (Radix Rehmanniae Glutinosae) nourish the Blood and emolliate the Liver, invigorate the Blood and reduce macules.
- *Fu Ling* (Sclerotium Poriae Cocos) and *Bai Zhu* (Rhizoma Atractylodis Macrocephalae) support the Spleen and transform Dampness.

LIVER-FIRE FLAMING UPWARD
If Liver-Fire flames upward, the macules are likely to be dark brown and located on the cheeks and around the eyes. Accompanying symptoms include headache and a bitter taste in the mouth.

Treatment principle
Clear the Liver to drain Fire.

Prescription
HUA GAN JIAN JIA JIAN
Decoction for Transforming the Liver, with modifications

Qing Pi (Pericarpium Citri Reticulatae Viride) 10g
Chen Pi (Pericarpium Citri Reticulatae) 10g
Chao Mu Dan Pi (Cortex Moutan Radicis, stir-fried) 10g
Jiao Zhi Zi (Fructus Gardeniae Jasminoidis, scorch-fried) 10g
Ze Xie (Rhizoma Alismatis Orientalis) 15g
Bai Shao (Radix Paeoniae Lactiflorae) 10g
Tu Bei Mu (Tuber Bolbostemmatis) 15g
Ling Xiao Hua (Flos Campsitis) 10g
Ji Guan Hua (Flos Celosiae Cristatae) 10g
Mei Gui Hua (Flos Rosae Rugosae) 10g

Explanation
- *Qing Pi* (Pericarpium Citri Reticulatae Viride) and *Chen Pi* (Pericarpium Citri Reticulatae) move Qi and relieve Depression.
- *Chao Mu Dan Pi* (Cortex Moutan Radicis, stir-fried), *Jiao Zhi Zi* (Fructus Gardeniae Jasminoidis, scorch-fried) and *Ze Xie* (Rhizoma Alismatis Orientalis) clear Heat and cool the Blood.
- *Tu Bei Mu* (Tuber Bolbostemmatis) and *Bai Shao* (Radix Paeoniae Lactiflorae) clear Heat and emolliate the Liver.
- *Ling Xiao Hua* (Flos Campsitis), *Ji Guan Hua* (Flos Celosiae Cristatae) and *Mei Gui Hua* (Flos Rosae Rugosae) cool the Blood and disperse macules.

SPLEEN-DAMP
This pattern is characterized by gray, grayish-black or light brown macules and patches, which gradually spread from the area around the eyes to the area around the mouth and nose, and possibly to the forehead. Accompanying symptoms and signs include shortness of breath, lassitude, listlessness, poor appetite, fullness and distension in the epigastrium and abdomen, or Phlegm-Fluids collecting internally, or thin clear vaginal discharge. The tongue body is pale red and slightly enlarged with a thin, yellow and slightly greasy coating; the pulse is soggy and thready.

Treatment principle
Support the Spleen and transform Dampness, invigorate the Blood and improve the complexion.

Prescription
REN SHEN JIAN PI WAN JIA JIAN
Ginseng Pill for Fortifying the Spleen, with modifications

Zhi Huang Qi (Radix Astragali seu Hedysari, mix-fried with honey) 12g
Dang Shen (Radix Codonopsitis Pilosulae) 12g
Bai Zhu (Rhizoma Atractylodis Macrocephalae) 12g
Fu Ling (Sclerotium Poriae Cocos) 12g

Dang Gui (Radix Angelicae Sinensis) 12g
Hong Hua (Flos Carthami Tinctorii) 6g
Ling Xiao Hua (Flos Campsitis) 6g
Sha Ren (Fructus Amomi) 6g, added 5 minutes before the end of the decoction process
Bai Fu Zi (Rhizoma Typhonii Gigantei) 6g
Sheng Ma (Rhizoma Cimicifugae) 6g
Shan Yao (Radix Dioscoreae Oppositae) 30g
Dong Gua Pi (Epicarpium Benincasae Hispidae) 30g
Zhi Gan Cao (Radix Glycyrrhizae, mix-fried with honey) 10g

Explanation
- *Zhi Huang Qi* (Radix Astragali seu Hedysari, mix-fried with honey), *Dang Shen* (Radix Codonopsitis Pilosulae), *Bai Zhu* (Rhizoma Atractylodis Macrocephalae), *Fu Ling* (Sclerotium Poriae Cocos), *Shan Yao* (Radix Dioscoreae Oppositae), *Zhi Gan Cao* (Radix Glycyrrhizae, mix-fried with honey), and *Sha Ren* (Fructus Amomi) augment Qi and fortify the Spleen, transform Dampness and disperse turbidity.
- *Dang Gui* (Radix Angelicae Sinensis), *Hong Hua* (Flos Carthami Tinctorii) and *Ling Xiao Hua* (Flos Campsitis) invigorate the Blood and reduce macules.
- *Bai Fu Zi* (Rhizoma Typhonii Gigantei) and *Sheng Ma* (Rhizoma Cimicifugae) dredge Wind and reduce color.
- *Dong Gua Pi* (Epicarpium Benincasae Hispidae) moistens the skin and improves the complexion.

YIN DEFICIENCY
Lesions are dull gray or grayish-black as if the face was covered by dust and are distributed symmetrically over the face centered on the nose. Accompanying symptoms and signs caused by Deficiency-Fire flaming upward due to Yin Deficiency of the Heart and Kidneys include aching in the lower back, weakness of the knees, dizziness, tinnitus, a feverish sensation in the palms, soles and center of the chest, frequent clear urination at night, and infertility or irregular menstruation. The tongue body is red with a scant coating; the pulse is thready and rapid.

Treatment principle
Enrich Yin and clear Heat, cool the Blood and disperse macules.

FOR PREDOMINANCE OF KIDNEY YIN DEFICIENCY

Prescription
ZHI BAI DI HUANG TANG JIA JIAN
Anemarrhena, Phellodendron and Rehmannia Decoction, with modifications

Zhi Mu (Rhizoma Anemarrhenae Asphodeloidis) 10g
Huang Bai (Cortex Phellodendri) 10g
Sheng Di Huang (Radix Rehmanniae Glutinosae) 15g

Shan Yao (Rhizoma Dioscoreae Oppositae) 15g
Shan Zhu Yu (Fructus Corni Officinalis) 10g
Fu Ling (Sclerotium Poriae Cocos) 10g
Mu Dan Pi (Cortex Moutan Radicis) 10g
Ling Xiao Hua (Flos Campsitis) 10g
Ji Guan Hua (Flos Celosiae Cristatae) 10g
Chai Hu (Radix Bupleuri) 6g

Explanation

- *Zhi Mu* (Rhizoma Anemarrhenae Asphodeloidis), *Huang Bai* (Cortex Phellodendri) and *Mu Dan Pi* (Cortex Moutan Radicis) nourish Yin, clear Heat and cool the Blood.
- *Sheng Di Huang* (Radix Rehmanniae Glutinosae), *Shan Yao* (Rhizoma Dioscoreae Oppositae), *Shan Zhu Yu* (Fructus Corni Officinalis), and Fu Ling (Sclerotium Poriae Cocos) nourish Yin and boost the Kidneys.
- *Ling Xiao Hua* (Flos Campsitis), *Ji Guan Hua* (Flos Celosiae Cristatae) and *Chai Hu* (Radix Bupleuri) cool the Blood and disperse macules.

FOR PREDOMINANCE OF HEART YIN DEFICIENCY

Prescription
HUANG LIAN E JIAO TANG JIA JIAN
Coptis and Donkey Hide Gelatin Decoction, with modifications

Huang Lian (Rhizoma Coptidis) 10g
Huang Qin (Radix Scutellariae Baicalensis) 10g
E Jiao‡ (Gelatinum Corii Asini) 10g
Sheng Di Huang (Radix Rehmanniae Glutinosae) 15g
Tong Cao (Medulla Tetrapanacis Papyriferi) 6g
Mai Men Dong (Radix Ophiopogonis Japonici) 15g
Ji Guan Hua (Flos Celosiae Cristatae) 10g
Ling Xiao Hua (Flos Campsitis) 10g

Explanation

- *Huang Lian* (Rhizoma Coptidis), *Huang Qin* (Radix Scutellariae Baicalensis) and *Tong Cao* (Medulla Tetrapanacis Papyriferi) clear Heat and eliminate irritability.
- *E Jiao*‡ (Gelatinum Corii Asini), *Sheng Di Huang* (Radix Rehmanniae Glutinosae) and *Mai Men Dong* (Radix Ophiopogonis Japonici) nourish Yin and quiet the Spirit.
- *Ji Guan Hua* (Flos Celosiae Cristatae) and *Ling Xiao Hua* (Flos Campsitis) cool and invigorate the Blood and disperse macules.

General modifications

1. For oppression in the chest and distension of the breasts, add *Yu Jin* (Radix Curcumae), *Chao Chuan Lian Zi* (Fructus Meliae Toosendan, stir-fried), *Jin Ju Ye* (Folium Fortunellae Margaritae), and *Bai Mei Hua* (Flos Mume Albus).

2. For abdominal distension and loose stools, add *Dang Shen* (Radix Codonopsitis Pilosulae), *Chao Shan Yao* (Radix Dioscoreae Oppositae, stir-fried) and *Chao Bai Bian Dou* (Semen Dolichoris Lablab, stir-fried).

3. For abdominal distension and lack of appetite, add *Chao Mai Ya* (Fructus Hordei Vulgaris Germinatus, stir-fried), *Chao Gu Ya* (Fructus Setariae Italicae Germinatus, stir-fried), *Mei Gui Hua* (Flos Rosae Rugosae), *Chen Pi* (Pericarpium Citri Reticulatae), and *Hou Po* (Cortex Magnoliae Officinalis).

4. For menstrual irregularities, add *Dan Shen* (Radix Salviae Miltiorrhizae) and *Yi Mu Cao* (Herba Leonuri Heterophylli).

5. For menstrual clots, add *Tao Ren* (Semen Persicae) and *Hong Hua* (Flos Carthami Tinctorii).

6. For insomnia and profuse dreaming, add *Long Gu*‡ (Os Draconis), *Mu Li*‡ (Concha Ostreae), *Suan Zao Ren* (Semen Ziziphi Spinosae) and *Gan Chao Suan Zao Ren* (Semen Ziziphi Spinosae, dry-fried), *Bai Zi Ren* (Semen Biotae Orientalis), and *He Huan Pi* (Cortex Albizziae Julibrissin).

PATENT HERBAL MEDICINES

- For Spleen Qi Deficiency, take *Ren Shen Jian Pi Wan* (Ginseng Pill for Fortifying the Spleen) 3g three times a day.
- For Kidney Deficiency, take *Liu Wei Di Huang Wan* (Six-Ingredient Rehmannia Pill) 3g with slightly salted boiled water three times a day.
- In the recuperation phase, take *Guo Lao Gao* (Licorice Syrup) 10ml twice a day.

EXTERNAL TREATMENT

- For extensive pigmentation, wash the face with warm water before going to bed and then mix *Xu Shi Yue Fu San* (Xu's Powder for Improving the Skin) into a paste with clean water. Apply evenly to the affected area. Leave the paste on for 45-60 minutes before washing off with warm water. Treat every other day.
- For limited pigmentation, apply *Yu Rong San* (Jade Countenance Powder) for 30 minutes each time before washing off with warm water. Treat every other day.

ACUPUNCTURE

Selection of points according to pattern identification
Liver Depression and Qi stagnation
Main points: ST-36 Zusanli, SP-6 Sanyinjiao and LR-3 Taichong.
Auxiliary points: SP-9 Yinlingquan, LR-2 Xingjian, BL-18 Ganshu, and BL-20 Pishu.

Spleen-Damp
Main points: CV-12 Zhongwan, ST-36 Zusanli and SP-6 Sanyinjiao.
Auxiliary points: BL-20 Pishu, CV-13 Shangwan and CV-10 Xiawan.

Kidney Yin Deficiency
Main points: KI-3 Taixi and SP-6 Sanyinjiao.
Auxiliary points: BL-23 Shenshu and SP-9 Yinling-quan.
Technique: Apply the reducing method for Excess patterns and the reinforcing method for Deficiency patterns. Retain the needles for 30 minutes after obtaining Qi. Treat once a day. A course consists of seven to ten treatment sessions.

Selection of adjacent points
Points: EX-HN-4 Yuyao,[i] EX-HN-5 Taiyang[ii] and SI-18 Quanliao.
Technique: Apply the even method and retain the needles for 30 minutes after obtaining Qi. Treat once a day. A course consists of ten treatment sessions.

Selection of points on the affected channels
Main points: GV-14 Dazhui, LI-11 Quchi, SP-10 Xuehai, ST-36 Zusanli, SP-6 Sanyinjiao, and GB-20 Fengchi.
Auxiliary points: KI-3 Taixi, GV-4 Mingmen, HT-7 Shenmen, PC-6 Neiguan, ST-18 Rugen, CV-3 Zhongji, and EX-B-2 Jiaji.[iii]
Technique: Apply the reinforcing method and retain the needles for 30 minutes after obtaining Qi. Treat every other day. A course consists of fifteen treatment sessions.

Explanation
- SP-6 Sanyinjiao, LR-2 Xingjian, LR-3 Taichong, PC-6 Neiguan, HT-7 Shenmen, and BL-18 Ganshu soothe the Liver and regulate Qi.
- CV-13 Shangwan, CV-12 Zhongwan, CV-10 Xiawan, BL-20 Pishu, ST-18 Rugen, SP-9 Yinlingquan, and ST-36 Zusanli support the Spleen and transform turbidity.
- BL-23 Shenshu, SP-6 Sanyinjiao, KI-3 Taixi, CV-3 Zhongji, and GV-4 Mingmen enrich the Liver and supplement the Kidneys.
- SP-10 Xuehai, EX-B-2 Jiaji and LI-11 Quchi invigorate the Blood and reduce macules.
- GV-14 Dazhui, GB-20 Fengchi and LI-11 Quchi dredge Wind and expel pathogenic factors.

MOXIBUSTION
Points: ST-36 Zusanli, CV-6 Qihai and BL-23 Shenshu.
Technique: Apply direct moxibustion for 5-10 minutes to each point twice a day. A course consists of ten treatment sessions.

EAR ACUPUNCTURE COMBINED WITH BODY ACUPUNCTURE

Selection of points according to disease differentiation
Main points: Liver, Kidney, Spleen, Face, and Endocrine.

Auxiliary points
- For painful menstruation, add Ovary.
- For lassitude, add Subcortex and Ear-Shenmen.
- For involvement of the forehead, add GV-23 Shangxing and GB-14 Yangbai.
- For involvement of the cheek and zygomatic region, add ST-6 Jiache and ST-2 Sibai.
- For involvement of the nose, add LI-20 Yingxiang and EX-HN-3 Yintang.[iv]
- For involvement of the upper lip, add ST-4 Dicang.
- For involvement of the lower lip, add CV-24 Chengjiang.
Technique: Retain the needles for 30 minutes. Treat every other day. A course consists of ten treatment sessions.

Empirical points
Points: Adrenal Gland, Endocrine, Uterus, Spleen, and Lung.
Technique: Retain the needles for 30 minutes. Treat every other day. A course consists of fifteen treatment sessions.

Pricking to bleed method
Ear points: Hot Point, Boils, Subcortex, Endocrine, and Spleen.
Technique: After routine sterilization, prick the points with a small gauge three-edged needle to cause slight bleeding. Treat once every three days. A course consists of five treatment sessions.

Pricking and cupping method
Ear points: Blood Pressure-Lowering Groove, Hot Point and Stomach.
Points on back: GV-14 Dazhui, GV-12 Shenzhu, GV-11 Shendao, GV-9 Zhiyang, GV-8 Jinsuo, and GV-4 Mingmen.

---

[i] M-HN-6 according to the system employed by the Shanghai College of Traditional Chinese Medicine.
[ii] M-HN-9 according to the system employed by the Shanghai College of Traditional Chinese Medicine.
[iii] M-BW-35 according to the system employed by the Shanghai College of Traditional Chinese Medicine.
[iv] M-HN-3 according to the system employed by the Shanghai College of Traditional Chinese Medicine.

Technique: Prick the ear points with a small gauge three-edged needle to cause slight bleeding. After bleeding the points on the back, apply flash-cupping and leave the cups in place for 15-20 minutes. Treat every other day. A course consists of ten treatment sessions.

Explanation

Melasma is related to dysfunction of the Liver, Spleen and Kidneys and both Deficiency and Excess patterns occur. Excess patterns result from Liver Depression and Qi stagnation causing stasis in the grandchild network vessels (*sun luo*), so that the face lacks proper nourishment and displays pronounced pigmentation. Deficiency patterns are associated with Yang Deficiency of the Spleen and Kidneys, resulting in the formation of Phlegm and Damp. These turbid pathogens may rush upward with Wind to attack the face, inducing a dark gray complexion.

The ear points detailed above are therefore determined on the basis of pattern identification. Liver, Spleen, Kidney, and Endocrine are selected as the main points because of their functions of soothing the Liver to relieve Depression, invigorating Yang to augment the Essence, fortifying the Spleen to supplement Qi, and regulating the endocrine function. The joint effect will enable Qi and Blood to be harmonized and a normal complexion to be restored.

Clinical notes

- Internal and external treatment should be combined for this disease. Internal treatment aims to dredge the Liver and boost the Kidneys, transform Blood stasis and reduce macules. External treatment focuses on the application of a medicated powder or mask as an adjuvant therapy.
- For non-pregnant women, particular emphasis should be laid on regulating menstruation.
- In some cases, pigmentation may fade or disappear postpartum or during recovery from liver diseases. Even where this does not happen, treatment based on proper pattern identification has a good prognosis.

Advice for the patient

- Try to avoid depression.
- Reduce exposure to the sun; wear a hat on sunny summer days.
- Keep to a light nutritious diet and avoid fatty and spicy foods and alcohol.
- Certain drugs, especially topical steroids, should be used with care.

- To reduce pigmentation and improve the complexion, add a dessertspoon of vinegar to warm water used for washing the face before going to bed; this water can also be used as a wet compress for 15-30 minutes each evening.

Case history

Patient
Female, aged 28.

Clinical manifestations
Two months previously, dark-colored macules started to appear on the patient's face, initially in the bilateral zygomatic regions and later spreading to the bilateral cheeks. Hyperpigmented macules with clearly defined margins were present on the cheeks and zygomatic regions in a symmetrical butterfly pattern, the largest patch measuring 8x6 cm.

Accompanying symptoms and signs included impatience and irritability, insomnia, profuse dreaming, and menstruation lasting ten days with small amounts of dark menstrual blood. The tongue body was pale with a thin white coating; the pulse was faint and slippery.

Pattern identification
Insufficiency of the Liver and Kidneys, Liver Depression and Qi stagnation.

Treatment principle
Enrich Yin and supplement the Kidneys, soothe the Liver and regulate Qi.

Prescription ingredients
Shu Di Huang (Radix Rehmanniae Glutinosae Conquita) 10g
Shan Zhu Yu (Fructus Corni Officinalis) 10g
Shan Yao (Rhizoma Dioscoreae Oppositae) 10g
Ze Xie (Rhizoma Alismatis Orientalis) 10g
Fu Ling (Sclerotium Poriae Cocos) 10g
Mu Dan Pi (Cortex Moutan Radicis) 10g
Bai Shao (Radix Paeoniae Lactiflorae) 10g
Dan Shen (Radix Salviae Miltiorrhizae) 10g
Chen Pi (Pericarpium Citri Reticulatae) 10g
Chai Hu (Radix Bupleuri) 10g
Han Lian Cao (Herba Ecliptae Prostratae) 15g
Nü Zhen Zi (Fructus Ligustri Lucidi) 15g
Ji Xue Teng (Caulis Spatholobi) 15g
Ye Jiao Teng (Caulis Polygoni Multiflori) 30g

One bag a day was used to prepare a decoction, taken twice a day.

Second visit
After one month (30 bags), the impatience and irritability, insomnia and profuse dreaming had all improved significantly. The prescription was modified by removing *Ye Jiao Teng* (Caulis Polygoni Multiflori) and adding *Yi Mu Cao* (Herba Leonuri Heterophylli) 10g.

Third visit
After another month, the melasma had lightened considerably, the patient was in a much better mood and the menses had

returned to a normal duration. *Yi Mu Cao* (Herba Leonuri Heterophylli) was removed from the prescription.

Outcome
After another month, the melasma had basically disappeared, leaving a faint trace.[1]

Modern clinical experience

TREATMENT BASED ON PATTERN IDENTIFICATION

1. **Yu**, **Jiang** and **Yang** reached similar conclusions in relation to pattern identification and treatment.[2, 3, 4]

Liver Depression and Qi stagnation
This pattern manifests as pale brown to deep brown pigmentation, with accompanying symptoms including distension and fullness in the chest and hypochondrium. The treatment principle focuses on soothing the Liver and regulating Qi with a prescription based on *Xiao Yao Wan* (Free Wanderer Pill).

Liver and Kidney Deficiency
This pattern manifests as a dull gray complexion, accompanied by dizziness, irritability and fever. The treatment principle focuses on enriching the Liver and supplementing the Kidneys with a prescription based on *Liu Wei Di Huang Wan* (Six-Ingredient Rehmannia Pill).

Qi stagnation and Blood stasis
This pattern manifests as dull brown pigmentation, accompanied by abdominal pain during menstruation or menstrual clots. The treatment principle focuses on regulating Qi and harmonizing the Blood with *Tao Hong Si Wu Tang* (Peach Kernel and Safflower Four Agents Decoction).

Spleen and Stomach Deficiency
This pattern manifests as a sallow complexion, accompanied by listlessness and poor appetite. The treatment principle focuses on fortifying the Spleen and harmonizing the Stomach with a prescription based on *Bu Zhong Yi Qi Tang* (Decoction for Supplementing the Middle and Augmenting Qi).

2. **Li** identified three patterns.[5]

- **Liver Depression**

Treatment principle
Clear the Liver and relieve Depression, regulate Qi and invigorate the Blood.

Prescription
QING GAN MI WAN
Honey Pill for Clearing the Liver

Chai Hu (Radix Bupleuri) 100g

Dang Gui (Radix Angelicae Sinensis) 100g
Bai Shao (Radix Paeoniae Lactiflorae) 120g
Sheng Di Huang (Radix Rehmanniae Glutinosae) 120g
Dan Shen (Radix Salviae Miltiorrhizae) 200g
Mu Dan Pi (Cortex Moutan Radicis) 150g
Zhi Zi (Fructus Gardeniae Jasminoidis) 100g
Ling Xiao Hua (Flos Campsitis) 100g
Yi Mu Cao (Herba Leonuri Heterophylli) 200g
Xiang Fu (Rhizoma Cyperi Rotundi) 100g
Bai Zhi (Radix Angelicae Dahuricae) 60g

- **Kidney Deficiency**

Treatment principle
Enrich Water to moisten Wood, nourish the Blood to moisten the skin.

Prescription
YU YI YIN MI WAN
Honey Pill for Boosting Yin

Tu Si Zi (Semen Cuscutae) 300g
Nü Zhen Zi (Fructus Ligustri Lucidi) 300g
Han Lian Cao (Herba Ecliptae Prostratae) 200g
Sheng Di Huang (Radix Rehmanniae Glutinosae) 150g
Shu Di Huang (Radix Rehmanniae Glutinosae Conquita) 150g
Mu Dan Pi (Cortex Moutan Radicis) 150g
Sang Ji Sheng (Ramulus Loranthi) 300g
Dang Gui (Radix Angelicae Sinensis) 120g
Ji Xue Teng (Caulis Spatholobi) 200g
Tian Hua Fen (Radix Trichosanthis) 120g
Fu Ling (Sclerotium Poriae Cocos) 120g

- **Spleen Deficiency**

Treatment principle
Fortify the Spleen and boost the Stomach, promote the movement of water and eliminate macules.

Prescription
YU SHI PI MI WAN
Honey Pill for Reinforcing the Spleen

Dang Shen (Radix Codonopsitis Pilosulae) 200g
Bai Zhu (Rhizoma Atractylodis Macrocephalae) 100g
Yi Yi Ren (Semen Coicis Lachryma-jobi) 300g
Dong Gua Pi (Epicarpium Benincasae Hispidae) 300g
Mu Xiang* (Radix Aucklandiae Lappae) 100g
Fu Ling (Sclerotium Poriae Cocos) 120g
Sheng Di Huang (Radix Rehmanniae Glutinosae) 120g
Dang Gui (Radix Angelicae Sinensis) 120g
Ji Xue Teng (Caulis Spatholobi) 200g
Ji Nei Jin‡ (Endothelium Corneum Gigeriae Galli) 100g

For all three patterns, the ingredients were ground into a fine powder, mixed with 250g of honey, simmered until sticky and then used to make honey pills, 10g per pill. One pill was taken three times a day for two months.

SPECIAL PRESCRIPTIONS

1. **Chen** recommended two different prescriptions depending on the time the melasma occurred. [6]

• **Melasma accompanied by irregular menstruation**

Prescription
YANG YAN QU BAN TANG YI HAO FANG
No. 1 Decoction Formula for Nourishing the Face and Dispelling Macules

Dang Gui (Radix Angelicae Sinensis) 10g
Shu Di Huang (Radix Rehmanniae Glutinosae Conquita) 15g
Chuan Xiong (Rhizoma Ligustici Chuanxiong) 10g
Bai Shao (Radix Paeoniae Lactiflorae) 10g
Dan Shen (Radix Salviae Miltiorrhizae) 10g
Chai Hu (Radix Bupleuri) 15g
Yin Yang Huo (Herba Epimedii) 10g
Huang Qin (Radix Scutellariae Baicalensis) 10g
He Shou Wu (Radix Polygoni Multiflori) 30g
Nü Zhen Zi (Fructus Ligustri Lucidi) 10g
Sang Zhi (Ramulus Mori Albae) 15g

• **Melasma postpartum**

Prescription
YANG YAN QU BAN TANG ER HAO FANG
No. 2 Decoction Formula for Nourishing the Face and Dispelling Macules

Dang Gui (Radix Angelicae Sinensis) 10g
Shu Di Huang (Radix Rehmanniae Glutinosae Conquita) 15g
Chuan Xiong (Rhizoma Ligustici Chuanxiong) 10g
Bai Shao (Radix Paeoniae Lactiflorae) 10g
Yi Mu Cao (Herba Leonuri Heterophylli) 15g
Tao Ren (Semen Persicae) 10g
Dan Shen (Radix Salviae Miltiorrhizae) 10g
Xian Tao Cao (Herba Veronicae Peregrinae) 6g
*Pao Chuan Shan Jia** (Squama Manitis Pentadactylae, blast-fried) 10g
Sang Bai Pi (Cortex Mori Albae Radicis) 30g
Ling Xiao Hua (Flos Campsitis) 6g

For both prescriptions, one bag a day was used to prepare a decoction, taken twice a day. Results were seen after two months.

2. **Xu** reported on the treatment of melasma with *Xiao Ban Jie Rong Wan* (Pill for Dispersing Macules and Cleansing the Countenance). [7]

Prescription ingredients

Bai Ji Li (Fructus Tribuli Terrestris) 15g
Dang Gui (Radix Angelicae Sinensis) 15g
Nü Zhen Zi (Fructus Ligustri Lucidi) 15g
Sheng Di Huang (Radix Rehmanniae Glutinosae) 30g
Chuan Xiong (Rhizoma Ligustici Chuanxiong) 10g

Gan Cao (Radix Glycyrrhizae) 10g

The ingredients were ground into a powder and made into pills with water. Nine grams were taken three times a day with warm water. Results were seen after two months.

3. **Peng** reported on the use of the classical formula *Xue Fu Zhu Yu Tang* (Decoction for Expelling Stasis from the House of Blood). [8]

Prescription ingredients

Sheng Di Huang (Radix Rehmanniae Glutinosae) 10g
Chi Shao (Radix Paeoniae Rubra) 10g
Chai Hu (Radix Bupleuri) 10g
Zhi Ke (Fructus Citri Aurantii) 10g
Niu Xi (Radix Achyranthis Bidentatae) 10g
Tao Ren (Semen Persicae) 10g
Dang Gui (Radix Angelicae Sinensis) 9g
Chuan Xiong (Rhizoma Ligustici Chuanxiong) 8g
Gan Cao (Radix Glycyrrhizae) 8g
Jie Geng (Radix Platycodi Grandiflori) 6g
Hong Hua (Flos Carthami Tinctorii) 6g

One bag a day was used to prepare a decoction, taken twice a day. A course of treatment consisted of ten bags followed by a five-day break. Results were generally seen after three courses.

4. **Wang** applied the method of cooling and invigorating the Blood to treat melasma. [9]

Prescription ingredients

Chi Shao (Radix Paeoniae Rubra) 9g
Chuan Xiong (Rhizoma Ligustici Chuanxiong) 6g
Dang Gui (Radix Angelicae Sinensis) 12g
Sheng Di Huang (Radix Rehmanniae Glutinosae) 12g
Mu Dan Pi (Cortex Moutan Radicis) 12g
Yi Mu Cao (Herba Leonuri Heterophylli) 12g
Ze Lan (Herba Lycopi Lucidi) 12g
Dan Shen (Radix Salviae Miltiorrhizae) 15g

One bag a day was used to prepare a decoction, taken warm twice a day. Results were seen within a range of 14 to 30 days.

EAR ACUPUNCTURE
Luan treated melasma with ear acupuncture using needles and seeds. [10]
Main points: Cheek, Lung, Endocrine, Pelvic Cavity, and Internal Genitals.
Auxiliary points:

• For Qi stagnation and Blood stasis, Diaphragm, Liver and Subcortex were added.

• For Yin Deficiency of the Liver and Kidneys, Kidney, Spleen and Liver were added.

Technique: Five or six points were selected for each treatment. After routine sterilization, 0.5 cun no. 30 stainless steel needles were used to find the sensitive spots in the area of the points chosen, then inserted quickly directly to the perichondrium. The needles were retained for 30 minutes after obtaining Qi and manipulated every 10 minutes. Ear seeds were attached to the same points on the other ear and the patient was told to press the seeds for five minutes three or four times a day. Treatment was given every other day, with each ear alternating between needling and pressure. A course of treatment consisted of ten sessions; courses were separated by a break of ten days. Results were seen after three courses.

TREATMENT WITH A COMBINATION OF TCM AND WESTERN MEDICINE

Pan treated melasma by combining TCM and Western medicine. [11]

Western medicine

Vitamin E capsules 100mg were prescribed for oral administration three times a day. For external application, the capsules were pricked with a needle and the oil applied to the melasma twice a day.

TCM prescription
XIAO YAO SAN
Free Wanderer Powder

Dang Gui (Radix Angelicae Sinensis) 15g
Bai Shao (Radix Paeoniae Lactiflorae) 15g
Bai Zhu (Rhizoma Atractylodis Macrocephalae) 15g
Fu Ling (Sclerotium Poriae Cocos) 10g
Chai Hu (Radix Bupleuri) 10g
Gan Cao (Radix Glycyrrhizae) 10g
Bo He (Herba Menthae Haplocalycis) 6g, added 5 minutes before the end of the decoction process
Wei Jiang (Rhizoma Zingiberis Officinalis Usta) 10g

One bag a day was used to prepare a decoction, taken warm twice a day. Results were seen within a range of 18 to 45 days.

Melanosis
黑变病

Melanosis is a skin disease marked by diffuse pigmentation of exposed areas due to an abnormal deposition of melanin in the skin. Although the cause of the disease has yet to be fully explained, inducing factors are considered to be long-term contact with tar, bitumen, petroleum products, and paint, external use of poor-quality cosmetics, environmental factors, and hypersensitivity to sunlight.

In TCM, this condition is known as *li hei bing* (soot-black complexion disease).

Clinical manifestations

- This disease occurs most frequently among the young and middle-aged, especially women.
- Yellowish-brown to grayish-black pigmentation on the face, forehead and neck frequently forms confluent patches without clear borders. In more serious cases, lesions spread to the chest, axillae, umbilicus, waist, abdomen, and back.
- The skin is dry with shedding of a few bran-like scales.
- Systemic symptoms include dizziness, poor appetite and emaciation.

- This disease usually develops slowly for several months and pigmentation persists for a long period. It may become lighter spontaneously in a few patients, but is unlikely to disappear completely.

Differential diagnosis

Melasma

This disease mainly involves the forehead, the cheeks, the perioral and perinasal areas, and the chin. Lesions manifest as light brown to dark brown hyperpigmented macules or patches of varying size and shape. Pigmentation evolves slowly and is more prevalent after exposure to sunlight.

Etiology and pathology

In TCM, melanosis is related to internal Fire and undernourishment of the skin. Depletion of Liver and Kidney Yin results in Water failing to control Fire. If this is accompanied by excessive thought and preoccupation, worry and depression, the Blood is weakened and cannot provide luster to the skin. Fire and Dryness combine to produce dark brown macules on the face, with the complexion gradually turning grayish-black. This color of the complexion can also result from Phlegm-Fluids in the Zang-Fu organs causing irregular movement of Qi and Blood.

Pattern identification and treatment

INTERNAL TREATMENT

LIVER DEPRESSION
This pattern is seen at the initial stage of the disease with brown or dark brown patches. The face has a grayish-black complexion that becomes more pronounced on exposure to the sun; a prickly itching sensation and flushing are also present. Accompanying symptoms and signs include irascibility, poor appetite, nausea, and a feverish sensation in the palms and soles. The tongue body is red with a thin yellow coating; the pulse is wiry and rapid.

Treatment principle
Dredge the Liver and relieve Depression.

Prescription
XIAO YAO SAN JIA JIAN
Free Wanderer Powder, with modifications

Cu Chai Hu (Radix Bupleuri, processed with vinegar) 6g
Qing Pi (Pericarpium Citri Reticulatae Viride) 6g
Gan Cao (Radix Glycyrrhizae) 6g
Shu Di Huang (Radix Rehmanniae Glutinosae Conquita) 10g
Bai Shao (Radix Paeoniae Lactiflorae) 10g
Fu Ling (Sclerotium Poriae Cocos) 10g
Chao Bai Zhu (Rhizoma Atractylodis Macrocephalae, stir-fried) 10g
Huang Qi (Radix Astragali seu Hedysari) 15g
Ji Xue Teng (Caulis Spatholobi) 15g
Qing Hao (Herba Artemisiae Chinghao) 15g
Di Gu Pi (Cortex Lycii Radicis) 12g
Chao Mai Ya (Fructus Hordei Vulgaris Germinatus, stir-fried) 12g
Chao Gu Ya (Fructus Setariae Italicae Germinatus, stir-fried) 12g
Dong Gua Pi (Epicarpium Benincasae Hispidae) 12g
Chao Bai Bian Dou (Semen Dolichoris Lablab, stir-fried) 12g

Explanation
* Cu Chai Hu (Radix Bupleuri, processed with vinegar), Qing Pi (Pericarpium Citri Reticulatae Viride), Chao Mai Ya (Fructus Hordei Vulgaris Germinatus, stir-fried), and Chao Gu Ya (Fructus Setariae Italicae Germinatus, stir-fried) soothe the Liver and relieve Depression.
* Shu Di Huang (Radix Rehmanniae Glutinosae Conquita), Bai Shao (Radix Paeoniae Lactiflorae), Fu Ling (Sclerotium Poriae Cocos), Chao Bai Zhu (Rhizoma Atractylodis Macrocephalae, stir-fried), and Huang Qi (Radix Astragali seu Hedysari) supplement Qi and nourish the Blood.
* Ji Xue Teng (Caulis Spatholobi) nourishes the Blood and frees the network vessels.
* Qing Hao (Herba Artemisiae Chinghao) and Di Gu Pi (Cortex Lycii Radicis) enrich Yin and boost the Kidneys.
* Dong Gua Pi (Epicarpium Benincasae Hispidae), Chao Bai Bian Dou (Semen Dolichoris Lablab, stir-fried) and Gan Cao (Radix Glycyrrhizae) support the Spleen and improve the complexion.

PHLEGM-DAMP
Lusterless dull gray or grayish-brown pigmentation in patches of various sizes and shapes mostly manifests around the bridge of the nose. Accompanying symptoms and signs include poor appetite, abdominal distension, profuse phlegm, and obesity. The tongue body is enlarged with tooth marks and a thin white coating; the pulse is soggy and rapid.

Treatment principle
Support the Spleen and transform Dampness, flush out Phlegm and improve the complexion.

Prescription
GUI LING GAN ZHU TANG JIA JIAN
Cinnamon Twig, Poria, Licorice, and White Atractylodes Decoction, with modifications

Fu Ling (Sclerotium Poriae Cocos) 15g
Tu Chao Bai Zhu (Rhizoma Atractylodis Macrocephalae, stir-fried with earth) 10g
Gan Cao (Radix Glycyrrhizae) 10g
Jiang Can ‡ (Bombyx Batryticatus) 10g
Shan Yao (Radix Dioscoreae Oppositae) 10g
Chao Bai Bian Dou (Semen Dolichoris Lablab, stir-fried) 10g
Chao Zhi Ke (Fructus Citri Aurantii, stir-fried) 6g
Hong Hua (Flos Carthami Tinctorii) 6g
Ling Xiao Hua (Flos Campsitis) 6g
Sheng Ma (Rhizoma Cimicifugae) 6g
Chen Pi (Pericarpium Citri Reticulatae) 6g
Zhu Ru (Caulis Bambusae in Taeniis) 6g
Dong Gua Ren (Semen Benincasae Hispidae) 30g
Ze Xie (Rhizoma Alismatis Orientalis) 12g

Explanation
* Fu Ling (Sclerotium Poriae Cocos), Tu Chao Bai Zhu (Rhizoma Atractylodis Macrocephalae, stir-fried with earth), Shan Yao (Radix Dioscoreae Oppositae), Chao Bai Bian Dou (Semen Dolichoris Lablab, stir-fried), Chao Zhi Ke (Fructus Citri Aurantii, stir-fried), Chen Pi (Pericarpium Citri Reticulatae), Zhu Ru (Caulis

Bambusae in Taeniis), and *Ze Xie* (Rhizoma Alismatis Orientalis) support the Spleen and transform Dampness; once Dampness has been eliminated, the skin will recover its luster.

- *Hong Hua* (Flos Carthami Tinctorii) and *Ling Xiao Hua* (Flos Campsitis) invigorate the Blood and free the network vessels.
- *Dong Gua Ren* (Semen Benincasae Hispidae), *Jiang Can*‡ (Bombyx Batryticatus) and *Gan Cao* (Radix Glycyrrhizae) moisten the skin and improve the complexion.
- *Sheng Ma* (Rhizoma Cimicifugae) bears the clear upward and the turbid downward, thus enhancing the effect of the other ingredients.

KIDNEY DEPLETION

This pattern is seen in diseases with a prolonged history and manifests with a grayish-black complexion. Accompanying symptoms and signs include aching and limpness of the lower back and knees, fatigue, dizziness, and tinnitus. The tongue body is pale red with a peeling coating; the pulse is deep and thready.

Treatment principle
Enrich the Kidneys and supplement Qi while improving the complexion.

Prescription
LIU WEI DI HUANG TANG JIA JIAN
Six-Ingredient Rehmannia Decoction, with modifications

Shu Di Huang (Radix Rehmanniae Glutinosae Conquita) 10g
Ze Xie (Rhizoma Alismatis Orientalis) 10g
Shan Zhu Yu (Fructus Corni Officinalis) 10g
Gou Qi Zi (Fructus Lycii) 10g
Xian Mao (Rhizoma Curculiginis Orchioidis) 10g
Yin Yang Huo (Herba Epimedii) 12g
Nü Zhen Zi (Fructus Ligustri Lucidi) 12g
Han Lian Cao (Herba Ecliptae Prostratae) 12g
Shan Yao (Radix Dioscoreae Oppositae) 12g
Chao Mu Dan Pi (Cortex Moutan Radicis, stir-fried) 6g
Dan Shen (Radix Salviae Miltiorrhizae) 10g
Qing Hao (Herba Artemisiae Chinghao) 30g

Explanation

- *Shu Di Huang* (Radix Rehmanniae Glutinosae Conquita), *Shan Zhu Yu* (Fructus Corni Officinalis), *Gou Qi Zi* (Fructus Lycii), *Xian Mao* (Rhizoma Curculiginis Orchioidis), *Yin Yang Huo* (Herba Epimedii), *Nü Zhen Zi* (Fructus Ligustri Lucidi), *Han Lian Cao* (Herba Ecliptae Prostratae), and *Shan Yao* (Radix Dioscoreae Oppositae) enrich the Kidneys and supplement Qi; when Kidney-Water is abundant, Liver-Blood is exuberant, which helps to disperse pigmentation.

- *Chao Mu Dan Pi* (Cortex Moutan Radicis, stir-fried) and *Dan Shen* (Radix Salviae Miltiorrhizae) invigorate the Blood and reduce macules, nourish Yin and clear Heat.

- *Qing Hao* (Herba Artemisiae Chinghao) clears Summerheat and repels brightness, thus helping to protect the skin from the effects of ultraviolet radiation.

- *Ze Xie* (Rhizoma Alismatis Orientalis) transforms Dampness and bears turbidity downward and therefore prevents congestion of Dampness caused by supplementing ingredients.

PATENT HERBAL MEDICINES

- For Kidney depletion, take *Liu Wei Di Huang Wan* (Six-Ingredient Rehmannia Pill) 3g three times a day.
- For Spleen Deficiency, take *Ren Shen Gui Pi Wan* (Ginseng Pill for Restoring the Spleen) 3g three times a day.
- For Liver Depression, take *Xiao Yao Wan* (Free Wanderer Pill) 1.5g three times a day.

EXTERNAL TREATMENT

For extensive pigmentation, wash the face with warm water before going to bed and then mix *Xu Shi Yue Fu San* (Xu's Powder for Improving the Skin) into a paste with clean water. Apply evenly to the affected area. Leave the paste on for 45-60 minutes before washing off with warm water. Treat every other day.

ACUPUNCTURE

Selection of points according to pattern identification
Liver depression
Main points: ST-36 Zusanli, SP-6 Sanyinjiao and LR-3 Taichong.
Auxiliary points: SP-9 Yinlingquan, LR-2 Xingjian, BL-18 Ganshu, and BL-20 Pishu.

Phlegm-Damp
Main points: CV-12 Zhongwan, ST-36 Zusanli, SP-6 Sanyinjiao, and GB-20 Fengchi.
Auxiliary points: BL-20 Pishu, CV-13 Shangwan and CV-10 Xiawan.

Kidney depletion
Main points: KI-3 Taixi and SP-6 Sanyinjiao.
Auxiliary points: BL-23 Shenshu and SP-9 Yinlingquan.

Technique
Apply the reducing method for Excess patterns and the reinforcing method for Deficiency patterns. Retain the needles for 30 minutes after obtaining Qi. Treat once a day. A course consists of ten treatment sessions.

Selection of points on the affected channels

Main points: GV-14 Dazhui, LI-11 Quchi, SP-10 Xuehai, ST-36 Zusanli, SP-6 Sanyinjiao, and GB-20 Fengchi.

Auxiliary points: KI-3 Taixi, GV-4 Mingmen, HT-7 Shenmen, PC-6 Neiguan, ST-18 Rugen, CV-3 Zhongji, and EX-B-2 Jiaji. v

Technique: Apply the reinforcing method and retain the needles for 30 minutes after obtaining Qi. Treat once a day. A course consists of ten treatment sessions.

Explanation

- SP-6 Sanyinjiao, LR-2 Xingjian, LR-3 Taichong, PC-6 Neiguan, HT-7 Shenmen, and BL-18 Ganshu soothe the Liver and regulate Qi.
- CV-13 Shangwan, CV-12 Zhongwan, CV-10 Xiawan, BL-20 Pishu, ST-18 Rugen, SP-9 Yinlingquan, and ST-36 Zusanli support the Spleen and transform turbidity.
- BL-23 Shenshu, SP-6 Sanyinjiao, KI-3 Taixi, CV-3 Zhongji, and GV-4 Mingmen enrich the Liver and supplement the Kidneys.
- SP-10 Xuehai, EX-B-2 Jiaji and LI-11 Quchi invigorate the Blood and reduce macules.
- GV-14 Dazhui, GB-20 Fengchi and LI-11 Quchi dredge Wind and expel pathogenic factors.

MOXIBUSTION

Points: BL-23 Shenshu, BL-20 Pishu and BL-17 Geshu.
Technique: Apply direct moxibustion with a moxa stick using the sparrow-pecking method for five minutes at each point. Treat once a day. A course consists of ten treatment sessions.

EAR ACUPUNCTURE

Main points: Liver, Kidney, Spleen, and Face.
Auxiliary points

- For painful menstruation, Ovary and Endocrine.
- For lassitude and fatigue, Subcortex and Ear-Shenmen.

Technique: Retain the needles for 30 minutes. Treat once a day. A course consists of ten treatment sessions.

Clinical notes

When treating melanosis, it is important to differentiate between Deficiency and Excess patterns. Deficiency patterns manifest as grayish-black pigmentation and treatment should focus on the Liver and Kidneys. Excess patterns manifest as brownish-black pigmentation and treatment should focus on the Liver and Spleen. Materia medica for transforming Blood stasis and freeing the network vessels can also be added for both patterns to enhance the result.

Advice for the patient

- Try to remain optimistic and avoid worry and fatigue.
- Avoid exposure to the sun and eat fewer ultraviolet spectrum-absorbing vegetables (see Phytophotodermatitis in Chapter 17).

Literature excerpt

In *Pu Ji Fang* [Prescriptions for Universal Relief], it says: "Phlegm-Fluids accumulating in the Zang-Fu organs or Wind entering through the interstices (*cou li*) will lead to disharmony between Qi and Blood. The skin is deprived of nourishment, thus giving rise to melanosis. Where there is invasion of Wind, treat by expelling Wind; treat retention of Phlegm-Fluids internally."

Modern clinical experience

INTERNAL TREATMENT

1. **Zhang** treated melanosis with a special prescription.[12]

Prescription
XING PI ZHU MAI TANG
Decoction for Arousing the Spleen and Expelling Haze

Huang Qi (Radix Astragali seu Hedysari) 30g
Cang Zhu (Rhizoma Atractylodis) 10g
Chao Bai Zhu (Rhizoma Atractylodis Macrocephalae, stir-fried) 10g
Zi Su Ye (Folium Perillae Frutescentis) 10g
Fa Ban Xia (Rhizoma Pinelliae Ternatae Praeparata) 10g
Huo Xiang (Herba Agastaches seu Pogostemi) 10g
Chen Pi (Pericarpium Citri Reticulatae) 7g
Cao Dou Kou (Semen Alpiniae Katsumadai) 5g
Sheng Jiang (Rhizoma Zingiberis Officinalis Recens) 6g

Modifications

- For headache and heavy head, *Xiang Ru* (Herba Elsholtziae seu Moslae) and *Bai Zhi* (Radix Angelicae Dahuricae) were added.
- For hiccoughs and vomiting, *Sha Ren* (Fructus Amomi) and *Hou Po Hua* (Flos Magnoliae Officinalis) were added.
- For alternating bitter and bland taste in the mouth, *Chao Huang Lian* (Rhizoma Coptidis, stir-fried) and *Zhu Ru* (Caulis Bambusae in Taeniis) were added.

---

v M-BW-35 according to the system employed by the Shanghai College of Traditional Chinese Medicine.

One bag a day was used to prepare a decoction, taken twice a day. Results began to be seen after two weeks.

2. **Li** also formulated a special prescription to treat melanosis. [13]

Prescription
SAN ZI QI BAI TANG
Three-Seed Seven-Whites Decoction

Lian Zi (Semen Nelumbinis Nuciferae) 20g
Bai Shao (Radix Paeoniae Lactiflorae) 20g
Bai Zhu (Rhizoma Atractylodis Macrocephalae) 10g
Fu Ling (Sclerotium Poriae Cocos) 15g
Bai Ji Li (Fructus Tribuli Terrestris) 15g
Bai Ju Hua (Flos Chrysanthemi Morifolii Albus) 15g
Bai Dou Kou (Fructus Amomi Kravanh) 4g
Gou Qi Zi (Fructus Lycii) 30g
Che Qian Zi (Semen Plantaginis) 9g, wrapped

Modifications

1. For constipation, *Feng Mi* ‡ (Mel) 30g was added to the prepared decoction.
2. For aversion to cold and cold limbs, *Gan Jiang* (Rhizoma Zingiberis Officinalis) 3g and *Fu Zi** (Radix Lateralis Aconiti Carmichaeli Praeparata) 7g were added.
3. For a feverish sensation in the chest, palms and soles, *Qing Hao* (Herba Artemisiae Chinghao) 10g and *Zhi Bie Jia** (Carapax Amydae Sinensis, mix-fried) 7g were added.
4. For red face and eyes and a painful and swollen inner ear with purulent discharge, *Jin Yin Hua* (Flos Lonicerae Japonicae) 30g and *Zhi Zi* (Fructus Gardeniae Jasminoidis) 12g were added.

One bag a day was used to prepare a decoction, taken warm twice a day. Results were seen within a range of 97 to 160 days.

3. **Yang** reported on his treatment of melanosis. [14]

Prescription
YI SHEN HUO XUE TANG
Decoction for Boosting the Kidneys and Invigorating the Blood

Shu Di Huang (Radix Rehmanniae Glutinosae Conquita) 20g
Shan Zhu Yu (Fructus Corni Officinalis) 15g
Shan Yao (Radix Dioscoreae Oppositae) 15g
Tao Ren (Semen Persicae) 10g
Fu Ling (Sclerotium Poriae Cocos) 10g
Mu Dan Pi (Cortex Moutan Radicis) 10g
Ze Lan (Herba Lycopi Lucidi) 10g
Ze Xie (Rhizoma Alismatis Orientalis) 6g
Hong Hua (Flos Carthami Tinctorii) 6g

Chuan Xiong (Rhizoma Ligustici Chuanxiong) 6g
Bai Fu Zi (Rhizoma Typhonii Gigantei) 6g
Jiang Can ‡ (Bombyx Batryticatus) 9g

One bag a day was used to prepare a decoction, taken twice a day. A course of treatment consisted of 30 bags. Results were seen after two courses.

EXTERNAL TREATMENT
Zhu prepared a facial mask to treat this condition. [15]

Prescription
ER ZI QU BAN GAO
Two-Seed Paste for Dispelling Macules

Bai Zhi (Radix Angelicae Dahuricae) 15g
Bai Fu Zi (Rhizoma Typhonii Gigantei) 10g
Jiang Can ‡ (Bombyx Batryticatus) 10g
Bai Ji (Rhizoma Bletillae Striatae) 10g
Fu Ling (Sclerotium Poriae Cocos) 15g
Bai Shao (Radix Paeoniae Lactiflorae) 10g
Dang Gui (Radix Angelicae Sinensis) 10g
Dong Gua Ren (Semen Benincasae Hispidae) 20g

The ingredients were ground to a very fine powder and made into a cold cream with *Zhen Zhu Mu* (Pearl Powder) and a base consisting of Vaseline®, white oil, beeswax, and water with an oil to water ratio of 2:1. After the face had been washed, the paste was massaged into the affected area for 10-15 minutes once a week and then washed off. Results were seen after 12 treatments.

TREATMENT WITH A COMBINATION OF TCM AND WESTERN MEDICINE
Hu combined Western medicine with TCM treatment according to pattern identification. Three different patterns were identified. [16]

- **Liver Depression and Qi stagnation**

Treatment principle
Dredge the Liver and relieve Depression, regulate Qi and invigorate the Blood.

Prescription ingredients

Chai Hu (Radix Bupleuri) 10g
Zhi Zi (Fructus Gardeniae Jasminoidis) 10g
Sheng Di Huang (Radix Rehmanniae Glutinosae) 10g
Tao Ren (Semen Persicae) 10g
Bai Zhi (Radix Angelicae Dahuricae) 10g
Dang Gui (Radix Angelicae Sinensis) 15g
Bai Shao (Radix Paeoniae Lactiflorae) 15g
Yi Mu Cao (Herba Leonuri Heterophylli) 15g
Chen Pi (Pericarpium Citri Reticulatae) 15g
Dan Shen (Radix Salviae Miltiorrhizae) 30g
Xiang Fu (Rhizoma Cyperi Rotundi) 12g

- **Insufficiency of Spleen Yang**

Treatment principle

Warm Spleen Yang, benefit the movement of Dampness and disperse macules.

Prescription ingredients

Dang Shen (Radix Codonopsitis Pilosulae) 12g
Ji Xue Teng (Caulis Spatholobi) 12g
Bai Zhu (Rhizoma Atractylodis Macrocephalae) 10g
Mu Xiang* (Radix Aucklandiae Lappae) 10g
Fu Ling (Sclerotium Poriae Cocos) 10g
Sheng Jiang Pi (Cortex Zingiberis Officinalis Recens) 10g
Dang Gui (Radix Angelicae Sinensis) 10g
Tao Ren (Semen Persicae) 10g
Ji Nei Jin‡ (Endothelium Corneum Gigeriae Galli) 10g
Bai Zhi (Radix Angelicae Dahuricae) 10g
Fu Zi* (Radix Lateralis Aconiti Carmichaeli Praeparata) 8g
Dong Gua Pi (Epicarpium Benincasae Hispidae) 15g

- **Yin Deficiency of the Liver and Kidneys**

Treatment principle

Enrich Kidney-Water to irrigate Liver-Wood, nourish the Blood and moisten the skin.

Prescription ingredients

Sheng Di Huang (Radix Rehmanniae Glutinosae) 10g
Shu Di Huang (Radix Rehmanniae Glutinosae Conquita) 10g
Mu Dan Pi (Cortex Moutan Radicis) 10g
Hong Hua (Flos Carthami Tinctorii) 10g
Tao Ren (Semen Persicae) 10g
Bai Zhi (Radix Angelicae Dahuricae) 10g
Fu Ling Pi (Cortex Poriae Cocos) 10g
Tu Si Zi (Semen Cuscutae) 15g
Nü Zhen Zi (Fructus Ligustri Lucidi) 15g
Sang Ji Sheng (Ramulus Loranthi) 15g
Tian Hua Fen (Radix Trichosanthis) 15g
Dang Gui (Radix Angelicae Sinensis) 12g
Han Lian Cao (Herba Ecliptae Prostratae) 12g
Ji Xue Teng (Caulis Spatholobi) 12g

For all patterns, one bag a day was used to prepare a decoction, taken twice a day.

Western medicine

Vitamin C 1.5g in 200ml of 5% glucose, administered by intravenous infusion once a day for 15 days.

Results began to be seen after 15 days.

Vitiligo
白癜风

Vitiligo is an acquired idiopathic disorder of circumscribed patches of depigmentation due to a complete loss of melanocytes from the affected areas. Many authorities consider that it is probably related to autoimmunity and auto-destruction of melanocytes. Additionally, it may also be associated with neurochemical factors, copper deficiency and genetic factors (generally about 30 percent of patients have a family history of the disorder). Up to 1 percent of the population may be affected. Vitiligo is usually more obvious in those with darker skin.

In TCM, vitiligo is known as *bai dian feng* or *bai bo feng* (white patch Wind).

Clinical manifestations

- Vitiligo can occur at any age without sex predilection, but is more common in adolescents and young adults and less likely in children.
- Lesions manifest as circumscribed depigmented patches of varying number and size and sharply demarcated borders. They appear inflamed with a sensation of burning heat after exposure to the sun. Hairs may be white in some affected areas.
- Autoimmune vitiligo manifests as small, usually symmetrically distributed, white patches with irregular but clearly defined margins on the hands (especially the dorsum), the wrists, the front of the knees, the neck, and around body orifices such as the mouth, eyes, genitals, anus, and umbilicus. Patients with this type of vitiligo often suffer from other autoimmune diseases such as thyroid disorder, pernicious anemia, alopecia, or diabetes mellitus.
- Segmental vitiligo, much less common than autoimmune vitiligo, is unilateral, with white patches in a segmental distribution, for example down a limb or dermatome.
- The disease progresses slowly or rapidly over a number of years.

Differential diagnosis

Pityriasis versicolor

This disease mainly occurs on the chest and back, but

may also spread to the upper arms, neck and abdomen. It occurs mainly in young adults, especially in summer. Lesions, which may be pale white, pale red, yellowish-brown, or dark brown, start with multiple small macules, which soon enlarge into round macular patches. Unlike vitiligo, there is fine, bran-like scaling.

Pityriasis alba

Pityriasis alba is most common in young adult women and children, and is particularly frequent in atopic individuals. It usually occurs in spring, but becomes more obvious in summer when the affected skin does not tan. The disease generally involves the face, but may occasionally affect other locations, such as the neck, shoulder or arm. Lesions usually manifest as white or very pale pink patches of varying size with indistinct borders. Their surface is usually covered by dry, fine scales.

Etiology and pathology

- Qi is the commander of Blood and Blood is the mother of Qi. If Qi and Blood are harmonious, the skin and flesh will be properly nourished and moistened, the skin will have its normal color and the hair will be lustrous and healthy. However, in circumstances of disharmony between Qi and Blood (several reasons for which are described below), the nourishing and moistening functions will be impaired and white patches may appear on the skin.

- Wind, Heat, Cold, or Dampness invading the skin and flesh will impair the diffusion of Lung Qi, which is retained in the channels and network vessels, thus affecting the movement of Wei Qi (Defensive Qi) and blocking the pores.

- Internal damage caused by the seven emotions disturbs the functional activities of Qi and leads to disharmony between Qi and Blood, which can no longer nourish and warm the body properly. If the body is then invaded by external Wind, Qi and Blood Deficiency result in Wind-Dryness disturbing upward, leading to obstruction of the channels and vessels and the appearance of white patches.

- Blood stasis resulting from knocks and falls (trauma) or from stagnation of Qi and Blood due to violent anger damaging the Liver will eventually obstruct the channels and impede the generation of Blood. A prolonged illness that is not treated properly can also lead to Blood stasis between the skin and membranes. Since the skin is not moistened or nourished adequately, vitiligo will develop.

- Insufficiency of the Kidneys may disturb the functions of other Zang-Fu organs; insufficiency of Kidney Yang results in impairment of the transpor-

tation and transformation functions of the Spleen leading to accumulation of Damp-Heat, which then steams upward; insufficiency of Kidney Yin results in hyperactivity of Heart-Fire with imbalance between Water and Fire and disharmony between Qi and Blood. In addition, improper nourishment during a prolonged illness consumes Blood and exhausts Essence. Disharmony between Qi and Blood or consumption of Blood and Essence impede the movement of Qi and Blood and deprive the skin of nourishment.

Pattern identification and treatment

INTERNAL TREATMENT

WIND-DRYNESS

This pattern mostly affects young people up to the mid-thirties and manifests as shiny white patches over the upper half of the body or throughout the body. These patches appear suddenly and develop rapidly. The tongue body is red with a scant coating; the pulse is surging and rapid.

Treatment principle
Dissipate Wind and moisten Dryness.

Prescription
ER ZHI WAN JIA JIAN
Double Supreme Pill, with modifications

Nü Zhen Zi (Fructus Ligustri Lucidi) 12g
Han Lian Cao (Herba Ecliptae Prostratae) 12g
Sang Shen (Fructus Mori Albae) 15g
Bai Ji Li (Fructus Tribuli Terrestris) 15g
Dan Shen (Radix Salviae Miltiorrhizae) 10g
Fang Feng (Radix Ledebouriellae Divaricatae) 10g
Fu Ping (Herba Spirodelae Polyrrhizae) 10g
Bai Fu Zi (Rhizoma Typhonii Gigantei) 6g
Gan Cao (Radix Glycyrrhizae) 6g
Hei Zhi Ma (Semen Sesami Indici) 30g

Explanation
- *Nü Zhen Zi* (Fructus Ligustri Lucidi), *Han Lian Cao* (Herba Ecliptae Prostratae), *Sang Shen* (Fructus Mori Albae), *Gan Cao* (Radix Glycyrrhizae), and *Hei Zhi Ma* (Semen Sesami Indici) enrich Yin and moisten Dryness.

- *Bai Ji Li* (Fructus Tribuli Terrestris), *Fang Feng* (Radix Ledebouriellae Divaricatae), *Fu Ping* (Herba Spirodelae Polyrrhizae), and *Bai Fu Zi* (Rhizoma Typhonii Gigantei) dredge Wind and expel pathogenic factors, and improve pigmentation by helping to increase the number of melanocytes.

- *Dan Shen* (Radix Salviae Miltiorrhizae) nourishes and

invigorates the Blood, thereby promoting the production of melanocytes.

DAMP-HEAT

This pattern mainly affects the young and early middle-aged, sometimes the elderly. It manifests as pale brown or pink patches around the seven orifices of the face or on the neck. These patches tend to develop fast in summer and autumn but remain static in winter and spring. Itching becomes severe on exposure to sunlight or heat. The tongue body is pale red with a thin or slightly greasy yellow coating; the pulse is soggy and rapid.

Treatment principle
Eliminate Dampness and clear Heat.

Prescription
HU MA WAN JIA JIAN
Black Sesame Seed Pill, with modifications

Hei Zhi Ma (Semen Sesami Indici) 15g
Ku Shen (Radix Sophorae Flavescentis) 10g
Fang Feng (Radix Ledebouriellae Divaricatae) 10g
Shi Chang Pu (Rhizoma Acori Graminei) 10g
Bai Fu Zi (Rhizoma Typhonii Gigantei) 6g
Cang Zhu (Rhizoma Atractylodis) 6g
Chong Lou (Rhizoma Paridis) 6g
Hong Hua (Flos Carthami Tinctorii) 6g
Chan Tui‡ (Periostracum Cicadae) 6g
Xi Xian Cao (Herba Siegesbeckiae) 15g

Explanation
* *Ku Shen* (Radix Sophorae Flavescentis), *Chong Lou* (Rhizoma Paridis), *Cang Zhu* (Rhizoma Atractylodis), and *Xi Xian Cao* (Herba Siegesbeckiae) clear Heat and eliminate Dampness.
* *Fang Feng* (Radix Ledebouriellae Divaricatae), *Bai Fu Zi* (Rhizoma Typhonii Gigantei), *Chan Tui*‡ (Periostracum Cicadae), and *Shi Chang Pu* (Rhizoma Acori Graminei) dredge Wind and dissipate the Blood, free the network vessels and increase pigmentation.
* *Hong Hua* (Flos Carthami Tinctorii) invigorates the Blood and dissipates Blood stasis.
* *Hei Zhi Ma* (Semen Sesami Indici) moistens Dryness and improves the complexion.

COLD CONGEALING

This pattern mainly affects the middle-aged and elderly and manifests as dull white patches on the lower part of the body and the extremities. The patches develop very slowly and may persist for years or throughout life. The tongue body is pale red with a thin white coating; the pulse is deep and thready.

Treatment principle
Dissipate Cold and free the network vessels.

Prescription
SHEN YING XIAO FENG SAN JIA JIAN
Wondrous Response Powder for Dispersing Wind, with modifications

Dang Shen (Radix Codonopsitis Pilosulae) 10g
Bai Zhi (Radix Angelicae Dahuricae) 10g
Cang Zhu (Rhizoma Atractylodis) 10g
He Shou Wu (Radix Polygoni Multiflori) 15g
Ji Xue Teng (Caulis Spatholobi) 15g
Ye Jiao Teng (Caulis Polygoni Multiflori) 15g
Dan Shen (Radix Salviae Miltiorrhizae) 15g
Hong Hua (Flos Carthami Tinctorii) 6g
Lu Lu Tong (Fructus Liquidambaris) 6g
*Ma Huang** (Herba Ephedrae) 6g
Guo Teng (Ramulus Uncariae cum Uncis) 6g
*Tian Ma** (Rhizoma Gastrodiae Elatae) 6g

Explanation
* *Dang Shen* (Radix Codonopsitis Pilosulae), *Bai Zhi* (Radix Angelicae Dahuricae), Cang Zhu (Rhizoma Atractylodis), and *Ma Huang** (Herba Ephedrae) augment Qi and warm Yang, dissipate Cold and free the network vessels.
* *He Shou Wu* (Radix Polygoni Multiflori), *Ji Xue Teng* (Caulis Spatholobi), *Ye Jiao Teng* (Caulis Polygoni Multiflori), and *Lu Lu Tong* (Fructus Liquidambaris) enrich and nourish the Liver and Kidneys, free the network vessels and increase pigmentation.
* *Dan Shen* (Radix Salviae Miltiorrhizae), *Hong Hua* (Flos Carthami Tinctorii), *Guo Teng* (Ramulus Uncariae cum Uncis), and *Tian Ma** (Rhizoma Gastrodiae Elatae) invigorate the Blood and transform Blood stasis, dredge Wind and expel pathogenic factors.

LIVER DEPRESSION

This pattern mostly affects women with irregular periods and manifests as pale pink patches, mostly limited to one location, but occasionally distributed throughout the body. As the lesions develop, the margins become more clearly defined. The evolution of the disease is often associated with excessive thought and preoccupation and depression. The tongue body is dark red with a scant coating; the pulse is wiry and rapid.

Treatment principle
Soothe the Liver and relieve Depression, invigorate the Blood and increase pigmentation.

Prescription
XIAO YAO SAN JIA JIAN
Free Wanderer Powder, with modifications

Dang Gui (Radix Angelicae Sinensis) 10g
Chao Bai Shao (Radix Paeoniae Lactiflorae, stir-fried) 12g

Fu Ling (Sclerotium Poriae Cocos) 10g
Gan Di Huang (Radix Rehmanniae Glutinosae Exsiccata) 10g
Yu Jin (Radix Curcumae) 6g
Ze Lan (Herba Lycopi Lucidi) 10g
Yi Mu Cao (Herba Leonuri Heterophylli) 15-30g
Cang Er Zi (Fructus Xanthii Sibirici) 12-15g
Ci Shi‡ (Magnetitum) 30g

Explanation

- *Dang Gui* (Radix Angelicae Sinensis), *Chao Bai Shao* (Radix Paeoniae Lactiflorae, stir-fried), *Fu Ling* (Sclerotium Poriae Cocos), *Gan Di Huang* (Radix Rehmanniae Glutinosae Exsiccata), and *Yu Jin* (Radix Curcumae) soothe the Liver and relieve Depression.
- *Ze Lan* (Herba Lycopi Lucidi) and *Yi Mu Cao* (Herba Leonuri Heterophylli) invigorate the Blood, dissipate Blood stasis and free the network vessels.
- *Cang Er Zi* (Fructus Xanthii Sibirici) dredges Wind and frees the orifices, conducting the effect of the other ingredients to the skin.
- *Ci Shi* ‡ (Magnetitum) settles the Liver and subdues Yang; the metal contained in this ingredient can promote the metabolism of pigment cells.

KIDNEY DEFICIENCY

This pattern manifests as porcelain-white patches with haphazard distribution. The evolution of the disease is closely related to overwork and/or excessive sexual activity. Men are more likely to be affected by this pattern with accompanying symptoms of impotence, dizziness and lassitude. The tongue body is pale red with a scant coating; the pulse is thready and weak.

Treatment principle

Enrich the Liver and supplement the Kidneys.

Prescription
WU ZI YAN ZONG WAN JIA JIAN

Five-Seed Progeny Decoction, with modifications

Sha Yuan Zi (Semen Astragali Complanati) 12g
She Chuang Zi (Fructus Cnidii Monnieri) 12g
Fu Pen Zi (Fructus Rubi Chingii) 12g
Gou Qi Zi (Fructus Lycii) 10g
Che Qian Zi (Semen Plantaginis) 10g
Sheng Di Huang (Radix Rehmanniae Glutinosae) 10g
Shu Di Huang (Radix Rehmanniae Glutinosae Conquita) 10g
Chi Shao (Radix Paeoniae Rubra) 10g
Dang Gui (Radix Angelicae Sinensis) 15g
He Shou Wu (Radix Polygoni Multiflori) 15g
Bai Ji Li (Fructus Tribuli Terrestris) 15g
Hei Zhi Ma (Semen Sesami Indici) 10-15g

Explanation

- *Sha Yuan Zi* (Semen Astragali Complanati), *She Chuang Zi* (Fructus Cnidii Monnieri), *Fu Pen Zi* (Fructus Rubi Chingii), *Gou Qi Zi* (Fructus Lycii), *Che Qian Zi* (Semen Plantaginis), and *Hei Zhi Ma* (Semen Sesami Indici) enrich the Liver and supplement the Kidneys.
- *Sheng Di Huang* (Radix Rehmanniae Glutinosae), *Shu Di Huang* (Radix Rehmanniae Glutinosae Conquita), *Chi Shao* (Radix Paeoniae Rubra), *Dang Gui* (Radix Angelicae Sinensis), and *He Shou Wu* (Radix Polygoni Multiflori) nourish the Blood and emolliate the Liver.
- *Bai Ji Li* (Fructus Tribuli Terrestris) dredges Wind and expels pathogenic factors, and stimulates the production of melanocytes.

General modifications

1. For impatience and irascibility, add *Mu Dan Pi* (Cortex Moutan Radicis), *Chong Lou* (Rhizoma Paridis) and *Jiao Zhi Zi* (Fructus Gardeniae Jasminoidis, scorch-fried).
2. For distending pain in the breasts or lumps in the breasts, add *Yuan Zhi* (Radix Polygalae Tenuifoliae), *Yan Hu Suo* (Rhizoma Corydalis Yanhusuo) and *Wang Bu Liu Xing* (Semen Vaccariae Segetalis).
3. For lesions on the face, add *Qiang Huo* (Rhizoma et Radix Notopterygii), *Sheng Ma* (Rhizoma Cimicifugae), *Jie Geng* (Radix Platycodi Grandiflori), and *Gao Ben* (Rhizoma et Radix Ligustici).
4. For lesions on the chest, add *Gua Lou Pi* (Pericarpium Trichosanthis) and *Xie Bai* (Bulbus Allii Macrostemi).
5. For lesions on the abdomen, add *Mu Xiang** (Radix Aucklandiae Lappae), *Wu Yao* (Radix Linderae Strychnifoliae) and *Xiang Fu* (Rhizoma Cyperi Rotundi).
6. For lesions on the lower limbs, add *Chuan Niu Xi* (Radix Cyathulae Officinalis), *Mu Gua* (Fructus Chaenomelis), *Bi Xie* (Rhizoma Dioscoreae Hypoglaucae seu Septemlobae), and *Can Sha*‡ (Excrementum Bombycis Mori).
7. For lesions on the upper limbs, add *Sang Zhi* (Ramulus Mori Albae) and *Jiang Huang* (Rhizoma Curcumae Longae).
8. For generalized lesions, add *Chan Tui* ‡ (Periostracum Cicadae), *Xi Xian Cao* (Herba Siegesbeckiae), *Pei Lan* (Herba Eupatorii Fortunei), *Fu Ping* (Herba Spirodelae Polyrrhizae), and *Cong Bai* (Bulbus Allii Fistulosi).
9. For prevalence of Wind, add *Qin Jiao* (Radix Gentianae Macrophyllae).
10. For prevalence of Cold, add *Gui Zhi* (Ramulus Cinnamomi Cassiae).
11. For prevalence of Damp, add *Huo Xiang* (Herba Agastaches seu Pogostemi) and *Pei Lan* (Herba Eupatorii Fortunei).
12. For prevalence of Blood stasis, add *Ze Lan* (Herba Lycopi Lucidi) and *Chuan Xiong* (Rhizoma Ligustici Chuanxiong).

13. For persistent lesions, add *Tan Xiang* (Lignum Santali Albi), *Chen Xiang* (Lignum Aquilariae Resinatum) and *Bai Zhi* (Radix Angelicae Dahuricae).
14. For prevalence of Blood Deficiency, add *E Jiao*‡ (Gelatinum Corii Asini) and *Sang Shen* (Fructus Mori Albae).
15. For knocks and falls, add *Ru Xiang* (Gummi Olibanum), *Mo Yao* (Myrrha) and *Su Mu* (Lignum Sappan).
16. For Qi Deficiency, add *Huang Qi* (Radix Astragali seu Hedysari).
17. For vaginal bleeding, add *E Jiao*‡ (Gelatinum Corii Asini).
18. For seminal emission, add *Long Gu*‡ (Os Draconis) and *Mu Li*‡ (Concha Ostreae).
19. Where there is a family history, take *Liu Wei Di Huang Wan* (Six-Ingredient Rehmannia Pill) with the prepared decoction.

EXTERNAL TREATMENT

- For lesions with widespread distribution or covering a large area, apply one of the following pastes:
1. Grind *Bai Fu Zi* (Rhizoma Typhonii Gigantei) 9g and *Liu Huang*‡ (Sulphur) 9g into a fine powder and mix with *Sheng Jiang Zhi* (Succus Rhizomatis Zingiberis Officinalis Recens).
2. Grind *Xi Xin** (Herba cum Radice Asari) 6g, *Bu Gu Zhi* (Fructus Psoraleae Corylifoliae)vi 10g and *Bai Zhi* (Radix Angelicae Dahuricae) 3g into a fine powder and mix with vinegar.
3. Grind *Jing Jie Sui* (Spica Schizonepetae Tenuifoliae) 3g, *Fang Feng* (Radix Ledebouriellae Divaricatae) 3g, *Qiang Huo* (Rhizoma et Radix Notopterygii) 3g, *Dang Gui Wei* (Extremitas Radicis Angelicae Sinensis) 3g, *Tou Gu Cao* (Herba Speranskiae seu Impatientis) 3g, *Bu Gu Zhi* (Fructus Psoraleae Corylifoliae) 10g, *Ku Fan*‡ (Alumen Praeparatum) 3g and *Di Fu Zi* (Fructus Kochiae Scopariae) 9g into a fine powder and mix with pork lard. Then wrap the mixture in a piece of cloth and apply it to the lesions.
- For circumscribed lesions or lesions on the face or at the transition zone between the skin and the mucosa, apply the juice of fresh eggplant/aubergine (*Qie Zi*, Radix Solani Melongenae) to the affected area two or three times a day.

ACUPUNCTURE

Selection of points according to pattern identification
Points

- For disharmony between Qi and Blood, select SP-10 Xuehai, SP-6 Sanyinjiao, ST-36 Zusanli, and LI-11 Quchi.
- For insufficiency of the Liver and Kidneys, select BL-18 Ganshu, BL-23 Shenshu, GV-4 Mingmen, LR-3 Taichong, KI-3 Taixi, and SP-6 Sanyinjiao.
- For Blood stasis, select SP-6 Sanyinjiao, SP-10 Xuehai, LR-2 Xingjian, GB-31 Fengshi, and BL-17 Geshu.

Technique: Apply the reinforcing method for insufficiency of the Liver and Kidneys, the even method for disharmony between Qi and Blood and the reducing method for Blood stasis. Retain the needles for 15-30 minutes. Treat once a day or every other day for three months.

Selection of adjacent points
Points

- For involvement of the head and face, select LI-4 Hegu and GB-20 Fengchi.
- For involvement of the abdomen, select CV-12 Zhongwan.
- For involvement of the chest, select CV-17 Danzhong.
- For involvement of the upper limb, select LI-11 Quchi.
- For involvement of the lower limb, select SP-10 Xuehai and SP-6 Sanyinjiao.

Technique: Apply the even method and retain the needles for 30 minutes after obtaining Qi. Treat once a day for three months.

Explanation

- LI-11 Quchi, GB-20 Fengchi, LR-3 Taichong, and GB-31 Fengshi dissipate Wind and free the network vessels.
- SP-10 Xuehai, BL-23 Shenshu, KI-3 Taixi, and GV-4 Mingmen enrich the Liver and supplement the Kidneys.
- SP-6 Sanyinjiao, BL-17 Geshu, BL-18 Ganshu, CV-17 Danzhong, and LR-2 Xingjian regulate Qi and invigorate the Blood.
- ST-36 Zusanli, CV-12 Zhongwan and LI-4 Hegu support the Spleen and consolidate the Root.

EAR ACUPUNCTURE

Points: Lung, Occiput, Endocrine, Adrenal Gland, and points corresponding to the area of the lesions.
Technique: Select two or three points for each session and stimulate the selected points with embedded needles. Change the needles once a week and embed in the other points.

---

vi External application of *Bu Gu Zhi* (Fructus Psoraleae Corylifoliae) results in photosensitivity and exposure to ultraviolet rays must be limited to avoid skin reaction.

SEVEN-STAR NEEDLING

Points: Ashi points (the site of the lesions).

Technique: After routine sterilization of the area, tap gently from the margins to the center in concentric circles until the skin becomes red without bleeding or until mild bleeding is induced. Treat every other day.

PRICKING AND CUPPING METHOD

Points: Ashi points (the site of the lesions).

Technique: Use a three-edged needle to prick the center of the lesions in the shape of a plum-blossom, then apply fire-cupping to drain the blood out. Treat once a week or once a fortnight.

Indication: Blood stasis obstructing the network vessels.

PRICKING AND MOXIBUSTION METHOD

Points: Xiaxia (located in the depression slightly above the junction of the middle third and lower third of the lateral aspect of the biceps brachii) and Dianfeng (located on the palmar aspect of the proximal side of the crease of the distal interphalangeal articulations of the hand).

Technique: First prick the points with a three-edged needle to induce slight bleeding. Then apply direct moxibustion to one of the Dianfeng points with three moxa cones prepared from the following ingredients:

Wu Bei Zi‡ (Galla Rhois Chinensis) 10g
Sang Ye (Folium Mori Albae) 10g
Wei Ling Xian (Radix Clematidis) 10g
Dang Gui (Radix Angelicae Sinensis) 10g
Chuan Xiong (Rhizoma Ligustici Chuanxiong) 10g
Bai Dou Kou (Fructus Amomi Kravanh) 10g
Shi Chang Pu (Rhizoma Acori Graminei) 30g
Bai Jie Zi (Semen Sinapis Albae) 30g
Guo Teng (Ramulus Uncariae cum Uncis) 10g
*Tian Ma** (Rhizoma Gastrodiae Elatae) 10g

Grind the ingredients into a fine powder to be used for moxibustion. Treat once a day, paying particular attention to avoid blistering.

Clinical notes

- The main focus in TCM is on Liver Depression, treated by dredging the Liver and regulating Qi; on Kidney Deficiency, treated by boosting the Kidneys and consolidating the Root; and on Qi Deficiency, treated by supplementing Qi with warmth and sweetness. Adding materia medica for invigorating pigmentation enhances the effectiveness of the treatment.

- Since this disease is prolonged and persistent, the patient must be encouraged to have confidence in the treatment and to persevere with it, sometimes for one year or more. The author's clinical experience suggests the treatment will bring results with the exception of lesions on the dorsum of the hand, which are very stubborn.

Advice for the patient

- Apply external medications containing heavy metals sparingly, as they may damage the skin, especially facial skin.
- Avoid eating seafood and stimulating food and cut down on acidy fruit and vegetables such as tomatoes.
- Do not take Vitamin C supplements.

Case histories

Case 1

Patient
Female, aged 18.

Clinical manifestations
When the patient was 10, a small white patch had appeared on her face, gradually enlarging to approximately 1cm in diameter. Two years ago, numerous small white patches began to appear on the limbs and trunk. There were no systemic symptoms. Although the patient was thin, she had a strong constitution and there was no history of chronic disorders. The tongue body was pale red with a scant coating; the pulse was deep and thready. Examination revealed a white patch 7.5 x 5 cm on the left temple, two hypopigmented patches (one large and one small) on each arm and a white patch approximately 10 x 6 cm on the neck.

Pattern identification
Yin Deficiency of the Liver and Kidneys, disharmony of Qi and Blood, Qi stagnation and Blood stasis.

Treatment principle
Enrich and supplement the Liver and Kidneys, nourish the Blood and augment Qi, invigorate the Blood and free the network vessels.

Prescription ingredients
Dang Gui (Radix Angelicae Sinensis) 10g
Nü Zhen Zi (Fructus Ligustri Lucidi) 10g
Shu Di Huang (Radix Rehmanniae Glutinosae Conquita) 15g
Shan Zhu Yu (Fructus Corni Officinalis) 10g
Chi Shao (Radix Paeoniae Rubra) 15g
Bai Shao (Radix Paeoniae Lactiflorae) 15g
Bei Sha Shen (Radix Glehniae Littoralis) 15g
Sang Shen (Fructus Mori Albae) 30g
Hei Zhi Ma (Semen Sesami Indici) 15g
Bu Gu Zhi (Fructus Psoraleae Corylifoliae) 10g
Bai Ji Li (Fructus Tribuli Terrestris) 15g
Gui Zhi (Ramulus Cinnamomi Cassiae) 10g

Hong Hua (Flos Carthami Tinctorii) 10g
Chuan Xiong (Rhizoma Ligustici Chuanxiong) 10g
*Mu Xiang** (Radix Aucklandiae Lappae) 8g
Dan Shen (Radix Salviae Miltiorrhizae) 10g

One bag a day was used to prepare a decoction, taken twice a day.

External treatment

Bu Gu Zhi (Fructus Psoraleae Corylifoliae) 15g, crushed and steeped in *Bai Bu Ding* (Stemona Root Tincture) for one week. The liquid was then used as a rub once a day.

Outcome

After three months, most of the lesions had shrunk, especially those on the face and neck, and spots of repigmentation had appeared around the hair follicles in the center of the lesions on the trunk. Repigmented areas were darker than before. The patient continued the treatment for another two months, after which the repigmented areas were larger. The patient then decided not to proceed with further treatment. [17]

Case 2
Patient

Female, aged 23.

Clinical manifestations

The patient had been suffering from white patches on the forehead for three or four years, but in the last six months these patches had developed rapidly and spread to the cheeks, expanding in size. The patient felt general malaise. The tongue body was red with a thin yellow coating; the pulse was calm.

Pattern identification

Wind and Dampness fighting each other, disharmony of Qi and Blood.

Treatment principle

Dispel Wind-Damp, regulate the Ying and Wei levels, harmonize Qi and Blood.

Prescription ingredients

Xi Xian Cao (Herba Siegesbeckiae) 9g
Cang Er Cao (Caulis et Folium Xanthii Sibirici) 9g
Fu Ping (Herba Spirodelae Polyrrhizae) 9g
Chuan Xiong (Rhizoma Ligustici Chuanxiong) 9g
Hong Hua (Flos Carthami Tinctorii) 9g
Bu Gu Zhi (Fructus Psoraleae Corylifoliae) 12g
Chi Shao (Radix Paeoniae Rubra) 12g
Bai Zhi (Radix Angelicae Dahuricae) 4.5g
Gui Zhi (Ramulus Cinnamomi Cassiae) 3g

Second visit

After one month, there was no obvious improvement. The white patches were bordered by a purple halo. The tongue body was red with a thin coating; the pulse was calm. This persistent disease had entered the network vessels, resulting in an amended treatment principle.

Amended treatment principle

Invigorate the Blood and dispel Blood stasis, dispel Wind and free the network vessels.

Prescription ingredients

Dang Gui Wei (Extremitas Radicis Angelicae Sinensis) 9g
Chuan Xiong (Rhizoma Ligustici Chuanxiong) 9g
Mu Dan Pi (Cortex Moutan Radicis) 9g
Gui Zhi (Ramulus Cinnamomi Cassiae) 9g
Wu Shao She‡ (Zaocys Dhumnades) 9g
Bai Xian Pi (Cortex Dictamni Dasycarpi Radicis) 9g
Di Fu Zi (Fructus Kochiae Scopariae) 9g
Xi Xian Cao (Herba Siegesbeckiae) 9g
Chi Shao (Radix Paeoniae Rubra) 15g

Outcome

After a further month, pigmentation had returned to 70 percent of the affected areas. The second prescription was continued for another month to consolidate recovery. [18]

Modern clinical experience

INTERNAL TREATMENT

1. **Tu** treated 195 vitiligo patients with a decoction. [19]

Prescription
KE BAI TANG
Overcoming Vitiligo Decoction

He Shou Wu (Radix Polygoni Multiflori) 10g
Chai Hu (Radix Bupleuri) 10g
Bu Gu Zhi (Fructus Psoraleae Corylifoliae) 10g
Shan Zhu Yu (Fructus Corni Officinalis) 10g
Gou Qi Zi (Fructus Lycii) 10g
Mu Dan Pi (Cortex Moutan Radicis) 10g
Chi Shao (Radix Paeoniae Rubra) 10g
Bai Zhi (Radix Angelicae Dahuricae) 10g
Dang Shen (Radix Codonopsitis Pilosulae) 15g
Gui Zhi (Ramulus Cinnamomi Cassiae) 6g
Sheng Jiang (Rhizoma Zingiberis Officinalis Recens) 3g

One bag a day was used to prepare a decoction, taken twice a day. A course of treatment lasted three months. After four courses, 23 patients had recovered, 41 had shown significant improvement, 81 some improvement and 50 no improvement.

2. **Zhu** treated vitiligo with tablets. [20]

Prescription
QU BAI PIAN
Dispelling Vitiligo Tablet

Dang Shen (Radix Codonopsitis Pilosulae) 10g
Huang Qin (Radix Scutellariae Baicalensis) 10g
Bai Zhu (Rhizoma Atractylodis Macrocephalae) 10g
Fu Ling (Sclerotium Poriae Cocos) 10g
Zi Cao (Radix Arnebiae seu Lithospermi) 10g
Bai Ji Li (Fructus Tribuli Terrestris) 15g
He Shou Wu (Radix Polygoni Multiflori) 15g

Cang Zhu (Rhizoma Atractylodis) 6g
Mai Men Dong (Radix Ophiopogonis Japonici) 15g
Han Lian Cao (Herba Ecliptae Prostratae) 10g
Dan Shen (Radix Salviae Miltiorrhizae) 10g
Tao Ren (Semen Persicae) 10g
Hong Hua (Flos Carthami Tinctorii) 10g
Bu Gu Zhi (Fructus Psoraleae Corylifoliae) 10g
Gan Cao (Radix Glycyrrhizae) 6g
Zi Ran Tong‡ (Pyritum) 6g

These ingredients were made into an extract with water and then pressed into tablets of 0.3g. The dosage for adults was six tablets three times a day. A course of treatment lasted three months and results were seen after one or two courses. This treatment proved more effective for circumscribed lesions than for other types of vitiligo. During treatment, a few patients complained of gastro-intestinal reaction and increased menstrual flow.

3. **Zhao** also preferred a pill form for treatment of this disease. [21]

Prescription
QU BAI WAN
Dispelling Vitiligo Pill

Ye Jiao Teng (Caulis Polygoni Multiflori) 300g
Huang Qi (Radix Astragali seu Hedysari) 300g
Cang Zhu (Rhizoma Atractylodis) 100g
Bai Zhu (Rhizoma Atractylodis Macrocephalae) 100g
Sheng Di Huang (Radix Rehmanniae Glutinosae) 100g
Dang Gui (Radix Angelicae Sinensis) 100g
Shan Yao (Radix Dioscoreae Oppositae) 100g
Bai Zhi (Radix Angelicae Dahuricae) 100g
Fang Feng (Radix Ledebouriellae Divaricatae) 100g
Fu Ling (Sclerotium Poriae Cocos) 150g
Ze Xie (Rhizoma Alismatis Orientalis) 150g
Dong Gua Pi (Epicarpium Benincasae Hispidae) 150g
Xi Xian Cao (Herba Siegesbeckiae) 150g
He Shou Wu (Radix Polygoni Multiflori) 150g
Chai Hu (Radix Bupleuri) 60g

These ingredients were ground into a fine powder and mixed with honey to make 6g pills. Treatment consisted of two pills twice a day, with the period of treatment ranging from 15 days to two years.

COMBINATION OF INTERNAL AND EXTERNAL TREATMENT

1. **Yin** treated circumscribed, widespread, discretely distributed, and unilateral vitiligo with one prescription. [22]

Prescription ingredients
Chao Chai Hu (Radix Bupleuri, stir-fried) 10g
Bai Shao (Radix Paeoniae Lactiflorae) 10g

Xiang Fu (Rhizoma Cyperi Rotundi) 10g
Chuan Xiong (Rhizoma Ligustici Chuanxiong) 10g
Dang Gui (Radix Angelicae Sinensis) 10g
Bai Ji Li (Fructus Tribuli Terrestris) 15g
Huang Qi (Radix Astragali seu Hedysari) 15g
Zi Ran Tong‡ (Pyritum) 6g
Hong Hua (Flos Carthami Tinctorii) 6g
Bu Gu Zhi (Fructus Psoraleae Corylifoliae) 10g
Fang Feng (Radix Ledebouriellae Divaricatae) 6g
Zhi He Shou Wu (Radix Polygoni Multiflori Praeparata) 15g
Cang Er Cao (Caulis et Folium Xanthii Sibirici) 6g

One bag a day was used to prepare a decoction, taken twice a day for two days. The decoction was also used externally; a piece of gauze dipped in the decoction was applied to the lesions four or five times a day. Results were seen after 6-18 weeks.

2. **Liu** treated vitiligo with a combination of a decoction and a tincture. [23]

Internal prescription
XIAO BAI TANG
Dispersing Vitiligo Decoction

Bai Xian Pi (Cortex Dictamni Dasycarpi Radicis) 16g
Dang Gui (Radix Angelicae Sinensis) 16g
Chuan Xiong (Rhizoma Ligustici Chuanxiong) 12g
Chi Shao (Radix Paeoniae Rubra) 12g
Mu Dan Pi (Cortex Moutan Radicis) 12g
Gou Qi Zi (Fructus Lycii) 12g
Han Lian Cao (Herba Ecliptae Prostratae) 12g
Fang Feng (Radix Ledebouriellae Divaricatae) 12g
Gui Zhi (Ramulus Cinnamomi Cassiae) 12g
Huang Qi (Radix Astragali seu Hedysari) 14g
He Shou Wu (Radix Polygoni Multiflori) 14g
Gan Cao (Radix Glycyrrhizae) 6g

One bag a day was used to prepare a decoction, taken three times a day. A course of treatment lasted 30 days.

External prescription
XIAO BAI DING
Dispersing Vitiligo Tincture

Bu Gu Zhi (Fructus Psoraleae Corylifoliae) 30g
Bai Zhi (Radix Angelicae Dahuricae) 20g
Rou Gui (Cortex Cinnamomi Cassiae) 10g

The ingredients were steeped in 100ml of 75 percent alcohol for 17 days. After filtering, the liquid was applied to the affected area once or twice a day.

Patients were told to expose the treated skin to sunlight. The combined treatment required five to 26 months with an average of 13 months. Young patients, vitiligo of recent onset and circumscribed vitiligo usually responded well to the treatment.

3. **Du** combined internal treatment with two alternating external applications. [24]

Internal prescription
GUI PI TANG
Decoction for Restoring the Spleen

Bai Zhu (Rhizoma Atractylodis Macrocephalae) 10g
Fu Ling (Sclerotium Poriae Cocos) 10g
Huang Qi (Radix Astragali seu Hedysari) 15g
Long Yan Rou (Arillus Euphoriae Longanae) 10g
Suan Zao Ren (Semen Ziziphi Spinosae) 10g
Dang Shen (Radix Codonopsitis Pilosulae) 10g
*Mu Xiang** (Radix Aucklandiae Lappae) 6g
Zhi Gan Cao (Radix Glycyrrhizae, mix-fried with honey) 6g
Dang Gui (Radix Angelicae Sinensis) 10g
Yuan Zhi (Radix Polygalae) 6g
Sheng Jiang (Rhizoma Zingiberis Officinalis Recens) 6g
Da Zao (Fructus Ziziphi Jujubae) 10g

Modifications

1. For Heat in the Blood, *Bai Mao Gen* (Rhizoma Imperatae Cylindricae), *Nü Zhen Zi* (Fructus Ligustri Lucidi) and *Huai Hua* (Flos Sophorae Japonicae) were added.
2. For Blood stasis, *Tao Ren* (Semen Persicae), *Hong Hua* (Flos Carthami Tinctorii) and *San Qi* (Radix Notoginseng) were added.
3. For Qi Deficiency, *Ren Shen* (Radix Ginseng) and *Huang Qi* (Radix Astragali seu Hedysari) were added.
4. For Damp-Heat, *Yin Chen Hao* (Herba Artemisiae Scopariae), *Zhi Zi* (Fructus Gardeniae Jasminoidis), *Long Dan Cao* (Radix Gentianae Scabrae), and *Huo*

Xiang (Herba Agastaches seu Pogostemi) were added.

External prescription 1
BAI DIAN YI HAO
No. 1 Vitiligo Prescription

Ding Xiang (Flos Caryophylli) 30g
Da Huang (Radix et Rhizoma Rhei) 30g
Bai Zhi (Radix Angelicae Dahuricae) 50g
Zi Cao (Radix Arnebiae seu Lithospermi) 30g
Hua Jiao (Pericarpium Zanthoxyli) 30g
Bu Gu Zhi (Fructus Psoraleae Corylifoliae) 50g
Zi Ran Tong ‡ (Pyritum) 30g

These ingredients were steeped in mature vinegar for five days before application to the affected area twice a day for one week.

External prescription 2
BAI DIAN ER HAO
No. 2 Vitiligo Prescription

Tou Gu Cao (Herba Speranskiae seu Impatientis) 50g
Lei Wan (Sclerotium Omphaliae Lapidescens) 30g
Ding Xiang (Flos Caryophylli) 30g
Hua Jiao (Pericarpium Zanthoxyli) 30g
Hong Hua (Flos Carthami Tinctorii) 30g
Bu Gu Zhi (Fructus Psoraleae Corylifoliae) 50g

These ingredients were steeped in 60 percent white alcohol for five days before application to the affected area once a day for the second week. The two external prescriptions were then used alternately. Results were seen between four and fifteen months.

References

1. An Jiafeng and Zhang Fan, *Zhang Zhi Li Pi Fu Bing Yi An Xuan Cui* [A Collection of Zhang Zhili's Skin Disease Cases] (Beijing: People's Medical Publishing House, 1994), 227.
2. Yu Youping, *Zhong Yi Yao Zhi Liao Huang He Ban 34 Li* [Treatment of 34 Cases of Melasma with Traditional Chinese Medicine and Materia Medica], *Xin Zhong Yi* [New Journal of Traditional Chinese Medicine] 29, 11 (1997): 39.
3. Jiang Ling, *Bian Zheng Fen Xing Zhi Liao Huang He Ban 60 Li* [Treatment of 60 Cases of Melasma Based on Pattern Identification], *Zhe Jiang Zhong Yi Za Zhi* [Zhejiang Journal of Traditional Chinese Medicine] 33, 1 (1998): 34.
4. Yang Wenxi, *124 Li Huang He Ban Lin Chuang Liao Xiao Fen Xi* [Analysis of the Clinical Efficacy of Treatment of 124 Cases of Melasma], *Tian Jin Zhong Yi* [Tianjin Journal of Traditional Chinese Medicine] 16, 1 (1999): 18.
5. Li Xiumin, *70 Li Huang He Ban De Bian Zheng Lun Zhi* [Treatment of 70 Cases of Melasma Based on Pattern Identification], *Zhong Yi Za Zhi* [Journal of Traditional Chinese Medicine] 3 (1986): 38.
6. Chen Yijing, *Yang Yan Qu Ban Tang Zhi Liao Huang He Ban* [Treatment of Melasma with *Yang Yan Qu Ban Tang* (Decoction for Nourishing the Face and Dispelling Macules)], *Shang Hai Zhong Yi Yao Za Zhi* [Shanghai Journal of Traditional Chinese Medicine and Materia Medica] 6 (1999): 33.
7. Xu Zhicheng, *Xiao Ban Jie Rong Wan Zhi Liao Fu Nü Huang He Ban 48 Li Liao Xiao Guan Cha* [Observation of the Effectiveness of Treatment of 48 Cases of Melasma in Women with *Xiao Ban Jie Rong Wan* (Pill for Dispersing Macules and Cleansing the Countenance)], *Hu Nan Zhong Yi* [Hunan Journal of Traditional Chinese Medicine] 19, 4 (1999): 37.
8. Peng Xuehai, *Xue Fu Zhu Yu Tang Zhi Liao Huang He Ban 46 Li* [Treatment of 46 Cases of Melasma with *Xue Fu Zhu Yu Tang* (Decoction for Expelling Stasis from the House of Blood)], *She Zhi* [Snake Journal] 11, 2 (1999): 58.
9. Wang Hongwei, *Liang Xue Huo Xue Fa Zhi Liao Huang He Ban 50 Li* [Treatment of 50 Cases of Melasma with the

Method of Cooling and Invigorating the Blood], *Shi Yong Zhong Yi Yao Za Zhi* [Journal of Practical Traditional Chinese Medicine and Materia Medica] 15, 3 (1999): 22-23.

10. Luan Yuhui, *Er Zhen Jia Er Xue Tie Ya Fa Zhi Liao Huang He Ban 60 Li Lin Chuang Guan Cha* [Clinical Observation of the Treatment of 60 Cases of Melasma with Ear Acupuncture and Ear Pressure], *Zhong Guo Zhen Jiu* [Chinese Journal of Acupuncture and Moxibustion] 16, 9 (1996): 17-18.

11. Pan Gui, *Zhong Xi Yi Jie He Zhi Liao Huang He Ban 100 Li* [Treatment of 100 Cases of Melasma with TCM and Western Medicine], *Xin Zhong Yi* [New Journal of Traditional Chinese Medicine] 26, 7 (1994): 50.

12. Zhang Guanrong, *Xing Pi Zhu Mai Tang Zhi Liao Rui Er Hei Bian Bing 110 Li* [Treatment of 110 Cases of Melanosis with *Xing Pi Zhu Mai Tang* (Decoction for Arousing the Spleen and Expelling Haze)], *Zhe Jiang Zhong Yi Za Zhi* [Zhejiang Journal of Traditional Chinese Medicine] 31, 11 (1996): 498.

13. Li Chuanyun, *San Zi Qi Bai Tang Zhi Liao Li Hei Ban 36 Li* [Treatment of 36 Cases of Melanosis with *San Zi Qi Bai Tang* (Three-Seed Seven-Whites Decoction)], *Hei Long Jiang Zhong Yi Yao* [Heilongjiang Journal of Traditional Chinese Medicine and Materia Medica] 1 (1997): 43.

14. Yang Jianzhen, *Yi Shen Huo Xue Tang Zhi Liao Pi Fu Hei Bian Bing 58 Li* [Treatment of 58 Cases of Melanosis with *Yi Shen Huo Xue Tang* (Decoction for Boosting the Kidneys and Invigorating the Blood)], *Hu Nan Zhong Yi Xue Yuan Xue Bao* [Journal of Hunan College of Traditional Chinese Medicine] 19, 1 (1999): 55.

15. Zhu Xiaohua, *Er Zi Qu Ban Gao He Mian Mo Zhi Liao Li Hei Ban 87 Li Liao Xiao Guan Cha* [Observation of the Effectiveness of Treatment of 87 Cases of Melanosis with *Er Zi Qu Ban Gao* (Two-Seed Paste for Dispelling Macules) Applied in a Facial Mask], *Hu Nan Zhong Yi Xue Yuan Xue Bao* [Journal of Hunan College of Traditional Chinese Medicine] 19, 3 (1999): 54.

16. Hu Yuling, *Zhong Xi Yi Jie He Zhi Liao Hei Bian Bing 18 Li Liao Xiao Guan Cha* [Observation of the Effectiveness of Treatment of 18 Cases of Melanosis with a Combination of TCM and Western Medicine], *Shi Yong Zhong Xi Yi Jie He Za Zhi* [Practical Journal of Integrated TCM and Western Medicine] 11, 6 (1998): 555.

17. Zhang Zhili, *Zhang Zhi Li Pi Fu Bing Lin Chuang Jing Yan Ji Yao* [A Collection of Zhang Zhili's Clinical Experiences in the Treatment of Skin Diseases] (Beijing: China Medical Science and Technology Publishing House, 2001), 320.

18. Gu Bohua, *Wai Ke Jing Yan Xuan* [A Selection of Gu Bohua's Experiences in the Treatment of External Diseases] (Shanghai: Shanghai People's Publishing House, 1977), 111.

19. Tu Fuhan, *Ke Bai Tang Zhi Liao Bai Dian Feng* [Treatment of Vitiligo with *Ke Bai Tang* (Overcoming Vitiligo Decoction)], *Shan Dong Zhong Yi Za Zhi* [Shandong Journal of Traditional Chinese Medicine] 17, 11 (1998): 499.

20. Zhu Tiejun, *Zhong Yao Qu Bai Pian Zhi Liao Bai Dian Feng 187 Li Lin Chuang Guan Cha* [Clinical Observation of the Treatment of 187 Cases of Vitiligo with the Herbal Medicine *Qu Bai Pian* (Dispelling Vitiligo Tablet)], *Zhong Guo Zhong Xi Yi Jie He Za Zhi* [Journal of Integrated TCM and Western Medicine] 14, 7 (1994): 441-2.

21. Zhao Xiurong, *Qu Bai Wan Zhi Liao Pi Xu Xing Bai Dian Feng Liao Xiao Guan Cha* [Observation of the Effectiveness of Treatment of Vitiligo due to Spleen Deficiency with *Qu Bai Wan* (Dispelling Vitiligo Pill)], *Pi Fu Bing Yu Xing Bing* [Skin Diseases and Venereal Diseases] 21, 3 (1999): 20-21.

22. Yin Ping, *Shu Gan Jie Du, Huo Xue Hua Yu Zhi Liao Bai Dian Feng 56 Li Liao Xiao Guan Cha* [Observation of the Effectiveness of Treatment of 56 Cases of Vitiligo by Dredging the Liver to Relieve Depression and Invigorating the Blood to Transform Stasis], *Bei Jing Zhong Yi* [Beijing Journal of Traditional Chinese Medicine] 3 (1998): 31.

23. Liu Yongxue, *Zhong Yao Xiao Bai Tang Yu Xiao Bai Ding Zhi Liao Bai Dian Feng Lin Chuang Guan Cha* [Clinical Observation of the Treatment of Vitiligo with *Xiao Bai Tang* (Dispersing Vitiligo Decoction) and *Xiao Bai Ding* (Dispersing Vitiligo Tincture)], *Zhong Hua Pi Fu Ke Za Zhi* [Chinese Journal of Dermatology] 32, 4 (1999): 268-9.

24. Du Ruiming, *Zhong Xi Yi Jie He Zhi Liao Bai Dian Feng 232 Li* [Treatment of 232 Cases of Vitiligo with TCM and Western Medicine], *Shan Xi Zhong Yi* [Shanxi Journal of Traditional Chinese Medicine] 12, 3 (1996): 22-23.

Disorders of keratinization

The four layers of the epidermis represent the stages of maturation of keratin by keratinocytes. Most of the basal cell layer (stratum basale) is comprised of dividing or non-dividing keratinocytes. Dividing keratinocytes migrate upward through the prickle cell layer (stratum spinosum) to the granular cell layer (stratum granulosum), where the cells lose their nuclei. These dead cells, known as corneocytes, are then pushed up into the horny layer (stratum corneum), where they are held together by intercellular lipids. Corneocytes are subsequently shed from the skin surface, a process that is usually invisible to the naked eye.

Under normal circumstances, the number of scales shed is balanced by the number of new cells reaching the horny layer so that its thickness does not change.

However, abnormalities of keratinization or cell cohesion can result in thickening of the horny layer or in the skin surface becoming dry and scaly. These changes may be local or generalized.

The disorders of keratinization included in this chapter also come into the category of inherited skin diseases, with the defect being related to a single gene. Other skin disorders such as psoriasis or corns also have abnormalities of keratinization as one of their features; these disorders are discussed in other chapters.

In TCM, disorders of keratinization are generally considered to be caused by the skin being deprived of nourishment as a result of insufficiency of Ying Qi (Nutritive Qi) and Blood or where the Spleen fails in its function of distributing Body Fluids.

Ichthyosis vulgaris
寻常性鱼鳞病

Ichthyosis vulgaris is an inherited abnormality of the skin, with those affected having fewer sweat and sebaceous glands than normal and a dry rough skin with pronounced scaling, giving the skin a fish-scale pattern. This disorder, which is autosomal dominant, is generally noted in early to middle childhood and occurs in varying degrees of severity. Around 1 in 300 people have the disorder, although mild cases may be barely noticeable.

In TCM, ichthyosis is also known as *she shen* (snake body), *she pi xuan* (snake-skin tinea) or *yu lin xuan* (fish-scale tinea).

Clinical manifestations

- A family history is likely, but may be hard to ascertain due to incomplete penetrance of the disorder. Onset generally occurs in early to middle childhood.
- Ichthyosis usually involves the extensor aspects of the limbs, and may become generalized in severe cases.
- Skin lesions vary in severity. Mild cases exhibit superficial coarse, thin, rectangular, dry scales in a net-like distribution. More serious cases present as dirty-looking, thicker squames arranged like fish scales; in severe cases, there may be keratinization and lichenification of the palms and soles, possibly with fissuring and accentuation of the skin creases.
- Keratosis pilaris may also be present on the limbs.
- Scales are more noticeable in winter and may become itchy. The condition tends to subside in summer or in warmer climates. It may improve in some patients in adulthood.
- Systemic symptoms are usually absent.

Etiology and pathology

- Congenital insufficiency of Kidney-Essence results in depletion of and damage to Ying Qi (Nutritive Qi) and Blood. Where this is combined with acquired disharmony of the Spleen and Stomach, it gives rise to Blood Deficiency, which generates Wind and Dryness, depriving the skin and flesh of nourishment. In addition, where Ying Qi and Blood are insufficient, an external invasion of Wind may also occur. In both instances, the appearance of dry scales (ichthyosis vulgaris) will result.

- The combination of insufficiency of Ying Qi (Nutritive Qi) and Blood with fetal Heat that has not been cleared also gives rise to Blood Deficiency generating Wind and Dryness, resulting in Qi stagnation and Blood stasis in the channels and vessels. This can impair the generation of new Blood, depriving the skin of nourishment and making it dry and scaly.

Pattern identification and treatment

INTERNAL TREATMENT

QI STAGNATION AND BLOOD STASIS

The disease generally appears in early childhood and there is normally a family history. The skin is dry with symmetrical scaling, which is more pronounced on the extensor aspects of the limbs. Rough skin or diffuse keratinization of the palms and soles may occur, with fissuring in severe conditions. Symptoms are exacerbated in winter and alleviated in summer, or may vary intermittently. The tongue body is dull purple with stasis spots or marks; the pulse is rough.

Treatment principle
Augment Qi and nourish the Blood, diffuse the Lungs and moisten the skin.

Prescription
YU LIN TANG JIA JIAN
Fish Scale Decoction, with modifications[i]

Huang Qi (Radix Astragali seu Hedysari) 50g
Hei Zhi Ma (Semen Sesami Indici) 40g
Dan Shen (Radix Salviae Miltiorrhizae) 25g
Di Fu Zi (Fructus Kochiae Scopariae) 25g
Dang Gui (Radix Angelicae Sinensis) 20g
Sheng Di Huang (Radix Rehmanniae Glutinosae) 20g
Shu Di Huang (Radix Rehmanniae Glutinosae Conquita) 20g
He Shou Wu (Radix Polygoni Multiflori) 20g
Shan Yao (Radix Dioscoreae Oppositae) 15g
Fang Feng (Radix Ledebouriellae Divaricatae) 15g
Gan Cao (Radix Glycyrrhizae) 10g
Gou Qi Zi (Fructus Lycii) 12g

Explanation
- *Huang Qi* (Radix Astragali seu Hedysari), *Hei Zhi Ma* (Semen Sesami Indici), *Dang Gui* (Radix Angelicae Sinensis), *Sheng Di Huang* (Radix Rehmanniae Glutinosae), *Shu Di Huang* (Radix Rehmanniae Glutinosae Conquita), and *He Shou Wu* (Radix Polygoni Multiflori) augment Qi and nourish the Blood, enrich Yin and moisten Dryness.
- *Shan Yao* (Radix Dioscoreae Oppositae), *Gou Qi Zi* (Fructus Lycii), *Gan Cao* (Radix Glycyrrhizae), and *Di Fu Zi* (Fructus Kochiae Scopariae) nourish Yin and moisten the skin, dispel Wind and alleviate itching.
- *Fang Feng* (Radix Ledebouriellae Divaricatae) diffuses the Lungs and moistens the skin.
- *Dan Shen* (Radix Salviae Miltiorrhizae) invigorates the Blood and frees the network vessels to promote nourishment of the skin by Qi and Blood.

INSUFFICIENCY OF YING QI AND BLOOD

This syndrome occurs in early to middle childhood. The skin is dry and rough. The skin surface is covered by a layer of dirty or grayish-white scales separated by white, reticular grooves. Calluses may appear on the hands and feet, which may also become fissured. The hair is lusterless, dry and thinning, and the nails become brittle. The skin is mildly pruritic, with the itching usually exacerbating in winter. Patients are thin and weak with a pale, lusterless complexion. The tongue body is pale red with a thin white coating; the pulse is wiry and thready.

Treatment principle
Nourish and invigorate the Blood, moisten and soften the skin.

Prescription
YANG XUE RUN FU YIN JIA JIAN
Decoction for Nourishing the Blood and Moistening the Skin, with modifications

Dang Gui (Radix Angelicae Sinensis) 10g
Chi Shao (Radix Paeoniae Rubra) 10g
Bai Shao (Radix Paeoniae Lactiflorae) 10g
Tian Men Dong (Radix Asparagi Cochinchinensis) 10g
Mai Men Dong (Radix Ophiopogonis Japonici) 10g
Sheng Di Huang (Radix Rehmanniae Glutinosae) 10g
Shu Di Huang (Radix Rehmanniae Glutinosae Conquita) 10g
Huang Qi (Radix Astragali seu Hedysari) 10g
Chen Pi (Pericarpium Citri Reticulatae) 10g
Dang Shen (Radix Codonopsitis Pilosulae) 10g
Dan Shen (Radix Salviae Miltiorrhizae) 15g

---

[i] This formula was created by Dr. Zhou Mingqi. Although the dosages are larger than normal, it has proved very effective in the author's clinical practice.

Ji Xue Teng (Caulis Spatholobi) 15g

Shan Yao (Radix Dioscoreae Oppositae) 15g

Nan Sha Shen (Radix Adenophorae) 15g

Fu Ling (Sclerotium Poriae Cocos) 12g

He Shou Wu (Radix Polygoni Multiflori) 12g

Explanation

- *Tian Men Dong* (Radix Asparagi Cochinchinensis), *Mai Men Dong* (Radix Ophiopogonis Japonici), *Sheng Di Huang* (Radix Rehmanniae Glutinosae), and *Nan Sha Shen* (Radix Adenophorae) nourish the skin and moisten Dryness with cold and sweetness.

- *Chi Shao* (Radix Paeoniae Rubra), *Bai Shao* (Radix Paeoniae Lactiflorae), *He Shou Wu* (Radix Polygoni Multiflori), *Dang Gui* (Radix Angelicae Sinensis), *Ji Xue Teng* (Caulis Spatholobi), *Shu Di Huang* (Radix Rehmanniae Glutinosae Conquita), and *Dan Shen* (Radix Salviae Miltiorrhizae) nourish and invigorate the Blood.

- *Shan Yao* (Radix Dioscoreae Oppositae), *Huang Qi* (Radix Astragali seu Hedysari), *Chen Pi* (Pericarpium Citri Reticulatae), *Dang Shen* (Radix Codonopsitis Pilosulae), and *Fu Ling* (Sclerotium Poriae Cocos) augment Qi and support the Spleen; when Spleen Qi is fortified, Yin-Blood is distributed throughout the body.

General modifications

1. For Blood Deficiency, add *E Jiao*‡ (Gelatinum Corii Asini) and *Sang Shen* (Fructus Mori Albae).

2. For Blood stasis, add *Shui Zhi*‡ (Hirudo seu Whitmania) and *Meng Chong*‡ (Tabanus).

3. For insomnia, add *Suan Zao Ren* (Semen Ziziphi Spinosae) and *Bai Zi Ren* (Semen Biotae Orientalis).

4. For constipation with dry stools, add *Rou Cong Rong* (Herba Cistanches Deserticolae), *Huo Ma Ren* (Semen Cannabis Sativae) and *Hai Shen*‡ (Stichopus Japonicus).

5. For a weak constitution, take *Shi Quan Da Bu Wan* (Perfect Major Supplementation Pill) with the prepared decoction.

EXTERNAL TREATMENT

- For dry, rough and scaly skin, wash the affected area with a warm decoction of *Xing Ren Xi Fang* (Apricot Kernel Wash Formula) and then apply *Hua Jiao You* (Chinese Prickly Ash Oil).

- For severe keratinization or fissuring, apply *Run Ji Gao* (Flesh-Moistening Paste) to the affected area.

ACUPUNCTURE

Main points: SP-10 Xuehai, GB-20 Fengchi and BL-23 Shenshu.

Auxiliary points: LI-11 Quchi, GB-39 Xuanzhong and SP-9 Yinlingquan.

Technique: Apply the reducing method for Qi stagnation and Blood stasis and the reinforcing method for insufficiency of Ying Qi (Nutritive Qi) and Blood. Retain the needles for 30 minutes and manipulate them once every 15 minutes. Treat once a day. A course consists of ten treatment sessions.

Explanation

- SP-10 Xuehai and BL-23 Shenshu warm the Kidneys and nourish the Blood.

- GB-20 Fengchi, LI-11 Quchi, GB-39 Xuanzhong, and SP-9 Yinlingquan move Qi and free the network vessels, dispel Wind and alleviate itching.

NEEDLE EMBEDDING TREATMENT

Points: Sympathetic Nerve, Endocrine, Adrenal Gland, Lung, Upper Limb, and Lower Limb.

Technique: Treat alternate ears each time. Embed the thumbtack needles after routine disinfection of the points. Change the needles once every seven days. Ask the patient to press the needles gently three to five times a day for one minute each time.

Clinical notes

- Ichthyosis vulgaris is best treated with a combination of internal and external medication. In overall terms, internal treatment aims at augmenting Qi, nourishing and enriching Yin, moistening Dryness, harmonizing the Blood, transforming Blood stasis, eliminating Wind, and freeing the network vessels, thus employing a method of attacking and supplementing simultaneously. External treatment is based on the application of skin-moistening ointments, which can alleviate the sensation of dryness and discomfort.

- The condition is not usually present at birth, but develops in the first few years of childhood. It tends to deteriorate slowly and progressively until the age of 15. It then stabilizes, usually improving with age and only occasionally resolving completely.

- Ichthyosis vulgaris is very difficult to cure, although symptoms can be alleviated and progress moderated.

Advice for the patient

- Avoid exposure to wind and cold; wear enough clothing to keep the body warm.

- Do not eat spicy and stimulating food, and increase intake of fruit and vegetables.

- Take warm baths or showers and apply skin-moistening oil afterwards; this will help to soften the skin, reduce scaling and alleviate itching.

Case history

Patient
Male, aged 14.

Clinical manifestations
The skin on the extensor aspects of the patient's lower limbs became dry two weeks after birth. As the patient grew older, the condition became generalized with dry, rough, fissured, and itchy skin, usually worsening in winter. The patient had already been to several hospitals and received internal and external treatment with various Western medicines, but without any significant improvement being seen.

On examination, the limbs, chest, abdomen, and back were covered by a layer of dry, coarse, grayish-brown squames resembling fish scales. The hair was also dry and lusterless. The only systemic complaint mentioned was one of general discomfort. Appetite, urine and stool were all normal. The tongue body was pale with a white coating; the pulse was deficient and moderate.

Pattern identification
Congenital (Earlier Heaven) Deficiency and acquired (Later Heaven) impairment of nourishment with the result that Qi, Blood, Essence, and Body Fluids were unable to nourish and moisten the skin and flesh adequately.

Treatment principle
Free the channels and network vessels, supplement the Blood and move Qi.

Prescription
YU LIN TANG JIA JIAN
Fish Scale Decoction, with modifications

Huang Qi (Radix Astragali seu Hedysari) 50g
Hei Zhi Ma (Semen Sesami Indici) 40g
Dan Shen (Radix Salviae Miltiorrhizae) 25g
Di Fu Zi (Fructus Kochiae Scopariae) 25g
Dang Gui (Radix Angelicae Sinensis) 20g
Sheng Di Huang (Radix Rehmanniae Glutinosae) 20g
Shu Di Huang (Radix Rehmanniae Glutinosae Conquita) 20g
Gou Qi Zi (Fructus Lycii) 20g
He Shou Wu (Radix Polygoni Multiflori) 20g
Bai Xian Pi (Cortex Dictamni Dasycarpi Radicis) 20g
Shan Yao (Radix Dioscoreae Oppositae) 15g
Ku Shen (Radix Sophorae Flavescentis) 15g
Fang Feng (Radix Ledebouriellae Divaricatae) 15g
Chuan Xiong (Rhizoma Ligustici Chuanxiong) 10g
Gui Zhi (Ramulus Cinnamomi Cassiae) 10g
Chan Tui‡ (Periostracum Cicadae) 10g
Gan Cao (Radix Glycyrrhizae) 10g

One bag was decocted three times. The liquids were mixed and divided into six equal portions. One portion was taken twice a day. Nine bags were prescribed initially.

Second visit
After four weeks, the dry skin had improved slightly but there was still some desquamation. The patient complained of epigastric discomfort after eating, with mild distension and fullness, this discomfort being caused by the cloying nature of the supplementing herbs. The prescription was therefore modified by adding Ji Nei Jin‡ (Endothelium Corneum Gigeriae Galli) 15g and Chao Bai Zhu (Rhizoma Atractylodis Macrocephalae, stir-fried) 15g. Eight bags were prescribed, taken as before.

Outcome
After 24 days, the skin was moister and the scales were greatly reduced. The epigastric discomfort had disappeared, allowing the patient to eat normally. Therefore, the treatment returned to the original prescription, Yu Lin Tang (Fish Scale Decoction), this time in the form of 10g pills. The patient took one pill twice a day for four months to consolidate the improvement. [1]

Modern clinical experience

1. **Liu** divided ichthyosis into three different types. [2]

- **Mild type**
The condition had occurred within the previous year. Clinical manifestations included grayish-brown bran-like scales on parts of the chest and abdomen and the extensor aspect of the limbs. The skin was still soft and lesions were barely noticeable. Sweating occurred from time to time. The tongue coating was thin and white; the pulse was thready and rapid.

Treatment principle
Harmonize the Ying and Wei levels, promote sweating, and relax the skin and flesh to reduce scaling.

Prescription ingredients
Ma Huang* (Herba Ephedrae) 15g
Gui Zhi (Ramulus Cinnamomi Cassiae) 25g
Xing Ren (Semen Pruni Armeniacae) 20g
Gan Cao (Radix Glycyrrhizae) 20g
Tao Ren (Semen Persicae) 25g
Hong Hua (Flos Carthami Tinctorii) 15g
Sang Ye (Folium Mori Albae) 20g
Xuan Shen (Radix Scrophulariae Ningpoensis) 50g
Chan Tui‡ (Periostracum Cicadae) 15g

- **Moderate type**
The condition had persisted for between one and five years. Clinical manifestations included dry, scaly skin on the trunk and the extensor aspects of the limbs with patches of thick, dark scale separated by fissured margins. The skin felt uneven and hard. Sweating rarely occurred. The tongue body was crimson with a dry and slightly yellow coating; the pulse was thready and rapid, or rough.

Treatment principle
Regulate the Ying level, promote sweating, transform

Blood stasis, and loosen the skin and flesh to cause the scales to be shed.

Prescription ingredients

*Ma Huang** (Herba Ephedrae) 20g
Gui Zhi (Ramulus Cinnamomi Cassiae) 30g
Xing Ren (Semen Pruni Armeniacae) 20g
Gan Cao (Radix Glycyrrhizae) 20g
Tao Ren (Semen Persicae) 25g
Da Huang (Radix et Rhizoma Rhei) 15g
Shui Zhi‡ (Hirudo seu Whitmania) 20g
Di Long‡ (Lumbricus) 30g
*Chuan Shan Jia** (Squama Manitis Pentadactylae) 20g
Chan Tui‡ (Periostracum Cicadae) 20g

- **Severe type**

The condition had persisted for more than five years. Clinical manifestations included patches of thick, dark, dry, and scaly skin densely distributed over the chest, abdomen, back, and limbs with deep fissuring at the margins of the patches. The skin felt as hard as wood. Sweating was absent and stiffness was felt in extension, pronation and supination. The tongue body was crimson or covered with stasis marks with a dry white or dry yellow coating; the pulse was rough, or slow and wiry.

Treatment principle

Regulate the Ying level, moisten Dryness, transform Blood stasis, and dispel dead Blood to generate new skin, shed dead scale and return Qi that had been consumed.

Prescription ingredients

*Ma Huang** (Herba Ephedrae) 30g
Gui Zhi (Ramulus Cinnamomi Cassiae) 30g
Xing Ren (Semen Pruni Armeniacae) 25g
Shui Zhi‡ (Hirudo seu Whitmania) 20g
Xuan Shen (Radix Scrophulariae Ningpoensis) 50g
Mai Men Dong (Radix Ophiopogonis Japonici) 50g
Sang Ye (Folium Mori Albae) 25g
Di Long‡ (Lumbricus) 30g
*Chuan Shan Jia** (Squama Manitis Pentadactylae) 20g
Tu Bie Chong‡ (Eupolyphaga seu Steleophaga) 15g
Da Huang (Radix et Rhizoma Rhei) 20g
She Tui‡ (Exuviae Serpentis) 20g
Chan Tui‡ (Periostracum Cicadae) 10g

When the severe type of the disease is halfway toward recovery, the treatment method of enriching the Liver and regulating the Spleen and Stomach to nourish Lung Yin should be added. This is the stage when Vital Qi (Zheng Qi) should be supported. Therefore, in the later stages, *Shu Di Huang* (Radix Rehmanniae Glutinosae Conquita), *Sheng Di Huang* (Radix Rehmanniae Glutinosae), *Chuan Lian Zi* (Fructus Meliae Toosendan), *Bai*

Shao (Radix Paeoniae Lactiflorae), *Rou Cong Rong* (Herba Cistanches Deserticolae), *Shan Yao* (Rhizoma Dioscoreae Oppositae), *Bai Zi Ren* (Semen Biotae Orientalis), and *Bai He* (Bulbus Lilii) should be added.

2. **Wang** used a combination of internal and external treatments. [3]

Internal prescription
CANG ZHU GAO
Concentrated Atractylodes Syrup

Cang Zhu (Rhizoma Atractylodis) 1000g
Ji Xue Teng (Caulis Spatholobi) 1000g
Yi Yi Ren (Semen Coicis Lachryma-jobi) 500g
Dang Gui (Radix Angelicae Sinensis) 500g
Feng Mi‡ (Mel) 500g

Preparation

Cang Zhu (Rhizoma Atractylodis) was steeped overnight in enough rice water to cover the herb and then steamed for one hour. *Ji Xue Teng* (Caulis Spatholobi) and *Dang Gui* (Radix Angelicae Sinensis) were cut into thin slices and *Yi Yi Ren* (Semen Coicis Lachryma-jobi) was crushed; they were then steeped in 7.5 liters of tap water overnight. All the ingredients were decocted for two hours over a mild heat. The residue was filtered out, the liquid set aside and the ingredients decocted again with the same method. The two liquids were mixed and boiled down to make an extract of 500ml before 500g of honey was added. After a thorough stirring, the mixture was boiled again for 15 minutes, left to cool and poured into a bottle.

Administration

40ml twice a day, in the morning and evening; 20ml for children younger than 10 years.

External prescription
GAN CAO YOU
Licorice Oil

Gan Cao (Radix Glycyrrhizae) 50g
Xiang You (Oleum Sesami Seminis) 500g
Cod-liver oil‡ 50ml

Preparation

Gan Cao (Radix Glycyrrhizae) was cut into slices and steeped in *Xiang You* (Oleum Sesami Seminis) for 24 hours. It was then deep-fried in the oil over a mild heat until it turned a deep yellow color. The oil was filtered and the residue removed. The cod-liver oil‡was added and mixed thoroughly. *Gan Cao You* (Licorice Oil) was applied to the affected area twice a day.

Results were seen after six months.

Keratosis pilaris
毛发角化症

Keratosis pilaris is characterized by small follicular papules, surmounted by keratotic spines, and rough skin. The lesions occur in patches, and tend to develop symmetrically. In TCM, this condition is also known as *ji pi zheng* (chicken skin syndrome).

Clinical manifestations

- The rate of incidence is highest among boys; adults are rarely affected. This condition is inherited as an autosomal dominant trait.
- Lesions commonly involve posterolateral aspects of the upper arms and the anterior thighs; the side of the face and the buttocks are affected less frequently. Generalized involvement is rare.
- Lesions initially manifest as pinpoint follicular papules with grayish-white, filiform, dry keratotic spines in the center; the papules are usually surrounded by red areolae. The skin feels rough.
- The disease may persist for several months before spontaneous remission. In some cases, it can continue into adult life.

Differential diagnosis

Acne
Keratosis pilaris involving the face should be differentiated from acne. The uniform small size of the follicular papules, the dry skin and the absence of comedones in keratosis pilaris normally allow differentiation.

Etiology and pathology

Keratosis pilaris is caused by constitutional insufficiency or failure of the Spleen to distribute Body Fluids, resulting in Blood-Dryness or shortage of Body Fluids, thus depriving the skin and flesh of nourishment.

Pattern identification and treatment

INTERNAL TREATMENT

LACK OF NOURISHMENT DUE TO BLOOD-DRYNESS
This pattern occurs in the progressive phase of the disease. Follicular keratotic papules appear on the upper arms, thighs, face, or neck. The skin looks like plucked chicken flesh, feels hard to the touch and is slightly itchy. The tongue body is pale red with a scant coating; the pulse is deficient and thready.

Treatment principle
Nourish the Blood and moisten Dryness.

Prescription
SHI LIU WEI DI HUANG YIN ZI JIA JIAN
Sixteen-Ingredient Rehmannia Drink, with modifications

Dang Gui (Radix Angelicae Sinensis) 10g
Bai Shao (Radix Paeoniae Lactiflorae) 10g
Bai Zhu (Rhizoma Atractylodis Macrocephalae) 10g
Gan Di Huang (Radix Rehmanniae Glutinosae Exsiccata) 12g
He Shou Wu (Radix Polygoni Multiflori) 12g
Sha Yuan Zi (Semen Astragali Complanati) 12g
Shan Yao (Radix Dioscoreae Oppositae) 12g
Gou Qi Zi (Fructus Lycii) 12g
Chuan Xiong (Rhizoma Ligustici Chuanxiong) 6g
Wu Wei Zi (Fructus Schisandrae) 6g
Gan Cao (Radix Glycyrrhizae) 6g

Explanation
- *Dang Gui* (Radix Angelicae Sinensis), *Bai Shao* (Radix Paeoniae Lactiflorae), *Gan Di Huang* (Radix Rehmanniae Glutinosae Exsiccata), and *He Shou Wu* (Radix Polygoni Multiflori) nourish the Blood and moisten Dryness.
- *Sha Yuan Zi* (Semen Astragali Complanati), *Gou Qi Zi* (Fructus Lycii) and *Wu Wei Zi* (Fructus Schisandrae) enrich Yin and boost the Kidneys.
- *Chuan Xiong* (Rhizoma Ligustici Chuanxiong), *Bai Zhu* (Rhizoma Atractylodis Macrocephalae), *Shan Yao* (Radix Dioscoreae Oppositae), and *Gan Cao* (Radix Glycyrrhizae) regulate Qi and boost the Spleen.

THE SPLEEN FAILING TO DISTRIBUTE BODY FLUIDS
This pattern occurs in the quiescent phase. Keratotic papules are evident on the limbs and occasionally on the face and buttocks; some coalesce to form oval plaques. Accompanying symptoms and signs include a preference for certain foods rather than a variety of foods, a pale tongue body with a scant coating, and a soggy and thready pulse.

Treatment principle
Fortify the Spleen to reinforce its transportation function.

Prescription
SHEN LING BAI ZHU SAN JIA JIAN
Ginseng, Poria, and White Atractylodes Powder, with modifications

Dang Shen (Radix Codonopsitis Pilosulae) 10g
Fu Ling (Sclerotium Poriae Cocos) 10g
Bai Zhu (Rhizoma Atractylodis Macrocephalae) 10g
Chao Bai Bian Dou (Semen Dolichoris Lablab, stir-fried) 10g
Chen Pi (Pericarpium Citri Reticulatae) 10g
Shan Yao (Radix Dioscoreae Oppositae) 12g
Nan Sha Shen (Radix Adenophorae) 12g
Tian Men Dong (Radix Asparagi Cochinchinensis) 12g
Mai Men Dong (Radix Ophiopogonis Japonici) 12g
Tian Hua Fen (Radix Trichosanthis) 12g
Fo Shou (Fructus Citri Sarcodactylis) 6g
Shan Zha (Fructus Crataegi) 6g
Sha Ren (Fructus Amomi) 6g, added 5 minutes before the end of the decoction process

Explanation

- *Dang Shen* (Radix Codonopsitis Pilosulae), *Fu Ling* (Sclerotium Poriae Cocos), *Bai Zhu* (Rhizoma Atractylodis Macrocephalae), *Chen Pi* (Pericarpium Citri Reticulatae), *Fo Shou* (Fructus Citri Sarcodactylis), and *Sha Ren* (Fructus Amomi) augment Qi and harmonize the Stomach.
- *Shan Yao* (Radix Dioscoreae Oppositae), *Chao Bai Bian Dou* (Semen Dolichoris Lablab, stir-fried), *Tian Men Dong* (Radix Asparagi Cochinchinensis), and *Mai Men Dong* (Radix Ophiopogonis Japonici) enrich Yin and support the Spleen.
- *Tian Hua Fen* (Radix Trichosanthis) and *Shan Zha* (Fructus Crataegi) generate Body Fluids and transform Blood stasis.
- *Nan Sha Shen* (Radix Adenophorae) harmonizes the Stomach, nourishes Yin and generates Body Fluids.

PATENT HERBAL MEDICINES
- At the initial stage, take two or three 3g tablets of *Wu She Pian* (Black-Tail Snake Tablet), two or three times a day.
- Once the main pathogenic factors have been cleared and the patient's condition is stable, take *Cang Zhu Gao* (Concentrated Atractylodes Syrup) 10ml twice a day with boiled water.
- For Blood-Dryness, take two or three 3g tablets of *Dang Gui Pian* (Chinese Angelica Root Tablet) two or three times a day.

EXTERNAL TREATMENT
Apply *Hei Bu Yao Gao* (Black Cloth Medicated Paste) if the keratotic papules tend to spread and there is slight itching.

Clinical notes

- It is essential to fortify the Spleen and augment Qi. In addition, special attention should also be given to managing the relationship between Dryness and Dampness.
- *Cang Zhu Gao* (Concentrated Atractylodes Syrup) has both therapeutic and preventive effects.

Advice for the patient

- Avoid excessive intake of spicy, oily and fried foods and alcohol and stick to a light diet with plenty of vitamin A (carrots).
- Do not wash the affected areas with hot water.

Keratosis follicularis (Darier's disease)
毛囊角化症

Keratosis follicularis, also known as Darier's disease, is a relatively rare chronic skin disease due to dyskeratosis of the epidermal cells and usually begins in the teenage years. Since it may manifest as hypertrophic lesions, it is also known as proliferative follicular keratosis or proliferative follicular dyskeratosis.

Keratosis follicularis is inherited as an autosomal dominant condition with variable penetrance.

Clinical manifestations

- This disease usually presents in teenagers or young adults, sometimes after sunburn, and varies from mild and unobtrusive in some individuals to severe and widespread in others.
- Skin eruptions usually involve the hands, chest,

upper back, scalp, face (especially the forehead), neck, flexor aspects of the limbs, axillae, and groin.

- At the initial stage, lesions manifest as pinpoint to 3mm hard follicular papules, capped by dirty-looking greasy, grayish or brown scale. The skin is dry and rough. Papules subsequently coalesce into plaques with a wart-like appearance.
- If eruptions occur in folds such as the axillae, the groin or behind the ear, they usually manifest as papillomatous or verruciform hypertrophic lesions.
- On the scalp, heavy crusting resembles seborrheic eczema.
- If the lips are involved, lesions usually manifest with scabs, fissuring or ulceration.
- If the palm and sole are involved, lesions usually present as hyperkeratotic papules or pits, with diffuse thickening of the stratum corneum.
- Nail changes are common, including broad longitudinal white bands, broad translucent longitudinal red bands and a combination of red and white bands, which is frequently associated with a V-shaped defect at the free margin of the nail. Splitting of the nail plate is common.
- Mucosal lesions are uncommon, but occur in a high proportion of affected subjects in certain families. If the oral mucosa is involved, small, smooth, flat nodules can be seen with erosion and superficial ulceration.
- If the disease involves the esophagus, the mucosa may be red with white keratotic papules and there may be difficulty in swallowing. A few patients may also have bullous lesions (known as bullous-type Darier's disease).
- Some patients may develop widespread herpes simplex or bacterial infections.
- This disease tends to be exacerbated in summer as a result of ultraviolet radiation.

Differential diagnosis

Keratosis pilaris
The rate of incidence of this condition is highest among boys. Lesions manifest as pinpoint follicular papules with grayish-white, filiform, dry keratotic spines in the center and commonly involve the posterolateral aspects of the upper arms and the anterior thighs rather than the areas favored by Darier's disease.

Acne
Lesions on the face may be confused with acne. The small size of the lesions and the dry, rough skin in keratosis follicularis permit differentiation. Comedones are absent in keratosis follicularis.

Plane warts (verruca plana)
These occur most commonly in young people. Lesions manifest as flat-topped papules with a shiny surface, and usually involve the face and the dorsum of the hand. Warts do not have the greasy scale characteristic of Darier's disease.

Etiology and pathology

- Constitutional insufficiency of Yin-Blood tends to transform into Dryness and generate Wind. Blood-Dryness deprives the skin and flesh of nourishment and Qi and Blood cannot supply adequate moisture, leading to dry and scaly skin.
- The Spleen transforms and transports Water and Dampness and distributes Body Fluids. If the Spleen cannot move the Body Fluids produced by the Stomach, the Essence of Water and Grain will not be transported to the skin and flesh, which after a period will be deprived of nourishment.

Pattern identification and treatment

INTERNAL TREATMENT

BLOOD-DRYNESS IMPAIRING NOURISHMENT OF THE SKIN
This pattern is usually seen at the initial stage of the disease. Eruptions occur on the scalp, face, neck, chest, groin, and the flexor aspects of the limbs. A layer of greasy, dirty-looking scabs covers the surface of the eruptions. The 1-2mm hyperkeratotic lesions feel hard and dry. The fingernails and sometimes the toenails are brittle, thin and ridged, or split. Dry mouth and tongue are often accompanying symptoms. The tongue body is red with a scant coating; the pulse is thready and rapid.

Treatment principle
Nourish the Blood and moisten Dryness.

Prescription
QING ZAO JIU FEI TANG JIA JIAN
Decoction for Clearing Dryness and Rescuing the Lungs, with modifications

Bei Sha Shen (Radix Glehniae Littoralis) 12g
Mai Men Dong (Radix Ophiopogonis Japonici) 12g
Pi Pa Ye (Folium Eriobotryae Japonicae) 12g
Xing Ren (Semen Pruni Armeniacae) 12g
Shan Yao (Radix Dioscoreae Oppositae) 15g
Chao Bai Bian Dou (Semen Dolichoris Lablab, stir-fried) 15g
Huo Ma Ren (Semen Cannabis Sativae) 15g
E Jiao ‡ (Gelatinum Corii Asini) 10g
Sang Ye (Folium Mori Albae) 10g

*Shi Hu** (Herba Dendrobii) 10g
Yu Zhu (Rhizoma Polygonati Odorati) 10g
Gan Cao (Radix Glycyrrhizae) 10g

Explanation

- *Bei Sha Shen* (Radix Glehniae Littoralis), *Mai Men Dong* (Radix Ophiopogonis Japonici), *Pi Pa Ye* (Folium Eriobotryae Japonicae), *Xing Ren* (Semen Pruni Armeniacae), and *Sang Ye* (Folium Mori Albae) clear the Lungs and moisten Yin.

- *Shan Yao* (Radix Dioscoreae Oppositae), *Chao Bai Bian Dou* (Semen Dolichoris Lablab, stir-fried), *Shi Hu** (Herba Dendrobii), *Yu Zhu* (Rhizoma Polygonati Odorati), and *Gan Cao* (Radix Glycyrrhizae) moisten Spleen Yin.

- *Huo Ma Ren* (Semen Cannabis Sativae) and *E Jiao* ‡ (Gelatinum Corii Asini) nourish the Blood and moisten the skin. As these materia medica are sweet, neutral and moistening, they can moisten the Lungs and Spleen and nourish the Blood, but they are included in this prescription to nourish and moisten the skin and flesh.

THE SPLEEN FAILING TO DISTRIBUTE BODY FLUIDS

This pattern occurs in the quiescent stage of the disease. Eruptions cover a large area, involving the cheeks, shoulders, back, axillae, hypochondrium, and groin. The 2-3 mm lesions feel as hard as a callus. Accompanying symptoms and signs include a sensation of heaviness throughout the body, no desire to speak, abdominal distension, and loose stools. The tongue body is pale red with tooth marks and a scant coating; the pulse is thready and forceless.

Treatment principle
Fortify the Spleen to reinforce its transportation function.

Prescription
SHEN LING BAI ZHU SAN JIA JIAN
Ginseng, Poria and White Atractylodes Powder, with modifications

Dang Shen (Radix Codonopsitis Pilosulae) 10g
Bai Zhu (Rhizoma Atractylodis Macrocephalae) 10g
Chen Pi (Pericarpium Citri Reticulatae) 10g
Gan Cao (Radix Glycyrrhizae) 10g
Cang Zhu (Rhizoma Atractylodis) 15g
Shan Yao (Radix Dioscoreae Oppositae) 15g
Fa Ban Xia (Rhizoma Pinelliae Ternatae Praeparata) 12g
Chao Zhi Ke (Fructus Citri Aurantii, stir-fried) 12g
Chao Gu Ya (Fructus Setariae Italicae Germinatus, stir-fried) 12g
Chao Mai Ya (Fructus Hordei Vulgaris Germinatus, stir-fried) 12g
Chao Bai Bian Dou (Semen Dolichoris Lablab, stir-fried) 12g
Ji Nei Jin ‡ (Endothelium Corneum Gigeriae Galli) 12g
Sha Ren (Fructus Amomi) 8g, added 5 minutes before the end of the decoction process

Explanation

- *Dang Shen* (Radix Codonopsitis Pilosulae), *Bai Zhu* (Rhizoma Atractylodis Macrocephalae), *Gan Cao* (Radix Glycyrrhizae), *Chen Pi* (Pericarpium Citri Reticulatae), *Cang Zhu* (Rhizoma Atractylodis), *Chao Zhi Ke* (Fructus Citri Aurantii, stir-fried), and *Fa Ban Xia* (Rhizoma Pinelliae Ternatae Praeparata) augment Qi and support the Spleen.

- *Chao Bai Bian Dou* (Semen Dolichoris Lablab, stir-fried), *Shan Yao* (Radix Dioscoreae Oppositae), *Ji Nei Jin* ‡ (Endothelium Corneum Gigeriae Galli), *Chao Gu Ya* (Fructus Setariae Italicae Germinatus, stir-fried), *Chao Mai Ya* (Fructus Hordei Vulgaris Germinatus, stir-fried), and *Sha Ren* (Fructus Amomi) nourish the Stomach with cold and sweetness.

- By supporting Spleen Yang and moistening Stomach Yin, the Body Fluids will be properly distributed.

General modifications
1. For low-grade afternoon fever, add *Di Gu Pi* (Cortex Lycii Radicis), *Sheng Di Huang* (Radix Rehmanniae Glutinosae), *Shu Di Huang* (Radix Rehmanniae Glutinosae Conquita), and *Mu Dan Pi* (Cortex Moutan Radicis).
2. For dry mouth and tongue, add *Tian Hua Fen* (Radix Trichosanthis) and *Yu Zhu* (Rhizoma Polygonati Odorati).
3. For lesions with purulent mucus and a foul smell, add *Huo Xiang* (Herba Agastaches seu Pogostemi) and *Pei Lan* (Herba Eupatorii Fortunei).
4. For a persistent condition and hard lesions, *Da Huang Zhe Chong Wan* (Rhubarb and Wingless Cockroach Pill) should be taken with the decoction.
5. For a family history of the illness, *Liu Wei Di Huang Wan* (Six-Ingredient Rehmannia Pill) should be taken with the decoction.

EXTERNAL TREATMENT
- For lesions manifesting as papules with fissuring and desquamation, apply *Hei Bu Yao Gao* (Black Cloth Medicated Paste) to the affected area.
- For lesions with exudation, erosion and a foul smell, decoct *Wu Mei Shui Xi Ji* (Black Plum Wash Preparation) and apply as a wet compress on the affected area for 15 minutes two or three times a day.

ACUPUNCTURE
Main points: GB-20 Fengchi, LI-11 Quchi, ST-36 Zusanli, and SP-10 Xuehai.

Auxiliary points: SP-6 Sanyinjiao, GB-39 Xuanzhong, ST-40 Fenglong, ST-38 Tiaokou, CV-12 Zhongwan, and BL-20 Pishu.

Technique: Select one or two of the main points and two or three of the auxiliary points for each treatment session. Apply the reinforcing or even method and retain the needles for ten minutes after obtaining Qi. Treat once a day. A course consists of ten treatment sessions.

Explanation

- ST-36 Zusanli, SP-10 Xuehai, SP-6 Sanyinjiao, ST-40 Fenglong, ST-38 Tiaokou, BL-20 Pishu, and CV-12 Zhongwan fortify the Spleen and nourish the Blood.
- LI-11 Quchi, GB-20 Fengchi and GB-39 Xuanzhong dispel Wind and alleviate itching.

EAR ACUPUNCTURE

Points: Endocrine, Spleen, Liver, Brain Stem, Sympathetic Nerve, and areas corresponding to the sites of the lesions.

Technique: Select two to four points for each treatment session. Retain the needles for 30 minutes. Treat once a day. A course consists of six treatment sessions.

NEEDLE EMBEDDING TREATMENT

Points: Endocrine, Spleen, Liver, and Sympathetic Nerve.

Technique: Embed the thumbtack needles after routine disinfection of the points. Change the needles once every seven days. Tell the patient to press the needles gently three to five times a day for one minute each time.

Clinical notes

- In treating this disease, the emphasis must be put on treating Dryness and Dampness patterns and the materia medica used in the prescription should focus on regulating the Spleen and Stomach. If these two organs can function properly, keratosis follicularis can be alleviated.
- Do not apply moxibustion or prescribe medication that may produce Damp-Heat.
- An improvement can be obtained if patients persist with the treatment for several months and maintain a proper diet.

Advice for the patient

- Reduce intake of spicy, fried and greasy food and alcohol; eat more carrots and bland food.
- Try to avoid getting stressed, worried or angry.
- Do not wash the affected area with hot water.

Keratoderma of the palms and soles
掌跖角化症

This condition covers a group of diseases, mostly inherited, characterized by hyperkeratosis of the palms and soles. The most common type, which is discussed in this section and is also known as tylosis, manifests as symmetrical diffuse thickening of the horny layer of the epidermis. Other types manifest with punctate papular lesions on the palms and soles or as a mutilating variety that strangulates the fingers and toes. The acquired type may also be a clinical manifestation of other skin diseases such as pityriasis rubra pilaris and lichen planus.

Clinical manifestations

- Lesions manifest as thick, dry, hard, shiny pale yellow skin on the palms and soles; the skin may fissure in winter, causing pain when walking.
- In mild cases, lesions have a scattered distribution, but in severe conditions, verrucous proliferation may occur.

- The condition usually alleviates in summer and exacerbates in winter.

Etiology and pathology

Insufficiency of Ying Qi (Nutritive Qi) and Blood due to Spleen Deficiency deprives the extremities of nourishment, thus causing dry and thick skin.

Pattern identification and treatment

INTERNAL TREATMENT

BLOOD DEFICIENCY AND WIND-DRYNESS
The skin on the palms and soles becomes semi-transparent and thickened like the bark of a pine tree. In summer, it may turn white due to maceration with sweat; in winter it may be painful due to fissuring and chapping.

The tongue body is pale with a scant coating; the pulse is thready and weak.

Treatment principle
Fortify the Spleen and harmonize the Ying level, nourish the Blood and moisten Dryness.

Prescription
LI ZHONG WAN JIA JIAN
Regulating the Middle Pill, with modifications

Dang Shen (Radix Codonopsitis Pilosulae) 10g
Bai Zhu (Rhizoma Atractylodis Macrocephalae) 10g
Dang Gui (Radix Angelicae Sinensis) 10g
Chuan Xiong (Rhizoma Ligustici Chuanxiong) 10g
Bai Shao (Radix Paeoniae Lactiflorae) 10g
Gan Jiang (Rhizoma Zingiberis Officinalis) 6g
Gan Cao (Radix Glycyrrhizae) 6g

Explanation
- *Dang Shen* (Radix Codonopsitis Pilosulae), *Bai Zhu* (Rhizoma Atractylodis Macrocephalae), *Gan Jiang* (Rhizoma Zingiberis Officinalis), and *Gan Cao* (Radix Glycyrrhizae) fortify the Spleen and harmonize the Ying level, dispel Dampness and fortify the skin.
- *Dang Gui* (Radix Angelicae Sinensis), *Chuan Xiong* (Rhizoma Ligustici Chuanxiong) and *Bai Shao* (Radix Paeoniae Lactiflorae) nourish the Blood and moisten the skin. Only when Qi and Blood are abundant can the skin become soft and moist.

Modifications
1. For pronounced Blood Deficiency, double the dosage of *Dang Gui* (Radix Angelicae Sinensis) and add *Shu Di Huang* (Radix Rehmanniae Glutinosae Conquita) and *He Shou Wu* (Radix Polygoni Multiflori).
2. For pronounced Qi Deficiency, add *Shan Yao* (Radix Dioscoreae Oppositae).
3. For dry and cracked skin, add *Hei Zhi Ma* (Semen Sesami Indici) and *E Jiao*‡ (Gelatinum Corii Asini).

EXTERNAL TREATMENT
If the skin is dry or there is slight fissuring or itching, apply *Hei Bu Yao Gao* (Black Cloth Medicated Paste) twice a day.

Clinical notes

- Since insufficiency of Spleen Yin depriving the skin of nourishment leads to keratinization of the skin on the palms and soles with fissuring in serious cases, the prescription should be made up principally of sweet and moistening herbs, with channel conductors such as *Chuan Xiong* (Rhizoma Ligustici Chuanxiong) as assistants.
- Since the cause of the disease is related to hereditary factors, symptoms can be alleviated, but a cure is very difficult to achieve.

Advice for the patient

- Try to avoid the palms and soles coming into contact with gasoline, alcohol, ether, benzene, or other chemical substances.
- Eat plenty of fresh vegetables and fruits and avoid spicy or greasy food.
- Avoid using alkaline soap.

Porokeratosis of Mibelli
汗管角化症

Porokeratosis of Mibelli is a rare chronic progressive skin disease with lesions characterized by a slightly atrophied center surrounded by a raised hyperkeratotic margin. The name for this disease was first suggested by Mibelli, who considered that the condition resulted from dyskeratosis of the sweat pores. However, other authorities have disputed this view and consider that the keratotic layer is related to the hair follicle. In addition, lesions can involve the mucosa, the penis, the glans penis, and other areas with no eccrine ducts, and so this name is probably incorrect. This disease usually shows autosomal dominant inheritance, but acquired cases occur sporadically. Males are more commonly affected than females.

Clinical manifestations

- Lesions commonly involve the limbs, neck, shoulders, face, and genitalia. However, any site can be involved, including the oral mucosa and cornea.
- At the initial stage, eruptions manifest as small, crater-like polygonal papules, which slowly expand

centrifugally into circular or irregular shapes surrounded by a raised dam-like border. Lesions may be grayish-yellow, light brown or skin-colored.

- The number of lesions varies between individuals, ranging from one to several hundred.

- New eruptions often occur around sites of external trauma.

- Lesions may remain quiescent for long periods in some cases, whereas in other cases, they may develop slowly and irregularly. When they disappear, they may leave permanent atrophic patches or no marks at all.

- There is an association with squamous cell carcinoma, and less frequently with basal cell carcinoma, in the atrophic patches.

Differential diagnosis

Lichen planus
Eruptions usually involve the wrists, forearms and lower legs, although they may sometimes appear in the oral cavity, on the lips and tongue, or in the genital region. Lesions manifest as intensely pruritic, waxy, purplish-red, flat-topped polygonal papules with an irregular, angulated border, and can therefore be differentiated from the crater-like papules of this porokeratosis.

Common warts (verruca vulgaris)
Common warts grow on the fingers, the dorsum of the hand, the edge of the foot, the face, or the genitals. The warts start with pinpoint papules, which grow gradually to a round or polygonal shape with a rough surface and obvious hyperkeratosis. They are firm, elevated and grayish-yellow, dirty yellow or dirty brown in color and their surface breaks up skin lines. Warts are likely to bleed when rubbed or knocked.

Etiology and pathology

- Congenital Deficiency means that Wei Qi (Defensive Qi) fails to protect the body from external pathogenic factors. Wind-Damp can therefore invade the skin and interstices (cou li) and obstruct the circulation of Ying Qi (Nutritive Qi) and Wei Qi (Defensive Qi). When the skin and flesh are deprived of proper nourishment, this disease can result.

- A weak constitution impairs the circulation of Qi and Blood, which leads to Qi stagnation and Blood stasis in the skin and flesh, thus impeding the generation of new Blood and preventing the skin and interstices (cou li) from receiving adequate nourishment.

- The Liver regulates the smooth flow of Qi. Emotional disturbances lead to Depression and binding of Liver Qi, and obstruction of Water and Body Fluids. If this situation is complicated by condensation of internal Heat, Phlegm turbidity or Phlegm stasis will gradually result. Phlegm congealing in the skin and flesh can then lead to this disease.

Pattern identification and treatment

INTERNAL TREATMENT

INVASION BY EXTERNAL WIND-DAMP
This pattern is usually seen at the initial stage of the disease and occurs more frequently in adults. Eruptions usually involve locations on the limbs, particularly the hand, foot, forearm, or thigh; lesions in these areas generally have a distinct margin. However, lesions between the toes look more like corns. Lesions on the face and neck have a central brown macule or patch with distinct, non-elevated margins and may resemble isolated keratoses; alternatively, the margins may be sinuous, spreading outward slowly to form a reticulate pattern. The tongue body is pale red with a white coating; the pulse is wiry and thready.

Treatment principle
Dispel Wind and eliminate Dampness, nourish the Blood and moisten Dryness.

Prescription
CANG ZHU GAO JIA JIAN
Concentrated Atractylodes Syrup, with modifications

Cang Zhu (Rhizoma Atractylodis) 1000g
Dang Gui (Radix Angelicae Sinensis) 200g
He Shou Wu (Radix Polygoni Multiflori) 200g
Bai Xian Pi (Cortex Dictamni Dasycarpi Radicis) 200g

Decoct the herbs three times in 4000ml of water, then mix the liquids and boil down to make an extract of 1000ml. Add *Feng Mi*‡ (Mel) 500g and cook until a concentrate is obtained; take two teaspoonfuls (10ml) twice a day.

Explanation
- *Cang Zhu* (Rhizoma Atractylodis) is acrid and strongly aromatic and is very effective for dispelling Wind and drying Dampness.

- *He Shou Wu* (Radix Polygoni Multiflori) enriches and nourishes the Liver and Kidneys, and moistens the skin and flesh.

- *Bai Xian Pi* (Cortex Dictamni Dasycarpi Radicis) clears Heat and relieves Toxicity, eliminates Dampness and alleviates itching.

- *Dang Gui* (Radix Angelicae Sinensis) supplements the Blood and moistens Dryness.
- When these herbs are used together, they can support each other to dispel Wind and eliminate Dampness to alleviate itching, and nourish the Blood and moisten the flesh to soften the skin.

OBSTRUCTION BY BLOOD STASIS

This pattern generally starts at an early age and has a family history. Lesions manifest as dark brown, roundish or irregularly-shaped keratinized macules surrounded by a raised margin. The affected skin feels rough and prickly. Once stabilized, the condition remains quiescent and seldom spreads. The tongue body is dark red or has stasis marks with a scant coating; the pulse is rough.

Treatment principle
Invigorate the Blood and transform Blood stasis, free the channels and network vessels.

Prescription
TONG QIAO HUO XUE TANG JIA JIAN
Decoction for Freeing the Orifices and Invigorating the Blood, with modifications

Dang Gui (Radix Angelicae Sinensis) 12g
Chi Shao (Radix Paeoniae Rubra) 12g
Sheng Di Huang (Radix Rehmanniae Glutinosae) 12g
Chuan Xiong (Rhizoma Ligustici Chuanxiong) 10g
Tao Ren (Semen Persicae) 10g
Qing Pi (Pericarpium Citri Reticulatae Viride) 10g
Chen Pi (Pericarpium Citri Reticulatae) 10g
Si Gua Luo (Fasciculus Vascularis Luffae) 10g
*Chuan Shan Jia** (Squama Manitis Pentadactylae) 10g
Zao Jiao Ci (Spina Gleditsiae Sinensis) 10g
Bai Zhi (Radix Angelicae Dahuricae) 6g

Explanation
- *Dang Gui* (Radix Angelicae Sinensis), *Chi Shao* (Radix Paeoniae Rubra), *Chuan Xiong* (Rhizoma Ligustici Chuanxiong), and *Tao Ren* (Semen Persicae) invigorate the Blood and transform Blood stasis to soften keratotic skin.
- *Qing Pi* (Pericarpium Citri Reticulatae Viride), *Chen Pi* (Pericarpium Citri Reticulatae), *Si Gua Luo* (Fasciculus Vascularis Luffae), *Chuan Shan Jia** (Squama Manitis Pentadactylae), and *Zao Jiao Ci* (Spina Gleditsiae Sinensis) regulate Qi and free the network vessels.
- *Sheng Di Huang* (Radix Rehmanniae Glutinosae) cools the Blood and moistens the skin.
- *Bai Zhi* (Radix Angelicae Dahuricae) dissipates Wind and alleviates itching.

INSUFFICIENCY OF THE LIVER AND KIDNEYS WITH CONGEALING AND BINDING OF PHLEGM STASIS

This pattern mainly involves the oral cavity, with lesions manifesting as milky-white patches. It may also occasionally involve the genitals, in which case it will be complicated by erosion. This pattern usually develops slowly and persists for a long time. The tongue body is pale red with a scant coating; the pulse is thready and rapid.

Treatment principle
Supplement and boost the Liver and Kidneys, transform Phlegm and soften hardness.

Prescription
YANG HE TANG JIA JIAN
Harmonious Yang Decoction, with modifications

Shu Di Huang (Radix Rehmanniae Glutinosae Conquita) 10g
Shan Zhu Yu (Fructus Corni Officinalis) 6g
Shan Yao (Radix Dioscoreae Oppositae) 10g
Ju Hua (Flos Chrysanthemi Morifolii) 10g
Gou Qi Zi (Fructus Lycii) 10g
Fu Ling (Sclerotium Poriae Cocos) 3g
Xia Ku Cao (Spica Prunellae Vulgaris) 6g
Bai Jie Zi (Semen Sinapis Albae) 6g
Xuan Shen (Radix Scrophulariae Ningpoensis) 6g
Mu Li‡ (Concha Ostreae) 3g
Chuan Xiong (Rhizoma Ligustici Chuanxiong) 6g
Zao Jiao Ci (Spina Gleditsiae Sinensis) 3g

Explanation
- *Shu Di Huang* (Radix Rehmanniae Glutinosae Conquita), *Gou Qi Zi* (Fructus Lycii) and *Ju Hua* (Flos Chrysanthemi Morifolii) supplement and boost the Liver and Kidneys, enrich Yin and moisten the skin.
- *Bai Jie Zi* (Semen Sinapis Albae) dispels Phlegm between the skin and membranes.
- *Shan Yao* (Radix Dioscoreae Oppositae) nourishes Yin and supplements the Kidneys.
- *Fu Ling* (Sclerotium Poriae Cocos) clears Heat and transforms Dampness.
- *Xuan Shen* (Radix Scrophulariae Ningpoensis), *Xia Ku Cao* (Spica Prunellae Vulgaris) and *Mu Li‡* (Concha Ostreae) clear Heat and dissipate the binding of Phlegm-Fire.
- *Zao Jiao Ci* (Spina Gleditsiae Sinensis) and *Chuan Xiong* (Rhizoma Ligustici Chuanxiong) invigorate the Blood and free the network vessels to disperse sores.
- This prescription enriches and supplements the Liver and Kidneys to treat the Root, while transforming Dampness and freeing the network vessels to treat the Manifestations.

General modifications

1. For Blood Deficiency, add *He Shou Wu* (Radix Polygoni Multiflori) and double the dosage of *Dang Gui* (Radix Angelicae Sinensis).
2. For Spleen Deficiency, take *Shen Ling Bai Zhu Wan* (Ginseng, Poria and White Atractylodes Pill) with the decoction.
3. For Phlegm congealing, take *Nei Xiao Luo Li Wan* (Scrofula Internal Dispersion Pill) with the decoction.

PATENT HERBAL MEDICINES

- For Deficiency of Vital Qi (Zheng Qi) and Excess of pathogenic factors, take *Da Huang Zhe Chong Wan* (Rhubarb and Wingless Cockroach Pill) 4.5g twice a day.
- For insufficiency of the Liver and Kidneys, take *Xin Liu Wei Pian* (New Six-Ingredient Tablet) five tablets three times a day in addition to the decoction listed under the pattern.

EXTERNAL TREATMENT

For circumscribed skin lesions and relatively severe itching, apply *Hong Ling Jiu* (Red Spirit Wine) to the affected area one to three times a day.

ACUPUNCTURE

Main points: GB-31 Fengshi, SP-10 Xuehai and SP-6 Sanyinjiao.
Auxiliary points: ST-36 Zusanli, BL-23 Shenshu, LI-11 Quchi, and ST-40 Fenglong.
Technique: Apply the even method and retain the needles for 30 minutes after obtaining Qi. Treat once every two days. A course consists of ten treatment sessions.

Explanation

- SP-10 Xuehai, ST-36 Zusanli, ST-40 Fenglong, and SP-6 Sanyinjiao nourish the Blood, fortify the Spleen and eliminate Dampness.
- BL-23 Shenshu warms the Kidneys and dissipates Cold.
- GB-31 Fengshi and LI-11 Quchi dispel Wind, free the network vessels and alleviate itching.

EAR ACUPUNCTURE

Points: Adrenal Gland, Ear-Shenmen, Sympathetic Nerve, and areas corresponding to the sites of the lesions.
Technique: Retain the needles for 30 minutes. Treat once every two days. A course consists of six treatment sessions.

Clinical notes

- Treatment of this disease should focus on the characteristics of the skin lesions on the basis of eliminating Phlegm turbidity and transforming Blood stasis. Therefore, materia medica for augmenting Qi and transforming Phlegm, invigorating the Blood and softening hardness will normally bring good results.
- Better results are obtained by keeping the prescription unchanged during the treatment. If the cause of the disease is related to hereditary factors, symptoms can be alleviated, but a cure is very difficult to achieve.

Advice for the patient

- Avoid exposure to humidity and cold and increase the intake of foods rich in vitamin A such as squashes and carrots.
- Do not wash the affected area frequently with hot water.

References

1. Zhou Mingqi, *Yu Lin Bing Zhi Yan* [Experiences in the Treatment of Ichthyosis], *Liao Ning Zhong Yi Za Zhi* [Liaoning Journal of Traditional Chinese Medicine] 3 (1980): 12.
2. Liu Xiangfa, *Qian Tan Yu Lin Bing Bian Zheng Lun Zhi* [Discussion on the Treatment of Ichthyosis Based on Pattern Identification], *Zhong Yi Yao Xue Bao* [Journal of Traditional Chinese Medicine and Materia Medica] 4 (1987): 21.
3. Wang Penghui, *Cang Zhu Gao Wei Zhu Zhi Liao Xun Chang Xing Yu Lin Bing 60 Li* [Treatment of 60 Cases of Ichthyosis Vulgaris with *Cang Zhu Gao* (Concentrated Atractylodes Syrup)], *Zhe Jiang Zhong Yi Za Zhi* [Zhejiang Journal of Traditional Chinese Medicine] 26, 11 (1991): 495.

Chapter 15

Regional disorders

This chapter covers disorders of the hair and mucocutaneous diseases of the mouth. Disorders of the nails are discussed in the relevant chapters – psoriasis in Chapter 4, pyogenic paronychia (whitlow) in Chapter 10, tinea unguium (ringworm of the nail) in Chapter 11, and hangnail in Chapter 17.

Alopecia areata
斑秃

A hair follicle is defined as an invagination of the epidermis containing a hair, with the density of hair follicles being greatest on the head. The hair grows from germinative cells in the hair bulb in the dermis; the number and type of melanocytes associated with these cells are responsible for the color of the hair. The cycle of each follicle is independent of its neighbors and passes through three phases – a growth phase (anagen), lasting for three to five years, a short conversion phase (catagen), and a resting phase (telogen), lasting for up to three months, after which the hair is shed. One possible cause of alopecia areata has been suggested as premature termination of the anagen phase.

Alopecia areata is sudden-onset patchy hair loss in one or more circumscribed round or oval areas, primarily on the scalp. The condition appears to have an immunologic basis, occurring in association with autoimmune and atopic disorders. Although the exact pathogenesis has yet to be definitively identified, the disease is often associated with emotional factors and endocrine dysfunction.

Alopecia areata usually appears as patchy baldness, but occasionally causes all hair to be lost. Although total baldness is often permanent, regrowth is possible in cases with limited involvement.

In TCM, alopecia areata is known as *gui ti tou* (ghost-shaved hair) or *you feng* (glossy scalp Wind).

Clinical manifestations

- The highest incidence of alopecia occurs among the young and middle-aged.
- The disease is characterized by the sudden appearance of one or several clearly defined round or oval patches of hair loss, generally 1-4 cm in size.
- In severe cases, there may be loss of eyebrow, moustache, beard, axillary, or genital hair. A few patients lose all the hair on the scalp (alopecia totalis); complete baldness of the head and body is known as alopecia universalis.
- The skin is smooth and white or may have short stubs of hair at the margins of lesions (so-called "exclamation mark hairs", about 4mm in length and tapering toward the scalp). Inflammation and scaling are absent.
- Hair loss may be accompanied by fine pitting of the nails.
- New hair growth is usually the same color and texture as existing hair, but may be fine and white, particularly in older patients.
- The outcome is variable. A first episode usually results in regrowth within a few months. Further episodes often result in more extensive patches of hair loss, with slower regrowth.

Differential diagnosis

Tinea capitis
This condition occurs most frequently in prepubertal children. Alopecia areata should be differentiated from the "gray patch ringworm" pattern, which is characterized by round or irregular scaly lesions of grayish-white

patches. The hair is dry and brittle and usually breaks off 3-4 mm above the skin surface with white sheaths left at the root of the affected hairs. Although hair loss may occur in persistent conditions, the disease normally disappears spontaneously during adolescence.

Other conditions

Alopecia can also be caused by habitual hair-pulling (trichotillomania) or traction from tight hair rollers or pulling the hair tightly into a bun or pony-tail. These causes need to be eliminated from the diagnosis.

Etiology and pathology

- Alopecia areata can result from Excess or Deficiency patterns:
  - Excess patterns are caused by excessive intake of spicy, hot or fried food or by a depressed mental state transforming into Fire, thus consuming Yin and Blood and generating Wind due to Blood-Heat. Another Excess pattern is caused by Blood stasis in the hair orifices, depriving the hair root of nourishment by Yin and Blood. Both patterns manifest as unexpected hair loss.
  - Deficiency patterns include Qi and Blood Deficiency and Liver and Kidney Deficiency. Depletion of Blood and damage to Yin results in lack of transformation and generation of Qi and Blood. The hair root is empty and the hair has no source of growth, leading to large areas of hair loss.
- Overindulgence in spicy, greasy or fried foods, or a depressed mental state transforming into Fire, or plentiful Qi and Blood in young people, or Liver-Wood transforming into Fire can consume Yin and Blood or cause Blood-Heat to transform into internal Wind. Wind-Heat then follows Qi upward to the vertex, preventing the hair root from being nourished by Yin and Blood. Sudden loss of hair, yellow discoloration of the hair or premature graying can then result.
- Overeating of sweet and fatty food tends to damage the Spleen and Stomach, leading to internal accumulation of Damp-Heat. If this Damp-Heat steams upward to the vertex along the channels and attacks the hair root, the hair will thin or fall out.
- Looseness of the pores in the scalp allows external Wind to attack, thus making the hair root less secure and depriving it of proper nourishment, resulting in patches of hair loss.
- Blood stasis in the hair orifices (follicles) obstructs the movement of Qi in the channels, making it difficult for new Blood to irrigate and nourish the hair root, thus leading to rapid hair loss over a large area.
- Qi and Blood Deficiency due to prolonged illness, or debilitation of the Chong and Ren vessels mean that the hair is no longer nourished properly, resulting in dry hair or thinning and lusterless hair, and eventually to hair loss.
- Internal damage due to the emotions, such as disappointment or excessive thought and preoccupation, can injure the Heart and Spleen, impairing the transformation and transportation function of the Spleen and leading to loss of the source for transforming and generating Qi and Blood. This manifests in the exterior as gray hair and hair loss and in the interior as Deficiency-Heat due to restlessness and overstrain.
- When Lung Qi is abundant, it promotes the diffusion and distribution of Body Fluids and Blood to nourish the Zang-Fu organs internally and moisten and enrich the skin, flesh, hair, and orifices externally. Damage to the Lungs can lead to various hair disorders, including thinning hair, dry or gray hair, or hair loss.
- The Kidneys store the Essence of the Zang-Fu organs. If the Essence is Deficient, the Kidneys cannot transform and generate Yin and Blood, causing depletion of the source for generating hair. This results in hair loss or premature graying of hair.
- Excessive sexual activity drains the Kidney Essence, damaging the Liver and Kidneys. Yang Qi is also discharged with the sperm. Apart from hair loss, this also causes cold in the glans penis, dizziness and blurred vision.
- Congenital Deficiency of Kidney Qi is also responsible for late growth of hair, thin hair, or lusterless dry yellowing hair.

Pattern identification and treatment

INTERNAL TREATMENT

BLOOD-HEAT GENERATING WIND

This pattern manifests as sudden hair loss, rapidly evolving into large round or oval bare patches with occasional itching. A few patients may experience loss of hair in the eyebrows, moustache and beard. In some cases, accompanying symptoms and signs include a sensation of heat in the scalp, irritability, irascibility, and restlessness. The tongue body is red with a scant coating; the pulse is thready and rapid.

Treatment principle

Cool the Blood and extinguish Wind, nourish Yin and protect the hair.

Prescription
SI WU TANG HE LIU WEI DI HUANG WAN JIA JIAN

Four Agents Decoction Combined With Six-Ingredient Rehmannia Pill, with modifications

Sheng Di Huang (Radix Rehmanniae Glutinosae) 15g
Nü Zhen Zi (Fructus Ligustri Lucidi) 15g
Sang Shen (Fructus Mori Albae) 15g
Chao Mu Dan Pi (Cortex Moutan Radicis, stir-fried) 10g
Chi Shao (Radix Paeoniae Rubra) 10g
Bai Shao (Radix Paeoniae Lactiflorae) 10g
Shan Zhu Yu (Fructus Corni Officinalis) 10g
Xuan Shen (Radix Scrophulariae Ningpoensis) 12g
Hei Zhi Ma (Semen Sesami Indici) 12g
Tu Si Zi (Semen Cuscutae) 12g
Fu Shen (Sclerotium Poriae Cocos cum Ligno Hospite) 18g
Dang Gui (Radix Angelicae Sinensis) 18g
Ce Bai Ye (Cacumen Biotae Orientalis) 18g
Dai Zhe Shi‡ (Haematitum) 18g

Explanation

- *Sheng Di Huang* (Radix Rehmanniae Glutinosae), *Nü Zhen Zi* (Fructus Ligustri Lucidi), *Sang Shen* (Fructus Mori Albae), *Xuan Shen* (Radix Scrophulariae Ningpoensis), and *Hei Zhi Ma* (Semen Sesami Indici) nourish Yin and protect the hair, clear Heat and cool the Blood.
- *Tu Si Zi* (Semen Cuscutae) and *Shan Zhu Yu* (Fructus Corni Officinalis) enrich the Liver and supplement the Kidneys.
- *Dai Zhe Shi*‡ (Haematitum) and *Fu Shen* (Sclerotium Poriae Cocos cum Ligno Hospite) extinguish Wind and quiet the Spirit.
- *Dang Gui* (Radix Angelicae Sinensis), *Ce Bai Ye* (Cacumen Biotae Orientalis), *Chi Shao* (Radix Paeoniae Rubra), *Chao Mu Dan Pi* (Cortex Moutan Radicis, stir-fried), and *Bai Shao* (Radix Paeoniae Lactiflorae) nourish and invigorate the Blood, because the hair can only grow when the Blood is abundant.

BLOOD STASIS IN THE HAIR FOLLICLES

Headache or a stabbing pain in the scalp precedes alopecia, which manifests initially as sudden patches of hair loss and may persist to develop into complete baldness. Accompanying symptoms and signs include frequent nightmares, difficulty in getting to sleep, restlessness with a feverish sensation, and grinding of the teeth. The tongue body is dark red or has stasis marks and a scant coating; the pulse is deep and rough.

Treatment principle
Free the orifices and invigorate the Blood.

Prescription
TONG QIAO HUO XUE TANG JIA JIAN

Decoction for Freeing the Orifices and Invigorating the Blood, with modifications

Dang Gui Wei (Extremitas Radicis Angelicae Sinensis) 12g
Chi Shao (Radix Paeoniae Rubra) 12g
Sheng Di Huang (Radix Rehmanniae Glutinosae) 12g
Chuan Xiong (Rhizoma Ligustici Chuanxiong) 10g
Gan Cao (Radix Glycyrrhizae) 10g
Tao Ren (Semen Persicae) 10g
Hong Hua (Flos Carthami Tinctorii) 10g
Suan Zao Ren (Semen Ziziphi Spinosae) 10g
Ju Hua (Flos Chrysanthemi Morifolii) 10g
Sang Ye (Folium Mori Albae) 10g
Bai Zhi (Radix Angelicae Dahuricae) 6g
Man Jing Zi (Fructus Viticis) 6g
Yuan Zhi (Radix Polygalae) 6g

Explanation

- *Dang Gui Wei* (Extremitas Radicis Angelicae Sinensis), *Chi Shao* (Radix Paeoniae Rubra), *Chuan Xiong* (Rhizoma Ligustici Chuanxiong), *Tao Ren* (Semen Persicae), *Hong Hua* (Flos Carthami Tinctorii), *Bai Zhi* (Radix Angelicae Dahuricae), *Man Jing Zi* (Fructus Viticis), and *Yuan Zhi* (Radix Polygalae) free the orifices and invigorate the Blood to increase local blood circulation.
- *Ju Hua* (Flos Chrysanthemi Morifolii), *Sang Ye* (Folium Mori Albae) and *Gan Cao* (Radix Glycyrrhizae) dredge Wind and clear Heat.
- *Sheng Di Huang* (Radix Rehmanniae Glutinosae) and *Suan Zao Ren* (Semen Ziziphi Spinosae) nourish Yin and quiet the Spirit.

QI AND BLOOD DEFICIENCY

This pattern generally occurs in patients with a weak constitution, or after a prolonged illness or postpartum. Hair loss gradually becomes increasingly serious with bald patches growing in size and number, especially in areas that may be rubbed frequently such as the occiput. The scalp is shiny and soft; short stubs of hair scattered unevenly over the affected area may fall off on rubbing. Accompanying symptoms and signs include pale lips, palpitations, shortness of breath, weak voice, dizziness, sleepiness, and lassitude. The tongue body is pale red with a thin white coating; the pulse is thready and weak.

Treatment principle
Augment Qi and supplement the Blood.

Prescription
BA ZHEN TANG JIA JIAN

Eight Treasure Decoction, with modifications

Dang Gui (Radix Angelicae Sinensis) 12g
Shu Di Huang (Radix Rehmanniae Glutinosae Conquita) 12g
Chao Bai Shao (Radix Paeoniae Lactiflorae, stir-fried) 12g
Dang Shen (Radix Codonopsitis Pilosulae) 12g
Bai Zhu (Rhizoma Atractylodis Macrocephalae) 12g
Huang Qi (Radix Astragali seu Hedysari) 15g
Fu Shen (Sclerotium Poriae Cocos cum Ligno
   Hospite) 15g
Nü Zhen Zi (Fructus Ligustri Lucidi) 15g
He Shou Wu (Radix Polygoni Multiflori) 15g
Sang Shen (Fructus Mori Albae) 15g
Huang Jing (Rhizoma Polygonati) 15g
Chuan Xiong (Rhizoma Ligustici Chuanxiong) 6g
Bai Fu Zi (Rhizoma Typhonii Gigantei) 6g
Zhi Gan Cao (Radix Glycyrrhizae, mix-fried with honey) 6g

Explanation

* *Dang Gui* (Radix Angelicae Sinensis), *Shu Di Huang* (Radix Rehmanniae Glutinosae Conquita), *Chao Bai Shao* (Radix Paeoniae Lactiflorae, stir-fried), *Dang Shen* (Radix Codonopsitis Pilosulae), *Bai Zhu* (Rhizoma Atractylodis Macrocephalae), *Huang Qi* (Radix Astragali seu Hedysari), *Chuan Xiong* (Rhizoma Ligustici Chuanxiong), *Fu Shen* (Sclerotium Poriae Cocos cum Ligno Hospite), and *Zhi Gan Cao* (Radix Glycyrrhizae, mix-fried with honey) augment Qi and supplement the Blood.
* *Nü Zhen Zi* (Fructus Ligustri Lucidi), *He Shou Wu* (Radix Polygoni Multiflori), *Sang Shen* (Fructus Mori Albae), and *Huang Jing* (Rhizoma Polygonati) enrich the Liver and supplement the Kidneys.
* *Bai Fu Zi* (Rhizoma Typhonii Gigantei) dissipates Wind and alleviates itching, while conducting the other ingredients upward to bring Qi, Blood, Yin, and Body Fluids directly to the diseased area to reinforce hair growth.

INSUFFICIENCY OF THE LIVER AND KIDNEYS

This pattern usually affects patients aged over 40 with a history of yellowing or graying hair. The hair generally falls out, leaving large bald patches with no hair stubs; in severe cases, there may be loss of eyebrow, axillary and genital hair. Accompanying symptoms and signs include a pale facial complexion, cold limbs, aversion to cold, dizziness, tinnitus, limpness and aching of the lower back and knees, and a cold sensation in the glans penis. The tongue body is pale red with fissures and a scant coating or no coating; the pulse is deep, thready and forceless.

Treatment principle
Enrich the Liver and boost the Kidneys.

Prescription
QI BAO MEI RAN DAN JIA JIAN
Seven Treasure Special Pill for Beautifying the Whiskers, with modifications

He Shou Wu (Radix Polygoni Multiflori) 15g
Gou Qi Zi (Fructus Lycii) 15g
Tu Si Zi (Semen Cuscutae) 15g
Dang Gui (Radix Angelicae Sinensis) 15g
Nü Zhen Zi (Fructus Ligustri Lucidi) 12g
Hei Zhi Ma (Semen Sesami Indici) 12g
Hu Tao Ren (Semen Juglandis Regiae) 12g
Huai Niu Xi (Radix Achyranthis Bidentatae) 12g
Huang Jing (Rhizoma Polygonati) 10g
Sang Shen (Fructus Mori Albae) 10g
Yuan Zhi (Radix Polygalae) 10g
Shi Chang Pu (Rhizoma Acori Graminei) 10g

Explanation

* *He Shou Wu* (Radix Polygoni Multiflori), *Gou Qi Zi* (Fructus Lycii), *Tu Si Zi* (Semen Cuscutae), *Sang Shen* (Fructus Mori Albae), *Nü Zhen Zi* (Fructus Ligustri Lucidi), *Huai Niu Xi* (Radix Achyranthis Bidentatae), and *Huang Jing* (Rhizoma Polygonati) enrich the Liver and boost the Kidneys to nourish the Essence and generate Blood.
* *Dang Gui* (Radix Angelicae Sinensis), *Hei Zhi Ma* (Semen Sesami Indici) and *Hu Tao Ren* (Semen Juglandis Regiae) moisten and blacken the hair.
* *Yuan Zhi* (Radix Polygalae) and *Shi Chang Pu* (Rhizoma Acori Graminei) free the orifices and invigorate the network vessels.

Alternative prescription
SHENG FA YIN
Generating Hair Beverage

Zhi He Shou Wu (Radix Polygoni Multiflori Praeparata) 15g
Sang Shen (Fructus Mori Albae) 15g
Huang Qi (Radix Astragali seu Hedysari) 15g
Gou Qi Zi (Fructus Lycii) 15g
Tu Si Zi (Semen Cuscutae) 15g
Xuan Shen (Radix Scrophulariae Ningpoensis) 15g
Jiu Dang Gui (Radix Angelicae Sinensis, processed
   with wine) 9g
Jiu Chuan Xiong (Rhizoma Ligustici Chuanxiong,
   processed with wine) 3g
Bu Gu Zhi (Fructus Psoraleae Corylifoliae) 12g
Sheng Di Huang (Radix Rehmanniae Glutinosae) 12g
Shu Di Huang (Radix Rehmanniae Glutinosae Conquita) 12g
Dang Shen (Radix Codonopsitis Pilosulae) 12g
Hei Zhi Ma (Semen Sesami Indici) 24g

Explanation

* *Huang Qi* (Radix Astragali seu Hedysari), *Xuan Shen*

(Radix Scrophulariae Ningpoensis), *Jiu Dang Gui* (Radix Angelicae Sinensis, processed with wine), *Jiu Chuan Xiong* (Rhizoma Ligustici Chuanxiong, processed with wine), *Sheng Di Huang* (Radix Rehmanniae Glutinosae), *Shu Di Huang* (Radix Rehmanniae Glutinosae Conquita), and *Dang Shen* (Radix Codonopsitis Pilosulae) augment Qi and nourish the Blood to generate hair.

- *Sang Shen* (Fructus Mori Albae), *Gou Qi Zi* (Fructus Lycii), *Tu Si Zi* (Semen Cuscutae), and *Bu Gu Zhi* (Fructus Psoraleae Corylifoliae) enrich and supplement the Liver and Kidneys.
- *Zhi He Shou Wu* (Radix Polygoni Multiflori Praeparata) and *Hei Zhi Ma* (Semen Sesami Indici) generate and blacken the hair.

General modifications

1. For palpitations and insomnia, add *Wu Wei Zi* (Fructus Schisandrae), *Bai He* (Bulbus Lilii), *Mai Men Dong* (Radix Ophiopogonis Japonici), *Bai Zi Ren* (Semen Biotae Orientalis), and *Lian Zi* (Semen Nelumbinis Nuciferae).
2. For emotional depression and self-pity, add *He Huan Pi* (Cortex Albizziae Julibrissin), *He Huan Hua* (Flos Albizziae Julibrissin), *Yu Jin* (Radix Curcumae), and *Xiang Fu* (Rhizoma Cyperi Rotundi).
3. For reduced appetite and abdominal distension, add *Chao Gu Ya* (Fructus Setariae Italicae Germinatus, stir-fried), *Ji Nei Jin* ‡ (Endothelium Corneum Gigeriae Galli), *Mei Gui Hua* (Flos Rosae Rugosae), *Hou Po Hua* (Flos Magnoliae Officinalis), and *Fo Shou* (Fructus Citri Sarcodactylis).
4. For prevalence of Wind-Heat with sudden and severe alopecia, add *Tian Ma** (Rhizoma Gastrodiae Elatae), *Bai Fu Zi* (Rhizoma Typhonii Gigantei) and *Chong Wei Zi* (Semen Leonuri Heterophylli).

PATENT HERBAL MEDICINES

- For Qi and Blood Deficiency, take *Sheng Fa Wan* (Generating Hair Pill), one 9g honeyed pill, three times a day.
- For Blood-Heat generating Wind, take *Ce Bai Wan* (Biota Pill), one 9g honeyed pill, twice a day.
- For insufficiency of the Liver and Kidneys, take *Yi Ma Er Zhi Wan* (Black Sesame Double Supreme Pill) 6g twice a day; or *Yi Shen Rong Fa Wan* (Pill for Boosting the Kidneys and Nourishing the Hair) 10g with water before meals, two or three times a day.

EXTERNAL TREATMENT

Apply *Sheng Fa Ding* (Generating Hair Tincture), *Gui Zhi Ban Mao Ding* (Cinnamon Twig and Mylabris Tincture) or *Dong Chong Xia Cao Jiu* (Cordyceps Wine) to the affected area.

ACUPUNCTURE

Selection of points according to pattern identification

- For Blood-Heat patterns, select GB-20 Fengchi, SP-10 Xuehai and ST-36 Zusanli.
- For Blood stasis patterns, select LR-3 Taichong, PC-6 Neiguan joined to TB-5 Waiguan, SP-6 Sanyinjiao, and BL-17 Geshu.
- For Blood Deficiency patterns, select BL-18 Ganshu, BL-23 Shenshu and ST-36 Zusanli.
- For Liver and Kidney insufficiency patterns, select BL-23 Shenshu, BL-18 Ganshu, KI-3 Taixi, SP-10 Xuehai, and SP-6 Sanyinjiao.

Selection of points on the affected channels
Main points: ST-36 Zusanli and SP-6 Sanyinjiao.
Auxiliary points: ST-8 Touwei, GB-41 Zulinqi, GB-43 Xiaxi, BL-60 Kunlun, LR-3 Taichong, and KI-3 Taixi.

Selection of adjacent points
Main points: GV-20 Baihui, GV-23 Shangxing and GV-19 Houding.
Auxiliary points

- For severe itching, add GB-20 Fengchi and GV-14 Dazhui.
- For insomnia, add EX-HN-1 Sishencong [i] and HT-7 Shenmen.
- For hair loss on the temples, add ST-8 Touwei and GB-8 Shuaigu.
- For poor appetite, add CV-12 Zhongwan and ST-36 Zusanli.
- For hair loss on the eyebrows, join EX-HN-4 Yuyao [ii] to TB-23 Sizhukong.

Empirical points
Main points: Fanglao (1 cun posterior to GV-20 Baihui) and Jiannao (0.5 cun inferior to GB-20 Fengchi).
Auxiliary points

- For severe itching, add GV-14 Dazhui.
- For greasy hair, add GV-23 Shangxing.
- For hair loss on the temples, add ST-8 Touwei.

Technique
Apply the reducing method for Excess patterns and the reinforcing method for Deficiency patterns. Retain the

---

[i] M-HN-1 according to the system employed by the Shanghai College of Traditional Chinese Medicine.
[ii] M-HN-6 according to the system employed by the Shanghai College of Traditional Chinese Medicine.

needles for 30 minutes after obtaining Qi; during this period, manipulate the needles three to five times. Treat once every two days. A course consists of ten treatment sessions.

Explanation

- ST-36 Zusanli, SP-6 Sanyinjiao and CV-12 Zhongwan fortify the Spleen, augment Qi and nourish the Blood.
- BL-60 Kunlun and KI-3 Taixi nourish and supplement the Liver and Kidneys.
- ST-8 Touwei, GB-41 Zulinqi, GB-43 Xiaxi, and LR-3 Taichong dissipate Wind, move Qi and free the network vessels.
- GB-20 Fengchi and GV-14 Dazhui dispel Wind and alleviate itching.
- EX-HN-1 Sishencong and HT-7 Shenmen clear Heat from the Heart and drain Fire.

EAR ACUPUNCTURE

Points: Lung, Kidney, Ear-Shenmen, Sympathetic Nerve, Endocrine, and Spleen.
Technique: Retain the needles for 30 minutes; during this period, manipulate the needles five or six times. Treat once every two days. A course consists of ten treatment sessions.

SCALP ACUPUNCTURE

Points: Upper three-fifths of the Motor and Sensory Areas.
Technique: Insert the needles quickly under the skin and rotate lightly and quickly for three to five minutes. Retain the needles for 30 minutes. Treat once a day. A course consists of ten treatment sessions.

PRICKING TO BLEED METHOD

Point: BL-40 Weizhong.
Technique: After routine sterilization of the point, prick with a three-edged needle to cause slight bleeding. Treat once every five days. A course consists of five treatment sessions.
Indication: Excess patterns such as Blood stasis in the hair follicles.

PLUM-BLOSSOM NEEDLING

Selection of points according to disease differentiation

Main points: Ashi points (hair loss sites).
Auxiliary points
- For hair loss on the temples, add ST-8 Touwei.
- For hair loss at the vertex, add GV-20 Baihui, GV-19 Houding and CV-21 Qianding.

- For severe itching, add GB-20 Fengchi and GV-16 Fengfu.
- For insomnia, add Anmian (located at the midpoint between SJ-17 Yifeng and GB-20 Fengchi).[iii]
- For Kidney Deficiency, add KI-3 Taixi and BL-23 Shenshu.

Selection of points along the affected channels
Points: Ashi points (hair loss sites), GB-20 Fengchi, LU-9 Taiyuan, PC-6 Neiguan, neck, sacrum, and lumbar region.

Local points
Points: Ashi points (hair loss sites).

Technique
Apply medium stimulation with the hand. Treat for ten minutes, once every two days. A course consists of fourteen treatment sessions.

POINT LASER THERAPY
Points: Ashi points (hair loss sites).
Technique: Apply a helium-neon laser to the Ashi points for 10 minutes in each treatment session. If there are several patches, treat each for five minutes. Treat once a day. Interrupt the treatment for one day after six treatment sessions before continuing. A course consists of thirty treatment sessions.

Clinical notes

- Although there are many treatments for alopecia areata, the disease is rather slow to respond. It is therefore important to bear in mind the classical adage of keeping a prescription relatively unchanged if it is reasonable, thus allowing it a certain time to work. Treatment will not be effective unless pattern identification is correct.
- Offer reassurance to patients to stop them worrying about the condition and increase their confidence in the treatment.
- Treatment can be accompanied by dietary therapy. Walnuts, sesame seeds and seafood are all beneficial to regeneration of the hair follicles.
- Alopecia areata may resolve spontaneously. However, total baldness is usually very difficult to treat.

Advice for the patient

- Eat a wide variety of foods.
- Look after the hair properly; do not wash it with

[iii] M-HN-54 according to the system employed by the Shanghai College of Traditional Chinese Medicine.

strongly alkaline soap or shampoo. Avoid using electric hair dryers or dyeing the hair.

Case history

Patient
Female, aged 28.

Clinical manifestations
The patient's hair started to fall out in clumps three months previously. The scalp was occasionally itchy. She rubbed fresh ginger into the affected areas, but this did not make any difference. She also used *Sheng Fa Jing* (a hair growth lotion) externally, again without any obvious effect. Examination revealed numerous patches of hair loss on the vertex, temples and occiput, covering approximately two-thirds of the scalp. The skin was shiny in the affected areas; fine soft hairs had appeared in some areas. Hair loss on the eyebrows and eyelashes had also started. Accompanying symptoms and signs included lack of appetite, sleeplessness with profuse dreaming, and late periods. The tongue body was pale with a thin coating; the pulse was deep and moderate.

Pattern identification
Insufficiency of the Liver and Kidneys and Blood Deficiency leading to hair loss.

Treatment principle
Enrich and supplement the Liver and Kidneys, nourish the Blood and promote hair growth.

Prescription ingredients
Shu Di Huang (Radix Rehmanniae Glutinosae Conquita) 10g
Ye Jiao Teng (Caulis Polygoni Multiflori) 30g
Huang Qi (Radix Astragali seu Hedysari) 15g
Dang Gui (Radix Angelicae Sinensis) 10g
Chuan Xiong (Rhizoma Ligustici Chuanxiong) 10g
Dan Shen (Radix Salviae Miltiorrhizae) 15g
Bai Shao (Radix Paeoniae Lactiflorae) 10g
Nü Zhen Zi (Fructus Ligustri Lucidi) 30g
Tu Si Zi (Semen Cuscutae) 15g
Sang Shen (Fructus Mori Albae) 30g
Hei Zhi Ma (Semen Sesami Indici) 15g
*Tian Ma** (Rhizoma Gastrodiae Elatae) 10g
Zhen Zhu Mu ‡ (Concha Margaritifera) 30g
Shi Chang Pu (Rhizoma Acori Graminei) 30g
Gou Teng (Ramulus Uncariae cum Uncis) 10g

One bag a day was used to prepare a decoction, taken twice a day.

Second visit
After 30 bags, the patient's appetite and sleep had improved, and menstruation was not late this month. Some new hair was growing and no new area of hair loss had appeared. The prescription was continued for another two months, with the following modifications according to symptoms:

- for palpitations, *He Huan Pi* (Cortex Albizziae Julibrissin) 10g, *He Huan Hua* (Flos Albizziae Julibrissin) 10g, *Mai Men Dong* (Radix Ophiopogonis Japonici) 10g, and *Wu Wei Zi* (Fructus Schisandrae) 5g were added;

- for poor appetite and diarrhea, *Hou Po* (Cortex Magnoliae Officinalis) 10g and *Bai Bian Dou* (Semen Dolichoris Lablab) 10g were added.

Outcome
After two months, most of the hair and eyelashes had grown back.

Discussion
Alopecia areata is often caused by insufficiency of the Essence and Blood, Deficiency of the Liver and Kidneys, and non-interaction of the Heart and Kidneys. Blood Deficiency means that the hair cannot be nourished. Insecurity of the interstices (*cou li*) leads to pathogenic Wind taking advantage of Deficiency to cause Blood-Dryness due to exuberant Wind. Accompanying symptoms and signs include restlessness with a feverish sensation in the palms, soles and the center of the chest, limpness and aching in the lower back and knees, and restless sleep.

In the prescription, *Shu Di Huang* (Radix Rehmanniae Glutinosae Conquita), *Ye Jiao Teng* (Caulis Polygoni Multiflori), *Sang Shen* (Fructus Mori Albae), *Nü Zhen Zi* (Fructus Ligustri Lucidi), and *Tu Si Zi* (Semen Cuscutae) enrich and supplement the Liver and Kidneys, replenish the Essence and supplement the Marrow; *Dang Gui* (Radix Angelicae Sinensis), *Dan Shen* (Radix Salviae Miltiorrhizae) and *Bai Shao* (Radix Paeoniae Lactiflorae) nourish and transform the Blood; *Tian Ma** (Rhizoma Gastrodiae Elatae), *Gou Teng* (Ramulus Uncariae cum Uncis) and *Chuan Xiong* (Rhizoma Ligustici Chuanxiong) invigorate the Blood and dispel Wind; *Huang Qi* (Radix Astragali seu Hedysari) regulates the Spleen and augments Qi; *Hei Zhi Ma* (Semen Sesami Indici) supplements and boosts the Essence and Blood; *Zhen Zhu Mu* ‡ (Concha Margaritifera) and *Shi Chang Pu* (Rhizoma Acori Graminei) quiet the Spirit. The overall prescription achieved the effect of promoting hair growth. [1]

Literature excerpt

In *Wai Ke Yi An Hui Bian* [A Collection of Case Histories Relating to External Diseases], it says: "Exuberance of Kidney Qi promotes the growth of the hair, whereas debilitation of Kidney Qi loosens the root of the hair and exhaustion of Yang Qi makes the hair turn gray, thus resulting in bald patches and hair loss. Treatment should therefore focus on the Kidneys and the three Yang channels.

"When Yang Qi is Deficient, it cannot protect the exterior and the interstices (*cou li*) will be loose; external Wind can then invade. This is an external pattern and should be treated by cooling the Blood and dispelling Wind.

"If the Blood cannot ascend and Qi and Blood cannot flow properly in the channels, this leads to Blood stasis in the hair orifices and impairs nourishment of the hair. This condition should be treated internally by strongly supplementing the Liver and Kidneys and externally by application of *Zhi Zhu Hua You* (Yellow Azalea Flower Oil) and other materia medica for moistening Dryness and cooling the Blood.

"If hair loss is due to Blood Deficiency and invasion of Wind, treat by supplementing the Blood and dissipating Wind; for premature graying of the hair, treat by nourishing the Blood and dispelling Wind.

"Materia medica for replenishing and supplementing the Liver and Kidneys should be combined with others for bearing Yang upward and dissipating Wind; materia medica for nourishing the Blood can be combined with others for freeing Yang Qi."

Modern clinical experience

TREATMENT BASED ON PATTERN IDENTIFICATION

1. **Pei** identified three patterns for this disease. [2]

- **Qi Deficiency of the Spleen and Stomach**

Accompanying symptoms and signs
Emaciation, a sallow yellow facial complexion, poor appetite, lassitude, a pale and swollen tongue body, and a deep and thready pulse.

Treatment principle
Supplement the Middle Burner and augment Qi.

Prescription ingredients
Dang Shen (Radix Codonopsitis Pilosulae) 10g
Bai Zhu (Rhizoma Atractylodis Macrocephalae) 10g
Fu Ling (Sclerotium Poriae Cocos) 10g
He Shou Wu (Radix Polygoni Multiflori) 10g
Dang Gui (Radix Angelicae Sinensis) 10g
Nü Zhen Zi (Fructus Ligustri Lucidi) 10g
Han Lian Cao (Herba Ecliptae Prostratae) 10g
Gan Cao (Radix Glycyrrhizae) 6g
Chen Pi (Pericarpium Citri Reticulatae) 6g
Huang Qi (Radix Astragali seu Hedysari) 20g
Mu Xiang* (Radix Aucklandiae Lappae) 3g
Cao Dou Kou (Semen Alpiniae Katsumadai) 3g
Sheng Di Huang (Radix Rehmanniae Glutinosae) 12g
Gou Qi Zi (Fructus Lycii) 12g

One bag a day was used to prepare a decoction, taken twice a day. A course of treatment consisted of 20 bags. Results were seen after two to three courses.

- **Liver Depression and Kidney Deficiency**

Accompanying symptoms and signs
Dizziness, aching in the lower back, weak legs, a bitter taste in the mouth, a sensation of fullness in the chest and hypochondrium, irritability and restlessness, a red tongue body, and a wiry pulse.

Treatment principle
Dredge the Liver and supplement the Kidneys.

Prescription ingredients
Shan Zhu Yu (Fructus Corni Officinalis) 6g
Chuan Xiong (Rhizoma Ligustici Chuanxiong) 6g
Gan Cao (Radix Glycyrrhizae) 6g
Bai Shao (Radix Paeoniae Lactiflorae) 15g
Dang Gui (Radix Angelicae Sinensis) 10g
Sheng Di Huang (Radix Rehmanniae Glutinosae) 10g
Dang Shen (Radix Codonopsitis Pilosulae) 10g
Bai Zhu (Rhizoma Atractylodis Macrocephalae) 10g
Fu Ling (Sclerotium Poriae Cocos) 10g
Nü Zhen Zi (Fructus Ligustri Lucidi) 10g
Chai Hu (Radix Bupleuri) 10g
Han Lian Cao (Herba Ecliptae Prostratae) 10g
He Shou Wu (Radix Polygoni Multiflori) 20g

One bag a day was used to prepare a decoction, taken twice a day. A course of treatment consisted of 20 bags. Results were seen after two to three courses.

- **Damage to Qi and Yin**

Accompanying symptoms and signs
A dark facial complexion, lassitude, dry mouth, Deficiency-type irritability, a pale tongue body, and a deep and thready pulse in a prolonged illness.

Treatment principle
Augment Qi and nourish Yin.

Prescription ingredients
Bu Gu Zhi (Fructus Psoraleae Corylifoliae) 100g
He Shou Wu (Radix Polygoni Multiflori) 100g
Dan Shen (Radix Salviae Miltiorrhizae) 100g
Chi Shao (Radix Paeoniae Rubra) 70g
Sheng Di Huang (Radix Rehmanniae Glutinosae) 70g
Shu Di Huang (Radix Rehmanniae Glutinosae Conquita) 70g
Han Lian Cao (Herba Ecliptae Prostratae) 70g
Dang Shen (Radix Codonopsitis Pilosulae) 70g
Dang Gui (Radix Angelicae Sinensis) 70g
Mai Men Dong (Radix Ophiopogonis Japonici) 70g
Wu Wei Zi (Fructus Schisandrae) 70g
Bai Xian Pi (Cortex Dictamni Dasycarpi Radicis) 70g
Mu Gua (Fructus Chaenomelis) 70g
Nü Zhen Zi (Fructus Ligustri Lucidi) 70g
Qiang Huo (Rhizoma et Radix Notopterygii) 70g

These ingredients were ground into a powder and mixed with honey to make 9g pills (approximately 120 pills). One pill was taken with boiled water twice a day, one in the morning and one in the evening. A course of treatment lasted for three months.

All patients were given a decoction of *Ce Bai Ye* (Cacumen Biotae Orientalis) 60g and *Sheng Jiang* (Rhizoma Zingiberis Officinalis Recens) 3g to be used to wash the affected areas once a day, with each bag being used for two days.

2. **Li** considered that alopecia was pathologically related to dysfunction of the Liver, Spleen and Kidneys. He employed three principles to treat alopecia areata (including alopecia totalis and alopecia universalis). [3]

- **Augment Qi and nourish the Blood**

Prescription
SHENG FA YIN
Generating Hair Beverage

Huang Qi (Radix Astragali seu Hedysari) 20g
Dang Gui (Radix Angelicae Sinensis) 15g
Bai Zhu (Rhizoma Atractylodis Macrocephalae) 15g
Huang Jing (Rhizoma Polygonati) 12g
Sang Shen (Fructus Mori Albae) 12g
Fu Shen (Sclerotium Poriae Cocos cum Ligno Hospite) 12g
Mu Gua (Fructus Chaenomelis) 12g
*Tian Ma** (Rhizoma Gastrodiae Elatae) 10g
Yuan Zhi (Radix Polygalae) 10g
Da Zao (Fructus Ziziphi Jujubae) 15g
Gan Cao (Radix Glycyrrhizae) 6g

- **Dredge the Liver and transform Blood stasis**

Prescription
TAO HONG XIAO YAO SAN JIA JIAN
Peach Kernel and Safflower Free Wanderer Powder, with modifications

Ji Xue Teng (Caulis Spatholobi) 30g
Dang Gui (Radix Angelicae Sinensis) 12g
Chi Shao (Radix Paeoniae Rubra) 12g
Han Lian Cao (Herba Ecliptae Prostratae) 12g
Tao Ren (Semen Persicae) 12g
Chai Hu (Radix Bupleuri) 10g
Yu Jin (Radix Curcumae) 10g
Hong Hua (Flos Carthami Tinctorii) 10g
Qing Pi (Pericarpium Citri Reticulatae Viride) 6g
Chen Pi (Pericarpium Citri Reticulatae) 6g
Chuan Xiong (Rhizoma Ligustici Chuanxiong) 6g

- **Enrich the Kidneys and nourish Yin**

Prescription
FU FANG SHOU WU TANG
Compound Fleeceflower Decoction

Zhi He Shou Wu (Radix Polygoni Multiflori Praeparata) 15g
Shu Di Huang (Radix Rehmanniae Glutinosae Conquita) 12g
Shan Yao (Radix Dioscoreae Oppositae) 12g
Gou Qi Zi (Fructus Lycii) 12g
Du Zhong (Cortex Eucommiae Ulmoidis) 12g

Hu Tao Ren (Semen Juglandis Regiae) 12g
Huang Jing (Rhizoma Polygonati) 12g
Tu Si Zi (Semen Cuscutae) 12g
Qiang Huo (Rhizoma et Radix Notopterygii) 10g
Chen Pi (Pericarpium Citri Reticulatae) 10g
Di Gu Pi (Cortex Lycii Radicis) 10g
Gan Cao (Radix Glycyrrhizae) 3g

For all prescriptions, one bag a day was used to prepare a decoction, taken twice a day. Results were seen at the earliest after 16 days and at the latest after six months. The best responses were achieved with alopecia areata and alopecia totalis; results for alopecia universalis were not as good.

3. **Hu** identified four patterns. [4]

- ***Yin Deficiency of the Liver and Kidneys***, treated with *Zuo Gui Yin* (Restoring the Left [Kidney Yin] Beverage) and *Er Zhi Wan* (Double Supreme Pill), with the addition of *Zhi He Shou Wu* (Radix Polygoni Multiflori Praeparata) 30g, *Zi He Che*‡ (Placenta Hominis) 30g and *E Jiao*‡ (Gelatinum Corii Asini) 30g.

- ***Blood-Dryness due to exuberant Wind***, treated with *Tian Ma Gou Teng Yin* (Gastrodia and Uncaria Beverage) with the addition of *Sheng Di Huang* (Radix Rehmanniae Glutinosae) 10g, *Xuan Shen* (Radix Scrophulariae Ningpoensis) 10g and *Dai Zhe Shi*‡ (Haematitum) 15g.

- ***Yin-Cold congealing due to Kidney Yang Deficiency***, treated with *Jin Kui Shen Qi Wan* (Kidney Qi Pill from the Golden Cabinet), or *Yang He Tang Jia Ma Huang Fu Zi Xi Xin Tang* (Harmonious Yang Decoction Plus Ephedra, Asarum and Prepared Aconite Decoction). If Cold congealing was due to Spleen Yang Deficiency, the pattern was treated with *Gui Zhi Ren Shen Tang He Ma Huang Fu Zi Xi Xin Tang* (Cinnamon Twig and Ginseng Decoction Combined With Ephedra, Asarum and Prepared Aconite Decoction).

- ***Blood stasis obstructing the channels and network vessels***, treated by freeing the network vessels and invigorating the Blood.

Prescription ingredients

Yi Mu Cao (Herba Leonuri Heterophylli) 10g
Chi Shao (Radix Paeoniae Rubra) 10g
Tao Ren (Semen Persicae) 10g
Chuan Xiong (Rhizoma Ligustici Chuanxiong) 10g
Hong Hua (Flos Carthami Tinctorii) 6g
Di Gu Pi (Cortex Lycii Radicis) 15g
Tu Bie Chong‡ (Eupolyphaga seu Steleophaga) 6g
Bai Zhi (Radix Angelicae Dahuricae) 10g
Qian Cao Gen (Radix Rubiae Cordifoliae) 10g
Sheng Di Huang (Radix Rehmanniae Glutinosae) 15g
Cong Bai (Bulbus Allii Fistulosi) 6g

SPECIAL PRESCRIPTIONS

1. **Ma** reported on his own formulation of a basic prescription plus modifications. [5]

Prescription
SHOU WU SHENG FA YIN
Fleeceflower Root Beverage for Generating Hair

He Shou Wu (Radix Polygoni Multiflori) 15g
Shan Zhu Yu (Fructus Corni Officinalis) 15g
Gou Qi Zi (Fructus Lycii) 15g
Tu Si Zi (Semen Cuscutae) 15g
Shu Di Huang (Radix Rehmanniae Glutinosae Conquita) 18g
Hei Zhi Ma (Semen Sesami Indici) 30g
Bai Shao (Radix Paeoniae Lactiflorae) 30g
Dang Gui (Radix Angelicae Sinensis) 12g
Chuan Xiong (Rhizoma Ligustici Chuanxiong) 10g
Qiang Huo (Rhizoma et Radix Notopterygii) 6g

Modifications
1. For Blood-Heat, *Sheng Di Huang* (Radix Rehmanniae Glutinosae) 15g and *Mu Dan Pi* (Cortex Moutan Radicis) 12g were added.
2. For Liver Depression, *Yu Jin* (Radix Curcumae) 15g and *Xiang Fu* (Rhizoma Cyperi Rotundi) 12g were added.
3. For Kidney Deficiency, *Lu Jiao Jiao*‡ (Gelatinum Cornu Cervi) 15g, melted in the prepared decoction, and *Sang Shen* (Fructus Mori Albae) 15g were added.
4. For insomnia, *He Huan Hua* (Flos Albizziae Julibrissin) 15g and *Ye Jiao Teng* (Caulis Polygoni Multiflori) 30g were added.

One bag a day was used to prepare a decoction, taken twice a day. Initial results were seen after one month.

2. **Liu** employed the treatment principle of freeing the orifices and invigorating the Blood to treat alopecia areata.[6]

Prescription
SHENG FA LING
Efficacious Remedy for Generating Hair

Dang Gui (Radix Angelicae Sinensis) 30g
Chi Shao (Radix Paeoniae Rubra) 30g
Chuan Xiong (Rhizoma Ligustici Chuanxiong) 30g
Tao Ren (Semen Persicae) 20g
Hong Hua (Flos Carthami Tinctorii) 20g
He Shou Wu (Radix Polygoni Multiflori) 60g
Hei Da Dou (Semen Glycines Atrum) 30g
Huang Qi (Radix Astragali seu Hedysari) 30g
Shi Chang Pu (Rhizoma Acori Graminei) 20g

The ingredients were decocted in one liter of water until 500ml of liquid was left. This liquid was stored in a bottle, with 70ml being taken twice a day. Patients with pronounced Liver-Fire symptoms accompanied by irritability and restlessness and yellow urine were also given *Long Dan Xie Gan Wan* (Chinese Gentian Pill for Draining the Liver).

External treatment
SHENG FA DING
Generating Hair Tincture

Ren Shen (Radix Ginseng) 20g
He Shou Wu (Radix Polygoni Multiflori) 30g
Gu Sui Bu (Rhizoma Drynariae) 30g
Bu Gu Zhi (Fructus Psoraleae Corylifoliae) 10g

The ingredients were steeped in wine for one month and then applied to the affected area two or three times a day. Results were seen at the earliest after 14 days and at the latest after six months.

COMBINATION OF INTERNAL AND EXTERNAL TREATMENT

Gong combined internal and external treatment. [7]

Internal prescription
SHENG FA YIN
Generating Hair Beverage

Dang Gui (Radix Angelicae Sinensis) 12g
Zhi Shou Wu (Radix Polygoni Multiflori Praeparata) 12g
Sang Shen (Fructus Mori Albae) 12g
Nü Zhen Zi (Fructus Ligustri Lucidi) 12g
Han Lian Cao (Herba Ecliptae Prostratae) 12g
Yu Jin (Radix Curcumae) 12g
Zhi Ke (Fructus Citri Aurantii) 12g
Huang Qi (Radix Astragali seu Hedysari) 15g
Dan Shen (Radix Salviae Miltiorrhizae) 15g
Yuan Zhi (Radix Polygalae) 9g
Si Gua Luo (Fasciculus Vascularis Luffae) 9g
Sheng Ma (Rhizoma Cimicifugae) 6g

One bag a day was used to prepare a decoction, taken twice a day.

External prescription
SHENG FA DING
Generating Hair Tincture

He Shou Wu (Radix Polygoni Multiflori) 200g
Bu Gu Zhi (Fructus Psoraleae Corylifoliae) 200g
Gan Jiang (Rhizoma Zingiberis Officinalis) 100g
Hong Hua (Flos Carthami Tinctorii) 100g
Chuan Xiong (Rhizoma Ligustici Chuanxiong) 100g
Rou Gui (Cortex Cinnamomi Cassiae) 100g
She Chuang Zi (Fructus Cnidii Monnieri) 100g

The ingredients were cut up and crushed, then soaked for ten days in 3000ml of a 75 percent alcohol solution. The liquid was filtered off for application to the affected area twice a day. Results were seen after two months.

Mucocutaneous diseases of the mouth
口腔粘膜皮肤病

There are many types of mucous membranes in the body, some of which are connected to the skin, such as the conjunctiva, the nasal cavity, the oral cavity, and the anus. This chapter deals only with diseases of the oral mucosa closely associated with the skin. Mucosal diseases may be an independent disease involving the mucosa alone (for example, stomatitis) or be a part of the manifestations of systemic or skin diseases (for example, oral candidiasis, discussed in this chapter, or lichen planus and pemphigus vulgaris, discussed in Chapters 4 and 8 respectively).

TCM recognizes three types of mucocutaneous diseases of the mouth:

- those occurring in the area around the mouth, often due to retention of Heat in the Spleen and Stomach channels (for example, perioral dermatitis in Chapter 6).
- those occurring on the lips, which are the consequence of long-term accumulation of Damp-Heat, which eventually transforms into Fire, thus damaging Yin and generating Dryness; these diseases can also be caused by Wind pathogenic factors settling in the exterior (for example, cheilitis).
- those occurring in the oral cavity, involving the tongue or the buccal mucosa (for example, recurrent aphthous stomatitis or herpetic stomatitis). These diseases are mainly caused by the external factors of Wind, Fire and Dryness and overindulgence in spicy food, and internally as a result of Heat in the Heart and Spleen or disharmony of the seven emotions.

Cheilitis
唇炎

Cheilitis is acute or chronic inflammation of the oral mucosa caused by exposure to ultraviolet rays from the sun or artificial sources (actinic cheilitis), or by irritants or sensitizers such as application of external medications or lipsticks (allergic cheilitis). It may occur alone or as part of general stomatitis or in connection with other skin disorders such as erythema multiforme, eczema, psoriasis, or urticaria.

In TCM, cheilitis is known as *chun feng* (lip Wind).

Clinical manifestations

- Cheilitis is most commonly seen among children and young women.
- The disease starts in the middle of the lower lip, gradually spreading to the whole lip. Sometimes it may also involve the upper lip.
- At the initial stage, the lower lip is slightly red and swollen, but it soon becomes dry and cracked with desquamation. Once all the scales peel off, a moist surface is exposed, followed by scab formation. This process may occur repeatedly.
- The patient may feel a sensation of burning heat and pain.

Differential diagnosis

Cancer of the lip
At the initial stage, the lesion may be white and scaly, gradually increasing in size. The margins may be indistinct, with a dry, fissured and itchy surface. In the long run, the affected area becomes indurated and ulcerates, taking on a spongy, fungus-like appearance. In the later stages, the lesion may become painful, ooze pus and blood, and give off a foul odor. At an advanced stage, the cervical lymph nodes are swollen and immobile. By this stage, a cure is unlikely. Where cancer of the lip is suspected, the patient should be referred immediately to doctors of Western medicine for treatment of the tumor.

Etiology and pathology

- This disease is closely related to overindulgence in spicy, rich and greasy food, which produces Heat in the Stomach. When Heat accumulates over a prolonged period, it will transform into Fire. If during this time, there is an invasion of external Wind-Heat, Wind and Fire will fight one another to steam and scorch the lips, leading to stagnation of Qi and Blood and red and swollen lips.

- Excessive thought and preoccupation damages the Spleen and depression damages Yin since depression can easily transform into Fire that surreptitiously damages Liver Yin; the Yin Liquids of the Liver and Spleen are therefore scorched, resulting in Blood-Heat, which transforms into Dryness and generates Wind. When Wind is exuberant, trembling will occur, whereas Dryness-Heat will steam and scorch the lips, leading to dry and fissured lips followed by exudation. In severe cases, the lips appear to have been peeled bare.

- Constitutional Deficiency impairs Spleen Qi in its transformation and transportation function and leads to accumulation of Dampness. If the body is then invaded by external Wind, Wind and Dampness ascend to harass the lips, making them red, swollen and fissured.

- Other factors such as exposure to the sun or wind, or habits such as constantly licking or biting the lips can also induce or aggravate this disease.

Pattern identification and treatment

INTERNAL TREATMENT

WIND-FIRE IN THE STOMACH CHANNEL

This syndrome is characterized by a rapid onset and manifests initially as red, swollen, painful, and itchy lips. The lips gradually become dry and fissured followed by exudation; the lips are constantly trembling. Accompanying symptoms and signs include thirst with a liking for cold drinks, bad breath and constipation. The tongue body is red with a thin yellow coating; the pulse is slippery and rapid.

Treatment principle
Clear Heat and drain Fire, cool the Blood and dredge Wind.

Prescription
SHUANG JIE TONG SHENG SAN
Double Relief Sage-Inspired Powder

Fang Feng (Radix Ledebouriellae Divaricatae) 10g
Jing Jie (Herba Schizonepetae Tenuifoliae) 10g
Lian Qiao (Fructus Forsythiae Suspensae) 10g
Bai Zhu (Rhizoma Atractylodis Macrocephalae) 10g
Huang Qin (Radix Scutellariae Baicalensis) 10g
Bai Shao (Radix Paeoniae Lactiflorae) 10g
Dang Gui (Radix Angelicae Sinensis) 6g
Jie Geng (Radix Platycodi Grandiflori) 6g
Gan Cao (Radix Glycyrrhizae) 6g

Zhi Zi (Fructus Gardeniae Jasminoidis) 6g
Sheng Ma (Rhizoma Cimicifugae) 6g
Shi Gao‡ (Gypsum Fibrosum) 15g
Hua Shi‡ (Talcum) 15g, wrapped in *He Ye* (Folium Nelumbinis Nuciferae) for decoction

Explanation
- *Fang Feng* (Radix Ledebouriellae Divaricatae), *Jing Jie* (Herba Schizonepetae Tenuifoliae), *Jie Geng* (Radix Platycodi Grandiflori), and *Gan Cao* (Radix Glycyrrhizae) dissipate Wind and disperse swelling.
- *Lian Qiao* (Fructus Forsythiae Suspensae), *Huang Qin* (Radix Scutellariae Baicalensis), *Zhi Zi* (Fructus Gardeniae Jasminoidis), and *Sheng Ma* (Rhizoma Cimicifugae) clear Heat and drain Fire.
- *Shi Gao*‡ (Gypsum Fibrosum) clears intense Heat from the Yangming channels.
- *Bai Shao* (Radix Paeoniae Lactiflorae) and *Dang Gui* (Radix Angelicae Sinensis) nourish Yin and invigorate the Blood.
- *Bai Zhu* (Rhizoma Atractylodis Macrocephalae) supports the Spleen and transforms Dampness.
- *Hua Shi*‡ (Talcum) clears Heat and benefits the movement of Dampness so that Damp-Heat can be relieved through urination.

BLOOD-DRYNESS IN THE SPLEEN CHANNEL

This pattern has a slow onset and is characterized by hot, dry and swollen lips with fissuring and scaling, or fissuring and exudation. Once all the scales peel off, a moist surface is exposed. Accompanying symptoms and signs include a sweet and sticky sensation in the mouth and yellow or reddish urine. The tongue body is red with a dry coating; the pulse is rapid.

Treatment principle
Cool the Blood and moisten Dryness, dispel Wind and clear Heat.

Prescription
SI WU XIAO FENG YIN JIA JIAN
Four Agents Beverage for Dispersing Wind, with modifications

Sheng Di Huang (Radix Rehmanniae Glutinosae) 30g
Dang Gui (Radix Angelicae Sinensis) 10g
Chi Shao (Radix Paeoniae Rubra) 10g
Fang Feng (Radix Ledebouriellae Divaricatae) 10g
Huang Qin (Radix Scutellariae Baicalensis) 10g
Chai Hu (Radix Bupleuri) 6g
Jing Jie (Herba Schizonepetae Tenuifoliae) 6g
Gan Cao (Radix Glycyrrhizae) 6g
Sheng Ma (Rhizoma Cimicifugae) 6g

Explanation

- *Sheng Di Huang* (Radix Rehmanniae Glutinosae), *Dang Gui* (Radix Angelicae Sinensis) and *Chi Shao* (Radix Paeoniae Rubra) cool the Blood and moisten Dryness.
- *Fang Feng* (Radix Ledebouriellae Divaricatae), *Huang Qin* (Radix Scutellariae Baicalensis), *Chai Hu* (Radix Bupleuri), *Gan Cao* (Radix Glycyrrhizae), and *Sheng Ma* (Rhizoma Cimicifugae) dredge Wind and clear Heat.
- *Jing Jie* (Herba Schizonepetae Tenuifoliae) dispels Wind and alleviates itching.
- By eliminating Blood-Dryness and expelling Wind, this prescription relieves both interior and exterior patterns.

EXUBERANT WIND DUE TO SPLEEN QI DEFICIENCY

This pattern is chronic. The lips are inflamed and swollen, with fissuring and exudation. Accompanying symptoms and signs include shortness of breath, fatigue, poor appetite, abdominal distension, loose stools, and emaciation. The tongue body is pale red with a thin white coating; the pulse is thready and rapid.

Treatment principle

Fortify the Spleen, augment Qi and dredge Wind.

Prescription
SHEN LING BAI ZHU SAN JIA JIAN
Ginseng, Poria and White Atractylodes Powder, with modifications

Dang Shen (Radix Codonopsitis Pilosulae) 10g
Bai Zhu (Rhizoma Atractylodis Macrocephalae) 10g
Fu Ling (Sclerotium Poriae Cocos) 10g
Chen Pi (Pericarpium Citri Reticulatae) 10g
Chao Bai Bian Dou (Semen Dolichoris Lablab, stir-fried) 10g
Shan Yao (Radix Dioscoreae Oppositae) 30g
Yi Yi Ren (Semen Coicis Lachryma-jobi) 30g
Sha Ren (Fructus Amomi) 8g, added 5 minutes before the end of the decoction process
Jie Geng (Radix Platycodi Grandiflori) 6g
Gan Cao (Radix Glycyrrhizae) 6g

Explanation

- *Dang Shen* (Radix Codonopsitis Pilosulae), *Bai Zhu* (Rhizoma Atractylodis Macrocephalae), *Fu Ling* (Sclerotium Poriae Cocos), *Gan Cao* (Radix Glycyrrhizae), and *Chao Bai Bian Dou* (Semen Dolichoris Lablab, stir-fried) augment Qi and support the Spleen.
- *Yi Yi Ren* (Semen Coicis Lachryma-jobi), *Shan Yao* (Radix Dioscoreae Oppositae), *Sha Ren* (Fructus Amomi), and *Chen Pi* (Pericarpium Citri Reticulatae) regulate Qi and fortify the Spleen, dissipate Wind and disperse swelling.

- *Jie Geng* (Radix Platycodi Grandiflori) bears Lung Qi upward so that the effect of the other materia medica reaches the lips.

EXTERNAL TREATMENT
For dry, fissured, painful, and itchy lips, apply *Gan Lan San* (Chinese Olive Powder) mixed with sesame oil, *Gan Cao You* (Licorice Oil) or *Zi Cao You* (Gromwell Root Oil) once or twice a day.

Clinical notes

When determining treatment, both local symptoms and general causes should be taken into consideration:

- Dry and fissured lips are generally caused by Fire pathogenic factors. Bitter and cold materia medica should be employed for Excess patterns; sweet, cold and moistening materia medica for Deficiency patterns.
- Lips with exudation and erosion are signs of Damp-Heat accumulating internally, and materia medica for clearing Heat and eliminating Dampness should therefore be added.
- Where lips are swollen or granulomatous, this is usually associated with stagnation of Phlegm-Damp, and treatment should concentrate on eliminating Dampness and transforming Phlegm, and transforming stasis and dispersing swelling.

In all of these cases, the Deficiency or Excess condition of the Spleen and Stomach must also be taken into account.

Advice for the patient

- Reduce irritation of the lips by avoiding alcohol, cigarettes, lipstick, and spicy and rich food.
- Abandon the habit of constantly licking or biting the lips, or peeling loose skin or scale from the lips. If the lip fissures and oozes, wash it with a dilute hydrogen peroxide solution rather than cold tap water.
- Drink a soup made from *Yi Yi Ren* (Semen Coicis Lachryma-jobi), *Qian Shi* (Semen Euryales Ferocis), *Bi Qi* (Cormus Heleocharitis), and *Chi Xiao Dou* (Semen Phaseoli Calcarati) from time to time.

Case history

Patient
Female, aged 47.

Clinical manifestations
The lower lip was red, swollen, ulcerated and oozing, with focal necrosis and punctate bleeding. Accompanying symptoms and

signs included a sensation of burning heat and pain, which was worse on eating or exposure to wind, thirst with a desire for drinks, yellow urine, and dry stools. The tongue coating was thin, greasy and slightly yellow; the pulse was slippery and rapid.

Pattern identification
Wind-Fire in the Stomach channel and Blood-Dryness in the Spleen Channel.

Treatment principle
Clear Heat, cool the Blood and moisten Dryness.

Prescription ingredients
Sheng Di Huang (Radix Rehmanniae Glutinosae) 15g
Mai Men Dong (Radix Ophiopogonis Japonici) 10g
Zhi Mu (Rhizoma Anemarrhenae Asphodeloidis) 10g
*Shi Hu** (Herba Dendrobii) 10g
Huang Qin (Radix Scutellariae Baicalensis) 10g
Yin Chen Hao (Herba Artemisiae Scopariae) 15g
Zhi Ke (Fructus Citri Aurantii) 10g
Gan Cao (Radix Glycyrrhizae) 6g
Deng Xin Cao (Medulla Junci Effusi) 6g
Lü Dou Yi (Testa Phaseoli Radiati) 6g
Dan Zhu Ye (Herba Lophatheri Gracilis) 6g
Da Huang (Radix et Rhizoma Rhei) 6g
Shi Gao ‡ (Gypsum Fibrosum) 15g
Tian Hua Fen (Radix Trichosanthis) 10g

One bag a day was used to prepare a decoction, taken twice a day.

External treatment
Application of *Huang Lian Ruan Gao* (Coptis Ointment) and *Xi Gua Shuang* (Watermelon Frost) twice a day.

Second visit
After five days, the local redness, swelling, burning pain, and exudation had obviously decreased, but the ulceration was still there. The prescription was therefore modified by adding *Xuan Shen* (Radix Scrophulariae Ningpoensis) 10g and *Pu Gong Ying* (Herba Taraxaci cum Radice) 10g. For the external treatment, *Huang Lian Ruan Gao* (Coptis Ointment) and *Zhu Huang San* (Pearl and Bezoar Powder) were applied twice a day.

Third visit
One week later, the symptoms of internal Heat such as thirst and constipation had been relieved and the urine was clear again. The second prescription was modified by removing *Da Huang* (Radix et Rhizoma Rhei), *Shi Gao* ‡ (Gypsum Fibrosum) and *Xuan Shen* (Radix Scrophulariae Ningpoensis); the external treatment was not changed.

Outcome
After another week, new skin had been generated and local swelling had disappeared. The patient had no discomfort while eating and her energy level had improved. The patient was prescribed one more week of internal and external treatment to consolidate the effect. [8]

Modern clinical experience

TREATMENT BASED ON PATTERN IDENTIFICATION

1. **Lai** identified three patterns. [9]

- **Damp-Heat in the Spleen and Stomach**
This pattern presented as fissured and erosive lips with purulent or bloody exudate, accompanied by bad breath, thirst with no desire for drinks, constipation, hot and reddish urine, a red tongue body with a thick and greasy yellow coating, and a slippery and rapid pulse.

Treatment principle
Clear Heat from the Spleen, benefit the movement of Dampness and relieve Toxicity.

Prescription
QING PI CHU SHI YIN JIA JIAN
Beverage for Clearing Heat from the Spleen and Eliminating Dampness, with modifications

Sheng Di Huang (Radix Rehmanniae Glutinosae) 12g
Huang Qin (Radix Scutellariae Baicalensis) 12g
Fu Ling (Sclerotium Poriae Cocos) 12g
Bai Zhu (Rhizoma Atractylodis Macrocephalae) 12g
Cang Zhu (Rhizoma Atractylodis) 12g
Zhi Zi (Fructus Gardeniae Jasminoidis) 12g
Mu Dan Pi (Cortex Moutan Radicis) 12g
Mai Men Dong (Radix Ophiopogonis Japonici) 12g
Ze Xie (Rhizoma Alismatis Orientalis) 12g
Yin Chen Hao (Herba Artemisiae Scopariae) 12g
Ye Ju Hua (Flos Chrysanthemi Indici) 15g
Gan Cao (Radix Glycyrrhizae) 6g

- **Yin Deficiency complicated by Dampness**
This pattern presented as recurrent ulcerating lip sores with fissuring and bloody exudate, accompanied by irritability and restlessness, thirst, dry throat, a red tongue body with a yellow coating, and a thready and rapid pulse.

Treatment principle
Nourish Yin, clear Heat and benefit the movement of Dampness.

Prescription
ZHI BAI DI HUANG WAN JIA JIAN
Anemarrhena, Phellodendron and Rehmannia Pill, with modifications

Sheng Di Huang (Radix Rehmanniae Glutinosae) 12g
Tian Hua Fen (Radix Trichosanthis) 12g
Zhi Mu (Rhizoma Anemarrhenae Asphodeloidis) 12g
Huang Bai (Cortex Phellodendri) 12g
Mai Men Dong (Radix Ophiopogonis Japonici) 12g

Nü Zhen Zi (Fructus Ligustri Lucidi) 12g
Di Gu Pi (Cortex Lycii Radicis) 12g
Mu Dan Pi (Cortex Moutan Radicis) 12g
Gou Qi Zi (Fructus Lycii) 12g
Xuan Shen (Radix Scrophulariae Ningpoensis) 15g
Ban Lan Gen (Radix Isatidis seu Baphicacanthi) 15g
Gan Cao (Radix Glycyrrhizae) 6g

- **Blood Deficiency transforming into Dryness**

This pattern presented as fissured lips with bleeding, dryness, itching, and scaling, accompanied by a pallid, lusterless complexion, poor appetite, loose stools, dizziness, blurred vision, shortness of breath, no desire to speak, a pale tongue body with a thin and slightly yellow coating, and a thready and weak pulse.

Treatment principle
Augment Qi and fortify the Spleen, nourish the Blood and moisten Dryness.

Prescription
GUI PI TANG JIA JIAN
Decoction for Restoring the Spleen, with modifications

Dang Shen (Radix Codonopsitis Pilosulae) 15g
Huang Qi (Radix Astragali seu Hedysari) 15g
Bai Zhu (Rhizoma Atractylodis Macrocephalae) 12g
Fu Ling (Sclerotium Poriae Cocos) 12g
Dang Gui (Radix Angelicae Sinensis) 12g
Chuan Xiong (Rhizoma Ligustici Chuanxiong) 12g
Bai Shao (Radix Paeoniae Lactiflorae) 12g
Sheng Di Huang (Radix Rehmanniae Glutinosae) 12g
Mu Dan Pi (Cortex Moutan Radicis) 12g
Huang Qin (Radix Scutellariae Baicalensis) 9g
Gan Jiang (Rhizoma Zingiberis Officinalis) 6g
Gan Cao (Radix Glycyrrhizae) 6g

For each pattern, one bag a day of the ingredients was used to prepare a decoction, taken three times a day. In addition, chlortetracycline (aureomycin) ointment was applied after washing the affected area with 30 percent hydrogen peroxide solution. A course of treatment lasted six days. Results were seen after three courses.

2. **Xu** identified two patterns in the treatment of cheilitis. [10]

- **Accumulated Heat in the Spleen and Stomach**

Prescription ingredients

Bo He (Herba Menthae Haplocalycis) 10g, added 5 minutes before the end of the decoction process
Bai Shao (Radix Paeoniae Lactiflorae) 10g
Sang Ye (Folium Mori Albae) 10g
Zhi Zi (Fructus Gardeniae Jasminoidis) 10g
Fang Feng (Radix Ledebouriellae Divaricatae) 10g

Chan Tui‡ (Periostracum Cicadae) 10g
Xuan Shen (Radix Scrophulariae Ningpoensis) 10g
Huang Qin (Radix Scutellariae Baicalensis) 15g
Huang Lian (Rhizoma Coptidis) 15g
Shi Gao‡ (Gypsum Fibrosum) 15g
Zhi Mu (Rhizoma Anemarrhenae Asphodeloidis) 12g
Gan Cao (Radix Glycyrrhizae) 6g

- **Prevalence of Wind due to Blood-Dryness**

Prescription ingredients

Mu Dan Pi (Cortex Moutan Radicis) 10g
Chi Shao (Radix Paeoniae Rubra) 10g
Sheng Di Huang (Radix Rehmanniae Glutinosae) 10g
Dang Gui (Radix Angelicae Sinensis) 10g
Bai Xian Pi (Cortex Dictamni Dasycarpi Radicis) 10g
Wu Shao She‡ (Zaocys Dhumnades) 10g
Xuan Shen (Radix Scrophulariae Ningpoensis) 10g
Zi Cao (Radix Arnebiae seu Lithospermi) 10g
Chen Pi (Pericarpium Citri Reticulatae) 10g
Chan Tui‡ (Periostracum Cicadae) 10g
Gan Cao (Radix Glycyrrhizae) 6g

For both patterns, one bag a day of the herbs was decocted in 700ml of water to obtain 300 ml of liquid, divided into 100ml portions and taken three times a day.

External prescription

Zi Cao (Radix Arnebiae seu Lithospermi) 10g
Bai Zhi (Radix Angelicae Dahuricae) 10g
Xiang You (Oleum Sesami Seminis) 30ml

The two herbs were cooked in the sesame oil over a mild heat until scorched; the oil was then filtered and stored in a bottle for application to the affected area on the lips twice a day with cotton buds.

Results were seen after three weeks.

SPECIAL PRESCRIPTIONS

1. **Wang** treated chronic cheilitis with a basic prescription with modifications. [11]

Prescription
ZHONG HE TANG
Harmonizing the Middle Decoction

Dang Shen (Radix Codonopsitis Pilosulae) 15g
Bai Zhu (Rhizoma Atractylodis Macrocephalae) 15g
Shan Yao (Radix Dioscoreae Oppositae) 15g
Yi Yi Ren (Semen Coicis Lachryma-jobi) 15g
Huang Qi (Radix Astragali seu Hedysari) 30g
Fu Ling (Sclerotium Poriae Cocos) 10g
Chen Pi (Pericarpium Citri Reticulatae) 10g
Sha Ren (Fructus Amomi) 3g, infused in the prepared decoction

Modifications

1. For accumulation of exuberant Heat in the Stomach, manifesting as a bitter taste in the mouth, dry tongue and a dry, eroded lower lip, *Lian Qiao* (Fructus Forsythiae Suspensae) 10g and *Bo He* (Herba Menthae Haplocalycis) 3g were added to clear Excess-Heat from the Upper Burner. *Dan Zhu Ye* (Herba Lophatheri Gracilis) 10g and *Sheng Ma* (Rhizoma Cimicifugae) 6g were also added to bear Excess-Heat downward; *Dan Zhu Ye* (Herba Lophatheri Gracilis) bears downward and *Sheng Ma* (Rhizoma Cimicifugae) has a strong ascending action so that together they promote the movement of Qi to assist in eliminating Heat.

2. For lesions with scabs and bleeding, *Sheng Di Huang* (Radix Rehmanniae Glutinosae) 15g, *Chi Shao* (Radix Paeoniae Rubra) 10g and *Bai Mao Gen* (Rhizoma Imperatae Cylindricae) 15g were added to cool the Blood and stop bleeding.

One bag a day was used to prepare a decoction, taken twice a day. Results were seen on average after three weeks.

2. **Zou** formulated her own prescription for erosive cheilitis. [12]

Prescription
YU CHUN FANG
Lip-Healing Formula

Da Huang (Radix et Rhizoma Rhei) 10g

Huang Lian (Rhizoma Coptidis) 10g
Huang Qin (Radix Scutellariae Baicalensis) 10g
Pei Lan (Herba Eupatorii Fortunei) 10g
Mu Dan Pi (Cortex Moutan Radicis) 10g
Tian Hua Fen (Radix Trichosanthis) 30g
Shi Gao‡ (Gypsum Fibrosum) 30g, decocted for 30 minutes before adding the other ingredients
Jin Yin Hua (Flos Lonicerae) 60g
Dang Gui (Radix Angelicae Sinensis) 45g
Xuan Shen (Radix Scrophulariae Ningpoensis) 15g
Pu Gong Ying (Herba Taraxaci cum Radice) 15g
Chan Tui‡ (Periostracum Cicadae) 9g

One bag a day of the ingredients was decocted in one liter of water to obtain 500 ml of liquid, taken twice a day. A small amount of the decoction was also set aside for use as a wash for the lips, once a day. Patients were advised to avoid spicy and other irritating food during the treatment. Results were seen after two weeks.

EXTERNAL TREATMENT

Wu treated exfoliative cheilitis with a wet compress. He steeped *Huang Lian* (Rhizoma Coptidis) 10g and *Huang Bai* (Cortex Phellodendri) 5g in 50ml of water for 30 minutes and then decocted them to produce the compress, which was used to dress the lesion for five to ten minutes three times a day. Results were seen after three to five days. [13]

Recurrent aphthous stomatitis (mouth ulcers)
复发性阿弗他口腔炎

Recurrent aphthous stomatitis is repeated superficial ulceration of the oral mucosa, onset of which may be associated with mechanical or physical irritation, digestive dysfunction, mental stress, fatigue, anemia, deficiency of vitamins or trace elements (such as zinc), immunologic function defects, and viral infection.

In TCM, this disease is also known as *kou chuang* (mouth sores).

Clinical manifestations

- One or several small, slightly raised papules occur on the lips, tongue, cheeks, or gums before rupturing to form superficial, oval, yellowish-white or grayish-white ulcers with a red areola.
- The lesions may be painful, with the pain worsening

when eating or drinking.
- The condition generally resolves spontaneously in seven to ten days, but tends to recur.
- Accompanying symptoms vary in severity and frequently include thirst, irritability, listlessness, or poor appetite.

Differential diagnosis

Table 15-1 in the Oral candidiasis (thrush) section of this chapter compares various types of common mouth sores.

Lichen planus
Although the eruptions in lichen planus usually involve the flexor surfaces of the wrists and forearms and the lower legs around and above the ankles, the mucous membranes

are involved in 40-60 percent of cases, sometimes as the only manifestation of the disease. Lichen planus on the oral mucosa commonly manifests as grayish-white papules, which can be distinguished from the lesions of recurrent aphthous stomatitis by the presence of Wickham's striae, a lacy white pattern of lines on their surface.

Erythema multiforme

In severe cases of erythema multiforme, the lips, oral mucosa or the surface of the tongue may become eroded and ulcerated, with the eroded areas frequently becoming confluent and malodorous. Other areas of the skin will also be affected.

Etiology and pathology

- This disease manifests as Excess or Deficiency patterns. Excess patterns are generally caused by the flaming upward of Heart-Fire or exuberant Heat in the Spleen and Stomach; Deficiency patterns result from effulgent Yin Deficiency-Fire or Yang Deficiency of the Spleen and Kidneys.

- Excessive intake of spicy or greasy food can produce Heat, leading to accumulation of Heat in the Spleen and Stomach, whereas emotional depression can cause hyperactivity of Heart Yang. Heat and Fire in the Heart or Spleen channels may rush along the channels, steaming upward to the mouth and scorching the flesh and membranes, resulting in ulcerating sores of the mouth.

- If accumulated internal Heat due to constitutional reasons is complicated by external Wind-Heat or if Toxic pathogenic factors attack an oral cavity where basic hygiene has been ignored, the external pathogenic factors will fight with Fire from the internal organs, damaging the flesh and membranes of the mouth.

- Yin Deficiency following an illness or insufficiency of Yin-Fluids of the Heart, Spleen and Kidneys due to overstrain can stir up Deficiency-Fire, which flames upward to the mouth and tongue, scorching and ulcerating the flesh and membranes.

- Constitutional Yang Deficiency, excessive intake of cold or raw foods or materia medica with bitter and cold properties, or overindulgence in sexual activities can damage Original Qi (Yuan Qi), resulting in Yang Deficiency of the Spleen and Kidneys. In this case, these organs are impaired in their warming and transforming function, leading to stagnation of Body Fluids. Damp pathogenic factors spread upward to the mouth and tongue, where Cold and Dampness are trapped in the mouth, rotting the flesh and membranes and forming ulcers.

Pattern identification and treatment

INTERNAL TREATMENT

FLAMING UPWARD OF HEART-FIRE

This pattern involves the tongue with ulcerating sores of different sizes; sores may become confluent in serious cases. The area around the sores is obviously red and swollen. There is a sensation of burning heat and pain, which worsens when speaking or eating. Accompanying symptoms include thirst and irritability. The tongue body is red with a yellow coating; the pulse is rapid.

Treatment principle

Clear Heat from the Heart and cool the Blood, disperse swelling and alleviate pain.

Prescription

DAO CHI SAN JIA JIAN

Powder for Guiding Out Reddish Urine, with modifications

Sheng Di Huang (Radix Rehmanniae Glutinosae) 15-30g
Jin Yin Hua (Flos Lonicerae) 15-30g
Dan Zhu Ye (Herba Lophatheri Gracilis) 10g
Zhi Zi (Fructus Gardeniae Jasminoidis) 10g
Gan Cao (Radix Glycyrrhizae) 10g
Tong Cao (Medulla Tetrapanacis Papyriferi) 6g
Deng Xin Cao (Medulla Junci Effusi) 6g
Hu Po‡ (Succinum) 4.5g
Che Qian Zi (Semen Plantaginis) 12g, wrapped
Che Qian Cao (Herba Plantaginis) 12g
Hua Shi‡ (Talcum) 15g, wrapped in *He Ye* (Folium Nelumbinis Nuciferae) for decoction

Explanation

- *Sheng Di Huang* (Radix Rehmanniae Glutinosae), *Zhi Zi* (Fructus Gardeniae Jasminoidis), *Gan Cao* (Radix Glycyrrhizae), *Tong Cao* (Medulla Tetrapanacis Papyriferi), *Dan Zhu Ye* (Herba Lophatheri Gracilis), and *Deng Xin Cao* (Medulla Junci Effusi) clear Heat from the Heart, cool the Blood and guide Heat downward to relieve the sensation of burning heat and pain in the tongue.

- *Jin Yin Hua* (Flos Lonicerae), *Che Qian Zi* (Semen Plantaginis) and *Che Qian Cao* (Herba Plantaginis) disperse swelling and alleviate pain.

- *Hu Po*‡ (Succinum) protects the Heart and quiets the Spirit.

- *Hua Shi*‡ (Talcum), when wrapped in *He Ye* (Folium Nelumbinis Nuciferae), clears Spleen Yang and removes Damp-Heat by promoting urination, enabling Heart-Fire Toxins to be eliminated at the same time as the urine.

EXUBERANT HEAT IN THE SPLEEN AND STOMACH

This pattern usually involves the lips, gums, cheeks, and palate. Lesions are red, swollen and painful and usually coalesce into patches on ulceration. Accompanying symptoms and signs include hot saliva, thirst and constipation. The tongue body is red with a yellow coating; the pulse is slippery and rapid.

Treatment principle

Clear Heat from the Stomach and drain Fire, disperse swelling and alleviate pain.

Prescription

QING WEI SAN JIA JIAN

Powder for Clearing Heat from the Stomach, with modifications

Dang Gui (Radix Angelicae Sinensis) 10g
Sheng Di Huang (Radix Rehmanniae Glutinosae) 10g
Tian Hua Fen (Radix Trichosanthis) 10g
Ju Hua (Flos Chrysanthemi Morifolii) 10g
Chao Mu Dan Pi (Cortex Moutan Radicis, stir-fried) 10g
Shi Gao ‡ (Gypsum Fibrosum) 15g, decocted for
  30 minutes before adding the other ingredients
Ge Gen (Radix Puerariae) 6g
Ku Shen (Radix Sophorae Flavescentis) 6g
Shu Da Huang (Radix et Rhizoma Rhei Conquitum) 6g
Sheng Ma (Rhizoma Cimicifugae) 6g

Explanation

- *Dang Gui* (Radix Angelicae Sinensis), *Chao Mu Dan Pi* (Cortex Moutan Radicis, stir-fried), *Sheng Di Huang* (Radix Rehmanniae Glutinosae), *Tian Hua Fen* (Radix Trichosanthis), and *Ju Hua* (Flos Chrysanthemi Morifolii) nourish Yin and clear Heat, cool the Blood and disperse swelling.
- *Shi Gao* ‡ (Gypsum Fibrosum), *Ge Gen* (Radix Puerariae), *Ku Shen* (Radix Sophorae Flavescentis), and *Shu Da Huang* (Radix et Rhizoma Rhei Conquitum) clear Heat from the Stomach and drain Fire to drive out Heat Toxins from the Spleen and Stomach and relieve redness, swelling and pain in the lips, gums and palate.
- *Sheng Ma* (Rhizoma Cimicifugae) guides the effect of the other ingredients up to the affected area and clears Heat Toxins.

EFFULGENT YIN DEFICIENCY-FIRE

This pattern is characterized by relatively few ulcerating sores in the oral cavity; ulcers have a pale red and slightly swollen margin or areola, but are only mildly painful. Recurrence is frequent. Accompanying symptoms and signs include palpitations, irritability due to Deficiency, insomnia, limpness and aching in the lower back and knees, a feverish sensation in the palms and soles, tinnitus, reddening of the cheeks, and yellow urine. The tongue body is dry with a red tip; the pulse is thready and rapid.

Treatment principle

Moisten Yin, clear Heat and nourish the Blood.

Prescription

GUI SHAO TIAN DI JIAN JIA JIAN

Angelica Root, Peony, Asparagus, and Rehmannia Brew, with modifications

Dang Gui (Radix Angelicae Sinensis) 10g
Chao Bai Shao (Radix Paeoniae Lactiflorae, stir-fried) 12g
Tian Men Dong (Radix Asparagi Cochinchinensis) 12g
Shu Di Huang (Radix Rehmanniae Glutinosae Conquita) 15g

Explanation

- *Dang Gui* (Radix Angelicae Sinensis) and *Chao Bai Shao* (Radix Paeoniae Lactiflorae, stir-fried) nourish the Blood and moisten Yin.
- *Tian Men Dong* (Radix Asparagi Cochinchinensis) clears Deficiency-Heat from the Lungs and Stomach, whereas *Shu Di Huang* (Radix Rehmanniae Glutinosae Conquita) enriches the Liver and supplements the Kidneys. When the Lungs and Kidneys are treated at the same time, mouth sores can be eliminated.

YANG DEFICIENCY OF THE SPLEEN AND KIDNEYS

This pattern manifests as relatively few, discretely distributed ulcers on the oral mucosa. Lesions are pale and slightly painful. Redness and swelling are absent from the surrounding area. Accompanying symptoms and signs include cold limbs, no desire for food or drink, loose stools, and long voidings of clear urine. The tongue body is pale red with a white and slightly greasy coating; the pulse is deep.

Treatment principle

Warm the Middle Burner and dissipate Cold, fortify the Spleen and augment Qi.

Prescription

FU ZI LI ZHONG TANG JIA JIAN

Aconite Decoction for Regulating the Middle, with modifications

Dang Shen (Radix Codonopsitis Pilosulae) 10g
Chao Bai Zhu (Rhizoma Atractylodis Macrocephalae,
  stir-fried) 10g
Gan Cao (Radix Glycyrrhizae) 10g
Fu Pen Zi (Fructus Rubi Chingii) 12g
Gan Jiang (Rhizoma Zingiberis Officinalis) 6g

Explanation

- *Dang Shen* (Radix Codonopsitis Pilosulae) and *Chao Bai Zhu* (Rhizoma Atractylodis Macrocephalae, stir-fried) warm Yang and boost the Spleen.

- *Fu Pen Zi* (Fructus Rubi Chingii) and *Gan Jiang* (Rhizoma Zingiberis Officinalis) warm the Middle Burner and dissipate Cold.
- *Gan Cao* (Radix Glycyrrhizae) harmonizes the properties of the other ingredients.
- This prescription focuses on treatment of both the Spleen and the Kidneys, thus making it very effective for mouth sores, especially persistent sores.

General modifications

1. For dry mouth and reduced appetite due to Spleen Yin Deficiency, add *Shi Hu** (Herba Dendrobii) and *Yin Chen Hao* (Herba Artemisiae Scopariae).
2. For fatigue due to Qi Deficiency, add *Tai Zi Shen* (Radix Pseudostellariae Heterophyllae) and *Fu Ling* (Sclerotium Poriae Cocos).
3. For Kidney Yin Deficiency, add *Shan Zhu Yu* (Fructus Corni Officinalis), *Shan Yao* (Radix Dioscoreae Oppositae) and *Zhi Mu* (Rhizoma Anemarrhenae Asphodeloidis).
4. For persistent, non-healing mouth sores, add *Wu Bei Zi‡* (Galla Rhois Chinensis) and *Cang Zhu* (Rhizoma Atractylodis).
5. For diarrhea, thirst and acid regurgitation, add *Huang Lian* (Rhizoma Coptidis).
6. For aversion to cold in the lower body, long voidings of clear urine and a deep and weak pulse in the Kidney position, add *Gan Di Huang* (Radix Rehmanniae Glutinosae Exsiccata), *Shan Zhu Yu* (Fructus Corni Officinalis), *Shan Yao* (Radix Dioscoreae Oppositae), *Mu Dan Pi* (Cortex Moutan Radicis), *Fu Ling* (Sclerotium Poriae Cocos), and *Ze Xie* (Rhizoma Alismatis Orientalis).

EXTERNAL TREATMENT

- A decoction of *Qiang Wei Gen* (Radix Rosae Multiflorae) 30g or *Shi Hu** (Herba Dendrobii) 30g prepared in 200ml of water can be used as a mouthwash for disinfecting or cleansing the affected area in all patterns.
- For Excess-Fire patterns, apply *Bing Shi San* (Borneol and Gypsum Powder); for Deficiency-Fire patterns, apply *Xi Gua Shuang* (Watermelon Frost); for Yang Deficiency patterns, apply *Shou Gan Sheng Ji Yao Fen* (Medicated Powder for Promoting Contraction and Generating Flesh); and for persistent, non-healing sores, apply *Zhu Huang San* (Pearl and Bezoar Powder). In all cases, the medication is rubbed into the affected area.

ACUPUNCTURE

Prescription 1: CV-24 Chengjiang, LI-4 Hegu, GV-26 Shuigou, and CV-4 Guanyuan.

Prescription 2: BL-40 Weizhong and SI-3 Houxi.

Technique: Apply the even method and retain the needles for 30 minutes after obtaining Qi. Treat once every two days. A course consists of seven treatment sessions.

Explanation

- CV-4 Guanyuan warms the Kidneys and returns Fire to its source.
- CV-24 Chengjiang, LI-4 Hegu and GV-26 Shuigou clear Heat and relieve Toxicity.
- BL-40 Weizhong and SI-3 Houxi clear Heat and cool the Blood.

EAR ACUPUNCTURE

Points: Ear-Shenmen, Heart, Spleen, Stomach, Liver, Kidney, and Endocrine.
Technique: Retain the needles for 30 minutes. Treat once every three days. Embedding needling can also be used at these points; change the needles once a week.

POINT DRESSING METHOD

For mouth sores due to Excess-Fire, grind *Wu Zhu Yu* (Fructus Evodiae Rutaecarpae) 10g into a fine powder, mix with vinegar and then apply the mixture as a dressing to KI-1 Yongquan. Change the dressing daily. A course of treatment lasts for five days

Clinical notes

- Differentiation must be made between Excess and Deficiency patterns when treating this disease. For Excess patterns, treat the Heart and Spleen; for Deficiency patterns, treat the Spleen and Kidneys. However, stubborn non-healing ulcers may be a combined Excess-Deficiency pattern.
- Any underlying chronic diseases should be treated to reduce the likelihood of mouth ulcers.
- This disease is self-limiting and most patients recover seven to ten days after onset. Lesions heal without scarring. However, aphthous stomatitis tends to recur, especially when it is caused by effulgent Yin Deficiency-Fire, in which case the condition may persist for years or decades.

Advice for the patient

- Oral hygiene is extremely important.
- Reduce intake of spicy, rich, greasy, or fried food.
- Exercise more frequently.
- Avoid overwork or stressful situations.

Case history

Patient
Female, aged 48.

Clinical manifestations
The patient had suffered from swollen gums and ulceration of the oral cavity and tongue for a number of months. The ulceration was painful and caused salivation; the patient had a poor appetite because of the difficulty in chewing resulting from the pain. Some of the ulcers were festering.

Accompanying symptoms and signs included a feeling of obstruction and oppression in the throat, disturbed sleep, dizziness, dry stools, and yellow urine. The tip of the tongue was red and the tongue coating was yellow; the pulse was wiry and rapid.

Pattern identification
Accumulation of Heat in the Spleen and Stomach, with Heart-Fire flaming upward.

Treatment principle
Clear Heat and drain Fire.

Prescription
YIN QIAO SAN HE HUANG LIAN JIE DU TANG JIA JIAN
Honeysuckle and Forsythia Powder Combined With Coptis Decoction for Relieving Toxicity, with modifications

Sheng Ma (Rhizoma Cimicifugae) 3g
Xi Xin* (Herba cum Radice Asari) 3g
Jiu Chao Huang Qin (Radix Scutellariae Baicalensis, stir-fried in wine) 10g
Jiu Chao Huang Bai (Cortex Phellodendri, stir-fried in wine) 10g
Huang Lian (Rhizoma Coptidis) 10g
Zhi Zi Yi (Testa Gardeniae Jasminoidis) 6g
Jiu Zhi Da Huang (Radix et Rhizoma Rhei, processed with wine) 6g
Niu Bang Zi (Fructus Arctii Lappae) 6g
Lian Qiao (Fructus Forsythiae Suspensae) 10g
Jie Geng (Radix Platycodi Grandiflori) 5g
Chao Zhi Ke (Fructus Citri Aurantii, stir-fried) 5g
Jin Yin Hua (Flos Lonicerae) 15g
Zhi Gan Cao (Radix Glycyrrhizae, mix-fried with honey) 3g

One bag a day was used to prepare a decoction, taken twice a day.

External treatment
Pu Huang (Pollen Typhae), 30g a day, was rubbed into the ulcerated areas four or five times a day.

Second visit
After two bags of the herbs, the swollen gums and the mouth and tongue ulcers had been significantly reduced. The prescription was modified by removing Huang Bai (Cortex Phellodendri) and Zhi Ke (Fructus Citri Aurantii) and adding Zhi Shi (Fructus Immaturus Citri Aurantii) 6g and Pu Gong Ying

(Herba Taraxaci cum Radice) 15g. The external treatment continued as before.

Third visit
After two more bags of the modified prescription and the same external treatment, the mouth and tongue ulcers had disappeared completely. Stools had become normal and sleep had improved. In order to prevent recurrence, the patient was told to take another two bags of the modified prescription (one bag to last two days) without the external treatment.

Discussion
The author of this report frequently used Yin Qiao San He Huang Lian Jie Du Tang Jia Jian (Honeysuckle and Forsythia Powder Combined With Coptis Decoction for Relieving Toxicity) to treat superficial mouth ulcers by clearing Heat in the Spleen and Stomach and draining Fire in the Heart. Jiu Zhi Da Huang (Radix et Rhizoma Rhei, processed with wine) and Chao Zhi Ke (Fructus Citri Aurantii, stir-fried) were added to free the bowels and drain Heat. He also found that using Pu Huang (Pollen Typhae) either externally or internally to treat mouth and tongue sores was very effective.

Sheng Ma (Rhizoma Cimicifugae) and Xi Xin* (Herba cum Radice Asari) are channel conductors. Sheng Ma (Rhizoma Cimicifugae) clears Heat and relieves Toxicity and enters the Yangming channels; Xi Xin* (Herba cum Radice Asari) eliminates swelling and alleviates pain and enters the Shaoyin channels. This represents the relationship between the mouth belonging to the Spleen and Stomach and the tongue belonging to the Heart and Kidneys. The addition of Sheng Ma (Rhizoma Cimicifugae) and Xi Xin* (Herba cum Radice Asari) to cold or cool herbs with the function of clearing Heat allows retention of Fire to be treated by moving outward. [14]

Literature excerpt

In Feng Shi Jin Nang Mi Lu [Feng's Secret Records of the Best Counsels], it says: "At the initial stage of mouth and tongue sores, cooling materia medica should not be applied, otherwise Cold will congeal and cannot be dissipated, and ulcers will burst forth and persist. It is best to use slightly acrid upward-bearing and dissipating materia medica at first and then to employ clearing and cooling ingredients to thrust retained Fire out to the exterior.

"When there is insufficiency of Qi in the Middle Burner, the Spleen and Stomach are Deficient and fail to astringe and contain the Lower Burner; Yin-Fire will then be forced to flame upward, thus causing Yang Deficiency mouth sores. Zhu Danxi said: 'Overstrain will result in Deficiency-Fire flaming upward and wandering out of control, thus causing sores in the mouth and on the tongue. It should be treated by Li Zhong Tang (Decoction for Regulating the Middle) plus Fu Zi* (Radix Lateralis Aconiti Carmichaeli Praeparata). For Excess-Heat patterns, do not add cool materia medica, otherwise the sores will not heal.'"

Modern clinical experience

TREATMENT BASED ON PATTERN IDENTIFICATION

1. **Zang Kuntang** identified three patterns for treating recurrent aphthous stomatitis. [15]

- **Accumulation of Heat in the Heart and Spleen**

Treatment principle
Clear Heat and drain Fire.

Prescription ingredients

Guang Huo Xiang (Herba Pogostemi) 10g
Zhi Zi (Fructus Gardeniae Jasminoidis) 10g
Tong Cao (Medulla Tetrapanacis Papyriferi) 10g
Dan Zhu Ye (Herba Lophatheri Gracilis) 10g
Chi Shao (Radix Paeoniae Rubra) 10g
Gan Cao (Radix Glycyrrhizae) 10g
Shi Gao‡ (Gypsum Fibrosum) 15g

- **Spleen and Kidney Deficiency**

Treatment principle
Fortify the Spleen and warm the Kidneys.

Prescription ingredients

Huang Qi (Radix Astragali seu Hedysari) 15g
Dang Shen (Radix Codonopsitis Pilosulae) 10g
Bai Zhu (Rhizoma Atractylodis Macrocephalae) 10g
Gan Cao (Radix Glycyrrhizae) 10g
Chen Pi (Pericarpium Citri Reticulatae) 10g
Yi Yi Ren (Semen Coicis Lachryma-jobi) 10g
Bu Gu Zhi (Fructus Psoraleae Corylifoliae) 10g
Sheng Ma (Rhizoma Cimicifugae) 4g
Chai Hu (Radix Bupleuri) 6g
Dang Gui (Radix Angelicae Sinensis) 6g
Gan Jiang (Rhizoma Zingiberis Officinalis) 3g

- **Effulgent Yin Deficiency-Fire**

Treatment principle
Enrich Yin and bear Fire downward.

Prescription ingredients

Zhi Mu (Rhizoma Anemarrhenae Asphodeloidis) 10g
Huang Bai (Cortex Phellodendri) 10g
Sheng Di Huang (Radix Rehmanniae Glutinosae) 10g
Shu Di Huang (Radix Rehmanniae Glutinosae Conquita) 10g
Shan Zhu Yu (Fructus Corni Officinalis) 10g
Mu Dan Pi (Cortex Moutan Radicis) 10g
Ze Xie (Rhizoma Alismatis Orientalis) 10g
Tian Men Dong (Radix Asparagi Cochinchinensis) 10g
Mai Men Dong (Radix Ophiopogonis Japonici) 10g
Xuan Shen (Radix Scrophulariae Ningpoensis) 20g
Ye Jiao Teng (Caulis Polygoni Multiflori) 30g
Huang Lian (Rhizoma Coptidis) 5g
Rou Gui (Cortex Cinnamomi Cassiae) 2g

Modifications for this pattern

1. For severe Deficiency-Fire, *Nan Sha Shen* (Radix Adenophorae) 15g, *Shi Hu** (Herba Dendrobii) 10g, and *Bai Shao* (Radix Paeoniae Lactiflorae) 10g or *Chuan Niu Xi* (Radix Cyathulae Officinalis) 10g were added to guide Fire downward.
2. For irritability and restlessness due to Deficiency, *Mu Li*‡ (Concha Ostreae) 30g and *Long Gu*‡ (Os Draconis) 15g were added.

For all patterns, one bag a day was used to prepare a decoction, taken twice a day for one week.

2. **Wang** treated patients according to two different patterns. [16]

- **Effulgent Yin Deficiency-Fire**
This pattern presented as one or two painful and recurrent grayish-white ulcerative spots on the oral mucosa. Accompanying symptoms and signs included dizziness, aching of the lower back, poor sleep with profuse dreaming, and menstrual irregularities in women patients. The tongue body was red with a scant coating; the pulse was thready and rapid.

Treatment principle
Nourish Yin, boost the Kidneys, and return Fire to its source.

Prescription ingredients

Huang Bai (Cortex Phellodendri) 10g
Shan Zhu Yu (Fructus Corni Officinalis) 10g
Mu Dan Pi (Cortex Moutan Radicis) 10g
Gan Cao (Radix Glycyrrhizae) 10g
Sheng Di Huang (Radix Rehmanniae Glutinosae) 15g
Shan Yao (Radix Dioscoreae Oppositae) 15g
Fu Ling (Sclerotium Poriae Cocos) 15g
Sha Ren (Fructus Amomi) 6g
Ze Xie (Rhizoma Alismatis Orientalis) 6g
Long Gu‡ (Os Draconis) 30g
Mu Li‡ (Concha Ostreae) 30g
Rou Gui (Cortex Cinnamomi Cassiae) 3g

Modifications

1. For menstrual irregularities, *Dang Gui* (Radix Angelicae Sinensis) 15g was added.
2. For insomnia, *Huang Lian* (Rhizoma Coptidis) 6g was added.

- **Spleen Deficiency**
This pattern presented as recurrent, slightly painful single ulcerative spots deep inside the oral mucosa; the pain worsened on eating. Accompanying symptoms and

signs included weak limbs, lassitude, a dehydrated complexion, and loose stools. The tongue body was pale with a white and greasy or yellow and greasy coating; the pulse was deep and thready.

Treatment principle
Fortify the Spleen and augment Qi, bear Yang upward and Fire downward.

Prescription ingredients
Huang Bai (Cortex Phellodendri) 6g
Sheng Ma (Rhizoma Cimicifugae) 6g
Sha Ren (Fructus Amomi) 10g
Zhi Gan Cao (Radix Glycyrrhizae, mix-fried with honey) 10g
Dang Shen (Radix Codonopsitis Pilosulae) 30g
Huang Qi (Radix Astragali seu Hedysari) 30g
Bai Zhu (Rhizoma Atractylodis Macrocephalae) 15g
Dang Gui (Radix Angelicae Sinensis) 15g
Hai Piao Xiao‡ (Os Sepiae seu Sepiellae) 20g

Modifications
1. For severe Yang Deficiency, *Rou Gui* (Cortex Cinnamomi Cassiae) 6g was added.
2. For prevalence of Dampness, *Bai Bian Dou* (Semen Dolichoris Lablab) 15g was added.

Results were seen after one week.

3. **Tu** treated 90 cases of recurrent ulcerating sores in the oral cavity. For pattern identification, he emphasized the importance of the color of the surrounding mucosa, the severity of the pain and the duration of the illness. He then differentiated between Deficiency-Fire and Excess-Fire before deciding on the treatment to be administered. He treated Excess-Fire by draining Fire and Deficiency-Fire by enriching Yin. [17]

• Heart-Fire flaming upward
This pattern manifested as red mucosa around the ulcer, a sensation of burning heat and obvious pain, with a dry mouth, a red tongue tip and a rapid pulse.

Treatment principle
Clear Heat from the Heart and drain Fire.

Prescription
DAO CHI SAN JIA JIAN
Powder for Guiding Out Reddish Urine, with modifications

Sheng Di Huang (Radix Rehmanniae Glutinosae) 10g
Dan Zhu Ye (Herba Lophatheri Gracilis) 10g
Mai Men Dong (Radix Ophiopogonis Japonici) 10g
Tong Cao (Medulla Tetrapanacis Papyriferi) 5g
Gan Cao (Radix Glycyrrhizae) 5g
Huang Lian (Rhizoma Coptidis) 2g
Deng Xin Cao (Medulla Junci Effusi) 1g

• Effulgent Yin Deficiency-Fire
This pattern manifested as pale red surrounding mucosa, mild pain and frequent recurrence, accompanied by palpitations, insomnia, a bare tongue with a scant coating, and a thready, slightly rapid pulse.

Treatment principle
Enrich Yin and bear Fire downward.

Prescription
ZI YIN BA WEI WAN JIA JIAN
Eight-Ingredient Pill for Enriching Yin, with modifications

Sheng Di Huang (Radix Rehmanniae Glutinosae) 15g
Shu Di Huang (Radix Rehmanniae Glutinosae Conquita) 10g
Shan Zhu Yu (Fructus Corni Officinalis) 12g
Mu Dan Pi (Cortex Moutan Radicis) 10g
Zhi Mu (Rhizoma Anemarrhenae Asphodeloidis) 10g
Huang Bai (Cortex Phellodendri) 10g
Nü Zhen Zi (Fructus Ligustri Lucidi) 10g
Xuan Shen (Radix Scrophulariae Ningpoensis) 15g

Modifications
1. For insomnia, *Ye Jiao Teng* (Caulis Polygoni Multiflori) 20g and *Suan Zao Ren* (Semen Ziziphi Spinosae) 10g were added.
2. For a persistent and lingering condition, *Rou Gui* (Cortex Cinnamomi Cassiae) 3g was added 5 minutes before the end of the decoction process.

External application
Yang Yin Sheng Ji San (Powder for Nourishing Yin and Generating Flesh) or *Xi Lei San* (Tin-Like Powder) was also applied locally.

Results were seen after one week.

SPECIAL PRESCRIPTIONS

1. **Li** reported on the treatment of 35 cases of recurrent aphthous stomatitis. [18]

Prescription
JIA WEI JIAO TAI WAN
Augmented Peaceful Interaction Pill

Huang Lian (Rhizoma Coptidis) 10g
Sha Ren (Fructus Amomi) 10g, added 5 minutes before the end of the decoction process
Rou Gui (Cortex Cinnamomi Cassiae) 10g
Bai Bian Dou (Semen Dolichoris Lablab) 20g
Tai Zi Shen (Radix Pseudostellariae Heterophyllae) 20g
Bai Zhu (Rhizoma Atractylodis Macrocephalae) 15g
Sheng Di Huang (Radix Rehmanniae Glutinosae) 15g
Mai Men Dong (Radix Ophiopogonis Japonici) 15g
Shan Yao (Radix Dioscoreae Oppositae) 30g
*Bie Jia** (Carapax Amydae Sinensis) 30g

Mu Dan Pi (Cortex Moutan Radicis) 12g
Gan Cao (Radix Glycyrrhizae) 6g

Modifications

1. For severe Qi Deficiency, *Huang Qi* (Radix Astragali seu Hedysari) 30g was added.
2. For severe Dampness, *Cang Zhu* (Rhizoma Atractylodis) 15g and *Yi Yi Ren* (Semen Coicis Lachrymajobi) 20g were added.

One bag a day was used to prepare a decoction, taken three times a day. Results were seen after seven days.

2. **Lu** treated aphthous stomatitis with a decoction used for internal treatment and as a mouthwash. [19]

Prescription
XIAO CHAI HU TANG JIA JIAN
Minor Bupleurum Decoction, with modifications

Chai Hu (Radix Bupleuri) 12g
Huang Qin (Radix Scutellariae Baicalensis) 9g
Da Zao (Fructus Ziziphi Jujubae) 9g
Huang Lian (Rhizoma Coptidis) 8g
Fa Ban Xia (Rhizoma Pinelliae Ternatae Praeparata) 10g
Dang Shen (Radix Codonopsitis Pilosulae) 10g
Sheng Jiang (Rhizoma Zingiberis Officinalis Recens) 9g

One bag a day was used to prepare a decoction, taken twice a day. Some of the decoction was also set aside to be used as a mouthwash several times a day. Patients were advised not to drink any water for half an hour after using the mouthwash. Results were seen within 3 to 15 days.

3. **Wang** treated stubborn recurrent aphthous stomatitis by augmenting Qi in the Middle Burner. This method is indicated for Spleen and Stomach Deficiency, sinking of Qi in the Middle Burner and upward floating of Deficiency-Fire. [20]

Treatment principle
Augment Qi and bear Yang upward, eliminate Heat with warmth and sweetness.

Prescription
BU ZHONG YI QI TANG JIA JIAN
Decoction for Supplementing the Middle and Augmenting Qi, with modifications

Huang Qi (Radix Astragali seu Hedysari) 15g
Bai Zhu (Rhizoma Atractylodis Macrocephalae) 10g
Dang Shen (Radix Codonopsitis Pilosulae) 10g
Fu Ling (Sclerotium Poriae Cocos) 10g
Chen Pi (Pericarpium Citri Reticulatae) 10g
Sheng Ma (Rhizoma Cimicifugae) 10g
Chai Hu (Radix Bupleuri) 10g

Dang Gui (Radix Angelicae Sinensis) 6g
Gan Jiang (Rhizoma Zingiberis Officinalis) 6g
Rou Gui (Cortex Cinnamomi Cassiae) 3g
Wu Bei Zi‡ (Galla Rhois Chinensis) 6g

Results were evaluated after one month with recurrence of the ulcers being halted in the majority of patients.

4. **Xie** treated recurrence of this condition by enriching the Kidneys and invigorating the Blood. [21]

Prescription ingredients

Shu Di Huang (Radix Rehmanniae Glutinosae Conquita) 15g
Nü Zhen Zi (Fructus Ligustri Lucidi) 10g
Shan Yao (Radix Dioscoreae Oppositae) 10g
Mu Dan Pi (Cortex Moutan Radicis) 10g
Huang Qi (Radix Astragali seu Hedysari) 10g
Dang Gui (Radix Angelicae Sinensis) 10g
Niu Xi (Radix Achyranthis Bidentatae) 10g
Chuan Xiong (Rhizoma Ligustici Chuanxiong) 10g
Shan Zhu Yu (Fructus Corni Officinalis) 10g
Fu Ling (Sclerotium Poriae Cocos) 10g

One bag a day was used to prepare a decoction, taken twice a day. Results were evaluated after four weeks with recurrence of the ulcers being halted in the majority of patients.

EXTERNAL TREATMENT

1. **Lu** applied *Kou Chuang San* (Mouth Sores Powder) to the umbilicus to treat the disease. The powder was composed of *Xuan Ming Fen*‡ (Mirabilitum Depuratum), *Huang Lian* (Rhizoma Coptidis), *Xi Xin** (Herba cum Radice Asari), and *Bing Pian* (Borneolum) in the proportions of 5:3:1:1. Each ingredient was ground separately into a powder with *Huang Lian* (Rhizoma Coptidis) and *Xi Xin** (Herba cum Radice Asari) then being sieved through a 100-mesh screen. The four powders were mixed thoroughly and stored in a bottle.

Prior to application, the patient's umbilicus was cleaned with a 75 percent alcohol solution with a small amount being left inside. The umbilicus was then filled with 1-2g of the mixture and covered with adhesive tape. The powder was changed once a day. With certain patients, pain was alleviated within 20 hours and the ulcer healed two days later, but in most cases seven days were needed for results. [22]

2. **Yang** employed a similar technique, applying 6g of powdered *Xi Xin** (Herba cum Radice Asari) mixed with vinegar to CV-8 Shenque and covering with adhesive tape. The dressing was changed once a day. Results were seen within five to seven days. [23]

EAR ACUPUNCTURE

Li treated aphthous stomatitis with ear acupuncture. [24]
Main points: Tooth 1 or 2, Mouth and Tongue.
Auxiliary points

- For Liver Qi stagnation and Heat in the Stomach, Stomach, Spleen, Liver, and Gallbladder were added.
- For accumulation of Heat in the Heart and Spleen, Heart, Spleen and Endocrine were added.
- For Heart-Fire flaming upward, Heart and Small Intestine were added.
- For disharmony between the Heart and Kidneys, Heart, Kidney, Ear-Shenmen, and Adrenal Gland were added.
- For intense pain, Sympathetic Nerve and Ear-Shenmen were added.
- For obvious Damp signs, Triple Burner, Ear Apex and Adrenal Gland were added.

Technique: After routine disinfection, 0.5 cun filiform needles were inserted in the points and retained for 30 minutes. Treatment took place once a day and ten treatment sessions made up a course. There was a break of three days between courses if a second course was needed.

COMBINED TREATMENT WITH TCM AND WESTERN MEDICINE

Ye treated a group of patients who had been suffering from this disease for periods ranging from 10 to 25 years. For the TCM treatment, he identified four patterns. [25]

- **Accumulation of Heat in the Heart and Spleen**

Prescription ingredients

Jin Yin Hua (Flos Lonicerae) 15g
Ban Lan Gen (Radix Isatidis seu Baphicacanthi) 15g
Zi Hua Di Ding (Herba Violae Yedoensitis) 12g
Lian Qiao (Fructus Forsythiae Suspensae) 10g
Sheng Di Huang (Radix Rehmanniae Glutinosae) 10g
Mu Dan Pi (Cortex Moutan Radicis) 10g
Huang Qin (Radix Scutellariae Baicalensis) 9g
Tong Cao (Medulla Tetrapanacis Papyriferi) 9g
Huang Lian (Rhizoma Coptidis) 9g
Gan Cao (Radix Glycyrrhizae) 6g
Da Huang (Radix et Rhizoma Rhei) 6g
Dan Zhu Ye (Herba Lophatheri Gracilis) 5g

- **Pathogenic Heat in the Lungs and Stomach**

Prescription ingredients

Ban Lan Gen (Radix Isatidis seu Baphicacanthi) 15g
Jin Yin Hua (Flos Lonicerae) 12g
Zhi Zi (Fructus Gardeniae Jasminoidis) 10g

Huang Qin (Radix Scutellariae Baicalensis) 10g
Lian Qiao (Fructus Forsythiae Suspensae) 10g
Jie Geng (Radix Platycodi Grandiflori) 10g
Da Huang (Radix et Rhizoma Rhei) 10g
Mang Xiao ‡ (Mirabilitum) 10g
Niu Bang Zi (Fructus Arctii Lappae) 10g
Xuan Shen (Radix Scrophulariae Ningpoensis) 10g
Bo He (Herba Menthae Haplocalycis) 9g, added 5 minutes before the end of the decoction process
Gan Cao (Radix Glycyrrhizae) 3g

- **Effulgent Yin Deficiency-Fire**

Prescription ingredients

Bei Sha Shen (Radix Glehniae Littoralis) 12g
Sheng Di Huang (Radix Rehmanniae Glutinosae) 10g
Xuan Shen (Radix Scrophulariae Ningpoensis) 10g
Mai Men Dong (Radix Ophiopogonis Japonici) 10g
Yu Zhu (Rhizoma Polygonati Odorati) 10g
Zhi Mu (Rhizoma Anemarrhenae Asphodeloidis) 10g
Bai Shao (Radix Paeoniae Lactiflorae) 10g
Niu Xi (Radix Achyranthis Bidentatae) 10g
Zi Cao (Radix Arnebiae seu Lithospermi) 8g
Gan Cao (Radix Glycyrrhizae) 6g

- **Floating Fire due to Yang Deficiency** [iv]

Prescription ingredients

Huang Qi (Radix Astragali seu Hedysari) 15g
Dang Shen (Radix Codonopsitis Pilosulae) 10g
Dang Gui (Radix Angelicae Sinensis) 10g
Shu Di Huang (Radix Rehmanniae Glutinosae Conquita) 10g
Gou Qi Zi (Fructus Lycii) 10g
Bu Gu Zhi (Fructus Psoraleae Corylifoliae) 10g
Shan Yao (Radix Dioscoreae Oppositae) 10g
Bai Zhu (Rhizoma Atractylodis Macrocephalae) 9g
Fu Ling (Sclerotium Poriae Cocos) 9g
Tu Si Zi (Semen Cuscutae) 9g
Ba Ji Tian (Radix Morindae Officinalis) 9g
Chuan Xiong (Rhizoma Ligustici Chuanxiong) 8g
Gan Cao (Radix Glycyrrhizae) 6g

In all patterns, one bag a day was used to prepare a decoction, taken twice a day.

Western medicine
Prednisone 30mg three times a day and four tablets of sulfamethoxazole 200mg twice a day for three days during the acute phase.

Results were evaluated after one month with recurrence of the ulcers being halted in the majority of patients.

---

iv See the literature excerpt above for an explanation of Yang Deficiency mouth sores.

Herpetic stomatitis
疱疹性口腔炎

Herpetic stomatitis is a type of acute infectious stomatitis due to the herpes simplex virus, of which it may be the primary infection.

In TCM, this condition is also known as *kou gan* (mouth Gan).

Clinical manifestations

- This disease mainly involves the mouth, tongue, internal cheeks, and palate; the throat may also be affected in severe conditions.
- At the initial stage, lesions manifest as 1-2 mm vesicles, but they may break several hours later and become ulcerative; ulcers are subsequently covered by yellowish-white fibrinous exudate.
- A sensation of burning heat and stabbing pain is felt.
- Accompanying systemic symptoms may include swelling and tenderness of the submaxillary lymph nodes, dry mouth and constipation.

Differential diagnosis

Table 15-1 in the Oral candidiasis (thrush) section of this chapter compares various types of common mouth sores.

Lichen planus
Although the eruptions in lichen planus usually involve the flexor surfaces of the wrists and forearms and the lower legs around and above the ankles, the mucous membranes are involved in 40-60 percent of cases, sometimes as the only manifestation of the disease. Lichen planus on the oral mucosa commonly manifests as grayish-white papules, which can be distinguished from the lesions of herpetic stomatitis by the presence of Wickham's striae, a lacy white pattern of lines on their surface.

Etiology and pathology

- Overintake of fatty, sweet or spicy food leads to Heat accumulating in the Spleen and Stomach, which tends to steam upward to scorch the mouth.
- Excessive thought and preoccupation may consume Yin and lead to Heat accumulating in the Heart and Spleen. If Heat due to Yin Deficiency is retained for a lengthy period, it will transform into Deficiency-Fire, which then flames upward to cause the disease.

Pattern identification and treatment

INTERNAL TREATMENT

EXCESS-FIRE
This pattern is seen more often in infants and children and manifests as redness of the oral mucosa and ulcers all over the tongue and mouth, with the throat being involved in more serious cases. Accompanying symptoms and signs include aversion to cold, fever, morbid crying, dry mouth, constipation, and refusal to eat. The tongue body is red with a yellow coating; the pulse is floating and rapid.

Treatment principle
Clear Heat and relieve Toxicity, dissipate Wind and alleviate pain.

Prescription
XUAN SHEN LIAN QIAO YIN JIA JIAN
Figwort and Forsythia Beverage, with modifications

Xuan Shen (Radix Scrophulariae Ningpoensis) 12g
Lian Qiao (Fructus Forsythiae Suspensae) 12g
Jin Yin Hua (Flos Lonicerae) 10g
Zi Hua Di Ding (Herba Violae Yedoensitis) 10g
Chao Niu Bang Zi (Fructus Arctii Lappae, stir-fried) 10g
Jiang Can ‡ (Bombyx Batryticatus) 10g
Chao Mu Dan Pi (Cortex Moutan Radicis, stir-fried) 10g
Ban Lan Gen (Radix Isatidis seu Baphicacanthi) 20g
Sheng Di Huang (Radix Rehmanniae Glutinosae) 15g
Bo He (Herba Menthae Haplocalycis) 6g, added 5 minutes before the end of the decoction process
Deng Xin Cao (Medulla Junci Effusi) 5g
Hu Po ‡ (Succinum) 4.5g

Explanation
- *Xuan Shen* (Radix Scrophulariae Ningpoensis), *Lian Qiao* (Fructus Forsythiae Suspensae), *Jin Yin Hua* (Flos Lonicerae), *Zi Hua Di Ding* (Herba Violae Yedoensitis), and *Ban Lan Gen* (Radix Isatidis seu Baphicacanthi) clear Heat, relieve Toxicity and nourish Yin.
- *Chao Niu Bang Zi* (Fructus Arctii Lappae, stir-fried), *Jiang Can* ‡ (Bombyx Batryticatus) and *Bo He* (Herba Menthae Haplocalycis) dredge Wind and disperse swelling.
- *Chao Mu Dan Pi* (Cortex Moutan Radicis, stir-fried), *Sheng Di Huang* (Radix Rehmanniae Glutinosae), *Deng*

Xin Cao (Medulla Junci Effusi), and *Hu Po*‡ (Succinum) nourish Yin and clear Heat, quiet the Heart and alleviate pain.

DEFICIENCY-FIRE

This pattern is seen more often in adults and manifests as relatively numerous pale red ulcers on the tongue and inner cheeks. Accompanying symptoms and signs include absence of thirst, restless sleep and loose stools. The tongue body is pale red with a thin coating; the pulse is thready and rapid.

Treatment principle

Nourish Yin and clear Heat, relieve Toxicity and alleviate pain.

Prescription

ZENG YE TANG JIA JIAN

Decoction for Increasing Body Fluids, with modifications

Sheng Di Huang (Radix Rehmanniae Glutinosae) 15-30g
Tian Men Dong (Radix Asparagi Cochinchinensis) 10g
Mai Men Dong (Radix Ophiopogonis Japonici) 10g
Yu Zhu (Rhizoma Polygonati Odorati) 10g
Shi Hu* (Herba Dendrobii) 10g
Xuan Shen (Radix Scrophulariae Ningpoensis) 10g
Tian Hua Fen (Radix Trichosanthis) 10g
Chao Bai Shao (Radix Paeoniae Lactiflorae, stir-fried) 10g
Dang Gui (Radix Angelicae Sinensis) 10g
Chao Huang Bai (Cortex Phellodendri, stir-fried) 6g
Chao Zhi Mu (Rhizoma Anemarrhenae Asphodeloidis, stir-fried) 6g
Chao Mu Dan Pi (Cortex Moutan Radicis, stir-fried) 6g
Shan Yao (Radix Dioscoreae Oppositae) 15g
Shan Zhu Yu (Fructus Corni Officinalis) 15g

Explanation

- *Sheng Di Huang* (Radix Rehmanniae Glutinosae), *Tian Men Dong* (Radix Asparagi Cochinchinensis), *Mai Men Dong* (Radix Ophiopogonis Japonici), *Yu Zhu* (Rhizoma Polygonati Odorati), *Shi Hu** (Herba Dendrobii), and *Xuan Shen* (Radix Scrophulariae Ningpoensis) nourish Yin and clear Heat to treat Deficiency.
- *Chao Huang Bai* (Cortex Phellodendri, stir-fried), *Chao Zhi Mu* (Rhizoma Anemarrhenae Asphodeloidis, stir-fried) and *Chao Mu Dan Pi* (Cortex Moutan Radicis, stir-fried) relieve Toxicity with cold and bitterness to treat the Manifestations.
- *Tian Hua Fen* (Radix Trichosanthis), *Chao Bai Shao* (Radix Paeoniae Lactiflorae, stir-fried), *Dang Gui* (Radix Angelicae Sinensis), *Shan Yao* (Radix Dioscoreae Oppositae), and *Shan Zhu Yu* (Fructus Corni Officinalis) enrich the Liver and supplement the Kidneys, support Vital Qi (Zheng Qi) and consolidate the Root to prevent recurrence.

General modifications

1. For constipation, add *Liang Ge San* (Powder for Cooling the Diaphragm), wrapped.
2. For short voidings of yellow urine, add *Che Qian Zi* (Semen Plantaginis), wrapped.
3. For insomnia and profuse dreaming, add *Suan Zao Ren* (Semen Ziziphi Spinosae), *Wu Wei Zi* (Fructus Schisandrae) and *Bai Zi Ren* (Semen Biotae Orientalis); or powdered *Rou Gui* (Cortex Cinnamomi Cassiae) to lead Fire back to its source.
4. For aching of the lower back and knees, add *Xu Duan* (Radix Dipsaci), *Niu Xi* (Radix Achyranthis Bidentatae) and *Chao Du Zhong* (Cortex Eucommiae Ulmoidis, stir-fried).

EXTERNAL TREATMENT

- For Excess-Fire patterns, apply *Kou Gan San* (Mouth Gan Powder) or *Qing Dai San* (Indigo Powder) to the affected area three to five times a day.
- For Deficiency-Fire patterns, apply *Qing Chui Kou San* (Indigo Mouth Insufflation Powder) to the affected area two or three times a day.
- *Qing Guo Shui Xi Ji* (Chinese Olive Wash Preparation) can be used as a mouthwash three to five times a day in either pattern.

Clinical notes

- A clear differentiation between Excess and Deficiency patterns is the key to treating this disease. Excess patterns are generally due to Heat in the Stomach and are usually treated with acrid and cool or bitter and cold materia medica. Deficiency patterns are generally caused by Deficiency of the Spleen and Kidneys and are usually treated by supporting the Spleen and augmenting Qi, and warming Yang and supplementing the Kidneys.
- Prevention of recurrence is closely associated with early diagnosis, prompt treatment and continuation of patent medicines for enriching the Liver and supplementing the Kidneys such as *Zhi Bai Di Huang Wan* (Anemarrhena, Phellodendron and Rehmannia Pill) after the condition has resolved.

Advice for the patient

- Eat less fatty, sweet and fried food, and increase intake of vegetables and fruit.
- Follow a light, semi-liquid diet during an attack.

- A cheerful mood and proper rest can prevent or reduce recurrence.

Literature excerpt

In *Wai Ke Bai Xiao Quan Shu* [A Compendium of Effective Treatments for External Diseases], it says: "If mouth sores refuse to respond to cool herbs, this must surely be due to Qi Deficiency in the Middle Burner, thus resulting in failure to restrict the Ministerial Fire. This can usually be treated effectively by a decoction of *Gan Jiang* (Rhizoma Zingiberis Officinalis), *Ren Shen* (Radix Ginseng) and *Bai Zhu* (Rhizoma Atractylodis Macrocephalae). In serious cases, add *Fu Zi** (Radix Lateralis Aconiti Carmichaeli Praeparata) or powdered *Guan Gui* (Cortex Tubiformis Cinnamomi Cassiae) to the decoction or add a powdered mixture of *Gan Jiang* (Rhizoma Zingiberis Officinalis) and *Huang Lian* (Rhizoma Coptidis). When the patient starts to salivate, this is a sign that the treatment has been effective."

Modern clinical experience

TREATMENT BASED ON PATTERN IDENTIFICATION

Zhang identified four patterns with corresponding treatment principles. [26]

- **Spleen and Stomach Deficiency**

Treatment principle
Fortify the Spleen, bear Yang upward and augment Qi.

Prescription ingredients
Dang Shen (Radix Codonopsitis Pilosulae) 12g
Dang Gui (Radix Angelicae Sinensis) 12g
Huang Qi (Radix Astragali seu Hedysari) 18g
Bai Zhu (Rhizoma Atractylodis Macrocephalae) 15g
Fu Ling (Sclerotium Poriae Cocos) 15g
Chai Hu (Radix Bupleuri) 6g
Chen Pi (Pericarpium Citri Reticulatae) 9g
Sheng Ma (Rhizoma Cimicifugae) 9g
Zhi Gan Cao (Radix Glycyrrhizae, mix-fried with honey) 9g

- **Stomach-Heat attacking upward**

Treatment principle
Clear Heat, relieve Toxicity and drain the Spleen.

Prescription ingredients
Shi Gao‡ (Gypsum Fibrosum) 30g, decocted for 30 minutes before adding the other ingredients
Zhi Zi (Fructus Gardeniae Jasminoidis) 12g
Huang Qin (Radix Scutellariae Baicalensis) 9g
Huo Xiang Geng (Caulis Agastaches seu Pogostemi) 9g
Fang Feng (Radix Ledebouriellae Divaricatae) 9g
Tian Hua Fen (Radix Trichosanthis) 9g
*Shi Hu** (Herba Dendrobii) 9g
Da Huang (Radix et Rhizoma Rhei) 9g
Dan Zhu Ye (Herba Lophatheri Gracilis) 6g
Gan Cao (Radix Glycyrrhizae) 6g

- **Damp-Heat accumulating internally with Dampness predominating over Heat**

Treatment principle
Fortify the Spleen, benefit the movement of Dampness and clear Heat.

Prescription ingredients
Xing Ren (Semen Pruni Armeniacae) 12g
Yi Yi Ren (Semen Coicis Lachryma-jobi) 15g
Hua Shi‡ (Talcum) 15g
Bai Dou Kou (Fructus Amomi Kravanh) 6g
Dan Zhu Ye (Herba Lophatheri Gracilis) 6g
Huang Lian (Rhizoma Coptidis) 6g
Cang Zhu (Rhizoma Atractylodis) 9g
Hou Po (Cortex Magnoliae Officinalis) 9g
Chen Pi (Pericarpium Citri Reticulatae) 9g
Fa Ban Xia (Rhizoma Pinelliae Ternatae Praeparata) 9g

- **Heart and Spleen Deficiency**

Treatment principle
Fortify the Spleen, quiet the Spirit and nourish the Blood.

Prescription ingredients
Dang Shen (Radix Codonopsitis Pilosulae) 12g
Bai Zhu (Rhizoma Atractylodis Macrocephalae) 9g
Fu Ling (Sclerotium Poriae Cocos) 9g
Dang Gui (Radix Angelicae Sinensis) 9g
Huang Qi (Radix Astragali seu Hedysari) 9g
Bai Shao (Radix Paeoniae Lactiflorae) 9g
Yuan Zhi (Radix Polygalae) 9g
Long Yan Rou (Arillus Euphoriae Longanae) 9g
Chao Suan Zao Ren (Semen Ziziphi Spinosae, stir-fried) 9g
*Mu Xiang** (Radix Aucklandiae Lappae) 6g
Zhi Gan Cao (Radix Glycyrrhizae, mix-fried with honey) 6g
Gan Jiang (Rhizoma Zingiberis Officinalis) 6g
Da Zao (Fructus Ziziphi Jujubae) 12g

INTERNAL TREATMENT

1. **Cen** combined two classical formulae to treat herpetic stomatitis. [27]

Prescription
SI NI SAN HE FENG SUI DAN
Counterflow Cold Powder Combined With Sealing the Marrow Special Pill

Chai Hu (Radix Bupleuri) 6g
Shen Qu (Massa Fermentata) 6g
Sha Ren (Fructus Amomi) 6g
Gan Cao (Radix Glycyrrhizae) 6g
Zhi Shi (Fructus Immaturus Citri Aurantii) 9g
Huang Bai (Cortex Phellodendri) 9g
Zhi Zi (Fructus Gardeniae Jasminoidis) 9g
Bai Shao (Radix Paeoniae Lactiflorae) 12g

One bag a day was used to prepare a decoction, taken twice a day. Results were seen after ten days

2. **Chen** combined internal treatment with application of a powder. [28]

Prescription
YANG XUE GAN LU YIN
Sweet Dew Beverage for Nourishing the Blood

Tian Men Dong (Radix Asparagi Cochinchinensis) 15g
Mai Men Dong (Radix Ophiopogonis Japonici) 15g
Sheng Di Huang (Radix Rehmanniae Glutinosae) 15g
Shu Di Huang (Radix Rehmanniae Glutinosae Conquita) 15g
Dang Gui (Radix Angelicae Sinensis) 15g
Huang Qin (Radix Scutellariae Baicalensis) 10g
Zhi Ke (Fructus Citri Aurantii) 10g
Gan Cao (Radix Glycyrrhizae) 10g
Yin Chen Hao (Herba Artemisiae Scopariae) 10g
Chuan Xiong (Rhizoma Ligustici Chuanxiong) 10g
Huang Bai (Cortex Phellodendri) 10g
*Shi Hu** (Herba Dendrobii) 30g
Bai Shao (Radix Paeoniae Lactiflorae) 12g
Huang Lian (Rhizoma Coptidis) 4.5g

One bag was used to prepare a decoction, taken twice a day. Additionally, *Xi Lei San* (Tin-Like Powder) was applied to the affected area four to six times a day. Results were seen after six days.

3. **Huang** steamed *Mu Zei* (Herba Equiseti Hiemalis), 50g of the fresh herb or 20g of the dried herb, in a double boiler with 200ml of water for 20 minutes. Children were given half the adult dose. After the residues were removed, *Bing Tang* (Saccharon Crystallinum) was dissolved in the decoction, which was then taken twice a day after meals. Results were usually seen after two or three days. [29]

4. **Liu** treated herpetic stomatitis with a modified classical formula. [30]

Prescription
YU NÜ JIAN JIA WEI
Jade Lady Brew, with additions

Shu Di Huang (Radix Rehmanniae Glutinosae Conquita) 20g

Chao Shi Gao ‡ (Gypsum Fibrosum, stir-fried) 20g
Zhi Mu (Rhizoma Anemarrhenae Asphodeloidis) 10g
Nan Sha Shen (Radix Adenophorae) 10g
Mai Men Dong (Radix Ophiopogonis Japonici) 12g
Qing Hao (Herba Artemisiae Chinghao) 12g
Niu Xi (Radix Achyranthis Bidentatae) 8g
Gan Cao (Radix Glycyrrhizae) 3g

One bag a day was used to prepare a decoction, taken twice a day. Results were seen after seven days.

5. **Zhang** reported on an empirical formula. [31]

Prescription
QING CHUANG TANG
Clearing Sores Decoction

Tai Zi Shen (Radix Pseudostellariae Heterophyllae) 15g
Sha Ren (Fructus Amomi) 9g
Zhi Gan Cao (Radix Glycyrrhizae, mix-fried with honey) 20g
Shan Zha (Fructus Crataegi) 20g
Lian Qiao (Fructus Forsythiae Suspensae) 12g
Huang Bai (Cortex Phellodendri) 12g
Huang Lian (Rhizoma Coptidis) 3g
Dan Zhu Ye (Herba Lophatheri Gracilis) 10g
Fa Ban Xia (Rhizoma Pinelliae Ternatae Praeparata) 10g
Shan Yao (Radix Dioscoreae Oppositae) 10g
Zhi Mu (Rhizoma Anemarrhenae Asphodeloidis) 10g
Xuan Shen (Radix Scrophulariae Ningpoensis) 10g

One bag a day was used to prepare a decoction, taken twice a day. Results were seen after ten days.

EXTERNAL TREATMENT

1. **Li** reported on his use of *Kou Chuang Ling* (Efficacious Remedy for Mouth Sores). The medication was made from *Ji Nei Jin* ‡ (Endothelium Corneum Gigeriae Galli), *Qie Di* (Pedicellus Solani Melongenae) and *Bing Pian* (Borneolum) in the proportions of 3:6:1. After washing and drying the first two ingredients, they were put into a porcelain jar, which was sealed and heated over a mild flame until the contents became carbonized. After the carbonized ingredients had cooled, they were ground into a fine powder, mixed with *Bing Pian* (Borneolum) and stored in an airtight bottle. The mixture was mixed with egg white or applied directly to the ulcers three or four times a day. Usually one application was sufficient to alleviate the pain and the sores healed in three or four days. [32]

2. **Chen** prepared a mouthwash with *Ye Ju Hua* (Flos Chrysanthemi Indici) 120g and *Qiang Wei Hua* (Flos Rosae Multiflorae) 120g by decocting the herbs in 1000ml of water for 30 minutes and then removing the

residue. The treatment consisted of washing the mouth with 100ml of the liquid twice a day. Alternatively, a cotton bud dipped in the mouthwash was used to clean the oral cavity. Results were seen after seven days. [33]

Oral candidiasis (thrush)
口腔念珠菌病

Thrush is a disease of the mucous membranes of the mouth due to infection with species of yeast of the genus *Candida*, generally *Candida albicans*. These organisms are normally present in the mouth and the yeast becomes pathogenic, particularly in debilitated children or adults, where the bacteria that normally suppress *Candida* are eliminated by antibiotic treatment. Dentures or poor oral hygiene may be a contributory factor, and the infection is more common in patients with diabetes mellitus.

In TCM, this condition is also known as *e kou chuang* (goose-mouth sore).

Table 15-1 Differential diagnosis of various common mouth sores

Western medicine name	Recurrent aphthous stomatitis	Herpetic stomatitis	Thrush
TCM name	*Kou chuang* (mouth sore)	*Kou gan* (mouth Gan)	*E kou chuang* (goose-mouth sore)
Age affected	Mainly the young and early middle-aged	Infants and children	Mainly infants and children, and debilitated adults
Type of illness	Chronic, without fever	Acute, with aversion to cold and heat	Acute or subacute, sometimes with fever
Overall health condition	Normal	Normal	Normal, or may occur in malnourished infants and children, debilitation after a severe illness, or after long-term use of antibiotics
Etiology and pathology	Exuberant Heat in the Spleen and Stomach, flaming upward of Heart-Fire, invasion by external pathogenic factors, dietary irregularities, Yin Deficiency after an illness	Excessive thought and preoccupation, Deficiency-Fire flaming upward, dietary irregularities, accumulation of Heat in the Spleen and Stomach	Accumulation of Heat in the Heart and Spleen channels, Deficiency-Fire flaming upward
Characteristics of lesions	Initially, one or several small, slightly raised papules, which rupture to form superficial, oval yellowish-white or grayish-white ulcers with a red areola; no bleeding	Initially, 1-2 mm vesicles, which may break several hours later and become ulcerative; ulcers are subsequently covered by yellowish-white fibrinous exudate; no bleeding	Tiny white raised spots or velvety macules on a red or pale mucous membrane; no bleeding unless removed by force
Type of pain	Pain affects eating	Stabbing pain	Burning hot pain
Course	Spontaneous healing in 7-10 days	Spontaneous healing in 7-10 days	Continuous development if not treated
Recurrence	Frequent	Possible	Occasional
Prognosis	Good	Generally good	Generally good, but on rare occasions dangerous or fatal if not treated and the infection becomes systemic

Clinical manifestations

- Thrush occurs most often in debilitated infants and children and persons not receiving appropriate care after an illness. However, some 15 percent of infants suffer from thrush on the tongue, lips or buccal mucosa, usually related to an infection contracted while passing through the birth canal.
- Lesions may appear in any part of the mouth, but are more common on the tongue, the inside of the cheeks, the soft palate, and the floor of the mouth.
- In the affected area, lesions manifest as adherent, milky-white, velvety membranes that resemble clotted milk. If they are removed by force, the base is red and tends to bleed.
- Some patients may also have redness, maceration, desquamation or, in more serious cases, erosion and fissuring of the angle of the mouth.
- In some cases, a sensation of burning heat may be felt; infants and children may drool at the mouth, refuse to eat, and suffer from irritability and low-grade fever.

Differential diagnosis

Mouth sores
Table 15-1 compares the characteristics of various common mouth sores.

Lichen planus
Although the eruptions in lichen planus usually involve the flexor surfaces of the wrists and forearms and the lower legs around and above the ankles, the mucous membranes are involved in 40-60 percent of cases, sometimes as the only manifestation of the disease. Lichen planus on the oral mucosa commonly manifests as grayish-white papules, which can be distinguished from the lesions of thrush by the presence of Wickham's striae, a lacy white pattern of lines on their surface.

Etiology and pathology

- Residual fetal Heat accumulated in the Heart and Spleen channels steams upward along the channels to the mouth, leading to snow-white macules and patches all over the mouth.
- Deficiency of Qi and Yin due to improper care after an illness, especially a febrile disease, predisposes to invasion by external pathogenic factors, resulting in Deficiency-Fire flaming upward and binding of Fire and Heat, which steam upward to the mouth.

Pattern identification and treatment

INTERNAL TREATMENT

EXCESS-FIRE
This pattern is seen in infants and children and manifests as snow-white macules and patches over a reddened mucous membrane. Accompanying symptoms and signs include increased saliva due to outward movement of pathogenic Heat, restlessness, persistent crying, difficulty in feeding, short voidings of reddish urine, constipation, and red lips. The tongue body is red with a yellow coating; a dark purple venule crosses the three gates.

Treatment principle
Clear and drain Excess-Fire.

Prescription
HUANG LIAN JIE DU TANG JIA JIAN
Coptis Decoction for Relieving Toxicity, with modifications

Chao Huang Lian (Rhizoma Coptidis, stir-fried) 3g
Tong Cao (Medulla Tetrapanacis Papyriferi) 3g
Lian Zi Xin (Plumula Nelumbinis Nuciferae) 3g
Chao Huang Qin (Radix Scutellariae Baicalensis, stir-fried) 6g
Chao Huang Bai (Cortex Phellodendri, stir-fried) 6g
Jiao Zhi Zi (Fructus Gardeniae Jasminoidis, scorch-fried) 6g
Jin Yin Hua (Flos Lonicerae) 10g
Lian Qiao (Fructus Forsythiae Suspensae) 10g
Chi Fu Ling (Sclerotium Poriae Cocos Rubrae) 10g
Deng Xin Cao (Medulla Junci Effusi) 4.5g
Dan Zhu Ye (Herba Lophatheri Gracilis) 4.5g

Explanation

- *Chao Huang Lian* (Rhizoma Coptidis, stir-fried), *Tong Cao* (Medulla Tetrapanacis Papyriferi), *Lian Zi Xin* (Plumula Nelumbinis Nuciferae), and *Lian Qiao* (Fructus Forsythiae Suspensae) clear Heat from the Heart and drain Fire.
- *Chao Huang Qin* (Radix Scutellariae Baicalensis, stir-fried) clears Heat from the Lungs and drains Fire; *Chao Huang Bai* (Cortex Phellodendri, stir-fried) clears Heat from the Kidneys and drains Fire; and *Jiao Zhi Zi* (Fructus Gardeniae Jasminoidis, scorch-fried) clears and drains Excess-Fire from the Triple Burner. These herbs function together to put out Fire with cold and bitterness in Excess patterns.
- *Chi Fu Ling* (Sclerotium Poriae Cocos Rubrae), *Deng Xin Cao* (Medulla Junci Effusi) and *Dan Zhu Ye* (Herba Lophatheri Gracilis) conduct Heat downward, providing a way for pathogenic factors to exit the body with the urine.
- *Jin Yin Hua* (Flos Lonicerae) aromatically clears Heat and relieves Toxicity, and protects the Heart from invasion.

DEFICIENCY-FIRE

This pattern is more common in adults and those suffering from prolonged chronic diseases such as wasting and thirsting (diabetes), abdominal masses or leukemia, or during long-term treatment with antibiotics. Lesions manifest as tiny white macules forming patches discretely distributed over a pale oral mucous membrane; in severe cases, distribution can take on a tortoiseshell pattern. Accompanying symptoms and signs include loss of appetite, a lusterless facial complexion, and constipation or loose stools. The tongue coating is white or thick and greasy; the pulse is deficient and small.

Treatment principle
Support Vital Qi (Zheng Qi) and supplement Deficiency.

Prescription
BAO YUAN TANG JIA JIAN
Preserving the Origin Decoction, with modifications

Zhi Huang Qi (Radix Astragali seu Hedysari, mix-fried with honey) 10g
Dang Shen (Radix Codonopsitis Pilosulae) 10g
Fu Ling (Sclerotium Poriae Cocos) 10g
Chao Bai Zhu (Rhizoma Atractylodis Macrocephalae, stir-fried) 10g
Rou Gui (Cortex Cinnamomi Cassiae) 1.5g
Huang Lian (Rhizoma Coptidis) 6g
Hu Po ‡ (Succinum) 6g
Shan Yao (Radix Dioscoreae Oppositae) 12g
Sheng Di Huang (Radix Rehmanniae Glutinosae) 12g
Shu Di Huang (Radix Rehmanniae Glutinosae Conquita) 12g
Chao Bai Shao (Radix Paeoniae Lactiflorae, stir-fried) 12g
Bai Wei (Radix Cynanchi Atrati) 4.5g
Gan Cao (Radix Glycyrrhizae) 4.5g

Explanation
- *Huang Qi* (Radix Astragali seu Hedysari), *Dang Shen* (Radix Codonopsitis Pilosulae), *Fu Ling* (Sclerotium Poriae Cocos), *Bai Zhu* (Rhizoma Atractylodis Macrocephalae), and *Shan Yao* (Radix Dioscoreae Oppositae) augment Qi and support the Spleen.
- *Shu Di Huang* (Radix Rehmanniae Glutinosae Conquita) and *Bai Shao* (Radix Paeoniae Lactiflorae) nourish the Liver and enrich the Kidneys.
- *Rou Gui* (Cortex Cinnamomi Cassiae) and *Huang Lian* (Rhizoma Coptidis) promote interaction of the Heart and Kidneys since they can clear Heat from the Heart and drain Fire, warm Yang and supplement the Kidneys.
- *Bai Wei* (Radix Cynanchi Atrati) clears and transforms Deficiency-Heat.
- *Hu Po* ‡ (Succinum) clears Heat from the Heart and quiets the Spirit to prevent the inward invasion of pathogenic factors.

- *Sheng Di Huang* (Radix Rehmanniae Glutinosae) quenches the upward flaming of Fire.
- *Gan Cao* (Radix Glycyrrhizae) harmonizes the actions of the other ingredients.

General modifications
1. For severe Heat, add *Di Gu Pi* (Cortex Lycii Radicis) and *Shi Gao* ‡ (Gypsum Fibrosum).
2. For severe Dampness, add *Cang Zhu* (Rhizoma Atractylodis), *Zhi Ke* (Fructus Citri Aurantii) and *Chen Pi* (Pericarpium Citri Reticulatae), or add *Yang Wei Tang* (Nourishing the Stomach Decoction) or *Ping Wei San* (Quieting the Stomach Powder) to the prepared decoction.
3. For bloating, add *Gua Lou* (Fructus Trichosanthis), *Zhi Shi* (Fructus Immaturus Citri Aurantii) and *Shan Zha* (Fructus Crataegi), or take *Liang Ge San* (Powder for Cooling the Diaphragm) with the decoction.

EXTERNAL TREATMENT
- For Excess-Fire patterns, use *Ye Qiang Wei Lu* (Multiflora Rose Distillate), *Jin Yin Hua Lu* (Honeysuckle Flower Distillate) or a decoction of *Yi Zhi Huang Hua* (Herba Solidaginis) 30g to wash the affected area or spread over the white spots.
- For Deficiency-Fire patterns, wash the affected area with warm boiled water or a weak saline solution, then apply *Qing Chui Kou San* (Indigo Mouth Insufflation Powder), *Xi Gua Shuang* (Watermelon Frost) or *Qing Ye San* (Indigo Fluid Powder).
- At the initial stage, apply powdered *Tian Nan Xing* (Rhizoma Arisaematis) or *Wu Zhu Yu* (Fructus Evodiae Rutaecarpae) mixed with vinegar to the center of the sole.
- For numerous white spots in the mouth, grind *Qing Dai* (Indigo Naturalis) 1.5g, *Peng Sha* ‡ (Borax) 1.5g, *Huang Bai* (Cortex Phellodendri) 3g, and *Bing Pian* (Borneolum) 0.3g to a fine powder and apply to the affected area.
- For a sensation of burning heat and pain in the mouth, prepare a paste with *Bing Shi San* (Borneol and Gypsum Powder) 250g and *Feng Mi* ‡ (Mel) 450g and apply to the lesions.

Clinical notes

- In terms of TCM pattern identification, Damp-Heat in the Heart and Spleen is relatively common, especially in newborns. However, for cases due to overuse of antibiotics or debilitation, effulgent Yin Deficiency-Fire patterns are frequently seen. Materia medica for clearing Heat and drying Dampness such as *Huang Lian* (Rhizoma Coptidis), *Huang Bai* (Cortex Phellodendri), *Huang Qin* (Radix Scutellariae

Baicalensis), and *Cang Zhu* (Rhizoma Atractylodis) are all effective in inhibiting and destroying the yeast.

- The disease occurs much more frequently in undernourished infants, in patients with diarrhea and renal failure, and during long-term treatment with antibiotics, corticosteroids and immunosuppressants. Clinically, correct treatment of the primary disease is very important and is a major factor in preventing the disease.
- The prognosis for this disease is good with prompt treatment and appropriate diet and exercise to strengthen the body. However, in serious cases, care should be taken to prevent the risk of critical or life-threatening conditions.

Advice for the patient

- Oral hygiene is very important at all ages, but particularly so for infants and children, whose mouth should be washed frequently with warm boiled water or a weak saline solution.
- During lactation, the hygiene of mother and baby should be emphasized and feeding utensils sterilized.

References

1. Zhang Zhili, *Zhang Zhi Li Pi Fu Bing Lin Chuang Jing Yan Ji Yao* [A Collection of Zhang Zhili's Clinical Experiences in the Treatment of Skin Diseases] (Beijing: China Medical Science and Technology Publishing House, 2001), 314.
2. Pei Zhengxue, *Bian Zheng Zhi Liao Ban Tu He Cao Tu 73 Li Chu Bu Bao Gao* [Preliminary Report on the Treatment of 73 Cases of Alopecia Areata and Premature Baldness Based on Pattern Identification], *Zhong Yi Za Zhi* [Journal of Traditional Chinese Medicine] 28, 7 (1987): 63.
3. Li Zhilao, *Tuo Fa Xing Pi Fu Bing Bian Zheng Lun Zhi De Tan Tao: Fu 100 Li Lin Chuang Fen Xi* [Study of the Treatment of Hair Loss Disorders Based on Pattern Identification with an Appendix Discussing the Clinical Analysis of 100 Cases], *Shan Xi Zhong Yi Xue Yuan Xue Bao* [Journal of Shaanxi College of TCM] 14, 4 (1991): 15-17.
4. Hu Guojun, *Tuo Fa Zheng Zhi Chu Tan* [Investigation into the Treatment of Hair Loss], *Xin Zhong Yi* [New Journal of Traditional Chinese Medicine] 10 (1991): 10-12.
5. Ma Guiqin, *Shou Wu Sheng Fa Yin Zhi Liao Ban Tu 36 Li* [Treatment of 36 Cases of Alopecia Areata with *Shou Wu Sheng Fa Yin* (Fleeceflower Root Beverage for Generating Hair)], *Shan Dong Zhong Yi Za Zhi* [Shandong Journal of Traditional Chinese Medicine] 13, 6 (1994): 259.
6. Liu Daihong, *Tong Qiao Huo Xue Fa Zhi Liao Tuo Fa 100 Li* [Treatment of 100 Cases of Hair Loss by the Method of Freeing the Orifices and Invigorating the Blood], *Xin Zhong Yi* [New Journal of Traditional Chinese Medicine] 29, 6 (1997): 45-46.
7. Gong Yiyun, *Nei Fu Sheng Fa Yin Wai Yong Sheng Fa Ding Zhi Liao Ban Tu 126 Li* [Treatment of 126 Cases of Alopecia Areata by Internal Administration of *Sheng Fa Yin* (Generating Hair Beverage) and External Application of *Sheng Fa Ding* (Generating Hair Tincture)], *Yun Nan Zhong Yi Zhong Yao Za Zhi* [Yunnan Journal of Traditional Chinese Medicine and Materia Medica] 18, 4 (1997): 14.
8. Li Jinjue, *Qing Liang Gan Lu Yin Zhi Liao Chun Feng 33 Li Liao Xiao Guan Cha* [Clinical Observation of *Qing Liang Gan Lu Yin* (Cool Clearing Sweet Dew Beverage) in the Treatment of 33 Cases of Cheilitis], *Fu Jian Zhong Yi Yao* [Fujian Journal of Traditional Chinese Medicine and Materia Medica] 1 (1985): 27.
9. Lai Zongyu, *Bian Zheng Zhi Liao Yao Wu Guo Min Xing Man Xing Chun Yan 35 Li* [Treatment of 35 Cases of Chronic Cheilitis due to Drug Allergy Based on Pattern Identification], *Si Chuan Zhong Yi* [Sichuan Journal of Traditional Chinese Medicine] 10 (1994): 43.
10. Xu Taishan, *Zhong Yi Bian Zheng Zhi Liao Xiao Er Chun Feng 12 Li* [TCM Treatment of 12 Cases of Infantile Cheilitis Based on Pattern Identification], *Zhong Yi Yao Xin Xi* [Traditional Chinese Medicine and Materia Medica News] 14, 6 (1997): 32.
11. Wang Jun, *Zhong He Tang Zhi Liao Man Xing Chun Yan 279 Li* [Treatment of 279 Cases of Chronic Cheilitis with *Zhong He Tang* (Harmonizing the Middle Decoction)], *Zhe Jiang Zhong Yi Za Zhi* [Zhejiang Journal of Traditional Chinese Medicine] 33, 10 (1998): 437.
12. Zou Mei, *Zhong Yao Zhi Liao Mi Lan Xing Chun Yan Lin Chuang Guan Cha* [Clinical Observation of the Treatment of Erosive Cheilitis with Chinese Materia Medica], *Shan Xi Zhong Yi Xue Yuan Xue Bao* [Journal of Shaanxi College of Traditional Chinese Medicine] 22, 3 (1999): 29.
13. Wu Jianfeng, *Zhong Yi Zhi Liao Bo Luo Xing Chun Yan* [TCM Treatment of Exfoliative Cheilitis], *Pi Fu Bing Yu Xing Bing* [Skin Diseases and Venereal Diseases] 14, 6 (1997): 32.
14. Xiang Ping, *Nan Jing Zhong Yi Yao Da Xue Zhong Yi Xue Jia Zhuan Ji* [Collected Experiences of Experts from Nanjing University of TCM], (Beijing: People's Medical Publishing House, 1999), 238.
15. Wu Xuxiang, *Zang Kun Tang Bian Zhi Fu Fa Xing Kou Chuang De Jing Yan* [Zang Kuntang's Experiences in Treating Recurrent Mouth Sores Based on Pattern Identification], *Liao Ning Zhong Yi Za Zhi* [Liaoning Journal of Traditional Chinese Medicine] 26, 8 (1999): 343.
16. Wang Jiying, *San Cai Feng Sui Dan Jia Wei Zhi Liao Fu Fa Xing Kou Chuang 20 Li* [Treatment of 20 Cases of Recurrent Mouth Sores with Augmented *San Cai Feng Sui Dan* (Heaven, Human and Earth Special Pill for Sealing the

Marrow)], *Yun Nan Zhong Yi Zhong Yao Za Zhi* [Yunnan Journal of Traditional Chinese Medicine and Materia Medica] 18, 3 (1997): 43.

17. Tu Ting, *Zhong Yi Zhi Liao Fu Fa Xing Kou Qiang Kui Yang Zhi Kui Jian* [Opinion on TCM Treatment of Recurrent Ulcerative Stomatitis], *Kou Qiang Yi Xue* [Stomatology Journal] 18, 2 (1998): 106-107.

18. Li Mingcui, *Jia Wei Jiao Tai Wan Zhi Liao Fu Fa Xing Kou Qiang Kui Yang 35 Li* [Treatment of 35 Cases of Recurrent Ulcerative Stomatitis with *Jia Wei Jiao Tai Wan* (Augmented Peaceful Interaction Pill)], *Yun Nan Zhong Yi Zhong Yao Za Zhi* [Yunnan Journal of Traditional Chinese Medicine and Materia Medica] 20, 3 (1999): 29-30.

19. Lu Jiangtao, *Xiao Chai Hu Tang Jia Huang Lian Zhi Liao Fu Fa Xing Kou Qiang Kui Yang 40 Li* [Treatment of 40 Cases of Recurrent Ulcerative Stomatitis with *Xiao Chai Hu Tang* (Minor Bupleurum Decoction) plus *Huang Lian* (Rhizoma Coptidis)], *Shan Xi Zhong Yi Xue Yuan Xue Bao* [Journal of Shaanxi College of Traditional Chinese Medicine] 22, 4 (1999): 39.

20. Wang Chonghua, *Bu Zhong Yi Qi Fa Zhi Liao Wan Gu Xing, Fu Fa Xing Kou Qiang Kui Yang Bing 35 Li* [Treatment of 35 Cases of Stubborn Recurrent Ulcerative Stomatitis by Supplementing the Middle and Augmenting Qi], *Bei Jing Zhong Yi* [Beijing Journal of Traditional Chinese Medicine] 2 (1999): 40.

21. Xie Jie, *Zi Shen Huo Xue Fa Zhi Liao Fu Fa Xing Kou Qiang Kui Yang 52 Li* [Treatment of 52 Cases of Recurrent Ulcerative Stomatitis by Enriching the Kidneys and Invigorating the Blood], *Hu Nan Zhong Yi Za Zhi* [Hunan Journal of Traditional Chinese Medicine] 15, 1 (1999): 30-31.

22. Lu Jianzhong, *Kou Chuang San Fu Qi Zhi Liao Fu Fa Xing Kou Qiang Kui Yang 30 Li* [Treatment of 30 Cases of Recurrent Ulcerative Stomatitis with Application of *Kou Chuang San* (Mouth Sores Powder) to the Umbilicus], *Jiang Su Zhong Yi* [Jiangsu Journal of Traditional Chinese Medicine] 18, 10 (1997): 14.

23. Yang Jianlu, *Bian Zheng Qu Xue Zhi Liao Fu Fa Xing Kou Chuang 39 Li* [Acupuncture Treatment of 39 Cases of Recurrent Mouth Sores Based on Syndrome Differentiation], *Zhong Guo Zhong Xi Yi Jie He Za Zhi* [Journal of Integrated TCM and Western Medicine] 17, 10 (1997): 633.

24. Li Lian, *Er Zhen Zhi Liao Man Xing Kou Qiang Kui Yang 52 Li* [Ear Acupuncture Treatment of 52 Cases of Chronic Ulcerative Stomatitis], *Zhong Guo Zhen Jiu* [Chinese Journal of Acupuncture and Moxibustion] 15, 4 (1995): 51.

25. Ye Minghua, *Zhong Xi Yi Jie He Zhi Liao Fu Fa Xing Kou Chuang 53 Li* [Treatment of 53 Cases of Recurrent Mouth Sores with a Combination of Chinese and Western Medicine], *Yun Nan Zhong Yi Zhong Yao Za Zhi* [Yunnan Journal of Traditional Chinese Medicine and Materia Medica] 18, 2 (1997): 10-11.

26. Zhang Guirong, *Kou Qiang Kui Yang Cong Pi Lun Zhi* [Ulcerative Stomatitis Treated According to Spleen Theory], *Zhong Guo Nong Cun Yi Xue* [Chinese Rural Medicine] 25, 12 (1997): 39-40.

27. Cen Daihui, *Si Ni San He Feng Sui Dan Zhi Liao Kou Chuang 47 Li* [Treatment of 47 Cases of Mouth Sores with *Si Ni San He Feng Sui Dan* (Counterflow Cold Powder Combined With Sealing the Marrow Special Pill)], *Guang Xi Zhong Yi Yao* [Guangxi Journal of Traditional Chinese Medicine and Materia Medica] 12, 6 (1997): 14.

28. Chen Xiaoqiong, *Yang Xue Gan Lu Yin Zhi Liao Kou Chuang 80 Li* [Treatment of 80 Cases of Mouth Sores with *Yang Xue Gan Lu Yin* (Sweet Dew Beverage for Nourishing the Blood)], *Zhong Hua Shi Yong Zhong Xi Yi Jie He Za Zhi* [Practical Journal of Integrated TCM and Western Medicine] 12, 11 (1999): 55.

29. Huang Zhongping, *Mu Zei Zhi Liao Kou Qiang Nian Mo Kui Yang* [Treatment of Ulcers of the Oral Mucosa with *Mu Zei* (Herba Equiseti Hiemalis)], *Zhe Jiang Zhong Yi Za Zhi* [Zhejiang Journal of Traditional Chinese Medicine] 31, 10 (1996): 467.

30. Liu Hongfang, *Yu Nü Jian Jia Wei Zhi Liao Kou Qiang Kui Yang 30 Li* [Treatment of 30 Cases of Ulcerative Stomatitis with Augmented *Yu Nü Jian* (Jade Lady Brew)], *Zhong Yi Yan Jiu* [Traditional Chinese Medicine Research] 12, 1 (1999): 33.

31. Zhang Zhenxian, *Qing Chuang Tang Zhi Liao Kou Qiang Nian Mo Kui Yang 200 Li* [Treatment of 200 Cases of Ulcers of the Oral Mucosa with *Qing Chuang Tang* (Clearing Sores Decoction)], *Hu Bei Zhong Yi Za Zhi* [Journal of Hubei Journal of Traditional Chinese Medicine] 18, 1 (1996): 33.

32. Li Bogang, *Kou Chuang Ling Zhi Liao Kou Chuang* [Treatment of Mouth Sores with *Kou Chuang Ling* (Efficacious Remedy for Mouth Sores)], *Xin Zhong Yi* [New Journal of Traditional Chinese Medicine] 31, 11 (1999): 7.

33. Chen Jun, *Zhong Yao Shu Kou Shui Dui Kou Chuang De Yu Fang Ji Zhi Liao* [Prevention and Treatment of Mouth Sores with a Herbal Mouthwash], *Zhong Hua Hu Li Za Zhi* [Chinese Journal of Nursing] 22, 9 (1987): 404.

Chapter 16

Drug eruptions

Drug eruptions
药疹

Cutaneous eruptions are a common form of adverse reaction to drugs. These reactions may also involve the mucous membranes, and visceral lesions are possible in severe cases. Virtually any drug can cause a skin reaction, irrespective of the route of administration – oral, inhalation, parenteral, or topical routes. Common drugs that can cause eruptions include:

- antipyretics and analgesics
- antibiotics, such as sulfonamides, penicillins, macrolides, cefalosporins, and tetracyclines
- hypnotics, sedatives and anti-epileptics
- steroids
- certain Chinese materia medica

Drug eruptions are not only allergic reactions, but may also result from overdosage, cumulative effects, pharmacological side-effects (for example, skin stretch marks from systemic steroids), facilitative effects (for example, where drugs aggravate psoriasis), or idiosyncratic effects restricted to a particular individual.

Clinical manifestations

- Drugs may be taken for a considerable period of time without adverse effect, but once the patient reacts, an eruption can appear within minutes to 48 hours from the time of exposure. In allergic drug reactions, the initial sensitizing time usually ranges from seven to ten days; subsequent exposure results in an eruption appearing much more rapidly.
- Cutaneous drug eruptions can mimic almost any type of skin disease with the result that drug reaction forms the differential diagnosis of virtually every skin disease. The commonest patterns of reaction are maculopapular (exanthematous eruptions, similar to viral exanthems), urticarial and angioedematous, erythema multiforme-type, and fixed drug eruptions.

- Cutaneous drug eruptions vary in appearance (see Table 16-1).
- There may be accompanying symptoms such as fever, malaise, headache, dizziness, decreased appetite, nausea, vomiting, and diarrhea.
- A full blood count may show eosinophilia.
- Visceral lesions may also develop including abnormal changes in the liver, kidney, lung, and blood.

According to classical TCM books such as *Zhu Bing Yuan Hou Lu* [A General Treatise on the Causes and Symptoms of Disease] and *Zheng Zhi Zhun Sheng: Yang Ke* [Standards of Diagnosis and Treatment: External Diseases], Chinese materia medica that may cause skin eruptions include:

Ai Ye (Folium Artemisiae Argyi)
Bai Ji Li (Fructus Tribuli Terrestris)
Bai Jie Zi (Semen Sinapis Albae)
Ban Lan Gen (Radix Isatidis seu Baphicacanthi)
Bi Ma Zi (Semen Ricini)
Chu Tao Ye (Folium Broussonetiae)
Chuan Bei Mu (Bulbus Fritillariae Cirrhosae)
Chuan Xin Lian (Herba Andrographitis Paniculatae)
Da Qing Ye (Folium Isatidis seu Baphicacanthi)
Da Suan (Bulbus Allii Sativi)
Dan Shen (Radix Salviae Miltiorrhizae)
Dang Gui (Radix Angelicae Sinensis)
Di Long‡ (Lumbricus)
Fang Feng (Radix Ledebouriellae Divaricatae)
Ge Gen (Radix Puerariae)
Hai Piao Xiao‡ (Os Sepiae seu Sepiellae)
Hong Hua (Flos Carthami Tinctorii)
Huai Hua (Flos Sophorae Japonicae)
Jin Gu Cao (Herba Ajugae Decumbentis)
Ma Chi Xian (Herba Portulacae Oleraceae)
Qian Li Guang (Herba Senecionis Scandentis)
Qing Hao (Herba Artemisiae Chinghao)

Table 16-1 Types of cutaneous drug eruptions

Exanthematous type
Maculopapular eruptions may resemble those of scarlet fever (scarlatiniform) or measles (morbilliform) and present as symmetrically distributed, generalized, usually itchy red macules and papules. Eruptions start seven to ten days after starting the drug and last for one or two weeks. Common causes among Western drugs include ampicillin, sulfonamides and barbiturates.

Urticarial and angioedematous type
Characteristic urticarial reactions may occur anywhere on the body (see Chapter 5) within minutes to hours after taking the drug, although they may only appear up to three weeks afterward in cases of serum sickness (circulating immune complex disease). Common causes among Western drugs include aspirin and penicillin.

Erythema multiforme type
Characteristic "target" lesions appear, mainly on the limbs (see Chapter 7); in severe cases, bullae may also form. Common causes among Western drugs include sulfonamides, barbiturates and NSAIDs.

Fixed drug eruptions
Single or multiple, clearly demarcated, round red or purplish plaques appear soon after a drug is administered and recur at the same site each time the same drug is taken. Lesions may blister and erode, leaving pigmentation on healing. The glans penis is a common site, but lesions may occur anywhere. Common causes among Western drugs include antibiotics, tranquilizers, paracetamol, and NSAIDs.

Small-vessel vasculitis type (palpable purpura)
Characteristic purpuric lesions appear most commonly on the lower legs (see Chapter 7). Common causes among Western drugs include sulfonamides, penicillin and thiazides.

Acneiform type
Common causes among Western drugs of characteristic acneiform eruptions (see Chapter 6) include bromides, lithium and steroids.

Lichenoid type
Lesions mimic those of lichen planus (see Chapter 4). Common causes among Western drugs include antimalarials and beta-blockers.

Eczematous type
This relatively uncommon pattern is generally only seen when systemic treatment follows sensitization by topical application. Causes among Western drugs include neomycin, sulfonamides and penicillin.

Photosensitivity type
Phototoxic reactions are concentration-related and can occur in any individual; an erythematous eruption appears within 24 hours of exposure to light after administration of the drug involved and fades when the drug is stopped (see also Phytophotodermatitis in Chapter 17). Photoallergic reactions occur in sensitized individuals and have a delayed onset. Common causes among Western drugs include psoralens, griseofulvin and thiazides.

Pigmentation
Among Western drugs, phenothiazines and amiodarone can result in the skin turning a blue-gray color, clofazimine can turn the skin red and mepacrine can make it yellow (see disorders of pigmentation in Chapter 13).

Exfoliative dermatitis (erythroderma) type
In this uncommon condition, the entire skin becomes red and scaly, constituting a medical emergency. Common causes among Western drugs include isoniazid, phenylbutazone and gold salts.

Toxic epidermal necrolysis
This rare, life-threatening condition presents with a red "scalded skin" appearance and is usually drug-induced. Common causes among Western drugs include sulfonamides, barbiturates and phenylbutazone.

Ren Shen (Radix Ginseng)
Sheng Ban Xia (Rhizoma Pinelliae Ternatae Cruda)
Tian Hua Fen (Radix Trichosanthis)
Wei Ling Xian (Radix Clematidis)
Ya Dan Zi (Fructus Bruceae Javanicae)
Yu Xing Cao (Herba Houttuyniae Cordatae)
Zi Cao (Radix Arnebiae seu Lithospermi)
Zi Zhu (Folium Callicarpae)

Examples of reports in modern literature on materia medica causing drug eruptions include:

- *San Qi* (Radix Notoginseng): One to three hours after oral administration of 2-3g of *San Qi* (Radix Notoginseng), three patients began to suffer from skin rash and pruritus, which disappeared after intake of the medicine ceased. [1]

- *Shan Yao* (Rhizoma Dioscoreae Oppositae): External

application of raw *Shan Yao* (Rhizoma Dioscoreae Oppositae) caused severe itching in the neck, chest and back. [2]

- *Wu Wei Zi Tang Jiang* (Schisandra Syrup): After taking 10ml of *Wu Wei Zi Tang Jiang* (Schisandra Syrup) twice a day for three days, a female patient began to experience generalized pruritus and urticaria. She stopped taking the medicine for one week, then restarted, resulting in recurrence of urticaria on the same day. [3]

According to *Chang Yong Zhong Cao Yao Bu Liang Fan Ying Ji Qi Fang Zhi* [Adverse Effects Induced by Commonly Used Chinese Materia Medica and Their Prevention and Treatment], there are recent reports on drug eruptions caused by a number of Chinese materia medica in addition to those mentioned in older literature. In many instances, these relate only to isolated cases. In these reports, materia medica that have caused drug eruptions in three or more individual cases in recent years include:

Bing Pian (Borneolum)
Bu Gu Zhi (Fructus Psoraleae Corylifoliae)
*Chuan Shan Jia** (Squama Manitis Pentadactylae)
Da Huang (Radix et Rhizoma Rhei)
Dong Chong Xia Cao‡ (Cordyceps Sinensis)
Gua Lou Pi (Pericarpium Trichosanthis)
He Shou Wu (Radix Polygoni Multiflori)
Jiang Can‡ (Bombyx Batryticatus)
Ku Lian Pi (Cortex Meliae Radicis)
Lang Du (Radix Euphorbiae Fischerianae)
Mo Yao (Myrrha)
*Mu Xiang** (Radix Aucklandiae Lappae)
*Qing Fen** (Calomelas)
Sang Ji Sheng (Ramulus Loranthi)
*She Xiang** (Secretio Moschi)
Shi Chang Pu (Rhizoma Acori Graminei)
Tian Nan Xing (Rhizoma Arisaematis)
Tu Bie Chong‡ (Eupolyphaga seu Steleophaga)
Xia Ku Cao (Spica Prunellae Vulgaris)
Xue Jie (Resina Draconis)
Yan Hu Suo (Rhizoma Corydalis Yanhusuo)
Yin Chen Hao (Herba Artemisiae Scopariae)
Yuan Hua (Flos Daphnes Genkwa)

It has also been reported that patent herbal medicines such as *Liu Shen Wan* (Six Spirits Pill), *Yun Nan Bai Yao* (Yunnan White), *Yi Mu Cao Gao* (Motherwort Extract), *Ling Yang Jie Du Wan* (Antelope Horn Pill for Relieving Toxicity), *Shuang Jie Wan* (Double Relief Pill), and *Niu Huang Jie Du Pian* (Bovine Bezoar Tablet for Relieving Toxicity) and external medications such as *Wu Hu Dan* (Five Tiger Special Powder) may also induce drug eruptions.

Differential diagnosis

Differential diagnosis for drug eruptions basically depends on the disease being mimicked. Patients presenting with an atypical eruption should always be asked about current medication, particularly any drugs introduced recently.

With viral exanthemata, multiple transient, usually red or pink, macules are a feature of numerous systemic, toxic or idiosyncratic drug reactions. Identical eruptions can occur as a response to several infective agents, particularly viral illnesses. Some eruptions are entirely macular, others entirely papular, but most commonly are a mixture of both. In patients with a maculopapular eruption, it may be impossible to determine whether a drug, an infection or a combination of the two is the cause of the rash.

In adults with acute onset of widespread skin pustules, differentiation between pustular psoriasis, viral infections and a drug eruption should be considered.

Etiology and pathology

Drug eruption arises due to a combination in some individuals of constitutional weakness and reaction to intake of certain drugs, plants or mineral ingredients with a strong action or of a very acrid, warm or dry nature. Since patients have different constitutions and different disease patterns (for example, some may have exuberant Heat in the Blood, others may have exuberant Damp-Heat), a given drug may produce different clinical manifestations in different patients or different drugs may produce similar clinical manifestations in different patients.

Constitutional weakness
Turbid Qi and Heat Toxins may accumulate in the Xue level in patients with a congenitally weak constitution due to Heat retained from the fetal stage. Where this is complicated by repeated exposure to attack by drug Toxins, these Toxins bind with the turbid Qi and Heat Toxins and move outward to the skin and flesh, resulting in maculopapular eruptions.

Retention of Wind-Heat in the flesh and interstices (*cou li*)
Drug Toxins entering the Ying level will give rise to exuberant Heat in the Xue level. Extreme Heat generates Wind; Wind and Heat then fight one another and are retained in the skin and flesh to cause wheals (urticaria). If Wind-Heat moves up to the upper part of the body, there may be redness and swelling on the head and face with swollen eyelids forcing the eyes closed, as in angioedema.

Drug Toxins entering the Ying level and consuming Body Fluids

Preparations with mineral ingredients often have a strong action and contain materia medica that are acrid, warm, dry, and drastic. Misuse or overdosage of such ingredients will allow Fire Toxins to attack the interior. As a result, Heat Toxins will disturb the Ying level and enter the Xue level, causing exuberant Heat in both the Qi and Xue levels, gradually leading to maculopapular eruptions. If the disease persists, Heat Toxins will progressively scorch Yin-Liquids and consume Body Fluids, thus depriving the skin of nourishment and resulting in desquamation.

In *Zheng Zhi Zhun Sheng* [Standards of Diagnosis and Treatment], it says: "This disease is caused by accumulation of Heat in the interior due to overintake of metal or mineral ingredients with a strong action. As a result, Heat accumulates in the Upper Burner, and stirs up Qi and Blood. Finally, skin eruptions occur."

Spleen Qi Deficiency leading to impairment of transportation and transformation

Overintake of rich, greasy or sweet food leads to Spleen Qi Deficiency and impairs the Spleen's transportation and transformation function, resulting in internal generation of Damp-Heat that cannot be drained internally or thrust outward to the exterior. Damp-Heat binds with the drug Toxins and pours downward to the genitals, causing maceration, erosion, swelling, and a sensation of scorching heat and burning pain, as in *shi huo dan* (stone erysipelas, or fixed drug eruption). If Damp-Heat obstructs the network vessels, Qi stagnation and Blood stasis will occur, manifesting as dark purple or purplish-red skin eruptions. If blood spills out of the vessels, clusters of purpuric lesions will appear.

Pattern identification and treatment

INTERNAL TREATMENT

HEAT TOXINS COMPLICATED BY WIND

Lesions are exanthematous (scarlatiniform or morbilliform) or urticarial and are usually widespread, manifesting principally as erythema, wheals or papules. Erythema can be generalized or circumscribed in location. Wheals appear and disappear swiftly, frequently being diffuse and swollen. Accompanying symptoms include raging fever and constipation. The tongue body is red with a thin yellow coating; the pulse is floating and rapid.

Western drugs commonly causing this pattern include penicillin, sulfonamides and salicylic acid preparations; Chinese materia medica include *Tian Hua Fen* (Radix

Trichosanthis), *Ai Ye* (Folium Artemisiae Argyi), *Ban Lan Gen* (Radix Isatidis seu Baphicacanthi), *Chu Tao Ye* (Folium Broussonetiae), and *Chuan Xin Lian* (Herba Andrographitis Paniculatae).

Treatment principle

Clear Heat from the Qi level, relieve Toxicity, cool the Blood, and reduce erythema.

Prescription

YIN QIAO SAN HE BAI HU TANG JIA JIAN
Honeysuckle and Forsythia Powder Combined With White Tiger Decoction, with modifications

Jin Yin Hua (Flos Lonicerae) 12g
Lian Qiao (Fructus Forsythiae Suspensae) 10g
Chi Shao (Radix Paeoniae Rubra) 10g
Huang Qin (Radix Scutellariae Baicalensis) 10g
Shi Gao ‡ (Gypsum Fibrosum) 30-60g, decocted for 30 minutes before adding the other ingredients
Chao Zhi Mu (Rhizoma Anemarrhenae Asphodeloidis, stir-fried) 6g
Chao Niu Bang Zi (Fructus Arctii Lappae, stir-fried) 6g
Jing Jie (Herba Schizonepetae Tenuifoliae) 6g
Fang Feng (Radix Ledebouriellae Divaricatae) 6g
Shan Yao (Radix Dioscoreae Oppositae) 15g
Sheng Di Huang (Radix Rehmanniae Glutinosae) 15g
Bai Mao Gen (Rhizoma Imperatae Cylindricae) 30g

Explanation

- *Jin Yin Hua* (Flos Lonicerae), *Lian Qiao* (Fructus Forsythiae Suspensae) and *Huang Qin* (Radix Scutellariae Baicalensis) clear Heat and relieve Toxicity.
- *Shi Gao* ‡ (Gypsum Fibrosum), *Chao Zhi Mu* (Rhizoma Anemarrhenae Asphodeloidis, stir-fried) and *Shan Yao* (Radix Dioscoreae Oppositae) clear the Qi level and cool the Ying level.
- *Chao Niu Bang Zi* (Fructus Arctii Lappae, stir-fried), *Jing Jie* (Herba Schizonepetae Tenuifoliae) and *Fang Feng* (Radix Ledebouriellae Divaricatae) dredge Wind and alleviate itching.
- *Sheng Di Huang* (Radix Rehmanniae Glutinosae), *Bai Mao Gen* (Rhizoma Imperatae Cylindricae) and *Chi Shao* (Radix Paeoniae Rubra) cool the Blood and reduce erythema.

BLOOD-HEAT

Lesions are exanthematous (scarlatiniform or morbilliform) or represent a photosensitive reaction. Large areas of the skin become inflamed; a dense distribution of pinpoint red papules that blanch on pressure may also appear. Accompanying symptoms include generalized fever and aching joints. The tongue body is red with a thin yellow coating; the pulse is thready, slippery and rapid.

Western drugs commonly causing this pattern include sulfonamides, tetracyclines, aspirin, and phenylbutazone; Chinese materia medica include *Dang Gui* (Radix Angelicae Sinensis), *Bai Ji Li* (Fructus Tribuli Terrestris) and *Chuan Bei Mu* (Bulbus Fritillariae Cirrhosae).

Treatment principle

Cool the Blood and relieve Toxicity, invigorate the Blood and reduce erythema.

Prescription

PI YAN TANG JIA JIAN

Dermatitis Decoction, with modifications

Sheng Di Huang (Radix Rehmanniae Glutinosae) 15g
Shi Gao ‡ (Gypsum Fibrosum) 15g
Mu Dan Pi (Cortex Moutan Radicis) 12g
Chi Shao (Radix Paeoniae Rubra) 12g
Jin Yin Hua (Flos Lonicerae) 12g
Lian Qiao (Fructus Forsythiae Suspensae) 12g
Chao Zhi Mu (Rhizoma Anemarrhenae Asphodeloidis, stir-fried) 6g
Dan Zhu Ye (Herba Lophatheri Gracilis) 6g
Gan Cao (Radix Glycyrrhizae) 6g
Zi Cao (Radix Arnebiae seu Lithospermi) 10g
Lü Dou Yi (Testa Phaseoli Radiati) 10g

Explanation

- *Sheng Di Huang* (Radix Rehmanniae Glutinosae), *Chi Shao* (Radix Paeoniae Rubra), *Mu Dan Pi* (Cortex Moutan Radicis), and *Zi Cao* (Radix Arnebiae seu Lithospermi) cool the Blood and relieve Toxicity, invigorate the Blood and reduce erythema.
- *Jin Yin Hua* (Flos Lonicerae Japonicae) and *Lian Qiao* (Fructus Forsythiae Suspensae) clear Heat and relieve Toxicity.
- *Chao Zhi Mu* (Rhizoma Anemarrhenae Asphodeloidis, stir-fried), *Dan Zhu Ye* (Herba Lophatheri Gracilis), *Gan Cao* (Radix Glycyrrhizae), *Lü Dou Yi* (Testa Phaseoli Radiati), and *Shi Gao* ‡ (Gypsum Fibrosum) clear Heat in the Qi level and reduce fever.

BLOOD-HEAT COMPLICATED BY DAMPNESS

Lesions, which can be widespread or circumscribed in location, manifest as erythema, papulovesicles or vesicles with exudation and erosion. They are more likely to be seen in the erythema multiforme, fixed drug eruption and erythroderma types of cutaneous drug reaction. Accompanying symptoms include poor appetite and abdominal distension. The tongue body is red with a yellow and slightly greasy coating; the pulse is soggy and rapid.

Western drugs commonly causing this pattern include antipyretics, analgesics, sulfonamides, iodine preparations (either as topical preparations or X-ray contrast media), barbiturates, and penicillin; Chinese materia medica include *Liu Shen Wan* (Six Spirits Pill), *Bai Ji Li* (Fructus Tribuli Terrestris) and *Ma Chi Xian* (Herba Portulacae Oleraceae).

Treatment principle

Cool the Blood and relieve Toxicity, clear Heat and transform Dampness.

Prescription

XI JIAO DI HUANG TANG JIA JIAN

Rhinoceros Horn and Rehmannia Decoction with modifications

Shui Niu Jiao ‡ (Cornu Bubali) 30g, decocted for 30 minutes before adding the other ingredients
Lü Dou Yi (Testa Phaseoli Radiati) 30g
Sheng Di Huang Tan (Radix Rehmanniae Glutinosae Carbonisata) 30g
Jin Yin Hua Tan (Flos Lonicerae Japonicae Carbonisatus) 30g
Yi Yi Ren (Semen Coicis Lachryma-jobi) 30g
Dan Shen (Radix Salviae Miltiorrhizae) 12g
Chao Mu Dan Pi (Cortex Moutan Radicis, stir-fried) 12g
Zi Cao (Radix Arnebiae seu Lithospermi) 12g
Fu Ling Pi (Cortex Poriae Cocos) 12g
Chi Xiao Dou (Semen Phaseoli Calcarati) 15g
Pu Gong Ying (Herba Taraxaci cum Radice) 15g

Explanation

- *Shui Niu Jiao* ‡ (Cornu Bubali), *Pu Gong Ying* (Herba Taraxaci cum Radice), *Sheng Di Huang Tan* (Radix Rehmanniae Glutinosae Carbonisata), *Jin Yin Hua Tan* (Flos Lonicerae Japonicae Carbonisatus), and *Lü Dou Yi* (Testa Phaseoli Radiati) clear Heat, cool the Blood and relieve Toxicity.
- *Dan Shen* (Radix Salviae Miltiorrhizae), *Chao Mu Dan Pi* (Cortex Moutan Radicis, stir-fried) and *Zi Cao* (Radix Arnebiae seu Lithospermi) cool the Blood and reduce erythema.
- *Chi Xiao Dou* (Semen Phaseoli Calcarati), *Fu Ling Pi* (Cortex Poriae Cocos) and *Yi Yi Ren* (Semen Coicis Lachryma-jobi) clear Heat and transform Dampness, disperse swelling and reduce erythema.

BLOOD STASIS

This pattern is likely to produce lesions of the vasculitis (purpura) type. Eruptions are dark red or purplish-red in color; blood-filled vesicles or subcutaneous nodules may also occur. Lesions may be painful, possibly with itching. The tongue body is dark red or has stasis marks; the pulse is thready and choppy.

Western drugs commonly causing this pattern include allopurinol, thiazides, sulfonamides, and bismuth preparations; Chinese materia medica include *Tian Hua Fen* (Radix Trichosanthis) and *Di Long‡* (Lumbricus).

Treatment principle

Invigorate the Blood and transform Blood stasis, free the network vessels and reduce erythema.

Prescription

TONG QIAO HUO XUE TANG JIA JIAN

Decoction for Freeing the Orifices and Invigorating the Blood, with modifications

Dang Gui (Radix Angelicae Sinensis) 10g
Chi Shao (Radix Paeoniae Rubra) 10g
Sheng Di Huang (Radix Rehmanniae Glutinosae) 10g
Su Mu (Lignum Sappan) 10g
Bai Zhi (Radix Angelicae Dahuricae) 6g
Chuan Xiong (Rhizoma Ligustici Chuanxiong) 6g
Xiang Fu (Rhizoma Cyperi Rotundi) 6g
Zi Cao (Radix Arnebiae seu Lithospermi) 12g
Mu Dan Pi (Cortex Moutan Radicis) 12g
Chuan Niu Xi (Radix Achyranthis Bidentatae) 12g
Jin Yin Hua (Flos Lonicerae) 12g
Bai Mao Gen (Rhizoma Imperatae Cylindricae) 12g
Chuan Shan Jia* (Squama Manitis Pentadactylae) 4.5g
Zao Jiao Ci (Spina Gleditsiae Sinensis) 4.5g
Si Gua Luo (Fasciculus Vascularis Luffae) 4.5g

Explanation

- *Dang Gui* (Radix Angelicae Sinensis), *Chi Shao* (Radix Paeoniae Rubra), *Su Mu* (Lignum Sappan), *Zao Jiao Ci* (Spina Gleditsiae Sinensis), and *Chuan Shan Jia** (Squama Manitis Pentadactylae) invigorate the Blood and free the network vessels, dissipate lumps and alleviate pain.

- *Zi Cao* (Radix Arnebiae seu Lithospermi), *Mu Dan Pi* (Cortex Moutan Radicis), *Sheng Di Huang* (Radix Rehmanniae Glutinosae), *Jin Yin Hua* (Flos Lonicerae), and *Bai Mao Gen* (Rhizoma Imperatae Cylindricae) cool the Blood and free the network vessels.

- *Xiang Fu* (Rhizoma Cyperi Rotundi), *Chuan Xiong* (Rhizoma Ligustici Chuanxiong), *Bai Zhi* (Radix Angelicae Dahuricae), *Chuan Niu Xi* (Radix Achyranthis Bidentatae) and *Si Gua Luo* (Fasciculus Vascularis Luffae) regulate Qi and invigorate the Blood, free the network vessels and dissipate Blood stasis.

DAMP-HEAT POURING DOWN

Since Dampness has a tendency to flow downward, lesions in this pattern, which usually occurs as part of eczematous or fixed drug eruptions, are concentrated in the genital region and lower limbs and manifest as papulovesicles or vesicles with exudation, erosion or crusting. Lesions are usually itchy. Short voidings of yellow urine is a frequent accompanying symptom. The tongue body is red with a yellow and greasy coating; the pulse is soggy and rapid.

Western drugs commonly causing this pattern include aspirin and sulfonamides; Chinese materia medica include *Qing Hao* (Herba Artemisiae Chinghao) and *Da Suan* (Bulbus Allii Sativi).

Treatment principle

Clear Heat and benefit the movement of Dampness, guide out reddish urine and reduce macules.

Prescription

LONG DAN XIE GAN TANG JIA JIAN

Chinese Gentian Decoction for Draining the Liver, with modifications

Chao Long Dan Cao (Radix Gentianae Scabrae, stir-fried) 6g
Chai Hu (Radix Bupleuri) 6g
Huang Qin (Radix Scutellariae Baicalensis) 6g
Chao Zhi Zi (Fructus Gardeniae Jasminoidis, stir-fried) 6g
Sheng Di Huang (Radix Rehmanniae Glutinosae) 15g
Ren Dong Teng (Caulis Lonicerae Japonicae) 15g
Chi Xiao Dou (Semen Phaseoli Calcarati) 15g
Chi Fu Ling (Sclerotium Poriae Cocos Rubrae) 15g
Che Qian Zi (Semen Plantaginis) 12g, wrapped
Bai Mao Gen (Rhizoma Imperatae Cylindricae) 12g
Lian Qiao (Fructus Forsythiae Suspensae) 12g
Gan Cao (Radix Glycyrrhizae) 4.5g
Deng Xin Cao (Medulla Junci Effusi) 6g

Explanation

- *Chao Long Dan Cao* (Radix Gentianae Scabrae, stir-fried), *Chai Hu* (Radix Bupleuri), *Chao Zhi Zi* (Fructus Gardeniae Jasminoidis, stir-fried), and *Huang Qin* (Radix Scutellariae Baicalensis) clear Heat from the Liver and drain Fire from the Gallbladder.

- *Chi Fu Ling* (Sclerotium Poriae Cocos Rubrae), *Che Qian Zi* (Semen Plantaginis), *Chi Xiao Dou* (Semen Phaseoli Calcarati), and *Bai Mao Gen* (Rhizoma Imperatae Cylindricae) clear Heat and transform Dampness.

- *Ren Dong Teng* (Caulis Lonicerae Japonicae), *Sheng Di Huang* (Radix Rehmanniae Glutinosae), *Lian Qiao* (Fructus Forsythiae Suspensae), *Gan Cao* (Radix Glycyrrhizae), and *Deng Xin Cao* (Medulla Junci Effusi) clear Heat from the Heart and relieve Toxicity.

QI AND YIN DEFICIENCY

This pattern is seen in the recovery phase of severe erythema multiforme or erythroderma types of drug eruptions as the eruptions gradually subside and peeling or scaling occurs. Itching is severe, especially at night. Accompanying symptoms and signs include thirst with a desire for drinks, shortness of breath, fatigue, and mental listlessness. The tongue body is pale red with a scant coating or no coating; the pulse is deficient and thready.

Treatment principle
Augment Qi and nourish Yin, support Vital Qi (Zheng Qi) and relieve Toxicity.

Prescription
ZENG YE TANG JIA JIAN
Decoction for Increasing Body Fluids, with modifications

Xian Di Huang (Radix Rehmanniae Glutinosae Recens) 30-60g
Jin Yin Hua (Flos Lonicerae) 12g
Nan Sha Shen (Radix Adenophorae) 12g
Xuan Shen (Radix Scrophulariae Ningpoensis) 12g
Huang Qi (Radix Astragali seu Hedysari) 12g
Lü Dou Yi (Testa Phaseoli Radiati) 30g
Shi Hu* (Herba Dendrobii) 30g
Shan Yao (Radix Dioscoreae Oppositae) 30g
Tian Men Dong (Radix Asparagi Cochinchinensis) 15g
Mai Men Dong (Radix Ophiopogonis Japonici) 15g
Yu Zhu (Rhizoma Polygonati Odorati) 15g
Chi Xiao Dou (Semen Phaseoli Calcarati) 15g
Ling Yang Jiao Fen* (Cornu Antelopis, powdered) 0.6g

Explanation
- *Yu Zhu* (Rhizoma Polygonati Odorati), *Xian Di Huang* (Radix Rehmanniae Glutinosae Recens), *Nan Sha Shen* (Radix Adenophorae), *Xuan Shen* (Radix Scrophulariae Ningpoensis), *Tian Men Dong* (Radix Asparagi Cochinchinensis), *Mai Men Dong* (Radix Ophiopogonis Japonici), *Shan Yao* (Radix Dioscoreae Oppositae), and *Shi Hu** (Herba Dendrobii) nourish Yin and protect Body Fluids.
- *Jin Yin Hua* (Flos Lonicerae), *Lü Dou Yi* (Testa Phaseoli Radiati) and *Chi Xiao Dou* (Semen Phaseoli Calcarati) relieve Toxicity and transform Blood stasis.
- *Ling Yang Jiao Fen** (Cornu Antelopis, powdered) calms the Liver and subdues Yang, extinguishes Wind and alleviates itching.
- *Huang Qi* (Radix Astragali seu Hedysari) supports Vital Qi (Zheng Qi) and consolidates the Root in order to prevent pathogenic factors from reaching the interior.

General modifications
1. For severe itching, add *Gou Teng* (Ramulus Uncariae cum Uncis), *Ku Shen* (Radix Sophorae Flavescentis) and *Bai Xian Pi* (Cortex Dictamni Dasycarpi Radicis).
2. For Heat in the Upper, Middle and Lower Burners, add *Lian Zi Xin* (Plumula Nelumbinis Nuciferae), *Chao Zhi Zi* (Fructus Gardeniae Jasminoidis, stir-fried) and *Huang Lian* (Rhizoma Coptidis).

3. For constipation, add *Da Huang* (Radix et Rhizoma Rhei) 10 minutes before the end of the decoction process.

EXTERNAL TREATMENT
- For papules and inflammation, apply *San Huang Xi Ji* (Three Yellows Wash Preparation), *San Shi Shui* (Three Stones Lotion) or *Lu Hu Xi Ji* (Calamine and Giant Knotweed Wash Preparation) as a rub twice a day.
- For papulovesicles and vesicles with exudation and erosion, use *Ma Chi Xian Shui Xi Ji* (Purslane Wash Preparation) or prepare a decoction with *Huang Bai* (Cortex Phellodendri) 15g and *Di Yu* (Radix Sanguisorbae Officinalis) 15g to apply as a wet compress for 10-15 minutes twice a day.
- For dry lesions with scaling and severe itching, apply a thin coating of *Qing Dai Gao* (Indigo Paste), *Huang Lian Ruan Gao* (Coptis Ointment) or *Hei Dou Liu You Ruan Gao* (Black Soybean and Vaseline® Ointment) twice a day.

ACUPUNCTURE

Selection of points on the affected channels
Main points: PC-6 Neiguan, LI-11 Quchi, SP-10 Xuehai, and ST-36 Zusanli.
Auxiliary points: LI-4 Hegu, LU-5 Chize, PC-3 Quze, SP-6 Sanyinjiao, and BL-40 Weizhong.
Technique: Apply the reinforcing method at PC-6 Neiguan. For SP-6 Sanyinjiao and ST-36 Zusanli, apply the reducing method first and then the reinforcing method. Apply the reducing method at all the other points. Retain the needles for 30 minutes. Treat once a day for two weeks.

Selection of points according to disease

Itchy urticaria due to penicillin allergy
Points: PC-6 Neiguan, LI-11 Quchi, LI-4 Hegu, ST-36 Zusanli, SP-10 Xuehai, and SP-6 Sanyinjiao.
Technique: Apply the reinforcing method and retain the needles for 30 minutes after obtaining Qi. Treat once a day. A course consists of five treatment sessions.

Nausea, vomiting and skin rashes due to chlorpromazine hydrochloride allergy
Points: LI-4 Hegu, SP-10 Xuehai, LI-11 Quchi, and SP-6 Sanyinjiao.
Technique: Apply the even method and retain the needles for 30 minutes after obtaining Qi. Treat once a day. A course consists of seven treatment sessions.

Urinary retention due to sulfonamides
Points: CV-4 Guanyuan (needled toward CV-6 Qihai) and GV-4 Mingmen.

Technique: Apply the reducing method once or twice a day until urination occurs. After Qi is obtained, patients should feel the needling sensation go up to the area above the umbilicus and then down to the perineum so as to induce urination.

Selection of points according to pattern identification
Points
- For Wind, Heat or Damp Toxins (as may be seen in urticarial or erythema multiforme type drug eruptions), select GB-20 Fengchi, GV-14 Dazhui, LI-11 Quchi, LI-4 Hegu, and SP-10 Xuehai.
- For Damp Toxins and exuberant Heat (as may be seen in fixed drug eruptions or eruptions with bullous lesions), select BL-17 Geshu, BL-15 Xinshu, ST-36 Zusanli, SP-10 Xuehai, and LI-11 Quchi.
- Where the Ying and Xue levels are both ablaze (as may be seen with drug eruptions of the erythroderma type), select GV-20 Baihui, SP-6 Sanyinjiao, GV-26 Shuigou, SP-10 Xuehai, GB-20 Fengchi, and EX-UE-11 Shixuan.[i]

Technique: Apply the reducing method to all the points. Treat once a day.

Explanation
- GB-20 Fengchi, GV-14 Dazhui and LI 4 Hegu dissipate Wind and alleviate itching.
- SP-10 Xuehai, LI-11 Quchi, BL-15 Xinshu, and BL-17 Geshu cool the Blood and reduce erythema.
- ST-36 Zusanli, SP-6 Sanyinjiao, CV-4 Guanyuan, CV-6 Qihai, and GV-4 Mingmen support Vital Qi (Zheng Qi) and consolidate the Root.
- BL-40 Weizhong, PC-3 Quze, EX-UE-11 Shixuan, and GV-26 Shuigou clear Heat and relieve Toxicity.
- HT-7 Shenmen, GV-20 Baihui and PC-6 Neiguan quiet the Spirit and alleviate itching.

ELECTRO-ACUPUNCTURE

Prescription 1
Points: ST-37 Shangjuxu and LI-4 Hegu.
Technique: Apply the reducing method and adjust the intensity of the current according to the patient's tolerance level. Retain the needles for 15 minutes. Treat once a day. A course consists of seven treatment sessions.
Indications: Drug eruptions of the urticarial type.

Prescription 2
Points: ST-36 Zusanli, KI-3 Taixi, LI-11 Quchi, and SI-19 Tinggong.
Technique: Apply the even method. After obtaining Qi at SI-19 Tinggong, point the needle tip horizontally toward TB-17 Yifeng. Adjust the intensity of the current according to the patient's tolerance level. Treat once a day. A course consists of seven treatment sessions.
Indications: This prescription can be used for all types of drug eruption.

Clinical notes

- For papular lesions, treatment should focus on dredging Wind and clearing Heat from the Ying level.
- For erythematous lesions, treatment should focus on cooling the Blood and clearing Heat from the Qi level.
- For vesicular lesions, treatment should focus on augmenting Qi and transforming Dampness.
- In the local management of lesions with vesicles, exudate and erosion, use ingredients with sour, bitter and astringent properties such as *Wu Mei* (Fructus Pruni Mume), *Huang Lian* (Rhizoma Coptidis) and *Ma Chi Xian* (Herba Portulacae Oleraceae).
- Cases of drug-induced dermatitis are relatively common, however some are very severe and a delay in treatment can be life-threatening. Treatment with Chinese materia medica can be effective for mild cases. Severe cases such as drug eruptions manifesting as erythroderma or toxic epidermal necrolysis must be considered as medical emergencies requiring Western medicine treatment. Chinese materia medica can be administered in the recovery phase.

Advice for the patient

Use drugs only when indicated and be aware of signs of potential allergic responses to medications.

Modern clinical experience

INTERNAL TREATMENT

1. **Wang** reported on the treatment of urticarial drug eruptions.[4]

Prescription
QING YING TANG JIA JIAN
Decoction for Clearing Heat from the Ying Level, with modifications

Shui Niu Jiao‡ (Cornu Bubali) 30g, decocted for 30 minutes before adding the other ingredients

---

[i] M-UE-1 according to the system employed by the Shanghai College of Traditional Chinese Medicine.

Xuan Shen (Radix Scrophulariae Ningpoensis) 10g
Mai Men Dong (Radix Ophiopogonis Japonici) 10g
Jin Yin Hua (Flos Lonicerae) 10g
Lian Qiao (Fructus Forsythiae Suspensae) 10g
Dan Shen (Radix Salviae Miltiorrhizae) 10g
Sheng Ma (Rhizoma Cimicifugae) 10g
Ge Gen (Radix Puerariae) 10g
Sheng Di Huang (Radix Rehmanniae Glutinosae) 15g
Huang Lian (Rhizoma Coptidis) 6g
Dan Zhu Ye (Herba Lophatheri Gracilis) 6g
Chan Tui‡ (Periostracum Cicadae) 6g

One bag a day was used to prepare a decoction, taken twice a day for three days.

2. **Song** treated various types of drug eruption, including the exanthematous, urticarial, purpuric, eczematoid and fixed drug reaction types, in some cases accompanied by glucocorticoids. [5]

Prescription
PI ZHEN TANG
Decoction for Skin Eruptions

Tu Fu Ling (Rhizoma Smilacis Glabrae) 60g
Sheng Di Huang (Radix Rehmanniae Glutinosae) 20g
Zi Cao (Radix Arnebiae seu Lithospermi) 12g
Di Fu Zi (Fructus Kochiae Scopariae) 12g
Chuan Xiong (Rhizoma Ligustici Chuanxiong) 10g
Bai Xian Pi (Cortex Dictamni Dasycarpi Radicis) 10g
Jing Jie (Herba Schizonepetae Tenuifoliae) 6g
Gan Cao (Radix Glycyrrhizae) 9g

One bag a day was used to prepare a decoction, taken twice a day. Results were seen after three to ten days.

3. **Li** formulated an empirical prescription for fixed drug eruptions in the genital region. [6]

Prescription
PI YAN LIANG XUE JIE DU TANG
Dermatitis Decoction for Cooling the Blood and Relieving Toxicity

Mu Dan Pi (Cortex Moutan Radicis) 15g
Lian Qiao (Fructus Forsythiae Suspensae) 15g
Tu Fu Ling (Rhizoma Smilacis Glabrae) 15g
Bai Xian Pi (Cortex Dictamni Dasycarpi Radicis) 15g

Sheng Di Huang (Radix Rehmanniae Glutinosae) 30g
Di Long‡ (Lumbricus) 10g

One bag a day was used to prepare a decoction, taken twice a day.

Externally a 3 percent boric acid solution was applied for ten minutes, once in the morning and evening, followed by *Tang Shang Gao* (Scald Paste). Results were seen after four to ten days, depending on the severity of the eruption.

COMBINATION OF MATERIA MEDICA AND ACUPUNCTURE

Shu combined internal and external treatment with acupuncture treatment. [7]

Prescription ingredients

Sheng Di Huang (Radix Rehmanniae Glutinosae) 24g
Dang Gui (Radix Angelicae Sinensis) 12g
Su Zi (Fructus Perillae Frutescentis) 12g
Chi Shao (Radix Paeoniae Rubra) 15g
Bai Shao (Radix Paeoniae Lactiflorae) 15g
Chuan Xiong (Rhizoma Ligustici Chuanxiong) 8g
Mu Dan Pi (Cortex Moutan Radicis) 10g
Huang Qin (Radix Scutellariae Baicalensis) 10g
Lian Qiao (Fructus Forsythiae Suspensae) 10g
Chan Tui‡ (Periostracum Cicadae) 10g
Gan Cao (Radix Glycyrrhizae) 10g
Jing Jie (Herba Schizonepetae Tenuifoliae) 10g
Fang Feng (Radix Ledebouriellae Divaricatae) 10g
Jin Yin Hua (Flos Lonicerae) 30g
Da Huang (Radix et Rhizoma Rhei) 3g, added 10 minutes before the end of the decoction process

One bag a day was used to prepare a decoction, taken twice a day. The ingredients were then decocted a third time and used to wash the affected area.

ACUPUNCTURE

Acupuncture was given at SP-10 Xuehai, LI-11 Quchi, KI-3 Taixi, SP-6 Sanyinjiao, LU-5 Chize, and TB-5 Waiguan using the reducing method. Results were seen between 3 and 20 days of daily treatments.

References

1. Lu Liping, *Kou Fu San Qi Fen Yin Qi Yao Zhen San Li Bao Dao* [Report on Three Cases of Drug Eruption after Oral Administration of Powdered *San Qi* (Radix Notoginseng)], *Xin Zhong Yi* [New Journal of Traditional Chinese Medicine] 35, 6 (1984): 43.

2. Guo Tingzan, *Sheng Shan Yao Wai Fu Zhi Guo Min* [Allergic Reaction Caused by External Application of Raw *Shan Yao* (Rhizoma Dioscoreae Oppositae)], *Si Chuan Zhong Yi* [Sichuan Journal of Traditional Chinese Medicine] 6 (1991): 41.

3. Song Hongqi, *Kou Fu Wu Wei Zi Tang Jiang Yin Qi Guo Min Fan Ying* [Allergic Reaction Caused by Oral Administration of *Wu Wei Zi Tang Jiang* (Schisandra Syrup)], *Zhong Guo Zhong Yao Za Zhi* [Journal of Chinese Materia Medica] 4 (1990): 51.

4. Wang Zongyuan, *Qing Ying Tang Hua Cai Zhi Liao Yao Wu Xing Pi Yan 38 Li* [Treatment of 38 Cases of Drug-Induced Dermatitis with Modified *Qing Ying Tang* (Decoction for Clearing Heat from the Ying Level)], *Jiang Su Zhong Yi* [Jiangsu Journal of Traditional Chinese Medicine] 20, 1 (1999): 29.

5. Song Zhenxing, *Pi Zhen Tang Zhi Liao Yao Wu Xing Pi Yan 10 Li* [Treatment of 10 Cases of Drug-Induced Dermatitis with *Pi Zhen Tang* (Decoction for Skin Eruptions)], *Zhong Guo Zhong Xi Yi Jie He Za Zhi* [Journal of Integrated TCM and Western Medicine] 18, 7 (1998): 428.

6. Li Huihua, *Wai Sheng Zhi Qi Yao Wu Xing Pi Yan De Zhong Yi Zhi Liao* [Treatment of Drug-Induced Dermatitis in the Genitalia with Traditional Chinese Medicine], *Zhong Yi Yao Xin Xi* [Traditional Chinese Medicine and Materia Medica News] 2 (1997): 41.

7. Shu Zhanjun, *Zhong Yi Zong He Zhi Liao Yao Zhen 12 Li* [Treatment of 12 Cases of Drug Eruptions with a Combination of Traditional Chinese Medicine Methods], *Xin Jiang Zhong Yi Yao* [Xinjiang Journal of Traditional Chinese Medicine and Chinese Materia Medica] 16, 4 (1998): 22.

Skin disorders
due to physical agents

The skin disorders in this chapter result from the skin reacting to such physical factors as temperature, light, radiation, and mechanical stimuli. Disorders may be local or generalized.

The resulting skin disorders may be classified as follows:

- those caused by cold, including chilblains and frostbite;
- those caused by direct contact with heat, such as burns, or by heat resulting from hot weather or high temperatures in the workplace, such as erythema ab igne;
- exposure to light may lead to acute or chronic skin lesions; exposure to strong light may result in sunburn, while exposure of photosensitive skin may lead to polymorphic light eruption or phytophotodermatitis;
- exposure to ionizing radiation (for example, from X-rays or gamma rays) can result in radiodermatitis;
- long-term or persistent friction or pressure on the skin can lead to disturbance of blood circulation locally, resulting in cornification, fissuring or necrosis of the skin, as for instance in corns or calluses.

TCM takes both internal and external factors into account in relation to the causes of the disorders discussed in this chapter.

Internal factors

Differentiation must be made between Deficiency and Excess patterns of the Zang-Fu organs. Excess patterns are more likely at the onset of the disorder and Deficiency patterns where the disorder persists.

External factors

Following an invasion of pathogenic factors such as Cold, Summerheat or Fire, they settle in the skin and flesh and affect the normal circulation of Qi and Blood, finally resulting in obstruction of the channels and network vessels or ulceration of the skin.

Chilblains
冻疮

Chilblains are circumscribed inflammatory skin lesions caused by exposure to cold. They generally heal spontaneously when the weather becomes warmer, but may recur the following winter when the weather turns cold again.

In TCM, this condition is also known as *dong feng* (frozen Wind).

Clinical manifestations

- Lesions mainly involve body parts that are often exposed to cold such as the hands, face, ears, and feet.
- The lesions initially manifest as circumscribed congestive edema, which feels cold on contact, blanches on pressure, and returns to a purple-pink and swollen state once pressure is removed. The lesions are usually self-limiting, resolving in 2-3 weeks. In severe cases, lesions may appear as vesicles or bullae, which ulcerate after rupture. Ulcerative lesions take much longer to heal.
- Heat provokes local itching.
- Chilblains mostly occur in children, women, people who sit with little movement for long periods, those working at low temperatures in contact with cold water, or those working for lengthy periods in a damp and cold environment.

Differential diagnosis

Erythema multiforme

Lesions typically manifest as symmetrically distributed erythematous papules, which evolve into concentric rings of varying color. Usually numerous, they commonly occur on the dorsum of the hands and feet, the palms and soles, and the extensor aspects of the forearms and legs, but may also be seen on the fingers and toes. Heat will not provoke itching. Erythema multiforme is commonly associated with a preceding infection, such as herpes simplex, tuberculosis or *Mycoplasma pneumoniae*, or with various drugs such as sulfonamides, barbiturates or salicylates.

Frostbite
After injury due to exposure to cold, initial symptoms appear as pallor of the skin, a sensation of freezing cold and pain, followed by numbness in the affected area, which becomes white and waxy in appearance. Skin color subsequently changes from white to blue or black depending on the severity of the condition.

Etiology and pathology

Failure to protect exposed skin adequately against cold winds, snow, frost, or freezing temperatures may allow strongly pathogenic Wind or Cold to attack the skin and flesh, leading to Qi stagnating and Blood congealing and the formation of chilblains.

Pattern identification and treatment

INTERNAL TREATMENT

QI AND BLOOD DEFICIENCY WITH PATHOGENIC COLD OBSTRUCTING THE CHANNELS
The affected area is swollen and red or dark red and feels cold on contact. Exposure to heat will provoke local itching. The tongue body is pale red with a thin white coating; the pulse is deep and thready.

Treatment principle
Augment Qi and warm Yang, free the network vessels and dissipate Cold.

Prescription
GUI ZHI JIA DANG GUI TANG JIA JIAN
Cinnamon Twig Decoction plus Chinese Angelica Root, with modifications

Dang Gui (Radix Angelicae Sinensis) 10g
Huang Qi (Radix Astragali seu Hedysari) 10g
Dang Shen (Radix Codonopsitis Pilosulae) 10g
Bai Zhu (Rhizoma Atractylodis Macrocephalae) 10g
Fu Ling Pi (Cortex Poriae Cocos) 10g
Gui Zhi (Ramulus Cinnamomi Cassiae) 6g
*Xi Xin** (Herba cum Radice Asari) 6g
Gan Jiang (Rhizoma Zingiberis Officinalis) 6g

Gan Cao (Radix Glycyrrhizae) 15g
Huo Xue Teng (Caulis seu Radix Schisandrae) 15g
Ji Xue Teng (Caulis Spatholobi) 15g
Dan Shen (Radix Salviae Miltiorrhizae) 15g
Jin Yin Hua (Flos Lonicerae) 15g

Explanation
- *Dang Gui* (Radix Angelicae Sinensis), *Huang Qi* (Radix Astragali seu Hedysari), *Dang Shen* (Radix Codonopsitis Pilosulae), and *Bai Zhu* (Rhizoma Atractylodis Macrocephalae) augment Qi and supplement the Blood.
- *Gui Zhi* (Ramulus Cinnamomi Cassiae) *Xi Xin** (Herba cum Radice Asari) and *Gan Jiang* (Rhizoma Zingiberis Officinalis) warm Yang and dissipate Cold.
- *Huo Xue Teng* (Caulis seu Radix Schisandrae), *Dan Shen* (Radix Salviae Miltiorrhizae), *Ji Xue Teng* (Caulis Spatholobi), *Jin Yin Hua* (Flos Lonicerae), *Gan Cao* (Radix Glycyrrhizae), and *Fu Ling Pi* (Cortex Poriae Cocos) free the network vessels and disperse swelling.

COLD TOXINS OBSTRUCTING THE CHANNELS DUE TO KIDNEY YANG DEFICIENCY
Lesions appear as purplish swellings with vesicles of various sizes. Ulceration follows rupture of the vesicles; ulcers may not heal. Other symptoms include aversion to cold, cold limbs and a lusterless, white facial complexion. The tongue body is pale with a thin white coating; the pulse is deep, thready and forceless.

Treatment principle
Support Yang and consolidate the Root, free the network vessels and close sores.

Prescription
SI MIAO TANG JIA WEI
Mysterious Four Decoction, with additions

Huang Qi (Radix Astragali seu Hedysari) 15-30g
Jin Yin Hua (Flos Lonicerae) 15-30g
Dang Shen (Radix Codonopsitis Pilosulae) 15-30g
Fu Ling (Sclerotium Poriae Cocos) 12g
Ji Xue Teng (Caulis Spatholobi) 12g
Shan Yao (Radix Dioscoreae Oppositae) 12g
Bai Zhu (Rhizoma Atractylodis Macrocephalae) 12g
Fu Pen Zi (Fructus Rubi Chingii) 12g
Shu Di Huang (Radix Rehmanniae Glutinosae Conquita) 12g
Zhi Gan Cao (Radix Glycyrrhizae, mix-fried with honey) 12g
Sheng Jiang (Rhizoma Zingiberis Officinalis Recens) 3g
Da Zao (Fructus Ziziphi Jujubae) 15g

Explanation
- *Huang Qi* (Radix Astragali seu Hedysari), *Dang Shen* (Radix Codonopsitis Pilosulae), *Shu Di Huang* (Radix Rehmanniae Glutinosae Conquita), and *Fu Pen Zi*

(Fructus Rubi Chingii) augment Qi and warm Yang, support Vital Qi (Zheng Qi) and consolidate the Root.

- *Shan Yao* (Radix Dioscoreae Oppositae), *Bai Zhu* (Rhizoma Atractylodis Macrocephalae), *Zhi Gan Cao* (Radix Glycyrrhizae, mix-fried with honey), *Sheng Jiang* (Rhizoma Zingiberis Officinalis Recens), *Fu Ling* (Sclerotium Poriae Cocos), and *Da Zao* (Fructus Ziziphi Jujubae) fortify the Spleen and harmonize the Stomach to consolidate the Middle Burner.

- *Ji Xue Teng* (Caulis Spatholobi) invigorates the network vessels and disperses swelling to assist the movement of Yang Qi.

- *Jin Yin Hua* (Flos Lonicerae) relieves Toxicity and closes sores.

General modifications

1. For patients with Yang Deficiency manifesting as aversion to cold, add *Ba Ji Tian* (Radix Morindae Officinalis), *Lu Jiao* ‡ (Cornu Cervi) or *Lu Jiao Jiao* ‡ (Gelatinum Cornu Cervi), *Pao Jiang* (Rhizoma Zingiberis Officinalis Praeparata), and *Jiu Xiang Chong* ‡ (Aspongopus).

2. For patients with Qi and Blood Deficiency, add *E Jiao* ‡ (Gelatinum Corii Asini) and *Gao Li Shen* (Radix Ginseng Coreensis).

3. For persistent non-healing of ulcerating chilblains, add *Rou Gui* (Cortex Cinnamomi Cassiae) and *Bai Lian* (Radix Ampelopsis Japonicae).

PATENT HERBAL MEDICINES

Take *Quan Lu Wan* (Whole Deer Pill) 3g with warm boiled water twice a day. This pill helps to prevent and treat chilblains.

EXTERNAL TREATMENT

- Apply *Zheng Hong Hua You* (Regular Safflower Oil) to the affected area two or three times a day.

- At the initial stage before ulceration, prepare a decoction with:

  Dang Gui (Radix Angelicae Sinensis) 10g
  Hong Hua (Flos Carthami Tinctorii) 10g
  Chuan Wu* (Radix Aconiti Carmichaeli) 10g
  Cao Wu* (Radix Aconiti Kusnezoffii) 10g
  Tou Gu Cao (Herba Speranskiae seu Impatientis) 12g

  Use first for steaming the lesions for 15 minutes, then for soaking them for a further 15 minutes. Treat once a day.

- If the lesions are red and swollen, apply *Hong Ling Jiu* (Red Spirit Wine) or *Du Sheng Gao* (Single Garlic Paste) to the affected area.

- If there is ulceration, use 20 percent *Dong Chuang Gao* (Chilblain Paste).

- If there are complications due to toxic infection and resulting abscess formation, use *Qing Dai San* (Indigo Powder) and cover it with *Ling Yi Gao* (Miraculous Difference Ointment) until the abscess heals and flesh is generated. Then use *Shou Gan Sheng Ji Yao Fen* (Medicated Powder for Promoting Contraction and Generating Flesh) and cover it with *Qing Liang Gao* (Cool Clearing Paste). Treat once a day until the lesion heals completely.

ACUPUNCTURE

Superficial needling
After routine disinfection, superficially needle Ashi points at the edge of the chilblains. Then insert needles slowly into healthy skin 0.2 cm from the border of the lesions and withdraw the needles immediately without causing bleeding.

Filiform needling
Points

- For lesions on the hand, select TB-4 Yangchi, LI-5 Yangxi, LI-4 Hegu, TB-5 Waiguan, and TB-3 Zhongzhu.

- For lesions on the foot, select ST-41 Jiexi, BL-66 Tonggu, GB-43 Xiaxi, and SP-4 Gongsun.

- For lesions on the ear, select Ashi points for bleeding.

Technique: Apply the even method and retain the needles for 5-15 minutes. Treat once every other day until the condition is resolved.

Explanation
Local points are used to treat chilblains on the hand and foot. The purpose of the treatment is to free the channels and network vessels, disperse swelling and alleviate pain. This treatment is effective for chilblains at the initial stage.

MOXIBUSTION

Direct moxibustion with a moxa stick
Ignite a moxa stick and apply to the lesion directly, moving it up and down two or three times per second. Treat once every day or every other day.

Indirect moxibustion
Cut fresh ginger into slices 0.5cm thick and place on the chilblains. Put a moxa cone on top of the ginger slices and ignite. When there is a pleasantly warm sensation in the chilblains, remove the ginger. Treat once a day.

Clinical notes

- More often than not, the patient's constitution is a major factor in the occurrence of chilblains. This condition is more common in people with Yang Deficiency. Internal treatment for chilblains should therefore follow the principle of augmenting Qi and warming Yang, invigorating the Blood and freeing the network vessels, while external treatment should focus on dissipating Cold and dispelling Dampness, transforming Blood stasis and dispersing swelling.

- Acupuncture and moxibustion are effective in dispersing swelling and freeing the network vessels, dissipating Blood stasis and alleviating pain.

Advice for the patient

- Wear a warm coat, hat and gloves when outside in sub-zero temperatures. Inside, keep the room temperature warm.
- Wear warm, dry and comfortable shoes and socks. People with sweaty hands and feet should change shoes and socks frequently and ensure that they are completely dry before wearing them again.
- A nutritious diet high in proteins and carbohydrates and rich in vitamins is important, especially for people with a weak constitution or those suffering from chronic illnesses.

Literature excerpt

In *Yang Yi Da Quan* [The Complete Book of External Diseases], it says: "Wind-Cold attacking warm flesh causes stagnation, which results in itching. This is the injury caused by frozen Wind (*dong feng*). It should not be warmed in front of a fire."

Modern clinical experience

INTERNAL TREATMENT
Rao proposed an internal treatment for chilblains. [1]

Prescription
HUANG QI DANG GUI SI NI TANG
Astragalus and Chinese Angelica Root Counterflow Cold Decoction

Huang Qi (Radix Astragali seu Hedysari) 30g

Dang Gui (Radix Angelicae Sinensis) 10g
Bai Shao (Radix Paeoniae Lactiflorae) 10g
Gui Zhi (Ramulus Cinnamomi Cassiae) 10g
*Xi Xin** (Herba cum Radice Asari) 10g
Gan Cao (Radix Glycyrrhizae) 6g
Tong Cao (Medulla Tetrapanacis Papyriferi) 6g
Da Zao (Fructus Ziziphi Jujubae) 20g

One bag a day of the ingredients was used to prepare a decoction, taken three times a day. Doses were reduced for children. Seven days made up a course. After one course of treatment, 80 of the 204 patients (39 percent) were cured, 120 (59 percent) experienced some improvement, and 4 (2 percent) showed no improvement. Follow-up visits to 150 patients indicated that 142 had no chilblains in the following three winters.

EXTERNAL APPLICATION OF POWDER PREPARATION
For ulcerative chilblains, **Yang** applied a mixture of powdered *Ru Xiang* (Gummi Olibanum) 10g and powdered *Mo Yao* (Myrrha) 10g directly to the affected area. For chilblains without ulceration, enough Vaseline® was added to make a paste before application. The treatment was applied four or five times a day. Five days made up one course. In patients with ulcerating chilblains, results were seen after one to three courses, and in those with red and swollen lesions, after one or two courses. [2]

EXTERNAL APPLICATION OF TINCTURE PREPARATIONS
1. **Yang** reported that external application three to four times a day of *Fu Fang Bai Yao Ding* (Compound Yunnan White Tincture), manufactured by Yunnan Baiyao Pharmaceutical Factory, proved effective after two to three days of treatment. [3]

2. **Hu** steeped 10g of *Fu Zi** (Radix Lateralis Aconiti Carmichaeli Praeparata) in 50ml of *Bai Jiu* (Spiritus Incolor Granorum). He warmed the medicated alcohol over a mild heat and applied it to the affected area while hot. Treatment took place over five consecutive days once a day before going to bed. Results were usually noted after one course of treatment. [4]

Chapped and fissured hands and feet
手足皲裂

Exposure to low temperatures, particularly in damp environments, results in erosion and cracking of the skin. Chapped and fissured hands and feet (*shou zu jun lie*) were first mentioned in *Zhu Bing Yuan Hou Lun* [A General Treatise on the Causes and Symptoms of Diseases]. It is also known in TCM as *cun lie chuang* (cracked chapping sore), *cun tong* (chapping pain), *lie gou chuang* (splitting sore), *lie shou lie zu* (cracked hands and feet), and *gan lie chuang* (dry cracked sore).

Clinical manifestations

- On the hand, lesions usually involve the thumb and the transverse crease overlying the joints of the extensor aspect of the index finger.
- On the foot, lesions generally involve the heel and its lateral and medial aspects.
- This condition is more common in adults and in winter.
- At the initial stage, the skin feels tight and hard; scaly plaques and superficial cracks are present. The skin gradually becomes rough and thick and deep linear fissures 2-3 mm or more in length appear. When the fissures reach the dermis, bleeding and crusting will occur.
- Pain accompanies movement of the hands and feet, making walking or working difficult.

Differential diagnosis

Tinea manuum
Lesions mainly involve the center of the palm and the palmar aspect of the fingers. Small vesicles appear initially, which rupture and then dry up to be covered by layers of white scale. The skin becomes dry, rough and thick, and may crack or fissure. The condition is worse in summer. There may be intolerable itching.

Tinea pedis
The hyperkeratotic form of tinea pedis infects the soles, which may be covered by fine, white scales; however, these do not develop into fissures.

Keratoderma of the palms and soles
This condition may be inherited or acquired. Lesions manifest as thick, dry, hard, shiny pale yellow skin on the palms and soles; the skin may fissure in winter, causing pain when walking.

Etiology and pathology

Internal factors
Constitutional Blood Deficiency leads to stagnation of Qi and Blood, which therefore fail to provide adequate nourishment to the skin and flesh, resulting in the skin becoming dry and cracked.

External factors
Exposure to Wind-Cold pathogenic factors leads to their retention in the skin and flesh. External pressure, repeated friction, frequent immersion in cold water, or maceration of the hands and feet reduce the ability of the skin and interstices (*cou li*) to resist pathogenic factors. Retention of these factors results in obstruction of Qi and Blood in the vessels, thus depriving the skin of nourishment and causing it to become dry.

Pattern identification and treatment

INTERNAL TREATMENT

EXTERNAL WIND-COLD OBSTRUCTING MOVEMENT OF QI AND BLOOD
The skin on the hands and feet is dry, accompanied by comparatively deep fissuring over the joints; in more severe cases, bleeding or crusting will occur. Contact with cold water or knocking into an object causes moderate to severe pain. The tongue body is pale red with a scant coating; the pulse is thready and rapid.

Treatment principle
Augment Qi and nourish the Blood, dispel Cold and moisten Dryness.

Prescription
BA ZHEN TANG JIA JIAN
Eight Treasure Decoction, with modifications

Dang Gui (Radix Angelicae Sinensis) 6g
Bai Shao (Radix Paeoniae Lactiflorae) 10g
Fu Ling (Sclerotium Poriae Cocos) 10g
Shu Di Huang (Radix Rehmanniae Glutinosae Conquita) 10g
Yi Yi Ren (Semen Coicis Lachryma-jobi) 10g
Bai Zhu (Rhizoma Atractylodis Macrocephalae) 3g
Gan Cao (Radix Glycyrrhizae) 3g
Huang Qi (Radix Astragali seu Hedysari) 15g
Ji Xue Teng (Caulis Spatholobi) 15g
Chuan Xiong (Rhizoma Ligustici Chuanxiong) 4.5g

Explanation

- *Bai Zhu* (Rhizoma Atractylodis Macrocephalae), *Huang Qi* (Radix Astragali seu Hedysari) and *Gan Cao* (Radix Glycyrrhizae) augment Qi and support the Spleen.
- *Dang Gui* (Radix Angelicae Sinensis), *Shu Di Huang* (Radix Rehmanniae Glutinosae Conquita) and *Bai Shao* (Radix Paeoniae Lactiflorae) nourish the Blood and moisten Dryness.
- *Yi Yi Ren* (Semen Coicis Lachryma-jobi) and *Fu Ling* (Sclerotium Poriae Cocos) fortify the Spleen and drain Dampness.
- *Chuan Xiong* (Rhizoma Ligustici Chuanxiong) invigorates the Blood and regulates Qi.
- *Ji Xue Teng* (Caulis Spatholobi) invigorates the Blood and frees the network vessels.

EXTERNAL TREATMENT

- Prepare *Cong Bai Tang* (Scallion Decoction) and allow the decoction to cool to a comfortable temperature before soaking the affected hand or foot in it for 10-15 minutes. Wipe dry and apply *Zi Cao You* (Gromwell Root Oil) or *Yu Ji Gao* (Jade Flesh Paste) to the affected areas.
- Apply *Hei Dou Liu You Ruan Gao* (Black Soybean and Vaseline® Ointment) to the affected areas twice a day.

Clinical notes

- If the lesions are triggered by an underlying condition, this should be treated first.
- The disease mainly occurs in cold and dry climates at the end of autumn or the beginning of winter. Soak the hands and feet in warm water before applying any external cream or paste to help absorption of the medication.

Advice for the patient

- Do not wash the hands or feet with detergent, medicated soap or alkaline powders.
- In winter, soak the hands and feet in warm water and use a moisturizing cream as soon as any cracks appear in the skin.
- Apply a protective cream immediately after a bath or shower.

Literature excerpts

In *Wai Ke Mi Lu* [Secret Records of External Diseases], it says: "*Cun lie chuang* (cracked chapping sore) affects those working with their hands. When the hands are red, but the interstices (*cou li*) loose, external Wind can attack to cause this condition, especially when the hands are wet. Where the skin is broken, pain is usually slight, but where cracks occur, pain will be much more intense."

In *Wai Ke Zheng Zong* [An Orthodox Manual of External Diseases], it says: "Chapped and fissured hands and feet appear as dry and cracked skin and are caused by Qi and Blood being deprived of nourishment. When hot flesh is suddenly attacked by Wind-Cold, Blood congeals in the vessels and the skin becomes dry and withered, resulting in cracks and fissures appearing. Where there is daily exposure to wind, Wind and Heat will fight, leading to pain."

Frostbite
冻伤

Frostbite is damage to body tissues induced by extremely cold conditions. Freezing of the tissues may result in irreversible tissue destruction. The tissue may become gangrenous and amputation may become necessary.

In TCM, this condition is also known as *dong lan chuang* (frozen ulcerating sore).

Clinical manifestations

- Lesions mainly involve the extremities and exposed parts of the body such as the fingers, toes, feet, ears, nose, and cheeks.
- Immediately after injury due to exposure to cold, symptoms initially appear as pallor of the skin, a sensation of freezing cold and pain, followed by numbness in the affected area, which becomes white and waxy in appearance. The characteristic manifestations of frostbite do not appear until the tissues thaw.
- The condition can be divided into four levels of severity according to the manifestations.

- **Mild frostbite:** The local skin color changes from pale white to mottled blue. Accompanying symptoms and signs include redness, localized edematous swelling, itching, stabbing pain, and altered sensation.
- **Moderate frostbite:** This level is characterized by local redness, edematous swelling, itching, and burning pain. Vesicles appear at the initial stage. Provided that there is no secondary infection, the vesicles will dry up to form black crusts.
- **Serious frostbite:** The local skin color changes from pale white to blue and then to black. Local sensation is lost. Swelling and blisters occur around the lesions, accompanied by severe pain. Necrotic tissue finally separates and the lesions heal slowly. Scars form, which may affect limb function.
- **Severe frostbite:** The skin appears dull gray in color. There is total loss of local motor and sensory functions. Dry or moist gangrene develops subsequently, resulting in deformity and disorders of function.

Etiology and pathology

- Cold pathogenic factors damage Yang Qi when they invade the skin and flesh. As a result, the circulation of Blood in the vessels will be impaired and Qi and Blood will stagnate. Externally, the limbs cannot be warmed up and the normal movement of Ying Qi (Nutritive Qi) and Wei Qi (Defensive Qi) will be interrupted. In mild cases, frostbite occurs with pain and swelling; in severe cases, there may be damage to the joints.
- Frostbite should not be treated with methods involving the sudden application of heat, otherwise Cold and Fire will fight and bind, leading to Qi and Blood stagnation that will accelerate the process of ulceration.

Pattern identification and treatment

FIRST AID PROCEDURES FOR EMERGENCY MANAGEMENT

- Move the patient from the cold environment as soon as possible to avoid further injury.
- Remove frozen and wet clothing and footwear.
- Take active measures to rewarm the patient, for example by immersing the patient in warm water (40-42°C) for up to 20 minutes.
- Emergency treatment with Western medicine is also likely to be required.

INTERNAL TREATMENT

BLOOD STASIS DUE TO COLD CONGEALING

This pattern manifests as local numbness and cold, swelling and lumps, with scorching pain and itching. The skin in the affected area of the hands and feet appears bluish-purple. The tongue body is pale red with a thin white coating; the pulse is deep or deep and thready.

Treatment principle

Warm the channels and dissipate Cold, dispel Blood stasis and free the vessels.

Prescription

DANG GUI SI NI TANG JIA JIAN

Chinese Angelica Root Counterflow Cold Decoction, with modifications

Dang Gui (Radix Angelicae Sinensis) 15g
Chi Shao (Radix Paeoniae Rubra) 15g
Bai Shao (Radix Paeoniae Lactiflorae) 15g
Huo Xue Teng (Caulis seu Radix Schisandrae) 15g
Ren Dong Teng (Caulis Lonicerae Japonicae) 15g
Shi Nan Teng (Caulis Photiniae) 15g
Gui Zhi (Ramulus Cinnamomi Cassiae) 10g
Chuan Xiong (Rhizoma Ligustici Chuanxiong) 10g
Sang Zhi (Ramulus Mori Albae) 10g
Zhi Gan Cao (Radix Glycyrrhizae, mix-fried with honey) 10g
Huang Qi (Radix Astragali seu Hedysari) 12g
Gan Jiang (Rhizoma Zingiberis Officinalis) 12g
Xi Xin* (Herba cum Radice Asari) 6g
Da Zao (Fructus Ziziphi Jujubae) 15g

Explanation

- *Dang Gui* (Radix Angelicae Sinensis), *Chi Shao* (Radix Paeoniae Rubra), *Bai Shao* (Radix Paeoniae Lactiflorae), *Gui Zhi* (Ramulus Cinnamomi Cassiae), *Huang Qi* (Radix Astragali seu Hedysari), *Chuan Xiong* (Rhizoma Ligustici Chuanxiong), *Zhi Gan Cao* (Radix Glycyrrhizae, mix-fried with honey), and *Sang Zhi* (Ramulus Mori Albae) augment Qi and warm Yang, dissipate Cold and free the network vessels.
- *Huo Xue Teng* (Caulis seu Radix Schisandrae), *Ren Dong Teng* (Caulis Lonicerae Japonicae) and *Shi Nan Teng* (Caulis Photiniae) free the network vessels and dissipate Blood stasis to speed up Blood circulation and improve microcirculation in the fingers and toes.
- *Gan Jiang* (Rhizoma Zingiberis Officinalis), *Xi Xin** (Herba cum Radice Asari) and *Da Zao* (Fructus Ziziphi Jujubae) warm Yang and dissipate Cold from the Spleen and Kidneys.

BLOOD DEFICIENCY DUE TO COLD CONGEALING

Symptoms include numbness, cold and pain, diffuse dull red swellings or vesicles, a dull sensation or local loss of sensation, lassitude, aversion to cold, and a pale, lusterless facial complexion. The tongue body is pale with a scant coating; the pulse is thready and weak, or deep and slow.

Treatment principle
Supplement and nourish Qi and Blood, warm and free the Blood vessels.

Prescription
REN SHEN YANG RONG TANG JIA JIAN
Ginseng Decoction for Nourishing Ying Qi, with modifications

Huang Qi (Radix Astragali seu Hedysari) 15g
Dang Shen (Radix Codonopsitis Pilosulae) 12g
Bai Zhu (Rhizoma Atractylodis Macrocephalae) 12g
Shu Di Huang (Radix Rehmanniae Glutinosae Conquita) 12g
Bai Shao (Radix Paeoniae Lactiflorae) 12g
Gui Zhi (Cortex Cinnamomi Cassiae) 6g
Wu Wei Zi (Fructus Schisandrae) 6g
Yuan Zhi (Radix Polygalae) 6g
Fu Pen Zi (Fructus Rubi Chingii) 10g
Gan Cao (Radix Glycyrrhizae) 10g
Lu Jiao‡ (Cornu Cervi) 10g
Huo Xue Teng (Caulis seu Radix Schisandrae) 10g
Ji Xue Teng (Caulis Spatholobi) 10g

Explanation
- *Huang Qi* (Radix Astragali seu Hedysari), *Dang Shen* (Radix Codonopsitis Pilosulae), *Bai Zhu* (Rhizoma Atractylodis Macrocephalae), *Bai Shao* (Radix Paeoniae Lactiflorae), *Shu Di Huang* (Radix Rehmanniae Glutinosae Conquita), *Huo Xue Teng* (Caulis seu Radix Schisandrae), and *Ji Xue Teng* (Caulis Spatholobi) augment Qi and nourish the Blood.
- *Fu Pen Zi* (Fructus Rubi Chingii), *Lu Jiao*‡ (Cornu Cervi), *Gan Cao* (Radix Glycyrrhizae), and *Gui Zhi* (Cortex Cinnamomi Cassiae) warm Yang and free the network vessels.
- *Wu Wei Zi* (Fructus Schisandrae) and *Yuan Zhi* (Radix Polygalae) hold the Qi of the five Zang organs, and also warm and free the network vessels.

COLD TRANSFORMING INTO HEAT TOXINS

This pattern manifests as ulcerating sores oozing serous fluid and pus. Lesions are surrounded by inflamed, swollen and painful areas; fever may be an accompanying symptom. The tongue body is red with a thin, yellow and slightly dry coating; the pulse is rapid.

Treatment principle
Nourish Yin and relieve Toxicity, invigorate the Blood and alleviate pain.

Prescription
SI MIAO YONG AN TANG JIA JIAN
Mysterious Four Resting Hero Decoction, with modifications

Huang Qi (Radix Astragali seu Hedysari) 15g
Dang Gui (Radix Angelicae Sinensis) 15g
Xuan Shen (Radix Scrophulariae Ningpoensis) 15g
Ren Dong Teng (Caulis Lonicerae Japonicae) 30g
Fu Ling (Sclerotium Poriae Cocos) 10g
Dang Shen (Radix Codonopsitis Pilosulae) 10g
Bai Zhu (Rhizoma Atractylodis Macrocephalae) 10g
Chuan Niu Xi (Radix Cyathulae Officinalis) 10g
Chi Xiao Dou (Semen Phaseoli Calcarati) 45g
Zhi Ru Xiang (Gummi Olibanum, processed with vinegar) 4.5g
Zhi Mo Yao (Myrrha, processed with vinegar) 4.5g
Zi Hua Di Ding (Herba Violae Yedoensitis) 6g

Explanation
- *Huang Qi* (Radix Astragali seu Hedysari), *Dang Shen* (Radix Codonopsitis Pilosulae), *Fu Ling* (Sclerotium Poriae Cocos), and *Bai Zhu* (Rhizoma Atractylodis Macrocephalae) supplement Original Qi (Yuan Qi).
- *Xuan Shen* (Radix Scrophulariae Ningpoensis), *Ren Dong Teng* (Caulis Lonicerae Japonicae), *Chi Xiao Dou* (Semen Phaseoli Calcarati), and *Zi Hua Di Ding* (Herba Violae Yedoensitis) nourish Yin and clear Heat, relieve Toxicity and alleviate pain.
- *Dang Gui* (Radix Angelicae Sinensis), *Chuan Niu Xi* (Radix Cyathulae Officinalis), *Zhi Ru Xiang* (Gummi Olibanum, processed with vinegar), and *Zhi Mo Yao* (Myrrha, processed with vinegar) invigorate the Blood, dissipate Blood stasis, disperse swelling and alleviate pain.

YANG DEBILITATION DUE TO EXUBERANT COLD

Symptoms include counterflow cold of the limbs, cold and painful extremities, sleepiness, numbness, and a pallid or slightly bluish facial complexion. The tongue body is pale purple with a scant coating; the pulse is deep and faint.

Treatment principle
Return Yang and stem counterflow, warm and free the Blood vessels.

Prescription
SI NI JIA REN SHEN TANG JIA JIAN
Counterflow Cold Decoction plus Ginseng, with modifications

Fu Pen Zi (Fructus Rubi Chingii) 10g

Gan Jiang (Rhizoma Zingiberis Officinalis) 10g
Dang Shen (Radix Codonopsitis Pilosulae) 10g
Bai Shao (Radix Paeoniae Lactiflorae) 10g
Gan Cao (Radix Glycyrrhizae) 10g
Gui Zhi (Ramulus Cinnamomi Cassiae) 12g
Huang Qi (Radix Astragali seu Hedysari) 12g
Zhi Chuan Shan Jia* (Squama Manitis Pentadactylae Praeparata) 12g
Lu Lu Tong (Fructus Liquidambaris) 12g
Shan Yao (Radix Dioscoreae Oppositae) 15g
Shan Zhu Yu (Fructus Corni Officinalis) 15g
Ba Ji Tian (Radix Morindae Officinalis) 15g
Sang Ji Sheng (Ramulus Loranthi) 15g
Dan Shen (Radix Salviae Miltiorrhizae) 15g

Explanation

- *Dang Shen* (Radix Codonopsitis Pilosulae), *Huang Qi* (Radix Astragali seu Hedysari), *Bai Shao* (Radix Paeoniae Lactiflorae), *Shan Yao* (Radix Dioscoreae Oppositae), and *Gan Cao* (Radix Glycyrrhizae) augment Qi.
- *Fu Pen Zi* (Fructus Rubi Chingii), *Gan Jiang* (Rhizoma Zingiberis Officinalis), *Gui Zhi* (Ramulus Cinnamomi Cassiae), *Zhi Chuan Shan Jia** (Squama Manitis Pentadactylae Praeparata), *Dan Shen* (Radix Salviae Miltiorrhizae), *Lu Lu Tong* (Fructus Liquidambaris), and *Sang Ji Sheng* (Ramulus Loranthi) warm Yang and free the network vessels, dissipate Cold and alleviate pain.
- *Shan Zhu Yu* (Fructus Corni Officinalis) and *Ba Ji Tian* (Radix Morindae Officinalis) warm and supplement the Liver and Kidneys, assisting *Gan Jiang* (Rhizoma Zingiberis Officinalis) and *Fu Pen Zi* (Fructus Rubi Chingii) to return Yang and stem counterflow.

EXTERNAL TREATMENT

- At the stage before ulceration, prepare a decoction with *Gan Cao* (Radix Glycyrrhizae) 15g and *Yuan Hua* (Flos Daphnes Genkwa) 15g to bathe the affected area. Then gently massage the area with *Hong Ling Jiu* (Red Spirit Wine) or *Sheng Jiang Zhi* (Succus Rhizomatis Zingiberis Officinalis Recens).
- If there are vesicles or bleeding vesicles, puncture the vesicles with acupuncture needles and squeeze the fluid out or refer to a practitioner of Western medicine to have the fluid drawn out. Then dress the lesions with *Zi Se Xiao Zhong Gao* (Purple Paste for Dispersing Swelling).
- For small ulcerating lesions, wash the lesions with *Jiao Ai Tang* (Chinese Prickly Ash and Mugwort Decoction) before applying *Dong Chuang Gao* (Chilblain Paste). Treat once a day.

ACUPUNCTURE

Treatment at adjacent points

Points

- For frostbite on the hand, select LI-4 Hegu, TB-5 Waiguan, TB-4 Yangchi, TB-3 Zhongzhu, and EX-UE-9 Baxie. [i]
- For frostbite on the foot, select LR-3 Taichong, LR-2 Xingjian, ST-41 Jiexi, BL-60 Kunlun, ST-44 Neiting, and GB-41 Zulinqi.

Technique: Select three or four points and treat with the even method. Retain the needles for 30 minutes and rotate once every 10 minutes. Treat once a day.

Treatment at Ashi points

After routine sterilization, insert one to four needles in the center of the red and swollen area (the number will depend on the extent of the lesion). Use the rotate, lift and thrust reinforcing method. The needles are not retained. Try to squeeze out a small amount of blood after the needles are withdrawn. Treat once every other day.

Explanation

The focus on local points for the treatment of frostbite on the hand and foot aims at dredging and freeing the channels and network vessels, dispersing swelling and alleviating pain. This treatment has a definite effect on frostbite at the initial stage.

MOXIBUSTION

Direct moxibustion with a moxa stick

Ignite a moxa stick and apply it to the affected area directly by moving it up and down two to three times per second. There will be a sensation of heat or mild burning pain in the area treated, but scarring will not occur. Treat once every day or every other day.

Moxibustion at acupuncture points

For generalized frostbite, apply moxibustion with a moxa stick to CV-8 Shenque and CV-4 Guanyuan for 15-30 minutes once or twice a day. A course consists of five treatment sessions. This treatment has the function of strengthening the Heart and adding warmth, returning Yang and stemming counterflow.

Warming with a moxa pole

Light a medicated moxa stick and insert in a moxa burner. Move the burner on the forearm in the area between SJ-8 Sanyangluo and SJ-5 Waiguan. Use one medicated moxa stick per session. Treat once a day. A course consists of seven treatment sessions.

---

[i] M-UE-22 according to the system employed by the Shanghai College of Traditional Chinese Medicine.

Clinical notes

- Treatment of frostbite should focus on reducing the possibility of deformity to a minimum.
- It is important to distinguish the degree of seriousness of the condition and treat accordingly. In TCM, the treatment principle for frostbite aims mainly at augmenting Qi, warming Yang, dissipating Cold, invigorating the Blood, and freeing the network vessels.
- Frostbitten areas must not be heated in front of a fire or placed in very hot water. Keep the room temperature steady and not too warm. Give the patient a hot drink such as tea prepared with ginger and sugar.
- Standard hygiene precautions must be taken against bacterial infection, to which frostbitten skin is highly susceptible.
- Immediate treatment for patients with non-gangrenous serious frostbite will help recovery. Tissue gangrene may necessitate surgery, preferably delayed for some weeks.

Advice for the patient

- Exposed parts of the body should be kept warm when outdoors in a cold climate.
- Keep shoes and socks dry. Change them as soon as possible if they become wet.
- Exercise appropriately to promote blood circulation.

Literature excerpts

In *Yi Xue Ru Men* [Elementary Medicine], it says: "In winter, the lower body is Deficient. If the body is exposed to Cold, Blood will stagnate and lead to the generation of sores. These sores will be persistent, but manifest without pain or itching. Internal treatment should be based on *Sheng Ma He Qi Yin* (Bugbane Beverage for Harmonizing Qi) with *Da Huang* (Radix et Rhizoma Rhei) removed. Externally, use a powder of *Mu Xiang** (Radix Aucklandiae Lappae), *Bing Lang** (Semen Arecae Catechu), *Liu Huang*‡ (Sulphur), *Wu Zhu Yu* (Fructus Evodiae Rutaecarpae), *Jiang Huang*

(Rhizoma Curcumae Longae) and *She Xiang** (Secretio Moschi) mixed with sesame oil."

In *Pi Fu Bing Zhong Yi Zhen Liao Xue* [Diagnosis and Treatment of Skin Diseases in Traditional Chinese Medicine], Xu Yihou states: "The basic cause of frostbite is Yang Deficiency due to exuberant Cold, accompanied by congealing of Qi, Blood and Water. Treatment should follow the general principle of warming to dissipate Cold, supplementing to reinforce Yang, and freeing to invigorate the vessels."

Modern clinical experience

EXTERNAL TREATMENT

1. **Shi** treated 87 patients with mild or moderate frostbite with a warm soak.[5]

Prescription
DONG SHANG TANG
Frostbite Decoction

Dang Gui (Radix Angelicae Sinensis) 40g
Hua Jiao (Pericarpium Zanthoxyli) 40g
Rou Gui (Cortex Cinnamomi Cassiae) 40g
*Fu Zi** (Radix Lateralis Aconiti Carmichaeli Praeparata) 30g
Gan Jiang (Rhizoma Zingiberis Officinalis) 30g
Er Cha (Pasta Acaciae seu Uncariae) 30g
Hong Hua (Flos Carthami Tinctorii) 20g
Hai Piao Xiao‡ (Os Sepiae seu Sepiellae) 20g
*Xi Xin** (Herba cum Radice Asari) 15g
Gui Zhi (Ramulus Cinnamomi Cassiae) 15g
Chi Shao (Radix Paeoniae Rubra) 15g
Gan Cao (Radix Glycyrrhizae) 10g

The ingredients were decocted and used while warm to soak the lesions for 20-30 minutes every evening before going to bed. One bag was sufficient for two applications. Six days of treatment made up one course. Results were seen after three courses.

2. *Shi Di Shui* (rheo-camphoradin, also popularly known as "ten drops"), produced by Hangzhou Tongjun Pharmaceutical Factory, can be used externally up to a dozen times a day for frostbite. Results are usually seen in three days for mild conditions of the first level of severity, and in four to ten days for moderate to serious conditions. No local pigmentation will remain.[6]

Sunburn

晒斑

Ultraviolet radiation (UVR) is the main cause of skin cancers and is also responsible for several other skin disorders. The UVR spectrum is divided into three sections. UVC is absorbed by the ozone layer in the atmosphere, whereas UVA and UVB both reach the earth's surface (see Figure 17-1). UVR is at its peak in the middle of the day and is intensified by reflection from sand, water or snow.

Some 90 percent of UVB is absorbed by the epider-mis, but approximately 30 percent of UVA reaches the dermis. UVB light in the 290-320 nm range causes sunburn, an acute inflammatory reaction of the skin due to overexposure to strong sunlight. These wavelengths are essentially blocked by window glass. UVA is long-wave ultraviolet light that tans the skin, but also contributes to skin aging. Sunbeds emit UVA radiation.

In TCM, sunburn is also known as *ri shai chuang* (sun exposure sore).

Figure 17-1 Ultraviolet radiation and skin disorders

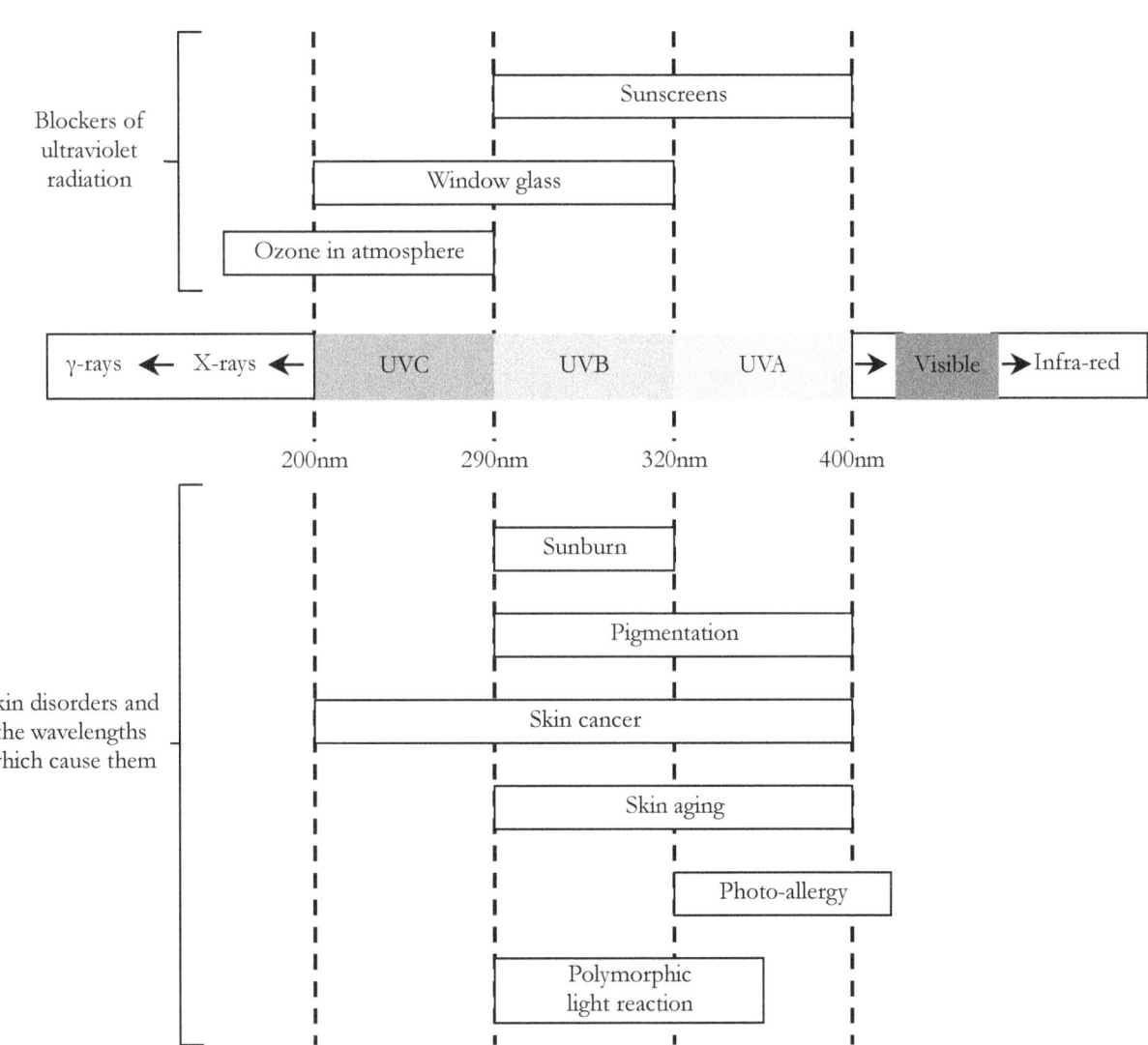

Clinical manifestations

- The main sites of involvement are exposed body parts such as the face, neck and limbs. In strong sunlight, burning can take place through thin clothing.
- Overexposure to sunlight results in a tingling sensation in the skin, which becomes red 2-12 hours later. Diffuse erythema and edema are noted in the sunburnt areas, where the skin appears smooth and shiny. The redness reaches its maximum after 24 hours and then fades over the next 48-60 hours to leave desquamation and pigmentation.
- In mild cases, there is localized burning and stabbing pain.
- In severe cases, red papules and vesicles appear; exudation follows rupture of the vesicles, which subsequently dry up and form crusts. If the sunburnt area is large, there may be accompanying symptoms such as fever, headache, nausea, and general malaise.

Differential diagnosis

Phytophotodermatitis
This condition occurs on exposure to sunlight after ingesting or coming into contact with plants (such as giant hogweed, carrot, parsnip, celery, fennel, or common rue) containing light-sensitizing substances known as psoralens (furanocoumarins). It is most common in spring and summer when furanocoumarins are highest and UV exposure is the greatest. Bizarre inflammatory patterns and linear streaks of hyperpigmentation are key clues to diagnosing phytophotodermatitis.

Contact dermatitis
This condition is unrelated to exposure to sunlight. Lesions present when the body is exposed to certain irritant substances. Erythema is associated with the pathogenic agents involved. Itching may also be present. Contact dermatitis may occur in any season.

Etiology and pathology

- Exposure to strong sunshine on hot summer days may result in the formation of Heat Toxins. If these Toxins attack the fleshy exterior, they can heat up Qi and Blood, damage the skin and putrefy the flesh, resulting in the temporary appearance of sore-like lesions.
- In summer, Summerheat often harbors Damp Toxins. These two pathogenic factors fight and combine to spread to the skin and flesh, causing erythema, blisters and peeling of the skin.

Pattern identification and treatment

INTERNAL TREATMENT

HEAT TOXINS
The sunburnt area is red and inflamed with diffuse edema. The skin may be shiny and feel tight, or the sunburn may manifest as a dense distribution of red papules. A local sensation of scorching heat may be present, possibly accompanied by itching or stabbing pain. The tongue body is red with a thin coating; the pulse is rapid.

Treatment principle
Clear Heat and dispel Summerheat, relieve Toxicity and disperse swelling.

Prescription
QING SHU TANG JIA JIAN
Decoction for Clearing Summerheat, with modifications

Jin Yin Hua (Flos Lonicerae) 12g
Lian Qiao (Fructus Forsythiae Suspensae) 12g
Che Qian Zi (Semen Plantaginis) 12g, wrapped
Zi Hua Di Ding (Herba Violae Yedoensitis) 12g
Pu Gong Ying (Herba Taraxaci cum Radice) 12g
Qing Hao (Herba Artemisiae Chinghao) 30g
Hua Shi‡ (Talcum) 30g, wrapped in *He Ye* (Folium Nelumbinis Nuciferae)
Chi Shao (Radix Paeoniae Rubra) 10g
Ze Xie (Rhizoma Alismatis Orientalis) 10g
Dan Zhu Ye (Herba Lophatheri Gracilis) 10g
Gan Cao (Radix Glycyrrhizae) 10g

Explanation
- *Jin Yin Hua* (Flos Lonicerae), *Lian Qiao* (Fructus Forsythiae Suspensae), *Pu Gong Ying* (Herba Taraxaci cum Radice), *Qing Hao* (Herba Artemisiae Chinghao), and *Zi Hua Di Ding* (Herba Violae Yedoensitis) clear Heat and relieve Toxicity.
- *Che Qian Zi* (Semen Plantaginis), *Hua Shi*‡ (Talcum) and *Ze Xie* (Rhizoma Alismatis Orientalis) benefit the movement of Dampness and flush out Summerheat.
- *Chi Shao* (Radix Paeoniae Rubra), *Dan Zhu Ye* (Herba Lophatheri Gracilis) and *Gan Cao* (Radix Glycyrrhizae) cool the Blood and reduce erythema.

DAMP TOXINS
Large, diffuse erythematous patches appear in the affected area, accompanied by obvious edema. Multiple densely distributed vesicles are also present. Exudation and erosion follow rupture of the vesicles. Accompanying symptoms and signs include itching, fever, thirst, red eyelids, profuse discharge from the eyes (due to Heat in the Liver channel), and short voidings of

yellow urine. The tongue body is red with a yellow coating; the pulse is slippery and rapid.

Treatment principle
Clear Heat and percolate Dampness, invigorate the Blood and relieve Toxicity.

Prescription
LONG DAN XIE GAN TANG JIA JIAN
Chinese Gentian Decoction for Draining the Liver, with modifications

Chao Long Dan Cao (Radix Gentianae Scabrae, stir-fried) 6g
Chai Hu (Radix Bupleuri) 6g
Jiao Zhi Zi (Fructus Gardeniae Jasminoidis, scorch-fried) 6g
Sheng Di Huang (Radix Rehmanniae Glutinosae) 15g
Che Qian Zi (Semen Plantaginis) 15g, wrapped
Ze Xie (Rhizoma Alismatis Orientalis) 12g
Fu Ling Pi (Cortex Poriae Cocos) 12g
Chi Shao (Radix Paeoniae Rubra) 12g
Chi Xiao Dou (Semen Phaseoli Calcarati) 12g
Lian Qiao (Fructus Forsythiae Suspensae) 10g
Gan Cao (Radix Glycyrrhizae) 10g

Explanation
- *Chao Long Dan Cao* (Radix Gentianae Scabrae, stir-fried), *Chai Hu* (Radix Bupleuri), *Jiao Zhi Zi* (Fructus Gardeniae Jasminoidis, scorch-fried), and *Lian Qiao* (Fructus Forsythiae Suspensae) clear and drain Damp-Heat from the Liver and Gallbladder.
- *Sheng Di Huang* (Radix Rehmanniae Glutinosae), *Chi Shao* (Radix Paeoniae Rubra) and *Chi Xiao Dou* (Semen Phaseoli Calcarati) cool the Blood and reduce erythema, percolate Dampness and relieve Toxicity.
- *Gan Cao* (Radix Glycyrrhizae) clears Heat and relieves Toxicity.
- *Fu Ling Pi* (Cortex Poriae Cocos), *Ze Xie* (Rhizoma Alismatis Orientalis) and *Che Qian Zi* (Semen Plantaginis) benefit the movement of Dampness and relieve Toxicity.

General modifications
1. For fever and fear of cold, add *Chai Hu* (Radix Bupleuri), *Shui Niu Jiao* ‡ (Cornu Bubali) and *Shi Gao* ‡ (Gypsum Fibrosum).
2. For redness, swelling and stabbing pain, add *Lü Dou Yi* (Testa Phaseoli Radiati) and *Zi Cao* (Radix Arnebiae seu Lithospermi).
3. For local edema, add *Dong Gua Pi* (Epicarpium Benincasae Hispidae), *Tong Cao* (Medulla Tetrapanacis Papyriferi) and *Chan Tui* ‡ (Periostracum Cicadae).
4. For obvious thirst, add *Tian Hua Fen* (Radix Trichosanthis), *Sang Ye* (Folium Mori Albae) and *Ju Hua* (Flos Chrysanthemi Morifolii).

5. For rupture and erosion of multiple vesicles, add *Cang Zhu* (Rhizoma Atractylodis), *Ma Chi Xian* (Herba Portulacae Oleraceae) and *Huang Bai* (Cortex Phellodendri).
6. For absence of thirst or thirst without a desire to drink, add *Huo Xiang* (Herba Agastaches seu Pogostemi), *Pei Lan* (Herba Eupatorii Fortunei) and *Zhu Ru* (Caulis Bambusae in Taeniis).
7. For clouded Spirit and delirious speech, add *Hu Po* ‡ (Succinum), *Shi Chang Pu* (Rhizoma Acori Graminei) and *Yuan Zhi* (Radix Polygalae).

EXTERNAL TREATMENT
- For red, swollen and itchy lesions, apply *Qing Liang Fen* (Cool Clearing Powder) externally; or use *San Huang Xi Ji* (Three Yellows Wash Preparation); or mix *Qing Bai San* (Green-White Powder) with water or sesame oil for application to the affected area two or three times a day.
- For clusters of unruptured vesicles, mix *Yu Lu San* (Jade Dew Powder) with sesame oil for external application, or apply *Yu Lu Gao* (Jade Dew Ointment) to the affected area once or twice a day.
- For exudation and erosion after rupture of vesicles, use *Ma Chi Xian Shui Xi Ji* (Purslane Wash Preparation), or select three or four herbs each time from *Ye Ju Hua* (Flos Chrysanthemi Indici), *Long Kui* (Herba Solani Nigri), *Chu Tao Ye* (Folium Broussonetiae), *Di Yu* (Radix Sanguisorbae Officinalis), *Qing Hao* (Herba Artemisiae Chinghao), and *Dong Gua Pi* (Epicarpium Benincasae Hispidae), and prepare a decoction to apply as a wet compress on the affected area for 30-45 minutes twice a day. Apply *Yu Lu Gao* (Jade Dew Ointment) after lesions dry up and crusts form.

Clinical notes

- For sunburnt skin due to severe Summerheat, it is important for treatment purposes to determine the relationship between external Heat pathogenic factors and weakness of the body due to Qi Deficiency. If Heat pathogenic factors are predominant, treatment should focus on clearing Heat from the Qi Level and relieving Toxicity (in other words, treating the Manifestations). If Qi Deficiency predominates, treatment should concentrate on augmenting Qi and protecting Yin (in other words treating the Root).
- Medications recommended for external application have the functions of reducing pain and diminishing the burning sensation.
- Erosion of the skin should be dealt with immediately to prevent the possibility of secondary infection.

Lesions should be disinfected and dressed and the patient referred to a doctor of Western medicine for further treatment including antibiotics.

Advice for the patient

- Wear broad-rimmed hats for outdoor activities and other appropriate clothing to protect the body from exposure.
- Avoid exposure to sunlight for long periods, especially between 10 a.m. and 3 p.m. when the sun is strongest.
- Start sun tanning by brief exposure periods (not exceeding 20 minutes) in the morning or late afternoon.
- Apply appropriate sunscreen skin creams with a high sun protection factor (SPF) on days of strong sunshine or on hot days with hazy sunshine.

Literature excerpt

In *Wai Ke Mi Lu* [Secret Records of External Diseases], it says: "*Ri shai chuang* (sun exposure sore) occurs because of exposure to strong sunshine on a hot summer's day. There will be pain followed by rupture of the lesions. The cause is external Heat rather than internal Heat. This condition often affects people working outdoors and farmers working in the fields. People leading an easy, comfortable life will not suffer from this problem. Treatment requires herbs for clearing Summerheat such as *Qing Hao* (Herba Artemisiae Chinghao) drunk as a decoction. Externally, powdered medications will help."

Polymorphic light eruption
多形日光疹

Polymorphic light eruption, often also referred to as "sun allergy", is a group of photosensitive skin disorders characterized by recurrent, polymorphic lesions with an acute onset, usually in spring or early summer. The eruption fades or disappears spontaneously in autumn and winter, only to recur the following year. The condition is triggered by exposure to ultraviolet radiation and so may also affect predisposed individuals on winter holidays to sunny regions.

Clinical manifestations

- Polymorphic light eruption occurs at any age, but is most common in younger women.
- Itchy, erythematous lesions mostly appear on sites exposed to the sun, such as the face, the neck, a V-shaped area on the upper chest, the extensor aspect of the forearms, the backs of the hands, and the lower legs.
- Manifestations vary according to type:
  - In acute eruptions, the rash appears a few hours after exposure to the sun and disappears spontaneously within one or two weeks after exposure ceases.
  - The chronic type usually develops as a result of recurrence of the acute type, but may have chronicity from the outset. It may recur for months or years, tending to be more extensive each time.

- The pruritic type manifests initially as patchy erythema or urticarial plaques. Dense clusters of papules subsequently appear on the erythema or groups of papulovesicles arise on the urticarial plaques. Lichenification may occur in chronic cases.
- The eczematous or actinic dermatitis type presents as an eczematous reaction and is characterized by erythema, swelling, papules, vesicles, erosion, and crusting. In serious cases, distribution may be generalized; in chronic cases, lichenification may occur.
- In the solar urticaria type, itchy wheals of various sizes appear within a short time at sites exposed to the sun.
- A combination of types may occur in some patients.

Differential diagnosis

See Table 17-1.

Etiology and pathology

- In spring and summer, the weather is warm and the skin, hair and interstices (*cou li*) are loose. If there is repeated exposure to sunlight, Heat pathogenic factors from the sun's rays fight and bind with Damp-Heat that has accumulated internally due to

Table 17-1 Differential diagnosis of skin disorders due to reaction to light

	Phototoxicity (including phytophotodermatitis)	Photoallergy	Polymorphic light eruption
History of contact with photosensitizing substances (e.g. drugs)	Yes	Yes	No
Family history of photosensitivity	No	No	Yes, rarely
Morbidity	Can affect anyone	Only involves certain sensitized individuals	Only involves certain sensitized individuals
Latency	None	Mostly occurs 5-20 days after exposure to the sun	None
Ultraviolet wavelengths causing sensitive reactions	UV wavelength of the sensitizing substance	Long UV wavelengths (UVA) and visible light	Medium UV wavelengths (UVB and shorter wavelength UVA)
Concentration of photosensitive substance	Comparatively high	Very low concentrations can trigger a reaction	Not relevant
Clinical manifestations	Erythema and vesicles	Eczematous, possibly with exudation (often similar to allergic contact dermatitis)	Polymorphic eruptions
Site of disease	Sites of sun exposure only	Mostly sites of sun exposure, occasionally elsewhere	Mostly sites of sun exposure, but may be generalized in severe cases
Duration of disease	Short, recovery within one or two weeks	Resolves several weeks after drug or exposure to sun is stopped	Chronic, recurrence for months or years
Photopatch testing	Negative	Positive, similar to eczema response	Negative

constitutional insufficiency, subsequently settling in the skin and flesh to cause the disease.

- Where Heat Toxins from sunlight invade the body at a time when there is excessive Heat in the Blood, Heat Toxins can draw Blood-Heat to the skin, where it congests, resulting in erythema and papules. Where Heat Toxins from sunlight and externally contracted Summerheat-Damp invade the body when there is existing Damp-Heat, the internal and external pathogenic factors combine and accumulate in the skin and flesh, giving rise to erythema, papules and vesicles.

Pattern identification and treatment

INTERNAL TREATMENT

CONGESTION OF BLOOD-HEAT
Flushed red skin at the sites of sun exposure gradually develops into bright or dull slightly raised erythema with clearly defined margins; symmetrically distributed clusters of 1-3 mm red papules then appear on the erythema. The eruption is itchy. Accompanying symptoms and signs include dry mouth and thirst, normal or dry stool, and short voidings of yellow urine. The tongue body is red with a thin yellow coating; the pulse is rapid.

Treatment principle
Clear Heat and cool the Blood.

Prescription
PI YAN TANG JIA WEI
Dermatitis Decoction, with additions

Sheng Di Huang (Radix Rehmanniae Glutinosae) 15g
Shi Gao‡ (Gypsum Fibrosum) 15g, decocted for 30 minutes before adding the other ingredients
Qing Hao (Herba Artemisiae Chinghao) 15g
Jin Yin Hua (Flos Lonicerae) 15g
Mu Dan Pi (Cortex Moutan Radicis) 10g

Chi Shao (Radix Paeoniae Rubra) 10g
Huang Qin (Radix Scutellariae Baicalensis) 10g
Lian Qiao (Fructus Forsythiae Suspensae) 10g
Dan Zhu Ye (Herba Lophatheri Gracilis) 6g
Gan Cao (Radix Glycyrrhizae) 6g
Zi Cao (Radix Arnebiae seu Lithospermi) 12g

Explanation

- *Sheng Di Huang* (Radix Rehmanniae Glutinosae), *Mu Dan Pi* (Cortex Moutan Radicis) and *Chi Shao* (Radix Paeoniae Rubra) cool and invigorate the Blood.
- *Shi Gao* ‡ (Gypsum Fibrosum) clears Heat from the Qi level.
- *Qing Hao* (Herba Artemisiae Chinghao), *Huang Qin* (Radix Scutellariae Baicalensis) and *Zi Cao* (Radix Arnebiae seu Lithospermi) clear Heat and cool the Blood.
- *Lian Qiao* (Fructus Forsythiae Suspensae), *Jin Yin Hua* (Flos Lonicerae), *Dan Zhu Ye* (Herba Lophatheri Gracilis), and *Gan Cao* (Radix Glycyrrhizae) clear Heat and relieve Toxicity.

ACCUMULATION AND OBSTRUCTION OF DAMP-HEAT

Erythema and papules appear initially at the sites of sun exposure; papulovesicles and vesicles subsequently appear on the red skin, becoming confluent to form plaques. Erosion and exudation may occur, with crusting and scaling in persistent conditions. The eruption is itchy. Accompanying symptoms and signs include poor appetite, listlessness and fatigued limbs. The tongue body is slightly red with a slightly yellow or greasy coating; the pulse is deep and soggy, or slippery and rapid.

Treatment principle

Clear Heat and benefit the movement of Dampness.

Prescription
XIE HUANG SAN JIA JIAN
Yellow-Draining Powder, with modifications

Shi Gao ‡ (Gypsum Fibrosum) 15-30g, decocted for
  30 minutes before adding the other ingredients
Sheng Di Huang (Radix Rehmanniae Glutinosae) 15g
Huo Xiang (Herba Agastaches seu Pogostemi) 15g
Yi Yi Ren (Semen Coicis Lachryma-jobi) 15g
Qing Hao (Herba Artemisiae Chinghao) 12g
Huang Qin (Radix Scutellariae Baicalensis) 10g
Jiao Zhi Zi (Fructus Gardeniae Jasminoidis, scorch-fried) 10g
Chi Fu Ling (Sclerotium Poriae Cocos Rubrae) 10g
Dan Zhu Ye (Herba Lophatheri Gracilis) 6g
Deng Xin Cao (Medulla Junci Effusi) 6g
Lian Zi Xin (Plumula Nelumbinis Nuciferae) 3g
Lü Dou (Semen Phaseoli Radiati) 30g

Chi Xiao Dou (Semen Phaseoli Calcarati) 30g

Explanation

- *Sheng Di Huang* (Radix Rehmanniae Glutinosae), *Qing Hao* (Herba Artemisiae Chinghao) and *Lian Zi Xin* (Plumula Nelumbinis Nuciferae) clear Heat and cool the Blood.
- *Jiao Zhi Zi* (Fructus Gardeniae Jasminoidis, scorch-fried), *Huang Qin* (Radix Scutellariae Baicalensis), *Deng Xin Cao* (Medulla Junci Effusi), *Dan Zhu Ye* (Herba Lophatheri Gracilis), and *Lü Dou* (Semen Phaseoli Radiati) clear Heat and benefit the movement of Dampness.
- *Yi Yi Ren* (Semen Coicis Lachryma-jobi), *Chi Fu Ling* (Sclerotium Poriae Cocos Rubrae) and *Chi Xiao Dou* (Semen Phaseoli Calcarati) promote urination and benefit the movement of Dampness.
- *Shi Gao* ‡ (Gypsum Fibrosum) clears Heat from the Qi level.
- *Huo Xiang* (Herba Agastaches seu Pogostemi) aromatically transforms Dampness.

EXTERNAL TREATMENT
- For reddened and itchy skin, apply *Lu Hu Xi Ji* (Calamine and Giant Knotweed Wash Preparation) two to four times a day.
- For erosion and exudation, prepare a decoction with equal proportions of *Sheng Di Yu* (Radix Sanguisorbae Officinalis Recens) and *Ma Chi Xian* (Herba Portulacae Oleraceae) and use as a cold wet compress on the affected areas for 15 minutes, two or three times a day.

FOLK REMEDY
Stew *Chi Xiao Dou* (Semen Phaseoli Calcarati) 30g, *Chao Bai Bian Dou* (Semen Dolichoris Lablab, stir-fried) 15g and *Lü Dou* (Semen Phaseoli Radiati) 15g until reduced to a pulp, then add *Bing Tang* (Saccharon Crystallinum) 5g and eat.

Clinical notes

- Treat patients with erosion and exudation immediately to avoid secondary infection.
- The prognosis is good if exposure to the sun is avoided.

Advice for the patient

- Avoid direct exposure to the sun and wear protective clothing such as wide-brimmed hats, long-sleeved shirts and long trousers.

- Sunscreens and sunblocks can also be used, but they should not be treated as a substitute for avoiding the sun and wearing protective clothing.

Case history

Patient
Female, aged 29.

Clinical manifestations
Papules had appeared at the beginning of summer for five consecutive years. Current examination revealed patches of erythema and papules on the right side of the back of the neck with slight infiltration and patches of 1-2 mm papules on the bilateral forearms.

Pattern identification
Looseness of the interstices (*cou li*) with external contraction of Summerheat.

Treatment principle
Cool the Blood and clear Heat, relieve Toxicity and dispel Summerheat.

Prescription ingredients
Sheng Di Huang (Radix Rehmanniae Glutinosae) 30g
Dan Shen (Radix Salviae Miltiorrhizae) 9g
Chi Shao (Radix Paeoniae Rubra) 9g
Zi Hua Di Ding (Herba Violae Yedoensitis) 9g
Lian Qiao (Fructus Forsythiae Suspensae) 9g
Chi Fu Ling (Sclerotium Poriae Cocos Rubrae) 9g
Ze Xie (Rhizoma Alismatis Orientalis) 9g
Er Miao Wan (Mysterious Two Pill) 9g, crushed and wrapped
Ren Dong Teng (Caulis Lonicerae Japonicae) 12g
Liu Yi San (Six-To-One Powder) 6g, wrapped

One bag a day was used to prepare a decoction, taken twice a day.

External treatment
Liu Yi San (Six-To-One Powder) 9g and *Ku Fan*‡ (Alumen Praeparatum) 1.5g were ground into a fine powder and applied to the affected areas.

Second visit
After four bags of the decoction, new papules appeared after the old ones disappeared. The treatment principle was amended to clearing Summerheat and relieving Toxicity. *Chi Fu Ling* (Sclerotium Poriae Cocos Rubrae), *Ze Xie* (Rhizoma Alismatis Orientalis) and *Er Miao Wan* (Mysterious Two Pill) were removed and *Qing Hao* (Herba Artemisiae Chinghao) 15g, *Zhi Zi* (Fructus Gardeniae Jasminoidis) 9g, *Dan Zhu Ye* (Herba Lophatheri Gracilis) 9g, and *Pei Lan* (Herba Eupatorii Fortunei) 9g added. The external treatment was not modified

Third visit
After five bags of the second prescription, no new papules had appeared despite one session of swimming in the open air. The patient was asked to continue with the second prescription for another five days to consolidate the improvement.[7]

Modern clinical experience

INTERNAL TREATMENT

1. **Shi** used a modified classical formula to treat polymorphic light eruption.[8]

Prescription
PU JI XIAO DU YIN JIA JIAN
Universal Salvation Beverage for Dispersing Toxicity, with modifications

Jiu Chao Huang Qin (Radix Scutellariae Baicalensis, stir-fried with wine) 10g
Jiu Chao Huang Lian (Rhizoma Coptidis, stir-fried with wine) 10g
Sheng Ma (Rhizoma Cimicifugae) 10g
Bo He (Herba Menthae Haplocalycis) 10g
Mu Dan Pi (Cortex Moutan Radicis) 10g
Jiang Can‡ (Bombyx Batryticatus) 10g
Tong Cao (Medulla Tetrapanacis Papyriferi) 10g
Niu Bang Zi (Fructus Arctii Lappae) 12g
Lian Qiao (Fructus Forsythiae Suspensae) 12g
Ban Lan Gen (Radix Isatidis seu Baphicacanthi) 15g
Xuan Shen (Radix Scrophulariae Ningpoensis) 15g
Gan Cao (Radix Glycyrrhizae) 6g
Che Qian Cao (Herba Plantaginis) 30g

One bag a day was used to prepare a decoction, taken three times a day. Some cases were additionally prescribed steroid creams. Treatment lasted for four weeks. Of 54 patients treated, only two showed no response. In follow-up visits one year later, the condition had recurred in 13 patients.

2. **Yang** prepared a decoction for internal use following the treatment principles of clearing Heat and cooling the Blood, eliminating Dampness and alleviating itching, arresting Wind and freeing the network vessels.[9]

Prescription ingredients
Bai Xian Pi (Cortex Dictamni Dasycarpi Radicis) 30g
Sheng Di Huang (Radix Rehmanniae Glutinosae) 20g
Di Fu Zi (Fructus Kochiae Scopariae) 15g
Zi Cao (Radix Arnebiae seu Lithospermi) 15g
Qing Hao (Herba Artemisiae Chinghao) 15g
Mu Dan Pi (Cortex Moutan Radicis) 10g
Wu Shao She‡ (Zaocys Dhumnades) 10g
Jing Jie (Herba Schizonepetae Tenuifoliae) 10g
Fang Feng (Radix Ledebouriellae Divaricatae) 10g
Feng Fang‡ (Nidus Vespae) 6g

One bag a day was used to prepare a decoction, taken twice a day. The ingredients were soaked in cold water for 30 minutes and then boiled for 20 minutes to prepare the decoction. Five days of treatment made up a course. Results were seen after a maximum of two courses.

3. **Qiao** infused *Qing Hao* (Herba Artemisiae Chinghao) 6g, *Yin Chen Hao* (Herba Artemisiae Scopariae) 9g and *Gan Cao* (Radix Glycyrrhizae) 3g in boiling water for 20 minutes, with the liquid then being drunk as a tea. One bag a day was used to make the tea, which was taken three or four times a day. Results were seen after three weeks. [10]

Phytophotodermatitis
植物日光性皮炎

Phytophotodermatitis is an acute phototoxic inflammatory reaction due to long-term exposure to the sun after overeating or contact with plants containing light-sensitizing substances known as psoralens (furanocoumarins).

According to TCM literature, plants that can trigger phytophotodermatitis include fat hen (also known as goosefoot or lamb's-quarters), Chinese milk vetch, three-colored amaranth, locust tree flower, birchleaf pear leaf, field thistle, radish leaf, colza, and purslane. Plants commonly recorded in Western literature as causing phytophotodermatitis include giant hogweed, carrot, parsnip, celery, fennel, cow parsley, and common rue.

Clinical manifestations

- This condition occurs in spring and summer (from March to August) when furanocoumarins are highest and UV exposure is the greatest; it is most frequent from March to May.
- Lesions mainly involve body parts often exposed to the sun such as the face and the dorsum of the hand. In severe cases, there is also involvement of the neck and limbs.
- Skin lesions generally manifest as diffuse parenchymal edema, which may be accompanied by petechiae, ecchymoses, vesicles, erosion, and ulceration. Bizarre inflammatory patterns and linear streaks of hyper-pigmentation are key clues to diagnosing phytophotodermatitis.
- Patients have subjective sensations at the fingertips such as numbness, pain (burning, stabbing or distending pain), itching, and formication. Systemic symptoms include headache and fever.
- In mild cases, the edema subsides in three to five days; in severe cases, this process may take ten days or more.

Differential diagnosis

Polymorphic light eruption
The itchy, erythematous or eczematous lesions of this condition tend to recur every spring on sites exposed to the sun. The bullous eruptions characteristic of phytophotodermatitis are absent and there is no history of contact with photosensitizing substances.

Sunburn
Overexposure to sunlight results in a tingling sensation in the skin, which becomes red 2-12 hours later; diffuse erythema and edema are noted in the sunburnt areas. The redness reaches its maximum after 24 hours and then fades over the next 48-60 hours to leave desquamation and pigmentation. In severe cases, red papules and vesicles appear; exudation follows rupture of the vesicles, which subsequently dry up and form crusts.

Angioedema
Lesions (urticarial plaques with diffuse swelling) are likely to involve the eyelids, lips, genitalia, palms, and soles. Exposure to the sun does not play a role in the occurrence of this skin condition.

Irritant contact dermatitis
This condition is unrelated to exposure to sunlight. Lesions present when the body is exposed to certain irritant substances. Erythema is associated with the pathogenic agents involved. Itching may also be present. Contact dermatitis may occur in any season.

Etiology and pathology

- Patients with congenital insufficiency are likely to have a weak exterior with looseness of the interstices (*cou li*). After excessive intake of certain vegetables, [ii]

[ii] In this case, vegetables that contain psoralens.

the normal transportation and transformation functions of the Spleen and Stomach will be impaired, and Dampness will result. Dampness accumulating inside the body will transform into Heat, giving rise to Damp-Heat. When the body is exposed to the sun, Yang Toxins can affect the exterior. Internal and external pathogenic factors then get mixed up with each other. As a result, pathogenic Wind and Heat Toxins are retained in the skin and flesh instead of being diffused and drained from the body, thus leading to phytophotodermatitis.

- In severe cases, Wind Toxins stream through the exterior to enter the Ying and Xue levels. Heat accumulates in the Xue level, resulting in exuberance of Toxins. Other symptoms appear such as large ecchymoses, severe swelling and mental confusion.

- In some cases, patients may develop the disease due to exposure to the sun after contact with or inhalation of pollen from vegetables such as common rue or giant hogweed. In such cases, Toxic pathogenic factors are transmitted to the Lungs through the skin and flesh.

Pattern identification and treatment

INTERNAL TREATMENT

RETENTION OF WIND-HEAT TOXINS IN THE SKIN AND FLESH

The disease has a sudden onset, but is relatively mild. It generally starts with slight, non-pitting edema on the face and the dorsum of the hand; the eyelids are swollen. Local numbness, slight itching and a feverish sensation are present. Accompanying symptoms and signs include dry mouth and yellow urine. The tongue body is slightly red with a greasy coating; the pulse is slippery.

Treatment principle
Disperse Wind and transform erythema, clear Heat and relieve Toxicity.

Prescription
HUA BAN JIE DU TANG JIA JIAN
Decoction for Transforming Macules and Relieving Toxicity, with modifications

Xuan Shen (Radix Scrophulariae Ningpoensis) 10g
Lian Qiao (Fructus Forsythiae Suspensae) 10g
Chao Niu Bang Zi (Fructus Arctii Lappae, stir-fried) 10g
Dan Zhu Ye (Herba Lophatheri Gracilis) 10g
Shi Gao‡ (Gypsum Fibrosum) 15g, decocted for 30 minutes before adding the other ingredients
Chao Zhi Mu (Rhizoma Anemarrhenae Asphodeloidis, stir-fried) 6g
Chao Huang Lian (Rhizoma Coptidis, stir-fried) 6g

Sheng Ma (Rhizoma Cimicifugae) 4.5g
Gan Cao (Radix Glycyrrhizae) 4.5g
Chan Tui‡ (Periostracum Cicadae) 4.5g

Explanation
- Chao Niu Bang Zi (Fructus Arctii Lappae, stir-fried), Chan Tui‡ (Periostracum Cicadae) and Sheng Ma (Rhizoma Cimicifugae) dredge Wind and alleviate itching.
- Shi Gao‡ (Gypsum Fibrosum), Chao Zhi Mu (Rhizoma Anemarrhenae Asphodeloidis, stir-fried), Gan Cao (Radix Glycyrrhizae), and Dan Zhu Ye (Herba Lophatheri Gracilis) clear Heat from the Qi level and relieve Toxicity.
- Xuan Shen (Radix Scrophulariae Ningpoensis), Lian Qiao (Fructus Forsythiae Suspensae) and Chao Huang Lian (Rhizoma Coptidis, stir-fried) clear Heat and relieve Toxicity, enrich Yin and reduce erythema.

WIND-HEAT TOXINS ENTERING THE XUE LEVEL

The condition develops quickly and is relatively severe. The skin becomes red, inflamed and swollen within a few hours, with lesions spreading from the head to the neck, chest, dorsum of the hand, forearm, dorsum of the foot, and ankle. The eyelids are closed and difficult to open. There is swelling and burning pain in the affected areas. Subsequent manifestations may involve petechiae, ecchymoses, Blood stasis and swelling under the nails, and incessant distending pain. Accompanying symptoms and signs include fever, dizziness, oppression in the chest, and poor appetite. The tongue body is red with a yellow coating; the pulse is rapid.

Treatment principle
Clear Heat and relieve Toxicity, dissipate Wind and disperse swelling.

Prescription
PU JI XIAO DU YIN JIA JIAN
Universal Salvation Beverage for Dispersing Toxicity, with modifications

Ban Lan Gen (Radix Isatidis seu Baphicacanthi) 12g
Da Qing Ye (Folium Isatidis seu Baphicacanthi) 12g
Pu Gong Ying (Herba Taraxaci cum Radice) 12g
Jin Yin Hua (Flos Lonicerae) 12g
Chao Niu Bang Zi (Fructus Arctii Lappae, stir-fried) 10g
Chao Huang Qin (Radix Scutellariae Baicalensis, stir-fried) 10g
Lian Qiao (Fructus Forsythiae Suspensae) 10g
Lü Dou Yi (Testa Phaseoli Radiati) 10g
Fu Ping (Herba Spirodelae Polyrrhizae) 6g
Sang Ye (Folium Mori Albae) 6g
Jiao Zhi Zi (Fructus Gardeniae Jasminoidis, scorch-fried) 6g
Che Qian Zi (Semen Plantaginis) 15g
Yi Yi Ren (Semen Coicis Lachryma-jobi) 15g

Explanation

- *Chao Huang Qin* (Radix Scutellariae Baicalensis, stir-fried), *Ban Lan Gen* (Radix Isatidis seu Baphicacanthi), *Da Qing Ye* (Folium Isatidis seu Baphicacanthi), *Pu Gong Ying* (Herba Taraxaci cum Radice), *Jin Yin Hua* (Flos Lonicerae), *Lian Qiao* (Fructus Forsythiae Suspensae), *Jiao Zhi Zi* (Fructus Gardeniae Jasminoidis, scorch-fried), and *Lü Dou Yi* (Testa Phaseoli Radiati) clear Heat and relieve Toxicity.
- *Chao Niu Bang Zi* (Fructus Arctii Lappae, stir-fried), *Fu Ping* (Herba Spirodelae Polyrrhizae) and *Sang Ye* (Folium Mori Albae) dredge Wind, disperse swelling and alleviate itching.
- *Che Qian Zi* (Semen Plantaginis) and *Yi Yi Ren* (Semen Coicis Lachryma-jobi) benefit the movement of Dampness and relieve Toxicity.

DEFICIENCY PATTERNS

This condition is characterized by gradual or recurrent onset and moderate edema. Skin lesions manifest as pale red maculopapular eruptions, papulovesicles or vesicles. Accompanying symptoms and signs include poor appetite, oppression in the chest and general malaise. The tongue body is pale red with a scant coating; the pulse is deficient and thready.

Treatment principle

Dredge Wind and relieve Toxicity, fortify the Spleen and benefit the movement of Dampness.

Prescription

SHEN LING BAI ZHU SAN HE MA HUANG LIAN QIAO CHI XIAO DOU TANG JIA JIAN

Ginseng, Poria and White Atractylodes Powder Combined With Ephedra, Forsythia Fruit and Aduki Bean Decoction, with modifications

Ma Huang* (Herba Ephedrae) 3g
Lian Qiao (Fructus Forsythiae Suspensae) 12g
Che Qian Zi (Semen Plantaginis) 12g, wrapped
Chi Xiao Dou (Semen Phaseoli Calcarati) 30g
Bai Mao Gen (Rhizoma Imperatae Cylindricae) 30g
Fu Ling Pi (Cortex Poriae Cocos) 15g
Chao Bai Bian Dou (Semen Dolichoris Lablab, stir-fried) 15g
Tu Chao Bai Zhu (Rhizoma Atractylodis Macrocephalae, stir-fried with earth) 15g
Yi Yi Ren (Semen Coicis Lachryma-jobi) 15g
Sang Ye (Folium Mori Albae) 10g
Ju Hua (Flos Chrysanthemi Morifolii) 10g
Fu Ping (Herba Spirodelae Polyrrhizae) 10g
Dang Shen (Radix Codonopsitis Pilosulae) 10g

Explanation

- *Ma Huang** (Herba Ephedrae), *Lian Qiao* (Fructus Forsythiae Suspensae), *Chi Xiao Dou* (Semen Phaseoli Calcarati), and *Che Qian Zi* (Semen Plantaginis) dissipate Wind and transform Dampness, clear Heat and alleviate itching.
- *Bai Mao Gen* (Rhizoma Imperatae Cylindricae) and *Fu Ling Pi* (Cortex Poriae Cocos) cool the Blood and transform Dampness.
- *Chao Bai Bian Dou* (Semen Dolichoris Lablab, stir-fried), *Tu Chao Bai Zhu* (Rhizoma Atractylodis Macrocephalae, stir-fried with earth), *Yi Yi Ren* (Semen Coicis Lachryma-jobi), and *Dang Shen* (Radix Codonopsitis Pilosulae) augment Qi and support the Spleen to consolidate the Root.
- *Sang Ye* (Folium Mori Albae), *Ju Hua* (Flos Chrysanthemi Morifolii) and *Fu Ping* (Herba Spirodelae Polyrrhizae) dredge Wind and clear Heat, relieve Toxicity and reduce erythema.

General modifications

1. For severe edema, add *Fang Feng* (Radix Ledebouriellae Divaricatae), *Chan Tui* ‡ (Periostracum Cicadae) and *Jiang Can* ‡ (Bombyx Batryticatus).
2. For ecchymoses or large patches of purplish-black petechiae, add *Xian Di Huang* (Radix Rehmanniae Glutinosae Recens), *Mu Dan Pi* (Cortex Moutan Radicis), *Zi Cao* (Radix Arnebiae seu Lithospermi), *Da Ji* (Herba seu Radix Cirsii Japonici), *Xiao Ji* (Herba Cephalanoploris seu Cirsii), and *Xian He Cao* (Herba Agrimoniae Pilosae).
3. For severe erosion or necrosis, add *Bai Lian* (Radix Ampelopsis Japonicae), *Zi Cao* (Radix Arnebiae seu Lithospermi), *Pu Gong Ying* (Herba Taraxaci cum Radice), *E Jiao* ‡ (Gelatinum Corii Asini), and *Bai Hua She She Cao* (Herba Hedyotidis Diffusae).
4. For shortness of breath and Phlegm-saliva congestion, add powdered *Chen Pi* (Pericarpium Citri Reticulatae), *Sang Bai Pi* (Cortex Mori Albae Radicis), *Ting Li Zi* (Semen Lepidii seu Descurainiae), and *Da Zao* (Fructus Ziziphi Jujubae).
5. For oppression in the chest and constipation, add *Chao Zhi Ke* (Fructus Citri Aurantii, stir-fried), *Jiu Zhi Da Huang* (Radix et Rhizoma Rhei, processed with wine) and *Jie Geng* (Radix Platycodi Grandiflori).

EXTERNAL TREATMENT

- For lesions with erythema, papules and papulovesicles, but without ulceration, select three or four herbs from *Pu Gong Ying* (Herba Taraxaci cum Radice), *Xu Chang Qing* (Radix Cynanchi Paniculati), *Ye Ju Hua* (Flos Chrysanthemi Indici), *Ma Chi Xian* (Herba Portulacae Oleraceae), and *Gan Cao* (Radix Glycyrrhizae) and prepare a decoction for use as a wet compress three to five times a day for 15-30 minutes each time.

- For ulcerating, eroded or necrotic lesions, apply *Qing Dai Gao* (Indigo Paste) or *Yu Lu Gao* (Jade Dew Ointment) to the affected area once a day.

ACUPUNCTURE
Points
- For lesions on the head and face, select CV-24 Chengjiang, ST-7 Xiaguan, ST-6 Jiache, EX-HN-5 Taiyang, [iii] BL-2 Cuanzhu, and ST-2 Sibai.
- For lesions on the upper limbs, select TB-5 Waiguan, PC-8 Laogong and LI-4 Hegu.
- For lesions on the lower limbs, select ST-36 Zusanli, KI-3 Taixi and BL-60 Kunlun.

Technique: The reducing method is applied to the points. The needles are retained for 15 minutes. Treat once a day. A course consists of five treatment sessions.

Explanation
Local points are used to dredge Wind and alleviate itching, relieve Toxicity and transform Dampness.

EAR ACUPUNCTURE
Points: Lung, Kidney, Heart, Spleen, Ear-Shenmen, and ear points corresponding to the location of lesions on the body.
Technique: Needle the points for 30 minutes, once a day. A course consists of five treatment sessions.

Clinical notes

- If there is severe local redness and swelling or erosion and exudation, it is necessary to use large dosages of materia medica for clearing Heat and relieving Toxicity, cooling the Blood and dispersing swelling. These materia medica can be used internally as a decoction or externally as a wet compress.
- If the condition is severe and the internal organs are involved, it is better to combine TCM treatment with Western medicine.
- Acupuncture is effective in dispersing swelling and alleviating itching.

Advice for the patient

- Avoid excessive intake of or contact with plants and vegetables that trigger the condition. At the same time, avoid exposure to strong sun.
- Change the method of cooking the vegetables. Add a little vinegar when preparing the food in order to destroy the toxins contained in the vegetables.

Case history

Patient
Male, aged 48.

Clinical manifestations
The patient ate cooked fat hen (*Chenopodium album*) and pies containing the plant on the two days before the condition appeared. He then worked outside in strong sunshine for several hours. He initially felt prickly itching on the face; obvious swelling later appeared on the face and hands. The eyelids were also swollen, making it difficult to open the eyes. Accompanying symptoms and signs included a burning sensation, stabbing pain, stifling oppression in the chest, dry throat, slight cough, and short voidings of reddish urine. The tongue coating was thin and white; the pulse was wiry and slippery.

Pattern identification
Accumulation of Damp Toxins complicated by external Yang Toxins after exposure to the sun.

Treatment principle
Clear Heat, relieve Toxicity and benefit the movement of Dampness.

Prescription ingredients
Jin Yin Hua (Flos Lonicerae) 18g
Lian Qiao (Fructus Forsythiae Suspensae) 18g
Fu Ping (Herba Spirodelae Polyrrhizae) 10g
Tong Cao (Medulla Tetrapanacis Papyriferi) 10g
Che Qian Zi (Semen Plantaginis) 10g, wrapped
Pu Gong Ying (Herba Taraxaci cum Radice) 15g
Yi Yi Ren (Semen Coicis Lachryma-jobi) 12g
Gan Cao (Radix Glycyrrhizae) 30g

External treatment
Huang Bai (Cortex Phellodendri) 60g was prescribed to prepare a decoction for use as a cold compress on the affected area.

Further visits
After two days, the swelling was significantly reduced. The patient was able to open his mouth and eyes more easily. However, he still had a cough with sputum that was difficult to expectorate, sore throat and constipation. The initial prescription was modified by adding *Zhe Bei Mu* (Bulbus Fritillariae Thunbergii) 10g, *Xing Ren* (Semen Pruni Armeniacae) 10g and *Da Huang* (Radix et Rhizoma Rhei) 10g.

The next day, the swelling had almost disappeared and the patient could open his eyes without any problem. The modified prescription was followed for one more day with the addition of *Gua Lou Ren* (Semen Trichosanthis) 10g, *Huang Qin* (Radix Scutellariae Baicalensis) 10g and *Jie Geng* (Radix Platycodi Grandiflori) 10g.

The following day, the swelling had disappeared completely although areas of painful, dull purple hemorrhagic spots remained on the face. The treatment principle was modified to include ingredients for cooling and invigorating the Blood.

[iii] M-HN-9 according to the system employed by the Shanghai College of Traditional Chinese Medicine.

Prescription ingredients

Sheng Di Huang (Radix Rehmanniae Glutinosae) 12g
Yi Yi Ren (Semen Coicis Lachryma-jobi) 12g
Mu Dan Pi (Cortex Moutan Radicis) 10g
Zi Cao (Radix Arnebiae seu Lithospermi) 10g
Fu Ping (Herba Spirodelae Polyrrhizae) 10g
Bai Xian Pi (Cortex Dictamni Dasycarpi Radicis) 10g
Che Qian Zi (Semen Plantaginis) 10g, wrapped
Tong Cao (Medulla Tetrapanacis Papyriferi) 10g
Lian Qiao (Fructus Forsythiae Suspensae) 10g
Gan Cao (Radix Glycyrrhizae) 10g
Jin Yin Hua (Flos Lonicerae) 18g

Externally, the cold wet compress was changed to a hot wet compress.

Outcome

After ten days, the hemorrhagic spots had almost gone. One 3x2 cm ulcer remained. Equal amounts of *Hua Du San* (Powder for Transforming Toxicity)[iv] and *Qing Dai San* (Indigo Powder) were mixed into a paste with groundnut oil for external application to treat the ulcer. [11]

Literature excerpt

In *Zhao Bing Nan Lin Chuang Jing Yan Ji* [A Collection of Zhao Bingnan's Clinical Experiences], the author states: "The symptoms of this disease resemble those of what is known in TCM as *ri shai chuang* (sun exposure sore). Spleen Deficiency results in failure to transform Water and Dampness. Accumulation of Water and Dampness over a long period gives rise to Heat, with Damp-Heat eventually being generated. If the body is affected externally by Heat Toxins due to exposure to the sun, the internal and external pathogenic factors combine to act on the body and trigger the condition of *shi du yang* or Damp Toxin sore (phytophotodermatitis). The treatment therefore focuses on clearing Heat, relieving Toxicity and benefiting the movement of Dampness."

Modern clinical experience

1. As described above, **Zhao Bingnan** followed the principles of clearing Heat, relieving Toxicity and benefiting the movement of Dampness to treat phytophotodermatitis. The materia medica he used most frequently included *Jin Yin Hua* (Flos Lonicerae), *Pu Gong Ying* (Herba Taraxaci cum Radice), *Lian Qiao* (Fructus Forsythiae Suspensae), *Yi Yi Ren* (Semen Coicis Lachryma-

jobi), *Che Qian Zi* (Semen Plantaginis), *Gan Cao* (Radix Glycyrrhizae), *Bai Xian Pi* (Cortex Dictamni Dasycarpi Radicis), and *Fu Ping* (Herba Spirodelae Polyrrhizae).

- For purple ecchymoses, he added *Sheng Di Huang* (Radix Rehmanniae Glutinosae), *Mu Dan Pi* (Cortex Moutan Radicis), *Zi Cao* (Radix Arnebiae seu Lithospermi), and *Chi Shao* (Radix Paeoniae Rubra).

- For non-transformation of Water and Dampness due to Spleen Deficiency, he added *Bai Zhu* (Rhizoma Atractylodis Macrocephalae) and increased the dosage of *Yi Yi Ren* (Semen Coicis Lachryma-jobi). [12]

2. **Cheng** recommended a combination of internal and external treatment for phytophotodermatitis. [13]

Internal treatment prescription
BAN LAN GEN TANG
Isatis Root Decoction

Ban Lan Gen (Radix Isatidis seu Baphicacanthi) 12g
Jin Yin Hua (Flos Lonicerae) 12g
Lian Qiao (Fructus Forsythiae Suspensae) 12g
Che Qian Zi (Semen Plantaginis) 12g
Dong Gua Pi (Epicarpium Benincasae Hispidae) 12g
Pu Gong Ying (Herba Taraxaci cum Radice) 15g
Fu Ling (Sclerotium Poriae Cocos) 9g
Xia Ku Cao (Spica Prunellae Vulgaris) 9g
Ze Xie (Rhizoma Alismatis Orientalis) 6g
Hou Po (Cortex Magnoliae Officinalis) 4g
Huang Qin (Radix Scutellariae Baicalensis) 3g

One bag a day was used to prepare a decoction, taken twice a day.

External treatment prescription
YE JU JIAN JI
Wild Chrysanthemum Decoction Preparation

Ye Ju Hua (Flos Chrysanthemi Indici) 750g
Qian Li Guang (Herba Senecionis Scandentis) 500g
Ce Bai Ye (Cacumen Biotae Orientalis) 500g
Tu Jing Jie (Herba Chenopodii Ambroisioidis) 250g
Shi Yan (Sal) 15g

The ingredients were covered with a double depth of water and boiled down until one-third of the liquid was left. The decoction was then applied as a wet compress for 15 minutes, three or four times a day until the condition cleared.

[iv] In those countries where the use of certain ingredients contained in this powder is not permitted, *Xin San Miao San* (New Mysterious Three Powder) can be applied instead.

Burns and scalds
烧伤与烫伤

A burn is an injury to tissues caused by heat (e.g. from a fire), electrical current or by chemical or physical agents that cause tissue damage similar to the effects of heat (e.g. strong acids or alkalis). A scald is a burn produced by a hot liquid or vapor.

Apart from the immediate damage to burnt tissue, burns cause blood vessels to leak plasma. With small burns, the leakage only results in local swelling or blistering. However, in children with more than 10% and adults with more than 15% of the skin area covered by burns, the volume of blood is reduced sufficiently to necessitate intravenous fluids, and there may be a possibility of shock. The amount of fluid loss depends on the extent rather than the depth of the burn. Infection is also a major risk with burns, since the damaged tissue is extremely vulnerable to bacterial superinfection.

Table 17-2 Classification of burns

Degree		Depth	Manifestations	Healing process where no infection is involved
First degree (erythema)		Involvement of the stratum corneum	Redness, swelling, heat and pain, hyperesthesia, dry skin, burnt skin very sensitive to the touch	Lesions heal in two to three days with scaling, but without scarring
Second degree (with blistering)	Superficial second degree	Involvement of the epidermis and superficial layers of the dermis with the stratum basale remaining partially unaffected	Severe pain, hyperesthesia, blisters, redness and moistness at the base of lesions, local swelling, burnt skin painfully sensitive to the touch	Lesions heal in one to two weeks with pigmentation but without scarring
	Deep second degree	Involvement of the deep layers of the dermis with skin appendages remaining	Dull pain, blisters, the base of the lesions are moist and white with red spots	Lesions heal in three to four weeks with scarring
Third degree (charring of the skin)		Involvement of all skin layers, extending to involvement of the subcutaneous flesh, sinews and bones	Loss of pain sensation; inelastic, waxy white, scorched yellow, or charred dry leathery skin; after lesions dry up, subcutaneous veins are arborescent as a result of obstruction	The charred crusts come off in two to four weeks with granulation tissue forming over lesions. Small lesions will heal, but a skin graft is necessary for larger lesions. Scarring or cicatricial contraction is possible

Clinical manifestations

The severity of the condition depends on the size of the area involved and the depth of the tissues affected (see Table 17-2).

Etiology and pathology

Reaction to intense heat attacking the body results in injuries to the skin and flesh. If exuberant Fire Toxins damage Yin Fluids or Heat Toxins attack the Zang-Fu organs, a variety of serious symptoms may occur.

Pattern identification and treatment

INTERNAL TREATMENT

HEAT AND FIRE DAMAGING YIN

Symptoms include fever, dry mouth with a desire for drinks, constipation, short voidings of reddish urine, and dry, red lips. The tongue body is red and dry with a yellow or yellow and rough coating, or smooth and bare with no coating; the pulse is surging and rapid, or wiry, rapid and thready.

Treatment principle
Nourish Yin and clear Heat.

Prescription
HUANG LIAN JIE DU TANG HE YIN HUA GAN CAO TANG JIA JIAN
Coptis Decoction for Relieving Toxicity Combined With Honeysuckle and Licorice Decoction, with modifications

Jin Yin Hua (Flos Lonicerae) 15g
Nan Sha Shen (Radix Adenophorae) 15g
Huang Qin (Radix Scutellariae Baicalensis) 10g
Huang Bai (Cortex Phellodendri) 10g
Sheng Di Huang (Radix Rehmanniae Glutinosae) 10g
Gan Cao (Radix Glycyrrhizae) 10g
Huang Lian (Rhizoma Coptidis) 6g
Zhi Zi (Fructus Gardeniae Jasminoidis) 6g
Chi Shao (Radix Paeoniae Rubra) 6g
Mu Dan Pi (Cortex Moutan Radicis) 6g
Lian Zi Xin (Plumula Nelumbinis Nuciferae) 3g
Hu Po‡ (Succinum) 3g

Explanation
- *Huang Lian* (Rhizoma Coptidis), *Huang Qin* (Radix Scutellariae Baicalensis), *Huang Bai* (Cortex Phellodendri), and *Zhi Zi* (Fructus Gardeniae Jasminoidis) are bitter and cold in nature and act directly on Fire Toxins.
- *Jin Yin Hua* (Flos Lonicerae), *Nan Sha Shen* (Radix Adenophorae) and *Gan Cao* (Radix Glycyrrhizae) augment Qi, nourish Yin and relieve Toxicity with cold and sweetness.
- *Sheng Di Huang* (Radix Rehmanniae Glutinosae), *Chi Shao* (Radix Paeoniae Rubra) and *Mu Dan Pi* (Cortex Moutan Radicis) cool the Blood and relieve Toxicity to reduce erythema.
- *Lian Zi Xin* (Plumula Nelumbinis Nuciferae) and *Hu Po*‡ (Succinum) clear Heat from the Heart and protect the Heart to prevent Fire Toxins from entering the interior.

INJURY TO YIN AND DESERTION OF YANG

Symptoms include a reduction in body temperature, faint breathing, indifferent expression, trance, sleepiness, delirium, cold limbs, and profuse perspiration. The tongue body is deep red or dull purple with a gray-black coating or no coating; the pulse is faint and verging on expiry, or hidden.

Treatment principle
Support Yang and stem counterflow, while assisting to protect Yin.

Prescription
SHEN FU TANG HE SHENG MAI SAN JIA JIAN
Ginseng and Aconite Decoction Combined With Pulse-Generating Powder, with modifications

Ren Shen (Radix Ginseng) 5-8g, decocted separately for 60 minutes and added to the prepared decoction
Fu Pen Zi (Fructus Rubi Chingii) 10-12g
Mai Men Dong (Radix Ophiopogonis Japonici) 12g
Nan Sha Shen (Radix Adenophorae) 12g
Shi Hu* (Herba Dendrobii) 12g
Yu Zhu (Rhizoma Polygonati Odorati) 12g
Gan Cao (Radix Glycyrrhizae) 6g

Explanation
- *Ren Shen* (Radix Ginseng), *Fu Pen Zi* (Fructus Rubi Chingii) and *Gan Cao* (Radix Glycyrrhizae) augment Qi and warm Yang to prevent desertion of Original Yang (Yuan Yang).
- *Mai Men Dong* (Radix Ophiopogonis Japonici), *Nan Sha Shen* (Radix Adenophorae), *Shi Hu** (Herba Dendrobii), and *Yu Zhu* (Rhizoma Polygonati Odorati) enrich Yin and protect Body Fluids.

HEAT TOXINS ENTERING THE INTERIOR

Symptoms include high fever, irritability and thirst, restlessness and disquiet, dry mouth and parched lips, constipation, and short voidings of reddish urine. The tongue body is red or deep red with a yellow, yellow and rough, or dry and prickly coating; the pulse is wiry and rapid.

Treatment principle
Clear Heat from the Ying level, cool the Blood and relieve Toxicity.

Prescription
QING YING TANG HE HUANG LIAN JIE DU TANG JIA JIAN
Decoction for Clearing Heat from the Ying Level Combined With Coptis Decoction for Relieving Toxicity, with modifications

Nan Sha Shen (Radix Adenophorae) 15g
Sheng Di Huang Tan (Radix Rehmanniae Glutinosae Carbonisata) 15g
Lü Dou Yi (Testa Phaseoli Radiati) 30g

Jin Yin Hua Tan (Flos Lonicerae Carbonisata) 15g

Mu Dan Pi (Cortex Moutan Radicis) 10g

Chi Shao (Radix Paeoniae Rubra) 10g

Huang Qin (Radix Scutellariae Baicalensis) 10g

Zhi Zi (Fructus Gardeniae Jasminoidis) 10g

Explanation

- *Sheng Di Huang Tan* (Radix Rehmanniae Glutinosae Carbonisata), *Jin Yin Hua Tan* (Flos Lonicerac Carbonisata) and *Lü Dou Yi* (Testa Phaseoli Radiati) cool the Blood and clear Heat from the Ying level, protect the Heart and relieve Toxicity.

- *Nan Sha Shen* (Radix Adenophorae) nourishes Yin and increases Body Fluids.

- *Mu Dan Pi* (Cortex Moutan Radicis) and *Chi Shao* (Radix Paeoniae Rubra) cool the Blood and reduce erythema.

- *Huang Qin* (Radix Scutellariae Baicalensis) and *Zhi Zi* (Fructus Gardeniae Jasminoidis) clear Heat and relieve Toxicity.

Modifications

1. If Heat Toxins pass to the Heart with such symptoms as irritability, restlessness and disquiet, mental confusion and delirious speech, add *Shui Niu Jiao*‡ (Cornu Bubali), *Xuan Shen* (Radix Scrophulariae Ningpoensis), *Dan Zhu Ye* (Herba Lophatheri Gracilis), and *Mai Men Dong* (Radix Ophiopogonis Japonici)

2. If Heat Toxins pass to the Lungs with such symptoms as rough breathing, flaring nostrils, and cough with Phlegm rale and blood-streaked sputum, add *Zi Wan* (Radix Asteris Tatarici), *Yu Xing Cao* (Herba Houttuyniae Cordatae), *Tian Zhu Huang* (Concretio Silicea Bambusae), *Dan Nan Xing*‡ (Pulvis Arisaematis cum Felle Bovis), and *Zhu Li* (Succus Bambusae).

3. If Heat Toxins pass to the Kidneys with such symptoms as scant urine or urinary block, add *Bai Mao Gen* (Rhizoma Impcratac Cylindricae), *Ze Xie* (Rhizoma Alismatis Orientalis), *Che Qian Zi* (Semen Plantaginis), and *Tong Cao* (Medulla Tetrapanacis Papyriferi); if there is profuse urination, add *Jin Ying Zi* (Fructus Rosae Laevigatae), *Sang Piao Xiao*‡ (Oötheca Mantidis) and *Shan Zhu Yu* (Fructus Corni Officinalis).

4. If Heat Toxins pass to the Liver with such symptoms as spasms and convulsions and a rigid neck, add *Ling Yang Jiao** (Cornu Antelopis), *Gou Teng* (Ramulus Uncariae cum Uncis), *Long Gu*‡ (Os Draconis), and *Shi Jue Ming*‡ (Concha Haliotidis).

5. If Heat Toxins pass to the Spleen with such symptoms as abdominal distension and constipation, or frequent, loose, sticky, foul-smelling stools, or vomiting of blood or blood in the stool, add *Da Huang* (Radix et Rhizoma Rhei), *Zhi Ke* (Fructus Citri Aurantii) and *Zhu Ru* (Caulis Bambusae in Taeniis).

6. For vomiting of blood, add *Shi Xiao San* (Sudden Smile Powder); for blood in the stool or black, loose stools, add *Di Yu Tan* (Radix Sanguisorbae Officinalis Carbonisata) and *Huai Hua Tan* (Flos Sophorae Japonicae Carbonisata); for blood in the urine, add *Ou Jie* (Nodus Nelumbinis Nuciferae Rhizomatis), *Bai Mao Gen* (Rhizoma Imperatae Cylindricae), *Da Ji* (Herba seu Radix Cirsii Japonici), and *Xiao Ji* (Herba Cephalanoploris seu Cirsii).

DAMAGE TO QI AND BLOOD

Symptoms include low-grade fever or absence of fever, emaciation, a lusterless facial complexion, lassitude, poor appetite, disturbed sleep, spontaneous sweating, night sweating, and non-generation of flesh at the lesions. The tongue body is pale and enlarged with a thin white or thin yellow coating, or is dull red with a white coating; the pulse is thready and rapid, or thready and weak.

Treatment principle

Regulate and supplement Qi and Blood.

Prescription
BA ZHEN TANG JIA JIAN

Eight Treasure Decoction, with modifications

Huang Qi (Radix Astragali seu Hedysari) 12g

Dang Shen (Radix Codonopsitis Pilosulae) 12g

Fu Ling (Sclerotium Poriae Cocos) 12g

Bai Zhu (Rhizoma Atractylodis Macrocephalae) 12g

Gan Cao (Radix Glycyrrhizae) 12g

Dang Gui (Radix Angelicae Sinensis) 10g

Gan Di Huang (Radix Rehmanniae Glutinosae Exsiccata) 10g

Bai Shao (Radix Paeoniae Lactiflorae) 10g

Chuan Xiong (Rhizoma Ligustici Chuanxiong) 6g

Explanation

- *Dang Shen* (Radix Codonopsitis Pilosulae), *Bai Zhu* (Rhizoma Atractylodis Macrocephalae), *Fu Ling* (Sclerotium Poriae Cocos), *Gan Cao* (Radix Glycyrrhizae), and *Huang Qi* (Radix Astragali seu Hedysari) augment Qi and support the Spleen to assist the source of generation of Blood.

- *Dang Gui* (Radix Angelicae Sinensis), *Chuan Xiong* (Rhizoma Ligustici Chuanxiong), *Bai Shao* (Radix Paeoniae Lactiflorae), and *Gan Di Huang* (Radix Rehmanniae Glutinosae Exsiccata) enrich Yin and nourish the Blood.

QI AND YIN DEFICIENCY OF THE SPLEEN AND STOMACH

Symptoms include ulceration of the mouth and tongue, dry mouth, belching, hiccups, poor appetite, abdominal distension, and loose stools. The tongue body is pale and enlarged and peeled bare of any coating; the pulse is thready and weak.

Treatment principle
Regulate the Spleen and Stomach.

Prescription
YI WEI TANG HE SHEN LING BAI ZHU SAN JIA JIAN
Decoction for Boosting the Stomach Combined With Ginseng, Poria and White Atractylodes Powder, with modifications

Nan Sha Shen (Radix Adenophorae) 12g
Tian Men Dong (Radix Asparagi Cochinchinensis) 12g
Mai Men Dong (Radix Ophiopogonis Japonici) 12g
Yu Zhu (Rhizoma Polygonati Odorati) 12g
Shi Hu* (Herba Dendrobii) 12g
Dang Shen (Radix Codonopsitis Pilosulae) 12g
Huang Qi (Radix Astragali seu Hedysari) 12g
Bai Zhu (Rhizoma Atractylodis Macrocephalae) 10g
Fu Ling (Sclerotium Poriae Cocos) 10g
Gan Cao (Radix Glycyrrhizae) 10g
Shan Yao (Radix Dioscoreae Oppositae) 15g

Explanation
- *Nan Sha Shen* (Radix Adenophorae), *Tian Men Dong* (Radix Asparagi Cochinchinensis), *Mai Men Dong* (Radix Ophiopogonis Japonici), *Shan Yao* (Radix Dioscoreae Oppositae), *Yu Zhu* (Rhizoma Polygonati Odorati), and *Shi Hu** (Herba Dendrobii) enrich Yin and nourish the Stomach.
- *Huang Qi* (Radix Astragali seu Hedysari), *Dang Shen* (Radix Codonopsitis Pilosulae), *Bai Zhu* (Rhizoma Atractylodis Macrocephalae), *Fu Ling* (Sclerotium Poriae Cocos), and *Gan Cao* (Radix Glycyrrhizae) support the Spleen with sweetness and warmth.
- Once the Spleen and Stomach perform their normal functions, the body will gradually recover.

EXTERNAL TREATMENT
Initial stage
After cleaning the lesions with saline, apply *Qing Liang Gao* (Cool Clearing Paste) or *Gan Cao You* (Licorice Oil); alternatively, mix equal amounts of powdered *Di Yu* (Radix Sanguisorbae Officinalis) and *Da Huang* (Radix et Rhizoma Rhei) to a paste with sesame oil for external application to the affected area.

Intermediate stage
If the lesions are infected, apply *Huang Lian Ruan Gao* (Coptis Ointment), *Fu Rong Gao* (Cotton Rose Flower Paste) or *Zi Se Xiao Zhong Gao* (Purple Paste for Dispersing Swelling) to the affected areas. If there is profuse exudation, apply a wet compress with 2 percent *Huang Lian Ye* (Coptis Lotion) or *Yin Hua Gan Cao Ye* (Honeysuckle and Licorice Lotion).

Final stage
When necrotic tissues are shed and new flesh is being generated, apply a mixture of *Sheng Ji Bai Yu Gao* (White Jade Paste for Generating Flesh) and *Shou Gan Sheng Ji Yao Fen* (Medicated Powder for Promoting Contraction and Generating Flesh) to the affected area. If keloids form, use *Hei Bu Yao Gao* (Black Cloth Medicated Paste) externally.

Clinical notes

- External treatment of burns with Chinese materia medica is highly effective in reducing exudation, healing lesions and preventing scarring.
- Internal treatment with Chinese materia medica at various stages of the healing process will help to clear Heat and relieve Toxicity, augment Qi and protect Yin, support Vital Qi (Zheng Qi) and close sores, thus assisting the body to recover more quickly.
- If burns are severe, combined treatment with TCM and Western medicine is necessary.

Advice for the patient

- Take appropriate action to prevent burns.
- Give patients comfort and encouragement so that they will be confident of recovery.
- Keep the patient's room well ventilated and quiet.

Case history

Patient
Boy, aged 2.

Clinical manifestations
The patient had been scalded on the lower left leg by boiling water 24 days previously. Blisters appeared on the day of the accident. The following day, the patient developed a fever, which was relieved after three days by an injection of penicillin. However, the scald on the leg did not improve. Western medicine doctors in the Surgery Department suggested a skin graft, but the patient's parents did not agree. The patient was therefore transferred to the TCM External Disease Department for treatment.

Physical examination on the first visit indicated an extensive formation of fresh red granulation with little secretion involving the extensor aspect of the lower left leg between the central tibia area and the dorsum of the foot.

Prescription
TANG SHANG YOU GAO
Oil Paste for Scalds
(for application to the entire affected area)

Bai Ji (Rhizoma Bletillae Striatae) 124g
Liu Ji Nu (Herba Artemisiae Anomalae) 124g
Ku Shen (Radix Sophorae Flavescentis) 62g
Zhi Zi (Fructus Gardeniae Jasminoidis) 62g
Qing Dai (Indigo Naturalis) 31g

The ingredients were ground and then processed into a very fine powder in a mortar. The powder was then mixed into a paste with unprocessed vegetable oil and applied to the affected area. It can be used for all types of scalds and burns with such symptoms as reddening of the skin, fever and local pain.

Further treatment
After three days, the secretion had decreased and there was moist red granulation without infection. *Ji Gao Dan* (Topmost Pill) was applied directly to the lesions and then covered by *Tang Shang You Gao* (Oil Paste for Scalds).

Prescription
JI GAO DAN
Topmost Pill

Zhu Sha ‡ (Cinnabaris) 6g ᵛ
Bai Ji (Rhizoma Bletillae Striatae) 30g
Duan Shi Gao ‡ (Gypsum Fibrosum Calcinatum) 18g
Qing Fen ‡ (Calomelas) 3g ᵛ
Ru Xiang (Gummi Olibanum) 9g
Yun Mu ‡ (Muscovitum) 12g
Bing Pian (Borneolum) 4.2g

The ingredients were ground and then processed into a very fine powder in a mortar prior to storage in a sterilized glass bottle. The medication can be used for sores after ulceration and for chronic fistulae after necrotic tissue has been shed and clean and fresh red granulation has appeared. The powder is applied directly to the lesions and covered with a medicated plaster or gauze.

Outcome
The scalded area gradually shrank. After 70 days of treatment, new skin had grown in most of the affected area on the lower leg; the only unhealed area was an ulcerating sore 2x2x5 cm on the dorsum of the foot. *Ji Gao Dan* (Topmost Pill) and *Tang Shang Gao* (Scald Paste) were applied externally. After another 15 days of treatment, the lesion healed completely. [14]

Modern clinical experience

APPLICATION OF ZI CAO YOU (GROMWELL ROOT OIL)
This oil is very effective in the treatment of burns, but the ingredients used for preparing the oil vary.

1. **Tang** prepared *Fu Fang Zi Cao You* (Compound Gromwell Root Oil).

Prescription ingredients
Zi Cao (Radix Arnebiae seu Lithospermi) 500g
Pu Gong Ying (Herba Taraxaci cum Radice) 400g
Jin Yin Hua (Flos Lonicerae) 400g
Huang Qin (Radix Scutellariae Baicalensis) 400g
Huang Lian (Rhizoma Coptidis) 400g
Sheng Di Huang (Radix Rehmanniae Glutinosae) 400g
Ru Xiang (Gummi Olibanum) 30g
Mo Yao (Myrrha) 30g
Bing Pian (Borneolum) 30g
Xiang You (Oleum Sesami Seminis) 3000ml

The ingredients were soaked in the sesame oil for 30 minutes and then simmered over a very low heat until all the herbs turned dark brown. The herbs were removed and the oil stored in a container ready for use.

For mild lesions covering a small area, treatment was given by the application of gauze soaked in the medicated oil. The gauze was kept wet by frequent spraying with the oil. Systemic treatment (such as supplementing body fluids to correct electrolyte imbalance) was also given to these patients. This treatment is successful in those who do not also suffer from multiple organ failure. [15]

2. **Jia** prepared *Zi Cao You Gao* (Gromwell Root Oil Paste) with the following basic ingredients:

Zi Cao (Radix Arnebiae seu Lithospermi) 500g
Dang Gui (Radix Angelicae Sinensis) 450g
Bing Pian (Borneolum) 50g
Xiang You (Oleum Sesami Seminis) 2000ml
Mi La ‡ (Cera) 200g

For first and second degree burns with reddening of the skin, heat, swelling, pain, and blisters, a prescription with the basic ingredients was used; for lesions with profuse exudation or characterized by severe Dampness and Blood stasis, *Di Yu* (Radix Sanguisorbae Officinalis) 400g was added; for lesions presenting with suppurating erosion due to Heat Toxins, *Da Huang* (Radix et Rhizoma Rhei) 200g and *Zhen Zhu Fen* ‡ (Pearl Powder) 200g were added.

The paste was prepared by heating the sesame oil to 135-140°C. Once smoke had been rising from the heated oil for about 10 minutes, the hard raw ingredients were put in and cooked for 15-18 minutes until the residues were scorch-fried to a yellow color. The residues were removed while the oil was hot. When the oil had cooled to around 125°C, *Zi Cao* (Radix Arnebiae

ᵛ In those countries where the use of *Zhu Sha* ‡ (Cinnabaris) and *Qing Fen* ‡ (Calomelas) is not permitted, they can be substituted by *Hu Po* ‡ (Succinum) 9g and *Lu Gan Shi* ‡ (Calamina) 15g.

seu Lithospermi) was added and cooked for five to eight minutes. Then the *Zi Cao* residue was removed and mixed with the residue of the other ingredients. A small amount of sesame oil was added to the residue mixture, heated to 125°C and cooked for 8-10 minutes. The residues were removed. The two oils were mixed while hot and allowed to cool to a paste at 50°C before storing in a container ready for use.

This paste can clear Heat and relieve Toxicity, eliminate putridity and alleviate pain, disperse inflammation and reduce swelling, cool and harmonize the Blood, and moisten the skin and generate flesh. The treatment period ranged from 13 to 36 days and no scarring resulted. [16]

Erythema ab igne
火激红斑

Erythema ab igne is a skin disease characterized by a reticular pattern of persistent erythema with supervening brown (melanin) pigmentation due to local long-term exposure to heat (without burning). It commonly develops because of chronic exposure to heat from a fire or stove, but can also occur from an electric blanket or heater, or from a hot-water bottle.

In TCM, this condition is also known as *huo ban chuang* (fire fleck sore).

Clinical manifestations

- Erythema ab igne usually affects cooks and other people often exposed to high temperatures at work. It may also occur in people who use a hot-water bottle as a hot compress, those who warm themselves too close to a fire (occurring most frequently on the leg), or those subjected to infrared radiation locally over a long period.
- Lesions start with local congestion of the skin in a reticular pattern. The color subsequently changes from pale red to deep red, purplish-red or purplish-brown, finally turning brown or black due to post-inflammatory hyperpigmentation with melanin.
- In a few cases, there may be blisters, telangiectasia, mild skin atrophy, or hyperkeratosis.
- Patients may also experience a burning sensation and stabbing pain.

Etiology and pathology

Looseness of the interstices (*cou li*) and weakness of Wei Qi (Defensive Qi) allow Heat and Fire pathogenic factors to attack the body. Even though these factors are relatively weak, over a long period they are still strong enough to heat up the skin and invade the interior to confront Qi and Blood, thus resulting in the formation of lesions.

Pattern identification and treatment

INTERNAL TREATMENT

FIRE TOXINS
The condition starts with well-defined erythema, which feels hot on palpation and blanches on pressure. Patients experience a local burning sensation and prickly itching. Accompanying symptoms and signs include dry mouth, irritability and thirst with a desire for cold drinks. The tongue body is red with a yellow coating; the pulse is wiry and rapid.

Treatment principle
Drain Fire and relieve Toxicity, cool the Blood and reduce erythema.

Prescription
LIANG XUE JIE DU TANG JIA JIAN
Decoction for Cooling the Blood and Relieving Toxicity, with modifications

Sheng Di Huang (Radix Rehmanniae Glutinosae) 30g
Shi Gao ‡ (Gypsum Fibrosum) 30g, decocted for 30 minutes before adding the other ingredients
Mu Dan Pi (Cortex Moutan Radicis) 10g
Chi Shao (Radix Paeoniae Rubra) 10g
Lian Qiao (Fructus Forsythiae Suspensae) 10g
Jin Yin Hua (Flos Lonicerae) 10g
Zhi Zi (Fructus Gardeniae Jasminoidis) 10g
Zhi Mu (Rhizoma Anemarrhenae Asphodeloidis) 10g
Dan Zhu Ye (Herba Lophatheri Gracilis) 6g

Explanation
- *Sheng Di Huang* (Radix Rehmanniae Glutinosae), *Zhi Mu* (Rhizoma Anemarrhenae Asphodeloidis), *Shi*

Gao ‡ (Gypsum Fibrosum), *Mu Dan Pi* (Cortex Moutan Radicis), *Chi Shao* (Radix Paeoniae Rubra), and *Zhi Zi* (Fructus Gardeniae Jasminoidis) clear Heat from the Qi level and cool the Blood, relieve Toxicity and reduce erythema.

- *Jin Yin Hua* (Flos Lonicerae), *Lian Qiao* (Fructus Forsythiae Suspensae) and *Dan Zhu Ye* (Herba Lophatheri Gracilis) relieve Toxicity and clear Heat.

CONSUMPTION OF YIN

The skin in the affected area is purplish-red, purplish-brown or purplish-black with vesicles; it may be atrophied and reticular. Accompanying symptoms and signs include a burning sensation, itching, pain, shortness of breath, lack of strength, dry stools, and short voidings of reddish urine. The tongue body is deep red with a scant coating; the pulse is thready and rapid.

Treatment principle

Relieve Toxicity and nourish Yin, cool the Blood and clear Heat.

Prescription

JIE DU YANG YIN TANG HUA CAI

Decoction for Relieving Toxicity and Nourishing Yin, with variations

Sheng Di Huang (Radix Rehmanniae Glutinosae) 30g
Bai Mao Gen (Rhizoma Imperatae Cylindricae) 30g
Mai Men Dong (Radix Ophiopogonis Japonici) 10g
Mu Dan Pi (Cortex Moutan Radicis) 10g
Jin Yin Hua (Flos Lonicerae) 10g
Nan Sha Shen (Radix Adenophorae) 10g
Gan Cao (Radix Glycyrrhizae) 10g
Da Huang (Radix et Rhizoma Rhei) 6g
Dan Shen (Radix Salviae Miltiorrhizae) 15g

Explanation

- *Sheng Di Huang* (Radix Rehmanniae Glutinosae), *Nan Sha Shen* (Radix Adenophorae) and *Mai Men Dong* (Radix Ophiopogonis Japonici) enrich Yin and protect Body Fluids.
- *Bai Mao Gen* (Rhizoma Imperatae Cylindricae) and *Mu Dan Pi* (Cortex Moutan Radicis) nourish Yin and cool the Blood.
- *Jin Yin Hua* (Flos Lonicerae), *Dan Shen* (Radix Salviae Miltiorrhizae) and *Da Huang* (Radix et Rhizoma Rhei) relieve Toxicity, invigorate the Blood, transform Blood stasis and reduce erythema.

EXTERNAL TREATMENT

- For erythema at the initial stage accompanied by a burning sensation and stabbing pain, use *Bo Jie Tang* (Peppermint and Schizonepeta Decoction) or prepare a decoction with *Jin Yin Hua* (Flos Lonicerae) 30g, *Bo He* (Herba Menthae Haplocalycis) 10g and *Lü Dou Yi* (Testa Phaseoli Radiati) 10g for use as a wet compress when lukewarm.
- If it appears that lesions are about to ulcerate, mix *Huang Bai* (Cortex Phellodendri) 15g and *Qing Dai* (Indigo Naturalis) 15g with vegetable oil and apply externally; or grind *Liu Yi San* (Six-To-One Powder) 30g, *Lü Dou Yi* (Testa Phaseoli Radiati) 15g, *Han Shui Shi* ‡ (Calcitum) 15g, *Huang Bai* (Cortex Phellodendri) 10g, and *Bing Pian* (Borneolum) 1g into a fine powder and apply to the affected area.

Clinical notes

- In the treatment of erythema ab igne, materia medica for transforming Blood stasis and invigorating the Blood should be used in addition to those for clearing Heat and relieving Toxicity. This will help promote local blood circulation and disperse erythema.
- The prognosis for this condition is good if patients keep away from fire and seek treatment at an early stage.

Advice for the patient

- Patients with erythema ab igne should rest and seek treatment as soon as possible.
- Keep the skin in the affected area dry, clean and free from infection. Avoid scratching the lesions, thus preventing secondary infection.
- Do not get too close to fires and do not expose the body to fire for lengthy periods.
- Avoidance of exposure to heat will help lesions to heal gradually.

Radiodermatitis
放射性皮炎

Radiodermatitis is inflammation of the skin due to exposure to ionizing radiation (mainly beta rays, gamma rays and X-rays). This may occur after a short dose of heavy radiation (for example, after radiotherapy or exposure to radioactive isotopes such as may occur in the nuclear industry) or as a result of prolonged exposure to small doses (as may happen, for example, to X-ray machine operators).

Clinical manifestations

Acute radiodermatitis
This condition is generally caused by single or repeated exposure to large doses of radiation. It can be classified into three levels of severity.

- Relatively mild cases: Lesions are initially bright red, subsequently evolving into dull red macules, possibly accompanied by mild edema. A sensation of scorching heat and itching may be present. Desquamation and pigmentation follow in three to six weeks.

- Moderate cases: Lesions manifest as acute inflammatory edematous erythema with a tense and glistening surface. Vesicles form, with erosion on rupture. A sensation of scorching heat or pain may be present. Lesions heal in one to three months, leaving pigmentation or depigmentation, telangiectasia and capillary atrophy.

- Severe cases: Erythema and edema are followed by the rapid progression of necrosis. Persistent ulcerating sores form subsequently, penetrating to different depths of the skin, flesh and, in serious cases, the bones. Accompanying symptoms and signs include headache, dizziness, listlessness, poor appetite, nausea and vomiting, abdominal pain, diarrhea, hemorrhage, and a decrease in the white blood cell count. In the most severe cases, this disease may prove fatal.

Chronic radiodermatitis
- This condition occurs due to prolonged and repeated exposure to small doses of radiation; it may also develop from an acute condition. The period from exposure to onset of clinical manifestations may range from a few months to several decades. Significant signs of inflammation are absent.

- Possible manifestations include dry, atrophic and sclerotic skin, and loss of hair, sebaceous glands and sweat glands. Radiation damage of the nails results in thickening or detachment of the nails or dark, lusterless nails with an uneven surface.

- Persistent lesions may lead to secondary complications of basal cell carcinomas (particularly on the scalp, face and trunk), squamous carcinomas (especially on the hands) or, in rare cases, fibroma or sarcoma.

Etiology and pathology

The disease develops because of injury to the skin and flesh by radiation. Radiation is a special form of pathogenic Toxin and, at the initial stage, burns and damages the flesh and interstices (*cou li*), giving rise to lesions that are similar in appearance to dermatitis. In the later stages, the Toxins combine with Deficiency of Vital Qi (Zheng Qi) to damage the muscles and bones, resulting in severe cases.

Pattern identification and treatment

INTERNAL TREATMENT

TOXIC PATHOGENIC FACTORS
Skin lesions manifest as erythema with deep infiltration and indistinct margins. Vesicles, erosion or ulceration may appear in relatively severe cases. Accompanying symptoms and signs include headache, reduced appetite, and nausea and vomiting. The tongue body is red with a scant coating or a yellow and greasy but dry coating; the pulse is thready and rapid.

Treatment principle
Support Vital Qi (Zheng Qi) and expel Toxicity, invigorate the Blood and reduce erythema.

Prescription
SI MIAO TANG JIA WEI
Mysterious Four Decoction, with additions

Huang Qi (Radix Astragali seu Hedysari) 12g
Bai Shao (Radix Paeoniae Lactiflorae) 12g
Chi Shao (Radix Paeoniae Rubra) 12g
Lian Qiao (Fructus Forsythiae Suspensae) 12g
Yi Yi Ren (Semen Coicis Lachryma-jobi) 30g
Shan Yao (Radix Dioscoreae Oppositae) 30g
Chi Xiao Dou (Semen Phaseoli Calcarati) 30g
Jin Yin Hua (Flos Lonicerae) 30g

Bai Hua She She Cao (Herba Hedyotidis Diffusae) 15g
Pu Gong Ying (Herba Taraxaci cum Radice) 15g
Gan Cao (Radix Glycyrrhizae) 6g
Zhu Ru (Caulis Bambusae in Taeniis) 6g
Fa Ban Xia (Rhizoma Pinelliae Ternatae Praeparata) 6g

Explanation

- *Huang Qi* (Radix Astragali seu Hedysari), *Gan Cao* (Radix Glycyrrhizac), *Shan Yao* (Radix Dioscoreae Oppositae), and *Yi Yi Ren* (Semen Coicis Lachryma-jobi) augment Qi and nourish Yin.
- *Jin Yin Hua* (Flos Lonicerae), *Bai Hua She She Cao* (Herba Hedyotidis Diffusae), *Pu Gong Ying* (Herba Taraxaci cum Radice), and *Lian Qiao* (Fructus Forsythiae Suspensae) clear Heat and relieve Toxicity.
- *Chi Xiao Dou* (Semen Phaseoli Calcarati), *Chi Shao* (Radix Paeoniae Rubra) and *Bai Shao* (Radix Paeoniae Lactiflorae) invigorate the Blood and reduce erythema.
- *Zhu Ru* (Caulis Bambusae in Taeniis) and *Fa Ban Xia* (Rhizoma Pinelliae Ternatae Praeparata) harmonize the Stomach and bear counterflow Qi downward to treat nausea and vomiting.

DEFICIENCY OF VITAL QI (ZHENG QI)

The duration of the disease is relatively long. Lesions manifest as pale red maculopapules. Dry skin, desquamation, depigmentation, and hair loss are likely. Accompanying symptoms and signs include dizziness, listlessness, shortness of breath, and sluggish speech. The tongue body is pale red with a scant coating or no coating; the pulse is deficient and thready.

Treatment principle

Augment Qi and protect Yin, fortify the Spleen and supplement the Kidneys.

Prescription
SAN CAI FENG SUI DAN JIA JIAN
Heaven, Human and Earth Pill for Sealing the Marrow, with modifications

Ren Shen (Radix Ginseng) 10g, decocted separately for 60 minutes and added to the prepared decoction
Tian Men Dong (Radix Asparagi Cochinchinensis) 15g
Shu Di Huang (Radix Rehmanniae Glutinosae Conquita) 15g
Shan Yao (Radix Dioscoreae Oppositae) 15g
Chao Huang Bai (Cortex Phellodendri, stir-fried) 12g
Gan Cao (Radix Glycyrrhizae) 12g
Huang Qi (Radix Astragali seu Hedysari) 12g
Chao Bai Shao (Radix Paeoniae Lactiflorae, stir-fried) 12g
Sha Ren (Fructus Amomi) 8g, added 5-10 minutes before the end of the decoction process

Explanation

- *Ren Shen* (Radix Ginseng), *Huang Qi* (Radix Astragali seu Hedysari), *Shan Yao* (Radix Dioscoreae Oppositae), *Tian Men Dong* (Radix Asparagi Cochinchinensis), *Chao Huang Bai* (Cortex Phellodendri, stir-fried), *Shu Di Huang* (Radix Rehmanniae Glutinosae Conquita), *Sha Ren* (Fructus Amomi), and *Gan Cao* (Radix Glycyrrhizae) augment Qi and nourish Yin, fortify the Spleen and supplement the Kidneys.
- *Chao Bai Shao* (Radix Paeoniae Lactiflorae, stir-fried) clears Heat from the Kidneys.

General modifications

1. For reduced appetite, nausea and vomiting, add *Shen Qu* (Massa Fermentata), *Jiang Zhi Chao Zhu Ru* (Caulis Bambusae in Taeniis, stir-fried with ginger juice), *Xian Zhu Li* (Succus Bambusae Recens), and *Ji Nei Jin*‡ (Endothelium Corneum Gigeriae Galli).
2. For abdominal pain and diarrhea, take *Xiang Lian Wan* (Aucklandia and Coptis Pill) with the decoction.
3. For lassitude and dizziness, add *Gui Ban Jiao** (Gelatinum Plastri Testudinis) and *Lu Jiao Jiao*‡ (Gelatinum Cornu Cervi).
4. For subcutaneous ecchymosis, add *E Jiao*‡ (Gelatinum Corii Asini) and *Da Zao* (Fructus Ziziphi Jujubae).
5. For persistent non-healing ulcers, add *Bai Lian* (Radix Ampelopsis Japonicae), *Zhe Bei Mu* (Bulbus Fritillariae Thunbergii) and *Bai Zhi* (Radix Angelicae Dahuricae).

EXTERNAL TREATMENT

- Prepare *Fang Zhuo Yi Hao* (No. 1 Medication for Radiation Burns) by decocting *Di Yu* (Radix Sanguisorbae Officinalis) 120g and *Huang Lian* (Rhizoma Coptidis) 18g in 1000ml of water to obtain 500ml of a medicated decoction for use as a cold wet compress.
- For lesions with erythema and desquamation, apply *Lu Hui Ru Ji* (Aloe Cream) externally two or three times a day.
- For vesicles and erosion, prepare a decoction with equal amounts of *Di Yu* (Radix Sanguisorbae Officinalis) and *Ma Chi Xian* (Herba Portulacae Oleraceae) and apply to the lesions as a cold compress for 15 minutes two or three times a day.
- For ulcerating lesions, apply *Dong Fang Yi Hao Yao Gao* (Oriental Medicated Plaster No. 1) externally once a day or *Dan Huang You* (Egg Yolk Oil) two or three times per day.

Clinical notes

- Skin lesions due to exposure to radiation are caused by a specific type of Toxin rather than Heat or Fire.

Internal treatment should focus on augmenting Qi and nourishing Yin to prevent Toxins from invading the interior. Externally, the treatment should follow the principles of clearing Heat and relieving Toxicity with mild materia medica.

- External application of erosive medications or medications containing heavy metals are contraindicated.
- In addition to paying close attention to the evolution of lesions, systemic changes should be strictly monitored.
- For mild cases, the prognosis is good, provided that appropriate treatment is given. Severe cases are difficult to cure and the underlying disease (such as cancer treated by radiotherapy) may prove fatal.

Modern clinical experience

There are relatively few clinical reports on the use of TCM in the treatment of radiodermatitis. Nevertheless, the literature that is available reflects the particular advantages of treatment with TCM.

1. **Zhang** used *Fu Fang Dan Qing Hu* (Compound Medicated Paste Prepared with Egg White) to treat 32 patients with second-degree acute radiodermatitis. The paste was prepared by mixing powdered *Da Huang* (Radix et Rhizoma Rhei), *Yun Nan Bai Yao* (Yunnan White) and egg white in the proportion of 1:0.5:8. The medicated paste was applied externally to the lesions and covered by a layer of gauze treated with Vaseline®. The treatment was given three times a day. Radiotherapy was stopped during treatment of radiodermatitis. Patients had less pain or burning sensation within 24-48 hours after beginning the medication, and less exudation from ulcerating skin lesions within 48-52 hours. Lesions took 6-17 days to heal. The author of the article considered that the three ingredients used in combination had the functions of improving the blood supply in the areas of the skin lesions, preventing infection and accelerating healing of the lesions. [17]

2. **Die** reported on the treatment of radiodermatitis due to radiotherapy with *Shuang Cao You* (Double Herb Oil) prepared with *Gan Cao* (Radix Glycyrrhizae) 200g and *Zi Cao* (Radix Arnebiae seu Lithospermi) 200g. After grinding the materia medica into a fine powder, it was filtered through an 80-100 mesh sieve and soaked in 1000 ml of sesame oil for one week. For first-degree radiodermatitis, treatment with the medicated oil was prescribed three times a day for three consecutive days; for second-degree conditions, it was used three times a day for five to seven consecutive days; and for third-degree conditions, treatment was initially applied at least four times a day. Once the symptoms were relieved or the skin lesions had healed, treatment continued once or twice a day until the end of the radiotherapy course, which all the patients were then able to finish. [18]

Intertrigo
擦烂

Intertrigo is an acute inflammatory skin condition involving the skin folds. It is caused by friction or sweating and is often complicated by bacterial infection or candidiasis.

In TCM, this condition is also known as *han xi chuang* (sweat immersion sore).

Clinical manifestations

- This condition generally occurs in obese individuals at all ages from infancy to old age. Other factors may predispose to this condition, such as tight clothing, poor personal hygiene, diabetes mellitus, and general debility from a variety of illnesses.

- Lesions usually involve the skin folds such as the inguinal grooves, the perianal area, the submammary folds, the axillae, and the neck. Where *Candida albicans* is the cause, the webs between the fingers can be involved in individuals whose hands are often immersed in water.

- The condition manifests initially as slight inflammation and swelling of the skin. Pustules form, subsequently macerating in the body folds and developing into red glazed plaques with moist scaling at the margin. Individual papules or pustules may be found beyond the opposing skin surfaces. Vesicles, erosion and exudation, or sores due to infection may also be present.

- Patients experience a burning sensation and itching. Stabbing pain occurs where there is erosion of the skin.

Differential diagnosis

Flexural psoriasis
This type of psoriasis, which usually affects older people, involves the axillae, submammary folds and anogenital region. Lesions manifest as well-demarcated, red, glistening plaques without scaling.

Seborrheic eczema of the flexures
Flexural involvement in seborrheic eczema is more common in the elderly. The condition manifests in the axillae, groins and submammary areas with a moist intertrigo, often colonized by *Candida albicans*. Differentiation is often difficult, but seborrheic eczema of the flexures is usually associated with other patterns of seborrheic eczema on the scalp, presternal and interscapular regions.

Tinea cruris (jock itch)
Lesions are clearly defined with spontaneous healing in the central area and desquamation and discrete papules at the periphery. Involvement of the scrotum is rare. Fungal examination is positive.

Etiology and pathology

In summer, if people neglect their personal hygiene or their clothing becomes soaked in sweat or they fail to change their clothes regularly, the skin will become sweaty and filthy. This is especially likely to be the case for obese women and children, who are more subject to profuse Dampness and Phlegm. Profuse sweating in the skin fold areas in obese women cannot easily be diffused and will result in intertrigo.

Pattern identification and treatment

INTERNAL TREATMENT

RETENTION OF HEAT IN THE EXTERIOR
The affected areas appear red, swollen and clearly defined. Friction and rubbing will cause the lesions to turn bright red or may produce superficial ulceration. Patients experience a local burning sensation with itching and stabbing pain. The tongue body is red with a thin yellow coating; the pulse is rapid.

Treatment principle
Clear Heat, cool the Blood and relieve Toxicity.

Prescription
LIANG XUE DI HUANG TANG JIA JIAN
Rehmannia Decoction for Cooling the Blood, with modifications

Sheng Di Huang (Radix Rehmanniae Glutinosae) 15g
Zi Cao (Radix Arnebiae seu Lithospermi) 15g
Ren Dong Teng (Caulis Lonicerae Japonicae) 15g
Ma Bian Cao (Herba cum Radice Verbenae) 15g
Huang Qin (Radix Scutellariae Baicalensis) 10g
Fang Feng (Radix Ledebouriellae Divaricatae) 10g
Fu Ling Pi (Cortex Poriae Cocos) 10g
Huang Bai (Cortex Phellodendri) 10g
Huang Lian (Rhizoma Coptidis) 6g
Zhi Mu (Rhizoma Anemarrhenae Asphodeloidis) 6g
Chai Hu (Radix Bupleuri) 6g
Gan Cao (Radix Glycyrrhizae) 6g

Explanation
- *Sheng Di Huang* (Radix Rehmanniae Glutinosae), *Zi Cao* (Radix Arnebiae seu Lithospermi), *Zhi Mu* (Rhizoma Anemarrhenae Asphodeloidis), *Huang Lian* (Rhizoma Coptidis), and *Huang Bai* (Cortex Phellodendri) clear Heat, cool the Blood, relieve Toxicity, and alleviate pain.
- *Ren Dong Teng* (Caulis Lonicerae Japonicae), *Fu Ling Pi* (Cortex Poriae Cocos) and *Ma Bian Cao* (Herba cum Radice Verbenae) transform Dampness and clear Heat.
- *Fang Feng* (Radix Ledebouriellae Divaricatae) dissipates Wind and alleviates itching.
- *Chai Hu* (Radix Bupleuri), *Huang Qin* (Radix Scutellariae Baicalensis) and *Gan Cao* (Radix Glycyrrhizae) dissipate Heat from the skin and clear retained Heat, thus relieving both the interior and the exterior.

DAMP TOXINS ACCUMULATING IN THE INTERIOR
Clusters of vesicles appear in the affected areas. Lesions are characterized by damp ulceration, exudation, swelling, and bright red erythema. Thick turbid fluid appears on rupture of the thin-walled vesicles, contributing to local maceration. Patients feel a burning sensation, itching and stabbing pain in the affected area. Accompanying symptoms and signs include irritability, thirst, yellow or reddish urine, and constipation. The tongue body is red with a greasy coating; the pulse is wiry, slippery and rapid.

Treatment principle
Clear Heat and benefit the movement of Dampness, cool the Blood and relieve Toxicity.

Prescription
TUI BAN TANG JIA JIAN
Decoction for Reducing Erythema, with modifications

Huang Lian (Rhizoma Coptidis) 6g
Jin Yin Hua (Flos Lonicerae) 10g

Lian Qiao (Fructus Forsythiae Suspensae) 10g
Gan Cao (Radix Glycyrrhizae) 10g
Mu Dan Pi (Cortex Moutan Radicis) 10g
Chi Shao (Radix Paeoniae Rubra) 10g
Zhi Zi (Fructus Gardeniae Jasminoidis) 10g
Che Qian Zi (Semen Plantaginis) 10g, wrapped
Lü Dou Yi (Testa Phaseoli Radiati) 12g
Hua Shi ‡ (Talcum) 15g
Bai Mao Gen (Rhizoma Imperatae Cylindricae) 15g
Chi Xiao Dou (Semen Phaseoli Calcarati) 30g

Explanation

- *Chi Shao* (Radix Paeoniae Rubra), *Mu Dan Pi* (Cortex Moutan Radicis), *Zhi Zi* (Fructus Gardeniae Jasminoidis), *Huang Lian* (Rhizoma Coptidis), and *Lü Dou Yi* (Testa Phaseoli Radiati) cool the Blood and relieve Toxicity, invigorate the Blood and reduce erythema.
- *Hua Shi* ‡ (Talcum), *Che Qian Zi* (Semen Plantaginis), *Bai Mao Gen* (Rhizoma Imperatae Cylindricae), and *Chi Xiao Dou* (Semen Phaseoli Calcarati) clear Heat and benefit the movement of Dampness.
- *Jin Yin Hua* (Flos Lonicerae), *Lian Qiao* (Fructus Forsythiae Suspensae) and *Gan Cao* (Radix Glycyrrhizae) clear Heat and relieve Toxicity.

General modifications

1. For thirst and reddish urine, add *Dan Zhu Ye* (Herba Lophatheri Gracilis) and *Gua Jin Deng* (Calyx Physalis Alkekengi).
2. For lesions that are red at the base and create a burning sensation, add *Mu Dan Pi* (Cortex Moutan Radicis), *Di Yu* (Radix Sanguisorbae Officinalis) and *Shi Gao* ‡ (Gypsum Fibrosum).
3. For constipation, add *Da Huang* (Radix et Rhizoma Rhei), *Chao Zhi Ke* (Fructus Citri Aurantii, stir-fried) and *Jie Geng* (Radix Platycodi Grandiflori).

EXTERNAL TREATMENT

- If the skin in the affected area is inflamed with an erosive tendency, apply *Zi Cao You* (Gromwell Root Oil) or *Gan Cao You* (Licorice Oil) directly to the lesions after routine cleaning with lukewarm water. Then spread *Qu Shi San* (Powder for Dispelling Dampness) on the top. Lesions should heal in three to four days in mild cases.
- For maceration and erosion, clean the affected areas with lukewarm water. Then apply *Gan Cao You* (Licorice Oil) and cover with *Qing Liang Fen* (Cool Clearing Powder).
- For severe erosion and exudation, it is better to use a local wet compress first, followed by the application of external medication. Prepare a decoction with *Ma Chi Xian* (Herba Portulacae Oleraceae) 30-60g, or *Gan Cao* (Radix Glycyrrhizae) 30g and *Jin Yin Hua* (Flos Lonicerae) 20g, and use as a wet compress for 20-30 minutes. Then apply *Huang Lian Ruan Gao* (Coptis Ointment) or *Qing Dai Gao* (Indigo Paste) and cover with *Qu Shi San* (Powder for Dispelling Dampness) or *Yan Kao San* (Buttock-Submerging Sore Powder).

Clinical notes

- The majority of patients with intertrigo are obese infants, children and women. It is important for these patients that the skin folds are kept clean and dry.
- Appropriate internal administration of materia medica to clear Heat and transform Dampness will help to eliminate Damp-Heat from the body, thus reducing the course of treatment.

Literature excerpt

In *Wai Ke Qi Xuan* [Revelations of the Mysteries of External Diseases], it says: "Obese people may find that their skin is immersed in sweat if they fail to take baths regularly in summer. This profuse sweating can lead to the formation of ulcerating sores characterized by unbearable pain. This condition is known as *han xi chuang* (sweat immersion sore)."

Corn (clavus)
鸡眼

A corn is an area of hard, thickened skin formed over bony prominences, principally on or between the toes or on the soles under prominent metatarsals. It occurs because of persistent local pressure and mechanical friction.

The circumscribed conical lesion resembles a chicken's eye in shape, hence its name in Chinese, *ji yan*. In TCM, it is also sometimes referred to as *rou ci* (flesh thorn).

Clinical manifestations

- Corns usually occur in areas subject to pressure and friction such as the toes, the area between the toes, and the soles and heels. Chronic pressure from ill-fitting footwear is the commonest predisposing factor.
- Lesions are a few millimeters in diameter and cylindrical in cross-section, extending down into the deeper skin layers. The hard core is surrounded by a semi-opaque area of hyperkeratosis.
- Corns are classified into two types – hard and soft. Hard corns manifest as pale yellow, hard, round or oval nodules with a smooth, flat surface. The skin lines are disrupted by the corn. Soft corns usually appear on the side of one of two adjacent toes; they are usually grayish-white as a result of maceration by moisture between the toes.
- Persistent pressure or sudden bumping will trigger pain, making locomotion difficult.
- Corns generally occur in adults and only rarely in those aged 16 or younger.
- Corns left untreated may not heal. Infection occasionally follows if the condition is not managed properly.

Differential diagnosis

Callus
A callus is a horny plate thicker at the center than at the edges. It covers a larger area than a corn, has no obvious border and does not extend into the deeper layers of the skin. The skin markings are preserved. Local tenderness is absent. Calluses generally occur at points of repeated friction, such as on the sole or palm.

Plantar warts (verruca plantaris)
Plantar warts occur on the sole of the foot or in the web between the toes, presenting with a keratinized, firm, uneven surface and a central depression. Removal of the horny layer reveals a soft milky-white cornified core with dark punctate dots representing thrombosed capillaries within the wart. When these lesions overlie a bony prominence, pain and tenderness may be severe on pressure.

Etiology and pathology

Wearing tight-fitting or narrow shoes, or deformity of the bones of the feet (as, for example, used to be the case in China for women with bound feet) will subject the toes to persistent friction or pressure. This inhibits the normal movement of Qi and Blood, and the skin and flesh will be deprived of nourishment, resulting in the growth of corns.

Treatment

EXTERNAL TREATMENT
For multiple corns of short duration, use *Gou Ji Shui Xi Ji* (Cibot Wash Preparation) or *Zhi Hou Tang* (Decoction for Treating Warts) to soak the affected areas for 10-15 minutes twice a day. When the superficial horny layer softens, protect the surrounding healthy skin with adhesive plaster leaving a central hole for the corn. Then apply one of the following to the corn – *Shui Jing Gao* (Crystal Paste), *Wu Mei Gao* (Black Plum Paste), *Ji Yan Gao Yi Hao* (Corn Plaster No. 1), *Ji Yan Gao Er Hao* (Corn Plaster No. 2), *Rou Ci San* (Flesh Thorn Powder), or *Ji Yan San* (Corn Powder) – and cover with another piece of adhesive plaster. Remove the plasters after two or three days, excise the corns and remove the residue. If heavy pressure does not result in pain, the corns are healed. Otherwise, the treatment should be continued.

ACUPUNCTURE
Perpendicular insertion
After sterilizing the surface of the lesion, insert a 1.0 cun needle in the center of the corn down to the root. Then heat the needle with a cigarette lighter for three to five minutes to conduct the heat to the affected area. Attach a piece of adhesive plaster to the corn after the needle is removed. Treat once every three days until the corn comes off. The patient's consent to this procedure must be obtained in advance.

Encirclement needling
Insert four 1.0 cun needles obliquely (superior to, inferior to, and to the right and left of the corn) with the tips of the needles all reaching the root of the corn; the needles thus form a cone shape. Retain the needles for 20-30 minutes, during which time the needles are rotated two or three times. Squeeze out a small amount of blood after the needles are removed. Cover the corn with disinfected gauze. Treat once every three days. The patient's consent to this procedure must be obtained in advance.

MOXIBUSTION
First apply Vaseline® or sesame oil to the surface of the corn. Then burn four or five moxa cones on the corn until it appears shriveled. Treat once a day. Remove the remnants of the corn after three to five days.

Clinical notes

Treatment for corns generally focuses on external applications. First soak the affected areas in warm water for 15-30 minutes to loosen and soften the hard horny layers and aid absorption of external medications. However, a complete cure for corns is very difficult and recurrence is not unusual.

Advice for the patient

- Avoid wearing tight-fitting or stiff shoes. Make sure that the feet are correctly positioned when walking.
- Avoid indiscriminate use of corrosive medications on the corns. Do not pare corns with dirty scissors or knives to avoid infection.

Literature excerpt

A detailed description of corns is found in *Yi Zong Jin Jian* [The Golden Mirror of Medicine] in the chapter relating to experiences with external diseases. It says: "Corns occur on the toes. They have the shape of a chicken's eye, are deep-rooted in the flesh, but are hard and elevated on top. Walking is difficult because of the pain. Corns may form for a number of reasons including the binding of feet, or wearing small, tight-fitting shoes when walking long distances."

Modern clinical experience

EXTERNAL TREATMENT

Li used *Wu Mei Gao* (Black Plum Paste) to treat 198 patients with corns. The medicated paste was prepared by mixing *Wu Mei* (Fructus Pruni Mume) to a paste-like consistency with an appropriate amount of white vinegar. The healthy skin surrounding the corn was protected by covering with reticular adhesive plaster. The paste was then applied to the corn and held in place by additional adhesive plaster. The dressing was changed every evening. Seven days made up a course of treatment. One to three courses were required. By the end of the third course, 178 patients had been treated successfully (89.9 percent). [19]

INTERNAL TREATMENT

Although most reports recommend external treatment for corns, internal treatment has also proved effective. Yan successfully treated corns with *Sha Shen Dan Shen Tang* (Adenophora and Red Sage Root Decoction) with no adverse effects. The prescription was made up of *Nan Sha Shen* (Radix Adenophorae) 50g and *Dan Shen* (Radix Salviae Miltiorrhizae) 50g. One bag per day was used to prepare the decoction, with half drunk in the morning and half in the evening. The course of treatment lasted for 30 days. This treatment is contraindicated for people with Deficiency-Cold patterns or during pregnancy. [20]

ACUPUNCTURE TREATMENT

Wang advocated acupuncture treatment with filiform needles to treat corns, similar to the method described in the treatment section above. He used five no. 30 needles, 1 cun in length. One needle was inserted perpendicularly in the center of the corn down to its base; the other four needles were inserted obliquely from the inferior, superior, right, and left sides of the corn. The tips of these needles met the tip of the central needle at the base of the corn. After strong stimulation, the needles were retained for 10-20 minutes. The effect was better when slight bleeding was produced on withdrawal. The bleeding was then stopped by pressure. The corn came out after one session. [21]

ACUPUNCTURE AND MOXIBUSTION

Qiu reported on the treatment of corns with a combination of acupuncture and moxibustion. He first pared the corns with a blade, eliciting little or no bleeding. After routine disinfection of the corns, he slowly inserted a 0.5 cun needle into the center of the corn to a depth of 0.3 cun. He then heated it with a moxa stick for 10-15 minutes before withdrawing the needle. This treatment was given once a day. Seven treatments made up a course. Results were seen within seven days (one course). [22]

Callus
胼胝

A callus, or callosity, is a circumscribed hardening and hyperkeratosis (thickening of the horny layer of the skin) due to persistent pressure or friction or shearing forces, usually on the hands or feet. Factors influencing the occurrence of the condition include the shape or structure of the foot or hand, and repeated friction such as may occur in certain occupations or recreations.

Clinical manifestations

- Calluses mostly affect those whose hands or feet are subjected to persistent pressure or friction when working.
- People with flat feet are particularly likely to have calluses on the feet. The lesion generally occurs on pressure areas of the sole, particularly on the heel, the big toe and the flexor aspect of the little toe. Lesions on the hand generally involve the palm where tools or implements exert long-term and repeated pressure.
- Lesions manifest as round or oval, flat or elevated, hard, smooth, semitransparent yellow or brownish-yellow horny plaques, thicker at the center and thinning toward the borders, which are not clearly demarcated. The number of lesions varies.
- Tenderness is felt in severe cases. Some lesions ulcerate and form abscesses with foul-smelling pus as a result of infection.

Differential diagnosis

Corns
Hard corns are characterized by a cylindrical hard nodule extending into deeper layers of the skin and a dull colored surface. The skin lines are disrupted by the corn. Walking on the corn causes pain.

Common wart (verruca vulgaris)
Common warts on the sole or palm have a rough surface and are round or polygonal in shape. Their surface breaks up skin lines. They are likely to bleed when rubbed or knocked.

Etiology and pathology

Inhibited movement of Qi and Blood
Persistent pressure or friction on the hands and feet leads to stagnation or inhibited movement of Qi and Blood. The skin is therefore deprived of nourishment and a callus will form. Additionally, profuse sweating or injury to the sinews when walking long distances can lead to Qi stagnation and Blood stasis. Ying Qi (Nutritive Qi) and Wei Qi (Defensive Qi) are not strong enough to nourish the skin and flesh with the result that the skin hardens and a callus forms.

Pattern identification and treatment

INTERNAL TREATMENT

INHIBITED MOVEMENT OF QI AND BLOOD
The skin becomes thickened, hardened and swollen. Where the callus is on the foot, local tenderness makes walking difficult. The tongue body is pale red with a scant coating; the pulse is thready and rough.

Treatment principle
Regulate Qi, invigorate the Blood and alleviate pain.

Prescription
XIAN FANG HUO MING YIN JIA JIAN
Immortal Formula Life-Giving Beverage, with modifications

Jin Yin Hua (Flos Lonicerae) 15g
Pu Gong Ying (Herba Taraxaci cum Radice) 15g
Dang Gui (Radix Angelicae Sinensis) 10g
Zhi Ru Xiang (Gummi Olibanum Praeparatum) 10g
Zhi Mo Yao (Myrrha Praeparata) 10g
Zi Hua Di Ding (Herba Violae Yedoensitis) 10g
Tian Hua Fen (Radix Trichosanthis) 10g
Chen Pi (Pericarpium Citri Reticulatae) 10g
*Chuan Shan Jia** (Squama Manitis Pentadactylae) 6g
Huai Niu Xi (Radix Achyranthis Bidentatae) 6g
Fu Ling (Sclerotium Poriae Cocos) 6g
Mu Gua (Fructus Chaenomelis) 6g
Chao Du Zhong (Cortex Eucommiae Ulmoidis, stir-fried) 6g

Explanation
- *Chen Pi* (Pericarpium Citri Reticulatae), *Dang Gui* (Radix Angelicae Sinensis), *Zhi Ru Xiang* (Gummi Olibanum Praeparatum), *Zhi Mo Yao* (Myrrha Praeparata), and *Chuan Shan Jia** (Squama Manitis Pentadactylae) regulate Qi and invigorate the Blood, dissipate Blood stasis and soften the skin.
- *Pu Gong Ying* (Herba Taraxaci cum Radice), *Jin Yin Hua* (Flos Lonicerae), *Zi Hua Di Ding* (Herba Violae

Yedoensitis), and *Tian Hua Fen* (Radix Trichosanthis) dissipate nodules and disperse swelling.

- *Huai Niu Xi* (Radix Achyranthis Bidentatae), *Mu Gua* (Fructus Chaenomelis), *Chao Du Zhong* (Cortex Eucommiae Ulmoidis, stir-fried), and *Fu Ling* (Sclerotium Poriae Cocos) transform Dampness and free the network vessels, and supplement the Kidneys to strengthen the sinews.

EXTERNAL TREATMENT

- At the initial stage of the callus with thick and hard skin, use *Gou Ji Shui Xi Ji* (Cibot Wash Preparation) to soak the affected area. Then apply *Pian Zhi Gao* (Callus Plaster).
- Where a chronic callus has an abscess that cannot rupture because of the thick skin, the abscess may be drained. Then apply *Qing Dai San* (Indigo Powder).
- If generation of flesh is difficult and the lesion remains unhealed, use *Shou Gan Sheng Ji Yao Fen* (Medicated Powder for Promoting Contraction and Generating Flesh) until the lesion heals completely.

ACUPUNCTURE

Perpendicular insertion

Locate the Ashi point at the site of the lesion. After sterilizing the surface of the lesion, insert a 1.0 cun filiform needle perpendicularly in the center of the callus. Manipulate the needle by lifting and thrusting; the needle is not retained. Treat once every three days. A course consists of five treatment sessions.

Encirclement needling

Locate the Ashi points around the site of the lesion. Insert four 1.0 cun filiform needles obliquely superior to, inferior to, and to the right and left of the callus with the tips of the needles pointing towards the center of the lesion. The even method is applied. The needles are retained for 30 minutes; during this period, they are stimulated three to five times. Treat once every three days. A course consists of five treatment sessions.

MOXIBUSTION

Soak the affected area in warm water. When the callus becomes soft, scrape off the thick surface layer with a blade. Then burn a moxa cone on top of a moxibustion device. Use two or three cones each time, once or twice a week. After moxibustion, apply *Wu Mei Gao* (Black Plum Paste) to the lesion.

FIRE NEEDLING AND MOXIBUSTION

Point: Ashi point (the site of the lesion).
Technique: Hold a needle in a flame until it turns red, then insert it quickly in the center of the Ashi point and withdraw it immediately. Slight bleeding may occur. Repeat the treatment once every five days. This treatment is accompanied by moxibustion. Burn two or three wedge-shaped moxa cones on top of the lesion once or twice a week. A course consists of three treatment sessions. The patient's consent to this procedure must be obtained in advance.

Clinical notes

External wash medications for calluses or corns have the function of softening the skin and removing the hardened, horny layer. Continuous use of such medications will bring good results.

Advice for the patient

- Calluses are often associated with mechanical pressure and friction. It is therefore important to prevent such stimuli, for example by not wearing tight-fitting or stiff shoes.
- Avoid indiscriminate use of corrosive medications. Pare calluses with sterile instruments only to avoid infection.

Hangnail
逆剥

Hangnail manifests as a torn strip of dry, broken skin at the side or base borders of the fingernails or toenails.

In TCM, this condition is also known as *ni lu* (retrograded skin).

Clinical manifestations

- Hangnail mostly affects children of school age, but can also be seen in adults with rough or dry skin.
- The epidermis splits and curls up at the sides of the nails and the nailbed. This is painless unless the split extends to the underlying dermis. Pulling the hangnail will cause pain and bleeding.

Etiology and pathology

Invasion of pathogenic Wind when the channels and vessels are empty leads to inhibited movement of Qi and Blood. The skin is therefore deprived of nourishment and becomes torn and curled up at the borders of the nails.

Treatment

EXTERNAL TREATMENT
Hangnail is best treated externally. Prepare a decoction of *Xi Xin** (Herba cum Radice Asari) 15g and *Ai Ye* (Folium Artemisiae Argyi) 30g and use it lukewarm to soak the affected finger or toe for 10-15 minutes. Cut off the torn skin and then, once or twice a day, apply a paste made from 1g of finely-powdered *Gan Jiang* (Rhizoma Zingiberis Officinalis) and 10g of pork lard ‡ (*Zhu Zhi*, Adeps Suis) or Vaseline®. The paste has the function of softening the skin and is therefore effective in the treatment and prevention of hangnail.

Advice for the patient

Do not pull off the torn strips of skin around the nail; use moisturizing ointment to soften the skin instead.

References

1. Rao Yong'an, *Huang Qi Dang Gui Si Ni Tang Zhi Liao Dong Chuang 204 Li* [Treatment of 204 Cases of Chilblains with *Huang Qi Dang Gui Si Ni Tang* (Astragalus and Chinese Angelica Root Counterflow Cold Decoction)], *He Bei Zhong Yi* [Hebei Journal of Traditional Chinese Medicine] 18, 1 (1996): 17.
2. Yang Bairu, *Ru Xiang He Mo Yao Zhi Liao Dong Chuang* [Treatment of Chilblains with *Ru Xiang* (Gummi Olibanum) and *Mo Yao* (Myrrha)], *Shan Xi Hu Li Za Zhi* [Shanxi Journal of Nursing] 12, 6 (1998): 265.
3. Yang Benxi, *Fu Fang Bai Yao Ding Zhi Liao Dong Chuang 30 Li* [Treatment of 30 Cases of Chilblains with *Fu Fang Bai Yao Ding* (Compound Yunnan White Tincture)], *Si Chuan Yi Xue* [Sichuan Journal of Medicine] 8, 5 (1987): 279.
4. Hu Rongting, *Fu Zi Wai Yong Zhi Liao Dong Chuang 32 Li* [External Treatment of 32 Cases of Chilblains with *Fu Zi* (Radix Lateralis Aconiti Carmichaeli Praeparata)], *Zhe Jiang Zhong Yi Za Zhi* [Zhejiang Journal of Traditional Chinese Medicine] 33, 10 (1998): 441.
5. Shi Huilin, *Dong Shang Tang Zhi Liao Dong Shang 87 Li* [Treatment of 87 Cases of Frostbite with *Dong Shang Tang* (Frostbite Decoction)], *Liao Ning Zhong Yi Za Zhi* [Liaoning Journal of Traditional Chinese Medicine] 18, 12 (1991): 32.
6. Xu Shunying, *Shi Di Shui Zhi Liao Dong Shang Xiao Guo Hao* [Effective Results Obtained in the Treatment of Frostbite with *Shi Di Shui* (Rheo-Camphoradin)], *Zhong Yi Za Zhi* [Journal of Traditional Chinese Medicine] 37, 6 (1996): 358.
7. Traditional Chinese Medicine Research Academy: Beijing Guang'anmen Hospital, *Zhu Ren Kang Lin Chuang Jing Yan Ji* [A Collection of Zhu Renkang's Clinical Experiences] (Beijing: People's Medical Publishing House, 1979), 215.
8. Shi Tianning, *Pu Ji Xiao Du Yin Jia Jian Zhi Liao Duo Xing Xing Ri Guang Zhen 54 Li* [Treatment of 54 Cases of Polymorphic Light Eruption with Modified *Pu Ji Xiao Du Yin* (Universal Salvation Beverage for Dispersing Toxicity)], *Zhong Guo Zhong Xi Yi Jie He Za Zhi* [Journal of Integrated TCM and Western Medicine] 18, 10 (1998): 630.
9. Yang Huaizhu, *Zhong Yao Zhi Liao Duo Xing Ri Guang Zhen 36 Li* [Treatment of 36 Cases of Polymorphic Light Eruption with Chinese Materia Medica], *Zhong Guo Pi Fu Xing Bing Xue Za Zhi* [Chinese Journal of Dermatology and Venereology] 13, 2 (1999): 114.
10. Qiao Jianhua, *Zhong Yao Dai Cha Yin Yong Zhi Liao Duo Xing Xing Ri Guang Zhen* [Treatment of Polymorphic Light Eruption with a Chinese Herbal Tea Preparation], *Zhong Hua Yi Xue Mei Rong Za Zhi* [Chinese Medical Cosmetology Journal] 4, 4 (1998): 215-216.
11. Beijing Hospital of Traditional Chinese Medicine, *Zhao Bing Nan Lin Chuang Jing Yan Ji* [A Collection of Zhao

Bingnan's Clinical Experiences] (Beijing: People's Medical Publishing House, 1975), 127.

12. Ibid., 129.

13. Cheng Yunqian, *Zhong Yi Pi Fu Bing Xue Jian Bian* [Dermatology in Traditional Chinese Medicine: Simplified Edition] (Xi'an: Shaanxi People's Publishing House, 1979), 198-9.

14. Wu Jiecheng, *Chuang Yang Jing Yan Lu* [Records of Experiences in the Treatment of Sores] (Beijing: People's Medical Publishing House, 1980), 82-83.

15. Tang Guorong, *Fu Fang Zi Cao You De Zhi Bei Ji Lin Chuang Ying Yong* [Preparation and Clinical Application of *Fu Fang Zi Cao You* (Compound Gromwell Root Oil)], *Zhong Guo Yi Yuan Yao Xue Za Zhi* [Chinese Journal of Hospital Pharmacology] 16, 10 (1996): 470.

16. Jia Xiaoguang, *Zi Cao You Gao Zhi Yu Shao Tang Shang 6 Li* [Six Cases of Burns and Scalds Treated with *Zi Cao You Gao* (Gromwell Root Oil Paste)], *Xin Jiang Zhong Yi Yao* [Xinjiang Journal of Traditional Chinese Medicine and Chinese Materia Medica] 16, 4 (1998): 39-40.

17. Zhang Fengxiang, *Fu Fang Dan Qing Hu Zhi Liao Er Du Ji Xing Fang She Xing Pi Yan 32 Li* [Treatment of 32 Cases of Second-Degree Acute Radiodermatitis with *Fu Fang Dan Qing Hu* (Compound Medicated Paste Prepared with Egg White)], *Ren Min Jun Yi* [Medical Journal of the People's Military] 7, 4 (1996): 60-61.

18. Die Xiaoping, *Zhong Yao Shuang Cao You Zhi Liao Fang She Xing Pi Yan* [Treatment of Radiodermatitis with *Shuang Cao You* (Double Herb Oil)], *Zhong Hua Hu Li Za Zhi* [Chinese Journal of Nursing] 31, 10 (1996): 602.

19. Li Zhihong, *Wu Mei Gao Zhi Liao 198 Li Ji Yan Lin Chuang Guan Cha* [Clinical Observation of the Treatment of 198 Cases of Corns with *Wu Mei Gao* (Black Plum Paste)], *Ling Nan Pi Fu Xing Bing Ke Za Zhi* [Lingnan Journal of Dermatology and Venereology] 2, 3 (1995): 20.

20. Yan Jiasun, *Sha Shen Dan Shen Tang Zhi Liao Ji Yan* [Treatment of Corns with *Sha Shen Dan Shen Tang* (Adenophora and Red Sage Root Decoction)], *Zhong Cheng Yao Yan Jiu* [Chinese Patent Herbal Medicine Research Journal] 7 (1986): 47.

21. Wang Youjun, *Zhen Ci Zhi Liao Ji Yan* [Treatment of Corns with Acupuncture], *Xin Jiang Zhong Yi Yao* [Xinjiang Journal of Traditional Chinese Medicine and Materia Medica] 16, 4 (1998): 63.

22. Qiu Zhihu, *Zhen Ci Jia Ai Jiu Zhi Liao Ji Yan* [Treatment of Corns with Acupuncture and Moxibustion], *Wu Jing Yi Xue* [People's Armed Police Journal of Medicine] 7, 3 (1996): 183.

Infestations and bites

Infestation is defined as the presence of insect or worm parasites on or in the body. Worms on or in the skin are usually only found in tropical countries and are not discussed in this chapter.

Insects can cause various skin reactions. An insect bite or other contact with an insect can induce a chemical effect or allergic reaction, for example after a bee or wasp sting, or an irritant reaction, for example after contact with certain caterpillars or beetles. Insects may also affect the skin directly by burrowing, as in scabies, or by sucking blood, as in pediculosis (lice infection).

Insect bites and stings
虫咬及蜇伤

Insect bites and stings can cause inflammation of the skin in humans. Bees, wasps and hornets inject minute quantities of poisons similar to snake venom. Generally, the amount is too small to be significant, but sensitized individuals who are allergic to the stings may have major systemic reactions. Scorpions, spiders, centipedes, and other insects can inject poison through their bites; some poisons may trigger toxic or allergic reactions in sensitized individuals, especially children.

Clinical manifestations

- Bites or stings usually involve the head, face, neck, hand, foot, or other exposed areas.
- Mild cases present with localized manifestations such as papules, small hemorrhagic spots, blisters, wheals, or swelling. Severe cases are often complicated by toxic symptoms such as chills, fever, dizziness, tinnitus, irritability, numbness, nausea and vomiting, poor appetite, and abdominal fullness.
- **Bee and wasp stings:** The sting discharges venom, leading to petechiae at the site of the wound and papules or wheals on a surrounding erythematous base. Itching, intense pain and a moderate burning sensation are likely. In some cases, allergic reactions or toxic systemic reactions may develop some time after the sting; these include dizziness, nausea, headache, muscle spasms, and loss of consciousness.

- **Mosquito, flea and bedbug bites:** Bites from these insects result in erythema or papular urticaria with central petechiae and intense itching. Flea bites are often clustered around the ankles.
- **Midge bites:** Bites give rise to petechiae, edematous erythema, wheals, and vesicles. Itching is often unbearable.
- **Tick bites:** As well as producing red, swollen, itchy, and painful skin, tick bites can also lead to tick fever, Lyme disease or tick paralysis.
- **Beetle bites:** These bites can cause band-like blisters and burning pain.
- **Centipede bites:** Two purplish spots appear at the location of the bite, surrounded by redness and swelling and accompanied by pain that seems to penetrate to the bone. In severe cases, other accompanying symptoms include numbness, headache, dizziness and vertigo, nausea, vomiting, palpitations, or possibly delirium and convulsions.
- **Scorpion stings:** Immediately after the sting enters the skin, a large swollen red patch appears accompanied by intense pain. In severe cases, symptoms may include salivation, nausea, vomiting, lethargy, chills, and high fever. In rare cases, spasms of the hands and feet and death due to asphyxiation may occur.
- **Leech bites:** Leeches suck blood from humans and animals. When they fall off, they leave papules or

wheals with petechiae in the center. If force is used to remove leeches, continuous bleeding is likely where the sucker was attached.

- **Caterpillar hairs:** Contact with the hair of certain caterpillars, particularly Arctiidae (tiger moths) and Saturniidae (emperor moths), can result in intense irritation and inflammation. Lesions manifest as urticarial patches or linear wheals. If lesions persist, they may become itchy, painful and ulcerated. In some cases, red eyes and lacrimation may occur.

Differential diagnosis

Papular urticaria
Papular urticaria is a reaction to bites of insects such as fleas, mites or bedbugs where the actual source of the bite is unknown. Lesions initially manifest as red, oval, infiltrative wheals with papulovesicles or vesicles at the center and mainly involve the lumbosacral region, buttocks, trunk, and limbs. Incidence is high among infants and children. The lesions characteristically occur in irregular lines and clusters, may last for up to two weeks and recur in crops. Itching is likely.

Scabies
Scabies usually involves the sides of the fingers, the webs between the fingers, the sides of the hands, the wrists, the elbows, the ankles and feet, the nipples, the lower abdomen around the umbilicus, and the genitals and buttocks. Insect bites lack the grayish linear, curved or serpiginous burrows characteristic of scabies.

Etiology and pathology

The bites and stings of Toxic insects allow Toxic fluids to enter the body through the wound. These fluids first attack the Ying and Xue levels or the sinews and vessels, and then the Zang-Fu organs, giving rise to a series of localized or generalized toxic symptoms of varying severity.

Pattern identification and treatment

INTERNAL TREATMENT

INTERNAL DAMP-HEAT WITH INVASION BY TOXINS
At the initial stage, the affected area is red and itching with small papules or larger wheals capped by pale vesicles. As the condition develops, itching and pain occur with inflammation and diffuse edema. The tongue body is red with a white coating; the pulse is slippery and rapid.

Treatment principle
Clear Heat and relieve Toxicity, eliminate Dampness and expel pathogenic factors.

Prescription
JIE DU CHU SHI TANG JIA JIAN
Decoction for Relieving Toxicity and Eliminating Dampness, with modifications

Lian Qiao (Fructus Forsythiae Suspensae) 12g
Pu Gong Ying (Herba Taraxaci cum Radice) 12g
Ban Zhi Lian (Herba Scutellariae Barbatae) 15g
Ma Chi Xian (Herba Portulacae Oleraceae) 15g
Mu Dan Pi (Cortex Moutan Radicis) 10g
Ye Ju Hua (Flos Chrysanthemi Indici) 10g
Niu Bang Zi (Fructus Arctii Lappae) 10g
Gan Cao (Radix Glycyrrhizae) 10g
Zhi Zi (Fructus Gardeniae Jasminoidis) 10g
Lü Dou Yi (Testa Phaseoli Radiati) 30g
Chi Xiao Dou (Semen Phaseoli Calcarati) 30g

Explanation
- *Lian Qiao* (Fructus Forsythiae Suspensae), *Pu Gong Ying* (Herba Taraxaci cum Radice), *Ban Zhi Lian* (Herba Scutellariae Barbatae), *Gan Cao* (Radix Glycyrrhizae), *Ma Chi Xian* (Herba Portulacae Oleraceae), and *Ye Ju Hua* (Flos Chrysanthemi Indici) clear Heat and relieve Toxicity.
- *Mu Dan Pi* (Cortex Moutan Radicis), *Chi Xiao Dou* (Semen Phaseoli Calcarati), *Zhi Zi* (Fructus Gardeniae Jasminoidis), and *Lü Dou Yi* (Testa Phaseoli Radiati) cool and harmonize the Blood, disperse swelling and alleviate pain.
- *Niu Bang Zi* (Fructus Arctii Lappae) dredges Wind and alleviates itching.

SCORCHING OF THE YING AND XUE LEVELS
This pattern manifests as unbearable pain around the bites, a sensation of burning heat on contact, huge areas of erythema and edema, turbid vesicles or bullae, or bloody blisters; vesicles and bullae are relatively flaccid and discharge a thick, turbid fluid when ruptured. Accompanying symptoms and signs include swollen lymph nodes, thirst, irritability, raging fever and delirium, constipation, difficult or painful urination, and yellow urine. The tongue body is dark red with a scant coating; the pulse is rapid.

Treatment principle
Clear Heat from the Ying level and cool the Blood, relieve Toxicity and expel pathogenic factors.

Prescription
QING YING TANG JIA JIAN
Decoction for Clearing Heat from the Ying Level, with modifications

Sheng Di Huang (Radix Rehmanniae Glutinosae) 30g
Mu Dan Pi (Cortex Moutan Radicis) 10g
Chi Shao (Radix Paeoniae Rubra) 10g
Ban Zhi Lian (Herba Scutellariae Barbatae) 10g
Da Huang (Radix et Rhizoma Rhei) 10g
Gan Cao (Radix Glycyrrhizae) 10g
Shui Niu Jiao ‡ (Cornu Bubali, powdered) 6g, infused in the prepared decoction
Lian Qiao (Fructus Forsythiae Suspensae) 12g
Lian Zi Xin (Plumula Nelumbinis Nuciferae) 4.5g

Explanation
- *Sheng Di Huang* (Radix Rehmanniae Glutinosae), *Mu Dan Pi* (Cortex Moutan Radicis) and *Chi Shao* (Radix Paeoniae Rubra) cool the Blood and reduce erythema.
- *Shui Niu Jiao* ‡ (Cornu Bubali), *Lian Zi Xin* (Plumula Nelumbinis Nuciferae) and *Gan Cao* (Radix Glycyrrhizae) clear Heat from the Ying level and protect the Heart.
- *Ban Zhi Lian* (Herba Scutellariae Barbatae), *Lian Qiao* (Fructus Forsythiae Suspensae) and *Da Huang* (Radix et Rhizoma Rhei) relieve Toxicity and alleviate pain.

General modifications
1. For prevalence of Fire Toxins, add *Huang Lian* (Rhizoma Coptidis) and *Huang Qin* (Radix Scutellariae Baicalensis).
2. For preponderance of Wind Toxins, add *Jing Jie* (Herba Schizonepetae Tenuifoliae), *Chan Tui* ‡ (Periostracum Cicadae), *Zi Su Ye* (Folium Perillae Frutescentis), and *Qing Hao* (Herba Artemisiae Chinghao).
3. For irritability, focal distension and vomiting in children, add *Xiao Er Jian Fu Tang Jiang* (Syrup for Fortifying Children's Skin) 10-20ml twice a day.
4. For convulsions or stiff neck, add *Jiang Can* ‡ (Bombyx Batryticatus), *Gou Teng* (Ramulus Uncariae cum Uncis) and *Tian Ma* * (Rhizoma Gastrodiae Elatae).

PATENT HERBAL MEDICINES
- Take three or four tablets of *Nan Tong She Yao Pian* (Nantong Snake Bite Tablet) two or three times a day; alternatively, dissolve 10-15 of these tablets in vinegar for external application three to five times a day.
- Take *Xiao Bai Du Gao* (Minor Toxicity-Vanquishing Syrup) 15g twice a day with warm water.

EXTERNAL TREATMENT

Bee and wasp stings
Pound *Xian Ma Chi Xian* (Herba Portulacae Oleraceae Recens), *Xian Ye Ju Hua* (Flos Chrysanthemi Indici Recens), *Xian Xia Ku Cao* (Spica Prunellae Vulgaris Recens), or *Xian Pu Gong Ying* (Herba Taraxaci cum Radice Recens) to a pulp and apply to the affected area. In addition, *Mi Cu* (Acetum Oryzae) can be used to wash the wound.

Mosquito, flea and bedbug bites
Treat as for bee and wasp stings.

Midge bites
First wash the bite with a decoction made from *Ye Ju Hua* (Flos Chrysanthemi Indici) 10g, *Pu Gong Ying* (Herba Taraxaci cum Radice) 10g and *Lü Cao* (Herba Humuli Scandentis) 10g; then apply *Sheng Jiang Zhi* (Succus Rhizomatis Zingiberis Officinalis) or *Dong Gua Ye* (Folium Benincasae Hispidae) pounded to a pulp.

Beetle bites
Treat as for midge bites.

Tick bites
Do not remove the tick from the skin by force; instead, spread paraffin or chilli oil over the tick's head and it will fall off after a few minutes. Then wash the bite with a decoction of *Cong Bai* (Bulbus Allii Fistulosi) 20g, *Gan Cao* (Radix Glycyrrhizae) 20g and *Han Lian Cao* (Herba Ecliptae Prostratae) 20g; or apply a medicinal wine made from *Bo He* (Herba Menthae Haplocalycis) 30g soaked in 70ml of *Bai Jiu* (Granorum Spiritus Incolor) for three days.

Centipede bites
Grind *Wu Ling Zhi* ‡ (Excrementum Trogopteri) into a fine powder, or pound *Xia Ku Cao* (Spica Prunellae Vulgaris) and *Xian Sang Ye* (Folium Mori Albae Recens) to a pulp for application to the lesion.

Scorpion stings
First try to extract the poisonous fluid with fire-cupping therapy, then pound *Xian Da Qing Ye* (Folium Isatidis seu Baphicacanthi Recens), *Xian Ma Chi Xian* (Herba Portulacae Oleraceae Recens) and *Xian He Ye* (Folium Nelumbinis Nuciferae Recens) to a pulp and apply to the affected area.

Leech bites
If the leech is tightly attached to the skin, gently pat the skin around the leech with the hand until it falls off. Then apply *Mi Cu* (Acetum Oryzae), *Bai Jiu* (Granorum Spiritus Incolor) or a salt solution to the bite. If the skin becomes ulcerated, apply *Zhu Huang San* (Pearl and Bovine Bezoar Powder) first, then cover with *Huang Lian Ruan Gao* (Coptis Ointment).

Caterpillar hairs
First wash the affected area with a warm decoction of *Bai Zhi* (Radix Angelicae Dahuricae). Then remove the hairs with adhesive plaster and spread a paste made from powdered *Wang Bu Liu Xing* (Semen Vaccariae Segetalis) mixed with cold boiled water. If the area is

Table 18-1 Folk remedies: treatment of bites and stings and methods of destroying insects

Bee stings	1. Apply powdered *Feng Fang*‡ (Nidus Vespae) mixed with pork lard‡ 2. Apply *Sheng Jiang Zhi* (Succus Rhizomatis Zingiberis Officinalis Recens) 3. Rub in *Qing Liang You* (Tiger Balm) 4. Apply salt
Mosquito bites	Soak *She Chuang Zi* (Fructus Cnidii Monnieri) 25g and *Bai Bu* (Radix Stemonae) 25g in 100ml of 50% surgical spirit for 24 hours, filter and apply the liquid to the affected areas twice a day
Flea bites	1. Scatter powdered *Shi Chang Pu* (Rhizoma Acori Graminei), dried in the shade, under the mattress 2. Cover the bites with ground fresh *Tao Ye* (Folium Persicae) that has been dried in the sun and spray a little water on top
Bedbug bites	1. Fumigation from burning sheep or goat bones can destroy the bugs 2. Drenching with a decoction of buckwheat straw can kill the bugs 3. Fumigation from burning pawpaw can make the bugs an empty shell
Centipede bites	1. Apply the juice of *Tian Nan Xing* (Rhizoma Arisaematis) 2. Apply powdered *Hu Jiao* (Fructus Piperis Nigri) 3. Apply a single bulb of *Da Suan* (Bulbus Allii Sativi)
Scorpion stings	1. Apply vinegar mixed with *Qian Dan*‡ (Minium) 2. Apply powdered *Ban Xia* (Rhizoma Pinelliae Ternatae) mixed with water
Caterpillar hairs	1. Apply *Bai Mi*‡ (Mel) 2. Wash the wound with a decoction of *Gan Cao* (Radix Glycyrrhizae) 3. Apply *Hai Piao Xiao*‡ (Os Sepiae seu Sepiellae) 4. Apply powdered *Dan Dou Chi* (Semen Sojae Praeparatum) mixed with vegetable oil
Spider bites	1. Fumigate with *Ai Ye* (Folium Artemisiae Argyi) 2. Apply slices of *Pao Jiang* (Rhizoma Zingiberis Officinalis Praeparata) 3. Apply *Tao Ye* (Folium Persicae) ground to a pulp 4. Apply slices of *Da Suan* (Bulbus Allii Sativi)

ulcerated, apply powdered *Hai Piao Xiao*‡ (Os Sepiae seu Sepiellae) instead.

FOLK REMEDIES
Table 18-1 lists folk remedies for a variety of bites and stings. The amount used will depend on the size and severity of the bite.

ACUPUNCTURE
Selection of points according to disease differentiation
- For insect bites and stings on the hands and feet, select EX-UE-9 Baxie [i] and EX-LE-10 Bafeng. [ii]
- For persistent raging fever, select EX-UE-11 Shixuan. [iii]
- For coma or syncope
  Main points: GV-20 Baihui, LI-4 Hegu and LR-3 Taichong.

Auxiliary points: GV-26 Shuigou, PC-6 Neiguan and ST-36 Zusanli.

Technique
Apply the reducing method, with rotation, lifting and thrusting, at all the points except EX-UE-11 Shixuan. The needles are not retained. EX-UE-11 Shixuan is pricked to cause bleeding. Treat once a day. A course consists of seven treatment sessions. Generally speaking, one course can achieve a good effect and a second course is not needed.

Selection of local points
Points
- For bites and stings on the hand, select PC-6 Neiguan, LI-4 Hegu and LI-11 Quchi.
- For bites and stings on the foot, select SP-6 Sanyinjiao, KI-3 Taixi and ST-36 Zusanli.

---

[i] M-UE-22 according to the system employed by the Shanghai College of Traditional Chinese Medicine.
[ii] M-LE-8 according to the system employed by the Shanghai College of Traditional Chinese Medicine.
[iii] M-UE-1 according to the system employed by the Shanghai College of Traditional Chinese Medicine.

Technique: Apply the even method to all points. Treat once a day. A course consists of seven treatment sessions. A second course is not normally needed.

Explanation

- GV-26 Shuigou and GV-20 Baihui free the orifices and arouse the brain.
- LI-11 Quchi, EX-UE-9 Baxie, EX-LE-10 Bafeng and EX-UE-11 Shixuan dredge Wind, disperse swelling, and alleviate pain and itching.
- LI-4 Hegu, LR-3 Taichong, PC-6 Neiguan, and ST-36 Zusanli clear Heat from the Heart and relieve Toxicity.
- SP-6 Sanyinjiao and KI-3 Taixi eliminate Dampness and relieve Toxicity.

EAR ACUPUNCTURE

Points: Lung, Liver, Kidney, Ear-Shenmen, and Sympathetic Region.

Technique: Retain the needles for 30 minutes and manipulate them three to five times during this period. Treat once a day.

Indication: Itching and slight redness and swelling after bites or stings from a poisonous insect.

PRICKING TO BLEED METHOD

Points: Ashi points (sites where the swelling is most obvious).

Technique: Prick the points with a three-edged needle to cause slight bleeding, then use the flash-cupping method for 5-10 minutes to drain Toxic Blood.

Clinical notes

- Insect bites and stings are essentially managed by external treatment with materia medica to relieve Toxicity, alleviate itching, free the network vessels, and dissipate lumps.
- The prognosis is generally good except in certain severe cases with multiple bites or stings or a violent allergic reaction; these may be fatal if there is no immediate treatment.

Advice for the patient

- Ensure that the breeding places of biting insects are thoroughly cleaned and, where possible, destroyed.
- Protect the body and avoid exposing the skin.
- When visiting areas where bites from poisonous insects are likely, take appropriate medication such as *Nan Tong She Yao Pian* (Nantong Snake Bite Tablet) for use in emergencies.

Papular urticaria
丘疹性荨麻疹

Despite the nomenclature, papular urticaria is not a variant of urticaria; rather it represents a reaction, possibly of allergic etiology, to bites of certain insects such as mosquitoes, fleas, mites, or bedbugs. Several people in one family may be affected at the same time, especially where the source of the bites is a garden insect or a parasite on a domestic pet.

In TCM, this condition is also known as *shui jie* (water scab).

Clinical manifestations

- Incidence is high among infants and young children, with the disease tending to occur in summer and autumn.
- The condition usually involves the lumbosacral region, the buttocks, the trunk, and the limbs.

- Lesions initially manifest as red, oval, infiltrative urticarial papules up to 5 mm in diameter with papulovesicles or vesicles at the center. Distribution is uneven in number and configuration. The lesions characteristically occur in irregular lines and clusters, may last for up to two weeks and recur in crops.
- Scratching may result in some lesions becoming infected and impetiginized; scabs may form.
- Pruritus is common and may result in difficulty in sleeping.

Differential diagnosis

Urticaria

This condition may affect people at any age and in any season. Lesions, which may occur on any part of the body, manifest as red, pink or white wheals of varying sizes without vesicles or papulovesicles in the center. They appear and disappear at irregular intervals. Once they disappear, no scar or other mark remains. Pruritus is normally intense.

Scabies

Scabies mainly involves the sides of the fingers, the webs between the fingers, the sides of the hands, and the wrists. It may develop in individuals of all ages. Papular urticaria lacks the grayish linear, curved or serpiginous burrows characteristic of scabies.

Varicella (chickenpox)

Systemic symptoms such as fever and aversion to cold usually occur initially prior to the appearance of large numbers of small vesicles, discretely distributed on the head, face, trunk, and limbs. No wheal-like lesions are to be found underneath the vesicles, but exudation and crusting may occur on rupture of blisters.

Etiology and pathology

- Repeated contraction of pathogenic Wind-Heat combines with congenital Heat from the fetal period that has accumulated in the skin and flesh.

- Constitutional sensitivity to certain foods that stir Wind, such as fish or seafood, results in impairment of the transportation and transformation function of the Spleen and Stomach, leading to retention of Damp-Heat in the skin and flesh.

- Toxins from mosquito, flea or other insect bites leads to Toxic juices combining with internally accumulated Damp-Heat to obstruct the skin and flesh and give rise to the condition.

Pattern identification and treatment

INTERNAL TREATMENT

BINDING OF WIND-HEAT

In this pattern, lesions manifest as red, infiltrative, itchy urticarial papules of different sizes, with papulovesicles or vesicles at the center. Lesions are discretely distributed on the upper body and usually appear in crops. The tongue body is red with a thin yellow coating; the pulse is rapid.

Treatment principle

Dredge Wind, clear Heat and alleviate itching.

Prescription

YIN QIAO SAN JIA JIAN

Honeysuckle and Forsythia Powder, with modifications

Jin Yin Hua (Flos Lonicerae) 10g
Lian Qiao (Fructus Forsythiae Suspensae) 10g
Chan Tui‡ (Periostracum Cicadae) 4.5g
Chao Niu Bang Zi (Fructus Arctii Lappae, stir-fried) 4.5g
Jing Jie (Herba Schizonepetae Tenuifoliae) 6g
Fang Feng (Radix Ledebouriellae Divaricatae) 6g
Huang Qin (Radix Scutellariae Baicalensis) 3g
Mu Dan Pi (Cortex Moutan Radicis) 3g

Explanation

- *Jin Yin Hua* (Flos Lonicerae), *Lian Qiao* (Fructus Forsythiae Suspensae), *Huang Qin* (Radix Scutellariae Baicalensis), and *Mu Dan Pi* (Cortex Moutan Radicis) clear Heat and relieve Toxicity, cool the Blood and reduce erythema.

- *Chan Tui*‡ (Periostracum Cicadae), *Chao Niu Bang Zi* (Fructus Arctii Lappae, stir-fried), *Jing Jie* (Herba Schizonepetae Tenuifoliae), and *Fang Feng* (Radix Ledebouriellae Divaricatae) dredge Wind and alleviate itching, dissipate pathogenic factors and disperse swelling.

RETENTION OF DAMP-HEAT

Lesions manifest as red or dark red, infiltrative, itchy urticarial papules involving the lower body. Vesicles at the center of the lesions give off exudation after rupture due to scratching. Some patients may have bullae or bloody blisters with a wet and erosive surface after rupture. The tongue body is red with a yellow and greasy coating; the pulse is slippery and rapid.

Treatment principle

Clear Heat and dispel Dampness, dredge Wind and alleviate itching.

Prescription

ZHI ZHU CHI DOU YIN JIA JIAN

Bitter Orange, White Atractylodes and Aduki Bean Beverage, with modifications

Chao Bai Zhu (Rhizoma Atractylodis Macrocephalae, stir-fried) 6g
Chao Zhi Ke (Fructus Citri Aurantii, stir-fried) 6g
Chan Tui‡ (Periostracum Cicadae) 6g
Chi Shao (Radix Paeoniae Rubra) 6g
Fang Feng (Radix Ledebouriellae Divaricatae) 6g
Fu Ling Pi (Cortex Poriae Cocos) 12g
Chi Xiao Dou (Semen Phaseoli Calcarati) 12g
Jing Jie (Herba Schizonepetae Tenuifoliae) 3g
Sha Ren (Fructus Amomi) 4.5g, added 5 minutes before the end of the decoction process
Yi Mu Cao (Herba Leonuri Heterophylli) 10g

Explanation

- *Chao Bai Zhu* (Rhizoma Atractylodis Macrocephalae, stir-fried), *Chao Zhi Ke* (Fructus Citri Aurantii, stir-fried), *Fu Ling Pi* (Cortex Poriae Cocos), *Chi Xiao Dou* (Semen Phaseoli Calcarati), and *Sha Ren* (Fructus

Amomi) transform Dampness and disperse swelling.

- *Chan Tui* ‡ (Periostracum Cicadae), *Chi Shao* (Radix Paeoniae Rubra), *Fang Feng* (Radix Ledebouriellae Divaricatae), *Jing Jie* (Herba Schizonepetae Tenuifoliae), and *Yi Mu Cao* (Herba Leonuri Heterophylli) disperse Wind and alleviate itching, invigorate the Blood and reduce erythema.

General modifications

1. For intense itching, add *Bai Ji Li* (Fructus Tribuli Terrestris), *Bai Xian Pi* (Cortex Dictamni Dasycarpi Radicis), *Cang Er Zi* (Fructus Xanthii Sibirici), and *Di Fu Zi* (Fructus Kochiae Scopariae).
2. For bullae or bloody blisters, add *Mu Dan Pi* (Cortex Moutan Radicis), *Zi Cao* (Radix Arnebiae seu Lithospermi), *Tong Cao* (Medulla Tetrapanacis Papyriferi), and *Che Qian Zi* (Semen Plantaginis).
3. For lesions with erosion and exudation, add *Di Yu* (Radix Sanguisorbae Officinalis), *Ma Chi Xian* (Herba Portulacae Oleraceae) and *Chi Shi Zhi* ‡ (Halloysitum Rubrum).
4. For infection by Toxins with formation of pus, add *Zi Hua Di Ding* (Herba Violae Yedoensitis), *Pu Gong Ying* (Herba Taraxaci cum Radice), *Bai Jiang Cao* (Herba cum Radice Patriniae), and *Lü Dou Yi* (Testa Phaseoli Radiati).
5. Where consumption of fish or seafood or dietary irregularities contribute to the appearance of wheals, add *Zi Su Ye* (Folium Perillae Frutescentis), *Jiao Shan Zha* (Fructus Crataegi, scorch-fried), *Jiao Shen Qu* (Massa Fermentata, scorch-fried), *Jiao Mai Ya* (Fructus Hordei Vulgaris Germinatus, scorch-fried), and *Hu Huang Lian* (Rhizoma Picrorhizae Scrophulariiflorae).

EXTERNAL TREATMENT

- If skin lesions manifest mainly as papules and papulovesicles, apply *Bai Bu Ding* (Stemona Root Tincture) or *Lu Hu Xi Ji* (Calamine and Giant Knotweed Wash Preparation).
- If blisters rupture and erode, prepare a decoction with equal amounts of *Ma Chi Xian* (Herba Portulacae Oleraceae) and *Di Yu* (Radix Sanguisorbae Officinalis) for application as a wet compress on the affected areas for 15-30 minutes, twice a day.
- If the lesions become infected with formation of pus, mix *Di Hu San* (Sanguisorba and Giant Knotweed Powder) into a paste with sunflower oil and apply to the affected area once or twice a day.

ACUPUNCTURE

Points: LI-11 Quchi, SP-10 Xuehai and ST-36 Zusanli.
Technique: Apply the reducing method without retaining the needles. Treat once a day. A course consists of five treatment sessions.
Explanation: These points clear Heat in the Blood and alleviate itching.

EAR ACUPUNCTURE

Points: Lung, Spleen and Heart.
Technique: Retain the needles for five minutes after insertion. Treat once a day. A course consists of five treatment sessions.

POINT LASER THERAPY

Point: LI-11 Quchi.
Technique: Expose a unilateral point to helium-neon laser therapy for 10 minutes; treat bilateral points alternately. Treat once a day. A course consists of five treatment sessions.

Clinical notes

- As this disease often involves the lumbar region, buttocks and lower limbs in children, the treatment principle of transforming Dampness, cooling the Blood, dissipating Wind and alleviating itching is generally the most appropriate. Personal clinical experience indicates that effective results are achieved with *Zhi Zhu Chi Dou Yin* (Bitter Orange, White Atractylodes and Aduki Bean Beverage) as the basic formula.
- If eruptions become infected and purulent after scratching, application of *Di Hu San* (Sanguisorba and Giant Knotweed Powder) mixed into a paste with sunflower oil will produce good results.

Advice for the patient

- Pay strict attention to personal and environmental hygiene.
- Take measures to get rid of offending insects such as fleas, or use protective creams or nets against mosquitoes.
- Avoid eating food that produces an allergic reaction.

Modern clinical experience

1. **Zhang** identified four patterns for papular urticaria. [1]

- **Eruptions due to insect Toxins**

Prescription ingredients

Dang Shen (Radix Codonopsitis Pilosulae) 10g
Bai Zhu (Rhizoma Atractylodis Macrocephalae) 10g
Fu Ling (Sclerotium Poriae Cocos) 10g

Shi Jun Zi (Fructus Quisqualis Indicae) 6g
Lu Hui* (Herba Aloes) 10g
Ku Lian Pi (Cortex Meliae Radicis) 6g
Yu Zhu (Rhizoma Polygonati Odorati) 6g
Jiao Shan Zha (Fructus Crataegi, scorch-fried) 10g
Chan Tui‡ (Periostracum Cicadae) 6g
Bai Xian Pi (Cortex Dictamni Dasycarpi Radicis) 15g
Zhi Gan Cao (Radix Glycyrrhizae, mix-fried with honey) 6g

Fifty out of ninety-four patients recovered completely with this treatment after a two-week course.

- **Spleen and Stomach Deficiency**

Prescription
WU WEI YI GONG SAN JIA WEI
Five-Ingredient Special Achievement Powder, with additions

Dang Shen (Radix Codonopsitis Pilosulae) 10g
Bai Zhu (Rhizoma Atractylodis Macrocephalae) 10g
Fu Ling (Sclerotium Poriae Cocos) 10g
Chen Pi (Pericarpium Citri Reticulatae) 6g
Da Fu Pi (Pericarpium Arecae Catechu) 10g
Wu Mei (Fructus Pruni Mume) 15g
Fang Feng (Radix Ledebouriellae Divaricatae) 6g
Zhi Gan Cao (Radix Glycyrrhizae, mix-fried with honey) 6g

Thirty-three out of sixty-one patients recovered completely with this treatment after a two-week course.

- **Accumulated Heat complicated by invasion of Wind**

Prescription
XIAO FENG DAO CHI SAN JIA WEI
Decoction for Dispersing Wind and Guiding Out Reddish Urine, with modifications

Bai Xian Pi (Cortex Dictamni Dasycarpi Radicis) 10g
Jin Yin Hua (Flos Lonicerae) 15g
Fang Feng (Radix Ledebouriellae Divaricatae) 6g
Chan Tui‡ (Periostracum Cicadae) 10g
Bo He (Herba Menthae Haplocalycis) 6g
Fu Ling (Sclerotium Poriae Cocos) 10g

Niu Bang Zi (Fructus Arctii Lappae) 10g
Sheng Di Huang (Radix Rehmanniae Glutinosae) 10g
Hu Huang Lian (Rhizoma Picrorhizae Scrophulariiflorae) 10g
Yu Zhu (Rhizoma Polygonati Odorati) 6g
Dan Zhu Ye (Herba Lophatheri Gracilis) 6g
Tong Cao (Medulla Tetrapanacis Papyriferi) 6g
Gan Cao Shao (Radix Tenuis Glycyrrhizae) 6g

Fourteen out of twenty-five patients recovered completely with this treatment after a two-week course.

- **External contraction of Wind-Heat**

Prescription
QIU MA YIN
Papular Urticaria Beverage

Jing Jie (Herba Schizonepetae Tenuifoliae) 10g
Fang Feng (Radix Ledebouriellae Divaricatae) 10g
Chan Tui‡ (Periostracum Cicadae) 6g
Jin Yin Hua (Flos Lonicerae) 10g
Zi Cao (Radix Arnebiae seu Lithospermi) 15g
Ku Shen (Radix Sophorae Flavescentis) 15g
Bai Xian Pi (Cortex Dictamni Dasycarpi Radicis) 30g
Shan Zha (Fructus Crataegi) 10g
Gan Cao (Radix Glycyrrhizae) 10g

Seventeen out of twenty-five patients recovered completely with this treatment after a two-week course.

2. **Lu** made a medicinal lotion with *Long Dan Cao* (Radix Gentianae Scabrae) by decocting 5000g of the herb with 20 liters of water and boiling for 40 minutes. The liquid was poured off and another 10 liters of water added and boiled for 40 minutes. The two decoctions were filtered and condensed to 10 liters; 1% carbolic acid was then added to prevent deterioration. The liquid was stored in 100ml bottles. During the treatment, the lotion was applied to the eruptions four or five times a day. Two to three days' application was normally sufficient to reduce the wheals, which disappeared completely after four to five days' treatment. [2]

Scabies
疥疮

Scabies is a chronic itchy contagious skin disease caused by the mite *Sarcoptes scabiei* var. *hominis*. It is characterized by the development of vesicles and burrows in the skin at any site, characteristically at the wrist, the web of the fin-

gers and the lower abdomen, with intense itching at night.

Scabies may develop in people of all ages, is likely to spread through households and is often endemic in institutions such as schools and kindergartens. The incidence of scabies rises and falls in cycles.

Mites are transmitted from person to person via bodily contact. Fertilized female mites burrow through the stratum corneum at a rate of about 2mm a day, laying two or three eggs per day, which mature in two to three weeks. The itchy scabies eruption is probably caused by sensitization to the mite saliva and feces.

In TCM, scabies is known as *wo chuang* (*wo* sore), *shi jie* (Damp scabies), *chong jie* (Worm scabies), *lai jie* (*lai* scabies), and *gan ba jie* (dry scar scabies).

Clinical manifestations

- Scabies usually involves the sides of the fingers, the webs between the fingers, the sides of the hands, the wrists, the elbows, the ankles and feet, the nipples, the lower abdomen around the umbilicus, and the genitals and buttocks. It seldom involves the face, head or neck (except in children).

- Skin lesions usually start from the web space between the fingers and may spread to the other areas within one to two weeks.

- Once infected by the scabies mite, severe itching develops after four to six weeks; itching is worse on exposure to heat or at night.

- The main manifestations of the disease are burrows, papules and vesicles. The grayish burrows of the scabies mites are linear, curved or serpiginous, 1-2 mm wide and up to 10mm long, and are not always visible. They are often located in the fingers, wrists and genital area where the skin is thinner. The closed end where the scabies mites retreat is known as the scabies spot. At the same time, the patient may develop red pinpoint papules, varying in number and density.

- The scabies mites or their eggs and the toxins they contain may cause pinpoint to 2mm pale red or skin-colored relatively thick-walled vesicles containing a small amount of serous fluid. Watery exudate or erosion may be seen after excoriation.

- Secondary infection after scratching may lead to pustules, often accompanied by lymphangitis or lymphadenitis.

- Red nodular lesions may occur on the penis and scrotum in some patients.

- Microscopic examination will find the mites and eggs. Prick open the skin at both ends of the burrow with a needle, scrape gently and place the burrow scrapings on a black surface. If a tiny moving spot is seen, this is the scabies mite.

- Even if scabies mites cannot be found, this diagnosis should not be ruled out, since misdiagnosis will lead to delayed treatment or the spread of infection. Diagnosis may be established through careful study of epidemic conditions, history of contact with scabies sufferers, and the site and pattern of skin lesions.

Differential diagnosis

Scabies can be identified by the characteristic burrows; when these are not evident, differentiation should include the following intensely pruritic disorders as well as pruritus without a primary rash.

Papular urticaria
This frequently occurs in children during summer and autumn, usually as a reaction to insect bites. Lesions manifest initially as red, oval wheals with papulovesicles or vesicles at the center. Distribution on the trunk or limbs varies in number and configuration. Pruritus is common.

Pediculosis
In infection by body lice, lesions presents with hemorrhagic spots and papules at the sites bitten and severe local itching. Lice or their egg cases can usually be found.

Lichen planus
Eruptions usually involve the flexor surfaces of the wrists and forearms, and the lower legs around and above the ankles. Lesions manifest as intensely pruritic 2-10 mm flat-topped shiny papules with an irregular, sharply defined angulated border. The surface of the lesions exhibits a lacy white pattern of lines (Wickham's striae).

Eczema
Eczema can occur at any age and is non-contagious. Skin lesions are polymorphous – inflamed, itchy, weeping, and erosive during the acute phase, thick and coarse during the chronic phase.

Pruritus
This condition affects large areas or the whole body and is more common in adults. There are no primary rashes associated with pruritus, which is paroxysmal and worse at night. Secondary lesions such as scratch marks, crusts, eczematoid lesions, or lichenification may occur as a result of scratching.

Etiology and pathology

- Prolonged accumulation of Toxins internally generates Worms; if this is complicated by contraction of Wind-Damp, which accumulates and transforms into

Damp-Heat, Worm Toxins fight with Damp-Heat, binding and gathering in the skin and flesh to cause Blood Deficiency due to Wind-Damp-Heat, leading to the disease.

- Direct infection from contact with patients with scabies or through using clothes, quilts, bed linen, or towels that have been contaminated is another frequent cause.

Pattern identification and treatment

Scabies is usually treated externally without internal medication. If the disease is prolonged and the patient very weak, internal treatment may be indicated to back up external treatment.

INTERNAL TREATMENT

STEAMING OF DAMP-HEAT
This pattern manifests at the initial stage with widespread vesicles, which discharge a watery exudate when broken by scratching. Itching is unbearable. Accompanying symptoms and signs include a dry mouth and throat with a bitter taste, constipation and reddish urine. The tongue body is red with a thin yellow coating; the pulse is slippery.

Treatment principle
Clear Heat and eliminate Dampness, kill Worms and alleviate itching.

Prescription
XIAO FENG SAN HE HUANG LIAN JIE DU TANG JIA JIAN
Powder for Dispersing Wind Combined with Coptis Decoction for Relieving Toxicity, with modifications

Jing Jie (Herba Schizonepetae Tenuifoliae) 6g
Chan Tui‡ (Periostracum Cicadae) 6g
Chao Cang Zhu (Rhizoma Atractylodis, stir-fried) 6g
Fang Feng (Radix Ledebouriellae Divaricatae) 10g
Dang Gui (Radix Angelicae Sinensis) 10g
Ku Shen (Radix Sophorae Flavescentis) 10g
Chao Niu Bang Zi (Fructus Arctii Lappae, stir-fried) 10g
Fu Ling Pi (Cortex Poriae Cocos) 12g
Bai Xian Pi (Cortex Dictamni Dasycarpi Radicis) 12g
Sheng Di Huang (Radix Rehmanniae Glutinosae) 12g
Lu Hui* (Herba Aloes) 4.5g
Gan Cao (Radix Glycyrrhizae) 3g

Explanation
- Ku Shen (Radix Sophorae Flavescentis), Bai Xian Pi (Cortex Dictamni Dasycarpi Radicis), Fu Ling Pi (Cortex Poriae Cocos), Fang Feng (Radix Ledebouriellae Divaricatae), and Chao Cang Zhu (Rhizoma Atractylodis, stir-fried), dispel Wind and eliminate Dampness to alleviate itching.
- Jing Jie (Herba Schizonepetae Tenuifoliae), Chan Tui ‡ (Periostracum Cicadae) and Chao Niu Bang Zi (Fructus Arctii Lappae, stir-fried) dissipate Wind, clear Heat and release the exterior to alleviate itching.
- Ku Shen (Radix Sophorae Flavescentis) and Lu Hui* (Herba Aloes) clear Heat and kill Worms.
- Dang Gui (Radix Angelicae Sinensis) and Sheng Di Huang (Radix Rehmanniae Glutinosae) clear Heat in the Blood.
- Bai Xian Pi (Cortex Dictamni Dasycarpi Radicis) and Gan Cao (Radix Glycyrrhizae) clear Heat and relieve Toxicity.

Modifications
1. For intense itching, add She Chuang Zi (Fructus Cnidii Monnieri) and Di Fu Zi (Fructus Kochiae Scopariae).
2. For pronounced Heat signs, add Huang Lian (Rhizoma Coptidis), Mu Dan Pi (Cortex Moutan Radicis) and Jin Yin Hua (Flos Lonicerae).
3. For exudation, add Huang Qi (Radix Astragali seu Hedysari) and Mu Li (Concha Ostreae).

EXTERNAL TREATMENT
- Apply 10%-20% Liu Huang Ruan Gao (Sulfur Ointment) for adults; for infants and young children, dilute the ointment to a 5% concentration by mixing with Qing Liang Gao (Cool Clearing Paste).
  Method: Take a bath or shower with hot water and soap before commencing the treatment. Apply the ointment all over the body below the neck including the webs of the fingers and toes, once in the morning and once in the evening. Do not have a shower or bath or change clothes until the fourth day. Disinfect clothes and sheets by high-temperature laundering and tumble-drying or drying in the sun. After two weeks, if the patient still has itching or scabies mites are found, repeat the treatment. Most patients will be cured after one or two treatments.
  Alternative application: For adults, mix Dian Dao San (Reversal Powder) with vinegar and apply as above.
- Prepare a decoction with Hua Jiao (Pericarpium Zanthoxyli) 9g, Ku Fan ‡ (Alumen Praeparatum) 15g and Di Fu Zi (Fructus Kochiae Scopariae) 30g and use as a steam-wash. Then mix powdered Liu Huang‡ (Sulphur) 20g with cooked pork lard‡ and apply to the affected area.
- Grind Liu Huang ‡ (Sulphur) 12g, Song Xiang (Resina Pini) 10g and Qian Dan ‡ (Minium) 3g into a fine powder, mix with Xiang You (Oleum Sesami Seminis) and apply to the affected area.

ACUPUNCTURE

Points: LI-11 Quchi, EX-UE-9 Baxie,[iv] SP-10 Xuehai, EX-LE-3 Baichongwo,[v] SP-9 Yinlingquan, and EX-LE-10 Bafeng.[vi]

Technique: Apply the reducing method. Retain the needles for 30 minutes after obtaining Qi. During this period, manipulate the needles three to five times. Treat once a day. A course consists of ten treatment sessions.

Explanation

- EX-UE-9 Baxie, EX-LE-10 Bafeng and EX-LE-3 Baichongwo dispel Wind, kill Worms and alleviate itching.
- LI-11 Quchi, SP-10 Xuehai and SP-9 Yinlingquan clear Heat and cool the Blood.

EAR ACUPUNCTURE

Points: Liver, Spleen and Ear-Shenmen.

Technique: Retain the needles for 30 minutes. Treat every two days. A course consists of seven treatment sessions.

FOLK REMEDIES

- Wash the affected area once a day with a decoction of *Hua Jiao* (Pericarpium Zanthoxyli) 10g and *Di Fu Zi* (Fructus Kochiae Scopariae) 30g; or *Xian Cai Gen* (Radix Amaranthi Tricoloris) 30g and *Fu Ping* (Herba Spirodelae Polyrrhizae) 30g; or *Bi Ba* (Fructus Piperis Longi) 3g; or *Nao Yang Hua* (Flos Rhododendri Mollis) 20g.
- Grind *Huang Lian* (Rhizoma Coptidis) 10g and *Cang Er Zi* (Fructus Xanthii Sibirici) 15g into a fine powder, add *Bing Pian* (Borneolum) 2.5g, grind again and mix well. Then make into a paste with Vaseline® and apply to the affected area once a day.
- Soak *Bai Bu* (Radix Stemonae) 50g in 500ml of *Bai Jiu* (Granorum Spiritus Incolor) for seven days, remove the herb and apply the liquid to the affected area twice a day.

Clinical notes

- Treatment is mainly external, based on the principle of killing Worms and alleviating itching. Sulfur preparations are recognized as an effective and safe treatment. Concentrations of preparations for external use should be 10-20% for adults and around 5% for children.
- Since scabies is a highly contagious disease, treatment should be complete. Observe patients for at least two weeks after cessation of treatment to see if there is any relapse. It takes about 15 days for the scabies egg to develop into the mite.
- Any patient identified with scabies should be treated promptly to stop the disease spreading to others. All household members and sexual partners should also be treated, irrespective of whether they are suffering from itching.

Advice for the patient

- Pay strict attention to personal hygiene.
- Patient's clothes, bedding and towels should be laundered to kill the mites.

Literature excerpts

Scabies was recorded very early. The ideogram *jie* (scabies) was already present in tortoiseshell characters as early as the 14th century BC. *Zhou Hou Bei Ji Fang* [A Handbook of Prescriptions for Emergencies] from the Western Jin dynasty (265-316) listed medicines for the treatment of scabies.

According to *Zhu Bing Yuan Hou Lun: Jie Hou* [A General Treatise on the Causes and Symptoms of Diseases: Scabies] from the Sui dynasty (582-618): "Scabies often develops in the hands and feet, then spreads all over the body. *Da jie* (large scabies) form sores containing pus, which are inflamed, itchy and painful. …. *Shi jie* (Damp scabies) are small and thin-skinned, often with exudate. Both are caused by parasites, which can often be picked up by a needle. *Wo* scabies often develop in the hands and feet, look like the new fruits of *Wu Zhu Yu* (Fructus Evodiae Rutaecarpae), and are painful and itchy. Scratching produces yellow exudate."

In *Wai Ke Da Cheng: Jie Chuang Lun* [A Compendium of External Diseases: On Scabies Sores] from the Ming dynasty (1368-1644), it says: "Scabies, hidden under the skin, passing through the skin and attacking, cause itching and boring pain."

Modern clinical experience

EXTERNAL TREATMENT

1. **Zou** et al prepared an empirical prescription for use as a rub.[3]

[iv] M-UE-22 according to the system employed by the Shanghai College of Traditional Chinese Medicine.
[v] M-LE-34 according to the system employed by the Shanghai College of Traditional Chinese Medicine.
[vi] M-LE-8 according to the system employed by the Shanghai College of Traditional Chinese Medicine.

Prescription
SHE CHUANG ZI BAI BU DING
Cnidium and Stemona Root Tincture

She Chuang Zi (Fructus Cnidii Monnieri) 250g
Bai Bu (Radix Stemonae) 250g

The ingredients were ground into a powder and moistened with cold boiled water for 30 minutes. Then 400ml of 75% alcohol was added and the mixture was sealed and steeped for 15 days. The liquid was strained and the tincture allowed to settle before being poured into 200ml bottles. Patients took a bath with warm water, then rubbed the tincture all over the body once a day for five days.

2. **Zeng** treated scabies with an external wash modified according to lesions. [4]

Prescription
XI JIE FANG
Scabies Wash Formula

Li Lu (Radix et Rhizoma Veratri) 20-30g
Da Feng Zi (Semen Hydnocarpi) 20-30g
Liu Huang‡ (Sulphur) 20-30g
Hua Jiao (Pericarpium Zanthoxyli) 8-10g

Modifications
1. For infection producing pustules, *Hua Jiao* (Pericarpium Zanthoxyli) was removed and *Yu Xing Cao* (Herba Houttuyniae Cordatae) 20-30g and *Pu Gong Ying* (Herba Taraxaci cum Radice) 20-30g added.
2. For nodules, *Zao Jiao Ci* (Spina Gleditsiae Sinensis) 20-30g and *Bai Ji Li* (Fructus Tribuli Terrestris) 20-30g were added.

The decoction was used as an external wash for about 20 minutes once a day. Improvements were seen within two to four days.

3. **Liu et al** also prepared a wash for external application. [5]

Prescription ingredients

Huang Bai (Cortex Phellodendri) 30g
Bai Bu (Radix Stemonae) 30g
Da Feng Zi (Semen Hydnocarpi) 30g
She Chuang Zi (Fructus Cnidii Monnieri) 30g
Ku Shen (Radix Sophorae Flavescentis) 30g
Hua Jiao (Pericarpium Zanthoxyli) 30g
Tu Jin Pi (Cortex Pseudolaricis) 30g
Bo He (Herba Menthae Haplocalycis) 15g

A decoction was prepared to wash the affected area or the whole body for 30 minutes once a day. Seven days made up a course of treatment. Results were seen after 5-14 days.

Pediculosis (lice infection)
虱病

Lice are flat, wingless, blood-sucking insects. Their eggs, known as nits, are laid on hair shafts and clothing. All types of lice induce severe itching; scratching subsequently results in excoriation and secondary infection. Two species of lice affect humans – *Pediculus humanus* (which has two varieties, *P. humanus capitis*, the head louse, and *P. humanus corporis*, the body louse) and *Phthirus pubis*, the pubic louse.

These species of lice are obligate human parasites; in other words, they cannot survive on other animals. Lice live for around one month and suck blood every three to six hours. Females lay seven to ten eggs a day; the nits hatch in eight to ten days. Nits are usually easier to see than lice. Lice infection results in itching due to a hypersensitivity reaction to louse saliva; in immunocompromised individuals, the itching response is muted.

Clinical manifestations

Head lice
- Head lice are common among schoolchildren, with girls more affected than boys.
- Lice infection is extremely contagious, spreading through head-to-head contact or by shared combs or hats.
- Examination of the hair reveals nits tightly bound to the hair shaft and difficult to remove.
- Itching caused by head lice usually starts at the sides and back of the scalp before becoming more general.
- Erythematous papules appear at the sites bitten and itching is severe.
- Scratching leads to secondary infection with exudation

and crusting. The condition may be complicated by impetigo or inflammation.

- In heavy infestations, exudation and crusting lead to the hair becoming matted and smelly. Cervical lymph nodes may enlarge.

Body lice

- Body lice usually affect those living in poor or unhygienic social conditions with little regard for personal hygiene. This condition is now relatively rare in developed countries.
- The lice are spread by direct contact or sharing infected clothes and bedding.
- Lice hide in the seams of clothes and bedding and usually suck blood from the shoulder, back or waist.
- The condition presents with hemorrhagic spots and papules at the sites bitten. Itching is severe, with scratching resulting in excoriations on the trunk, usually accompanied by exudation and crusting, possibly with impetigo.
- In chronic, untreated infections, lichenification and pigmentation is common.

Pubic lice

- Pubic lice (also known as crabs) are generally transmitted by sexual contact and are mostly found in young adults.
- The condition presents with papules at the sites bitten and intense itching. Scratching results in exudation and crusting with secondary eczema and infection. Inflammation is common in untreated cases.
- Lice and nits can be seen in the pubic hair.

Differential diagnosis

Head lice

Patients with chronic impetigo or crusting eczema on the scalp should be examined for lice and nits. The scales (dandruff) of seborrheic eczema are not as firmly attached to the hair shafts.

Body lice

Lesions should be inspected for similarity to the burrows characteristic of scabies. The presence of lice and nits excludes eczema.

Pubic lice

Genital eczema resembles lice infection and manifests as papules, papulovesicles, exudation, erosion, and crusting. When the condition becomes persistent, scratching results in excoriation, infiltration and lichenification. The presence of lice and nits excludes eczema.

Etiology and pathology

Pathogenic Toxins invade the skin and flesh after lice bites damage the skin.

Treatment

EXTERNAL TREATMENT
External treatment only is needed to kill the lice and nits.

Head lice
Apply 25% *Bai Bu Ding* (Stemona Root Tincture) and benzyl benzoate gel [vii] once a day and then wrap the head in a towel for 12 hours. Apply for three to five days. This procedure kills the lice. Comb the hair to get rid of the nits. Repeat the treatment after eight days to eliminate any remaining lice. Ordinary laundering, tumble-drying or dry-cleaning is usually sufficient to eliminate lice from hats, scarves, pillow cases, and any other infested items of clothing or bed linen. Combs should be disinfected.

Body lice
Disinfect clothes, bedding and any other infested items by laundering, tumble-drying or dry-cleaning. After a warm bath or shower, patients should rub 10% *Bai Bu Ding* (Stemona Root Tincture) into all affected areas for 30 minutes once a day for three to five days. Change to non-infested clothing.

Pubic lice
Rub in 10% *Bai Bu Ding* (Stemona Root Tincture) for 30 minutes once a day for three to five days. This treatment should be applied to all the trunk and limbs, not just the pubic area. The pubic hair can be shaved if necessary. Treat all sexual contacts. Disinfect clothes, bedding and any other infected items by laundering, tumble-drying or dry-cleaning. Change to non-infected clothes.

In addition, in all three types of lice infection, *San Huang Xi Ji* (Three Yellows Wash Preparation) or *Dian Dao San* (Reversal Powder) can be applied twice a day until the lesions disappear.

Clinical notes

- Once lice infection is found, thorough treatment is required. All infected items must be disinfected completely to get rid of the source of infestation.
- If infestations are complicated by other skin disorders such as impetigo and folliculitis, treatment for those diseases should be implemented.

[vii] In some countries, benzyl benzoate gel may only be available on a prescription basis.

Advice for the patient

Proper hygiene is paramount. Schoolchildren should be warned against sharing combs, headgear or earphones, and against head contact.

References

1. Zhang Xucang, *Bian Zheng Wei Zhu Zhi Liao Qiu Zhen Xing Qian Ma Zhen 203 Li* [Treatment of 203 Cases of Papular Urticaria Based on Pattern Identification], *Pi Fu Bing Yu Xing Bing* [Journal of Dermatology and Venereology] 17, 1 (1995): 80.
2. Lu Shubai, *Long Dan Jian Ji Zhi Liao Qiu Zhen Xing Qian Ma Zhen 60 Li* [Treatment of 60 Cases of Papular Urticaria with a *Long Dan Cao* (Radix Gentianae Scabrae) Decoction], *Yun Nan Zhong Yi Zhong Yao* [Yunnan Journal of Traditional Chinese Medicine and Materia Medica] 17, 6 (1996): 62-63.
3. Zou Mingxiang et al, *She Chuang Zi Bai Bu Ding Zhi Liao Cheng Ren Jie Chuang 280 Li* [Treatment of 280 Adult Cases of Scabies With *She Chuang Zi Bai Bu Ding* (Cnidium and Stemona Root Tincture)], *Zhe Jiang Zhong Yi Za Zhi* [Zhejiang Journal of Traditional Chinese Medicine] 1 (1990): 23.
4. Zeng Qingfa, *Zi Ni Xi Jie Fang Zhi Liao Jie Chuang 68 Li* [Treatment of 68 Cases of Scabies with the Empirical Prescription *Xi Jie Fang* (Scabies Wash Formula)], *Guang Xi Zhong Yi Yao* [Guangxi Journal of Traditional Chinese Medicine and Materia Medica] 10, 4 (1987): 3.
5. Liu Jian et al, *Jie Shao Yi Zhong Zhi Chuang De Zhong Yao Fang* [Description of a Chinese Materia Medica Formula for Treating Scabies], *Zhong Guo Yi Yuan Yao Xue Za Zhi* [Chinese Journal of Hospital Pharmacology] 9, 7 (1989): 331.

Chapter 19

Benign skin tumors

Tumors, also known as neoplasms, are an enlargement of the tissues to form a mass. This mass arises from existing body cells and is characterized by a tendency to autonomous and unrestricted growth. Tumors differ from inflammatory or other swellings because the cells they contain are abnormal in their appearance and other characteristics, having frequently resulted from hypertrophy, hyperplasia or dysplasia.

Some tumors are composed of cells that appear different from their parent cells in size, shape and structure – these tumors are usually malignant. All tumors, benign or malignant in type, can cause death by local effects depending on location. However, malignancy is normally taken to mean an inherent tendency of the cells in the tumor to disseminate widely both locally (local invasion) and throughout the body (metastasis) and finally to cause the patient to die unless all the malignant cells can be destroyed.

Cells in a benign tumor tend to remain in one solid mass centered on the site of origin and may be removed completely by surgery if the location allows. A benign tumor may undergo malignant transformation, and a malignant tumor may remain quiescent for long periods, mimicking a benign tumor. However, a malignant tumor will never regress to a benign tumor.

The major types of benign tumors relevant to skin diseases include lipomas, which are composed of fat cells; angiomas, composed of blood or lymphatic vessels; and adenomas, which arise from glands. This chapter discusses benign tumors of the dermis (hemangiomas, nevus flammeus, keloids, and lipomas) and the epidermis (benign melanocytic nevi).

In TCM, skin tumors have the following etiology:

- Internal damage can be caused by the seven emotions; for instance, worry or depression leads to Qi stagnation and Blood congealing, with binding of turbid Phlegm.
- External Wind can invade or attack ulcers or wounds.
- The five emotions can transform into Fire, generating Heat Toxins in the Xue level, which spread outward to the skin.

Hemangioma
血管瘤

Hemangioma is a benign tumor composed of blood vessels and is the most common vascular tumor in babies and infants. The most obvious symptom is a bright red macule or nodule, commonly situated on the head or neck.

In TCM, hemangioma is also known as *xue liu* (blood tumor).

Clinical manifestations

- These vascular tumors generally occur in the first year of life, with female patients outnumbering males.

Strawberry hemangioma

- Strawberry hemangiomas (or nevi), also known as capillary hemangiomas, usually appear on the head or neck within a few weeks of birth.
- They manifest initially as one or more pink vascular macules, growing over a few weeks or several months into bright red (strawberry-colored), firm, lobulated, compressible nodules that do not blanch on pressure.
- Lesions generally grow rapidly over weeks, stabilize over months and gradually regress over years, with the central part of the lesion whitening.

- Involution usually occurs by age 5-9 years.

Cavernous hemangioma
- This condition presents as soft subcutaneous lumps with an ill-defined skin-colored, red or blue surface. If expansion leads to ulceration, there will be secondary infection and subsequent scarring.
- Cavernous hemangiomas may extend quite deeply and compress underlying structures. Any organ system may be involved, with frequency of incidence noted as skin, bone, liver, skeleton, muscle, and intestines.

Etiology and pathology

- The Heart governs the Blood and vessels. Heat in the Blood caused by the frenetic stirring of Heart-Fire due to emotional dissatisfaction in the mother may be inherited; if this is complicated by external contraction of Cold, these pathogenic factors will congeal and bind in the skin and flesh, resulting in the condition.
- Where Qi stagnation and Blood binding is caused by insufficiency of Original Qi (Yuan Qi), movement of Qi and Blood in the channels and network vessels is impaired. If at the same time external pathogenic factors invade the body, they will fight with Qi and Blood, causing them to accumulate in the channels and network vessels.

Pattern identification and treatment

INTERNAL TREATMENT

BLOOD STASIS DUE TO BLOOD-HEAT
This pattern occurs with strawberry hemangioma. At the initial stage, a red swelling appears on the skin and increases gradually in size. There is often a sensation of heat in the affected area. The tongue body is red with a scant coating; the pulse is thready and rapid.

Treatment principle
Cool and invigorate the Blood, enrich Yin and repress Fire.

Prescription
QIN LIAN ER MU TANG JIA JIAN
Scutellaria, Coptis, Anemarrhena, and Fritillaria Decoction, with modifications

Huang Qin (Radix Scutellariae Baicalensis) 6g
Zhi Mu (Rhizoma Anemarrhenae Asphodeloidis) 6g
Zhe Bei Mu (Bulbus Fritillariae Thunbergii) 6g
Chao Bai Shao (Radix Paeoniae Lactiflorae, stir-fried) 10g

Jiu Chao Dang Gui (Radix Angelicae Sinensis, stir-fried with wine) 6g
Sheng Di Huang (Radix Rehmanniae Glutinosae) 10g
Shu Di Huang (Radix Rehmanniae Glutinosae Conquita) 10g
Di Gu Pi (Cortex Lycii Radicis) 10g
Chuan Xiong (Rhizoma Ligustici Chuanxiong) 4.5g
Gan Cao (Radix Glycyrrhizae) 4.5g
Pu Huang (Pollen Typhae) 4.5g
Ling Yang Jiao* (Cornu Antelopis) 4.5g
Zi Cao (Radix Arnebiae seu Lithospermi) 12g

Explanation
- Huang Qin (Radix Scutellariae Baicalensis), Zhi Mu (Rhizoma Anemarrhenae Asphodeloidis), Gan Cao (Radix Glycyrrhizae), and Ling Yang Jiao* (Cornu Antelopis) clear Heat retained in the Lungs and Stomach.
- Jiu Chao Dang Gui (Radix Angelicae Sinensis, stir-fried with wine), Chao Bai Shao (Radix Paeoniae Lactiflorae, stir-fried), Sheng Di Huang (Radix Rehmanniae Glutinosae), Shu Di Huang (Radix Rehmanniae Glutinosae Conquita), and Di Gu Pi (Cortex Lycii Radicis) regulate Qi and invigorate the Blood, constrain Yin and transform Blood stasis.
- Pu Huang (Pollen Typhae) and Zi Cao (Radix Arnebiae seu Lithospermi) cool the Blood and stop bleeding.
- Chuan Xiong (Rhizoma Ligustici Chuanxiong) moves Qi, invigorates the Blood and disperses tumors.
- Zhe Bei Mu (Bulbus Fritillariae Thunbergii) transforms Phlegm to dissipate lumps.
- The prescription contains ingredients to stop bleeding, regulate Qi and transform Phlegm, thus treating the Root, and ingredients to clear Heat, cool the Blood and dissipate lumps, thus treating the Manifestations. On the one hand, cooling the Blood and stopping bleeding reduces bleeding externally from the tumor into the skin and prevents the blood tumor (hemangioma) from expanding; on the other hand, blood tumors on the skin surface are considered in TCM as being caused by Blood stasis due to blood leaking outside the vessels and so Blood stasis must also be transformed.

BLOOD STASIS DUE TO COLD CONGEALING
This pattern occurs when strawberry hemangioma has persisted for a long period and usually manifests with dark purple tumors. Accompanying symptoms include aversion to cold and pain that worsens at night. The tongue body is dull red with a scant coating; the pulse is thready and rough.

Treatment principle
Warm the channels and supplement Qi, invigorate the Blood and transform Blood stasis.

Prescription
TONG QIAO HUO XUE TANG JIA JIAN
Decoction for Freeing the Orifices and Invigorating the Blood, with modifications

Dang Gui (Radix Angelicae Sinensis) 12g
Chi Shao (Radix Paeoniae Rubra) 12g
Huang Qi (Radix Astragali seu Hedysari) 12g
Sheng Di Huang (Radix Rehmanniae Glutinosae) 12g
Shu Di Huang (Radix Rehmanniae Glutinosae Conquita) 12g
Chuan Xiong (Rhizoma Ligustici Chuanxiong) 10g
Gui Zhi (Ramulus Cinnamomi Cassiae) 10g
Fu Pen Zi (Fructus Rubi Chingii) 10g
San Leng (Rhizoma Sparganii Stoloniferi) 6g
E Zhu (Rhizoma Curcumae) 6g
Gan Jiang (Rhizoma Zingiberis Officinalis) 6g
Chuan Shan Jia* (Squama Manitis Pentadactylae) 6g
Huo Xue Teng (Caulis seu Radix Schisandrae) 15g
Ji Xue Teng (Caulis Spatholobi) 15g
Ru Xiang (Gummi Olibanum) 4.5g
Mo Yao (Myrrha) 4.5g

Explanation
- *Huang Qi* (Radix Astragali seu Hedysari), *Sheng Di Huang* (Radix Rehmanniae Glutinosae), *Shu Di Huang* (Radix Rehmanniae Glutinosae Conquita), *Chuan Xiong* (Rhizoma Ligustici Chuanxiong), *Gui Zhi* (Ramulus Cinnamomi Cassiae), *Gan Jiang* (Rhizoma Zingiberis Officinalis), and *Fu Pen Zi* (Fructus Rubi Chingii) augment Qi and warm Yang, warm the channels and free the network vessels.
- *Dang Gui* (Radix Angelicae Sinensis), *Chi Shao* (Radix Paeoniae Rubra), *San Leng* (Rhizoma Sparganii Stoloniferi), *E Zhu* (Rhizoma Curcumae), *Chuan Shan Jia** (Squama Manitis Pentadactylae), *Huo Xue Teng* (Caulis seu Radix Schisandrae), *Ji Xue Teng* (Caulis Spatholobi), Ru Xiang (Gummi Olibanum), and *Mo Yao* (Myrrha) invigorate the Blood and transform Blood stasis, free the network vessels and alleviate pain.

BLOOD STASIS DUE TO QI DEFICIENCY

This pattern occurs with cavernous hemangioma. Lesions manifest as bright or dull red, soft, circular or semicircular protuberances with a complex reticular pattern of vessels. They shrink in size and height on pressure but are restored after release. The tongue body is pale red with a scant coating; the pulse is thready and weak.

Treatment principle
Augment Qi and cool the Blood, enrich Yin and free the network vessels.

Prescription
SI WU TANG JIA JIAN
Four Agents Decoction, with modifications

Sheng Di Huang (Radix Rehmanniae Glutinosae) 10g
Bai Shao (Radix Paeoniae Lactiflorae) 10g
Chi Shao (Radix Paeoniae Rubra) 10g
Chao Mu Dan Pi (Cortex Moutan Radicis, stir-fried) 10g
Zi Cao (Radix Arnebiae seu Lithospermi) 10g
Dan Shen (Radix Salviae Miltiorrhizae) 10g
Huang Qi (Radix Astragali seu Hedysari) 30g
Dang Shen (Radix Codonopsitis Pilosulae) 15g
Bai Ying (Herba Solani Lyrati) 15g
Mu Man Tou (Flos Fici Pumilae) 15g
Tu Fu Ling (Rhizoma Smilacis Glabrae) 15g

Explanation
- *Sheng Di Huang* (Radix Rehmanniae Glutinosae), *Bai Shao* (Radix Paeoniae Lactiflorae), *Chi Shao* (Radix Paeoniae Rubra), *Zi Cao* (Radix Arnebiae seu Lithospermi), *Dan Shen* (Radix Salviae Miltiorrhizae), and *Chao Mu Dan Pi* (Cortex Moutan Radicis, stir-fried) cool the Blood and free the network vessels.
- *Huang Qi* (Radix Astragali seu Hedysari) and *Dang Shen* (Radix Codonopsitis Pilosulae) augment Qi and warm Yang.
- *Bai Ying* (Herba Solani Lyrati), *Mu Man Tou* (Flos Fici Pumilae) and *Tu Fu Ling* (Rhizoma Smilacis Glabrae) relieve Toxicity and transform Dampness, disperse tumors and alleviate pain.

EXTERNAL TREATMENT
If the tumor is large, use the licorice tumor-shrinking method. Make a paste from decocted *Gan Cao* (Radix Glycyrrhizae) and spread it around the edge of the tumor three times with a small brush. Grind equal quantities of *Yuan Hua* (Flos Daphnes Genkwa), *Jing Da Ji* (Radix Euphorbiae Pekinensis) and *Gan Sui* (Radix Euphorbiae Kansui) into a powder and mix with vinegar for application to the center of the tumor. Make sure that the two preparations do not come into contact with one another.[i]

ACUPUNCTURE
Points: HT-7 Shenmen, PC-6 Neiguan and LR-3 Taichong.
Technique: Apply the reducing method and retain the needles for 15-30 minutes after obtaining Qi. Treat once every two days. A course consists of ten treatment sessions.

---

[i] According to the ancient classics, *Gan Cao* (Radix Glycyrrhizae) is incompatible with *Yuan Hua* (Flos Daphnes Genkwa), *Jing Da Ji* (Radix Euphorbiae Pekinensis) and *Gan Sui* (Radix Euphorbiae Kansui), these herbs being part of the Eighteen Incompatibilities. If they do come into contact, wash off with tap water.

Explanation
HT-7 Shenmen, PC-6 Neiguan and LR-3 Taichong clear the Heart and cool the Blood, move Qi and invigorate the Blood.

Clinical notes

- It is essential to achieve the right balance between cooling the Blood and transforming Blood stasis during treatment. The result will be better if materia medica for regulating Qi and invigorating the Blood are added to the prescription.
- Hemangiomas will normally have resolved by the age of 9. However, if the tumor is very enlarged or interfering with vital structures, the patient should be referred to a doctor of Western medicine for consideration of plastic surgery.

Advice for the patient

For cavernous hemangiomas especially, try to keep the child calm and prevent it from crying or shouting; this will reduce the amount of blood flowing into the tumor.

Literature excerpt

In *Dong Tian Ao Zhi (Wai Ke Mi Lu)* [Secret Records of External Diseases], it says: "*Xue liu* (blood tumor) is a wart generated on the outer surface of the skin and is caused by Blood stasis in the Zang-Fu organs combined with Damp pathogenic factors entering the Blood. At the initial stage, it may be as fine as a hair, but it enlarges as time passes. Small tumors look like a berry, larger ones resemble an eggplant."

Modern clinical experience

INTERNAL TREATMENT
Hu Anbang followed the principle of dredging the Liver and draining Fire, transforming Phlegm and dissipating lumps to treat both types of hemangioma. [1]

Prescription ingredients

Chai Hu (Radix Bupleuri) 5g
Long Dan Cao (Radix Gentianae Scabrae) 3g
Xia Ku Cao (Spica Prunellae Vulgaris) 3g
Ban Lan Gen (Radix Isatidis seu Baphicacanthi) 5g
*Zhi Bie Jia** (Carapax Amydae Sinensis, mix-fried with vinegar) 10g
Di Gu Pi (Cortex Lycii Radicis) 6g
Feng Wei Cao (Herba Pteridis Multifidi) 3g
Di Long‡ (Lumbricus) 3g
Chan Tui‡ (Periostracum Cicadae) 3g
Jiang Can‡ (Bombyx Batryticatus) 3g
Lou Lu (Radix Rhapontici seu Echinopsis) 3g
Sheng Jiang (Rhizoma Zingiberis Officinalis Recens) 3g

One bag a day was used to prepare a decoction, taken twice a day. Tumors had shrunk noticeably after intake of 45 bags of the prescription and disappeared after 124 bags.

EXTERNAL TREATMENT
Xie treated cavernous hemangioma externally. [2]

Prescription
XUE GUAN LIU CHA JI
Hemangioma Application

Hong Hua (Flos Carthami Tinctorii) 15g
Xue Jie (Resina Draconis) 15g
San Qi (Radix Notoginseng) 15g
Shui Zhi‡ (Hirudo seu Whitmania) 15g
Tao Ren (Semen Persicae) 20g
Dang Gui Wei (Extremitas Radicis Angelicae Sinensis) 20g
San Leng (Rhizoma Sparganii Stoloniferi) 20g
E Zhu (Rhizoma Curcumae) 20g

The ingredients were baked over a fire until dry, ground into a fine powder and steeped in 500ml of rice vinegar for a month. The mixture was then spread over the tumor three or four times a day. Results were seen after three months.

Nevus flammeus
鲜红斑痣

Nevus flammeus is caused by congenitally dilated mature dermal blood vessels. Lesions, usually present at birth, are normal tissue that is arranged or functions abnormally. These malformations present as two main types – salmon patches (also known as stork bites) and port-wine stains.

In TCM, nevus flammeus is also known as *chi ci* (red blemish).

Clinical manifestations

Salmon patches

- These patches are common at birth and may be present in one-third to one-half of all babies.
- They manifest as one or several pink or dull red macules or patches, with clear but irregularly defined margins. The color fades on pressure but returns on release. Emotional upsets may cause the color to deepen temporarily.
- Patches are found most frequently on the nape of the neck, especially between the occipital tuberosity and the fifth cervical vertebrae, the forehead and the upper eyelids.
- The long axis of lesions on the nape may point proximally or distally. Lesions in this region tend to persist.
- Lesions on the forehead and eyelids usually fade during childhood.

Port-wine stains

- This type of nevus is also present at birth and usually involves the face and neck, but may occasionally occur on the trunk.
- Lesions manifest as one or several dull red to purple macules or patches, with clear but irregularly defined margins. Pale lesions may hardly be noticeable, whereas deep-colored lesions may cause a significant cosmetic problem for the patient.
- Port-wine stains do not normally fade with age. In middle age, they may darken and become interspersed with nodules.
- Occasionally, a port-wine stain of the trigeminal area may be complicated by epilepsy. Port-wine stains near the eye may be associated with glaucoma.

Etiology and pathology

- Where Qi stagnation and Blood binding is caused by insufficiency of Original Qi (Yuan Qi), movement of Qi and Blood in the channels and network vessels is impaired. If at the same time external pathogenic factors invade the body, they will fight with Qi and Blood, causing them to accumulate in the channels and network vessels.
- Where disharmony of Qi and Blood is aggravated by Wind restricting the exterior, the channels and network vessels are obstructed and movement inhibited.

Pattern identification and treatment

INTERNAL TREATMENT

BLOOD STASIS OBSTRUCTING THE NETWORK VESSELS

The lesion, present at birth or appearing shortly afterward, manifests as a circumscribed bright red or crimson patch on the head or neck, especially the occipital region. The surface feels smooth and generally remains unchanged over time. The tongue body is normal or slightly dull with a scant coating; the pulse is thready and small.

Treatment principle
Invigorate the Blood and free the network vessels, cool the Blood and reduce patches.

Prescription
TAO HONG SI WU TANG JIA JIAN
Peach Kernel and Safflower Four Agents Decoction, with modifications

Tao Ren (Semen Persicae) 6g
Hong Hua (Flos Carthami Tinctorii) 6g
Chi Shao (Radix Paeoniae Rubra) 6g
Dang Gui Wei (Extremitas Radicis Angelicae Sinensis) 12g
Ji Xue Teng (Caulis Spatholobi) 12g
Ren Dong Teng (Caulis Lonicerae Japonicae) 12g
Chen Pi (Pericarpium Citri Reticulatae) 10g
Si Gua Luo (Fasciculus Vascularis Luffae) 10g
Gui Jian Yu (Lignum Suberalatum Euonymi) 15g

Explanation

- *Tao Ren* (Semen Persicae), *Hong Hua* (Flos Carthami Tinctorii), *Chi Shao* (Radix Paeoniae Rubra), and *Dang Gui Wei* (Extremitas Radicis Angelicae Sinensis) invigorate the Blood and transform Blood stasis.
- *Ji Xue Teng* (Caulis Spatholobi), *Ren Dong Teng* (Caulis Lonicerae Japonicae) and *Si Gua Luo* (Fasciculus Vascularis Luffae) cool the Blood and free the

network vessels, transform Blood stasis and reduce patches.

- *Chen Pi* (Pericarpium Citri Reticulatae) regulates Qi, thereby assisting the other ingredients to transform Blood stasis.
- *Gui Jian Yu* (Lignum Suberalatum Euonymi) invigorates the Blood and dissipates lumps, thereby strengthening the effect of the other ingredients in freeing the network vessels.

QI AND BLOOD STAGNATING IN THE CHANNELS AND VESSELS

Bright red or dull red patches with clearly defined borders are comparatively extensive and do not resolve spontaneously. The tongue body is dark red with a scant coating; the pulse is rough.

Treatment principle
Invigorate the Blood and transform Blood stasis, free the channels and invigorate the network vessels.

Prescription
TONG QIAO HUO XUE TANG JIA JIAN
Decoction for Freeing the Orifices and Invigorating the Blood, with modifications

Tao Ren (Semen Persicae) 10g
Hong Hua (Flos Carthami Tinctorii) 10g
Chuan Xiong (Rhizoma Ligustici Chuanxiong) 10g
Chi Shao (Radix Paeoniae Rubra) 10g
Chao Mu Dan Pi (Cortex Moutan Radicis, stir-fried) 10g
Dang Gui Wei (Extremitas Radicis Angelicae Sinensis) 12g
Bai Zhi (Radix Angelicae Dahuricae) 6g
Bai Fu Zi (Rhizoma Typhonii Gigantei) 6g
Huang Jiu (Vinum Aureum) 50ml

Explanation
- *Tao Ren* (Semen Persicae), *Hong Hua* (Flos Carthami Tinctorii), *Chuan Xiong* (Rhizoma Ligustici Chuanxiong), *Chi Shao* (Radix Paeoniae Rubra), *Chao Mu Dan Pi* (Cortex Moutan Radicis, stir-fried), and *Dang Gui Wei* (Extremitas Radicis Angelicae Sinensis) invigorate the Blood and transform Blood stasis.
- *Bai Zhi* (Radix Angelicae Dahuricae), *Bai Fu Zi* (Rhizoma Typhonii Gigantei) and *Huang Jiu* (Vinum Aureum) regulate Qi and free the network vessels, and conduct the other ingredients upward to the affected area.

DISHARMONY OF QI AND BLOOD

The pale red skin lesions are relatively small with a clear but irregular margin. The color fades on pressure but returns on release. The tongue body is pale red with a scant coating; the pulse is thready and rapid.

Treatment principle
Regulate Qi and harmonize the Blood, free the network vessels and reduce patches.

Prescription
XUE FU ZHU YU TANG JIA JIAN
Decoction for Expelling Stasis from the House of Blood, with modifications

Dang Gui (Radix Angelicae Sinensis) 10g
Sheng Di Huang (Radix Rehmanniae Glutinosae) 10g
Hong Hua (Flos Carthami Tinctorii) 10g
Chuan Xiong (Rhizoma Ligustici Chuanxiong) 10g
Chao Zhi Ke (Fructus Citri Aurantii, stir-fried) 6g
Chai Hu (Radix Bupleuri) 6g
Xiang Fu (Rhizoma Cyperi Rotundi) 6g
Tao Ren (Semen Persicae) 6g
Jie Geng (Radix Platycodi Grandiflori) 6g
Qiang Huo (Rhizoma et Radix Notopterygii) 6g
Chi Shao (Radix Paeoniae Rubra) 15g
Dan Shen (Radix Salviae Miltiorrhizae) 15g
Huo Xue Teng (Caulis seu Radix Schisandrae) 15g

Explanation
- *Dang Gui* (Radix Angelicae Sinensis), *Sheng Di Huang* (Radix Rehmanniae Glutinosae), *Hong Hua* (Flos Carthami Tinctorii), *Chuan Xiong* (Rhizoma Ligustici Chuanxiong), *Dan Shen* (Radix Salviae Miltiorrhizae), *Huo Xue Teng* (Caulis seu Radix Schisandrae), *Chi Shao* (Radix Paeoniae Rubra), *Qiang Huo* (Rhizoma et Radix Notopterygii), and *Tao Ren* (Semen Persicae) invigorate the Blood and dissipate Blood stasis, free the network vessels and reduce patches.
- *Chao Zhi Ke* (Fructus Citri Aurantii, stir-fried), *Chai Hu* (Radix Bupleuri), *Xiang Fu* (Rhizoma Cyperi Rotundi), and *Jie Geng* (Radix Platycodi Grandiflori) dredge the Liver and transform Blood stasis, regulate Qi and invigorate the Blood.

Clinical notes

- For this condition, the treatment principle of augmenting Qi and invigorating the Blood to transform Blood stasis and reduce patches should be applied for Deficiency patterns and that of cooling and invigorating the Blood to transform Blood stasis and reduce patches for Excess patterns. The relative balance depends on the severity of the causative factors.
- In addition, in my clinic, we sometimes apply the main treatment principle of nourishing Yin and clearing Heat supported by transforming Blood stasis and reducing patches to treat bright red lesions, and that of transforming Blood stasis and reducing patches supported by nourishing Yin and clearing

Heat for dull red lesions.

- If herbal treatment does not render satisfactory results, the patient should be referred to a doctor of Western medicine for pulsed dye laser treatment or electrodesiccation.

Literature excerpt

In *Zhu Bing Yuan Hou Lun* [A General Treatise on the Causes and Symptoms of Diseases], it says: "*Chi ci* (red blemish) manifests as coin to hand-sized patches of mottled pink or red skin on the face or body with no pain or itching. They are caused by Wind pathogenic factors attacking the skin, leading to disharmony of Qi and Blood. If disharmony of Qi and Blood occurs in children, the flesh will redden, with the red patches gradually extending."

Keloid
瘢痕疙瘩

Keloid results from hyperplasia of connective tissue in the skin of predisposed persons, usually induced in response to trauma, including surgical trauma, or suppurative inflammation. Keloids are more common in black Africans than Caucasians. The tendency to develop keloids is genetically inherited. Keloids can be differentiated from hypertrophic scars because they extend beyond the original site of the injury.

In TCM, this condition is also known as *huang gua yong* (cucumber abscess), *xie zu zhong* (crab claw swelling) or *ban hen ge da* (scar pimple).

Clinical manifestations

- Both sexes are affected by keloids, which can occur at any age, but are more frequent up to the age of 30.
- Keloids can occur on any skin site, but mostly involve the presternal area, the neck, the shoulders, the upper back, and areas over skin flexural creases.
- At the initial stage, an elevated scar forms over the site of the injury. As the condition persists, the scar becomes firm with a smooth, skin-colored, pink or red surface, extending beyond the original limits of the injury. Lesions vary in size and number, and may be linear, nodular or irregular in shape.
- A sensation of itching and stabbing pain may occur.

Etiology and pathology

- In persons with constitutional Deficiency, invasion by external pathogenic factors or external injury from impact, burns, scalds, or insect bites causes disharmony between Qi and Blood, resulting in Qi stagnating and Blood congealing, leading to Blood stasis in the skin and flesh.
- Disharmony between Qi and Blood may also occur where residual toxins are not completely eliminated after the healing of abscesses or clove sores. Qi and Blood will congeal and accumulate, being retained in the skin and flesh to cause the condition.

Pattern identification and treatment

INTERNAL TREATMENT

ACCUMULATION OF RESIDUAL TOXINS
This pattern is seen at the initial stage. Lesions manifest as pale red protruding lumps resembling crab claws, possibly accompanied by itching. The tongue body is red with a thin white coating; the pulse is wiry and slippery.

Treatment principle
Relieve toxicity and dissipate lumps, free the channels and network vessels.

Prescription
JIE DU TONG LUO YIN JIA JIAN
Beverage for Relieving Toxicity and Freeing the Network Vessels, with modifications

Lian Qiao (Fructus Forsythiae Suspensae) 10g
Jin Yin Hua (Flos Lonicerae) 10g
Mu Dan Pi (Cortex Moutan Radicis) 10g
Chi Shao (Radix Paeoniae Rubra) 10g
Xia Ku Cao (Spica Prunellae Vulgaris) 10g
Lu Lu Tong (Fructus Liquidambaris) 12g
Dang Gui (Radix Angelicae Sinensis) 15g
Shan Ci Gu (Pseudobulbus Shancigu) 15g
Zhi Xiang Fu (Rhizoma Cyperi Rotundi Praeparata) 6g
Chuan Xiong (Rhizoma Ligustici Chuanxiong) 6g
Zao Jiao Ci (Spina Gleditsiae Sinensis) 6g

Explanation

- *Lian Qiao* (Fructus Forsythiae Suspensae), *Jin Yin Hua* (Flos Lonicerae), *Mu Dan Pi* (Cortex Moutan Radicis), *Chi Shao* (Radix Paeoniae Rubra), and *Xia Ku Cao* (Spica Prunellae Vulgaris) relieve Toxicity and dissipate lumps.
- *Lu Lu Tong* (Fructus Liquidambaris), *Dang Gui* (Radix Angelicae Sinensis), *Chuan Xiong* (Rhizoma Ligustici Chuanxiong), and *Zao Jiao Ci* (Spina Gleditsiae Sinensis) invigorate the Blood and free the network vessels, transform Blood stasis and soften hardness.
- *Shan Ci Gu* (Pseudobulbus Shancigu) and *Zhi Xiang Fu* (Rhizoma Cyperi Rotundi Praeparata) regulate Qi and transform Phlegm.

QI STAGNATING AND BLOOD CONGEALING

This pattern occurs in persistent conditions. Lesions manifest as dull purple swellings with irregular margins extending beyond the original wound and resembling a centipede or tree root. Intermittent itching or stabbing pain may occur. The tongue body is dark red with stasis marks; the pulse is rough.

Treatment principle

Invigorate the Blood and regulate Qi, relieve Toxicity and soften hardness.

Prescription

TAO HONG SI WU TANG JIA JIAN

Peach Kernel and Safflower Four Agents Decoction, with modifications

Tao Ren (Semen Persicae) 6g
Hong Hua (Flos Carthami Tinctorii) 6g
Qing Pi (Pericarpium Citri Reticulatae Viride) 6g
Chen Pi (Pericarpium Citri Reticulatae) 6g
Dang Gui Wei (Extremitas Radicis Angelicae Sinensis) 6g
Chi Shao (Radix Paeoniae Rubra) 10g
Dang Shen (Radix Codonopsitis Pilosulae) 10g
San Leng (Rhizoma Sparganii Stoloniferi) 4.5g
E Zhu (Rhizoma Curcumae) 4.5g
Huang Qi (Radix Astragali seu Hedysari) 12g
Zao Jiao Ci (Spina Gleditsiae Sinensis) 12g
Fu Ling (Sclerotium Poriae Cocos) 12g
Chuan Xiong (Rhizoma Ligustici Chuanxiong) 4.5g
Zhi Ke (Fructus Citri Aurantii) 4.5g
*Mu Xiang** (Radix Aucklandiae Lappae) 4.5g
Tu Bie Chong‡ (Eupolyphaga seu Steleophaga) 9g

Explanation

- *Tao Ren* (Semen Persicae), *Hong Hua* (Flos Carthami Tinctorii), *Dang Gui Wei* (Extremitas Radicis Angelicae Sinensis), *Chi Shao* (Radix Paeoniae Rubra), *San Leng* (Rhizoma Sparganii Stoloniferi), *E Zhu* (Rhizoma Cur-

cumae), and *Tu Bie Chong*‡ (Eupolyphaga seu Steleophaga) transform Blood stasis and dissipate lumps.
- *Qing Pi* (Pericarpium Citri Reticulatae Viride), *Chen Pi* (Pericarpium Citri Reticulatae), *Zao Jiao Ci* (Spina Gleditsiae Sinensis), *Chuan Xiong* (Rhizoma Ligustici Chuanxiong), *Zhi Ke* (Fructus Citri Aurantii), and *Mu Xiang** (Radix Aucklandiae Lappae) regulate Qi and free the network vessels.
- *Dang Shen* (Radix Codonopsitis Pilosulae), *Huang Qi* (Radix Astragali seu Hedysari) and *Fu Ling* (Sclerotium Poriae Cocos) augment Qi and percolate Dampness, support Vital Qi (Zheng Qi) and consolidate the Root.

General modifications

1. For the initial stage of superficial, bright red scars, add *Qian Cao Gen* (Radix Rubiae Cordifoliae), *Gui Jian Yu* (Lignum Suberalatum Euonymi), *Ren Dong Teng* (Caulis Lonicerae Japonicae), and *Shi Nan Teng* (Caulis Photiniae).
2. For deep-seated, dull red scars, add *Tao Ren* (Semen Persicae), *San Qi* (Radix Notoginseng), *Gou Teng* (Ramulus Uncariae cum Uncis), *Tian Ma** (Rhizoma Gastrodiae Elatae), *Zao Jiao* (Fructus Gleditsiae Sinensis), *Tu Bei Mu* (Tuber Bolbostemmatis), and *Duan Mu Li*‡ (Concha Ostreae Calcinata).

EXTERNAL TREATMENT

- For keloids at the initial stage, grind the following ingredients into a powder and mix with vegetable oil to make a paste for application to the affected area.

  *Fu Zi** (Radix Lateralis Aconiti Carmichaeli Praeparata) 15g
  Hai Piao Xiao‡ (Os Sepiae seu Sepiellae) 15g
  Duan Mu Li‡ (Concha Ostreae Calcinata) 15g
  Chuan Xiong (Rhizoma Ligustici Chuanxiong) 15g
  Fu Ling (Sclerotium Poriae Cocos) 15g

- For persistent keloids, apply *Hei Bu Yao Gao* (Black Cloth Medicated Paste), *Ba Hen Ruan Hua Gao* (Softening Scar Paste) or *Du Jiao Lian Gao* (Giant Typhonium Paste).

ACUPUNCTURE

Points: Ashi points
Technique: Insert 1.5 cun needles obliquely at an angle of 70° towards the center of the keloid from positions 0.5 cm distant from the edge of the lesion. Retain the needles for 30 minutes; manipulate them three to five times during this period. Treat once every two days. A course consists of ten treatment sessions.

SEVEN-STAR NEEDLING

Points: Ashi points.

Technique: After routine sterilization, lightly tap the thickened tissue with a seven-star needle until it turns slightly red. Treat once every three days. A course consists of ten treatment sessions.

Clinical notes

- Internal treatment follows the principles of invigorating the Blood and transforming Blood stasis, softening hardness and dissipating lumps. External treatment emphasizes softening hardness and dissipating lumps and often uses vinegar as a basis (see also Modern clinical experience below). A combination of internal and external treatment usually produces the best results.
- For cases complicated by Heat Toxins, herbs for clearing Heat and relieving Toxicity should be added; for cases complicated by Qi and Yin Deficiency, herbs for augmenting Qi and nourishing Yin should be added.
- In some cases, the keloid may spread gradually before stopping; spontaneous recovery is rare, although not unknown.

Advice for the patient

- Avoid trauma and the application of caustic medication.
- Eat less spicy food.
- If a prickly itching sensation is experienced, seek medical help immediately rather than simply applying a caustic agent.

Literature excerpt

According to *Zhong Yi Da Ci Dian* [A Dictionary of Chinese Medicine], keloids are due to pathogenic factors invading the Heart and Kidney channels. It describes the lesion as tortoise-shaped with a head, tail and four feet, located on the intercostal regions of the chest and back, and rising 2 cun above the normal skin surface.

Modern clinical experience

Reports on the treatment of keloids mainly focus on external applications composed of materia medica that harmonize Ying Qi (Nutritive Qi), soften hardness, transform Blood stasis, and dissipate lumps.

1. **Zhao Bingnan** formulated a medicated paste to treat *xie zu zhong* (crab claw swelling) and other hyperplastic skin diseases by breaking up Blood stasis and softening hardness. [3]

Prescription
HEI BU YAO GAO
Black Cloth Medicated Paste

Lao Hei Cu (Acetum Atrum Vetum) 2500g
Wu Bei Zi‡ (Galla Rhois Chinensis) 860g
Wu Gong‡ (Scolopendra Subspinipes) 100g
Feng Mi‡ (Mel) 180g
Bing Pian (Borneolum) 3g

The medicated paste was prepared by boiling the black vinegar (*Lao Hei Cu*) in an earthenware cooking pot for 30 minutes, then adding *Feng Mi*‡ (Mel). When the mixture returned to the boil, powdered *Wu Bei Zi*‡ (Galla Rhois Chinensis) was sieved slowly into the pot and the mixture stirred in one direction. Once all the powdered *Wu Bei Zi*‡ (Galla Rhois Chinensis) had been added, the mixture was decocted over a mild heat until it became sticky and paste-like. Powdered *Wu Gong*‡ (Scolopendra Subspinipes) and *Bing Pian* (Borneolum) were added and the medicated paste was stored in a porcelain jar or glass bottle. Good-quality paste should be shiny, moist and black. The skin was cleaned with antiseptic before treatment, then a 2-3 cm layer of paste was applied over the keloid and covered with a thick cloth. The paste was changed every two or three days. On average, three months were required for treatment.

In the prescription, *Lao Hei Cu* (Acetum Atrum Vetum) softens hardness and relieves Toxicity, *Wu Bei Zi*‡ (Galla Rhois Chinensis) promotes contraction and relieves Toxicity, *Wu Gong*‡ (Scolopendra Subspinipes) breaks up Blood stasis to attack Toxins with toxin, *Bing Pian* (Borneolum) alleviates itching and pain and relieves Toxicity, and *Feng Mi*‡ (Mel) regulates and harmonizes the actions of the other ingredients.

2. **Luo et al** also recommended a paste for treating keloids. [4]

Prescription
RUAN JIAN GAO
Paste for Softening Hardness

Wu Gong‡ (Scolopendra Subspinipes) 30g
Wu Bei Zi‡ (Galla Rhois Chinensis) 30g
Bai Shao (Radix Paeoniae Lactiflorae) 15g
Huang La‡ (Cera Aurea) 20g
Feng Mi‡ (Mel) 60g

The paste was prepared by covering *Bai Shao* (Radix Paeoniae Lactiflorae) with *Mi Cu* (Acetum Oryzae) and leaving to soak for two days. The mixture was then decocted in an iron pot over a mild heat until the vinegar became concentrated. The herb residue was removed and *Huang La*‡ (Cera Aurea) and *Feng Mi*‡ (Mel) added. When the wax and honey were fully melted, the powdered *Wu Gong*‡(Scolopendra Subspinipes) and *Wu Bei Zi*‡ (Galla Rhois Chinensis) were beaten into the mixture, which was removed from the heat, left to cool and stored in a porcelain jar. During treatment, the paste was spread evenly to cover the keloid completely.

Treatment was given once a day or every two days for three months. This paste functioned to harmonize Ying Qi (Nutritive Qi), soften hardness, expel Wind, and alleviate itching and was indicated for all sizes of keloid irrespective of cause.

Lipoma
脂肪瘤

Lipomas are benign tumors in the subcutaneous tissue composed of mature fat cells. In TCM, lipomas are also known as *rou liu* (flesh tumors).

Clinical manifestations

- Lipomas are most common on the forearm and thigh, but can also involve the breast, back, abdomen, neck, shoulder, and axillae.

- The tumor manifests as one or several round or lobulated nodes, 2-10 cm in diameter, and with a soft, rubber-like consistency. The skin is normal in color and may feel slightly cool.

- Of the five types of lipoma seen in the clinic, multiple lipoma (the type discussed in this section) is the most frequently encountered. From two to one hundred confluent tumors can occur at any body site, but are most common on the trunk, neck and proximal extremities. They are not painful unless they grow rapidly. This type is more common in women.

Etiology and pathology

- Dietary irregularities such as overindulgence in fatty, sweet, rich, spicy, or fried food impairs the Spleen's transportation function, leading to Phlegm-Damp obstructing the network vessels and to binding of Qi and Blood.

- Depression binding the Spleen leads to Spleen Deficiency and impairment of the transformation and transportation function. This results in the accumulation of Phlegm turbidity in the flesh, giving rise to the swelling that is characteristic of this condition.

- Depression and anger damaging the Liver together with excessive thought and preoccupation damaging the Spleen mean that the free movement of Qi is not maintained, resulting in Qi stagnation and Blood stasis and the appearance of the tumor.

Pattern identification and treatment

INTERNAL TREATMENT

PHLEGM CONGEALING DUE TO QI STAGNATION

This pattern is usually seen at the initial stage in obese individuals or those with a robust constitution. The tumors involve the back, shoulder and abdomen and feel like silk floss to the touch; they may feel distended on pressure. The tongue body is enlarged and tender with a thin white coating; the pulse is slippery and full.

Treatment principle
Move Qi and dissipate lumps, dry Dampness and transform Phlegm.

Prescription
ER CHEN TANG JIA WEI
Two Matured Ingredients Decoction, with additions

Chen Pi (Pericarpium Citri Reticulatae) 10g
Jiang Ban Xia (Rhizoma Pinelliae Ternatae, processed with ginger) 10g
Chao Bai Jie Zi (Semen Sinapis Albae, stir-fried) 10g
Chao Zhi Ke (Fructus Citri Aurantii, stir-fried) 10g
Qing Meng Shi‡ (Lapis Chloriti) 15g
Fu Ling (Sclerotium Poriae Cocos) 15g
Long Gu‡ (Os Draconis) 15g
Mu Li‡ (Concha Ostreae) 15g
Zhi Nan Xing (Rhizoma Arisaematis Praeparata) 6g
Kun Bu (Thallus Laminariae seu Eckloniae) 6g
Hai Zao (Herba Sargassi) 6g
Cang Zhu (Rhizoma Atractylodis) 12g
Hou Po (Cortex Magnoliae Officinalis) 12g

Explanation
- *Chen Pi* (Pericarpium Citri Reticulatae), *Jiang Ban Xia* (Rhizoma Pinelliae Ternatae, processed with ginger), *Chao Bai Jie Zi* (Semen Sinapis Albae, stir-fried), *Qing*

Meng Shi‡ (Lapis Chloriti), *Fu Ling* (Sclerotium Poriae Cocos), and *Zhi Nan Xing* (Rhizoma Arisaematis Praeparata) regulate Qi and transform Phlegm, dissipate lumps and free the network vessels.

- *Kun Bu* (Thallus Laminariae seu Eckloniae) and *Hai Zao* (Herba Sargassi) soften hardness and disperse tumors.
- *Chao Zhi Ke* (Fructus Citri Aurantii, stir-fried), *Long Gu*‡ (Os Draconis), *Mu Li*‡ (Concha Ostreae), *Cang Zhu* (Rhizoma Atractylodis), and *Hou Po* (Cortex Magnoliae Officinalis) support the Spleen and dry Dampness.

PHLEGM TURBIDITY DUE TO QI DEFICIENCY

This pattern manifests as persistent tumors enlarging gradually, sometimes to several centimeters in diameter. The skin-colored tumors feel loose and soft when pinched. Accompanying symptoms and signs include reduced appetite, listlessness and lassitude, or puffy swelling and loose stools. The tongue body is pale red with a white and greasy coating; the pulse is soggy and moderate.

Treatment principle
Fortify the Spleen and augment Qi, loosen the Middle Burner and transform Phlegm.

Prescription
SHUN QI GUI PI WAN JIA JIAN
Pill for Normalizing Qi and Restoring the Spleen, with modifications

Chen Pi (Pericarpium Citri Reticulatae) 10g
Zhe Bei Mu (Bulbus Fritillariae Thunbergii) 10g
Xiang Fu (Rhizoma Cyperi Rotundi) 10g
Wu Yao (Radix Linderae Strychnifoliae) 10g
Fu Ling (Sclerotium Poriae Cocos) 12g
Huang Qi (Radix Astragali seu Hedysari) 12g
Dang Shen (Radix Codonopsitis Pilosulae) 12g
Bai Zhu (Rhizoma Atractylodis Macrocephalae) 6g
Mu Xiang* (Radix Aucklandiae Lappae) 6g
Chao Qian Niu Zi (Semen Pharbitidis, stir-fried) 6g
Gan Cao (Radix Glycyrrhizae) 6g
Yuan Zhi (Radix Polygalae) 4.5g
Zao Jiao Ci (Spina Gleditsiae Sinensis) 4.5g
Chuan Xiong (Rhizoma Ligustici Chuanxiong) 4.5g

Explanation
- *Chen Pi* (Pericarpium Citri Reticulatae), *Xiang Fu* (Rhizoma Cyperi Rotundi), *Wu Yao* (Radix Linderae Strychnifoliae), *Fu Ling* (Sclerotium Poriae Cocos), *Huang Qi* (Radix Astragali seu Hedysari), *Dang Shen* (Radix Codonopsitis Pilosulae), *Bai Zhu* (Rhizoma Atractylodis Macrocephalae), *Mu Xiang** (Radix Aucklandiae Lappae), and *Gan Cao* (Radix Glycyrrhizae) fortify the Spleen and augment Qi, move stagnation and dissipate lumps.

- *Zhe Bei Mu* (Bulbus Fritillariae Thunbergii) and *Chao Qian Niu Zi* (Semen Pharbitidis, stir-fried) expel turbidity and transform Phlegm.
- *Yuan Zhi* (Radix Polygalae), *Zao Jiao Ci* (Spina Gleditsiae Sinensis) and *Chuan Xiong* (Rhizoma Ligustici Chuanxiong) regulate Qi and free the orifices.

LIVER-SPLEEN DISHARMONY

In this pattern, the tumor is soft or pliable. Accompanying symptoms and signs include oppression in the chest, distension in the hypochondrium, restlessness, irritability and irascibility, and poor appetite. The tongue body is pale red with a white and slightly slippery coating; the pulse is wiry and thready.

Treatment principle
Dredge the Liver and harmonize the Spleen, regulate Qi and invigorate the Blood.

Prescription
SHI QUAN LIU QI YIN JIA JIAN
Perfect Major Qi Flow Beverage, with modifications

Wu Yao (Radix Linderae Strychnifoliae) 10g
Xiang Fu (Rhizoma Cyperi Rotundi) 10g
Mu Xiang* (Radix Aucklandiae Lappae) 10g
Qing Pi (Pericarpium Citri Reticulatae Viride) 10g
Fu Ling (Sclerotium Poriae Cocos) 12g
Bai Shao (Radix Paeoniae Lactiflorae) 12g
Dang Gui (Radix Angelicae Sinensis) 12g
Zhe Bei Mu (Bulbus Fritillariae Thunbergii) 12g
Shan Ci Gu (Pseudobulbus Shancigu) 12g
Xia Ku Cao (Spica Prunellae Vulgaris) 30g
Mei Gui Hua (Flos Rosae Rugosae) 6g
Yu Jin (Radix Curcumae) 6g

Explanation
- *Wu Yao* (Radix Linderae Strychnifoliae), *Xiang Fu* (Rhizoma Cyperi Rotundi), *Mu Xiang** (Radix Aucklandiae Lappae), and *Qing Pi* (Pericarpium Citri Reticulatae Viride) dredge the Liver and regulate Qi.
- *Fu Ling* (Sclerotium Poriae Cocos), *Bai Shao* (Radix Paeoniae Lactiflorae), *Dang Gui* (Radix Angelicae Sinensis), *Mei Gui Hua* (Flos Rosae Rugosae), and *Yu Jin* (Radix Curcumae) transform Blood stasis and harmonize the Spleen.
- *Zhe Bei Mu* (Bulbus Fritillariae Thunbergii), *Shan Ci Gu* (Pseudobulbus Shancigu) and *Xia Ku Cao* (Spica Prunellae Vulgaris) transform Phlegm and dissipate lumps.

PATENT HERBAL MEDICINES
- For pronounced Phlegm-Damp, take *Nei Xiao Lian Qiao Wan* (Forsythia Internal Dispersion Pill) 6g twice a day.

- For Qi stagnation and Blood stasis, take five tablets of *Dang Gui Pian* (Chinese Angelica Root Tablet) twice a day.
- For pronounced Phlegm turbidity, take *Meng Shi Gun Tan Wan* (Chlorite Pill for Rolling Phlegm) 3-6g, twice a day.

Clinical notes

- As this condition is chiefly caused by retained Phlegm due to Qi Deficiency binding with Damp turbidity to obstruct the channels and network vessels, treatment should emphasize the principles of supporting the Spleen and augmenting Qi, regulating Qi and transforming Phlegm, and softening hardness and dissipating lumps. Herbs with these functions are often prepared into pills for oral administration and the result is especially good for multiple lipoma.
- TCM is most effective for small tumors. Patients with large persistent tumors, especially where accompanied by pain or where diagnosis cannot exclude the possibility of malignancy, should be referred to a doctor of Western medicine for treatment.

Advice for the patient

- Avoid overindulgence in oily or greasy food.
- Eat more fresh vegetables and soybean products.

Modern clinical experience

1. **Wen Zhuozhi** prepared tablets from a powder to treat lipoma.[5]

Prescription
BIE JIA XIAO LIU FANG
Turtle Shell Formula for Dispersing Tumors

Xuan Shen (Radix Scrophulariae Ningpoensis) 12g
Mu Li‡ (Concha Ostreae) 12g
Chuan Bei Mu (Bulbus Fritillariae Cirrhosae) 9g
Bie Jia* (Carapax Amydae Sinensis) 9g
Mu Xiang* (Radix Aucklandiae Lappae) 9g
Kun Bu (Thallus Laminariae seu Eckloniae) 9g
Hai Zao (Herba Sargassi) 9g
Yu Jin (Radix Curcumae) 9g

Xia Ku Cao (Spica Prunellae Vulgaris) 9g
Ban Zhi Lian (Herba Scutellariae Barbatae) 15g
Bai Hua She She Cao (Herba Hedyotidis Diffusae) 15g
Dan Shen (Radix Salviae Miltiorrhizae) 15g

The ingredients were ground into a fine powder and made into 0.25g tablets with a suitable excipient. Two tablets were taken three times a day. A course of treatment lasted one month and results were usually seen after three courses.

2. **Sun** reported on the treatment of lipoma in female patients.[6]

Prescription
XIAO ZHI LIU FANG
Dispersing Lipoma Formula

Dang Shen (Radix Codonopsitis Pilosulae) 10-15g
Bai Zhu (Rhizoma Atractylodis Macrocephalae) 10-15g
Fu Ling (Sclerotium Poriae Cocos) 10-15g
Gan Cao (Radix Glycyrrhizae) 3g
Chen Pi (Pericarpium Citri Reticulatae) 10g
Ju He (Semen Citri Reticulatae) 10g
Fa Ban Xia (Rhizoma Pinelliae Ternatae Praeparata) 10-20g
Tu Bei Mu (Tuber Bolbostemmatis) 15-30g
Dang Gui (Radix Angelicae Sinensis) 6-10g
Lu Lu Tong (Fructus Liquidambaris) 6-10g
Bai Jie Zi (Semen Sinapis Albae) 10-30g

Modifications
1. For flushing prior to periods, *Shu Di Huang* (Radix Rehmanniae Glutinosae Conquita) and *He Shou Wu* (Radix Polygoni Multiflori) were added.
2. During the rest of the menstrual cycle, *Chuan Shan Jia** (Squama Manitis Pentadactylae) and *Hai Zao* (Herba Sargassi) were added.
3. For insomnia, *Ye Jiao Teng* (Caulis Polygoni Multiflori) and *Yuan Zhi* (Radix Polygalae) were added.
4. For profuse white vaginal discharge, *Yi Yi Ren* (Semen Coicis Lachryma-jobi) was added.
5. For indigestion, *Shan Zha* (Fructus Crataegi) and *Mai Ya* (Fructus Hordei Vulgaris Germinatus) were added.

One bag a day was used to prepare a decoction, taken twice a day. Small tumors disappeared after 50 bags, medium-sized tumors after 100 bags and larger tumors after 130 bags.

Benign melanocytic nevi (moles)
良性黑痣

A nevus is a benign proliferation of one or more of the cells that are normal constituents of the skin. Melanocytic nevi are localized benign skin tumors composed of melanocytes. Congenital melanocytic nevi are present at birth, whereas acquired nevi generally appear through childhood, adolescence and early adulthood (up to about 30 years old). Nevi may appear on any area of the skin, although most acquired nevi appear on skin exposed to the sun. Most adults have between 10 and 30 nevi.

In TCM, this condition is also known as *hei zhi* (black moles).

Clinical manifestations

- Melanocytic nevi generally start in childhood.
- At the initial stage, nevi appear as flat, round, uniformly colored light or dark brown papules, 2-10 mm in size. They tend to expand laterally, possibly darkening in color, and may disappear in old age.
- Symptomatic manifestations such as pain or itching are generally absent.
- Black spots developing within congenital melanocytic nevi in patients with a weak constitution may be an indication of malignant melanoma, especially if there are pigmentation changes and bleeding.

Differential diagnosis

Ephelides (freckles)
Freckles are reddish-tan to light brown clearly defined macules up to 5mm in diameter, generally involving the face, arms and upper trunk. They increase in number and darken in color after exposure to the sun, and are more common in fair-haired or red-haired people. Freckles do not require treatment.

Malignant melanoma
This type of tumor is most common in people with fair or red hair; incidence increases with exposure to the sun. Melanomas are asymmetrical with irregular borders, variable coloring and a diameter in excess of 5mm. They are single and rarely appear before adulthood. There is also a risk of congenital melanocytic nevi becoming malignant.

Etiology and pathology

- Wind pathogenic factors invading the body fight with Qi and Blood, causing Qi stagnation and Blood stasis and obstructing the channels and network vessels, thus causing moles to occur.
- In cases of weakness due to Deficiency, turbid Qi from the Kidneys steams upward to the face, leading to restriction of Yang Qi and black spots.

Pattern identification and treatment

INTERNAL TREATMENT

WIND PATHOGENIC FACTORS FIGHTING AND BINDING
Light brown, dark brown or gray-black spots of various sizes are seen on the face, limbs and trunk. Accompanying symptoms and signs can include pale and tender skin, photosensitivity, or patterns of disharmony between the Stomach and Large Intestine. The tongue body is pale red with a scant coating; the pulse is deficient and floating.

Treatment principle
Dredge Wind and clear Heat, regulate Qi and transform turbidity.

Prescription
QIANG HUO TANG JIA JIAN
Notopterygium Decoction, with modifications

Qiang Huo (Rhizoma et Radix Notopterygii) 6g
Chuan Xiong (Rhizoma Ligustici Chuanxiong) 6g
Chao Zhi Ke (Fructus Citri Aurantii, stir-fried) 6g
Huang Qin (Radix Scutellariae Baicalensis) 6g
Fu Ling (Sclerotium Poriae Cocos) 12g
Ju Hua (Flos Chrysanthemi Morifolii) 12g
Qing Hao (Herba Artemisiae Chinghao) 12g
Fang Feng (Radix Ledebouriellae Divaricatae) 12g
Sheng Di Huang (Radix Rehmanniae Glutinosae) 12g
Bai Zhi (Radix Angelicae Dahuricae) 6g
*Zhi Ma Huang** (Herba Ephedrae, mix-fried with honey) 4.5g
Man Jing Zi (Fructus Viticis) 4.5g
Bai He (Bulbus Lilii) 15g
Shan Yao (Radix Dioscoreae Oppositae) 15g
Bei Sha Shen (Radix Glehniae Littoralis) 15g

Explanation
- *Qiang Huo* (Rhizoma et Radix Notopterygii), *Ju Hua* (Flos Chrysanthemi Morifolii), *Qing Hao* (Herba Artemisiae Chinghao), *Zhi Ma Huang** (Herba Ephedrae, mix-fried with honey), and *Fang Feng* (Radix

Ledebouriellae Divaricatae), dredge Wind and clear Heat to eliminate external pathogenic factors.

- *Man Jing Zi* (Fructus Viticis) and *Chuan Xiong* (Rhizoma Ligustici Chuanxiong) dispel Wind and regulate Qi.
- *Sheng Di Huang* (Radix Rehmanniae Glutinosae), *Bai He* (Bulbus Lilii), *Shan Yao* (Radix Dioscoreae Oppositae), and *Bei Sha Shen* (Radix Glehniae Littoralis) enrich Yin and protect Body Fluids to offset the dryness caused by materia medica for expelling Wind.
- *Chao Zhi Ke* (Fructus Citri Aurantii, stir-fried), *Huang Qin* (Radix Scutellariae Baicalensis) and *Fu Ling* (Sclerotium Poriae Cocos) clear Heat and eliminate Dampness.
- *Bai Zhi* (Radix Angelicae Dahuricae) warms and transforms Cold-Damp.

KIDNEY TURBIDITY CONFUSING YANG

Darkly pigmented spots occur extensively over the body. When the constitution is weakened, they become even darker and there may be a mild itching sensation. The tongue body is pale red with a scant coating; the pulse is thready and rapid.

Treatment principle
Enrich Kidney Yin and invigorate the Blood to reduce moles.

Prescription
XIAO TU SI ZI WAN JIA JIAN
Minor Dodder Seed Pill, with modifications

Tu Si Zi (Semen Cuscutae) 15g
Shan Yao (Radix Dioscoreae Oppositae) 15g
Shu Di Huang (Radix Rehmanniae Glutinosae Conquita) 15g
Shan Zhu Yu (Fructus Corni Officinalis) 15g
Lian Zi (Semen Nelumbinis Nuciferae) 12g
Chao Mu Dan Pi (Cortex Moutan Radicis, stir-fried) 12g
Ze Lan (Herba Lycopi Lucidi) 12g
Hong Hua (Flos Carthami Tinctorii) 6g
Tao Ren (Semen Persicae) 6g
Chuan Xiong (Rhizoma Ligustici Chuanxiong) 6g
Dong Gua Ren (Semen Benincasae Hispidae) 30g

Explanation
- *Tu Si Zi* (Semen Cuscutae), *Shan Yao* (Radix Dioscoreae Oppositae), *Shu Di Huang* (Radix Rehmanniae Glutinosae Conquita), *Shan Zhu Yu* (Fructus Corni Officinalis), and *Lian Zi* (Semen Nelumbinis Nuciferae) enrich Kidney Yin.
- *Chao Mu Dan Pi* (Cortex Moutan Radicis, stir-fried), *Ze Lan* (Herba Lycopi Lucidi), *Hong Hua* (Flos Carthami Tinctorii), *Tao Ren* (Semen Persicae), and *Chuan Xiong* (Rhizoma Ligustici Chuanxiong) invigorate the Blood and reduce moles.

- *Dong Gua Ren* (Semen Benincasae Hispidae) cleanses the skin and moistens the face.

EXTERNAL TREATMENT
- Prepare *Shui Jing Gao* (Crystal Paste) by dissolving *Shi Hui‡* (Calx) 15g in water, then adding half a teacup of concentrated alkaline solution to cover the mixture to a depth of two finger-widths (about 50ml). Then sprinkle 50 grains of *Nuo Mi* (Semen Oryzae Glutinosae) into the liquid and leave for one day and one night (two days and one night in winter). Take the rice out and pound it into a cream for application. Spread a little directly on the nevus only; avoid normal skin as it may be injured by the application.
- Prepare *Yang Shi Ru Sheng Gao* (Yang's Sage-Like Paste) by grinding equal amounts of the ashes of *Hei Dou Geng* (Caulis Glycines Atrum), *Qiao Mai Geng* (Caulis Fagopyri), *Sang Bai Pi* (Cortex Mori Albae Radicis), and charcoal into a fine powder. Place the powder in a sieve and sprinkle 1000 ml of water over it three times. The liquid is then decocted over a mild heat to make a paste. Make a dimple in the nevus with a needle and apply a small amount each time.
- For light brown superficial nevi with a shallow root, break the head with a needle and apply the oil extracted from *Ya Dan Zi* (Fructus Bruceae Javanicae). A scab will form in three to four days and fall off spontaneously.

FIRE NEEDLING
Points: Ashi points (sites of nevi).
Technique: After routine sterilization of the area, select a no. 24-26 gauge needle (depending on the dimensions of the nevus), heat the needle over a flame until 2cm of the needle tip is red, then insert rapidly into the center of the nevus. The depth of insertion depends on the elevation of the nevus. If it is not raised above skin level, insertion should not go deeper than the subcutaneous layer; if the nevus is elevated above the skin surface, insertion can be a little deeper. It is crucial not to damage the normal tissues. After treatment, the area should be kept away from water or other liquids for one week to prevent infection. Scabs should not be removed by force, but allowed to fall off spontaneously (normally after about five days).

Clinical notes

- Melanocytic nevi are best treated externally with internal treatment playing a supporting role. This combination is effective in preventing recurrence and spread.

- If the condition deteriorates (for example, the lesion enlarges, turns a darker color or ulcerates – all indications of a possibility of malignant melanoma), the patient should be referred to a doctor of Western medicine immediately.
- If melanocytic nevi are treated for cosmetic purposes, the prognosis is usually good, subject to the usual warnings on malignancy.

Advice for the patient

According to the ancient physicians, soy sauce and vinegar are to be avoided during treatment.

References

1. Hu Ximing (ed.), *Zhong Guo Zhong Yi Mi Fang Da Quan* [A Compendium of TCM Secret Formulae] (Shanghai: Wen Hui Publishing House, 1991), 102.
2. Xie Zicheng, *Xue Guan Liu Cha Ji Wai Cha Zhi Liao Hai Mian Zhuang Xue Guan Liu* [External Treatment of Cavernous Hemangioma with *Xue Guan Liu Cha Ji* (Hemangioma Application)], *Tian Jin Zhong Yi* [Tianjin Journal of Traditional Chinese Medicine] 14, 5 (1997): 230.
3. Beijing Hospital of Traditional Chinese Medicine, *Zhao Bing Nan Lin Chuang Jing Yan Ji* [A Collection of Zhao Bingnan's Clinical Experiences] (Beijing: People's Medical Publishing House, 1975) 277.
4. Luo Yutian et al., *Zhong Yi Wai Ke Lin Zheng Ji Yao* [A Collection of Clinical Patterns in the Treatment of External Diseases with Traditional Chinese Medicine] (Chengdu: Sichuan Science and Technology Publishing House, 1987) 303-4.
5. Hu Ximing (ed.), *Zhong Guo Zhong Yi Mi Fang Da Quan: Zhong Juan* [A Compendium of Secret Prescriptions of Traditional Chinese Medicine, vol. 2] (Shanghai: Wen Hui Publishing House, 1991), 96.
6. Sun Huiwen, *Zhi Fang Liu Zhi Yan* [Experiences in the Treatment of Lipoma], *Si Chuan Zhong Yi* [Sichuan Journal of Traditional Chinese Medicine] 6 (1986): back cover.

1. Materia medica commonly used in the treatment of skin disorders

2. Less common materia medica used in the treatment of skin disorders

3. Acupuncture points commonly used in the treatment of skin disorders

4. TCM formulae and patent medicines used in the treatment of skin disorders

5. TCM external formulae used in the treatment of skin disorders

Materia medica commonly used in the treatment of skin disorders

The application of Chinese materia medica in internal and external medicine, gynecology and pediatrics is well covered in many ancient and contemporary works. However, a general overview of the application of these materia medica to skin disorders is generally not readily available. I have classified Chinese materia medica commonly used internally in the dermatology clinic into eight categories on the basis of a study of the classic works and my 40 years of clinical experience in the treatment of skin diseases. Full understanding and correct use of these materia medica will achieve a satisfactory effect in treatment provided that pattern identification has been properly applied.

MATERIA MEDICA FOR ALLEVIATING ITCHING

Itching is one of the most common symptoms seen in the dermatology clinic. There are no specific Chinese materia medica solely for alleviating itching. Itching is generally treated on the basis of pattern identification and the nature of the itching.

- Itching due to urticaria is more likely to belong to the category of Wind itch and treatment should focus on dispelling Wind to alleviate itching.
- If itching worsens when meeting Heat, it belongs more to the Wind-Heat category and treatment should focus on clearing Heat and dispelling Wind or cooling the Blood and dispelling Wind.
- Itching caused by Dampness, characterized by erosion and exudation, belongs to the Damp itch category and treatment should focus on eliminating Dampness to alleviate itching.
- Pruritus in old age and some types of itching found in lichen simplex chronicus (neurodermatitis) belong to the Blood Deficiency itching category and treatment should focus on nourishing the Blood and moistening the skin to alleviate itching.
- Itching caused by infectious diseases and parasites, for instance scabies or tinea, belongs essentially to the category of Worm itching and the treatment should focus on killing Worms.

Wind-type itching, Damp-type itching and Blood Deficiency-type itching are often seen in the dermatology clinic. It is convenient to divide materia medica for alleviating itching into two types – materia medica for dispelling Wind and eliminating Dampness to alleviate itching, and materia medica for nourishing the Blood and moistening the skin to alleviate itching.

MATERIA MEDICA FOR DISPELLING WIND AND ELIMINATING DAMPNESS TO ALLEVIATE ITCHING

Jing Jie (Herba Schizonepetae Tenuifoliae)
Functions: Dispels Wind, releases the exterior and regulates the Blood. This herb can dispel Wind between the skin and membranes and dissipate pathogenic Wind retained in the exterior. *Jing Jie Sui* (Spica Schizonepetae Tenuifoliae) is even more effective than *Jing Jie* (Herba Schizonepetae Tenuifoliae) in dispelling Wind and can be used for clearing Wind-Heat in the Blood.

Indications: This herb's functions of dispelling Wind and releasing the exterior mean that it is mainly used to alleviate itching in the treatment of conditions such as pruritus, urticaria, acute eczema, seborrheic eczema, lichen simplex chronicus (neurodermatitis), lichen planus, and pityriasis rosea.

Common dosage: 3-10g.

Combinations

- Often used in conjunction with *Fang Feng* (Radix Ledebouriellae Divaricatae), *Niu Bang Zi* (Fructus Arctii Lappae) or *Chan Tui* ‡ (Periostracum Cicadae) to increase its effectiveness in dispelling Wind and alleviating itching, for example in urticaria, pruritus, acute eczema, pityriasis rosea, lichen planus, and lichen simplex chronicus (neurodermatitis).

- In addition, it can be used in combination with *Bai Ji Li* (Fructus Tribuli Terrestris) to extinguish internal Wind and dispel external Wind simultaneously, for example in dermographism, pruritus or seborrheic eczema.

- Combined with *Sheng Ma* (Rhizoma Cimicifugae) and *Ge Gen* (Radix Puerariae), *Jing Jie Sui* (Spica Schizonepetae Tenuifoliae) releases the exterior and vents papules to treat measles.

Fang Feng (Radix Ledebouriellae Divaricatae)
Functions: Dispels Wind, releases the exterior and overcomes Dampness; among materia medica with the function of dispelling Wind, it is one of those with more pronounced moistening properties. *Fang Feng* (Radix Ledebouriellae Divaricatae) can be used to treat all types of pathogenic Wind and is more effective than *Jing Jie* (Herba Schizonepetae Tenuifoliae) in dispelling Wind. It can enter the bones and flesh and is good at arresting Wind in the sinews and bones.

Indications: This herb's functions of dispelling Wind and releasing the exterior mean that it is mainly used to alleviate itching in the treatment of conditions such as acute eczema, contact dermatitis, lichen simplex chronicus (neurodermatitis), urticaria, pityriasis rosea, lichen planus, and psoriasis.

Since it also overcomes Dampness, it is often used for Damp patterns with itching in such conditions as pruritus, contact dermatitis, lichen simplex chronicus (neurodermatitis), scabies, and psoriatic arthritis.

Common dosage: 3-10g.

Combinations

- Often used in conjunction with *Jing Jie* (Herba Schizonepetae Tenuifoliae), *Niu Bang Zi* (Fructus Arctii Lappae) or *Chan Tui*‡ (Periostracum Cicadae) to increase its effectiveness in dispelling Wind and alleviating itching.
- In addition, it can be used in combination with *Bai Ji Li* (Fructus Tribuli Terrestris) to extinguish internal Wind and dispel external Wind simultaneously, for example in papular eczema, pruritus or lichen planus.
- Combined with *Qiang Huo* (Rhizoma et Radix Notopterygii) and *Ku Shen* (Radix Sophorae Flavescentis), it dissipates Wind and dispels Dampness to treat lichen simplex chronicus (neurodermatitis).
- Combined with *Gou Teng* (Ramulus Uncariae cum Uncis) and *Bai Xian Pi* (Cortex Dictamni Dasycarpi Radicis), it dredges Wind, eliminates Dampness and relieves Toxicity to treat nipple eczema or pruritus.
- Combined with *Sheng Di Huang* (Radix Rehmanniae Glutinosae) and *Mu Dan Pi* (Cortex Moutan Radicis), it dredges Wind and cools the Blood to treat pityriasis rosea.
- Combined with *Gan Jiang* (Rhizoma Zingiberis Officinalis), *Gui Zhi* (Ramulus Cinnamomi Cassiae) and *Zi Su Ye* (Folium Perillae Frutescentis), it warms Yang and dispels Wind-Cold to treat cold urticaria.

Qiang Huo (Rhizoma et Radix Notopterygii)

Functions: Dispels Wind and overcomes Dampness, dissipates exterior Cold, frees the Blood vessels, expels pus and generates flesh.

Indications: Itching and pain due to Wind-Cold-Damp, abscesses and sores without ulceration.

Common dosage: 3-10g.

Combinations

- Combined with *Fang Feng* (Radix Ledebouriellae Divaricatae) and *Jing Jie* (Herba Schizonepetae Tenuifoliae), it treats urticaria and pruritus.
- Combined with *Du Huo* (Radix Angelicae Pubescentis), *Sang Ji Sheng* (Ramulus Loranthi) and *Qin Jiao* (Radix Gentianae Macrophyllae), it treats psoriatic arthritis.
- Combined with *Sheng Di Huang* (Radix Rehmanniae Glutinosae), *Dong Gua Ren* (Semen Benincasae Hispidae), *Mu Dan Pi* (Cortex Moutan Radicis), and *Ju Hua* (Flos Chrysanthemi Morifolii), it treats seborrhea.
- Combined with *Chi Shao* (Radix Paeoniae Rubra), *Jin Yin Hua* (Flos Lonicerae) and *Pu Gong Ying* (Herba Taraxaci cum Radice), it treats folliculitis.

*Ma Huang** (Herba Ephedrae)

Functions: Induces sweating, calms wheezing and dissipates Wind-Cold. This herb can dissipate pathogenic factors from the exterior when Wind-Cold-Damp settles in the skin and hair.

Indications: Itching due to disharmony between the Ying and Wei levels caused by Wind-Cold invading the flesh.

Common dosage: 1-6g. ᶦ

Combinations

Ma Huang* (Herba Ephedrae) can be combined with *Gui Zhi* (Ramulus Cinnamomi Cassiae) and *Da Zao* (Fructus Ziziphi Jujubae) to harmonize the Ying and Wei levels:

- When *Sheng Jiang* (Rhizoma Zingiberis Officinalis Recens) is added, the combination can treat urticaria.
- When *Sheng Jiang* (Rhizoma Zingiberis Officinalis Recens) and *Xing Ren* (Semen Pruni Armeniacae) are added, the combination can treat psoriasis.
- When *Bai Shao* (Radix Paeoniae Lactiflorae), *Gan Cao* (Radix Glycyrrhizae) and *Gan Jiang* (Rhizoma Zingiberis Officinalis) are added, the combination can treat pruritus.

Ju Hua (Flos Chrysanthemi Morifolii)

Functions: Dredges Wind and dissipates Heat, calms the Liver and brightens the eyes, and relieves Toxicity. *Huang Ju Hua* (Flos Aureus Chrysanthemi Morifolii) is used more often in the dermatology clinic as it is more effective in dissipating Wind-Heat than *Bai Ju Hua* (Flos Albus Chrysanthemi Morifolii), which is better for calming the Liver and brightening the eyes.

Indications: Pruritus, phytophotodermatitis, urticaria due to Wind-Heat, seborrhea, and alopecia areata.

Common dosage: 10g.

Combinations

- Combined with *Sheng Di Huang* (Radix Rehmanniae Glutinosae) and *Mu Dan Pi* (Cortex Moutan Radicis), it clears Heat and cools the Blood to treat seborrhea and mouth ulcers.
- Combined with *Sang Ye* (Folium Mori Albae) and *Gan Cao* (Radix Glycyrrhizae), it dredges Wind and clears Heat to treat alopecia areata.
- Combined with *Ma Huang** (Herba Ephedrae), *Lian Qiao* (Fructus Forsythiae Suspensae) and *Chi Xiao Dou* (Semen Phaseoli Calcarati), it dissipates Wind and clears Heat to alleviate itching in the treatment of phytophotodermatitis.

Ye Ju Hua (Flos Chrysanthemi Indici)

Functions: Clears Heat, relieves Toxicity, disperses swelling.

Indications: Impetigo, folliculitis, furuncles (boils), erysipelas, and diaper dermatitis (nappy rash); external application as a wash for acute eczema, perianal eczema and genital eczema.

Common dosage: 10g.

Combinations

- Combined with *Jin Yin Hua* (Flos Lonicerae), *Lian Qiao* (Fructus Forsythiae Suspensae), *Pu Gong Ying* (Herba Taraxaci cum Radice), and *Gan Cao* (Radix Glycyrrhizae), it clears Heat, relieves Toxicity and eliminates swelling to treat impetigo, folliculitis and furuncles
- Combined with *Niu Bang Zi* (Fructus Arctii Lappae), *Sang Ye* (Folium Mori Albae), *Chan Tui*‡ (Periostracum Cicadae), and *Jin Yin Hua* (Flos Lonicerae), it dissipates Wind and disperses swelling to treat erysipelas.

ᶦ In the UK, the dosage of *Ma Huang* (Herba Ephedrae) is restricted to 0.6g three times a day.

- Combined with *Pu Gong Ying* (Herba Taraxaci cum Radice), it can be used to prepare a wet compress for application in acute eczema or diaper dermatitis (nappy rash).
- Combined with *She Chuang Zi* (Fructus Cnidii Monnieri), *Cang Er Zi* (Fructus Xanthii Sibirici) and *Ku Shen* (Radix Sophorae Flavescentis), it can be used to steam the affected area to treat genital or perianal eczema.

Niu Bang Zi (Fructus Arctii Lappae)
Functions: Dispels Wind and clears Heat, diffuses Lung Qi and vents papules, relieves Toxicity and disperses swelling.
Indications: Eczema, contact dermatitis, lichen simplex chronicus (neurodermatitis), urticaria due to Wind-Heat, pityriasis rosea, and lichen planus.
Common dosage: 3-10g.
Combinations

- Often used in conjunction with *Jing Jie* (Herba Schizonepetae Tenuifoliae), *Fang Feng* (Radix Ledebouriellae Divaricatae) or *Chan Tui*‡ (Periostracum Cicadae) to increase its effectiveness in dispelling Wind and alleviating itching in such skin disorders as eczema, urticaria, lichen planus, psoriasis, and scabies.
- Combined with *Shi Gao*‡ (Gypsum Fibrosum), *Chai Hu* (Radix Bupleuri) and *Jing Jie* (Herba Schizonepetae Tenuifoliae), it clears Heat, dissipates Wind and relieves Toxicity to treat small vessel vasculitis.
- Combined with *Sheng Ma* (Rhizoma Cimicifugae) and *Qiang Huo* (Rhizoma et Radix Notopterygii), it dredges Wind and clears Heat to treat folliculitis.
- Combined with *Ge Gen* (Radix Puerariae) and *Lian Qiao* (Fructus Forsythiae Suspensae), it relieves Toxicity and vents papules to treat measles.

Fu Ping (Herba Spirodelae Polyrrhizae)
Functions: Dispels Wind and releases the exterior, vents papules and alleviates itching, moves water and disperses swelling.
Indications: Urticaria, angioedema, contact dermatitis, lichen simplex chronicus (neurodermatitis), pityriasis alba, and vitiligo.
Common dosage: 10-15g.
Combinations

- Combined with *Jing Jie* (Herba Schizonepetae Tenuifoliae), *Chai Hu* (Radix Bupleuri) and *Chan Tui*‡ (Periostracum Cicadae), it dissipates Wind and alleviates itching to treat angioedema.
- Combined with *Lian Zi Xin* (Plumula Nelumbinis Nuciferae) and *Bai Mao Gen* (Rhizoma Imperatae Cylindricae), it clears Heat, eliminates Dampness, dredges Wind and alleviates itching to treat contact dermatitis.
- Combined with *Bai Ji Li* (Fructus Tribuli Terrestris), *Fang Feng* (Radix Ledebouriellae Divaricatae) and *Bai Fu Zi* (Rhizoma Typhonii Gigantei), it dredges Wind, expels pathogenic factors and increases pigmentation to treat vitiligo.
- Combined with *Jing Jie* (Herba Schizonepetae Tenuifoliae), *Niu Bang Zi* (Fructus Arctii Lappae) and *Mu Dan Pi* (Cortex Moutan Radicis), it disperses Wind and clears Heat to treat pityriasis alba.

Chan Tui‡ (Periostracum Cicadae)
Functions: Dispels Wind and diffuses the Lungs, vents papules and alleviates itching.
Indications: Urticaria due to Wind-Heat, pruritus, eczema, lichen simplex chronicus (neurodermatitis), pityriasis rosea, lichen planus, and measles.
Common dosage: 3-10g.
Combinations

- Often used in conjunction with *Fang Feng* (Radix Ledebouriellae Divaricatae), *Niu Bang Zi* (Fructus Arctii Lappae) or *Jing Jie* (Herba Schizonepetae Tenuifoliae) to increase its effectiveness in dispelling Wind and alleviating itching, for example in urticaria, pruritus, acute eczema, pityriasis rosea, lichen planus, and lichen simplex chronicus (neurodermatitis).
- Combined with *Chen Pi* (Pericarpium Citri Reticulatae), it dissipates Heat and alleviates itching to treat angioedema.
- Combined with *Lian Zi Xin* (Plumula Nelumbinis Nuciferae), *Sheng Di Huang* (Radix Rehmanniae Glutinosae) and *Mai Ya* (Fructus Hordei Vulgaris Germinatus), it clears Heat, fortifies the Spleen and enriches Yin to treat atopic eczema.
- Combined with *Sheng Ma* (Rhizoma Cimicifugae), *Ge Gen* (Radix Puerariae) and *Xi He Liu* (Cacumen Tamaricis), it releases the exterior and vents papules to treat measles.

Ku Shen (Radix Sophorae Flavescentis)
Functions: Clears Heat and eliminates Dampness, dispels Wind and kills Worms to alleviate itching.
Indications: Urticaria, pruritus due to Wind-Damp-Heat, genital eczema, asteatotic eczema, lichen simplex chronicus (neurodermatitis), psoriasis, lichen planus, tinea cruris (jock itch), and scabies.
Common dosage: 5-10g.
Combinations

- Combined with *Bai Xian Pi* (Cortex Dictamni Dasycarpi Radicis) and *Di Fu Zi* (Fructus Kochiae Scopariae), it clears Heat and dispels Dampness to alleviate itching in the treatment of urticaria, asteatotic eczema and lichen simplex chronicus (neurodermatitis).
- Combined with *Gou Teng* (Ramulus Uncariae cum Uncis), *Bai Ji Li* (Fructus Tribuli Terrestris) and *Huang Qin* (Radix Scutellariae Baicalensis), it clears Heat, dries Dampness and extinguishes Wind to alleviate itching in the treatment of perianal eczema.
- Combined with *Huang Bai* (Cortex Phellodendri), *Long Dan Cao* (Radix Gentianae Scabrae), *Zhi Zi* (Fructus Gardeniae Jasminoidis), *Bai Xian Pi* (Cortex Dictamni Dasycarpi Radicis), and *Wei Ling Xian* (Radix Clematidis), it clears Heat and relieves Toxicity, kills Worms and alleviates itching to treat tinea cruris (jock itch).
- Combined with *Jing Jie* (Herba Schizonepetae Tenuifoliae), *Fang Feng* (Radix Ledebouriellae Divaricatae) and *Che Qian Zi* (Semen Plantaginis), it clears Heat, dries Dampness, dissipates Wind and alleviates itching to treat nodular prurigo.

- *Ku Shen* (Radix Sophorae Flavescentis) can also be used on its own or in combination with other ingredients as a wash or soak to treat urticaria, genital eczema, asteatotic eczema, tinea pedis (athlete's foot), or localized pruritus.

Bai Xian Pi (Cortex Dictamni Dasycarpi Radicis)

Functions: Dispels Wind and dries Dampness, clears Heat and relieves Toxicity.

Indications: Acute or chronic eczema, atopic eczema, pompholyx, asteatotic eczema, lichen simplex chronicus (neurodermatitis), pruritus due to Wind-Damp-Heat, lichen planus, tinea cruris (jock itch), and scabies.

Common dosage: 15-30g.

Combinations

- Combined with *Ren Dong Teng* (Caulis Lonicerae Japonicae), *Xi Xian Cao* (Herba Siegesbeckiae), *Hai Tong Pi* (Cortex Erythrinae), and *Di Fu Zi* (Fructus Kochiae Scopariae), it relieves Toxicity, eliminates Dampness and dissipates Wind to alleviate itching in the treatment of acute eczema.
- Combined with *Ze Xie* (Rhizoma Alismatis Orientalis) and *She Chuang Zi* (Fructus Cnidii Monnieri), it transforms Dampness to alleviate itching in the treatment of chronic eczema.
- Combined with *Di Fu Zi* (Fructus Kochiae Scopariae) and/or *Ku Shen* (Radix Sophorae Flavescentis), it alleviates itching, relieves Toxicity and dissipates Wind to treat asteatotic eczema, lichen simplex chronicus (neurodermatitis), pruritus, or bullous pemphigoid.
- Combined with *Fu Ling Pi* (Cortex Poriae Cocos), *Cang Zhu* (Rhizoma Atractylodis), and *Fang Feng* (Radix Ledebouriellae Divaricatae), it dispels Wind and eliminates Dampness to alleviate itching in the treatment of scabies.

Jiang Can‡ (Bombyx Batryticatus)

Functions: Dispels Wind, alleviates tetany, transforms Phlegm, dissipates lumps.

Indications: Lichen planus, psoriasis, urticaria, furuncles, hidradenitis suppurativa, and plantar warts (verruca plantaris).

Common dosage: 5-10g.

Combinations

- Combined with *Fu Ping* (Herba Spirodelae Polyrrhizae) and *Chan Tui*‡ (Periostracum Cicadae), it dispels Wind and alleviates itching to treat urticaria.
- Combined with *Fang Feng* (Radix Ledebouriellae Divaricatae), *Qiang Huo* (Rhizoma et Radix Notopterygii) and *Bai Xian Pi* (Cortex Dictamni Dasycarpi Radicis), it expels Wind, eliminates Dampness and alleviates itching to treat lichen planus.
- Combined with *Du Zhong* (Cortex Eucommiae Ulmoidis), *Xu Duan* (Radix Dipsaci) and *Tu Fu Ling* (Rhizoma Smilacis Glabrae), it supplements the Liver and Kidneys, dredges Wind and alleviates itching to treat chronic psoriasis.
- Combined with *Zhe Bei Mu* (Bulbus Fritillariae Thunbergii), *Xia Ku Cao* (Spica Prunellae Vulgaris), *Jie Geng* (Radix Platycodi Grandiflori), and *Fu Ling* (Sclerotium Poriae Cocos), it transforms Phlegm and dissipates nodules in the treatment of hidradenitis suppurativa.

Bai Ji Li (Fructus Tribuli Terrestris)

Functions: Dissipates Wind and alleviates itching, calms the Liver and brightens the eyes.

Indications: Pruritus, urticaria due to Blood stasis, seborrheic eczema, lichen planus, psoriasis, and vitiligo.

Common dosage: 10-15g.

Combinations

- Combined with *Fang Feng* (Radix Ledebouriellae Divaricatae) and *Chan Tui*‡ (Periostracum Cicadae), or with *Gou Teng* (Ramulus Uncariae cum Uncis), *Qiang Huo* (Rhizoma et Radix Notopterygii) and *Jing Jie* (Herba Schizonepetae Tenuifoliae), it dissipates Wind and alleviates itching to treat pruritus.
- Combined with *Chuan Xiong* (Rhizoma Ligustici Chuanxiong), *Xiang Fu* (Rhizoma Cyperi Rotundi) and *Qing Pi* (Pericarpium Citri Reticulatae Viride), it regulates Qi, invigorates the Blood and dispels Wind to treat urticaria.
- Combined with *Xu Chang Qing* (Radix Cynanchi Paniculati), *Fang Feng* (Radix Ledebouriellae Divaricatae) and *He Shou Wu* (Radix Polygoni Multiflori), it nourishes the Blood, arrests Wind and alleviates itching to treat lichen planus.
- Combined with *Nü Zhen Zi* (Fructus Ligustri Lucidi), *Hei Zhi Ma* (Semen Sesami Indici), *Fang Feng* (Radix Ledebouriellae Divaricatae) and *Fu Ping* (Herba Spirodelae Polyrrhizae), it enriches Yin, moistens Dryness, dredges Wind and increases pigmentation to treat vitiligo.

MATERIA MEDICA FOR NOURISHING THE BLOOD AND MOISTENING THE SKIN TO ALLEVIATE ITCHING

He Shou Wu (Radix Polygoni Multiflori)

Functions: Nourishes the Blood and dispels Wind, supplements the Liver and boosts the Kidneys, blackens the hair and beard.

Indications: Urticaria or pruritus due to Blood Deficiency; Blood-Dryness patterns of atopic eczema, lichen simplex chronicus (neurodermatitis), tinea manuum (ringworm of the hands), and dermatitis herpetiformis; premature graying.

Common dosage: 10-15g.

Combinations

This herb is frequently combined with *Dang Gui* (Radix Angelicae Sinensis), *Bai Shao* (Radix Paeoniae Lactiflorae), and *Sheng Di Huang* (Radix Rehmanniae Glutinosae) or *Shu Di Huang* (Radix Rehmanniae Glutinosae Conquita) to nourish the Blood and moisten Dryness:

- with the addition of *Fang Feng* (Radix Ledebouriellae Divaricatae), the combination also dissipates Wind and alleviates itching to treat atopic eczema.
- with the addition of *Gou Teng* (Ramulus Uncariae cum Uncis), the combination also extinguishes Wind and alleviates itching to treat pruritus or lichen simplex chronicus (neurodermatitis).
- with the addition of *Mai Men Dong* (Radix Ophiopogonis Japonici) and *Shan Yao* (Rhizoma Dioscoreae Oppositae), the combination also enriches Yin and fortifies the Spleen to treat tinea manuum due to Blood-Dryness.

- with the addition of *Nü Zhen Zi* (Fructus Ligustri Lucidi), *Sang Shen* (Fructus Mori Albae) and *Huang Jing* (Rhizoma Polygonati), the combination also enriches the Liver and supplements the Kidneys to treat alopecia areata; and with the addition of *Sha Yuan Zi* (Semen Astragali Complanati), *She Chuang Zi* (Fructus Cnidii Monnieri), *Fu Pen Zi* (Fructus Rubi Chingii), *Gou Qi Zi* (Fructus Lycii), *Che Qian Zi* (Semen Plantaginis), and *Hei Zhi Ma* (Semen Sesami Indici), it has the same functions in the treatment of vitiligo.

Ye Jiao Teng (Caulis Polygoni Multiflori)

Functions: Nourishes the Blood and quiets the Spirit, dispels Wind and frees the network vessels to alleviate itching.

Indications: Pain and itching due to Blood Deficiency, insomnia, alopecia areata, vitiligo.

Common dosage: 15-30g.

Combinations

- Combined with *Fang Feng* (Radix Ledebouriellae Divaricatae), *Bai Ji Li* (Fructus Tribuli Terrestris), *Ku Shen* (Radix Sophorae Flavescentis), and *Dang Gui* (Radix Angelicae Sinensis), it expels Wind, dispels Dampness and nourishes the Blood to alleviate itching and treat pruritus due to Wind-Damp.

- Combined with *Gui Zhi* (Ramulus Cinnamomi Cassiae), *Gan Jiang* (Rhizoma Zingiberis Officinalis) and *Dang Gui* (Radix Angelicae Sinensis), it nourishes the Blood and dissipates Cold to treat urticaria due to Blood Deficiency.

- Combined with *Shu Di Huang* (Radix Rehmanniae Glutinosae Conquita), *Nü Zhen Zi* (Fructus Ligustri Lucidi), *Dan Shen* (Radix Salviae Miltiorrhizae), and *Bai Shao* (Radix Paeoniae Lactiflorae), it supplements the Liver and Kidneys and nourishes the Blood to treat alopecia areata.

- Combined with *Bai Ji Li* (Fructus Tribuli Terrestris), it nourishes the Blood, quiets the Spirit and dredges Wind to alleviate itching in the treatment of asteatotic eczema.

Bai Shao (Radix Paeoniae Lactiflorae)

Functions: Nourishes the Blood and calms the Liver, alleviates pain and constrains sweating.

Indications: Urticaria due to Qi and Blood Deficiency, pruritus due to Wind-Cold, atopic, nummular and asteatotic eczema, Blood-Dryness patterns of psoriasis or pityriasis rosea, herpes zoster, radiodermatitis, hyperhidrosis, and vitiligo.

Common dosage: 10-15g.

Combinations

- Combined with *Dang Shen* (Radix Codonopsitis Pilosulae), *Bai Zhu* (Rhizoma Atractylodis Macrocephalae), *Dang Gui* (Radix Angelicae Sinensis), and *Sheng Di Huang* (Radix Rehmanniae Glutinosae), it augments Qi and supplements the Blood to treat urticaria due to Qi and Blood Deficiency.

- Combined with *Dang Gui* (Radix Angelicae Sinensis), *Shu Di Huang* (Radix Rehmanniae Glutinosae Conquita), *He Shou Wu* (Radix Polygoni Multiflori), and *Fang Feng* (Radix Ledebouriellae Divaricatae), it nourishes the Blood and moistens Dryness to alleviate itching and treat atopic eczema.

- Combined with *Chai Hu* (Radix Bupleuri), *Qing Pi* (Pericarpium Citri Reticulatae Viride) and *Zi Cao* (Radix Arnebiae seu Lithospermi), it regulates Qi and frees the network vessels to alleviate lingering pain in herpes zoster.

- Combined with *Tian Men Dong* (Radix Asparagi Cochinchinensis), *Mai Men Dong* (Radix Ophiopogonis Japonici), *Chi Shao* (Radix Paeoniae Rubra), and *Dan Shen* (Radix Salviae Miltiorrhizae), it invigorates the Blood, nourishes the skin and moistens Dryness to treat ichthyosis vulgaris.

- Combined with *Huang Qi* (Radix Astragali seu Hedysari), *Bai Zhu* (Rhizoma Atractylodis Macrocephalae), *Shu Di Huang* (Radix Rehmanniae Glutinosae Conquita), and *E Jiao*‡ (Gelatinum Corii Asini), it fortifies the Spleen and augments Qi to contain the Blood and stop bleeding in the treatment of anaphylactoid purpura.

Chi Shao (Radix Paeoniae Rubra)

Functions: Clears Heat and cools the Blood, dissipates Blood stasis and disperses swelling to alleviate pain.

Indications: Blood-Heat or Blood stasis patterns in skin disorders such as psoriasis, pityriasis rosea, acne, rosacea, pruritus, alopecia areata, anaphylactoid purpura, exanthematous or purpuric drug eruptions, and polymorphic light eruption; also used for erythema multiforme, folliculitis, furuncles (boils), and herpes zoster (shingles).

Common dosage: 10-15g.

Combinations

- Combined with *Sheng Di Huang* (Radix Rehmanniae Glutinosae) and *Mu Dan Pi* (Cortex Moutan Radicis), it clears Heat and cools the Blood to treat psoriasis, pityriasis rosea, acne, rosacea, or alopecia areata due to Blood-Heat.

- Combined with *Bai Mao Gen* (Rhizoma Imperatae Cylindricae), *Zi Cao* (Radix Arnebiae seu Lithospermi), *Mu Dan Pi* (Cortex Moutan Radicis), and *Chi Xiao Dou* (Semen Phaseoli Calcarati), it cools and invigorates the Blood to disperse swelling and transform purpura.

- Combined with *Dang Gui* (Radix Angelicae Sinensis), *Bai Shao* (Radix Paeoniae Lactiflorae), *Huo Xue Teng* (Caulis Schisandrae), and *Ji Xue Teng* (Caulis Spatholobi), it invigorates the Blood and frees the network vessels to treat erythema multiforme.

- Combined with *Huang Qin* (Radix Scutellariae Baicalensis), *Zhi Zi* (Fructus Gardeniae Jasminoidis), *Ze Xie* (Rhizoma Alismatis Orientalis), and *Fang Feng* (Radix Ledebouriellae Divaricatae), it clears Heat, cools the Blood, transforms Dampness, and dissipates Wind to treat acute eczema.

- Combined with *Dang Gui* (Radix Angelicae Sinensis), *Ze Lan* (Herba Lycopi Lucidi), *Qian Cao Gen* (Radix Rubiae Cordifoliae), *Tao Ren* (Semen Persicae), and *Hong Hua* (Flos Carthami Tinctorii), it invigorates and cools the Blood to free the network vessels in the treatment of erythema induratum.

Ji Xue Teng (Caulis Spatholobi)

Functions: Strongly invigorates and supplements the Blood, soothes the sinews and alleviates pain. It can remove static Blood to generate new Blood.

Indications: Cold patterns in skin disorders such as vitiligo, erythema multiforme, chilblains, and Raynaud's disease; Blood Deficiency patterns in psoriasis or ichthyosis vulgaris; and asteatotic eczema due to Blood-Dryness.

Common dosage: 15-30g.

Combinations

- Combined with *Dang Gui* (Radix Angelicae Sinensis), *Shu Di Huang* (Radix Rehmanniae Glutinosae Conquita), *Chi Shao* (Radix Paeoniae Rubra), *Bai Shao* (Radix Paeoniae Lactiflorae), and *Dan Shen* (Radix Salviae Miltiorrhizae), it nourishes and invigorates the Blood to treat asteatotic eczema or ichthyosis vulgaris.

- Combined with *Bai Zhu* (Rhizoma Atractylodis Macrocephalae), *Huang Qi* (Radix Astragali seu Hedysari), *Gui Zhi* (Ramulus Cinnamomi Cassiae), and *Gan Jiang* (Rhizoma Zingiberis Officinalis), it supplements the Blood, warms Yang and frees the network vessels to treat chilblains and Raynaud's disease.

- Combined with *Sheng Di Huang* (Radix Rehmanniae Glutinosae), *Mu Dan Pi* (Cortex Moutan Radicis), *Zi Cao* (Radix Arnebiae seu Lithospermi), and *Dan Shen* (Radix Salviae Miltiorrhizae), it cools the Blood, transforms Blood stasis and reduces erythema to treat psoriasis.

MATERIA MEDICA FOR CLEARING HEAT, DRAINING FIRE AND COOLING THE BLOOD

MATERIA MEDICA FOR CLEARING HEAT AND DRAINING FIRE

Shi Gao ‡ (Gypsum Fibrosum)

Functions: Clears Heat and drains Fire, eliminates irritability and alleviates thirst. It is particularly effective for clearing Excess-Heat in the Qi level and for clearing Heat from the Lungs and Stomach.

Indications: Heat Toxin patterns in skin disorders such as urticaria, exanthematous or urticarial drug eruptions, allergic contact dermatitis, and recurrent aphthous stomatitis; Blood-Heat patterns in conditions such as rosacea, lichen simplex chronicus (neurodermatitis), anaphylactoid purpura, and polymorphic light eruption; Damp-Heat patterns in skin disorders such as contact dermatitis, seborrheic eczema, pustular psoriasis, pemphigus vulgaris, and hyperhidrosis; also for measles and varicella (chickenpox).

Common dosage: 15-30g.

Combinations

- Combined with *Sheng Di Huang* (Radix Rehmanniae Glutinosae), *Chi Shao* (Radix Paeoniae Rubra) and *Mu Dan Pi* (Cortex Moutan Radicis), it cools and invigorates the Blood, clears Heat and reduces erythema to treat urticaria, exanthematous or urticarial drug eruptions, and polymorphic light eruption.

- Combined with *Huang Qin* (Radix Scutellariae Baicalensis), *Zhi Mu* (Rhizoma Anemarrhenae Asphodeloidis), *Pi Pa Ye* (Folium Eriobotryae Japonicae), *Di Gu Pi* (Cortex Lycii Radicis), and *Sang Bai Pi* (Cortex Mori Albae Radicis), it clears accumulated Heat from the Lungs and Stomach to treat rosacea.

- Combined with *Ge Gen* (Radix Puerariae), *Ku Shen* (Radix Sophorae Flavescentis), *Da Huang* (Radix et Rhizoma Rhei), and *Sheng Ma* (Rhizoma Cimicifugae), it clears Heat from the Spleen and Stomach to treat recurrent aphthous stomatitis (mouth ulcers).

- Combined with *Qing Dai* (Indigo Naturalis), *Huang Lian* (Rhizoma Coptidis), *Xuan Shen* (Radix Scrophulariae Ningpoensis), and *Lü Dou Yi* (Testa Phaseoli Radiati), it clears Heat from the Qi level, relieves Toxicity, and cools the Blood to reduce purpura.

- Combined with *Pu Gong Ying* (Herba Taraxaci cum Radice), *Mu Dan Pi* (Cortex Moutan Radicis) and *Che Qian Zi* (Semen Plantaginis), it clears Heat, benefits the movement of Dampness, cools the Blood, and relieves Toxicity to treat pustular psoriasis.

Zhi Mu (Rhizoma Anemarrhenae Asphodeloidis)

Functions: Clears Heat and drains Fire, enriches Yin and moistens Dryness. This herb is very effective for clearing Heat in the Qi level and for clearing Heat from the Lungs and Stomach.

Indications: Heat Toxin patterns in skin disorders such as exanthematous drug eruptions, allergic contact dermatitis and urticaria; Dryness patterns in atopic or seborrheic eczema; Heat retention patterns in intertrigo and phytophotodermatitis; other Heat patterns in rosacea, anaphylactoid purpura, psoriasis, pemphigus, varicella (chickenpox), and measles.

Common dosage: 10g.

Combinations

- *Zhi Mu* (Rhizoma Anemarrhenae Asphodeloidis) can be combined with *Shi Gao* ‡ (Gypsum Fibrosum) and *Dan Zhu Ye* (Herba Lophatheri Gracilis) or *Xuan Shen* (Radix Scrophulariae Ningpoensis) to clear Heat and treat skin disorders accompanied by fever such as exanthematous drug eruptions, phytophotodermatitis and varicella (chickenpox).

- Combined with *Sheng Di Huang* (Radix Rehmanniae Glutinosae), *Shi Hu** (Herba Dendrobii) and *Xuan Shen* (Radix Scrophulariae Ningpoensis), it treats mouth and tongue sores due to Deficiency-Fire flaming upward.

- Combined with *Dang Gui* (Radix Angelicae Sinensis), *Bai Shao* (Radix Paeoniae Lactiflorae) and *Huang Qin* (Radix Scutellariae Baicalensis), it clears Heat, nourishes the Blood and moistens Dryness to treat atopic eczema.

- Combined with *Huang Qin* (Radix Scutellariae Baicalensis), *Huang Lian* (Rhizoma Coptidis) and *Tong Cao* (Medulla Tetrapanacis Papyriferi), it drains Fire, clears Heat and eliminates Dampness to treat pemphigus.

Huang Qin (Radix Scutellariae Baicalensis)

Functions: Clears Heat and dries Dampness, drains Fire and relieves Toxicity. This herb is very effective at clearing Heat from the Lungs and draining Fire from the Upper Burner.

Indications: Damp-Heat patterns in acute eczema, seborrheic eczema, herpes simplex, impetigo, pemphigus, psoriasis, and fixed drug eruptions; Blood-Heat patterns in acne, rosacea, pruritus, and pityriasis rosea; and other Heat patterns in urticaria, herpes zoster (shingles), intertrigo, and hyperhidrosis.

Common dosage: 10g.

Combinations

- Combined with *Pi Pa Ye* (Folium Eriobotryae Japonicae), *Sang Bai Pi* (Cortex Mori Albae Radicis), *Chao Mu Dan Pi* (Cortex Moutan Radicis, stir-fried), and *Hong Hua* (Flos Carthami Tinctorii), it clears Heat from the Lungs, cools the Blood, relieves Toxicity, and reduces erythema to treat acne and rosacea.

- Combined with *Long Dan Cao* (Radix Gentianae Scabrae), *Zhi Zi* (Fructus Gardeniae Jasminoidis), *Che Qian Zi* (Semen Plantaginis), and *Chai Hu* (Radix Bupleuri), it clears Heat, transforms Dampness and relieves Toxicity to treat acute eczema or fixed drug eruptions.
- Combined with *Jing Jie* (Herba Schizonepetae Tenuifoliae), *Fang Feng* (Radix Ledebouriellae Divaricatae), *Ku Shen* (Radix Sophorae Flavescentis), and *Lian Qiao* (Fructus Forsythiae Suspensae), it dissipates Wind, dispels Dampness, clears Heat, and relieves Toxicity to treat psoriasis due to Wind-Heat.

Huang Lian (Rhizoma Coptidis)
Functions: Drains Fire and relieves Toxicity, clears Heat and dries Dampness. This herb is very effective at draining Stomach-Fire and clearing Heat in the Heart channel.

Indications: Perioral dermatitis due to Fire in the Spleen and Stomach; urticaria due to Heat in the Heart channel; Damp-Heat patterns in erythema multiforme, pompholyx and pemphigus; Wind-Heat patterns in erysipelas, dermographism and phytophotodermatitis.

Common dosage: 5-10g.

Combinations

- Combined with *Huang Qin* (Radix Scutellariae Baicalensis) and *Zhi Zi* (Fructus Gardeniae Jasminoidis), it clears Heat in the Triple Burner to treat Damp-Heat patterns of pompholyx, impetigo, pemphigus, and hyperhidrosis; this combination also drains Excess-Fire to treat perioral dermatitis and oral candidiasis (thrush).
- Combined with *Ze Xie* (Rhizoma Alismatis Orientalis), *Yi Yi Ren* (Semen Coicis Lachryma-jobi), *Chen Pi* (Pericarpium Citri Reticulatae), and *Zhi Zi* (Fructus Gardeniae Jasminoidis), it fortifies the Spleen, dries Dampness, clears Heat, and relieves Toxicity to treat erythema multiforme.
- Combined with *Jing Jie* (Herba Schizonepetae Tenuifoliae), *Fang Feng* (Radix Ledebouriellae Divaricatae), *Ku Shen* (Radix Sophorae Flavescentis), *Lian Qiao* (Fructus Forsythiae Suspensae), and *Huang Qin* (Radix Scutellariae Baicalensis), it drains Fire, disperses Wind and alleviates itching to treat dermographism due to Wind-Heat.

Huang Bai (Cortex Phellodendri)
Functions: Clears Heat and drains Fire, dries Dampness and relieves Toxicity. This herb is very effective at clearing Excess-Heat in the Lower Burner and draining Fire at the Gate of Vitality.

Indications: Damp-Heat patterns in skin disorders such as genital and perianal eczema, vulval pruritus, stasis eczema, tinea cruris (jock itch), erysipelas, and palmoplantar pustulosis; Yin Deficiency patterns in lichen planus and melasma (chloasma); also for herpetic stomatitis due to Deficiency-Fire and oral candidiasis (thrush) due to Excess-Fire.

Common dosage: 10-15g.

Combinations

- Combined with *Mu Dan Pi* (Cortex Moutan Radicis), *Che Qian Zi* (Semen Plantaginis), *Ze Xie* (Rhizoma Alismatis Orientalis), and *Fu Ling* (Sclerotium Poriae Cocos), it

clears Heat, percolates Dampness and relieves Toxicity to treat atopic eczema and vulval and scrotal pruritus.

- Combined with *Sheng Di Huang* (Radix Rehmanniae Glutinosae), *Fu Ling* (Sclerotium Poriae Cocos) and *Cang Zhu* (Rhizoma Atractylodis), it clears Heat and transforms Dampness to treat genital eczema and tinea cruris (jock itch).
- Combined with *Huang Lian* (Rhizoma Coptidis), *Huang Qin* (Radix Scutellariae Baicalensis) and *Zhi Zi* (Fructus Gardeniae Jasminoidis), it clears Heat and drains Excess-Fire from the Triple Burner to treat oral candidiasis (thrush).
- Combined with *Gan Di Huang* (Radix Rehmanniae Glutinosae Exsiccata), *Mu Dan Pi* (Cortex Moutan Radicis) and *Shan Zhu Yu* (Fructus Corni Officinalis), it nourishes the Liver, supplements the Kidneys and enriches Yin to treat lichen planus involving the buccal mucosa.

Zhi Zi (Fructus Gardeniae Jasminoidis)
Functions: Drains Fire and eliminates irritability, clears Heat and benefits the movement of Dampness, cools the Blood and relieves Toxicity. This herb is very effective at draining Heart-Fire and clearing Damp-Heat from the Triple Burner.

Indications: Damp-Heat patterns in skin disorders such as acute eczema, seborrheic eczema, pompholyx, fixed drug eruptions, erythema multiforme, impetigo, and herpes simplex; Heart-Fire patterns in mouth ulcers and bullous pemphigoid; Liver-Fire patterns in melasma (chloasma) and erysipelas; and Lung-Heat patterns in acne and rosacea.

Common dosage: 5-10g.

Combinations

- Combined with *Long Dan Cao* (Radix Gentianae Scabrae), *Chai Hu* (Radix Bupleuri), *Huang Qin* (Radix Scutellariae Baicalensis), and *Che Qian Zi* (Semen Plantaginis), it clears Heat, drains Fire and transforms Dampness to treat acute eczema, ear eczema, fixed drug eruptions, herpes simplex, impetigo, and hyperhidrosis.
- Combined with *Sheng Di Huang* (Radix Rehmanniae Glutinosae), *Tong Cao* (Medulla Tetrapanacis Papyriferi), *Dan Zhu Ye* (Herba Lophatheri Gracilis), *Deng Xin Cao* (Medulla Junci Effusi), and *Jin Yin Hua* (Flos Lonicerae), it clears Heat from the Heart, cools the Blood and guides Heat downward, enabling Heart-Fire Toxins to be eliminated to treat mouth ulcers and bullous pemphigoid.
- Combined with *Mu Dan Pi* (Cortex Moutan Radicis), *Sheng Di Huang* (Radix Rehmanniae Glutinosae), *Chi Shao* (Radix Paeoniae Rubra), and *Sang Bai Pi* (Cortex Mori Albae Radicis), it drains the Lungs, clears Heat, cools the Blood, and reduces erythema to treat rosacea and pityriasis rosea.

Long Dan Cao (Radix Gentianae Scabrae)
Functions: Drains Excess-Fire in the Liver and Gallbladder channels, clears Heat and dries Dampness. This herb is very effective at clearing Damp-Heat from the Lower Burner.

Indications: Damp-Heat patterns in skin disorders such as acute eczema, flexural psoriasis, tinea cruris (jock itch), herpes simplex, fixed drug eruptions, and hyperhidrosis.

Common dosage: 5-10g.

Combinations

- Combined with *Huang Qin* (Radix Scutellariae Baicalensis), *Zhi Zi* (Fructus Gardeniac Jasminoidis), *Chai Hu* (Radix

Bupleuri), and *Che Qian Zi* (Semen Plantaginis), it clears Heat, cools the Blood, transforms Dampness, and relieves Toxicity to treat acute eczema, fixed drug eruptions, herpes simplex, and hyperhidrosis.

- Combined with *Bai Xian Pi* (Cortex Dictamni Dasycarpi Radicis), *Ku Shen* (Radix Sophorae Flavescentis), *Che Qian Zi* (Semen Plantaginis), *Sheng Di Huang* (Radix Rehmanniae Glutinosae), and *Bai Mao Gen* (Rhizoma Imperatae Cylindricae), it clears Heat, benefits the movement of Dampness, cools the Blood, and reduces erythema to treat contact dermatitis and tinea cruris (jock itch).

- Combined with *Chai Hu* (Radix Bupleuri), *Zhi Zi* (Fructus Gardeniae Jasminoidis), *Huang Lian* (Rhizoma Coptidis), and *Huang Qin* (Radix Scutellariae Baicalensis), it clears Heat and drains Fire to treat erysipelas and hyperhidrosis.

MATERIA MEDICA FOR CLEARING HEAT AND COOLING THE BLOOD

Huai Hua (Flos Sophorae Japonicae)
Functions: Clears Heat, cools the Blood and stops bleeding. This herb is very effective at clearing Heat from the Large Intestine.

Indications: Blood-Heat patterns in skin disorders such as acne, psoriasis and pityriasis rosea; rosacea due to Blood stasis; Damp patterns in allergic contact dermatitis and annular erythema.

Common dosage: 10-15g.

Combinations

- Combined with *Sheng Di Huang* (Radix Rehmanniae Glutinosae), *Mu Dan Pi* (Cortex Moutan Radicis), *Chi Shao* (Radix Paeoniae Rubra), and *Ling Xiao Hua* (Flos Campsitis), it cools the Blood and clears Heat to treat acne, rosacea, psoriasis, and pityriasis rosea.

- Combined with *Fu Ling* (Sclerotium Poriae Cocos), *Chen Pi* (Pericarpium Citri Reticulatae), *Zhi Zi* (Fructus Gardeniae Jasminoidis), and *Huang Qin* (Radix Scutellariae), it cools the Blood, eliminates Dampness and relieves Toxicity.

Qian Cao Gen (Radix Rubiae Cordifoliae)
Functions: Cools the Blood and stops bleeding, invigorates the Blood and dispels stasis, frees the channels and invigorates the network vessels.

Indications: Blood Heat patterns in psoriasis and pityriasis rosea; Blood stasis patterns in erythema induratum and dermographism.

Common dosage: 10-15g.

Combinations

- Combined with *Chi Shao* (Radix Paeoniae Rubra), *Ling Xiao Hua* (Flos Campsitis) and *Zi Cao* (Radix Arnebiae seu Lithospermi), it cools the Blood, frees the network vessels and reduces erythema to treat pityriasis rosea.

- Combined with *Dang Gui* (Radix Angelicae Sinensis), *Chi Shao* (Radix Paeoniae Rubra), *Tao Ren* (Semen Persicae), and *Hong Hua* (Flos Carthami Tinctorii), it invigorates and cools the Blood to free the network vessels and treat erythema induratum and dermographism.

Zi Cao (Radix Arnebiae seu Lithospermi)
Functions: Cools and invigorates the Blood, clears Heat and relieves Toxicity to vent papules. This herb is very effective at clearing Heat in the Xue level to treat Excess-Fire due to the frenetic movement of hot Blood.

Indications: Blood-Heat patterns in skin disorders such as psoriasis, pityriasis rosea, exanthematous drug eruptions, dermographism, and polymorphic light eruption; Damp-Heat patterns in anaphylactoid purpura, irritant contact dermatitis and varicella (chickenpox); Blood stasis patterns in herpes zoster and purpuric drug eruptions. *Zi Cao You* (Gromwell Root Oil) is used externally in the treatment of burns, intertrigo, chapped and fissured hands and feet, diaper dermatitis (nappy rash), and herpes zoster.

Common dosage: 10-15g.

Combinations

- Combined with *Chi Shao* (Radix Paeoniae Rubra), *Sheng Di Huang* (Radix Rehmanniae Glutinosae) and *Mu Dan Pi* (Cortex Moutan Radicis), it strengthens the effect of cooling the Blood, relieving Toxicity and reducing erythema to treat psoriasis, pityriasis rosea, exanthematous drug eruptions, and polymorphic light eruption.

- Combined with *Mu Dan Pi* (Cortex Moutan Radicis), *Qian Cao Gen* (Radix Rubiae Cordifoliae) and *Bai Mao Gen* (Rhizoma Imperatae Cylindricae), it cools and invigorates the Blood to stop bleeding, transform Blood stasis and disperse purpura.

- Combined with *Ma Chi Xian* (Herba Portulacae Oleraceae) and *Da Qing Ye* (Folium Isatidis seu Baphicacanthi) or *Ban Lan Gen* (Radix Isatidis seu Baphicacanthi), it can be used to treat plane warts (verruca plana).

Mu Dan Pi (Cortex Moutan Radicis)
Functions: Clears Heat and cools the Blood, invigorates the Blood and dissipates Blood stasis. This herb is widely used for clearing Heat in the treatment of skin disorders.

Indications: Blood-Heat patterns in skin disorders such as psoriasis, pityriasis rosea, lichen simplex chronicus (neurodermatitis), acne, rosacea, exanthematous drug eruptions, and alopecia areata; Damp-Heat patterns in acute eczema, genital eczema, anaphylactoid purpura, pemphigus vulgaris, pustular psoriasis, and tinea pedis (athlete's foot); Wind-Heat patterns in seborrheic eczema, pruritus, urticaria, and erysipelas; and other Heat patterns in erythema multiforme, recurrent aphthous stomatitis (mouth ulcers) and herpes zoster (shingles).

Common dosage: 10-15g.

Combinations

- Combined with *Sheng Di Huang* (Radix Rehmanniae Glutinosae), *Chi Shao* (Radix Paeoniae Rubra), *Huai Hua* (Flos Sophorae Japonicae), and *Zi Cao* (Radix Arnebiae seu Lithospermi), it cools the Blood, relieves Toxicity and reduces erythema to treat psoriasis and pityriasis rosea.

- Combined with *Sheng Di Huang* (Radix Rehmanniae Glutinosae), *Chi Shao* (Radix Paeoniae Rubra), and *Huang Qin* (Radix Scutellariae Baicalensis), it clears Heat from the Stomach, cools and invigorates the Blood, and reduces erythema to treat rosacea, acne and polymorphic light eruption.

- Combined with *Yi Yi Ren* (Semen Coicis Lachryma-jobi), *Hua Shi‡* (Talcum), *Bai Mao Gen* (Rhizoma Imperatae Cylindricae), and *Zi Cao* (Radix Arnebiae seu Lithospermi), it clears Heat, transforms Dampness, and cools and invigorates the Blood to transform purpura and disperse swelling.

- Combined with *Huang Bai* (Cortex Phellodendri), *Yi Yi Ren* (Semen Coicis Lachryma-jobi), *Chi Xiao Dou* (Semen Phaseoli Radiati), *Gou Teng* (Ramulus Uncariae cum Uncis), and *Ku Shen* (Radix Sophorae Flavescentis), it clears Heat, transforms Dampness, dissipates Wind, and alleviates itching to treat pruritus.
- Combined with *Dang Gui* (Radix Angelicae Sinensis), *Chi Shao* (Radix Paeoniae Rubra), *Chuan Xiong* (Rhizoma Ligustici Chuanxiong), *Zi Cao* (Radix Arnebiae seu Lithospermi), and *Xiang Fu* (Rhizoma Cyperi Rotundi), it invigorates the Blood and dissipates Blood stasis, frees the network vessels and dissipates lumps to treat drug eruptions due to Blood stasis.

Sheng Di Huang (Radix Rehmanniae Glutinosae)
Functions: Clears Heat and cools the Blood, nourishes Yin and generates Body Fluids. The fresh herb, *Xian Di Huang* (Radix Rehmanniae Glutinosae Recens) has a stronger effect in clearing Heat and cooling the Blood, whereas the dried herb, *Gan Di Huang* (Radix Rehmanniae Glutinosae Exsiccata) has a stronger effect in nourishing Yin and cooling the Blood.
Indications: Blood-Heat patterns in skin disorders such as psoriasis, pityriasis rosea, acne, rosacea, pruritus, anaphylactoid purpura, alopecia areata, exanthematous drug eruptions, and furuncles (boils); Blood-Dryness patterns in acute eczema, pityriasis rosea, psoriasis, dermatitis herpetiformis, plane warts (verruca plana), and tinea manuum (ringworm of the hands); Blood stasis patterns in acne, rosacea, lichen planus, alopecia areata, and nodular prurigo; Yin Deficiency patterns in herpes simplex, erythema induratum, melasma (chloasma), and vitiligo.
Common dosage: 15-30g.
Combinations

- Combined with *Xuan Shen* (Radix Scrophulariae Ningpoensis), *Huang Qin* (Radix Scutellariae Baicalensis), *Fang Feng* (Radix Ledebouriellae Divaricatae), *Chan Tui* ‡ (Periostracum Cicadae), and *Bai Ji Li* (Fructus Tribuli Terrestris), it clears Heat and cools the Blood, dissipates Wind and alleviates itching to treat pruritus.
- Combined with *Shan Yao* (Rhizoma Dioscoreae Oppositae), *Yi Yi Ren* (Semen Coicis Lachryma-jobi), *Dang Gui* (Radix Angelicae Sinensis), and *Dan Shen* (Radix Salviae Miltiorrhizae), it enriches Yin, protects Body Fluids, moistens Dryness, invigorates the Blood, and alleviates itching to treat chronic eczema.
- Combined with *Tao Ren* (Semen Persicae), *Hong Hua* (Flos Carthami Tinctorii), *Dan Shen* (Radix Salviae Miltiorrhizae), *Dang Gui* (Radix Angelicae Sinensis), and *He Shou Wu* (Radix Polygoni Multiflori), it transforms Blood stasis, softens hardness, nourishes the Blood, and moistens Dryness to treat lichen planus.
- Combined with *Long Dan Cao* (Radix Gentianae Scabrae), *Huang Qin* (Radix Scutellariae Baicalensis), *Zhi Zi* (Fructus Gardeniae Jasminoidis), *Che Qian Zi* (Semen Plantaginis), and *Bai Xian Pi* (Cortex Dictamni Dasycarpi Radicis), it clears Heat, cools the Blood and transforms Dampness to treat acute eczema.

- Combined with *Nü Zhen Zi* (Fructus Ligustri Lucidi), *Sang Shen* (Fructus Mori Albae), *Xuan Shen* (Radix Scrophulariae Ningpoensis), and *Hei Zhi Ma* (Semen Sesami Indici), it clears Heat and cools the Blood, nourishes Yin and protects the hair to treat alopecia areata.
- Combined with *Ling Xiao Hua* (Flos Campsitis) and *Ji Guan Hua* (Flos Celosiae Cristatae), it nourishes Yin, cools the Blood and disperses macules to treat melasma (chloasma).

Ling Xiao Hua (Flos Campsitis)
Functions: Cools the Blood, breaks up Blood stasis and dispels Wind. This herb can clear deeply lying Fire in the Blood to treat itching due to Blood-Heat generating Wind.
Indications: Used in skin disorders for cooling the Blood to treat cosmetic dermatitis, psoriasis, pityriasis rosea, erythema multiforme, acne, and rosacea; and for invigorating the Blood to treat melasma (chloasma).
Common dosage: 3-9g.
Combinations

- Combined with *Huang Qin* (Radix Scutellariae Baicalensis), *Sheng Di Huang* (Radix Rehmanniae Glutinosae), *Hong Hua* (Flos Carthami Tinctorii), and *Jin Yin Hua* (Flos Lonicerae), it clears Heat from the Lungs and Spleen, cools the Blood and alleviates itching to treat perioral dermatitis.
- Combined with *Mu Dan Pi* (Cortex Moutan Radicis), *Chi Shao* (Radix Paeoniae Rubra), *Zi Cao* (Radix Arnebiae seu Lithospermi), *Fang Feng* (Radix Ledebouriellae Divaricatae), and *Zhi Zi* (Fructus Gardeniae Jasminoidis), it cools the Blood, reduces erythema, dissipates Wind, and alleviates itching to treat pityriasis rosea.

MATERIA MEDICA FOR INVIGORATING THE BLOOD AND TRANSFORMING BLOOD STASIS

Hong Hua (Flos Carthami Tinctorii)
Functions: Invigorates the Blood and frees the channels, dispels Blood stasis and alleviates pain, dissipates swelling and disperses macules.
Indications: This herb is frequently used in the dermatology clinic to invigorate the Blood and treat Blood stasis patterns in conditions such as pruritus, lichen planus, dermographism, alopecia areata, and erythema induratum; and to cool the Blood to treat Heat patterns in psoriasis, pityriasis rosea, acne, and rosacea.
Common dosage: 10g.
Combinations

- Combined with *Sheng Di Huang* (Radix Rehmanniae Glutinosae), *Mu Dan Pi* (Cortex Moutan Radicis) and *Ling Xiao Hua* (Flos Campsitis), it cools the Blood and reduces erythema to treat psoriasis, pityriasis rosea, acne, and rosacea.
- Combined with *Tao Ren* (Semen Persicae), *E Zhu* (Rhizoma Curcumae), *Dan Shen* (Radix Salviae Miltiorrhizae), *Niu Xi* (Radix Achyranthis Bidentatae), and *Dang Gui* (Radix Angelicae Sinensis), it transforms Blood stasis and frees the network vessels, softens hardness and dissipates lumps to treat lichen planus.
- Combined with *Dang Gui* (Radix Angelicae Sinensis), *Tao Ren* (Semen Persicae), *Chi Shao* (Radix Paeoniae Rubra), *Jing Jie* (Herba Schizonepetae Tenuifoliae), and *Bai Ji Li*

(Fructus Tribuli Terrestris), it invigorates the Blood, frees the network vessels, disperses Wind, and alleviates itching to treat pruritus.

- Combined with *Dang Gui* (Radix Angelicae Sinensis), *Bai Shao* (Radix Paeoniae Lactiflorae), *Sheng Di Huang* (Radix Rehmanniae Glutinosae), and *Ling Xiao Hua* (Flos Campsitis), it nourishes and invigorates the Blood, emolliates the Liver, and disperses macules to treat melasma (chloasma).

Tao Ren (Semen Persicae)
Functions: Invigorates the Blood and breaks up Blood stasis, moistens the Intestines and promotes bowel movement.

Indications: Blood stasis patterns in skin disorders such as lichen planus, urticaria, pruritus, nodular prurigo, acne, rosacea, alopecia areata, and erythema induratum.

Common dosage: 6-10g.

Combinations

- Combining *Tao Ren* (Semen Persicae) with *Hong Hua* (Flos Carthami Tinctorii), *Dang Gui* (Radix Angelicae Sinensis) and *Chi Shao* (Radix Paeoniae Rubra) strengthens the effect in invigorating the Blood, breaking up Blood stasis and alleviating itching to treat pruritus due to Blood-Heat.

- Combined with *Mu Li* ‡ (Concha Ostreae), *Ci Shi* ‡ (Magnetitum), *Hong Hua* (Flos Carthami Tinctorii), and *Chuan Niu Xi* (Radix Cyathulae Officinalis), it invigorates the Blood and softens hardness to treat plantar warts (verruca plantaris).

- Combined with *Dang Gui* (Radix Angelicae Sinensis), *Chi Shao* (Radix Paeoniae Rubra), *Qian Cao Gen* (Radix Rubiae Cordifoliae), *Qing Pi* (Pericarpium Citri Reticulatae Viride), and *Xiang Fu* (Rhizoma Cyperi Rotundi), it invigorates the Blood and regulates Qi to free the network vessels and treat erythema induratum.

Dan Shen (Radix Salviae Miltiorrhizae)
Functions: Invigorates the Blood and dispels Blood stasis, clears Heart-Fire and eliminates irritability, expels pus to alleviate pain.

Indications: This herb is frequently used in the dermatology clinic to invigorate the Blood to treat Blood-Dryness patterns in skin disorders such as psoriasis, chronic eczema, asteatotic eczema, pityriasis rosea, and plane warts (verruca plana); Blood-Heat patterns in psoriasis, pruritus and lichen simplex chronicus (neurodermatitis); and Blood stasis patterns in lichen planus, nodular prurigo and ichthyosis vulgaris.

Common dosage: 10-20g.

Combinations

- Combined with *Sheng Di Huang* (Radix Rehmanniae Glutinosae), *Xuan Shen* (Radix Scrophulariae Ningpoensis), *Yi Yi Ren* (Semen Coicis Lachryma-jobi), *Dang Gui* (Radix Angelicae Sinensis), and *Bai Xian Pi* (Cortex Dictamni Dasycarpi Radicis), it enriches Yin, protects Body Fluids, transforms Dampness, and invigorates the Blood to alleviate itching and treat chronic eczema and pityriasis rosea.

- Combined with *Dang Gui* (Radix Angelicae Sinensis), it invigorates the Blood and frees the network vessels to assist *Fang Feng* (Radix Ledebouriellae Divaricatae), *Chan Tui* ‡ (Periostracum Cicadae) and *Bai Ji Li* (Fructus Tribuli Terrestris) to dissipate Wind and alleviate itching to treat pruritus.

- Combined with *Huang Qi* (Radix Astragali seu Hedysari), *Hei Zhi Ma* (Semen Sesami Indici), *Dang Gui* (Radix Angelicae Sinensis), *Sheng Di Huang* (Radix Rehmanniae Glutinosae), *Shu Di Huang* (Radix Rehmanniae Glutinosae Conquita), and *He Shou Wu* (Radix Polygoni Multiflori), it invigorates the Blood and frees the network vessels to promote nourishment of the skin by Qi and Blood in the treatment of Raynaud's disease.

- *Dan Shen* (Radix Salviae Miltiorrhizae) is also used in the treatment of vitiligo to nourish and invigorate the Blood, thereby promoting the production of melanocytes.

Da Huang (Radix et Rhizoma Rhei)
Functions: Invigorates the Blood and transforms Blood stasis, drains Fire, clears Heat and cools the Blood, attacks accumulation and guides out stagnation, disperses swelling and alleviates pain.

Indications: Patterns of Heat in the Lungs, Spleen or Stomach in skin disorders such as acne, rosacea, perioral dermatitis, and recurrent aphthous stomatitis (mouth ulcers); also for nodular prurigo, perianal eczema and insect bites. *Da Huang* (Radix et Rhizoma Rhei) is frequently used where constipation is an accompanying symptom, for example in herpes zoster (shingles), furuncles, drug eruptions, pemphigus vulgaris, and varicella (chickenpox); in these circumstances, it is generally added 10 minutes before the end of the decoction process.

Common dosage: 3-12g.

Combinations

- Combined with *Shi Gao* ‡ (Gypsum Fibrosum), *Huang Qin* (Radix Scutellariae Baicalensis) and *Hong Hua* (Flos Carthami Tinctorii), it clears Heat from the Lungs and Spleen, cools the Blood and reduces erythema to treat rosacea and perioral dermatitis.

- Combined with *Tao Ren* (Semen Persicae), *Chi Shao* (Radix Paeoniae Rubra), *Dan Shen* (Radix Salviae Miltiorrhizae), and *Chuan Xiong* (Rhizoma Ligustici Chuanxiong), *Jiu Da Huang* (Radix et Rhizoma Rhei, prepared with wine) transforms Blood stasis and dissipates nodules to treat nodular prurigo.

Chuan Xiong (Rhizoma Ligustici Chuanxiong)
Functions: Invigorates the Blood and moves Qi, dispels Wind and alleviates pain.

Indications: Blood stasis patterns in skin disorders such as rosacea, urticaria, nodular prurigo, purpuric drug eruptions, and alopecia areata; Qi stagnation patterns in erythema induratum, hidradenitis suppurativa and carbuncles; Dryness patterns in stasis eczema, seborrhea and tinea manuum (ringworm of the hands); and Cold patterns in psoriasis, chapped hands and feet, nummular eczema, and Raynaud's disease.

Common dosage: 3-10g.

Combinations

- Combined with *Dang Gui* (Radix Angelicae Sinensis), *Chi Shao* (Radix Paeoniae Rubra), *Tao Ren* (Semen Persicae), and *Bai Zhi* (Radix Angelicae Dahuricae), it transforms Blood stasis, dissipates lumps, frees the network vessels, and reduces erythema to treat rosacea and purpuric drug eruptions.

- Combined with *Dang Gui* (Radix Angelicae Sinensis), *Huang Qi* (Radix Astragali seu Hedysari), *Gui Zhi* (Ramulus

Cinnamomi Cassiae), *Hong Hua* (Flos Carthami Tinctorii), and *Dan Shen* (Radix Salviae Miltiorrhizae), it invigorates the Blood, frees the network vessels, warms Yang, and dissipates Cold to treat Raynaud's disease.

- Combined with *Xiang Fu* (Rhizoma Cyperi Rotundi), *Qing Pi* (Pericarpium Citri Reticulatae Viride) and *Chen Pi* (Pericarpium Citri Reticulatae), it soothes the Liver and regulates Qi to disperse swelling and alleviate pain at the initial stage of hidradenitis suppurativa.

Yi Mu Cao (Herba Leonuri Heterophylli)
Functions: Invigorates the Blood and dispels Blood stasis, clears Heat and relieves Toxicity, regulates the Chong and Ren vessels.

Indications: Blood-Dryness patterns in skin disorders such as chronic eczema, atopic eczema and plane warts (verruca plana); Blood stasis patterns in pruritus and acne; and vitiligo due to Liver Depression. This herb is also used where eruptions may be exacerbated before periods, as can be seen with psoriasis, acne and rosacea.

Common dosage: 3-10g.
Combinations

- Combined with *Dang Gui* (Radix Angelicae Sinensis), *Xu Chang Qing* (Radix Cynanchi Paniculati) and *Dan Shen* (Radix Salviae Miltiorrhizae), it invigorates the Blood to alleviate itching and treat chronic eczema.
- Combined with *Dang Gui* (Radix Angelicae Sinensis), *Tao Ren* (Semen Persicae), *Hong Hua* (Flos Carthami Tinctorii), and *Chi Shao* (Radix Paeoniae Rubra), it invigorates the Blood, transforms Blood stasis, frees the network vessels, and alleviates itching to treat pruritus.

MATERIA MEDICA FOR ELIMINATING DAMPNESS AND BENEFITING THE MOVEMENT OF WATER

MATERIA MEDICA FOR FORTIFYING THE SPLEEN AND ELIMINATING DAMPNESS

Bai Zhu (Rhizoma Atractylodis Macrocephalae)
Functions: Fortifies the Spleen and nourishes the Stomach, dries Dampness and promotes urination, consolidates the exterior and stops sweating. This herb is mainly used for Qi Deficiency of the Spleen and Stomach, which therefore fail to move and transform food and water, and for dispelling Dampness in all channels in order to regulate the Spleen and Stomach.

Indications: Spleen Deficiency patterns in skin disorders such as chronic eczema, atopic eczema, asteatotic eczema, angioedema, pruritus, lichen planus, and recurrent aphthous stomatitis (mouth ulcers); Spleen-Damp patterns in pemphigus, bullous pemphigoid and dermatitis herpetiformis; patterns involving impairment of the Spleen's functions in keratosis follicularis (Darier's disease), pityriasis alba, anaphylactoid purpura, and keratosis pilaris; and Qi and Blood Deficiency patterns in urticaria, alopecia areata and chilblains.

Common dosage: 5-10g.
Combinations

- Combined with *Cang Zhu* (Rhizoma Atractylodis), *Chen Pi* (Pericarpium Citri Reticulatae), *Zhu Ling* (Sclerotium Polypori Umbellati), *Ze Xie* (Rhizoma Alismatis Orientalis),

and *Fu Ling* (Sclerotium Poriae Cocos), it fortifies the Spleen and Stomach and eliminates Dampness to treat atopic eczema.
- Combined with *Chi Fu Ling* (Sclerotium Poriae Cocos Rubrae), *Yin Chen Hao* (Herba Artemisiae Scopariae), *Zhi Ke* (Fructus Citri Aurantii), *Cang Zhu* (Rhizoma Atractylodis), and *Ze Xie* (Rhizoma Alismatis Orientalis), it clears Heat, transforms Dampness, fortifies the Spleen, and harmonizes the Stomach to treat pemphigus.
- Combined with *Zhi Shi* (Fructus Immaturus Citri Aurantii), *Mu Xiang** (Radix Aucklandiae Lappae), *Xiang Fu* (Rhizoma Cyperi Rotundi), *Da Zao* (Fructus Ziziphi Jujubae), and *Sheng Jiang* (Rhizoma Zingiberis Officinalis Recens), it fortifies the Spleen, harmonizes the Stomach, loosens the Middle Burner, and regulates Qi to treat urticaria.
- Combined with *Huang Qi* (Radix Astragali seu Hedysari), *Dang Shen* (Radix Codonopsitis Pilosulae), *Dang Gui* (Radix Angelicae Sinensis), *Bai Shao* (Radix Paeoniae Lactiflorae), *Shu Di Huang* (Radix Rehmanniae Glutinosae Conquita), and *E Jiao*‡ (Gelatinum Corii Asini), it fortifies the Spleen and augments Qi to contain the Blood and stop bleeding to treat anaphylactoid purpura.
- Combined with *Huang Qi* (Radix Astragali seu Hedysari), *Duan Long Gu*‡ (Os Draconis Calcinatum), *Duan Mu Li*‡ (Concha Ostreae Calcinata), and *Dang Shen* (Radix Codonopsitis Pilosulae), it augments Qi and consolidates the exterior to constrain sweating.

Cang Zhu (Rhizoma Atractylodis)
Functions: Fortifies the Spleen and dries Dampness, dispels Wind and eliminates Dampness. This herb is very effective for treating Dampness in the Upper, Middle and Lower Burners, but it is contraindicated for patients with Heat patterns due to Yin Deficiency.

Indications: Damp-Heat patterns in skin disorders such as subacute eczema, stasis eczema, genital eczema, erythema multiforme, seborrhea, flexural psoriasis, erysipelas, tinea cruris (jock itch), and palmoplantar pustulosis; Spleen-Damp patterns in pemphigus and bullous pemphigoid; and atopic eczema due to Spleen and Stomach Deficiency.

Common dosage: 5-10g.
Combinations

- Combined with *Chen Pi* (Pericarpium Citri Reticulatae), *Hou Po* (Cortex Magnoliae Officinalis), *Zhi Ke* (Fructus Citri Aurantii), *Che Qian Zi* (Semen Plantaginis), and *Sha Ren* (Fructus Amomi), it clears Heat, fortifies the Spleen and regulates Dampness to treat subacute eczema.
- Combined with *Ku Shen* (Radix Sophorae Flavescentis), *Fu Ling* (Sclerotium Poriae Cocos), *Ze Xie* (Rhizoma Alismatis Orientalis), and *Bi Xie* (Rhizoma Dioscoreae Hypoglaucae seu Septemlobae), it clears Heat and dries Dampness to treat flexural psoriasis.
- Combined with *Huang Qi* (Radix Astragali seu Hedysari), *Dang Shen* (Radix Codonopsitis Pilosulae), *Shan Yao* (Radix Dioscoreae Oppositae), and *Chen Pi* (Pericarpium Citri Reticulatae), it augments Qi, supports the Spleen, transforms Dampness, and disperses eruptions to treat palmoplantar pustulosis.

Fu Ling (Sclerotium Poriae Cocos)

Functions: Fortifies the Spleen and harmonizes the Stomach, percolates Dampness and benefits the movement of water.

Indications: *Fu Ling* (Sclerotium Poriae Cocos) is employed to support the Spleen and transform Dampness in a variety of patterns in skin disorders such as chronic eczema, atopic, nummular, asteatotic and stasis eczema, lichen planus, bullous pemphigoid, erythema multiforme, flexural psoriasis, and vulval pruritus; *Chi Fu Ling* (Sclerotium Poriae Cocos Rubrae) treats Damp-Heat patterns in skin disorders such as seborrheic eczema, folliculitis, fixed drug eruptions, and ecthyma; *Fu Ling Pi* (Cortex Poriae Cocos) transforms Dampness and disperses swelling to treat disorders such as impetigo, herpes zoster (shingles) and chronic venous ulcer of the lower leg.

Common dosage: 10-15g.

Combinations

- Combined with *Dang Shen* (Radix Codonopsitis Pilosulae), *Bai Zhu* (Rhizoma Atractylodis Macrocephalae) and *Gan Cao* (Radix Glycyrrhizae), *Fu Ling* (Sclerotium Poriae Cocos) augments Qi and supports the Spleen to treat urticaria.

- Combined with *Sheng Di Huang* (Radix Rehmanniae Glutinosae), *Xuan Shen* (Radix Scrophulariae Ningpoensis), *Shan Yao* (Rhizoma Dioscoreae Oppositae), and *Yi Yi Ren* (Semen Coicis Lachryma-jobi), *Fu Ling* (Sclerotium Poriae Cocos) enriches Yin, transforms Dampness and moistens Dryness to treat chronic eczema due to damage to Yin.

- Combined with *Pu Gong Ying* (Herba Taraxaci cum Radice), *Zi Hua Di Ding* (Herba Violae Yedoensitis), *Yi Yi Ren* (Semen Coicis Lachryma-jobi), *Che Qian Zi* (Semen Plantaginis), and *Chi Xiao Dou* (Semen Phaseoli Calcarati), *Chi Fu Ling* (Sclerotium Poriae Cocos Rubrae) percolates Dampness, clears Heat and relieves Toxicity to treat ecthyma.

- Combined with *Yi Yi Ren* (Semen Coicis Lachryma-jobi), *Huo Xiang* (Herba Agastaches seu Pogostemi), *Chi Xiao Dou* (Semen Phaseoli Calcarati), and *Di Fu Zi* (Fructus Kochiae Scopariae), *Fu Ling Pi* (Cortex Poriae Cocos) clears Heat and transforms Dampness to treat herpes zoster (shingles).

Yi Yi Ren (Semen Coicis Lachryma-jobi)

Functions: Fortifies the Spleen and benefits the movement of water, stops diarrhea, clears Heat and expels pus.

Indications: Damp-Heat patterns in skin disorders such as subacute eczema, pompholyx, herpes zoster (shingles), erythema multiforme, erysipelas, palmoplantar pustulosis, anaphylactoid purpura, and plantar warts (verruca plantaris); Wind-Heat patterns in lichen planus and phytophotodermatitis; and Wind-Heat-Damp patterns in pruritus, herpes simplex and chronic venous ulcer of the lower leg.

Common dosage: 10-30g.

Combinations

- Combined with *Dang Shen* (Radix Codonopsitis Pilosulae), *Fu Ling* (Sclerotium Poriae Cocos), *Bai Zhu* (Rhizoma Atractylodis Macrocephalae), and *Cang Zhu* (Rhizoma Atractylodis), it augments Qi and supports the Spleen to treat bullous pemphigoid.

- Combined with *Fu Ling Pi* (Cortex Poriae Cocos), *Bai Zhu* (Rhizoma Atractylodis Macrocephalae), *Yin Chen Hao* (Herba Artemisiae Scopariae), and *Bai Xian Pi* (Cortex Dictamni Dasycarpi Radicis), it supports the Spleen, transforms Dampness and clears Heat to treat chronic eczema due to Damp obstruction.

- Combined with *Da Qing Ye* (Folium Isatidis seu Baphicanthi), *Huang Qin* (Radix Scutellariae Baicalensis), *Pi Pa Ye* (Folium Eriobotryae Japonicae), *Xin Yi Hua* (Flos Magnoliae), and *Mai Men Dong* (Radix Ophiopogonis Japonici), it clears Heat, transforms Dampness, nourishes Yin, and supplements the Lungs to treat herpes simplex.

- Combined with *Sheng Di Huang* (Radix Rehmanniae Glutinosae), *Mu Dan Pi* (Cortex Moutan Radicis), *Dang Gui* (Radix Angelicae Sinensis), *Bai Zhu* (Rhizoma Atractylodis Macrocephalae), and *Fu Ling* (Sclerotium Poriae Cocos), it supports the Spleen, nourishes the Blood, emolliates the Liver, and dissipates lumps to treat plane warts (verruca plana) caused by Blood-Dryness due to Liver Deficiency.

Bai Bian Dou (Semen Dolichoris Lablab)

Functions: Fortifies the Spleen and harmonizes the Middle Burner, disperses Summerheat and transforms Dampness.

Indications: Spleen Deficiency patterns in skin disorders such as lichen planus, dermatitis herpetiformis, nipple eczema, and tinea manuum (ringworm of the hands); and patterns of the Spleen failing to distribute Body Fluids as in keratosis pilaris or keratosis follicularis (Darier's disease).

Common dosage: 10-20g.

Combinations

- Combined with *Sheng Di Huang* (Radix Rehmanniae Glutinosae), *Xuan Shen* (Radix Scrophulariae Ningpoensis), *Shan Yao* (Rhizoma Dioscoreae Oppositae), *Fu Ling* (Sclerotium Poriae Cocos), and *Yi Yi Ren* (Semen Coicis Lachryma-jobi), it transforms Dampness, moistens Dryness, enriches Yin, and protects Body Fluids to treat chronic eczema due to Blood-Dryness.

- Combined with *Dang Shen* (Radix Codonopsitis Pilosulae), *Bai Zhu* (Rhizoma Atractylodis Macrocephalae), *Chen Pi* (Pericarpium Citri Reticulatae), *Shan Yao* (Radix Dioscoreae Oppositae), and *Sha Ren* (Fructus Amomi), it augments Qi, enriches Yin, supports the Spleen, and harmonizes the Stomach to treat keratosis pilaris or keratosis follicularis (Darier's disease).

- Combined with *Huo Xiang* (Herba Agastaches seu Pogostemi), *Pei Lan* (Herba Eupatorii Fortunei), *Shan Yao* (Radix Dioscoreae Oppositae), *Ze Xie* (Rhizoma Alismatis Orientalis), and *Huang Qin* (Radix Scutellariae Baicalensis), it dries Dampness, transforms turbidity, augments Qi, and supports the Spleen to treat dermatitis herpetiformis.

MATERIA MEDICA FOR CLEARING HEAT AND ELIMINATING DAMPNESS

Bi Xie (Rhizoma Dioscoreae Hypoglaucae seu Septemlobae)

Functions: Eliminates Dampness and dispels Wind to treat Wind-Damp Bi syndrome pain.

Indications: Damp-Heat patterns in skin disorders such as erysipelas, flexural psoriasis, nodular prurigo, and tinea cruris; also for bromhidrosis and for Bi syndrome in psoriatic arthritis.

Common dosage: 10-15g.

Combinations

- Combined with *Qiang Huo* (Rhizoma et Radix Notopterygii), *Du Huo* (Radix Angelicae Pubescentis), *Sang Ji Sheng* (Ramulus Loranthi), *Wu Jia Pi* (Cortex Acanthopanacis Gracilistyli Radicis), and *Luo Shi Teng* (Caulis Trachelospermi Jasminoidis), it dissipates Wind, eliminates Dampness, disperses swelling, and alleviates pain to treat psoriatic arthritis.

- Combined with *Huo Xiang* (Herba Agastaches seu Pogostemi), *Ding Xiang* (Flos Caryophylli), *Mu Xiang** (Radix Aucklandiae Lappae), and *Xiang Fu* (Rhizoma Cyperi Rotundi), it clears Heat, transforms Dampness and repels foulness to treat bromhidrosis.

Yin Chen Hao (Herba Artemisiae Scopariae)

Functions: Clears Heat and promotes the movement of Dampness to alleviate itching.

Indications: Damp-Heat patterns in skin disorders such as seborrhea, seborrheic eczema and bromhidrosis; Spleen-Damp patterns in chronic eczema, pemphigus and bullous pemphigoid.

Common dosage: 15-30g.

Combinations

- Combined with *Chi Fu Ling* (Sclerotium Poriae Cocos Rubrae), *Zhi Ke* (Fructus Citri Aurantii), *Cang Zhu* (Rhizoma Atractylodis), *Bai Zhu* (Rhizoma Atractylodis Macrocephalae), and *Ze Xie* (Rhizoma Alismatis Orientalis), it clears Heat, transforms Dampness, fortifies the Spleen, and harmonizes the Stomach to treat pemphigus.

- Combined with *Huo Xiang* (Herba Agastaches seu Pogostemi), *Huang Qin* (Radix Scutellariae Baicalensis), *Jing Jie* (Herba Schizonepetae Tenuifoliae), *Fang Feng* (Radix Ledebouriellae Divaricatae), and *Sheng Di Huang* (Radix Rehmanniae Glutinosae), it clears Heat, transforms Dampness, dissipates Wind, and alleviates itching to treat seborrheic eczema.

Di Fu Zi (Fructus Kochiae Scopariae)

Functions: Clears Heat and benefits the movement of Dampness to alleviate itching.

Indications: This herb can dispel Heat accumulated in the skin and flesh and eliminate itching due to external Dampness to treat acute eczema, impetigo, herpes zoster (shingles), lichen planus, and lichen simplex chronicus (neurodermatitis).

Common dosage: 10-15g.

Combinations

- Combined with *Niu Bang Zi* (Fructus Arctii Lappae), *Fang Feng* (Radix Ledebouriellae Divaricatae), *Jing Jie* (Herba Schizonepetae Tenuifoliae), *Cang Er Zi* (Fructus Xanthii Sibirici), and *Ku Shen* (Radix Sophorae Flavescentis), it percolates Dampness, clears Heat, dredges Wind, and alleviates itching to treat lichen planus.

- Combined with *Yi Yi Ren* (Semen Coicis Lachryma-jobi), *Chi Xiao Dou* (Semen Phaseoli Calcarati), *Fu Ling Pi* (Cortex Poriae Cocos), and *Huo Xiang* (Herba Agastaches seu Pogostemi) it clears Heat and transforms Dampness to treat impetigo.

- Combined with *Ku Shen* (Radix Sophorae Flavescentis), *Ku Fan*‡ (Alumen Praeparatum) and *Bai Bu* (Radix Stemonae),

it can be used to prepare an external wash to treat chronic eczema, atopic eczema and asteatotic eczema.

AROMATIC MATERIA MEDICA FOR TRANSFORMING DAMPNESS

Huo Xiang (Herba Agastaches seu Pogostemi)

Functions: Aromatically transforms Dampness, relieves Summerheat and repels foulness, harmonizes the Middle Burner to stop vomiting, and fortifies the Spleen to reinforce Vital Qi (Zheng Qi) in the Spleen and Stomach.

Indications: Damp-Heat patterns in herpes zoster (shingles), impetigo, seborrheic eczema, and pompholyx; Summerheat-Damp patterns in miliaria rubra (prickly heat) and annular erythemas; and for foul turbidity in bromhidrosis.

Common dosage: 3-10g.

Combinations

- Combined with *Pei Lan* (Herba Eupatorii Fortunei) and *Qing Hao* (Herba Artemisiae Chinghao), it clears Summerheat and aromatically transforms turbidity to flush out Dampness and treat miliaria rubra (prickly heat).

- Combined with *Pei Lan* (Herba Eupatorii Fortunei), *Shan Yao* (Radix Dioscoreae Oppositae), *Bai Bian Dou* (Semen Dolichoris Lablab), *Ze Xie* (Rhizoma Alismatis Orientalis), and *Bai Zhu* (Rhizoma Atractylodis Macrocephalae), it aromatically transforms turbidity, augments Qi and supports the Spleen to treat dermatitis herpetiformis.

- Combined with *Ding Xiang* (Flos Caryophylli), *Mu Xiang** (Radix Aucklandiae Lappae), *Da Fu Pi* (Pericarpium Arecae Catechu), *Xiang Fu* (Rhizoma Cyperi Rotundi), and *Fu Ling* (Sclerotium Poriae Cocos), it aromatically repels foulness, clears Heat and transforms Dampness to treat bromhidrosis.

Pei Lan (Herba Eupatorii Fortunei)

Functions: Fortifies the Spleen and transforms Dampness, clears Summerheat and repels foulness, generates Body Fluids, alleviates thirst and moistens the skin.

Indications: Damp-Heat patterns in herpes zoster (shingles), impetigo, pompholyx, and bromhidrosis; miliaria rubra (prickly heat) due to Summerheat-Damp; dermatitis herpetiformis due to Dampness encumbering the Spleen.

Common dosage: 10-15g.

Combinations

- Combined with *Huo Xiang* (Herba Agastaches seu Pogostemi), *Yi Yi Ren* (Semen Coicis Lachryma-jobi), *Zhi Zi* (Fructus Gardeniae Jasminoidis), *Huang Qin* (Radix Scutellariae Baicalensis), and *Shan Yao* (Radix Dioscoreae Oppositae), it clears Heat, transforms Dampness, supports the Spleen, and transforms turbidity to treat pompholyx.

- Combined with *Huo Xiang* (Herba Agastaches seu Pogostemi) and *Qing Hao* (Herba Artemisiae Chinghao), it clears Summerheat and aromatically transforms turbidity to flush out Dampness and treat miliaria rubra (prickly heat).

MATERIA MEDICA FOR BENEFITING THE MOVEMENT OF WATER AND DISPERSING SWELLING

Ze Xie (Rhizoma Alismatis Orientalis)

Functions: Benefits the movement of water and percolates Dampness, clears Heat and drains Fire.

Indications: Damp-Heat patterns in skin disorders such as acute eczema, pompholyx, erythema multiforme, folliculitis, flexural psoriasis, herpes simplex, impetigo, and vulval pruritus; patterns of Blood-Dryness due to Yin Deficiency in chronic eczema, atopic eczema and pityriasis rosea; and patterns involving Fire in melasma (chloasma) and anaphylactoid purpura.

Common dosage: 10-15g.

Combinations

- Combined with *Chi Fu Ling* (Sclerotium Poriae Cocos Rubrae), *Zhi Ke* (Fructus Citri Aurantii), *Cang Zhu* (Rhizoma Atractylodis), and *Bai Zhu* (Rhizoma Atractylodis Macrocephalae), it clears Heat, transforms Dampness, fortifies the Spleen and harmonizes the Stomach to treat pemphigus.

- Combined with *Huang Bai* (Cortex Phellodendri), *Zhi Mu* (Rhizoma Anemarrhenae Asphodeloidis), *Sheng Di Huang* (Radix Rehmanniae Glutinosae), *Che Qian Zi* (Semen Plantaginis), and *Fu Ling* (Sclerotium Poriae Cocos), it clears Heat, percolates Dampness and transforms turbidity to treat vulval pruritus.

- Combined with *Xuan Shen* (Radix Scrophulariae Ningpoensis), *Shan Yao* (Rhizoma Dioscoreae Oppositae), *Fu Ling* (Sclerotium Poriae Cocos), *Yi Yi Ren* (Semen Coicis Lachryma-jobi), and *Bai Xian Pi* (Cortex Dictamni Dasycarpi Radicis), it enriches Yin, protects Body Fluids, transforms Dampness, and moistens Dryness to treat chronic eczema.

- Combined with *Da Ji* (Herba seu Radix Cirsii Japonici), *Xiao Ji* (Herba Cephalanoploris seu Cirsii), *Zi Cao* (Radix Arnebiae seu Lithospermi), and *Xuan Shen* (Radix Scrophulariae Ningpoensis), it cools the Blood, enriches Yin and bears Fire downward to treat purpura.

Che Qian Zi (Semen Plantaginis)

Functions: Benefits the movement of water, percolates Dampness, clears Heat, brightens the eyes, and dispels Phlegm.

Indications: Damp-Heat patterns in skin disorders such as acute eczema, pompholyx, impetigo, herpes zoster (shingles), pemphigus, vulval pruritus, tinea cruris (jock itch), sunburn, and hyperhidrosis.

Common dosage: 10-15g.

Combinations

- Combined with *Long Dan Cao* (Radix Gentianae Scabrae), *Zhi Zi* (Fructus Gardeniae Jasminoidis), *Chai Hu* (Radix Bupleuri), *Huang Qin* (Radix Scutellariae Baicalensis), and *Tong Cao* (Medulla Tetrapanacis Papyriferi), it clears and drains Damp-Heat from the Liver and Gallbladder to treat ear eczema.

- Combined with *Jin Yin Hua* (Flos Lonicerae), *Lian Qiao* (Fructus Forsythiae Suspensae), *Qing Hao* (Herba Artemisiae Chinghao), *Hua Shi* ‡ (Talcum), and *Ze Xie* (Rhizoma Alismatis Orientalis), it benefits the movement of Dampness and clears Summerheat to treat sunburn.

- Combined with *Yi Yi Ren* (Semen Coicis Lachryma-jobi), *Chi Xiao Dou* (Semen Phaseoli Calcarati), *Fu Ling Pi* (Cortex Poriae Cocos), *Che Qian Cao* (Herba Plantaginis), and *Ma Chi Xian* (Herba Portulacae Oleraceae), it clears Heat, transforms Dampness and relieves Toxicity to treat herpes zoster (shingles).

Dong Gua Pi (Epicarpium Benincasae Hispidae)

Functions: *Dong Gua Pi* (Epicarpium Benincasae Hispidae) benefits the movement of water, disperses swelling, dispels Dampness, and expels Wind; *Dong Gua Ren* (Semen Benincasae Hispidae) clears Heat and expels pus.

Indications: Acne, miliaria rubra (prickly heat), urticaria, melasma (chloasma).

Common dosage: 15-30g.

Combinations

- Combined with *Pi Pa Ye* (Folium Eriobotryae Japonicae), *Zhi Zi* (Fructus Gardeniae Jasminoidis), *Sang Bai Pi* (Cortex Mori Albae Radicis), *Huang Qin* (Radix Scutellariae Baicalensis), and *Lian Qiao* (Fructus Forsythiae Suspensae), *Dong Gua Pi* (Epicarpium Benincasae Hispidae) and *Dong Gua Ren* (Semen Benincasae Hispidae) clear Lung-Heat, transform Dampness and moisten the skin to treat acne.

- Combined with *Tian Men Dong* (Radix Asparagi Cochinchinensis), *Sheng Di Huang* (Radix Rehmanniae Glutinosae), *Yi Yi Ren* (Semen Coicis Lachryma-jobi), and *Chi Xiao Dou* (Semen Phaseoli Calcarati), *Dong Gua Pi* (Epicarpium Benincasae Hispidae) benefits the movement of water, moistens Dryness and generates Body Fluids to treat keratolysis exfoliativa.

Chi Xiao Dou (Semen Phaseoli Calcarati)

Functions: Benefits the movement of water, eliminates Dampness, disperses swelling, relieves Toxicity, and expels pus.

Indications: This herb is often used for skin disorders manifesting with vesicles or bullae, treating Damp-Heat patterns in erythema multiforme, herpes zoster (shingles), impetigo, fixed drug eruptions, and hand and foot eczema, and Heart-Fire patterns in bullous pemphigoid and dermatitis herpetiformis; it is also used for Heat Toxin patterns in urticaria, palmoplantar pustulosis and pyogenic paronychia (whitlow).

Common dosage: 10-30g.

Combinations

- Combined with *Chi Fu Ling* (Sclerotium Poriae Cocos Rubrae), *Che Qian Zi* (Semen Plantaginis) and *Bai Mao Gen* (Rhizoma Imperatae Cylindricae), it clears Heat and transforms Dampness to treat fixed drug eruptions due to Damp-Heat pouring down.

- Combined with *Lian Qiao* (Fructus Forsythiae Suspensae), *Jin Yin Hua* (Flos Lonicerae), *Lü Dou Yi* (Cortex Phaseoli Radiati), and *Gan Cao* (Radix Glycyrrhizae), it clears Heat, relieves Toxicity, invigorates the Blood, and reduces erythema to treat urticaria due to Heat Toxins setting the Ying level ablaze.

- Combined with *Jin Yin Hua* (Flos Lonicerae), *Zhi Zi* (Fructus Gardeniae Jasminoidis), *Lian Qiao* (Fructus Forsythiae Suspensae), *Tong Cao* (Medulla Tetrapanacis Papyriferi), and *Dan Zhu Ye* (Herba Lophatheri Gracilis), it clears Heat from the Heart and disperses swelling to treat bullous pemphigoid.

MATERIA MEDICA FOR CLEARING HEAT AND RELIEVING TOXICITY

Pu Gong Ying (Herba Taraxaci cum Radice)

Functions: Clears Heat and relieves Toxicity, benefits the movement of Dampness and dissipates lumps. This is an important herb for relieving Toxicity and cooling the Blood.

Indications: Skin disorders caused by Toxins (principally Heat Toxins) such as folliculitis, furuncles and carbuncles, palmoplantar pustulosis, tinea capitis (kerion), plantar warts (verruca plantaris), pityriasis lichenoides, pyogenic paronychia (whitlow), insect bites, sunburn, and radiodermatitis.

Common dosage: 10-30g.

Combinations

- *Pu Gong Ying* (Herba Taraxaci cum Radice) is often combined with *Jin Yin Hua* (Flos Lonicerae), *Zi Hua Di Ding* (Herba Violae Yedoensitis) and/or *Lian Qiao* (Fructus Forsythiae Suspensae) to reinforce the Toxicity-relieving effect in various infectious or pyogenic skin disorders such as folliculitis, furuncles and carbuncles, impetigo, ecthyma, palmoplantar pustulosis, tinea capitis (kerion), and radiodermatitis.

- Combined with *Da Qing Ye* (Folium Isatidis seu Baphicacanthi), *Ban Lan Gen* (Radix Isatidis seu Baphicacanthi), *San Leng* (Rhizoma Sparganii Stoloniferi), *E Zhu* (Rhizoma Curcumae), and *Tao Ren* (Semen Persicae), it clears Heat, relieves Toxicity, invigorates the Blood, and softens hardness to treat plantar warts (verruca plantaris).

Jin Yin Hua (Flos Lonicerae)

Functions: Clears Heat and relieves Toxicity, dissipates Wind-Heat.

Indications: Skin disorders caused by Toxins (principally Heat Toxins) such as herpes zoster (shingles), folliculitis, furuncles and carbuncles, urticaria, drug eruptions, palmoplantar pustulosis, hidradenitis suppurativa, sunburn, and radiodermatitis; Wind-Heat patterns in pityriasis rosea, erysipelas, common warts (verruca vulgaris), and phytophotodermatitis; Excess-Fire patterns in recurrent aphthous stomatitis and herpetic stomatitis; and for varicella (chickenpox) and measles.

Common dosage: 10-30g.

Combinations

- *Jin Yin Hua* (Flos Lonicerae) is often combined with *Lian Qiao* (Fructus Forsythiae Suspensae), *Pu Gong Ying* (Herba Taraxaci cum Radice), *Zi Hua Di Ding* (Herba Violae Yedoensitis), and *Chi Shao* (Radix Paeoniae Rubra) to clear Heat and relieve Toxicity to treat a variety of skin disorders (mostly infectious or pyogenic).

- Combined with *Qing Hao* (Herba Artemisiae Chinghao), *Nan Sha Shen* (Radix Adenophorae), *Lü Dou Yi* (Testa Phaseoli Radiati), *Xi Gua Pi* (Epicarpium Citrulli Vulgaris), and *Dong Gua Pi* (Epicarpium Benincasae Hispidae), it clears Summerheat, relieves Toxicity and alleviates itching to treat miliaria rubra (prickly heat).

- Combined with *Lian Qiao* (Fructus Forsythiae Suspensae), *Da Qing Ye* (Folium Isatidis seu Baphicacanthi), *Jing Jie* (Herba Schizonepetae Tenuifoliae), and *Fang Feng* (Radix Ledebouriellae Divaricatae), it dissipates Wind-Heat and alleviates itching to treat urticaria.

- Combined with *Sheng Di Huang* (Radix Rehmanniae Glutinosae), *Zhi Zi* (Fructus Gardeniae Jasminoidis), *Tong Cao* (Medulla Tetrapanacis Papyriferi), *Dan Zhu Ye* (Herba Lophatheri Gracilis), and *Deng Xin Cao* (Medulla Junci Effusi), it clears Heat from the Heart, cools the Blood, disperses swelling, and alleviates pain to treat mouth ulcers.

Lian Qiao (Fructus Forsythiae Suspensae)

Functions: Clears Heat and relieves Toxicity, dissipates Wind-Heat, disperses abscesses and expels pus. This herb is very effective at clearing Heart-Fire.

Indications: Skin disorders caused by Toxins (principally Heat Toxins) such as herpes zoster (shingles), urticaria, hidradenitis suppurativa, pyoderma faciale, erythema multiforme, intertrigo, erythema ab igne, and sunburn; Wind-Heat patterns in folliculitis, pityriasis rosea, erysipelas, and phytophotodermatitis; Heart-Fire patterns in bullous pemphigoid and oral candidiasis (thrush); and for varicella (chickenpox) and measles.

Common dosage: 10-15g.

Combinations

- *Lian Qiao* (Fructus Forsythiae Suspensae) is often combined with *Jin Yin Hua* (Flos Lonicerae), *Pu Gong Ying* (Herba Taraxaci cum Radice), *Zi Hua Di Ding* (Herba Violae Yedoensitis), and *Chi Shao* (Radix Paeoniae Rubra) to clear Heat and relieve Toxicity to treat a variety of skin disorders (mostly infectious or pyogenic).

- Combined with *Sheng Ma* (Rhizoma Cimicifugae), *Qiang Huo* (Rhizoma et Radix Notopterygii), *Fang Feng* (Radix Ledebouriellae Divaricatae), *Jin Yin Hua* (Flos Lonicerae), *Ye Ju Hua* (Flos Chrysanthemi Indici), and *Chong Lou* (Rhizoma Paridis), it dredges Wind, clears Heat, relieves Toxicity, and dissipates lumps to treat folliculitis.

- Combined with *Mu Dan Pi* (Cortex Moutan Radicis), *Huang Lian* (Rhizoma Coptidis), *Huang Qin* (Radix Scutellariae Baicalensis), *Zhi Zi* (Fructus Gardeniae Jasminoidis), *Chai Hu* (Radix Bupleuri), and *Long Dan Cao* (Radix Gentianae Scabrae), it drains Fire and relieves Toxicity to treat erysipelas.

- Combined with *Huang Lian* (Rhizoma Coptidis), *Tong Cao* (Medulla Tetrapanacis Papyriferi), *Lian Zi Xin* (Plumula Nelumbinis Nuciferae), and *Jin Yin Hua* (Flos Lonicerae), it clears Heat from the Heart, drains Fire and relieves Toxicity to treat oral candidiasis (thrush).

Zi Hua Di Ding (Herba Violae Yedoensitis)

Functions: Clears Heat and relieves Toxicity, eliminates Dampness and disperses swelling.

Indications: This herb is often used for treating skin disorders manifesting with pustular lesions such as folliculitis, furuncles and carbuncles, pyogenic paronychia (whitlow), ecthyma, pustular psoriasis, palmoplantar pustulosis, tinea capitis (kerion), and hidradenitis suppurativa.

Common dosage: 10-15g.

Combinations

- *Zi Hua Di Ding* (Herba Violae Yedoensitis) is often combined with *Jin Yin Hua* (Flos Lonicerae), *Pu Gong Ying* (Herba Taraxaci cum Radice), *Lian Qiao* (Fructus Forsythiae Suspensae), *Bai Hua She She Cao* (Herba Hedyotidis Diffusae), and *Chi Shao* (Radix Paeoniae Rubra) to clear Heat and relieve Toxicity to treat a variety of skin disorders manifesting with pustular lesions.

- Combined with *Chuan Xiong* (Rhizoma Ligustici Chuanxiong), *Zhe Bei Mu* (Bulbus Fritillariae Thunbergii), *Lian Qiao* (Fructus Forsythiae Suspensae), *Bai Zhi* (Radix

Angelicae Dahuricae), and *Jin Yin Hua* (Flos Lonicerae), it clears Heat, draws out Toxins and expels pus to treat hidradenitis suppurativa.

Bai Hua She She Cao (Herba Hedyotidis Diffusae)

Functions: Clears Heat and relieves Toxicity, invigorates the Blood, disperses abscesses, and promotes urination.

Indications: Skin disorders caused by Toxins such as folliculitis, sycosis barbae, ecthyma, tinea capitis (kerion), candidal balanitis, hand and foot eczema, erythrodermic psoriasis, palmoplantar pustulosis, and radiodermatitis; and Yin Deficiency patterns in pemphigus, dermatitis herpetiformis and parapsoriasis.

Common dosage: 15-30g.

Combinations

*   Combined with *Zi Hua Di Ding* (Herba Violae Yedoensitis), *Jin Yin Hua* (Flos Lonicerae) and *Pu Gong Ying* (Herba Taraxaci cum Radice), it clears Heat and relieves Toxicity to treat folliculitis, ecthyma and tinea capitis (kerion).

*   Combined with *Jin Yin Hua* (Flos Lonicerae), *Lü Dou Yi* (Testa Phaseoli Radiati), *Bai Hua She She Cao* (Herba Hedyotidis Diffusae), and *Bai Lian* (Radix Ampelopsis Japonicae), it clears Heat, relieves Toxicity, closes sores, and absorbs exudate to treat the later stages of pemphigus.

Ma Chi Xian (Herba Portulacae Oleraceae)

Functions: Clears Heat and relieves Toxicity, dissipates Blood stasis and disperses swelling. This herb is very effective for relieving Heat Toxins.

Indications: External use for acute eczema, irritant contact dermatitis, nummular and stasis eczema, herpes simplex, herpes zoster (shingles), impetigo, intertrigo, sunburn, and phytophotodermatitis.

Common dosage: 15-30g.

Combinations

In the dermatology clinic, *Ma Chi Xian* (Herba Portulacae Oleraceae) is usually applied externally as a wet compress or wash to treat weeping lesions or erosive lesions with profuse exudate.

*   *Ma Chi Xian Shui Xi Ji* (Purslane Wash Preparation) can be used as a wet compress to treat nummular eczema (discoid eczema), stasis eczema, sunburn, impetigo, herpes simplex, and varicella (chickenpox).

*   *Ma Chi Xian* (Herba Portulacae Oleraceae) can be combined with *Di Yu* (Radix Sanguisorbae Officinalis) to prepare a wet compress to treat acute eczema, pemphigus, papular urticaria, radiodermatitis, and polymorphic light eruption.

*   Combined with *Pu Gong Ying* (Herba Taraxaci cum Radice) and *Ye Ju Hua* (Flos Chrysanthemi Indici), *Ma Chi Xian* (Herba Portulacae Oleraceae) can be used to prepare a wet compress to treat ecthyma or phytophotodermatitis.

Tian Hua Fen (Radix Trichosanthis)

Functions: Clears Heat and generates Body Fluids, relieves Toxicity and expels pus.

Indications: Skin disorders with pustular lesions such as folliculitis, furuncles (boils), hidradenitis suppurativa, and

ecthyma; also for stomatitis, pruritus, dermatitis herpetiformis, and keratosis pilaris.

Common dosage: 10-15g.

Combinations

*   Combined with *Nan Sha Shen* (Radix Adenophorae), *Mai Men Dong* (Radix Ophiopogonis Japonici), *Xuan Shen* (Radix Scrophulariae Ningpoensis), and *Shan Yao* (Radix Dioscoreae Oppositae), it enriches Yin and generates Body Fluids to treat dermatitis herpetiformis.

*   Combined with *Jin Yin Hua* (Flos Lonicerae), *Lian Qiao* (Fructus Forsythiae Suspensae), *Ye Ju Hua* (Flos Chrysanthemi Indici), *Bai Zhi* (Radix Angelicae Dahuricae), and *Jie Geng* (Radix Platycodi Grandiflori), it relieves Toxicity, dissipates lumps and expels pus to treat folliculitis.

Da Qing Ye (Folium Isatidis seu Baphicacanthi)

Functions: Clears Heat and relieves Toxicity, cools the Blood and reduces erythema. This herb can be used to clear Heat Toxins in the Heart and Stomach as well as to drain Excess-Fire in the Liver and Gallbladder.

Indications: Heat Toxin patterns in skin disorders such as herpes zoster (shingles), palmoplantar pustulosis, plantar warts (verruca plantaris), and toxic erythema; Wind-Heat patterns in urticaria, pityriasis rosea, herpes simplex, phytophotodermatitis, and varicella (chickenpox).

Common dosage: 10-15g.

Combinations

*   Combined with *Jin Yin Hua* (Flos Lonicerae) and *Lian Qiao* (Fructus Forsythiae Suspensae), it dissipates Wind-Heat to treat urticaria, pityriasis rosea, varicella (chickenpox), phytophotodermatitis, and toxic erythema.

*   Combined with *Long Dan Xie Gan Tang* (Chinese Gentian Decoction for Draining the Liver), *Yi Yi Ren* (Semen Coicis Lachryma-jobi) and *Bai Mao Gen* (Rhizoma Imperatae Cylindricae), it clears Heat, transforms Dampness, cools the Blood, and reduces erythema to treat herpes simplex in the lower part of the body.

Ban Lan Gen (Radix Isatidis seu Baphicacanthi)

Functions: Clears Heat and relieves Toxicity, cools the Blood and reduces erythema.

Indications: Wind-Heat patterns in erysipelas, common warts (verruca vulgaris), phytophotodermatitis, and palpebral eczema; also used for herpes simplex, herpetic stomatitis and erythema multiforme.

Common dosage: 10-15g.

Combinations

*   Combined with *Huang Qin* (Radix Scutellariae Baicalensis), *Ma Bo* (Sclerotium Lasiosphaerae seu Calvatiae), *Huang Lian* (Rhizoma Coptidis), *Xuan Shen* (Radix Scrophulariae Ningpoensis), and *Niu Bang Zi* (Fructus Arctii Lappae), it dredges Wind, clears Heat and relieves Toxicity to treat palpebral eczema.

*   Combined with *Nan Sha Shen* (Radix Adenophorae), *Huang Qi* (Radix Astragali seu Hedysari), *Bai Shao* (Radix Paeoniae Lactiflorae), and *Sheng Di Huang* (Radix Rehmanniae Glutinosae), it augments Qi and nourishes Yin to consolidate the Root and treat herpes simplex.

MATERIA MEDICA FOR WARMING THE CHANNELS, DISSIPATING COLD AND FREEING THE NETWORK VESSELS

Gui Zhi (Ramulus Cinnamomi Cassiae)

Functions: Warms the channels and frees the network vessels, induces sweating and releases the exterior, regulates and harmonizes the Ying and Wei levels, frees Heart Yang, and dispels Wind-Damp in the skin and flesh, guiding materia medica to painful areas in the upper limbs and shoulders in order to eliminate Phlegm congealing and Blood stagnation between the joints.

Indications: Wind-Cold patterns in skin disorders such as urticaria, pruritus, psoriasis, and pityriasis lichenoides chronica; Yang Deficiency patterns in Raynaud's disease, cold urticaria and hyperhidrosis; other Cold patterns in erythema multiforme and chilblains.

Common dosage: 5-10g.

Combinations

- Combined with *Ma Huang** (Herba Ephedrae), *Da Zao* (Fructus Ziziphi Jujubae), *Sheng Jiang* (Rhizoma Zingiberis Officinalis Recens), *Qiang Huo* (Rhizoma et Radix Notopterygii), and *Zi Su Ye* (Folium Perillae Frutescentis), it harmonizes the Ying and Wei levels and dissipates Wind-Cold to treat urticaria due to Wind-Cold.

- Combined with *Gan Cao* (Radix Glycyrrhizae), *Bai Shao* (Radix Paeoniae Lactiflorae), *Ma Huang** (Herba Ephedrae), *Da Zao* (Fructus Ziziphi Jujubae), *Duan Long Gu* ‡ (Os Draconis Calcinatum), and *Duan Mu Li* ‡ (Concha Ostreae Calcinata), it regulates the Ying and Wei levels, augments Qi and consolidates the exterior to constrain sweating.

- Combined with *Huang Qi* (Radix Astragali seu Hedysari), *Dang Shen* (Radix Codonopsitis Pilosulae), *Dang Gui* (Radix Angelicae Sinensis), *Ji Xue Teng* (Caulis Spatholobi), and *Huo Xue Teng* (Caulis seu Radix Schisandrae), it augments Qi, warms Yang, nourishes the Blood, and frees the network vessels to treat Raynaud's disease.

Gan Jiang (Rhizoma Zingiberis Officinalis)

Functions: Warms the Middle Burner and dissipates Cold, returns Yang and frees the vessels.

Indications: Spleen Yang Deficiency patterns in skin disorders such as Raynaud's disease, cold urticaria, recurrent aphthous stomatitis (mouth ulcers), and nummular eczema (discoid eczema); Cold patterns in pruritus, erythema multiforme and chilblains.

Common dosage: 5-10g.

Combinations

- Combined with *Gui Zhi* (Ramulus Cinnamomi Cassiae), *Zi Su Ye* (Folium Perillae Frutescentis), *Bai Shao* (Radix Paeoniae Lactiflorae), *Dang Shen* (Radix Codonopsitis Pilosulae), *Huang Qi* (Radix Astragali seu Hedysari), and *Fang Feng* (Radix Ledebouriellae Divaricatae), it warms Yang, dissipates Cold, dispels Wind, augments Qi, and supports the Spleen to treat cold urticaria.

- Combined with *Huang Qi* (Radix Astragali seu Hedysari), *Dang Shen* (Radix Codonopsitis Pilosulae), *Bai Zhu* (Rhizoma Atractylodis Macrocephalae), *Gui Zhi* (Ramulus

Cinnamomi Cassiae), *Huo Xue Teng* (Caulis seu Radix Schisandrae), and *Ji Xue Teng* (Caulis Spatholobi), it augments Qi, supplements the Blood, warms Yang, and frees the network vessels to treat chilblains.

Rou Gui (Cortex Cinnamomi Cassiae)

Functions: Warms the Middle Burner and supplements Yang, dissipates Cold and alleviates pain, warms and frees the channels and vessels. This herb warms the Spleen and Stomach and enters the Xue level to free the Blood vessels and return Fire to its source.

Indications: Kidney Yang Deficiency patterns in skin disorders such as cold urticaria, hyperhidrosis and chronic venous ulcer of the lower leg.

Common dosage: 3-6g.

Combinations

- Combined with *Lu Jiao* ‡ (Cornu Cervi), *Fu Pen Zi* (Fructus Rubi Chingii), *Huang Qi* (Radix Astragali seu Hedysari), and *Xu Chang Qing* (Radix Cynanchi Paniculati), it augments Qi, warms the Kidneys, dissipates Cold, and alleviates itching to treat cold urticaria.

- Combined with *Fu Pen Zi* (Fructus Rubi Chingii), *Shan Zhu Yu* (Fructus Corni Officinalis), *Du Zhong* (Cortex Eucommiae Ulmoidis), *Shu Di Huang* (Radix Rehmanniae Glutinosae Conquita), and *Gou Qi Zi* (Fructus Lycii), it supports Vital Qi (Zheng Qi), reinforces Yang, and enriches and supplements the Liver and Kidneys to treat hyperhidrosis.

MATERIA MEDICA FOR ENRICHING YIN AND REINFORCING YANG

MATERIA MEDICA FOR ENRICHING YIN

Nan Sha Shen (Radix Adenophorae)

Functions: Clears Lung-Heat, drains Fire, relieves Toxicity, and dispels Phlegm to stop coughing.

Indications: Yin Deficiency patterns in skin disorders such as lichen simplex chronicus (neurodermatitis), lichen planus, furuncles (boils), herpes simplex, pityriasis rosea, erythema multiforme-type drug eruptions, and dermatitis herpetiformis; Blood Deficiency patterns in ichthyosis vulgaris and hand and foot eczema; and Blood-Heat patterns in psoriasis and anaphylactoid purpura.

Common dosage: 10-15g.

Combinations

- Combined with *Dang Gui* (Radix Angelicae Sinensis), *Bai Shao* (Radix Paeoniae Lactiflorae), *He Shou Wu* (Radix Polygoni Multiflori), *Hei Zhi Ma* (Semen Sesami Indici), *Shan Yao* (Radix Dioscoreae Oppositae), and *Gou Teng* (Ramulus Uncariae cum Uncis), it enriches Yin, nourishes the Blood, moistens Dryness, extinguishes Wind, and alleviates itching to treat lichen simplex chronicus (neurodermatitis).

- Combined with *Xuan Shen* (Radix Scrophulariae Ningpoensis), *Sheng Di Huang* (Radix Rehmanniae Glutinosae), *Zhi Mu* (Rhizoma Anemarrhenae Asphodeloidis), and *Jing Jie* (Herba Schizonepetae Tenuifoliae), it nourishes Yin, clears Heat, dissipates Wind, and protects Body Fluids to treat anaphylactoid purpura.

- Combined with *Tian Men Dong* (Radix Asparagi Cochinchinensis), *Mai Men Dong* (Radix Ophiopogonis Japonici), *He Shou Wu* (Radix Polygoni Multiflori), *Shu Di Huang* (Radix Rehmanniae Glutinosae Conquita), and *Dan Shen* (Radix Salviae Miltiorrhizae), it nourishes and invigorates the Blood, nourishes the skin and moistens Dryness to treat ichthyosis vulgaris.

Bei Sha Shen (Radix Glehniae Littoralis)
Functions: Clears Lung-Heat and nourishes Yin, boosts the Stomach and generates Body Fluids.
Indications: Urticaria, pityriasis rosea, furuncles (boils), and keratosis follicularis (Darier's disease).
Common dosage: 10-15g.
Combinations

- Combined with *Nan Sha Shen* (Radix Adenophorae), *Huang Qi* (Radix Astragali seu Hedysari), *Shan Yao* (Radix Dioscoreae Oppositae), *Shan Zhu Yu* (Fructus Corni Officinalis), *Tian Men Dong* (Radix Asparagi Cochinchinensis), and *Sheng Di Huang* (Radix Rehmanniae Glutinosae), it augments Qi and nourishes Yin to treat persistent furuncles.
- Combined with *Mai Men Dong* (Radix Ophiopogonis Japonici), *Shi Hu** (Herba Dendrobii), *Yu Zhu* (Rhizoma Polygonati Odorati), *Sheng Di Huang* (Radix Rehmanniae Glutinosae), *Shan Yao* (Rhizoma Dioscoreae Oppositae), and *Bai Bian Dou* (Semen Dolichoris Lablab), it supports the Spleen, nourishes the Stomach and moistens the skin to treat nipple eczema.

*Shi Hu** (Herba Dendrobii)
Functions: Enriches Yin and clears Heat, nourishes the Stomach and generates Body Fluids.
Indications: Yin Deficiency patterns in skin disorders such as furuncles (boils), lichen planus and erythema multiforme-type drug eruptions; Blood-Dryness patterns in pityriasis rosea, tinea manuum (ringworm of the hands), and keratosis follicularis (Darier's disease); also used for folliculitis, pityriasis rubra pilaris, erythema multiforme, and herpetic stomatitis.
Common dosage: 10-15g.
Combinations
- Combined with *Sheng Di Huang* (Radix Rehmanniae Glutinosae), *Tian Men Dong* (Radix Asparagi Cochinchinensis), *Mai Men Dong* (Radix Ophiopogonis Japonici), *Yu Zhu* (Rhizoma Polygonati Odorati), and *Xuan Shen* (Radix Scrophulariae Ningpoensis), it nourishes Yin and clears Heat to treat herpetic stomatitis due to Deficiency-Fire.
- Combined with *Gan Di Huang* (Radix Rehmanniae Glutinosae Exsiccata), *Shan Zhu Yu* (Fructus Corni Officinalis), *Gou Qi Zi* (Fructus Lycii), *Nan Sha Shen* (Radix Adenophorae), and *Xuan Shen* (Radix Scrophulariae Ningpoensis), it supplements the Liver and Kidneys, enriches Yin and bears Fire downward to treat oral lichen planus.
- Combined with *Nan Sha Shen* (Radix Adenophorae), *Tian Men Dong* (Radix Asparagi Cochinchinensis), *Yu Zhu* (Rhizoma Polygonati Odorati), *Bai Shao* (Radix Paeoniae Lactiflorae), and *Yi Yi Ren* (Semen Coicis Lachryma-jobi), it enriches Yin, nourishes the Stomach, moistens Dryness, and generates Body Fluids to treat keratolysis exfoliativa.

Nü Zhen Zi (Fructus Ligustri Lucidi)
Functions: Supplements Liver and Kidney Yin, strengthens the lower back and spine, brightens the eyes.
Indications: Alopecia areata, melanosis, vitiligo, and patterns of disharmony of the Chong and Ren vessels in urticaria and psoriasis.
Common dosage: 10-15g.
Combinations

- Combined with *He Shou Wu* (Radix Polygoni Multiflori), *Gou Qi Zi* (Fructus Lycii), *Tu Si Zi* (Semen Cuscutae), *Sang Shen* (Fructus Mori Albae), *Huang Jing* (Rhizoma Polygonati), and *Hei Zhi Ma* (Semen Sesami Indici), it enriches the Liver and supplements the Kidneys to nourish the Essence, generate Blood, and moisten and blacken the hair to treat alopecia areata.
- Combined with *Shu Di Huang* (Radix Rehmanniae Glutinosae Conquita), *Shan Zhu Yu* (Fructus Corni Officinalis), *Gou Qi Zi* (Fructus Lycii), *Han Lian Cao* (Herba Ecliptae Prostratae), and *Shan Yao* (Radix Dioscoreae Oppositae), it enriches the Kidneys and supplements Qi to disperse pigmentation and treat melanosis.
- *Xian Mao* (Rhizoma Curculiginis Orchioidis), *Yin Yang Huo* (Herba Epimedii), *Tu Si Zi* (Semen Cuscutae), *Dang Gui* (Radix Angelicae Sinensis), *Shu Di Huang* (Radix Rehmanniae Glutinosae Conquita), and *Han Lian Cao* (Herba Ecliptae Prostratae), it warms Yang, boosts the Kidneys and regulates the Chong and Ren vessels to treat urticaria and psoriasis.

Gou Qi Zi (Fructus Lycii)
Functions: Enriches the Kidneys, supplements the Liver, brightens the eyes, moistens the Lungs, supplements the Essence, and augments Qi.
Indications: Kidney Deficiency patterns in skin disorders such as lichen planus, alopecia areata, melanosis, vitiligo, cold urticaria, and hyperhidrosis; also for ichthyosis vulgaris, anaphylactoid purpura and tinea unguium (ringworm of the nail).
Common dosage: 10-15g.
Combinations

- Combined with *Dang Gui* (Radix Angelicae Sinensis), *Bai Shao* (Radix Paeoniae Lactiflorae), *Shu Di Huang* (Radix Rehmanniae Glutinosae Conquita), *He Shou Wu* (Radix Polygoni Multiflori), *Sang Shen* (Fructus Mori Albae), and *Mai Men Dong* (Radix Ophiopogonis Japonici), it enriches and moistens the Liver and Kidneys to treat tinea unguium (ringworm of the nail).
- Combined with *He Shou Wu* (Radix Polygoni Multiflori), *Nü Zhen Zi* (Fructus Ligustri Lucidi), *Tu Si Zi* (Semen Cuscutae), *Sang Shen* (Fructus Mori Albae), *Huang Jing* (Rhizoma Polygonati), and *Hei Zhi Ma* (Semen Sesami Indici), it enriches the Liver and supplements the Kidneys to nourish the Essence, generate Blood, and moisten and blacken the hair to treat alopecia areata.
- Combined with *Sha Yuan Zi* (Semen Astragali Complanati), *She Chuang Zi* (Fructus Cnidii Monnieri), *Che Qian Zi* (Semen Plantaginis), *Hei Zhi Ma* (Semen Sesami Indici), and *Bai Ji Li* (Fructus Tribuli Terrestris), it enriches the Liver and supplements the Kidneys to treat vitiligo.

Xuan Shen (**Radix Scrophulariae Ningpoensis**)
Functions: Enriches Yin and bears Fire downward, clears Heat and cools the Blood, relieves Toxicity and dissipates lumps.

Indications: Yin Deficiency patterns in furuncles and carbuncles, lichen planus, erythema multiforme-type drug eruptions, genital eczema, ear eczema, dermatitis herpetiformis, and erythema induratum; Blood-Heat patterns in pruritus, dermographism, alopecia areata, and anaphylactoid purpura; also used for chronic eczema, pityriasis rosea, urticaria, herpes simplex, and herpetic stomatitis.

Common dosage: 10-30g.

Combinations

- Combined with *Yu Zhu* (Rhizoma Polygonati Odorati), *Nan Sha Shen* (Radix Adenophorae), *Tian Men Dong* (Radix Asparagi Cochinchinensis), *Mai Men Dong* (Radix Ophiopogonis Japonici), *Shan Yao* (Radix Dioscoreae Oppositae), and *Huang Qi* (Radix Astragali seu Hedysari), it supports Vital Qi (Zheng Qi), nourishes Yin and protects Body Fluids to treat severe drug eruptions.

- Combined with *Sheng Di Huang* (Radix Rehmanniae Glutinosae), *Mai Men Dong* (Radix Ophiopogonis Japonici), *Xu Duan* (Radix Dipsaci), *Nü Zhen Zi* (Fructus Ligustri Lucidi), *Huang Qin* (Radix Scutellariae Baicalensis), and *Tu Si Zi* (Semen Cuscutae), it enriches Yin and clears Heat to supplement the Lungs and Kidneys and treat erythema induratum.

- Combined with *Lian Qiao* (Fructus Forsythiae Suspensae), *Jin Yin Hua* (Flos Lonicerae), *Zi Hua Di Ding* (Herba Violae Yedoensitis), *Ban Lan Gen* (Radix Isatidis seu Baphicacanthi), and *Niu Bang Zi* (Fructus Arctii Lappae), it clears Heat, dissipates Wind, relieves Toxicity, and nourishes Yin to treat Excess-Fire patterns of herpetic stomatitis.

- Combined with *Sheng Di Huang* (Radix Rehmanniae Glutinosae), *Nü Zhen Zi* (Fructus Ligustri Lucidi), *Sang Shen* (Fructus Mori Albae), and *Hei Zhi Ma* (Semen Sesami Indici), it clears Heat, cools the Blood, nourishes Yin, and protects the hair to treat alopecia areata.

Mai Men Dong (**Radix Ophiopogonis Japonici**)
Functions: Nourishes Yin and moistens the Lungs, boosts the Stomach and generates Body Fluids, clears Heat from the Heart and eliminates irritability.

Indications: Yin Deficiency patterns in skin disorders such as lichen planus, herpes simplex, furuncles and carbuncles, psoriasis, pemphigus, dermatitis herpetiformis, melasma (chloasma), erythema multiforme-type drug eruptions, erythema induratum, and hyperhidrosis; Blood Deficiency or Blood-Dryness patterns in pruritus, tinea unguium (ringworm of the nail), ichthyosis vulgaris, and keratosis follicularis (Darier's disease).

Common dosage: 10-15g.

Combinations

- Combined with *Huang Lian* (Rhizoma Coptidis), *Huang Qin* (Radix Scutellariae Baicalensis), *Tong Cao* (Medulla Tetrapanacis Papyriferi), *E Jiao* (Gelatinum Corii Asini), and *Sheng Di Huang* (Radix Rehmanniae Glutinosae), it nourishes Yin, clears Heat and eliminates irritability to treat melasma (chloasma).

- Combined with *Dang Gui* (Radix Angelicae Sinensis), *He Shou Wu* (Radix Polygoni Multiflori), *Shu Di Huang* (Radix Rehmanniae Glutinosae Conquita), *Tian Men Dong* (Radix Asparagi Cochinchinensis), *Dan Shen* (Radix Salviae Miltiorrhizae), and *Mu Dan Pi* (Cortex Moutan Radicis), it enriches Yin, moistens Dryness, clears Heat, and cools the Blood to treat persistent psoriasis.

- Combined with *Dang Shen* (Radix Codonopsitis Pilosulae), *Huang Qi* (Radix Astragali seu Hedysari), *Dang Gui* (Radix Angelicae Sinensis), *Tian Men Dong* (Radix Asparagi Cochinchinensis), and *Shi Hu** (Herba Dendrobii), it augments Qi and enriches Yin to treat folliculitis.

- Combined with *Sheng Di Huang* (Radix Rehmanniae Glutinosae), *Dang Gui* (Radix Angelicae Sinensis), *Tao Ren* (Semen Persicae), *Hong Hua* (Flos Carthami Tinctorii), *Tian Hua Fen* (Radix Trichosanthis), and *He Shou Wu* (Radix Polygoni Multiflori), it nourishes the Blood to disperse Wind, enriches Yin and moistens Dryness to treat pruritus in the elderly or in people with a weak constitution.

Tian Men Dong (**Radix Asparagi Cochinchinensis**)
Functions: Nourishes Yin and clears Heat, moistens Dryness and generates Body Fluids.

Indications: Yin Deficiency patterns in skin disorders such as impetigo, psoriasis, erythema multiforme-type drug eruptions, oral lichen planus, pemphigus, furuncles and carbuncles, and genital eczema; also used for pruritus, stomatitis and radiodermatitis.

Common dosage: 10-15g.

Combinations

- Combined with *Nan Sha Shen* (Radix Adenophorae), *Huang Qi* (Radix Astragali seu Hedysari), *Bai Shao* (Radix Paeoniae Lactiflorae), *Sheng Di Huang* (Radix Rehmanniae Glutinosae), *Mai Men Dong* (Radix Ophiopogonis Japonici), and *Yi Yi Ren* (Semen Coicis Lachryma-jobi), it augments Qi and nourishes Lung and Spleen Yin to consolidate the Root and treat impetigo.

- Combined with *Mai Men Dong* (Radix Ophiopogonis Japonici), *Bai Shao* (Radix Paeoniae Lactiflorae), *Zhi Mu* (Rhizoma Anemarrhenae Asphodeloidis), and *Shan Yao* (Radix Dioscoreae Oppositae), it nourishes Yin and protects Body Fluids to treat pemphigus.

- Combined with *Shu Di Huang* (Radix Rehmanniae Glutinosae Conquita), *Xuan Shen* (Radix Scrophulariae Ningpoensis), *Wu Wei Zi* (Fructus Schisandrae), *Dang Shen* (Radix Codonopsitis Pilosulae), *Fu Shen* (Sclerotium Poriae Cocos cum Ligno Hospite), and *Shan Yao* (Rhizoma Dioscoreae Oppositae), it supplements the Spleen and boosts the Kidneys to treat genital eczema.

MATERIA MEDICA FOR REINFORCING YANG

She Chuang Zi (**Fructus Cnidii Monnieri**)
Functions: Warms the Kidneys and reinforces Yang, dispels Wind and dissipates Cold (internal use); dries Dampness, kills Worms and alleviates itching (external use).

Indications: This herb is mainly used externally as a wash or wet compress for itchy skin disorders such as generalized or vulval pruritus, chronic eczema, asteatotic eczema, genital or

perianal eczema, or tinea cruris; it can also be used internally for vitiligo, chronic eczema, genital eczema, and vulval pruritus.
Common dosage: 5-10g.
Combinations

- Combined with *Shan Zhu Yu* (Fructus Corni Officinalis), *Xiao Hui Xiang* (Fructus Foeniculi Vulgaris), *Xu Duan* (Radix Dipsaci), and *Du Zhong* (Cortex Eucommiae Ulmoidis), it warms Yang, supplements the Kidneys, dissipates Cold, and alleviates itching to treat genital eczema.

- Combined with *Bai Xian Pi* (Cortex Dictamni Dasycarpi Radicis), *Di Fu Zi* (Fructus Kochiae Scopariae), *Ma Chi Xian* (Herba Portulacae Oleraceae), *Huang Bai* (Cortex Phellodendri), *Ku Shen* (Radix Sophorae Flavescentis), and *Bai Bu* (Radix Stemonae), it is used to prepare a sitz bath to treat vulval pruritus.

- Combined with *Huo Xiang* (Herba Agastaches seu Pogostemi), *Hu Zhang* (Radix et Rhizoma Polygoni Cuspidati), *Da Huang* (Radix et Rhizoma Rhei), *Ku Shen* (Radix Sophorae Flavescentis), and *Bai Bu* (Radix Stemonae), it is used to prepare a wash to treat tinea cruris (jock itch).

Tu Si Zi (Semen Cuscutae)
Functions: Supplements Kidney Yang and augments Kidney Yin, consolidates the Essence and replenishes the Marrow, nourishes the Liver and fortifies the Spleen.
Indications: Kidney Deficiency patterns in skin disorders such as alopecia areata, erythema induratum and anaphylactoid purpura; disharmony of the Chong and Ren vessels in psoriasis and urticaria.
Common dosage: 10-15g.
Combinations

- Combined with *Fu Pen Zi* (Fructus Rubi Chingii), *Zao Xin Tu* (Terra Flava Usta), *Bai Zhu* (Rhizoma Atractylodis Macrocephalae), *E Jiao*‡ (Gelatinum Corii Asini), and *Xian He Cao* (Herba Agrimoniae Pilosae), it warms Yang, supplements the Kidneys, fortifies the Spleen, and contains the Blood to treat purpura.

- Combined with *Xian Mao* (Rhizoma Curculiginis Orchioidis), *Yin Yang Huo* (Herba Epimedii), *Dang Gui* (Radix Angelicae Sinensis), and *Sheng Di Huang* (Radix Rehmanniae Glutinosae), it warms Yang, boosts the Kidneys and nourishes the Blood to treat psoriasis and urticaria due to disharmony of the Chong and Ren vessels.

MATERIA MEDICA FOR SUPPLEMENTING QI AND BLOOD

Huang Qi (Radix Astragali seu Hedysari)
Functions: *Huang Qi* (Radix Astragali seu Hedysari) is a key herb for supplementing Qi. The raw herb augments Wei Qi (Defensive Qi) and consolidates the exterior, promotes the movement of water and disperses swelling, draws out Toxins and generates flesh; the herb mix-fried with honey supplements the Middle Burner, augments Qi and bears Yang upward.
Indications: Qi Deficiency patterns in skin disorders such as impetigo, herpes simplex, folliculitis, plane warts (verruca plana), pemphigus, erythema multiforme-type drug eruptions, Raynaud's disease, chilblains, radiodermatitis; Blood Deficiency patterns in psoriasis, pruritus, alopecia areata, and ichthyosis

vulgaris; Spleen Deficiency patterns in pompholyx, angioedema, anaphylactoid purpura, and palmoplantar pustulosis; Kidney Deficiency patterns in oral lichen planus, tinea pedis (athlete's foot) and chronic venous ulcer of the lower leg.
Common dosage: 10-15g.
Combinations

- Combined with *Bai Zhu* (Rhizoma Atractylodis Macrocephalae), *Chen Pi* (Pericarpium Citri Reticulatae), *Mu Xiang** (Radix Aucklandiae Lappae), *Sha Ren* (Fructus Amomi), *Fang Feng* (Radix Ledebouriellae Divaricatae) and *Jing Jie* (Herba Schizonepetae Tenuifoliae), it augments Qi, fortifies the Spleen, dissipates Wind, and alleviates itching to treat pruritus.

- Combined with *Dang Shen* (Radix Codonopsitis Pilosulae), *Dang Gui* (Radix Angelicae Sinensis), *Gui Zhi* (Ramulus Cinnamomi Cassiae), *Ji Xue Teng* (Caulis Spatholobi), and *Huo Xue Teng* (Caulis seu Radix Schisandrae), it augments Qi, warms Yang, nourishes the Blood, and frees the network vessels to treat Raynaud's disease and chilblains.

- Combined with *Nan Sha Shen* (Radix Adenophorae), it augments Qi and protects Yin to support Vital Qi (Zheng Qi) and alleviate itching to treat impetigo at the final stages.

- Combined with *Dan Shen* (Radix Salviae Miltiorrhizae), *Ze Lan* (Herba Lycopi Lucidi), *Chi Shao* (Radix Paeoniae Rubra), *Xiang Fu* (Rhizoma Cyperi Rotundi), *Qing Pi* (Pericarpium Citri Reticulatae Viride), and *Chen Pi* (Pericarpium Citri Reticulatae), it augments Qi and invigorates the Blood to treat psoriasis.

- Combined with *Dang Shen* (Radix Codonopsitis Pilosulae), *Bai Zhu* (Rhizoma Atractylodis Macrocephalae), *Chai Hu* (Radix Bupleuri), and *Sheng Ma* (Rhizoma Cimicifugae), it bears Yang upward, augments Qi and supports the Spleen to treat angioedema.

- Combined with *Duan Long Gu*‡ (Os Draconis Calcinatum), *Duan Mu Li*‡ (Concha Ostreae Calcinata), *Dang Shen* (Radix Codonopsitis Pilosulae), and *Bai Zhu* (Rhizoma Atractylodis Macrocephalae), it augments Qi and consolidates the exterior to constrain sweating.

Dang Shen (Radix Codonopsitis Pilosulae)
Functions: Supplements the Middle Burner, augments Qi, generates Body Fluids, harmonizes the Spleen and Stomach, and nourishes the Blood. This herb is very effective at supplementing Qi in the Spleen and Lungs.
Indications: Qi and Blood Deficiency patterns in skin disorders such as urticaria, alopecia areata, Raynaud's disease, chilblains, and ichthyosis vulgaris; Spleen Deficiency patterns in pruritus, asteatotic eczema, perianal eczema, pompholyx, lichen planus, angioedema, and recurrent aphthous stomatitis (mouth ulcers); and patterns involving impairment of the Spleen's functions in anaphylactoid purpura, pityriasis alba, keratosis follicularis (Darier's disease), and keratosis pilaris.
Common dosage: 10-30g.
Combinations

- Combined with *Bai Zhu* (Rhizoma Atractylodis Macrocephalae), *Fu Ling* (Sclerotium Poriae Cocos), *Dang Gui* (Radix Angelicae Sinensis), *Bai Shao* (Radix Paeoniae Lactiflorae), and *Shu Di Huang* (Radix Rehmanniae Glutinosae

Conquita), it augments Qi, supports the Spleen, enriches Yin, and supplements the Blood to treat urticaria.

- Combined with *Tian Men Dong* (Radix Asparagi Cochinchinensis), *Xuan Shen* (Radix Scrophulariae Ningpoensis), *Wu Wei Zi* (Fructus Schisandrae), *Fu Shen* (Sclerotium Poriae Cocos cum Ligno Hospite), and *Shan Yao* (Rhizoma Dioscoreae Oppositae), it supplements the Spleen and boosts the Kidneys to treat genital eczema.
- Combined with *Fu Ling* (Sclerotium Poriae Cocos), *Bai Zhu* (Rhizoma Atractylodis Macrocephalae), *Cang Zhu* (Rhizoma Atractylodis), *Yi Yi Ren* (Semen Coicis Lachryma-jobi), *Yin Chen Hao* (Herba Artemisiae Scopariae), and *Che Qian Zi* (Semen Plantaginis), it augments Qi, fortifies the Spleen, clears Heat, and transforms Dampness to treat bullous pemphigoid.
- Combined with *Fu Ling* (Sclerotium Poriae Cocos), *Bai Zhu* (Rhizoma Atractylodis Macrocephalae), *Sha Ren* (Fructus Amomi), and *Mu Xiang** (Radix Aucklandiae Lappae), it supports the Spleen and harmonizes the Stomach to treat pityriasis alba.

Dang Gui (Radix Angelicae Sinensis)
Functions: Supplements and harmonizes the Blood, invigorates the Blood to alleviate pain, moistens the Intestines and frees the bowels.
Indications: Blood Deficiency patterns in skin disorders such as urticaria, pruritus, hand and foot eczema, chilblains, and Raynaud's disease; Blood-Dryness patterns in chronic eczema, lichen simplex chronicus (neurodermatitis), atopic eczema, asteatotic eczema, psoriasis, pityriasis rosea, and dermatitis herpetiformis; Blood stasis patterns in lichen planus, herpes zoster (shingles), acne, rosacea, erythema induratum, alopecia areata, and purpuric drug eruptions.
Common dosage: 5-15g.
Combinations

- Combined with *Bai Shao* (Radix Paeoniae Lactiflorae), *E Jiao* ‡ (Gelatinum Corii Asini), *Shu Di Huang* (Radix Rehmanniae Glutinosae Conquita), and *Sheng Di Huang* (Radix Rehmanniae Glutinosae), it supplements the Blood and enriches Yin to treat urticaria due to Blood Deficiency.
- Combined with *Huang Qi* (Radix Astragali seu Hedysari), *Dang Shen* (Radix Codonopsitis Pilosulae), *Bai Shao* (Radix Paeoniae Lactiflorae), *Shu Di Huang* (Radix Rehmanniae Glutinosae Conquita), *Ji Xue Teng* (Caulis Spatholobi), and *Bai Zhi* (Radix Angelicae Dahuricae), it augments Qi, nourishes the Blood and disperses Wind to treat psoriasis due to Blood Deficiency generating Wind.
- Combined with *Xuan Shen* (Radix Scrophulariae Ningpoensis), *Shan Yao* (Rhizoma Dioscoreae Oppositae), *Yi Mu Cao* (Herba Leonuri Heterophylli), *Xu Chang Qing* (Radix Cynanchi Paniculati), and *Dan Shen* (Radix Salviae Miltior-

rhizae), it enriches Yin, protects Body Fluids, and invigorates the Blood to alleviate itching in the treatment of chronic eczema.

- Combined with *Bai Shao* (Radix Paeoniae Lactiflorae), *Shu Di Huang* (Radix Rehmanniae Glutinosae Conquita), *Gan Cao* (Radix Glycyrrhizae), and *He Shou Wu* (Radix Polygoni Multiflori), it nourishes the Blood and moistens Dryness to treat adult atopic eczema.
- Combined with *Bai Shao* (Radix Paeoniae Lactiflorae), *Zi Cao* (Radix Arnebiae seu Lithospermi) and *Si Gua Luo* (Fasciculus Vascularis Luffae), it invigorates the Blood and frees the network vessels to treat herpes zoster in the elderly.

Shu Di Huang (Radix Rehmanniae Glutinosae Conquita)
Functions: Nourishes the Blood, enriches Yin, frees the Blood vessels, augments Qi, supplements the Essence, and replenishes the Marrow.
Indications: Qi Deficiency and/or Blood Deficiency patterns in skin disorders such as urticaria, pruritus, stasis eczema, angioedema, alopecia areata, and Raynaud's disease; Blood-Dryness patterns in psoriasis, atopic eczema, asteatotic eczema, and dermatitis herpetiformis; and Qi stagnation patterns in erythema induratum, hidradenitis suppurativa, hyperhidrosis, and ichthyosis vulgaris.
Common dosage: 10-20g.
Combinations

- Combined with *Shan Zhu Yu* (Fructus Corni Officinalis), *Gou Qi Zi* (Fructus Lycii), *Xian Mao* (Rhizoma Curculiginis Orchioidis), *Yin Yang Huo* (Herba Epimedii), *Nü Zhen Zi* (Fructus Ligustri Lucidi), and *Han Lian Cao* (Herba Ecliptae Prostratae), it enriches and supplements the Liver and Kidneys and augments Qi to disperse pigmentation and treat melanosis.
- Combined with *Dang Gui* (Radix Angelicae Sinensis), *He Shou Wu* (Radix Polygoni Multiflori), *Sheng Di Huang* (Radix Rehmanniae Glutinosae), *Tian Men Dong* (Radix Asparagi Cochinchinensis), and *Mai Men Dong* (Radix Ophiopogonis Japonici), it enriches Yin and moistens Dryness to treat psoriasis due to Yin damage resulting in Blood-Dryness.
- Combined with *Sheng Di Huang* (Radix Rehmanniae Glutinosae), *Dang Gui* (Radix Angelicae Sinensis), *Tao Ren* (Semen Persicae), and *Hong Hua* (Flos Carthami Tinctorii), it nourishes the Blood to disperse Wind and treat pruritus due to Blood Deficiency.
- Combined with *Bai Shao* (Radix Paeoniae Lactiflorae), *Dang Gui* (Radix Angelicae Sinensis), *Dang Shen* (Radix Codonopsitis Pilosulae), *Bai Zhu* (Rhizoma Atractylodis Macrocephalae), *Huang Qi* (Radix Astragali seu Hedysari), and *Chuan Xiong* (Rhizoma Ligustici Chuanxiong), it augments Qi and supplements the Blood to treat alopecia areata.

Note

Animal, insect and mineral materia medica are marked with the symbol ‡; materia medica whose use may be restricted in certain countries are marked with the symbol *. Please refer to the author's preface for further details.

Less common materia medica used in the treatment of skin disorders

This appendix provides a brief outline of less common materia medica referred to in this book for use in the treatment of skin disorders. These materia medica are not included in *Chinese Materia Medica: Combinations and Applications* by Xu Li and Wang Wei, which has been taken as the standard reference for the more common materia medica. [1]

Ba Qia (Rhizoma Smilacis Chinensis)
Properties: Bitter, astringent, neutral.
Channels entered: Liver, Kidney.
Functions: Dispels Wind and promotes the movement of Dampness, relieves Toxicity and disperses swelling.
Indications: Joint pain, muscle numbness, diarrhea, dysentery, Lin syndrome, red and white vaginal discharge, tonsillitis, scrofula, hemorrhoids, psoriasis, urticaria.
Common dosage: 9-30g.

Bai Cao Shuang (Fuligo Herbarum Ustarum)
Properties: Acrid, warm.
Channels entered: Lung, Stomach, Large Intestine.
Functions: Stops bleeding and diarrhea, absorbs Dampness.
Indications: Vomiting, nosebleeds, blood in the stool, profuse uterine bleeding, dysentery; external application for tinea capitis (ringworm of the scalp).
Common dosage: 0.9-4.5g.

Bai Cu (Acetum Album)
Properties: Sour, bitter, warm.
Channels entered: Liver, Stomach.
Functions: Dissipates Blood stasis and stops bleeding, fortifies the Spleen and disperses food accumulation, relieves Toxicity and kills Worms.
Indications: Pain in the chest and abdomen, jaundice, dysentery, Worm accumulation, blood in the stool.
Common dosage: 15-30ml.

Bai Mei Hua (Flos Mume Albus)
Properties: Sour, astringent, neutral.
Channels entered: Liver, Stomach.
Functions: Drains the Liver and relieves Depression, harmonizes the Stomach and transforms Phlegm.
Indications: Depression and binding of Liver Qi, pain in the stomach, oppression in the chest, poor appetite, plum-pit Qi (globus hystericus).
Common dosage: 3-6g.

Bai Yao Zi (Tuber Stephaniae Cepharanthae)
Properties: Bitter, acrid, cool, slightly toxic.
Channels entered: Spleen, Lung, Kidney.
Functions: Clears Heat and relieves Toxicity, disperses Phlegm and alleviates pain, cools the Blood and stops bleeding.
Indications: Hepatitis, acute gastroenteritis, sore throat, nosebleeds, vomiting of blood due to tuberculosis, hemorrhage of the digestive tract, and swelling due to Toxins (for example, in erythema induratum).
Common dosage: 6-9g.

Bai Ying (Herba Solani Lyrati)
Properties: Bitter, neutral, slightly toxic.
Channels entered: Liver, Stomach.
Functions: Clears Heat and benefits the movement of Dampness, relieves Toxicity and disperses swelling.
Indications: Fever due to the common cold, Damp-Heat jaundice, white vaginal discharge, cholecystitis, and benign skin tumors such as hemangioma.
Common dosage: 9-30g.
Cautions: Contraindicated for patients with constitutional Deficiency without Damp-Heat.

Ban Mao‡ (Mylabris)
Properties: Acrid, cold, toxic.
Channels entered: Liver, Large Intestine, Small Intestine.
Functions: Attacks Toxins and erodes sores, breaks up Blood stasis and dissipates lumps.
Indications: Non-healing abscesses and sores, scrofula, amenorrhea due to Blood stasis, focal distension.
Common dosage: 0.03-0.06g.
Cautions: This substance is very toxic and should only be administered in extremely small doses; it is highly irritating to the skin and must not be used long-term.

Ban Zhi Lian (Herba Scutellariae Barbatae)
Properties: Acrid, bitter, cold.
Channels entered: Lung, Liver, Kidney.
Functions: Clears Heat and relieves Toxicity, transforms Blood stasis, promotes urination.
Indications: Clove sores, abscesses, insect bites, severe patterns of psoriasis, swollen and painful throat, knocks and falls (trauma), edema, jaundice.
Common dosage: Dried, 15-30g; fresh, 30-60g.
Cautions: Long-term use can cause damage to the liver and kidneys.

Bei Dou Gen (Rhizoma Menispermi)
Properties: Bitter, cold.
Channels entered: Heart, Lung.

Functions: Clears Heat, relieves Toxicity and frees the bowels.
Indications: Tonsillitis, sore and swollen throat, cough due to Lung-Heat, dysentery, constipation due to binding of Heat, jaundice, Bi syndrome pain due to Wind-Damp.
Common dosage: 6-12g.
Cautions: Contraindicated for Deficiency-Heat or Excess-Heat.

Bi Ba (Fructus Piperis Longi)
Properties: Acrid, hot.
Channels entered: Stomach, Large Intestine.
Functions: Warms the Middle Burner, dissipates Cold and alleviates pain.
Indications: Vomiting, abdominal pain, diarrhea due to Deficiency-Cold.
Common dosage: 2-5g.
Cautions: Contraindicated for Deficiency-Heat or Excess-Heat.

Bi Hu‡ (Gekko Swinhoana)
Properties: Salty, cold, slightly toxic.
Functions: Dispels Wind and settles fright, dissipates lumps and relieves Toxicity.
Indications: Paralysis due to Wind-stroke, child fright Wind, epilepsy, tetanus, joint pain in arthritis.
Common dosage: 0.9-1.5g.

Bi Ma Zi (Semen Ricini)
Properties: Sweet, acrid, neutral, toxic.
Channels entered: Large Intestine, Lung.
Functions: Disperses swelling and relieves Toxicity, drains downward to free stagnation.
Indications: Abscesses, toxic swellings, scrofula, inflammation of the throat, sores due to scabies or tinea, edema, abdominal fullness, constipation.
Common dosage: 2-3 seeds (stir-fried).
Cautions: This herb must be stir-fried and must not be taken raw. It is contraindicated during pregnancy and for patients with diarrhea. Death can result from intake of 2-7 raw seeds by children aged 4-7 years and 20 seeds by adults. Intake of 1-2 raw seeds of certain types of this herb grown in Africa can be fatal. The main toxic symptoms include headache, enteritis, an increase in the white blood cell count, anuria, and jaundice.

Bi Qi (Cormus Heleocharitis)
Properties: Sweet, cold.
Channels entered: Lung, Stomach, Liver.
Functions: Clears Heat and cools the Blood, transforms Phlegm and disperses accumulation, eliminates eye screen.
Indications: Febrile diseases, wasting and thirsting, cough due to Phlegm-Heat, jaundice, red eyes, sore throat, short voidings of reddish urine, blood in the stool, scrofula.
Common dosage: 60-120g.

Can Sha‡ (Excrementum Bombycis Mori)
Properties: Sweet, acrid, warm.
Channels entered: Spleen, Stomach, Liver.
Functions: Dispels Wind and eliminates Dampness, harmonizes the Stomach and transforms turbidity.
Indications: Wind-Damp Bi syndrome pain, vomiting and diarrhea due to internal obstruction of Damp turbidity; generalized pruritus, and itching in eczema and urticaria.
Common dosage: 10-15g.

Cang Er Cao (Caulis et Folium Xanthii Sibirici)
Properties: Bitter, acrid, slightly cold, slightly toxic.
Channel entered: Lung.
Functions: Dispels Wind, clears Heat and relieves Toxicity.
Indications: Wind-Damp Bi syndrome, spasms of the limbs, pruritus, clove sores.
Common dosage: 6-15g.
Cautions: Contraindicated for patients with a weak constitution and for prolonged internal use.

Cha Shu Gen (Radix Camelliae Sinensis)
Properties: Bitter, neutral.
Channels entered: Heart, Lung.
Functions: Strengthens the Heart and promotes urination.
Indications: Heart failure, edema due to heart disease, hepatitis, mouth ulcers.
Common dosage: 30-60g.

Chong Wei Zi (Semen Leonuri Heterophylli)
Properties: Acrid, sweet, slightly cold, toxic.
Channels entered: Liver, Spleen.
Functions: Invigorates the Blood and regulates menstruation, clears the Liver and brightens the eyes.
Indications: Irregular menstruation, profuse uterine bleeding, vaginal discharge, abdominal pain due to Blood stasis postpartum, hypertension, red, sore and swollen eyes; palpebral eczema, alopecia and seborrhea.
Common dosage: 3-9g.
Cautions: Single dosages in excess of 30g can cause toxic side-effects with symptoms such as generalized limpness and aching.

Chu Shi Zi (Fructus Broussonetiae)
Properties: Sweet, cold.
Channels entered: Liver, Kidney.
Functions: Enriches the Kidneys, clears Heat from the Liver and brightens the eyes.
Indications: Deficiency taxation, blurred vision, eye screen, edema.
Common dosage: 9-15g.

Chu Tao Ye (Folium Broussonetiae)
Properties: Sweet, cool.
Channels entered: Liver, Kidney.
Functions: Cools the Blood, relieves Toxicity, and benefits the movement of water.
Indications: Vomiting of blood, nosebleed, uterine bleeding, dysentery, Shan disorder, edema; external use for sunburn, urticaria and dermatitis herpetiformis.
Common dosage: 3-6g.

Da Feng Zi (Semen Hydnocarpi)
Properties: Acrid, hot, toxic.
Channels entered: Liver, Spleen, Kidney.
Functions: Dispels Wind and dries Dampness, attacks Toxicity and kills Worms.
Indications: External application for leprosy, syphilis, scabies, tinea manuum, and tinea pedis.
Common dosage: 1.5-3g.
Cautions: This herb is usually applied externally; internal administration can cause headache, dizziness, nausea, and vomiting. Long-term use is contraindicated.

Da Suan (Bulbus Allii Sativi)
Properties: Acrid, warm.
Channels entered: Lung, Large Intestine, Spleen, Stomach.
Functions: Disperses swelling, relieves Toxicity, kills Worms.
Indications: Dysentery, diarrhea, hookworm, roundworm, influenza, seafood poisoning, carbuncles, scabies, and tinea.
Common dosage: 6-15g.
Cautions: Contraindicated for long-term external application or oral administration to patients with disorders of the mouth or throat.

Da Ye An Ye (Folium Eucalypti Globuli)
Properties: Bitter, acrid, cool.
Functions: Dredges Wind and clears Heat, relieves Toxicity and kills Worms.
Indications: Common cold, influenza, bronchitis, pneumonia, dysentery, urinary infections, filariasis, and hookworm; also used in skin disorders for pruritus and prurigo.
Common dosage: 9-15g.
Cautions: Contraindicated during pregnancy and for patients with ulcers of the digestive tract.

Dao Dou Zi (Semen Canavaliae)
Properties: Sweet, warm.
Channels entered: Stomach, Kidney.
Functions: Warms the Middle Burner, causes Qi to descend, and boosts the Kidneys.
Indications: Hiccoughs due to Deficiency-Cold, vomiting, abdominal distension, and pain in the lower back due to Kidney Deficiency.
Common dosage: 4.5-9g in a decoction.
Cautions: Contraindicated for patients with exuberant Stomach-Heat.

Dong Gua Ye (Folium Benincasae Hispidae)
Properties: Sweet, cool.
Channels entered: Large Intestine, Lung.
Functions: Clears Summerheat and relieves Toxicity.
Indications: Wasting and thirsting, malaria, diarrhea, dysentery.
Common dosage: 15-30g.

Duan Lü Fan‡ (Melanteritum Rubrum)
Properties: Sour, cold.
Channels entered: Liver, Spleen.
Functions: Supplements the Middle Burner and relaxes tension, moistens the Lungs and stops coughing, moistens the Intestines and frees the bowels, relieves Toxicity.
Indications: Spleen and Stomach Deficiency, pain in the stomach and abdomen, persistent cough due to Lung Deficiency, constipation; external use in pastes to treat a variety of skin disorders.

Feng Mi‡ (Mel)
Properties: Sweet, neutral.
Channels entered: Lung, Spleen, Large Intestine.
Functions: Supplements the Middle Burner and relaxes tension, moistens the Lungs and stops coughing, moistens the Intestines and frees the bowels, relieves Toxicity.
Indications: Spleen and Stomach Deficiency, pain in the stomach and abdomen, persistent cough due to Lung Deficiency, constipation; external use in pastes to treat a variety of skin disorders.

Common dosage: 15-30g.
Cautions: This substance is contraindicated for patients with internal accumulation of Phlegm-Damp, distension in the Middle Burner, or dysentery.

Feng Wei Cao (Herba Pteridis Multifidi)
Properties: Bland, slightly bitter, cool.
Channels entered: Liver, Kidney, Large Intestine.
Functions: Clears Heat and promotes the movement of Dampness, cools the Blood and stops bleeding, disperses swelling and relieves Toxicity.
Indications: Turbid Lin syndrome, vaginal discharge, icteric hepatitis, enteritis, vomiting of blood, nosebleed, blood in the stool, blood in the urine, suppurative abscesses.
Common dosage: 9-18g.
Cautions: This herb is contraindicated for patients with Deficiency-Cold patterns.

Feng Xian Hua (Flos Impatientis Balsaminae)
Properties: Sweet, warm, slightly toxic.
Functions: Invigorates the Blood and frees menstruation, dispels Wind and alleviates pain, disperses swelling and relieves Toxicity.
Indications: Amenorrhea, postpartum Blood stasis, knocks and falls, joint pain, external use for tinea unguium.
Common dosage: 3-6g.
Cautions: Contraindicated during pregnancy.

Fu Rong Ye (Folium Hibisci Mutabilis)
Properties: Bitter, acrid, slightly cold.
Channels entered: Lung, Liver.
Functions: Clears Heat and cools the Blood, disperses swelling and alleviates pain.
Indications: Cough due to Lung-Heat, vomiting of blood, leukorrhea, burns and scalds, abscesses and sores.
Common dosage: 15-30g.

Gan Lan You (Oleum Canarii Albi Fructi)
Properties: Sweet, sour, neutral.
Channel entered: Lung.
Functions: Clears the Lungs and benefits the throat, relieves Toxicity.
Indications: Sore and swollen throat due to Lung-Heat, irritability and thirst, expectoration of blood.
Common dosage: 10-15ml.

Gan Song (Rhizoma Nardostachydis)
Properties: Sweet, acrid, warm.
Channels entered: Spleen, Stomach.
Functions: Moves Qi and alleviates pain, relieves stagnation and arouses the Spleen.
Indications: Oppression in the chest, abdominal distension, loss of appetite, epigastric pain.
Common dosage: 3-6g.
Cautions: Contraindicated for patients with patterns of Qi Deficiency and Blood-Heat.

Ge Fen‡ (Concha Meretricis seu Cyclinae Pulverata)
Properties: Salty, cold.
Channels entered: Lung, Kidney.
Functions: Clears Heat and promotes the movement of Dampness, transforms Phlegm and softens hardness.

Indications: Coughing and wheezing due to accumulation of Phlegm-Fluids, stomach pain, vaginal discharge, scrofula, scalds.
Common dosage: 3-9g.

Gou Gan Cai (Herba Diclipterae Chinensis)
Properties: Sweet, bitter, cold.
Functions: Clears Heat, cools the Blood, promotes urination, relieves Toxicity.
Indications: Fever due to common colds or accompanying maculopapular eruptions, cough due to Lung-Heat, vomiting of blood, nosebleed, blood in the urine and stool, dribbling urination, dysentery, red and swollen eyes.
Common dosage: 15-30g.

Gou Qi Ye (Folium Lycii)
Properties: Bitter, cool.
Channels entered: Liver, Kidney.
Functions: Nourishes Yin and clears Heat, supplements and boosts the Liver and Kidneys, dispels Wind-Damp.
Indications: Expectoration of blood due to pulmonary tuberculosis, tidal fever and steaming bone disorder, dizziness, tinnitus, limpness and aching in the lumbar region and knees, Bi syndrome pain due to Wind-Damp.
Common dosage: 9-30g.

Gua Jin Deng (Calyx Physalis Alkekengi)
Properties: Sour, cold.
Channels entered: Lung, Spleen.
Functions: Clears Heat and relieves Toxicity, transforms Phlegm and benefits the throat, promotes urination.
Indications: Lung-Heat cough, sore throat, loss of voice, steaming bone disorder, jaundice, edema, painful urination.
Common dosage: 4.5-9g.
Cautions: Contraindicated during pregnancy.

Gui Jian Yu (Lignum Suberalatum Euonymi)
Properties: Bitter, cold.
Channel entered: Liver.
Functions: Breaks up Blood stasis, dispels Wind, kills Worms.
Indications: Amenorrhea, abdominal masses, abdominal pain due to Blood stasis postpartum or to Worm accumulation, joint pain due to Wind-Damp, knocks and falls, swelling and pain due to Blood stasis; used in skin disorders such as psoriatic arthritis and nevus flammeus to invigorate the Blood, and for joint pain accompanying erythema multiforme or small vessel vasculitis.
Common dosage: 4.5-9g.
Cautions: Contraindicated during pregnancy.

Hai Shen‡ (Stichopus Japonicus)
Properties: Sweet, salty, warm.
Channels entered: Heart, Kidney.
Functions: Supplements the Kidneys and augments the Essence, nourishes the Blood and moistens Dryness.
Indications: Seminal emission, impotence, frequent urination, enuresis, constipation, aplastic anemia.
Common dosage: 9-15g (usually eaten as food).

Han Shui Shi‡ (Calcitum)
Properties: Acrid, salty, very cold.
Channels entered: Heart, Stomach, Kidney.
Functions: Clears Heat and drains Fire.

Indications: Raging fever, irritability and thirst in febrile diseases such as chickenpox.
Common dosage: 5-15g.

He Shi (Fructus Carpesii)
Properties: Bitter, acrid, neutral, slightly toxic.
Channels entered: Spleen, Stomach.
Functions: Kills Worms and disperses accumulations.
Indications: Roundworm, hookworm, pinworm, abdominal pain due to Worm accumulation, child Gan accumulation; external application for perianal eczema.
Common dosage: 6-9g.
Cautions: This herb should be used with caution for patients with a weak constitution.

Hei Da Dou (Semen Glycines Atrum)
Properties: Sweet, neutral.
Channels entered: Spleen, Kidney.
Functions: Promotes the movement of water, dispels Wind, invigorates the Blood, relieves Toxicity.
Indications: Edema, distension and fullness in the abdomen, Wind Bi syndrome, leg Qi, jaundice, toxic sores (for example in subcorneal pustulosis).
Common dosage: 9-30g.

Hei Mian Shen (Radix Breyniae Fruticosae)
Properties: Bitter, cold, slightly toxic.
Functions: Clears Heat and relieves Toxicity, alleviates pain and itching.
Indications: Clove sores and toxic swellings, eczema, allergic contact dermatitis, pruritus, vaginitis, burns and scalds.
Common dosage: 4.5-9g.
Cautions: Contraindicated during pregnancy.

Hong Teng (Caulis Sargentodoxae Cuneatae)
Properties: Bitter, neutral.
Channels entered: Liver, Large Intestine.
Functions: Clears Heat and relieves Toxicity, invigorates the Blood and alleviates pain, disperses swelling.
Indications: Abdominal pain due to Intestinal abscess, Wind-Damp Bi syndrome pain, painful menstruation, knocks and falls, abscesses and swelling due to Heat Toxins.
Common dosage: 9-15g.
Cautions: Contraindicated during pregnancy.

Hou Po Hua (Flos Magnoliae Officinalis)
Properties: Bitter, warm, aromatic.
Channels entered: Spleen, Stomach.
Functions: Regulates Qi and loosens the Middle Burner, aromatically transforms turbidity.
Indications: Oppression in the chest, stomach pain, poor appetite.
Common dosage: 1.5-4.5g.

Hu Jiao (Fructus Piperis Nigri)
Properties: Acrid, hot.
Channels entered: Large Intestine, Stomach.
Functions: Warms the Middle Burner and alleviates pain.
Indications: Pain in the stomach and abdomen, vomiting and diarrhea due to Stomach-Cold.
Common dosage: 1.5-4.5g.

Huang Jing Gen (Radix Viticis Negundinis)
Properties: Acrid, warm.
Channel entered: Heart.
Functions: Releases the exterior, interrupts malaria, stabilizes wheezing, normalizes Qi, dispels Wind and Dampness.
Indications: Common cold, malaria, chronic bronchitis, gastric ulcers, Wind-Damp Bi syndrome pain, hepatitis.
Common dosage: 6-15g.

Huang Jing Ye (Folium Viticis Negundinis)
Properties: Bitter, neutral.
Channel entered: Lung.
Functions: Clears Heat, releases the exterior, benefits the movement of Dampness, relieves Toxicity.
Indications: Common cold, vomiting, diarrhea, dysentery, jaundice, malaria, painful urination.
Common dosage: 9-30g.

Huang Jiu (Vinum Aureum)
Properties: Sweet, bitter, acrid, warm.
Channels entered: Heart, Liver, Lung, Stomach.
Functions: Frees the Blood vessels and vanquishes Cold.
Indications: Cold and pain in the Heart and abdomen, Wind-Cold Bi syndrome pain, spasms of the sinews and vessels.
Common dosage: 15-30ml.

Huang La‡ (Cera Aurea)
See *Mi La‡* (Cera)

Huo Tan Mu (Herba Polygoni Chinensis)
Properties: Slightly sour, astringent, cool.
Functions: Clears Heat and relieves Toxicity, transforms stagnation and benefits the movement of Dampness, disperses swelling.
Indications: Common cold, sore throat, cough due to Lung-Heat, whooping cough, diphtheria, bacillary dysentery.
Common dosage: 15-30g.

Huo Xue Teng (Caulis seu Radix Schisandrae)
Properties: Acrid, sour, bitter, warm.
Channels entered: This herb enters the Xue level.
Functions: Invigorates the Blood and transforms Blood stasis, regulates Qi and transforms Dampness.
Indications: Vomiting of blood in consumptive diseases, Qi pain in the Heart and stomach, leg Qi, joint pain, irregular menstruation, knocks and falls; used in skin disorders for freeing the network vessels to treat chilblains, Raynaud's disease and lichen planus, and for invigorating the Blood to treat psoriasis and erythema multiforme.
Common dosage: 15-30g.
Cautions: Contraindicated during pregnancy.

Ji Guan Hua (Flos Celosiae Cristatae)
Properties: Sweet, astringent, cool.
Channels entered: Liver, Large Intestine.
Functions: Cools the Blood and stops bleeding.
Indications: Coughing or vomiting of blood, profuse uterine bleeding, bleeding due to hemorrhoids, Blood Lin syndrome, bloody dysentery; used in skin disorders for cooling the Blood to treat acne.
Common dosage: 9-15g.

Ji Xing Zi (Semen Impatientis Balsaminae)
Properties: Slightly bitter, acrid, warm, slightly toxic.
Channels entered: Lung, Liver, Kidney.
Functions: Invigorates the Blood and frees menstruation, softens hardness and disperses accumulations.
Indications: Menstrual block, accumulations and lumps.
Common dosage: 6-9g.
Cautions: Contraindicated during pregnancy.

Jin Gu Cao (Herba Ajugae Decumbentis)
Properties: Bitter, cold.
Functions: Clears Heat and cools the Blood, reduces fever and disperses swelling.
Indications: Coughing of blood due to Lung-Heat, tonsillitis, laryngitis, pharyngitis.
Common dosage: 15g.

Jin Guo Lan (Tuber Tinosporae)
Properties: Bitter, cold.
Channels entered: Lung, Stomach
Functions: Clears Heat and relieves Toxicity, benefits the throat and disperses swelling.
Indications: Tonsillitis, stomatitis, loss of voice, stomach pain, bacillary dysentery; also used for skin disorders involving the oral mucosa such as pemphigus vulgaris and lichen planus.
Common dosage: 3-9g.

Jin Ju Ye (Folium Fortunellae Margaritae)
Properties: Acrid, bitter, neutral.
Channels entered: Liver, Stomach.
Functions: Dredges the Liver, supports the Spleen, increases the appetite, dissipates lumps.
Indications: Dysphagia and diaphragmatic occlusion, scrofula, lumps in the breast.
Common dosage: 3-9g.

Jin Lian Hua (Flos Trollii)
Properties: Bitter, cold.
Functions: Clears Heat and relieves Toxicity.
Indications: Tonsillitis, otitis media, conjunctivitis, clove sores, mouth sores; also used for skin disorders involving the oral mucosa such as pemphigus vulgaris and lichen planus.
Common dosage: 3-6g.

Jin Que Hua (Flos Caraganae Sinicae)
Properties: Sweet, neutral.
Channels entered: Lung, Spleen, Liver.
Functions: Enriches Yin, fortifies the Spleen, harmonizes the Blood, dispels Wind.
Indications: Cough due to Lung Deficiency, dizziness, headache, tinnitus, blurred vision, limpness and aching in the lumbar region and knees, white vaginal discharge, knocks and falls; also used for skin disorders involving the oral mucosa such as pemphigus vulgaris and lichen planus.
Common dosage: 3-10g.

Jiu Cai (Folium Allii Tuberosi)
Properties: Acrid, warm.
Channels entered: Spleen, Stomach
Functions: Warms the Middle Burner, moves Qi, dissipates Blood, relieves Toxicity.

Indications: Acid reflux, nosebleeds, vomiting of blood, blood in the urine, stasis and swelling due to knocks and falls.
Common dosage: 20-60g.

Jiu Xiang Chong‡ (Aspongopus)
Properties: Salty, warm.
Channels entered: Liver, Kidney.
Functions: Regulates Qi and alleviates pain, warms the Middle Burner and strengthens Yang.
Indications: Qi stagnation, distension and oppression in the stomach, Spleen and Kidney Deficiency, limpness and aching in the lower back and knees, lack of strength, impotence.
Common dosage: 3-6g.

Lang Du (Radix Euphorbiae Fischerianae)
Properties: Acrid, bitter, neutral, slightly toxic.
Channels entered: Liver, Spleen.
Functions: Expels water, dispels Phlegm, dissipates lumps, alleviates pain, kills Worms.
Indications: Edema, abdominal distension, Worm accumulation, accumulation of Phlegm, and hiccoughs.
Common dosage: 1.0-2.5g.
Cautions: This herb should not be taken in large dosages or for long periods. Long-term use can cause damage to the liver. Overdosage can cause scorching pain in the mouth, tongue and throat, nausea, vomiting, abdominal pain, and diarrhea. When used in combination with *Dang Gui* (Radix Angelicae Sinensis) and *Gan Cao* (Radix Glycyrrhizae), there is less likelihood of damage to the liver and kidneys.

Lao Guan Cao (Herba Erodii seu Geranii)
Properties: Bitter, acrid, neutral.
Channels entered: Stomach, Large Intestine.
Functions: Dispels Wind-Damp, frees the channels and network vessels, stops diarrhea, clears Heat and relieves Toxicity.
Indications: Wind-Damp Bi syndrome pain, numbness and spasm of the limbs, aching of the sinews and bones, diarrhea, abscesses; also used for psoriatic arthritis.
Common dosage: 9-15g.

Lei Gong Teng (Radix Tripterygii Wilfordi)
Properties: Bitter, cold, extremely toxic.
Functions: Dispels Wind and eliminates Dampness, invigorates the Blood and frees the network vessels, disperses swelling and alleviates pain.
Indications: Arthritis, rheumatoid arthritis, small vessel vasculitis, erythromelalgia, psoriasis, and impetigo.
Common dosage: 6-9g.
Cautions: This herb is extremely toxic and great care should be exercised when taken internally.

Li Lu (Radix et Rhizoma Veratri)
Properties: Acrid, bitter, cold, toxic.
Channels entered: Lung, Liver, Stomach.
Functions: Induces vomiting, kills Worms.
Indications: Wind-stroke, epilepsy, throat Bi syndrome with exuberant Phlegm; external use for scabies and tinea.
Common dosage: 0.3-0.9g for internal use, 20-30g for external use.
Cautions: This herb is very toxic and internal use requires extreme caution.

Li Zhi Cao (Herba Salviae Plebeiae)
Properties: Acrid, cool.
Functions: Benefits the movement of water, cools the Blood, clears Heat, and relieves Toxicity.
Indications: Ascites, edema due to nephritis, inhibited urination, expectoration and vomiting of blood, blood in the urine and stool; external use for vaginitis.
Common dosage: 9-30g.

Lian Qiao Xin (Semen Forsythiae Suspensae)
Properties: Bitter, slightly cold.
Channel entered: Pericardium.
Functions: Clears Heat from the Heart and drains Fire.
Indications: High fever, irritability and restlessness due to pathogenic factors entering the Pericardium channel, clouded Spirit and delirious speech.
Common dosage: 6-15g.

Ling Xiao Hua (Flos Campsitis)
Properties: Acrid, sour, cold.
Channels entered: Liver, Pericardium.
Functions: Cools the Blood, breaks up Blood stasis, and dispels Wind.
Indications: Menstrual block due to Blood stasis, painful menstruation, abdominal masses, itchy skin due to Blood-Heat; used in skin disorders for cooling the Blood to treat cosmetic dermatitis, psoriasis, pityriasis rosea, erythema multiforme, acne, and rosacea.
Common dosage: 3-9g.
Cautions: Contraindicated during pregnancy.

Liu Ye (Folium Salicis)
Properties: Bitter, cold.
Channels entered: Lung, Bladder.
Functions: Clears Heat, vents eruptions, promotes urination, relieves Toxicity.
Indications: Varicella (chickenpox) with difficult expression of the lesions, white urinary turbidity, clove sores, boils, toothache.
Common dosage: 9-15g.

Long Kui (Herba Solani Nigri)
Properties: Bitter, cold, slightly toxic.
Channels entered: Liver, Stomach.
Functions: Clears Heat and relieves Toxicity, invigorates the Blood and disperses swelling, promotes urination.
Indications: Swollen abscesses, clove sores, knocks and falls (trauma), edema, inhibited urination; external use for sunburn and pemphigus.
Common dosage: 10-30g.
Cautions: Large dosages can reduce the white blood cell count and induce aversion to cold and night sweating.

Lu Bian Ju (Herba et Radix Kalimeridis)
Properties: Bitter, acrid.
Functions: Clears Heat and relieves Toxicity.
Indications: Common cold, influenza, headache due to Wind-Heat, sinusitis, bronchitis, sore throat, varicella (chickenpox); external use for furuncles (boils).
Common dosage: 9-15g.

Lü Cao (Herba Humuli Scandentis)
Properties: Sweet, bitter, cold.

Channels entered: Lung, Bladder.
Functions: Clears Heat, promotes urination, disperses Blood stasis, relieves Toxicity.
Indications: Lin syndrome, inhibited urination, malaria, diarrhea, pulmonary tuberculosis, Lung abscess, pneumonia, hemorrhoids, scrofula; external use for insect bites.
Common dosage: 9-30g.

Ma Bian Cao **(Herba cum Radice Verbenae)**
Properties: Bitter, cold.
Channels entered: Liver, Spleen.
Functions: Clears Heat and relieves Toxicity, promotes the movement of water and disperses swelling, invigorates the Blood and dissipates Blood stasis, kills Worms.
Indications: Fever due to the common cold, malaria, Damp-Heat jaundice, dysentery, diphtheria, Lin syndrome, menstrual block, abdominal masses; used in skin disorders for clearing Heat and relieving Toxicity to treat candidal balanitis, intertrigo, erysipelas, and annular erythemas.
Common dosage: 15-30g.

Ma Wei Lian **(Radix Thalictri)**
Properties: Bitter, cold.
Channels entered: Heart, Large Intestine, Liver, Bladder.
Functions: Clears Heat, dries Dampness, drains Fire, relieves Toxicity.
Indications: Mouth and tongue ulcers, dysentery, enteritis, infectious hepatitis, tonsillitis, conjunctivitis.
Common dosage: 3-9g.

Meng Chong‡ **(Tabanus)**
Properties: Bitter, slightly cold, toxic.
Channel entered: Liver.
Functions: Expels static Blood, disperses abdominal masses, dissipates lumps.
Indications: Amenorrhea, abdominal masses due to Cold or Heat, pain due to Blood stasis, knocks and falls (trauma).
Common dosage: 1.5-3g.
Cautions: Contraindicated during pregnancy.

Mi Cu **(Acetum Oryzae)**
Properties: Sour, bitter, warm.
Channels entered: Liver, Stomach.
Functions: Dissipates Blood stasis, stops bleeding, relieves Toxicity, and kills Worms.
Indications: Pain in the Heart and abdomen, jaundice, dysentery, Worm accumulation, vomiting of blood, blood in the stool, food poisoning; external use in pastes to treat a variety of skin disorders.
Common dosage: 15-30ml.

Mi La‡ **(Cera)**
Properties: Sweet, bland, neutral.
Functions: Promotes contraction, closes sores, generates flesh, alleviates pain.
Indications: Ulcerating sores that are slow to heal, erosive shank sores, wounds, burns and scalds.
Common dosage: 4.5-9g.

Mo Li Hua **(Flos Jasmini)**
Properties: Acrid, sweet, warm.
Functions: Regulates Qi and relieves Depression, expels turbidity and harmonizes the Middle Burner.
Indications: Abdominal pain due to dysentery, toxic swellings.
Common dosage: 4.5-9g.

Mu Bie Zi **(Semen Momordicae Cochinchinensis)**
Properties: Bitter, slightly sweet, warm, toxic.
Channels entered: Liver, Spleen, Stomach.
Functions: Dissipates lumps and disperses swelling, invigorates the Blood, alleviates pain and relieves Toxicity.
Indications: Abscesses, clove sores, scrofula, hemorrhoids, stasis and swelling due to trauma, Wind-Damp Bi syndrome; external application for tinea capitis (ringworm of the scalp).
Common dosage: 0.3-0.9g.
Cautions: The toxic nature of this herb means that great care should be exercised with internal administration.

Mu Jin Pi **(Cortex Hibisci Syriaci Radicis)**
Properties: Sweet, bitter, slightly cold.
Channels entered: Liver, Spleen, Large Intestine.
Functions: Clears Heat and promotes the movement of Dampness, kills Worms and alleviates itching.
Indications: Jaundice, dysentery, Lung abscess, Intestinal abscess, red and white vaginal discharge; external application for tinea capitis (ringworm of the scalp), pruritus and scabies.
Common dosage: 3-9g.

Mu Man Tou **(Flos Fici Pumilae)**
Properties: Sweet, acrid, bland.
Channel entered: Kidney.
Functions: Supplements the Kidneys and consolidates the Essence, invigorates the Blood and stops bleeding, relieves Toxicity and disperses swelling.
Indications: Aching in the lumbar region due to Kidney Deficiency, impotence, seminal emission, prolapse of the rectum due to enduring dysentery, blood in the stool, hemorrhoids.
Common dosage: 6-15g.

Nao Sha‡ **(Sal Ammoniacum)**
Properties: Salty, bitter, acrid, warm, slightly toxic.
Channels entered: Liver, Spleen, Stomach.
Functions: Disperses accumulations and softens hardness, breaks up Blood stasis and dissipates lumps, transforms Phlegm.
Indications: Abdominal masses, throat Bi syndrome, menstrual block, polyps, warts, clove sores, scrofula, painful swellings and boils.
Common dosage: 0.1-0.3g.
Cautions: Not suitable for long-term use; contraindicated for patients with a weak constitution and liver disease, those without exuberant pathogenic factors, and during pregnancy.

Nao Yang Hua **(Flos Rhododendri Mollis)**
Properties: Acrid, warm, extremely toxic.
Channel entered: Liver.
Functions: Dispels Wind, eliminates Dampness, settles pain.
Indications: Bi syndrome pain due to arthritis, pain due to trauma.
Common dosage: 0.3-0.6g.
Cautions: Contraindicated for internal use.

Nen Liu Zhi **(Ramulus Tener Salicis)**
Properties: Bitter, cold.

Channels entered: Liver, Stomach.
Functions: Dispels Wind, alleviates pain, promotes urination, disperses swelling.
Indications: Rheumatic arthritis, Lin syndrome, difficult urination, white turbid urine, vaginal discharge, Damp-Heat jaundice, swollen gums.
Common dosage: 30-60g.

Qian Dan‡ (Minium)
Properties: Acrid, cool, toxic.
Channels entered: Liver, Heart, Spleen.
Functions: Relieves Toxicity, generates flesh and alleviates itching, guides Phlegm downward, interrupts malaria.
Indications: Internal use for convulsions, insomnia and malaria; external use for non-healing ulcers and sores (for example, chronic venous ulcer of the lower leg), and burns.
Common dosage: 0.3-0.9g (internal use), 3-5g (external use).
Cautions: The toxic nature of this substance means that all uses (including external uses) are strictly controlled or prohibited in many countries.

Qian Li Guang (Herba Senecionis Scandentis)
Properties: Bitter, cold.
Functions: Clears Heat, relieves Toxicity, kills Worms, brightens the eyes.
Indications: Wind-Fire red eye (conjunctivitis), upper respiratory tract infection, tonsillitis, laryngopharyngitis, pneumonia, bacillary dysentery, enteritis, trichomoniasis; external application for chronic venous ulcer of the lower leg.
Common dosage: 15-30g.

Qian Nian Jian (Rhizoma Homalomenae)
Properties: Acrid, bitter, warm.
Channels entered: Liver, Kidney.
Functions: Dispels Wind-Damp, strengthens the sinews and bones.
Indications: Joint pain, pain in the lumbar region, limpness and aching in the sinews and bones, numbness of the arms and legs, pain and swelling due to knocks and falls.
Common dosage: 15-30g.

Qiang Wei Gen (Radix Rosae Multiflorae)
Properties: Bitter, astringent, cool.
Channels entered: Spleen, Stomach.
Functions: Clears Heat and benefits the movement of Dampness, expels Wind, invigorates the Blood, relieves Toxicity.
Indications: Lung abscess, wasting and thirsting, dysentery, arthritis, vomiting of blood, nosebleed, blood in the urine, frequent urination, irregular menstruation, knocks and falls; used as a mouthwash to treat recurrent aphthous stomatitis (mouth ulcers).
Common dosage: 4.5-12g.

Qiang Wei Hua (Flos Rosae Multiflorae)
Properties: Sweet, cool.
Channels entered: Stomach, Liver.
Functions: Clears Summerheat, harmonizes the Stomach, stops bleeding.
Indications: Vomiting of blood due to Summerheat, thirst, diarrhea, malaria, bleeding due to incised wounds; used as a mouthwash to treat herpetic stomatitis.

Common dosage: 3-6g.

Qiao Mai Geng (Caulis Fagopyri)
Properties: Sour, cold.
Functions: Lowers blood pressure, stops bleeding, bears Qi downward, relieves Toxicity.
Indications: High blood pressure, bleeding due to capillary fragility, deep pustules.
Common dosage: 30-60g (fresh).

Qie Di (Pedicellus Solani Melongenae)
Properties: Sweet, cool.
Channels entered: Spleen, Stomach, Large Intestine.
Functions: Stops bleeding and disperses swelling.
Indications: Intestinal bleeding; also external use to apply rubs or powders.
Common dosage: 6-9g.

Qie Zi (Fructus Solani Melongenae)
Properties: Sweet, cool.
Channels entered: Spleen, Stomach, Large Intestine.
Functions: Clears Heat, stops bleeding and disperses swelling.
Indications: Bleeding due to Intestinal Wind, hemorrhoids, toxic swellings.
Common dosage: 9g.

Qing Meng Shi‡ (Lapis Chloriti)
Properties: Sweet, salty, neutral.
Channels entered: Liver, Lung.
Functions: Causes Qi to descend and disperses Phlegm, calms the Liver and settles fright.
Indications: Binding of stubborn thick phlegm, Excess patterns of coughing and wheezing due to Qi counterflow, fright epilepsy due to Phlegm accumulation; also used for skin disorders due to congealing of Phlegm such as lipoma.
Common dosage: 6-9g.

Qing Xiang Zi (Semen Celosiae Argenteae)
Properties: Sweet, cool.
Channel entered: Liver.
Functions: Clears Heat and drains Fire from the Liver, brightens the eyes and eliminates eye screen.
Indications: Red, sore and swollen eyes due to Liver-Fire, eye screen, blurred vision, pruritus due to Wind-Heat; also used in skin disorders for herpes simplex involving the eyes.
Common dosage: 3-15g.
Cautions: Contraindicated in cases of glaucoma or Deficiency of the Liver or Kidneys.

Qing Yang Shu Ye (Folium Populi)
Properties: Bitter, cold.
Functions: Transforms Dampness.
Indications: Edema.
Common dosage: 50-100g.

Shan Cha Hua (Flos Camelliae Japonicae)
Properties: Sweet, slightly acrid, cool.
Channels entered: Liver, Stomach, Large Intestine.
Functions: Cools the Blood, and stops bleeding, dissipates Blood stasis and disperses swelling.
Indications: Vomiting of blood, nosebleeds, flooding and

spotting, blood in the stool, bloody dysentery, Blood Lin syndrome, knocks and falls (trauma), scalds.
Common dosage: 3-9g.
Cautions: This herb should be used with care in cases of Spleen and Stomach Deficiency-Cold.

Shan Ci Gu **(Pseudobulbus Shancigu)**
Properties: Sweet, slightly acrid, cold, slightly toxic.
Channels entered: Liver, Spleen.
Functions: Disperses swelling and dissipates lumps, transforms Phlegm and relieves Toxicity.
Indications: Used in dermatology to treat sores, abscesses and toxic swellings in such skin conditions as plantar warts, pyoderma faciale, erythema induratum, keloids, and lipoma.
Common dosage: 3-6g.
Cautions: This herb should be used with care for patients with a weak constitution.

Shang Lu **(Radix Phytolaccae)**
Properties: Bitter, cold, toxic.
Channels entered: Bladder, Kidney, Spleen, Large Intestine.
Functions: Drains downward and expels water, disperses swelling and dissipates lumps.
Indications: Edema, difficult urination, constipation, abdominal distension and fullness, and painful swellings; external use for sores.
Common dosage: 3-9g.
Cautions: This is a toxic herb with a drastic effect; usage is normally restricted to severe cases requiring purgation.

She Tui‡ **(Exuviae Serpentis)**
Properties: Sweet, salty, neutral, toxic.
Channel entered: Liver.
Functions: Dispels Wind and settles fright, relieves Toxicity and disperses swelling, eliminates eye screen, kills Worms.
Indications: Infantile convulsions, epilepsy, sore throat, inhibited urination, eye screen; also used in skin disorders to alleviate itching in various skin disorders such as chronic urticaria and palpebral eczema.
Common dosage: 1.5-3g.
Cautions: Contraindicated during pregnancy.

Shi Hua **(Parmelia)**
Properties: Sweet, cold.
Channel entered: Liver.
Functions: Nourishes the Blood and brightens the eyes, stops bleeding, clears Heat and relieves Toxicity, promotes the movement of Dampness.
Indications: Blurred vision, vomiting of blood, profuse uterine bleeding, painful voidings of hot urine, white vaginal discharge, pain in the lumbar region and knees, burns and scalds.
Common dosage: 6-9g.

Shi Hui‡ **(Calx)**
Properties: Acrid, warm.
Channels entered: Liver, Spleen.
Functions: External use for drying Dampness, killing Worms, stopping bleeding, alleviating pain, and removing necrotic tissue; internal use for stopping dysentery.
Indications: Damp sores, bleeding due to external trauma,

scalds, hemorrhoids, prolapse of the anus, dysentery; sometimes used as a corrosive agent in skin disorders.
Common dosage: 9g.

Shi Nan Teng **(Caulis Photiniae)**
Properties: Acrid, warm.
Channels entered: Liver, Kidney.
Functions: Dispels Wind and frees the network vessels, strengthens the lumbar region and alleviates pain, invigorates Yang.
Indications: Wind-Cold-Damp Bi syndrome, pain in the lumbar region due to Kidney Deficiency, painful menstruation, impotence, coughing and wheezing; also used in skin disorders for freeing the network vessels to treat erythema multiforme, Raynaud's disease and frostbite.
Common dosage: 9-15g.

Shi Shuang **(Saccharum Kaki)**
Properties: Sweet, cool.
Channels entered: Lung, Heart.
Functions: Clears Heat, dries Dampness and transforms Phlegm.
Indications: Cough due to Lung-Heat, dry and sore throat, mouth and tongue ulcers, vomiting of blood, wasting and thirsting.
Common dosage: 3-9g.
Cautions: Contraindicated for patients with a cough due to Wind-Cold.

Shu Qu Cao **(Herba Gnaphalii Affinis)**
Properties: Sweet, neutral.
Channel entered: Lung.
Functions: Transforms Phlegm, stops coughing, dispels Wind.
Indications: Cough with profuse phlegm, wheezing, common cold due to Wind-Cold, pain in the sinews and bones, white vaginal discharge, abscesses.
Common dosage: 2-5g.
Cautions: Overdosage may affect vision.

Shui Qin Cai **(Herba et Radix Oenanthes Benghalensis)**
Properties: Sweet, cool.
Channels entered: Lung, Stomach.
Functions: Clears Heat and relieves Toxicity, promotes urination, stops bleeding and reduces blood pressure.
Indications: Fever due to the common cold, cough due to Lung-Heat, whooping cough, jaundice, edema, painful urination, white vaginal discharge, blood in the urine and stool, hypertension.
Common dosage: 15-30g.

Si Gua Luo **(Fasciculus Vascularis Luffae)**
Properties: Sweet, neutral.
Channels entered: Lung, Stomach, Liver.
Functions: Dispels Wind and frees the network vessels, relieves Toxicity, and transforms Phlegm.
Indications: Oppression and pain in the chest and hypochondrium, Wind-Damp Bi syndrome, cough with profuse phlegm; used in skin disorders for freeing the network vessels to treat herpes zoster (shingles), measles, psoriasis, lichen planus, erythromelalgia, and hemangioma.
Common dosage: 6-15g.

Si Gua Tan (Fasciculus Vascularis Luffae Carbonisatus)
Properties: Bitter, slightly cold, toxic.
Channels entered: Heart, Spleen, Kidney.
Functions: Dredges the sinews, invigorates the Blood, fortifies the Spleen, kills Worms.
Indications: Numbness of the limbs, lumbar region and knees, irregular menstruation, nasal congestion.
Common dosage: 15-30g.

Song Xiang (Resina Pini)
Properties: Bitter, sweet, warm.
Channels entered: Liver, Spleen.
Functions: Dries Dampness, kills Worms, generates flesh, alleviates pain.
Indications: External application for swollen abscesses, boils, clove sores, scabies, bleeding due to trauma; also used for fumigation or moxibustion to treat lichen simplex chronicus (neurodermatitis) and chronic venous ulcer of the lower leg.
Common dosage: 6-12g (external use).

Tao Ye (Folium Persicae)
Properties: Bitter, neutral.
Channels entered: Spleen, Kidney.
Functions: Relieves Toxicity, dispels Wind, kills Worms.
Indications: External use for perianal eczema, urticaria, tinea pedis (athlete's foot), hemorrhoids, and insect bites.
Common dosage: 60g.

Teng Huang (Resina Garciniae)
Properties: Sour, astringent, toxic.
Functions: Disperses swelling, transforms Toxicity, stops bleeding, kills Worms.
Indications: Swollen abscesses such as furuncles, stubborn tinea (particularly tinea manuum and tinea pedis), bleeding due to trauma, burns and scalds.
Common dosage: 10-12g (for pills, powders or soaks).
Cautions: Overdosage can cause dizziness, vomiting, abdominal pain, or diarrhea.

Tian Kui Zi (Tuber Semiaquilegiae)
Properties: Sweet, bitter, cold, slightly toxic.
Channels entered: Liver, Kidney.
Functions: Clears Heat and relieves Toxicity, disperses swelling and dissipates lumps, promotes urination.
Indications: Swollen abscesses, clove sores, scrofula, turbid Lin syndrome, swelling and pain due to trauma, and snake bites.
Common dosage: 6-15g.
Cautions: This herb should be used with care for patients with Spleen and Stomach Deficiency-Cold and loose stools, and during pregnancy.
Note: *Tian Kui* (Herba Semiaquilegiae) has similar functions and indications, but is sweet, cold and slightly toxic.

Tian Xian Zi (Semen Hyoscyami)
Properties: Bitter, warm, very toxic.
Channels entered: Heart, Liver, Stomach.
Functions: Settles epilepsy, alleviates pain, calms wheezing, stops diarrhea.
Indications: Epilepsy, mania and withdrawal, pain in the stomach and abdomen, coughing and wheezing, persistent diarrhea and dysentery; external use for furuncles (boils).

Common dosage: 0.6-1.2g.
Cautions: Contraindicated for patients with glaucoma and heart disease. Overdosage can also cause drug poisoning, manifesting as blurred vision and mental confusion.

Tong You (Oleum Aleuritis Seminis)
Properties: Sweet, acrid, cold, toxic.
Functions: Kills worms and relieves Toxicity, closes sores and generates flesh.
Indications: External use for sores at the initial stage, burns and scalds, herpes zoster (shingles), erysipelas, scabies, and tinea; can be used on its own or as a vehicle.
Common dosage: 6-9g.

Tou Gu Cao (Herba Speranskiae seu Impatientis)
Properties: Acrid, bitter, warm.
Channels entered: Liver, Kidney.
Functions: Dispels Wind, soothes the sinews, eliminates Dampness, invigorates the Blood, alleviates pain.
Indications: Wind-Damp Bi syndrome pain, inhibited bending and stretching, amenorrhea, leg Qi due to Cold-Damp; also used internally for skin disorders involving Bi syndrome such as psoriatic arthritis, and externally to treat tinea manuum, chilblains, genital eczema, and erythema multiforme.
Common dosage: 6-9g.

Tu Bei Mu (Tuber Bolbostemmatis)
Properties: Bitter, slightly cold.
Channels entered: Lung, Spleen.
Functions: Clears Heat and relieves Toxicity, dissipates lumps and disperses swelling.
Indications: Breast abscess, breast cancer, scrofula, Phlegm nodes, sores, swellings; used in skin disorders for transforming Phlegm to treat erythema induratum and lipoma.
Common dosage: 3-9g.

Tu Da Huang (Radix Rumicis Madaio)
Properties: Bitter, acrid, cool.
Functions: Clears Heat and relieves Toxicity, cools the Blood and stops bleeding, frees the bowels and kills Worms.
Indications: Sore throat, Lung abscess, constipation, vomiting of blood, nosebleeds; external use for tinea capitis (ringworm of the scalp) and tinea unguium (ringworm of the hands).
Common dosage: 9-15g.

Tu Jin Pi (Cortex Pseudolaricis)
Properties: Bitter, acrid, warm, toxic.
Functions: Kills Worms and alleviates itching.
Indications: External use for scabies, tinea capitis (ringworm of the scalp), tinea manuum (ringworm of the hands), and tinea pedis (athlete's foot), and for itching in seborrheic eczema, asteatotic eczema and eczema of the scrotum.
Common dosage: Appropriate amount for external use.

Tu Jing Jie (Herba Chenopodii Ambroisioidis)
Properties: Acrid, bitter, warm, toxic.
Functions: Dispels Wind, kills Worms, frees the channels, alleviates pain.
Indications: Wind-Damp Bi syndrome pain, roundworm, painful menstruation, snake bites.
Common dosage: 3-6g.

Cautions: Overdosage when taken internally can lead to nausea, vomiting, constipation, tinnitus, and visual impairment. Contraindicated during pregnancy.

Wa Leng Zi‡ (Concha Arcae)
Properties: Sweet, salty, neutral.
Channels entered: Liver, Spleen, Stomach.
Functions: Inhibits acid and alleviates pain, disperses Phlegm and transforms stasis, soften hardness and dissipates lumps.
Indications: Stomach pain, acid vomiting, abdominal masses, accumulation of stubborn Phlegm, scrofula.
Common dosage: 9-15g.

Wu Shao She‡ (Zaocys Dhumnades)
Properties: Sweet, salty, neutral.
Channels entered: Liver, Lung.
Functions: Dispels Wind-Damp, frees the channels and network vessels, attacks Toxicity.
Indications: Wind-Damp Bi syndrome pain, numbness of the skin and flesh, tetanus, leprosy, tinea pedis (athlete's foot), stubborn pruritus, and itching in eczema, lichen simplex chronicus (neurodermatitis), lichen planus, and urticaria.
Common dosage: 4.5-12g in a decoction, 0.9-1.5g as a powder.

Wu Yi (Fructus Praeparatio Ulmi)
Properties: Bitter, acrid, warm.
Channels entered: Spleen, Stomach.
Function: Kills Worms.
Indications: Pain due to Worm accumulation, persistent diarrhea.
Common dosage: 3-9g.
Cautions: Contraindicated in cases of Spleen and Stomach Deficiency.

Xi Gua Pi (Epicarpium Citrulli Vulgaris)
Properties: Sweet, cool.
Channels entered: Heart, Stomach, Bladder.
Functions: Clears Heat and relieves Summerheat, alleviates thirst and promotes urination.
Indications: Vexation and thirst due to Summerheat, hypertension, edema due to nephritis, cystitis, short voidings of scant urine, dry and sore throat; used in skin disorders to treat miliaria rubra (prickly heat).
Common dosage: 15-30g.

Xi He Liu (Cacumen Tamaricis)
Properties: Sweet, salty, neutral.
Channels entered: Lung, Stomach, Heart.
Functions: Dredges Wind, releases the exterior and vents papules, promotes urination.
Indications: Facilitating expression of the measles rash, cough, irritability and restlessness, itching due to Wind papules, common cold, headache, chronic bronchitis, joint pain due to Wind-Damp, inhibited urination.
Common dosage: 4.5-9g.

Xian Cai Gen (Radix Amaranthi Tricoloris)
Properties: Sweet, cold.
Functions: Clears Heat and benefits the orifices.
Indications: Soreness and swelling in the scrotum, hemorrhoids, toothache, knocks and falls, vaginal discharge.
Common dosage: 4.5-9g.

Xian Ren Zhang (Radix et Caulis Opuntiae Dillenii)
Properties: Bitter, cold.
Channels entered: Stomach, Lung.
Functions: Invigorates the Blood and moves Qi, disperses swelling and alleviates pain, clears Heat and relieves Toxicity.
Indications: Qi pain in the Heart and stomach, focal distension, dysentery, bleeding from hemorrhoids, cough, sore throat, Lung abscess, breast abscess, clove sores, burns and scalds, snake bites.
Common dosage: 30-60g.
Cautions: Contraindicated during pregnancy.

Xian Tao Cao (Herba Veronicae Peregrinae)
Properties: Sweet, bland, warm.
Channels entered: Liver, Stomach.
Functions: Invigorate the Blood and stop bleeding, regulate Qi and alleviate pain.
Indications: Vomiting, expectoration of blood due to internal injury, nosebleed, blood in the stool, pain in the Liver and Stomach, Shan disorder, painful menstruation.
Common dosage: 9-15g.

Xiang You (Oleum Sesami Seminis)
Properties: Sweet, cool.
Functions: Moistens Dryness, frees the bowels, relieves Toxicity, generates flesh.
Indications: Constipation due to Intestinal Dryness, roundworm, abdominal pain due to food accumulation, ulcers, tinea and scabies, cracking of the skin.
Common dosage: 30-60ml.

Xiao Bo (Radix seu Caulis Berberidis)
Properties: Bitter, very cold.
Functions: Clears Heat and dries Dampness, drains Fire and relieves Toxicity.
Indications: Acute gastroenteritis, dysentery, jaundice, white vaginal discharge, swollen and painful joints, fever due to Yin Deficiency, steaming bone disorder, night sweating, mouth ulcers, folliculitis, impetigo.
Common dosage: 3-9g.

Xing Xing Cao (Herba Eragrosti)
Properties: Sweet, bland, cool.
Channels entered: Liver, Spleen, Stomach.
Functions: Clears Heat, dredges Wind, promotes urination, and expels stones.
Indications: Eye screen, conjunctivitis, keratitis, nephritis, pyelonephritis, cystitis, kidney and bladder stones.
Common dosage: 9-15g.

Xue Yu Tan‡ (Crinis Carbonisatus Hominis)
Properties: Bitter, neutral.
Channels entered: Heart, Liver, Kidney.
Functions: Stops bleeding and dissipates Blood stasis, supplements Yin and promotes urination.
Indications: Nosebleed, coughing of blood, Blood Lin syndrome, blood in the stool, uterine bleeding.
Common dosage: 1.5-9g.

Yang Qi Shi‡ (Actinolitum)
Properties: Salty, slightly warm.
Channel entered: Kidney.

Functions: Warms the Kidneys and strengthens Yang, warms the Uterus.

Indications: Impotence due to Kidney Yang Deficiency, cold in the Uterus, Deficiency-Cold in the Lower Burner, cold and aching in the lumbar region and knees.

Common dosage: 3-4.5g.

Cautions: Contraindicated for long-term use and in cases of Yin Deficiency with Heat signs.

Yang Ti Gen (Radix Rumicis Crispi)

Properties: Bitter, cold, slightly toxic.

Channel entered: Heart.

Functions: Cools the Blood and stops bleeding, kills Worms and treats tinea.

Indications: Bleeding due to Blood-Heat, stubborn tinea (notably tinea cruris, or jock itch).

Common dosage: 9-15g.

Cautions: Contraindicated for patients with Spleen and Stomach Deficiency-Cold or dysentery.

Yi Zhi Huang Hua (Herba Solidaginis)

Properties: Acrid, bitter, cool.

Channels entered: Liver, Gallbladder.

Functions: Dredges Wind and clears Heat, disperses swelling and relieves Toxicity.

Indications: Headache due to common colds, sore and swollen throat, jaundice, thrush, tinea capitis.

Common dosage: 3-4.5g.

Cautions: Contraindicated for long-term use and in cases of Yin Deficiency with Heat signs.

Yu Shu Ye (Folium Ulmi)

Properties: Sweet, neutral.

Channels entered: Bladder, Kidney.

Function: Promotes urination.

Indications: Stone Lin syndrome, edema.

Common dosage: 4.5-9g.

Yue Ji Hua (Flos et Fructus Rosae Chinensis)

Properties: Sweet, warm.

Channel entered: Liver.

Functions: Invigorates the Blood, regulates menstruation, disperses swelling.

Indications: Delayed or scant menstruation, distension and pain in the chest and abdomen, swollen and painful non-ulcerated scrofula.

Common dosage: 3-6g.

Cautions: Overuse may cause diarrhea in patients with Spleen and Stomach Deficiency; contraindicated during pregnancy.

Zang Qing Guo (Fructus Immaturus Terminaliae Chebulae)

Properties: Bitter, slightly sweet, astringent, cool.

Channels entered: Lung, Stomach, Large Intestine.

Functions: Generates Body Fluids, benefits the throat, astringes the Intestines.

Indications: Chronic laryngopharyngitis, hoarse voice, tonsillitis, acute enteritis, bacillary dysentery.

Common dosage: 3-9g.

Zhang Mu (Lignum Cinnamomi Camphorae)

Properties: Acrid, warm.

Channels entered: Liver, Spleen, Lung.

Functions: Dispels Wind and eliminates Dampness, invigorates the Blood and frees the network vessels, benefits the joints.

Indications: Distension and pain in the chest and abdomen, Wind-Damp Bi syndrome pain, knocks and falls, intense itching (for example in scabies or urticaria).

Common dosage: 9-15g.

Cautions: Contraindicated during pregnancy.

Zhang Nao (Camphora)

Properties: Acrid, hot, toxic.

Channels entered: Heart, Spleen.

Functions: Opens the orifices and repels turbidity, dispels Wind-Damp and kills Worms.

Indications: Loss of consciousness, delirium, scabies, tinea.

Common dosage: 0.1-0.2g (internal use); 5-15g (external use).

Cautions: Extreme care should be exercised when administered internally; contraindicated in cases of Qi Deficiency and during pregnancy.

Zi Bei Chi‡ (Concha Mauritiae)

Properties: Salty, bland.

Channel entered: Liver.

Functions: Clears Heat from the Liver and brightens the eyes, settles fright and quiets the Spirit.

Indications: Eye screen due to Heat Toxins, sore red and swollen eyes, dizziness, headache, insomnia, convulsions of the limbs.

Common dosage: 9-15g.

Note

Animal, insect and mineral materia medica are marked with the symbol ‡.

Reference

1. Xu Li and Wang Wei, *Chinese Materia Medica: Combinations and Applications*, London: Donica Publishing, 2002.

Acupuncture points commonly used in the treatment of skin disorders

POINTS FOR DREDGING WIND TO ALLEVIATE ITCHING

LU-7 Lieque
Functions: Dredges Wind to release the exterior and diffuses Lung Qi with the reducing method; supplements the Lungs to augment Qi with the reinforcing method.
Indications: Lichen planus, measles, plane warts.

LU-9 Taiyuan
Functions: Regulates Lung Qi with the reducing method; supplements the Lungs to augment Qi with the reinforcing method.
Indications: Lichen planus.

LI-4 Hegu
Functions: Dredges Wind to release the exterior, clears Heat and diffuses the Lungs with the reducing method; supplements the Spleen, enriches Yin, augments Qi, and bears Yang upward with the reinforcing method.
Indications: Acne, hyperhidrosis, insect bites, lichen planus, lichen simplex chronicus (neurodermatitis), mouth ulcers, pityriasis rosea, plane warts (verruca plana), pruritus, psoriasis, urticaria.

LI-11 Quchi
Functions: Dispels Wind, dissipates pathogenic factors, clears Heat, and releases the exterior with the reducing method; nourishes Yin, moistens the skin, strengthens the sinews, and supplements Deficiency with the reinforcing method.
Indications: Acne, urticarial or fixed drug eruptions, eczema, lichen planus, lichen simplex chronicus (neurodermatitis), pityriasis rosea, pruritus, psoriasis, scabies, urticaria.

LI-20 Yingxiang
Functions: Benefits the nose and clears retained Heat with the reducing method; strengthens the sinews and supplements Deficiency with the reinforcing method.
Indications: Acne, rosacea, urticaria.

SI-3 Houxi
Functions: Dispels pathogenic factors, dissipates stagnation, and dredges the channels to alleviate itching with the reducing method; strengthens the sinews and supplements Deficiency with the reinforcing method.
Indications: Hyperhidrosis, mouth ulcers, pompholyx, tinea pedis (athlete's foot).

BL-12 Fengmen
Functions: Dredges Wind, clears Heat, diffuses the Lungs, and dissipates pathogenic factors with the reducing method; warms Yang and consolidates Wei Qi (Defensive Qi) with the reinforcing method.
Indications: Psoriasis and rosacea.

BL-13 Feishu
Functions: Diffuses Lung Qi, expels Wind and dissipates pathogenic factors with the reducing method; supports Vital Qi (Zheng Qi), consolidates the exterior and warms Yang Qi with the reinforcing method.
Indications: Eczema, herpes simplex, pruritus, psoriasis, rosacea, urticaria.

GB-20 Fengchi
Functions: Dredges Wind, clears Heat, frees the channels, and dissipates pathogenic factors with the reducing method; fortifies the Brain and quiets the Spirit with the reinforcing method.
Indications: Alopecia areata, folliculitis, furuncles, pityriasis rosea, pruritus, psoriasis, seborrhea, urticaria.

GB-31 Fengshi
Functions: Dispels Wind and alleviates itching with the reducing method; strengthens the sinews and vessels with the reinforcing method.
Indications: Lichen planus, tinea corporis, urticaria, vitiligo.

GV-14 Dazhui
Functions: Dredges Wind, clears Heat and releases the exterior with the reducing method; augments Yang and consolidates the exterior with the reinforcing method.
Indications: Acne, acute eczema, folliculitis, furuncles (boils), hyperhidrosis, pityriasis rosea, pruritus, psoriasis, urticaria.

POINTS FOR CLEARING HEAT AND ALLEVIATING PAIN

LU-5 Chize
Functions: Clears and bears Lung-Heat downward, dispels stasis and frees the network vessels with the reducing method; strengthens the sinews and supplements Deficiency with the reinforcing method.
Indications: Contact dermatitis and drug eruptions.

ST-41 Jiexi
Functions: Clears and bears Stomach-Fire downward and invigorates the network vessels with the reducing method; supports the Spleen and nourishes the Stomach with the reinforcing method.
Indications: Chilblains, erythema multiforme, erythromelalgia, pompholyx.

ST-44 Neiting

Functions: Clears Fire and drains Heat, and frees the network vessels to alleviate pain with the reducing method; supplements the Spleen, warms the Middle Burner and returns Yang with the reinforcing method.

Indications: Erythromelalgia and herpes zoster (shingles).

BL-40 Weizhong

Functions: Clears Heat, relieves Toxicity, cools and invigorates the Blood, and dispels Blood stasis with the reducing method; strengthens the sinews and supplements Deficiency with the reinforcing method.

Indications: Anaphylactoid purpura, eczema, erysipelas, folliculitis, furuncles (boils), lichen planus, pruritus, tinea corporis.

BL-57 Chengshan

Functions: Clears Heat, relieves Toxicity, invigorates the Blood, and frees the network vessels with the reducing method; strengthens the sinews and supplements Deficiency with the reinforcing method.

Indications: Chronic venous ulcer of the lower leg, lichen planus, seborrhea, tinea pedis (athlete's foot).

BL-60 Kunlun

Functions: Clears Heat, invigorates the Blood, dredges Wind, and frees the network vessels with the reducing method; warms Cold and dispels Dampness with the reinforcing method.

Indications: Alopecia areata, furuncles, phytophotodermatitis, plantar warts (verruca plantaris), tinea manuum (ringworm of the hands), tinea pedis (athlete's foot).

PC-3 Quze

Functions: Clears Heat, cools the Blood, dispels Blood stasis, and relieves Toxicity with the reducing method; strengthens the sinews and supplements Deficiency with the reinforcing method.

Indications: Contact dermatitis, drug eruptions, eczema, tinea corporis (ringworm of the body).

TB-5 Waiguan

Functions: Clears Heat in the Triple Burner, bears Fire downward and harmonizes Shaoyang with the reducing method; warms Yang, dissipates Cold, supports Vital Qi (Zheng Qi), and consolidates the exterior with the reinforcing method.

Indications: Chilblains, erythema multiforme, erythromelalgia, furuncles (boils), herpes zoster (shingles), pompholyx.

GB-40 Qiuxu

Functions: Drains Heat to free the network vessels, dredges the Gallbladder and Liver, and clears and diffuses Qi in the Shaoyang channels with the reducing method; strengthens the sinews and supplements Deficiency with the reinforcing method.

Indications: Erythromelalgia, folliculitis, furuncles (boils).

LR-2 Xingjian

Functions: Clears and drains Liver-Fire, dredges the Liver and Gallbladder, and frees Qi in the Jueyin channels with the reducing method; supports Vital Qi (Zheng Qi) and supplements Deficiency with the reinforcing method.

Indications: Erythromelalgia, melasma, pruritus, urticaria, vitiligo.

LR-3 Taichong

Functions: Clears and drains Liver-Fire, dredges the Liver and benefits the movement of Qi with the reducing method; enriches and supplements Liver-Blood with the reinforcing method.

Indications: Alopecia areata, anaphylactoid purpura, erysipelas, erythromelalgia, pruritus, Raynaud's disease, vulval pruritus.

POINTS FOR TRANSFORMING TURBIDITY AND FREEING THE INTESTINES

ST-25 Tianshu

Functions: Frees the Intestines and guides out stagnation, clears Heat and frees the bowels with the reducing method; warms Yang and consolidates the Intestines with the reinforcing method.

Indications: Pruritus.

BL-25 Dachangshu

Functions: Frees the Intestines and guides out stagnation with the reducing method; fortifies and consolidates the Intestines with the reinforcing method.

Indications: Perianal eczema and urticaria.

TB-6 Zhigou

Functions: Clears Heat and frees the bowels, and clears and diffuses Qi in the Shaoyang channels with the reducing method; strengthens the sinews and supplements Deficiency with the reinforcing method.

Indications: Herpes zoster (shingles) and psoriasis.

CV-12 Zhongwan

Functions: Harmonizes the Stomach and guides out stagnation, dispels Phlegm and disperses accumulation, and frees Qi in the Fu organs with the reducing method; fortifies the Stomach and supplements the Middle Burner with the reinforcing method.

Indications: Annular erythemas, eczema, melasma (chloasma), pruritus, urticaria, vitiligo.

POINTS FOR MOVING QI AND TRANSFORMING DAMPNESS

SP-9 Yinlingquan

Functions: Clears Heat and transforms Dampness with the reducing method; warms and supplements Spleen Yang, augments Qi and supports the Spleen with the reinforcing method.

Indications: Chronic eczema, chronic venous ulcer of the lower leg, erysipelas, ichthyosis vulgaris, pruritus, scabies, vulval pruritus.

BL-18 Ganshu

Functions: Moves Qi, dispels Blood stasis, dredges the Liver, and relieves Depression with the reducing method; supplements and nourishes Liver-Blood with the reinforcing method.

Indications: Alopecia areata, herpes zoster (shingles), melasma (chloasma), psoriasis, seborrhea, vitiligo.

PC-6 Neiguan

Functions: Moves Qi and disperses stagnation, and harmonizes the Stomach to stop vomiting with the reducing method; strengthens the sinews and supplements Deficiency with the reinforcing method.

Indications: Alopecia areata, drug eruptions, insect bites, lichen simplex chronicus (neurodermatitis), melasma (chloasma), palmoplantar pustulosis.

GB-34 Yanglingquan
Functions: Dredges the Liver, relieves Depression, moves Qi, and frees the channels with the reducing method.

Indications: Erythema multiforme, herpes zoster (shingles), pruritus, psoriasis.

CV-3 Zhongji
Functions: Moves Qi, transforms turbidity and clears Heat from the Bladder with the reducing method; enriches the Liver, supplements the Kidneys and consolidates the Root with the reinforcing method.

Indications: Angioedema, eczema, melasma (chloasma), tinea cruris (jock itch), vulval pruritus.

POINTS FOR OPENING THE ORIFICES AND FREEING THE NETWORK VESSELS

KI-1 Yongquan
Functions: Opens the orifices, arouses the Brain, clears Heat, and supplements Yin with the reducing method.

Indications: Anaphylactoid purpura and pompholyx.

PC-7 Daling
Functions: Opens the orifices, frees the network vessels and clears Heat from the Ying and Xue levels with the reducing method; strengthens the sinews and supplements Deficiency with the reinforcing method.

Indications: Eczema and tinea pedis (athlete's foot).

GV-20 Baihui
Functions: Opens the orifices and frees the network vessels with the reducing method; dissipates Cold, supplements Yang and bears Spleen Qi upward with the reinforcing method.

Indications: Alopecia areata, drug eruptions, erythromelalgia, pruritus, urticaria.

POINTS FOR CONSOLIDATING THE ROOT AND CULTIVATING THE ORIGIN

ST-36 Zusanli
Functions: Harmonizes the Stomach, frees the Intestines, clears Heat, and eliminates Dampness with the reducing method; fortifies the Spleen, nourishes the Stomach, supplements the Middle Burner, and augments Qi with the reinforcing method.

Indications: Acne, anaphylactoid purpura, eczema, erythema multiforme, furuncles (boils), herpes zoster (shingles), insect bites, lichen planus, lichen simplex chronicus (neurodermatitis), pruritus, psoriasis, urticaria, warts (verrucae).

SP-6 Sanyinjiao
Functions: Cools the Blood, reduces erythema, dredges the Liver, and transforms Dampness with the reducing method; supports Vital Qi (Zheng Qi), consolidates the Root, fortifies the Spleen, contains the Blood, enriches the Liver, and supplements the Kidneys with the reinforcing method.

Indications: Acne, acute eczema, alopecia areata, anaphylactoid purpura, erysipelas, herpes zoster (shingles), insect bites, melasma (chloasma), psoriasis, tinea, urticaria, vulval pruritus.

SP-10 Xuehai
Functions: Moves Qi and dispels Blood stasis with the reducing method; boosts the Spleen and contains, generates and nourishes the Blood with the reinforcing method.

Indications: Alopecia areata, anaphylactoid purpura, chronic venous ulcer of the lower leg, eczema, ichthyosis vulgaris, lichen simplex chronicus (neurodermatitis), pruritus, psoriasis, scabies, urticaria.

HT-7 Shenmen
Functions: Clears the Heart and opens the orifices with the reducing method; supplements the Heart and quiets the Spirit with the reinforcing method.

Indications: Eczema, herpes zoster (shingles), melasma (chloasma).

BL-15 Xinshu
Functions: Invigorates the Blood, dissipates Blood stasis, frees the channels, and expels pathogenic factors with the reducing method; supplements the Heart, quiets the Spirit, nourishes the Blood, and boosts the Mind with the reinforcing method.

Indications: Fixed drug eruptions and psoriasis.

BL-17 Geshu
Functions: Dispels Blood stasis, frees the network vessels, loosens the diaphragm, and regulates Qi with the reducing method; supplements and nourishes Yin-Blood, contains the Blood and stops bleeding with the reinforcing method.

Indications: Alopecia areata, anaphylactoid purpura, drug eruptions, pruritus, psoriasis, vitiligo.

BL-20 Pishu
Functions: Expels pathogenic factors, disperses stagnation, regulates the Spleen, and transforms Dampness with the reducing method; supplements and augments Spleen Qi, fortifies the Spleen and boosts the Stomach with the reinforcing method.

Indications: Acne, anaphylactoid purpura, melasma (chloasma), psoriasis, seborrhea, urticaria.

BL-23 Shenshu
Functions: Dissipates Cold and dispels Dampness with the reducing method; supplements the Kidneys, augments the Essence, strengthens the lumbar region, and supplements Spleen Yang with the reinforcing method.

Indications: Acne, alopecia areata, genital herpes, pruritus, psoriasis, urticaria, vitiligo.

KI-3 Taixi
Functions: Soothes the sinews and invigorates the network vessels with the reducing method; supplements Kidney Qi and augments Kidney Yin with the reinforcing method.

Indications: Alopecia areata, erythromelalgia, lichen planus, melasma (chloasma), plantar warts (verruca plantaris), tinea.

KI-7 Fuliu
Functions: Expels pathogenic factors and dissipates stagnation with the reducing method; constrains sweating,

enriches Yin and supplements the Kidneys with the reinforcing method.

Indications: Chronic venous ulcer of the lower limb and hyperhidrosis.

GB-39 Xuanzhong

Functions: Frees Qi in the Shaoyang channels with the reducing method; supplements the Marrow and strengthens the bones with the reinforcing method.

Indications: Chronic venous ulcer of the lower limb, ichthyosis vulgaris, keratosis follicularis (Darier's disease).

CV-6 Qihai

Functions: Moves Qi, disperses stagnation, regulates Qi, and moves the Blood with the reducing method; cultivates and supplements Original Qi (Yuan Qi), warms Yang and augments Qi with the reinforcing method.

Indications: Genital herpes and pruritus.

GV-4 Mingmen

Functions: Frees Qi in the Governor Vessel with the reducing method; supplements the Kidneys, cultivates the Origin, strengthens the lumbar region, warms Yang, and boosts the Spleen with the reinforcing method.

Indications: Drug eruptions, melasma (chloasma), vitiligo.

EXTRA POINTS

EX-HN-5 Taiyang (M-HN-9)

Functions: Clears Heat and disperses swelling, dredges the network vessels and alleviates pain, dissipates Wind and alleviates itching.

Indications: Acne, angioedema, erysipelas (facial), herpes zoster (facial), melasma (chloasma), plane warts (verruca plana).

EX-UE-9 Baxie (M-UE-22)

Functions: Clears Heat and disperses swelling, invigorates the Blood and dissipates Blood stasis.

Indications: Insect bites, pompholyx, Raynaud's disease, scabies, tinea pedis (athlete's foot).

EX-UE-11 Shixuan (M-UE-1)

Functions: Opens the orifices and arouses the brain, clears Heat and settles convulsions.

Indications: Drug eruptions (erythrodermic type) and Raynaud's disease.

EX-LE-10 Bafeng (M-LE-8)

Functions: Clears Heat and disperses swelling, invigorates the Blood and dissipates Blood stasis.

Indications: Insect bites, pompholyx, Raynaud's disease, scabies.

TCM formulae and patent medicines used in the treatment of skin disorders

This appendix lists the ingredients of patent medicines or formulae referred to by name only in the text. The ingredients of formulae used in pattern identification are detailed under the pattern involved (see index for page numbers).

A small number of the patent medicines and classical formulae listed below may contain ingredients whose use may not be permitted in certain countries outside China (marked with *). Practitioners should always check the contents of any patent medicines to ensure that they comply with the legal requirements of the country in which they practice. Where possible, alternatives for these preparations have been suggested in the text. However, in certain instances, notably in case histories, modern clinical experience reports or literature excerpts, the original formulae have also been retained to give practitioners an insight into the way the particular condition involved would be treated in China.

An Shen Wan (Quieting the Kidney Pill)
Hu Lu Ba (Semen Trigonellae Foeni-graeci)
Bu Gu Zhi (Fructus Psoraleae Corylifoliae)
Chuan Lian Zi (Fructus Meliae Toosendan)
Xiao Hui Xiang (Fructus Foeniculi Vulgaris)
Xu Duan (Radix Dipsaci)
Xing Ren (Semen Pruni Armeniacae)
Tao Ren (Semen Persicae)
Shan Yao (Radix Dioscoreae Oppositae)
Fu Ling (Sclerotium Poriae Cocos)
Source: *Za Bing Yuan Liu Xi Zhu* [Enlightenment of the Origins of Miscellaneous Diseases]

Ba Wei Xiao Yao San (Eight-Ingredient Free Wanderer Powder)
Gan Cao (Radix Glycyrrhizae)
Dang Gui (Radix Angelicae Sinensis)
Bai Shao (Radix Paeoniae Lactiflorae)
Fu Ling (Sclerotium Poriae Cocos)
Bai Zhu (Rhizoma Atractylodis Macrocephalae)
Chai Hu (Radix Bupleuri)
Mu Dan Pi (Cortex Moutan Radicis)
Zhi Zi (Fructus Gardeniae Jasminoidis)
Source: *Xiao Zhu Fu Ren Liang Fang* [Proof and Explanation of Women's Formulae]

Ba Zhen Tang (Eight Treasure Decoction)
Dang Gui (Radix Angelicae Sinensis)
Chuan Xiong (Rhizoma Ligustici Chuanxiong)
Bai Shao (Radix Paeoniae Lactiflorae)
Shu Di Huang (Radix Rehmanniae Glutinosae Conquita)
Dang Shen (Radix Codonopsitis Pilosulae)
Bai Zhu (Rhizoma Atractylodis Macrocephalae)
Fu Ling (Sclerotium Poriae Cocos)
Zhi Gan Cao (Radix Glycyrrhizae, mix-fried with honey)
Source: *Rui Zhu Tang Jing Yan Fang* [Rui Zhutang's Empirical Formulae]

Bai He Gu Jin Tang (Lily Bulb Decoction for Consolidating Metal)
Sheng Di Huang (Radix Rehmanniae Glutinosae)
Shu Di Huang (Radix Rehmanniae Glutinosae Conquita)
Mai Men Dong (Radix Ophiopogonis Japonici)
Bai He (Bulbus Lilii)
Bai Shao (Radix Paeoniae Lactiflorae)
Dang Gui (Radix Angelicae Sinensis)
Chuan Bei Mu (Bulbus Fritillariae Cirrhosae)
Gan Cao (Radix Glycyrrhizae)
Xuan Shen (Radix Scrophulariae Ningpoensis)
Jie Geng (Radix Platycodi Grandiflori)
Source: *Yi Fang Ji Jie* [Collection of Prescriptions with Notes]

Bai Hu Jia Ren Shen Tang (White Tiger Decoction Plus Ginseng)
Shi Gao‡ (Gypsum Fibrosum)
Zhi Mu (Rhizoma Anemarrhenae Asphodeloidis)
Zhi Gan Cao (Radix Glycyrrhizae, mix-fried with honey)
Jing Mi (Semen Oryzae)
Ren Shen (Radix Ginseng)
Source: *Shang Han Lun* [On Cold Damage]

Bai Hu Tang (White Tiger Decoction)
Shi Gao‡ (Gypsum Fibrosum)
Zhi Mu (Rhizoma Anemarrhenae Asphodeloidis)
Zhi Gan Cao (Radix Glycyrrhizae, mix-fried with honey)
Jing Mi (Semen Oryzae)
Source: *Shang Han Lun* [On Cold Damage]

Ban Xia Xie Xin Tang (Pinellia Decoction for Draining the Heart)
Fa Ban Xia (Rhizoma Pinelliae Ternatae Praeparata)
Huang Qin (Radix Scutellariae Baicalensis)
Gan Jiang (Rhizoma Zingiberis Officinalis)
Ren Shen (Radix Ginseng)
Zhi Gan Cao (Radix Glycyrrhizae, mix-fried with honey)
Huang Lian (Rhizoma Coptidis)

Da Zao (Fructus Ziziphi Jujubae)
Source: *Shang Han Lun* [On Cold Damage]

Bao He Wan (Preserving Harmony Pill)
Shan Zha (Fructus Crataegi)
Shen Qu (Massa Fermentata)
Fa Ban Xia (Rhizoma Pinelliae Ternatae Praeparata)
Fu Ling (Sclerotium Poriae Cocos)
Chen Pi (Pericarpium Citri Reticulatae)
Lian Qiao (Fructus Forsythiae Suspensae)
Lai Fu Zi (Semen Raphani Sativi)
Source: *Dan Xi Xin Fa* [Dan Xi's Experiential Therapy]

Bi Yan Pian (Nasal Inflammation Tablet)
Qian Li Guang (Herba Senecionis Scandentis)
Xin Yi Hua (Flos Magnoliae)
Juan Bai (Herba Selaginellae)
Qiang Huo (Rhizoma et Radix Notopterygii)
Jue Ming Zi (Semen Cassiae)
*Ma Huang** (Herba Ephedrae)
Chuan Xiong (Rhizoma Ligustici Chuanxiong)
Bai Zhi (Radix Angelicae Dahuricae)
Source: Empirical formula

Bu Zhong Yi Qi Tang [Wan] (Decoction [Pill] for Supplementing the Middle and Augmenting Qi)
Huang Qi (Radix Astragali seu Hedysari)
Gan Cao (Radix Glycyrrhizae)
Dang Shen (Radix Codonopsitis Pilosulae)
Bai Zhu (Rhizoma Atractylodis Macrocephalae)
Dang Gui (Radix Angelicae Sinensis)
Sheng Ma (Rhizoma Cimicifugae)
Chen Pi (Pericarpium Citri Reticulatae)
Chai Hu (Radix Bupleuri)
Source: *Dong Yuan Shi Shu* [Li Dongyuan's Ten Works]

Cang Zhu Gao (Concentrated Atractylodes Syrup)
Cang Zhu (Rhizoma Atractylodis)
The herb is decocted three times and the liquids mixed together to produce a concentrate, to which sugar is added to make the syrup (see text for other preparation methods).
Source: Empirical formula

Ce Bai Wan (Biota Pill)
Ce Bai Ye (Cacumen Biotae Orientalis)
Dang Gui (Radix Angelicae Sinensis)
Source: *Jing Yan Nü Ke* [Empirical Gynecology]

Chai Hu Qing Gan Tang (Bupleurum Decoction for Clearing the Liver)
Chai Hu (Radix Bupleuri)
Sheng Di Huang (Radix Rehmanniae Glutinosae)
Chi Shao (Radix Paeoniae Rubra)
Chao Niu Bang Zi (Fructus Arctii Lappae, stir-fried)
Dang Gui (Radix Angelicae Sinensis)
Lian Qiao (Fructus Forsythiae Suspensae)
Chuan Xiong (Rhizoma Ligustici Chuanxiong)
Huang Qin (Radix Scutellariae Baicalensis)
Zhi Zi (Fructus Gardeniae Jasminoidis)
Tian Hua Fen (Radix Trichosanthis)
Gan Cao (Radix Glycyrrhizae)
Hua Shi‡ (Talcum)

Fang Feng (Radix Ledebouriellae Divaricatae)
Source: *Wai Ke Zheng Zong* [An Orthodox Manual of External Diseases]

Chai Hu Qing Gan Yin (Bupleurum Beverage for Clearing the Liver)
Chai Hu (Radix Bupleuri)
Zhi Zi (Fructus Gardeniae Jasminoidis)
Qing Pi (Pericarpium Citri Reticulatae Viride)
Zhi Ke (Fructus Citri Aurantii)
Su Geng (Caulis Perillae Frutescentis)
Gou Teng (Ramulus Uncariae cum Uncis)
*Mu Tong** (Caulis Mutong)
Huang Qin (Radix Scutellariae Baicalensis)
Zhi Mu (Rhizoma Anemarrhenae Asphodeloidis)
Gan Cao (Radix Glycyrrhizae)
Source: *Zheng Yin Mai Zhi* [On the Pulse and Treatment of Signs and Symptoms]
Note: In those countries where it is illegal to include *Mu Tong** (Caulis Mutong) in a prescription, *Tong Cao* (Medulla Tetrapanacis Papyriferi) may be substituted.

Chu Shi Wan (Pill for Eliminating Dampness)
Wei Ling Xian (Radix Clematidis)
Zhu Ling (Sclerotium Polypori Umbellati)
Zhi Zi (Fructus Gardeniae Jasminoidis)
Huang Qin (Radix Scutellariae Baicalensis)
Huang Lian (Rhizoma Coptidis)
Lian Qiao (Fructus Forsythiae Suspensae)
Dang Gui Wei (Extremitas Radicis Angelicae Sinensis)
Ze Xie (Rhizoma Alismatis Orientalis)
Zi Cao (Radix Arnebiae seu Lithospermi)
Qian Cao Gen (Radix Rubiae Cordifoliae)
Fu Ling Pi (Cortex Poriae Cocos)
Bai Xian Pi (Cortex Dictamni Dasycarpi Radicis)
Mu Dan Pi (Cortex Moutan Radicis)
Gan Di Huang (Radix Rehmanniae Glutinosae Exsiccata)
Source: *Zhao Bing Nan Lin Chuang Jing Yan Ji* [A Collection of Zhao Bingnan's Clinical Experiences]

Chu Shi Wei Ling Tang (Poria Five Decoction for Eliminating Dampness and Calming the Stomach)
Cang Zhu (Rhizoma Atractylodis)
Hou Po (Cortex Magnoliae Officinalis)
Chen Pi (Pericarpium Citri Reticulatae)
Zhu Ling (Sclerotium Polypori Umbellati)
Ze Xie (Rhizoma Alismatis Orientalis)
Chi Fu Ling (Sclerotium Poriae Cocos Rubrae)
Bai Zhu (Rhizoma Atractylodis Macrocephalae)
Hua Shi‡ (Talcum)
Fang Feng (Radix Ledebouriellae Divaricatae)
Zhi Zi (Fructus Gardeniae Jasminoidis)
*Mu Tong** (Caulis Mutong)
Rou Gui (Cortex Cinnamomi Cassiae)
Gan Cao (Radix Glycyrrhizae)
Deng Xin Cao (Medulla Junci Effusi)
Source: *Yi Zong Jin Jian* [The Golden Mirror of Medicine]
Note: In those countries where it is illegal to include *Mu Tong** (Caulis Mutong) in a prescription, *Tong Cao* (Medulla Tetrapanacis Papyriferi) may be substituted.

Da Bai Du Gao (Major Toxicity-Vanquishing Syrup)
Da Huang (Radix et Rhizoma Rhei)
Pu Gong Ying (Herba Taraxaci cum Radice)
Chen Pi (Pericarpium Citri Reticulatae)
Mu Bie Zi (Semen Momordicae Cochinchinensis)
Bai Zhi (Radix Angelicae Dahuricae)
Tian Hua Fen (Radix Trichosanthis)
Jin Yin Hua (Flos Lonicerae)
Huang Bai (Cortex Phellodendri)
Chi Shao (Radix Paeoniae Rubra)
Ru Xiang (Gummi Olibanum)
Gan Cao (Radix Glycyrrhizae)
Dang Gui (Radix Angelicae Sinensis)
She Tui‡ (Exuviae Serpentis)
Gan Chan‡ (Bufo Siccus)
Wu Gong‡ (Scolopendra Subspinipes)
Quan Xie‡ (Buthus Martensi)
Mang Xiao‡ (Mirabilitum)
Source: Empirical formula.

Da Huang Wan (Rhubarb Pill)
Pao Da Huang (Radix et Rhizoma Rhei, blast-fried)
Chao Jie Geng (Radix Platycodi Grandiflori, stir-fried)
Chao Zhi Ke (Fructus Citri Aurantii, stir-fried)
Chuan Xiong (Rhizoma Ligustici Chuanxiong)
Qiang Huo (Rhizoma et Radix Notopterygii)
*Mu Xiang** (Radix Aucklandiae Lappae)
Chai Hu (Radix Bupleuri)
Du Huo (Radix Angelicae Pubescentis)
Qian Niu Zi (Semen Pharbitidis)
Source: *Sheng Ji Zong Lu* [General Collection for Holy Relief]

Da Huang Zhe Chong Wan (Rhubarb and Wingless Cockroach Pill)
Da Huang (Radix et Rhizoma Rhei)
Tu Bie Chong‡ (Eupolyphaga seu Steleophaga)
Sheng Di Huang (Radix Rehmanniae Glutinosae)
Xing Ren (Semen Pruni Armeniacae)
Huang Qin (Radix Scutellariae Baicalensis)
Chi Shao (Radix Paeoniae Rubra)
Shui Zhi‡ (Hirudo seu Whitmania)
Gan Qi (Lacca Exsiccata)
Tao Ren (Semen Persicae)
Gan Cao (Radix Glycyrrhizae)
Meng Chong‡ (Tabanus)
Qi Cao‡ (Vermiculus Holotrichiae)
Source: *Yi Zong Jin Jian* [The Golden Mirror of Medicine]

Dan Shen Pian (Red Sage Root Tablet)
Dan Shen (Radix Salviae Miltiorrhizae)
Source: Empirical formula

Dan Shen Zhu She Ye (Red Sage Root Injection)
Dan Shen (Radix Salviae Miltiorrhizae)
Source: Commercial preparation (used for intravenous infusion preparations)

Dang Gui Bu Xue Tang (Chinese Angelica Root Decoction for Supplementing the Blood)
Huang Qi (Radix Astragali seu Hedysari)
Dang Gui (Radix Angelicae Sinensis)
Source: *Nei Wai Shang Bian Huo Lun* [Discussion on Difficult Problems Related to Internal and External Damage]

Dang Gui Ku Shen Wan (Chinese Angelica Root and Flavescent Sophora Root Pill)
Dang Gui (Radix Angelicae Sinensis)
Ku Shen (Radix Sophorae Flavescentis)
Source: *Gu Jin Ming Yi Lin Zheng Jin Jian* [The Golden Mirror of Clinical Practice of Famous Doctors Ancient and Modern]

Dang Gui Pian (Chinese Angelica Root Tablet)
Dang Gui (Radix Angelicae Sinensis)
Source: Empirical formula

Dang Gui Yin Zi (Chinese Angelica Root Drink)
Dang Gui (Radix Angelicae Sinensis)
Shu Di Huang (Radix Rehmanniae Glutinosae Conquita)
Bai Shao (Radix Paeoniae Lactiflorae)
Chuan Xiong (Rhizoma Ligustici Chuanxiong)
He Shou Wu (Radix Polygoni Multiflori)
Jing Jie Sui (Spica Schizonepetae Tenuifoliae)
Fang Feng (Radix Ledebouriellae Divaricatae)
Bai Ji Li (Fructus Tribuli Terrestris)
Huang Qi (Radix Astragali seu Hedysari)
Gan Cao (Radix Glycyrrhizae)
Source: *Yi Zong Jin Jian* [The Golden Mirror of Medicine]

Di Gu Pi Lu (Wolfberry Root Bark Distillate)
Di Gu Pi (Cortex Lycii Radicis)
The herb is steamed to produce 2500ml of distillate for every 500g of the dried material.
Source: *Shi Yong Zhong Cheng Yao Shou Ce* [A Compilation of Chinese Herbal Patent Medicines]

Di Huang Yin Zi (Rehmannia Drink)
Sheng Di Huang (Radix Rehmanniae Glutinosae)
Shu Di Huang (Radix Rehmanniae Glutinosae Conquita)
Dang Gui (Radix Angelicae Sinensis)
Xuan Shen (Radix Scrophulariae Ningpoensis)
Mu Dan Pi (Cortex Moutan Radicis)
Hong Hua (Flos Carthami Tinctorii)
Bai Ji Li (Fructus Tribuli Terrestris)
Jiang Can‡ (Bombyx Batryticatus)
He Shou Wu (Radix Polygoni Multiflori)
Gan Cao (Radix Glycyrrhizae)
Source: *Yi Zong Jin Jian* [The Golden Mirror of Medicine]

Di Long Pian (Earthworm Tablet)
Di Long‡ (Lumbricus)
Source: Empirical formula

Du Huo Ji Sheng Tang (Pubescent Angelica Root and Mistletoe Decoction)
Du Huo (Radix Angelicae Pubescentis)
Sang Ji Sheng (Ramulus Loranthi)
Du Zhong (Cortex Eucommiae Ulmoidis)
Huai Niu Xi (Radix Achyranthis Bidentatae)
*Xi Xin** (Herba cum Radice Asari)
Qin Jiao (Radix Gentianae Macrophyllae)
Fu Ling (Sclerotium Poriae Cocos)
Gui Zhi (Ramulus Cinnamomi Cassiae)
Fang Feng (Radix Ledebouriellae Divaricatae)

Chuan Xiong (Rhizoma Ligustici Chuanxiong)
Dang Shen (Radix Codonopsitis Pilosulae)
Gan Cao (Radix Glycyrrhizae)
Dang Gui (Radix Angelicae Sinensis)
Bai Shao (Radix Paeoniae Lactiflorae)
Sheng Di Huang (Radix Rehmanniae Glutinosae)
Source: *Qian Jin Yao Fang* [Prescriptions Worth a Thousand Gold Pieces for Emergencies]

E Han Fang (Forehead Sweating Formula)
Dan Shen (Radix Salviae Miltiorrhizae)
Dang Gui (Radix Angelicae Sinensis)
Fu Shen (Sclerotium Poriae Cocos cum Ligno Hospite)
Sheng Di Huang (Radix Rehmanniae Glutinosae)
Suan Zao Ren (Semen Ziziphi Spinosae)
Huang Qi (Radix Astragali seu Hedysari)
Bai Shao (Radix Paeoniae Lactiflorae)
Long Yan Rou (Arillus Euphoriae Longanae)
Source: Empirical formula

Er Dong Gao (Asparagus and Ophiopogon Syrup)
Tian Men Dong (Radix Asparagi Cochinchinensis)
Mai Men Dong (Radix Ophiopogonis Japonici)
Source: *She Sheng Zong Yao* [A Summary of Secret Prescriptions for Preserving Health]

Er Miao Wan (Mysterious Two Pill)
Huang Bai (Cortex Phellodendri)
Cang Zhu (Rhizoma Atractylodis)
Source: *Dan Xi Xin Fa* [Danxi's Experiential Therapy]

Er Zhi Wan (Double Supreme Pill)
Han Lian Cao (Herba Ecliptae Prostratae)
Nü Zhen Zi (Fructus Ligustri Lucidi)
Source: *Zheng Zhi Zhun Sheng* [Standards of Diagnosis and Treatment]

Fang Feng Tong Sheng San [Wan] (Ledebouriella Powder [Pill] that Sagely Unblocks)
Fang Feng (Radix Ledebouriellae Divaricatae)
Chuan Xiong (Rhizoma Ligustici Chuanxiong)
Dang Gui (Radix Angelicae Sinensis)
Chi Shao (Radix Paeoniae Rubra)
Da Huang (Radix et Rhizoma Rhei)
Mang Xiao‡ (Mirabilitum)
Lian Qiao (Fructus Forsythiae Suspensae)
Bo He (Herba Menthae Haplocalycis)
*Ma Huang** (Herba Ephedrae)
Shi Gao‡ (Gypsum Fibrosum)
Jie Geng (Radix Platycodi Grandiflori)
Huang Qin (Radix Scutellariae Baicalensis)
Bai Zhu (Rhizoma Atractylodis Macrocephalae)
Zhi Zi (Fructus Gardeniae Jasminoidis)
Jing Jie (Herba Schizonepetae Tenuifoliae)
Hua Shi‡ (Talcum)
Gan Cao (Radix Glycyrrhizae)
Source: *Su Wen: Xuan Ming Fang Lun* [Simple Questions: Discussion on Xuan Ming's Formulae]

Fang Ji Huang Qi Tang (Stephania and Astragalus Decoction)
*Fang Ji** (Radix Stephaniae Tetrandrae)

Gan Cao (Radix Glycyrrhizae)
Bai Zhu (Rhizoma Atractylodis Macrocephalae)
Huang Qin (Radix Astragali seu Hedysari)
Gui Zhi (Ramulus Cinnamomi Cassiae)
Source: *Jin Kui Yao Lue* [Synopsis of Prescriptions from the Golden Cabinet]
Note: In those countries where the supply and importation of *Fang Ji** (Radix Stephaniae Tetrandrae) is not permitted, *Ze Lan* (Herba Lycopi Lucidi) may be substituted.

Fu Fang Dan Shen Pian (Compound Red Sage Root Tablet)
Dan Shen (Radix Salviae Miltiorrhizae)
San Qi (Radix Notoginseng)
Bing Pian (Borneolum)
Source: *Zhong Hua Ren Ming Gong He Guo Yao Dian* [Pharmacopoeia of the People's Republic of China]

Fu Fang Kang Yin Ji (Compound Anti-Psoriasis Preparation)
Jin Gang Teng (Rhizoma Smilacis Bockii)
Ban Lan Gen (Radix Isatidis seu Baphicacanthi)
Ban Zhi Lian (Herba Scutellariae Barbatae)
Bai Hua She She Cao (Herba Hedyotidis Diffusae)
Bai Zhu (Rhizoma Atractylodis Macrocephalae)
He Huan Pi (Cortex Albizziae Julibrissin)
E Zhu (Rhizoma Curcumae)
San Leng (Rhizoma Sparganii Stoloniferi)
Dan Shen (Radix Salviae Miltiorrhizae)
Hong Hua (Flos Carthami Tinctorii)
Source: Empirical formula

Ge Hua Jie Cheng Tang (Kudzu Flower Decoction for Resolving the Effects of Alcohol)
Qing Pi (Pericarpium Citri Reticulatae Viride)
*Mu Xiang** (Radix Aucklandiae Lappae)
Chen Pi (Pericarpium Citri Reticulatae)
Ren Shen (Radix Ginseng)
Zhu Ling (Sclerotium Polypori Umbellati)
Fu Ling (Sclerotium Poriae Cocos)
Shen Qu (Massa Fermentata)
Ze Xie (Rhizoma Alismatis Orientalis)
Sheng Jiang (Rhizoma Zingiberis Officinalis Recens)
Bai Zhu (Rhizoma Atractylodis Macrocephalae)
Bai Dou Kou (Fructus Amomi Kravanh)
Ge Hua (Flos Puerariae)
Sha Ren (Fructus Amomi)
Source: *Pi Wei Lun* [A Treatise on the Spleen and Stomach]

Gui Fu Ba Wei Tang (Cinnamon Bark and Aconite Eight-Ingredient Decoction)
Rou Gui (Cortex Cinnamomi Cassiae)
*Fu Zi** (Radix Lateralis Aconiti Carmichaeli Praeparata)
Gan Di Huang (Radix Rehmanniae Glutinosae Exsiccata)
Shan Yao (Rhizoma Dioscoreae Oppositae)
Shan Zhu Yu (Fructus Corni Officinalis)
Ze Xie (Rhizoma Alismatis Orientalis)
Fu Ling (Sclerotium Poriae Cocos)
Mu Dan Pi (Cortex Moutan Radicis)
Source: *Jin Kui Yao Lue* [Synopsis of Prescriptions from the Golden Cabinet]

Note: In those countries where internal use of *Fu Zi** (Radix Lateralis Aconiti Carmichaeli Praeparata) is not permitted, *Gan Jiang* (Rhizoma Zingiberis Officinalis) may be substituted.

Gui Pi Tang (Decoction for Restoring the Spleen)
Bai Zhu (Rhizoma Atractylodis Macrocephalae)
Fu Shen (Sclerotium Poriae Cocos cum Ligno Hospite)
Huang Qi (Radix Astragali seu Hedysari)
Long Yan Rou (Arillus Euphoriae Longanae)
Dang Shen (Radix Codonopsitis Pilosulae)
Suan Zao Ren (Semen Ziziphi Spinosae)
*Mu Xiang** (Radix Aucklandiae Lappae)
Zhi Gan Cao (Radix Glycyrrhizae, mix-fried with honey)
Dang Gui (Radix Angelicae Sinensis)
Yuan Zhi (Radix Polygalae)
Sheng Jiang (Rhizoma Zingiberis Officinalis Recens)
Da Zao (Fructus Ziziphi Jujubae)
Source: *Fu Ren Liang Fang* [Best Prescriptions for Women]

Gui Zhi Ren Shen Tang (Cinnamon Twig and Ginseng Decoction)
Gui Zhi (Ramulus Cinnamomi Cassiae)
Zhi Gan Cao (Radix Glycyrrhizae, mix-fried with honey)
Bai Zhu (Rhizoma Atractylodis Macrocephalae)
Ren Shen (Radix Ginseng)
Gan Jiang (Rhizoma Zingiberis Officinalis)
Source: *Shang Han Lun* [On Cold Damage]

Gui Zhi Tang (Cinnamon Twig Decoction)
Gui Zhi (Ramulus Cinnamomi Cassiae)
Bai Shao (Radix Paeoniae Lactiflorae)
Sheng Jiang (Rhizoma Zingiberis Officinalis Recens)
Zhi Gan Cao (Radix Glycyrrhizae, mix-fried with honey)
Da Zao (Fructus Ziziphi Jujubae)
Source: *Shang Han Lun* [On Cold Damage]

Guo Lao Gao (Licorice Syrup)
Zhi Gan Cao (Radix Glycyrrhizae, mix-fried with honey)
Yin Chai Hu (Radix Stellariae Dichotomae)
Qin Jiao (Radix Gentianae Macrophyllae)
Wu Mei (Fructus Pruni Mume)
Source: *You You Xin Shu* [A New Book of Pediatrics]

Hao Qin Qing Dan Tang (Sweet Wormwood and Scutellaria Decoction for Clearing the Gallbladder)
Qing Hao (Herba Artemisiae Chinghao)
Dan Zhu Ye (Herba Lophatheri Gracilis)
Fa Ban Xia (Rhizoma Pinelliae Ternatae Praeparata)
Chi Fu Ling (Sclerotium Poriae Cocos Rubrae)
Huang Qin (Radix Scutellariae Baicalensis)
Zhi Ke (Fructus Citri Aurantii)
Chen Pi (Pericarpium Citri Reticulatae)
Hua Shi‡ (Talcum)
Zhi Gan Cao (Radix Glycyrrhizae, mix-fried with honey)
Qing Dai (Indigo Naturalis)
Source: *Chong Ding Tong Su Shang Han Lun* [Simplified Revision of On Cold Damage]

Hua Ban Tang (Decoction for Transforming Macules)
Shi Gao‡ (Gypsum Fibrosum)
Zhi Mu (Rhizoma Anemarrhenae Asphodeloidis)
Gan Cao (Radix Glycyrrhizae)
Xuan Shen (Radix Scrophulariae Ningpoensis)
Shui Niu Jiao‡ (Cornu Bubali)
Jing Mi (Semen Oryzae)
Source: *Wen Bing Tiao Bian* [Treatise on the Identification of Warm Diseases]

Hua Du Wan (Pill for Transforming Toxicity)
Jie Geng (Radix Platycodi Grandiflori)
Sheng Di Huang (Radix Rehmanniae Glutinosae)
Chi Shao (Radix Paeoniae Rubra)
Niu Bang Zi (Fructus Arctii Lappae)
Xuan Shen (Radix Scrophulariae Ningpoensis)
Lian Qiao (Fructus Forsythiae Suspensae)
Gan Cao (Radix Glycyrrhizae)
Qing Dai (Indigo Naturalis)
Mang Xiao‡ (Mirabilitum)
Huang Lian (Rhizoma Coptidis)
Source: *Shou Shi Bao Yuan* [Safeguarding the Origins of Longevity]

Huang Lian Jie Du Tang (Coptis Decoction for Relieving Toxicity)
Huang Lian (Rhizoma Coptidis)
Huang Qin (Radix Scutellariae Baicalensis)
Huang Bai (Cortex Phellodendri)
Zhi Zi (Fructus Gardeniae Jasminoidis)
Source: *Wai Ke Mi Yao* [Secret Records of External Diseases]

Huang Lian Shang Qing Wan (Coptis Pill for Clearing the Upper Body)
Da Huang (Radix et Rhizoma Rhei)
Huang Qin (Radix Scutellariae Baicalensis)
Zhi Zi (Fructus Gardeniae Jasminoidis)
Lian Qiao (Fructus Forsythiae Suspensae)
Chuan Xiong (Rhizoma Ligustici Chuanxiong)
Jing Jie Sui (Spica Schizonepetae Tenuifoliae)
Shi Gao‡ (Gypsum Fibrosum)
Huang Lian (Rhizoma Coptidis)
Bo He (Herba Menthae Haplocalycis)
Ju Hua (Flos Chrysanthemi Morifolii)
Jie Geng (Radix Platycodi Grandiflori)
Gan Cao (Radix Glycyrrhizae)
Huang Bai (Cortex Phellodendri)
Bai Zhi (Radix Angelicae Dahuricae)
Xuan Fu Hua (Flos Inulae)
Man Jing Zi (Fructus Viticis)
Fang Feng (Radix Ledebouriellae Divaricatae)
Source: *Zui Xin Zhong Cheng Yao Shou Ce* [A Manual of Current TCM Patent Medicines]

Huang Qi Jian Zhong Tang (Astragalus Decoction for Fortifying the Middle)
Huang Qi (Radix Astragali seu Hedysari)
Gui Zhi (Ramulus Cinnamomi Cassiae)
Zhi Gan Cao (Radix Glycyrrhizae, mix-fried with honey)
Da Zao (Fructus Ziziphi Jujubae)
Bai Shao (Radix Paeoniae Lactiflorae)
Sheng Jiang (Rhizoma Zingiberis Officinalis Recens)
Yi Tang (Saccharum Granorum)

Source: *Jin Kui Yao Lue* [Synopsis of Prescriptions from the Golden Cabinet]

Huang Tu Tang (Yellow Earth Decoction)
Zao Xin Tu (Terra Flava Usta)
Gan Di Huang (Radix Rehmanniae Glutinosae Exsiccata)
Bai Zhu (Rhizoma Atractylodis Macrocephalae)
E Jiao‡ (Gelatinum Corii Asini)
Pao Fu Zi* (Radix Lateralis Aconiti Carmichaeli Praeparata, blast-fried)
Gan Cao (Radix Glycyrrhizae)
Huang Qin (Radix Scutellariae Baicalensis)
Source: *Jin Kui Yao Lue* [Synopsis of Prescriptions from the Golden Cabinet]
Note: In those countries where internal use of *Pao Fu Zi** (Radix Lateralis Aconiti Carmichaeli Praeparata, blast-fried) is not permitted, *Pao Gan Jiang* (Rhizoma Zingiberis Officinalis Praeparata) may be substituted.

Huo Ma Wan (Hemp Seed Pill)
Huo Ma Ren (Semen Cannabis Sativae)
Bai Shao (Radix Paeoniae Lactiflorae)
Zhi Shi (Fructus Immaturus Citri Aurantii)
Da Huang (Radix et Rhizoma Rhei)
Hou Po (Cortex Magnoliae Officinalis)
Xing Ren (Semen Pruni Armeniacae)
Source: *Shang Han Lun* [On Cold Damage]

Huo Ming Yin (Life-Giving Beverage)
Zhi Chuan Shan Jia* (Squama Manitis Pentadactylae, mix-fried with honey)
Chao Zao Jiao Ci (Spina Gleditsiae Sinensis, stir-fried)
Dang Gui Wei (Extremitas Radicis Angelicae Sinensis)
Gan Cao (Radix Glycyrrhizae)
Jin Yin Hua (Flos Lonicerae)
Chi Shao (Radix Paeoniae Rubra)
Ru Xiang (Gummi Olibanum)
Mo Yao (Myrrha)
Tian Hua Fen (Radix Trichosanthis)
Chen Pi (Pericarpium Citri Reticulatae)
Bai Zhi (Radix Angelicae Dahuricae)
Fang Feng (Radix Ledebouriellae Divaricatae)
Chuan Bei Mu (Bulbus Fritillariae Cirrhosae)
Source: *Yi Zong Jin Jian* [The Golden Mirror of Medicine]

Huo Xue Xiao Yan Wan (Pill for Invigorating the Blood and Dispersing Inflammation)
Zhi Ru Xiang (Gummi Olibanum, mix-fried with honey)
Zhi Mo Yao (Myrrha, mix-fried with honey)
Shi Chang Pu (Rhizoma Acori Graminei)
Niu Huang‡ (Calculus Bovis)
Huang Mi (Semen Setariae)
Source: Empirical formula

Huo Xue Zhi Tong San (Powder for Invigorating the Blood and Alleviating Pain)
Tu Bie Chong‡ (Eupolyphaga seu Steleophaga)
Dang Gui (Radix Angelicae Sinensis)
Cu Zhi Ru Xiang (Gummi Olibanum, mix-fried with vinegar)
Duan Zi Ran Tong‡ (Pyritum Calcinatum)
San Qi (Radix Notoginseng)

Bing Pian (Borneolum)
Source: Empirical formula

Jia Wei Xiao Yao Wan (Augmented Free Wanderer Pill)
Chai Hu (Radix Bupleuri)
Dang Gui (Radix Angelicae Sinensis)
Bai Zhu (Rhizoma Atractylodis Macrocephalae)
Fu Ling (Sclerotium Poriae Cocos)
Zhi Gan Cao (Radix Glycyrrhizae, mix-fried with honey)
Mu Dan Pi (Cortex Moutan Radicis)
Zhi Zi (Fructus Gardeniae Jasminoidis)
Sheng Jiang (Rhizoma Zingiberis Officinalis Recens)
Bai Shao (Radix Paeoniae Lactiflorae)
Bo He (Herba Menthae Haplocalycis)
Source: *Nei Ke Zhai Yao* [A Digest of Internal Medicine]

Jie Du Yang Yin Tang (Decoction for Relieving Toxicity and Nourishing Yin)
Xi Yang Shen (Radix Panacis Quinquefolii)
Nan Sha Shen (Radix Adenophorae)
Bei Sha Shen (Radix Glehniae Littoralis)
Shi Hu* (Herba Dendrobii)
Xuan Shen (Radix Scrophulariae Ningpoensis)
Fo Shou (Fructus Citri Sarcodactylis)
Huang Qin (Radix Scutellariae Baicalensis)
Gan Di Huang (Radix Rehmanniae Glutinosae Exsiccata)
Dan Shen (Radix Salviae Miltiorrhizae)
Jin Yin Hua (Flos Lonicerae)
Pu Gong Ying (Herba Taraxaci cum Radice)
Mai Men Dong (Radix Ophiopogonis Japonici)
Tian Men Dong (Radix Asparagi Cochinchinensis)
Yu Zhu (Rhizoma Polygonati Odorati)
Source: *Zhao Bing Nan Lin Chuang Jing Yan Ji* [A Collection of Zhao Bingnan's Clinical Experiences]

Jin Kui Shen Qi Wan (Kidney Qi Pill from the Golden Cabinet)
Shu Di Huang (Radix Rehmanniae Glutinosae Conquita)
Shan Yao (Rhizoma Dioscoreae Oppositae)
Shan Zhu Yu (Fructus Corni Officinalis)
Mu Dan Pi (Cortex Moutan Radicis)
Fu Ling (Sclerotium Poriae Cocos)
Ze Xie (Rhizoma Alismatis Orientalis)
Gui Zhi (Ramulus Cinnamomi Cassiae)
Rou Gui (Cortex Cinnamomi Cassiae)
Source: *Jin Kui Yao Lue* [Synopsis of Prescriptions from the Golden Cabinet]

Jin Lian Hua Pian (Globeflower Tablet)
Jin Lian Hua (Flos Trollii)
Source: *Zhang Zhi Li Pi Fu Bing Lin Chuang Jing Yan Ji Yao* [A Collection of Zhang Zhili's Clinical Experiences in the Treatment of Skin Diseases]

Jin Ling Zi San (Sichuan Chinaberry Powder)
Chuan Lian Zi (Fructus Meliae Toosendan)
Yan Hu Suo (Rhizoma Corydalis Yanhusuo)
Source: *Tai Ping Sheng Hui Fang* [Peaceful Holy Benevolent Prescriptions]

Jin Yin Hua Lu (Honeysuckle Flower Distillate)
Jin Yin Hua (Flos Lonicerae)

The herb is steamed to produce 2500ml of distillate for every 500g of the dried material (also used as a mouthwash).
Source: *Shi Yong Zhong Cheng Yao Shou Ce* [A Compilation of Chinese Herbal Patent Medicines]

Jing Fang Bai Du San (Schizonepeta and Ledebouriella Powder for Vanquishing Toxicity)
Jing Jie (Herba Schizonepetae Tenuifoliae)
Fang Feng (Radix Ledebouriellae Divaricatae)
Qiang Huo (Rhizoma et Radix Notopterygii)
Du Huo (Radix Angelicae Pubescentis)
Qian Hu (Radix Peucedani)
Chai Hu (Radix Bupleuri)
Jie Geng (Radix Platycodi Grandiflori)
Zhi Ke (Fructus Citri Aurantii)
Fu Ling (Sclerotium Poriae Cocos)
Chuan Xiong (Rhizoma Ligustici Chuanxiong)
Gan Cao (Radix Glycyrrhizae)
Source: *Wai Ke Li Li* [Theory and Case Reports on External Diseases]

Kan Li Sha (Fire and Water Hexagram Granules)
Fang Feng (Radix Ledebouriellae Divaricatae)
Tou Gu Cao (Herba Speranskiae seu Impatientis)
Chuan Xiong (Rhizoma Ligustici Chuanxiong)
Dang Gui (Radix Angelicae Sinensis)
Mi Cu (Acetum Oryzae)
Sheng Tie Xie ‡ (Frusta Ferri)
Source: *Zui Xin Fang Ji Shou Ce* [A New Handbook of Chinese Materia Medica Formulae]

Kang Bing Du Kou Fu Ye (Antivirus Syrup)
Ban Lan Gen (Radix Isatidis seu Baphicacanthi)
Shi Gao ‡ (Gypsum Fibrosum)
Lu Gen (Rhizoma Phragmitis Communis)
Sheng Di Huang (Radix Rehmanniae Glutinosae)
Lian Qiao (Fructus Forsythiae Suspensae)
Huo Xiang (Herba Agastaches seu Pogostemi)
Source: Empirical formula

Ku Shen Wan (Flavescent Sophora Root Pill)
Ku Shen (Radix Sophorae Flavescentis)
Xuan Shen (Radix Scrophulariae Ningpoensis)
Huang Lian (Rhizoma Coptidis)
Chao Da Huang (Radix et Rhizoma Rhei, stir-fried)
Du Huo (Radix Angelicae Pubescentis)
Chao Zhi Ke (Fructus Citri Aurantii, stir-fried)
Fang Feng (Radix Ledebouriellae Divaricatae)
Huang Qin (Radix Scutellariae Baicalensis)
Zhi Zi (Fructus Gardeniae Jasminoidis)
Ju Hua (Flos Chrysanthemii Morifolii)
Source: *Zheng Zhi Zhun Sheng* [Standards of Diagnosis and Treatment]

La Fan Wan (Wax and Alum Pill)
Dan Nan Xing ‡ (Pulvis Arisaematis cum Felle Bovis)
Fa Ban Xia (Rhizoma Pinelliae Ternatae Praeparata)
Ming Fan ‡ (Alumen)
Huang La ‡ (Cera Aurea)
Source: *Huo Ren Xin Tong* [A Thorough Understanding of People]

Lei Gong Teng Pian (Thunder God Vine Tablet)
Lei Gong Teng (Radix Tripterygii Wilfordi)
Source: Empirical formula

Li Zhong Tang (Decoction for Regulating the Middle)
Dang Shen (Radix Codonopsitis Pilosulae)
Bai Zhu (Rhizoma Atractylodis Macrocephalae)
Gan Jiang (Rhizoma Zingiberis Officinalis)
Zhi Gan Cao (Radix Glycyrrhizae, mix-fried with honey)
Source: *Shang Han Lun* [On Cold Damage]

Lian Qiao Bai Du Wan (Forsythia Pill for Vanquishing Toxicity)
Lian Qiao (Fructus Forsythiae Suspensae)
Fang Feng (Radix Ledebouriellae Divaricatae)
Bai Zhi (Radix Angelicae Dahuricae)
Huang Lian (Rhizoma Coptidis)
Ku Shen (Radix Sophorae Flavescentis)
Bo He (Herba Menthae Haplocalycis)
Dang Gui (Radix Angelicae Sinensis)
Jing Jie Sui (Spica Schizonepetae Tenuifoliae)
Tian Hua Fen (Radix Trichosanthis)
Gan Cao (Radix Glycyrrhizae)
Huang Qin (Radix Scutellariae Baicalensis)
Chi Shao (Radix Paeoniae Rubra)
Chai Hu (Radix Bupleuri)
*Ma Huang** (Herba Ephedrae)
Qiang Huo (Rhizoma et Radix Notopterygii)
Jin Yin Hua (Flos Lonicerae)
Huang Bai (Cortex Phellodendri)
Zi Hua Di Ding (Herba Violae Yedoensitis)
Da Huang (Radix et Rhizoma Rhei)
Source: *Zhao Bing Nan Lin Chuang Jing Yan Ji* [A Collection of Zhao Bingnan's Clinical Experiences]

Liang Ge San (Powder for Cooling the Diaphragm)
Da Huang (Radix et Rhizoma Rhei)
Mang Xiao ‡ (Mirabilitum)
Gan Cao (Radix Glycyrrhizae)
Zhi Zi (Fructus Gardeniae Jasminoidis)
Bo He (Herba Menthae Haplocalycis)
Huang Qin (Radix Scutellariae Baicalensis)
Lian Qiao (Fructus Forsythiae Suspensae)
Dan Zhu Ye (Herba Lophatheri Gracilis)
Source: *Yi Zong Jin Jian* [The Golden Mirror of Medicine]

Liang Xue Si Wu Tang (Four Agents Decoction for Cooling the Blood)
Sheng Di Huang (Radix Rehmanniae Glutinosae)
Dang Gui (Radix Angelicae Sinensis)
Chi Shao (Radix Paeoniae Rubra)
Chuan Xiong (Rhizoma Ligustici Chuanxiong)
Hong Hua (Flos Carthami Tinctorii)
Fu Ling (Sclerotium Poriae Cocos)
Huang Qin (Radix Scutellariae Baicalensis)
Source: *Yi Zong Jin Jian* [The Golden Mirror of Medicine]

Liang Xue Wu Gen Tang (Five-Root Decoction for Cooling the Blood)
Bai Mao Gen (Rhizoma Imperatae Cylindricae)
Tian Hua Fen (Radix Trichosanthis)

Qian Cao Gen (Radix Rubiae Cordifoliae)
Zi Cao (Radix Arnebiae seu Lithospermi)
Ban Lan Gen (Radix Isatidis seu Baphicacanthi)
Source: *Zhao Bing Nan Lin Chuang Jing Yan Ji* [A Collection of Zhao Bingnan's Clinical Experiences]

Liang Xue Xiao Feng San (Powder for Cooling the Blood and Dispersing Wind)
Sheng Di Huang (Radix Rehmanniae Glutinosae)
Dang Gui (Radix Angelicae Sinensis)
Jing Jie (Herba Schizonepetae Tenuifoliae)
Chan Tui‡ (Periostracum Cicadae)
Ku Shen (Radix Sophorae Flavescentis)
Bai Ji Li (Fructus Tribuli Terrestris)
Zhi Mu (Rhizoma Anemarrhenae Asphodeloidis)
Shi Gao‡ (Gypsum Fibrosum)
Gan Cao (Radix Glycyrrhizae)
Source: *Zhu Ren Kang Lin Chuang Jing Yan Ji* [A Collection of Zhu Renkang's Clinical Experiences]

Ling Xiao Hua San (Campsis Flower Powder)
Ling Xiao Hua (Flos Campsitis)
Zhi Zi (Fructus Gardeniae Jasminoidis)
Source: Empirical formula

Ling Yang Gou Teng Tang (Antelope Horn and Uncaria Decoction)
*Ling Yang Jiao** (Cornu Antelopis)
Sang Ye (Folium Mori Albae)
Chuan Bei Mu (Bulbus Fritillariae Cirrhosae)
Sheng Di Huang (Radix Rehmanniae Glutinosae)
Gou Teng (Ramulus Uncariae cum Uncis)
Ju Hua (Flos Chrysanthemi Morifolii)
Fu Shen (Sclerotium Poriae Cocos cum Ligno Hospite)
Bai Shao (Radix Paeoniae Lactiflorae)
Gan Cao (Radix Glycyrrhizae)
Zhu Ru (Caulis Bambusae in Taeniis)
Source: *Shang Han Lun* [On Cold Damage]

Ling Yang Jiao San (Antelope Horn Powder)
*Ling Yang Jiao Fen** (Cornu Antelopis, powdered)
Fang Feng (Radix Ledebouriellae Divaricatae)
Mai Men Dong (Radix Ophiopogonis Japonici)
Xuan Shen (Radix Scrophulariae Ningpoensis)
Zhi Mu (Rhizoma Anemarrhenae Asphodeloidis)
Huang Qin (Radix Scutellariae Baicalensis)
Niu Bang Zi (Fructus Arctii Lappae)
Gan Cao (Radix Glycyrrhizae)
Source: *Wai Ke Zheng Zong* [An Orthodox Manual of External Diseases]

Liu Wei Di Huang Wan [Tang] (Six-Ingredient Rehmannia Pill [Decoction])
Shu Di Huang (Radix Rehmanniae Glutinosae Conquita)
Shan Zhu Yu (Fructus Corni Officinalis)
Mu Dan Pi (Cortex Moutan Radicis)
Shan Yao (Rhizoma Dioscoreae Oppositae)
Fu Ling (Sclerotium Poriae Cocos)
Ze Xie (Rhizoma Alismatis Orientalis)
Source: *Xiao Er Yao Zheng Zhi Jue* [Key to the Treatment of Children's Diseases]

Long Dan Xie Gan Tang [Wan] (Chinese Gentian Decoction [Pill] for Draining the Liver)
Long Dan Cao (Radix Gentianae Scabrae)
Zhi Zi (Fructus Gardeniae Jasminoidis)
Huang Qin (Radix Scutellariae Baicalensis)
Sheng Di Huang (Radix Rehmanniae Glutinosae)
Dang Gui (Radix Angelicae Sinensis)
Chai Hu (Radix Bupleuri)
Ze Xie (Rhizoma Alismatis Orientalis)
Che Qian Zi (Semen Plantaginis)
*Mu Tong** (Caulis Mutong)
Gan Cao (Radix Glycyrrhizae)
Source: *Yi Fang Ji Jie* [Collection of Prescriptions with Notes]
Note: In those countries where it is illegal to include *Mu Tong** (Caulis Mutong) in a prescription, *Tong Cao* (Medulla Tetrapanacis Papyriferi) will normally be substituted.

Lu Sun Pian (Asparagus Tablet)
Lu Sun (Herba Asparagi Officinalis)
Source: Empirical formula

Ma Gui Ge Ban Tang (Ephedra and Cinnamon Twig Half-and-Half Decoction)
*Ma Huang** (Herba Ephedrae)
Gui Zhi (Ramulus Cinnamomi Cassiae)
Bai Shao (Radix Paeoniae Lactiflorae)
Xing Ren (Semen Pruni Armeniacae)
Sheng Jiang (Rhizoma Zingiberis Officinalis Recens)
Da Zao (Fructus Ziziphi Jujubae)
Gan Cao (Radix Glycyrrhizae)
Source: Empirical formula

Ma Huang Fang (Ephedra Formula)
*Ma Huang** (Herba Ephedrae)
Gui Zhi (Ramulus Cinnamomi Cassiae)
Xing Ren (Semen Pruni Armeniacae)
Gan Cao (Radix Glycyrrhizae)
Source: *Shang Han Lun* [On Cold Damage]

Ma Huang Fu Zi Xi Xin Tang (Ephedra, Asarum and Prepared Aconite Decoction)
*Ma Huang** (Herba Ephedrae)
*Xi Xin** (Herba cum Radice Asari)
*Fu Zi** (Radix Lateralis Aconiti Carmichaeli Praeparata)
Source: *Shang Han Lun* [On Cold Damage]

Ma Huang Tang (Ephedra Decoction)
See *Ma Huang Fang* (Ephedra Formula).

Mai Wei Di Huang Tang (Ophiopogon and Rehmannia Decoction)
Mai Men Dong (Radix Ophiopogonis)
Wu Wei Zi (Fructus Schisandrae)
Shan Zhu Yu (Fructus Corni Officinalis)
Shan Yao (Rhizoma Dioscoreae Oppositae)
Mu Dan Pi (Cortex Moutan Radicis)
Ze Xie (Rhizoma Alismatis Orientalis)
Sheng Di Huang (Radix Rehmanniae Glutinosae)
Fu Ling (Sclerotium Poriae Cocos)
Source: *Yi Ji: Za Bing Lei Fang* [Medical Works: Prescriptions for Various Categories of Miscellaneous Diseases]

Meng Shi Gun Tan Wan (**Chlorite Pill for Rolling Phlegm**)
Qing Meng Shi ‡ (Lapis Chloriti)
Chen Xiang (Lignum Aquilariae Resinatum)
Da Huang (Radix et Rhizoma Rhei)
Huang Qin (Radix Scutellariae Baicalensis)
Source: *Jing Yue Quan Shu* [The Complete Works of Zhang Jingyue]

Nan Tong She Yao Pian (**Nantong Snake Tablet**)
Chong Lou (Rhizoma Paridis)
Ban Zhi Lian (Herba Scutellariae Barbatae)
Wu Gong ‡ (Scolopendra Subspinipes)
Source: *Zui Xin Zhong Cheng Yao Shou Ce* [A Manual of Current TCM Patent Medicines]

Nei Xiao Lian Qiao Wan (**Forsythia Internal Dispersion Pill**)
Lian Qiao (Fructus Forsythiae Suspensae)
Xia Ku Cao (Spica Prunellae Vulgaris)
She Gan (Rhizoma Belamcandae Chinensis)
Ze Lan (Herba Lycopi Lucidi)
Tian Hua Fen (Radix Trichosanthis)
Bai Ji (Rhizoma Bletillae Striatae)
Sha Shen (Radix Glehniae seu Adenophorae)
Lu Gen (Rhizoma Phragmitis Communis)
Hu Tao Ren (Semen Juglandis Regiae)
Source: *Zhao Bing Nan Lin Chuang Jing Yan Ji* [A Collection of Zhao Bingnan's Clinical Experiences]

Nei Xiao Luo Li Wan (**Scrofula Internal Dispersion Pill**)
Xia Ku Cao (Spica Prunellae Vulgaris)
Hai Zao (Herba Sargassi)
Tian Hua Fen (Radix Trichosanthis)
Lian Qiao (Fructus Forsythiae Suspensae)
Sheng Di Huang (Radix Rehmanniae Glutinosae)
Dang Gui (Radix Angelicae Sinensis)
Xuan Shen (Radix Scrophulariae Ningpoensis)
Zhe Bei Mu (Bulbus Fritillariae Thunbergii)
Hai Ge Ke (Concha Meretricis seu Cyclinae)
Jiu Zhi Da Huang (Radix et Rhizoma Rhei, mix-fried with alcohol)
Jie Geng (Radix Platycodi Grandiflori)
Xuan Ming Fen ‡ (Mirabilitum Depuratum)
Da Qing Yan ‡ (Halitum)
Bo He (Herba Menthae Haplocalycis)
Bai Lian (Radix Ampelopsis Japonicae)
Chao Zhi Ke (Fructus Citri Aurantii)
Mu Li ‡ (Concha Ostreae)
Source: *Zhao Bing Nan Lin Chuang Jing Yan Ji* [A Collection of Zhao Bingnan's Clinical Experiences]

Niu Huang Jie Du Wan (**Bovine Bezoar Pill for Relieving Toxicity**)
Niu Huang ‡ (Calculus Bovis)
Gan Cao (Radix Glycyrrhizae)
Jin Yin Hua (Flos Lonicerae)
Chong Lou (Rhizoma Paridis)
Source: *Bao Ying Cuo Yao* [Essentials for the Care of Infants]

Niu Huang Shang Qing Wan (**Bovine Bezoar Pill for Clearing the Upper Body**)
Huang Lian (Rhizoma Coptidis)

Jie Geng (Radix Platycodi Grandiflori)
Bai Zhi (Radix Angelicae Dahuricae)
Chuan Xiong (Rhizoma Ligustici Chuanxiong)
Chi Shao (Radix Paeoniae Rubra)
Jing Jie Sui (Spica Schizonepetae Tenuifoliae)
Shi Gao ‡ (Gypsum Fibrosum)
Da Huang (Radix et Rhizoma Rhei)
Huang Qin (Radix Scutellariae Baicalensis)
Dang Gui (Radix Angelicae Sinensis)
Zhi Zi (Fructus Gardeniae Jasminoidis)
Lian Qiao (Fructus Forsythiae Suspensae)
Bo He (Herba Menthae Haplocalycis)
Lian Zi Xin (Plumula Nelumbinis Nuciferae)
Ju Hua (Flos Chrysanthemi Morifolii)
Huang Bai (Cortex Phellodendri)
Gan Cao (Radix Glycyrrhizae)
Niu Huang ‡ (Calculus Bovis)
Bing Pian (Borneolum)
Source: *Zui Xin Zhong Cheng Yao Shou Ce* [A Manual of Current TCM Patent Medicines]

Pi Fu Bing Xue Du Wan (**Skin Disease Blood Toxicity Pill**)
Chi Shao (Radix Paeoniae Rubra)
Dang Gui (Radix Angelicae Sinensis)
Chan Tui ‡ (Periostracum Cicadae)
Bai Mao Gen (Rhizoma Imperatae Cylindricae)
Di Fu Zi (Fructus Kochiae Scopariae)
Lian Qiao (Fructus Forsythiae Suspensae)
Jin Yin Hua (Flos Lonicerae)
Zi Cao (Radix Arnebiae seu Lithospermi)
Zi Jing Pi (Cortex Cercis)
Source: Empirical formula from Shi Jinmo

Ping Wei San (**Quieting the Stomach Powder**)
Cang Zhu (Rhizoma Atractylodis)
Hou Po (Cortex Magnoliae Officinalis)
Chen Pi (Pericarpium Citri Reticulatae)
Zhi Gan Cao (Radix Glycyrrhizae, mix-fried with honey)
Source: *Tai Ping Hui Min He Ji Ju Fang* [Prescriptions from the Peaceful Benevolent Dispensary]

Qin Jiao Wan (**Large-Leaf Gentian Pill**)
Qin Jiao (Radix Gentianae Macrophyllae)
Ku Shen (Radix Sophorae Flavescentis)
Jiu Zheng Da Huang (Radix et Rhizoma Rhei, steamed with alcohol)
Huang Qi (Radix Astragali seu Hedysari)
Fang Feng (Radix Ledebouriellae Divaricatae)
Lou Lu (Radix Rhapontici seu Echinopsis)
Huang Lian (Rhizoma Coptidis)
Wu Shao She ‡ (Zaocys Dhumnades)
Source: *Zhao Bing Nan Lin Chuang Jing Yan Ji* [A Collection of Zhao Bingnan's Clinical Experiences]

Qin Lian Ping Wei San (**Scutellaria and Coptis Powder for Calming the Stomach**)
Huang Qin (Radix Scutellariae Baicalensis)
Huang Lian (Rhizoma Coptidis)
Chen Pi (Pericarpium Citri Reticulatae)
Chao Cang Zhu (Rhizoma Atractylodis, stir-fried)
Gan Cao (Radix Glycyrrhizae)

Sheng Jiang (Rhizoma Zingiberis Officinalis Recens)
Hou Po (Cortex Magnoliae Officinalis)
Source: *Yi Zong Jin Jian* [The Golden Mirror of Medicine]

Qing Gong Tang (Clearing the Palace Decoction)
Xuan Shen (Radix Scrophulariae Ningpoensis)
Lian Zi Xin (Plumula Nelumbinis Nuciferae)
Dan Zhu Ye (Herba Lophatheri Gracilis)
Mai Men Dong (Radix Ophiopogonis Japonici)
Lian Qiao (Fructus Forsythiae Suspensae)
Shui Niu Jiao‡ (Cornu Bubali)
Source: *Wen Bing Tiao Bian* [Treatise on the Identification of Warm Diseases]

Qing Hao Lu (Sweet Wormwood Distillate)
Qing Hao (Herba Artemisiae Chinghao)
The herb is steamed to produce 2500ml of distillate for every 500g of the dried material.
Source: Empirical formula

Qing Ji Shen Shi Tang (Decoction for Clearing Heat from the Flesh and Percolating Dampness)
Cang Zhu (Rhizoma Atractylodis)
Bai Zhu (Rhizoma Atractylodis Macrocephalae)
Sheng Ma (Rhizoma Cimicifugae)
Gan Cao (Radix Glycyrrhizae)
Ze Xie (Rhizoma Alismatis Orientalis)
Zhi Zi (Fructus Gardeniae Jasminoidis)
Huang Lian (Rhizoma Coptidis)
Che Qian Zi (Semen Plantaginis)
Hou Po (Cortex Magnoliae Officinalis)
Fu Ling (Sclerotium Poriae Cocos)
Dang Gui (Radix Angelicae Sinensis)
Chuan Xiong (Rhizoma Ligustici Chuanxiong)
Qing Pi (Pericarpium Citri Reticulatae Viride)
*Mu Tong** (Caulis Mutong)
Ku Shen (Radix Sophorae Flavescentis)
Chai Hu (Radix Bupleuri)
Source: *Chuang Yang Jing Yan Quan Shu* [A Complete Manual of Experience in the Treatment of Sores]
Note: In those countries where it is illegal to include *Mu Tong** (Caulis Mutong) in a prescription, *Tong Cao* (Medulla Tetrapanacis Papyriferi) may be substituted.

Qing Jie Pian (Clearing and Relieving Tablet)
Da Huang (Radix et Rhizoma Rhei)
Huang Qin (Radix Scutellariae Baicalensis)
Huang Bai (Cortex Phellodendri)
Cang Zhu (Rhizoma Atractylodis)
Source: Empirical formula

Qing Wen Bai Du Yin (Beverage for Clearing Scourge and Vanquishing Toxicity)
Shi Gao‡ (Gypsum Fibrosum)
Sheng Di Huang (Radix Rehmanniae Glutinosae)
Shui Niu Jiao‡ (Cornu Bubali)
Huang Lian (Rhizoma Coptidis)
Zhi Zi (Fructus Gardeniae Jasminoidis)
Jie Geng (Radix Platycodi Grandiflori)
Huang Qin (Radix Scutellariae Baicalensis)
Zhi Mu (Rhizoma Anemarrhenae Asphodeloidis)

Chi Shao (Radix Paeoniae Rubra)
Xuan Shen (Radix Scrophulariae Ningpoensis)
Lian Qiao (Fructus Forsythiae Suspensae)
Dan Zhu Ye (Herba Lophatheri Gracilis)
Gan Cao (Radix Glycyrrhizae)
Mu Dan Pi (Cortex Moutan Radicis)
Source: *Yi Zhen Yi De* [An Understanding of Epidemic Diseases with Eruptions]

Qing Ying Tang (Decoction for Clearing Heat from the Ying Level)
Shui Niu Jiao‡ (Cornu Bubali)
Sheng Di Huang (Radix Rehmanniae Glutinosae)
Dan Zhu Ye (Herba Lophatheri Gracilis)
Jin Yin Hua (Flos Lonicerae)
Lian Qiao (Fructus Forsythiae Suspensae)
Huang Lian (Rhizoma Coptidis)
Xuan Shen (Radix Scrophulariae Ningpoensis)
Mai Men Dong (Radix Ophiopogonis Japonici)
Dan Shen (Radix Salviae Miltiorrhizae)
Source: *Wen Bing Tiao Bian* [Treatise on the Identification of Warm Diseases]

Qu Feng Huan Ji Wan (Pill for Dispelling Wind and Regenerating the Flesh)
Wei Ling Xian (Radix Clematidis)
Shi Chang Pu (Rhizoma Acori Graminei)
He Shou Wu (Radix Polygoni Multiflori)
Ku Shen (Radix Sophorae Flavescentis)
Niu Xi (Radix Achyranthis Bidentatae)
Cang Zhu (Rhizoma Atractylodis)
Ya Ma Ren (Semen Lini)
Tian Hua Fen (Radix Trichosanthis)
Gan Cao (Radix Glycyrrhizae)
Chuan Xiong (Rhizoma Ligustici Chuanxiong)
Dang Gui (Radix Angelicae Sinensis)
Source: *Wai Ke Zheng Zong* [An Orthodox Manual of External Diseases]

Quan Lu Wan (Whole Deer Pill)
Quan Lu‡ (Cervus Integer)
Ren Shen (Radix Ginseng)
Chao Bai Zhu (Rhizoma Atractylodis Macrocephalae, stir-fried)
Fu Ling (Sclerotium Poriae Cocos)
Zhi Gan Cao (Radix Glycyrrhizae, mix-fried with honey)
Dang Gui (Radix Angelicae Sinensis)
Sheng Di Huang (Radix Rehmanniae Glutinosae)
Chuan Xiong (Rhizoma Ligustici Chuanxiong)
Shu Di Huang (Radix Rehmanniae Glutinosae Conquita)
Zhi Huang Qin (Radix Scutellariae Baicalensis, mix-fried with honey)
Tian Men Dong (Radix Asparagi Cochinchinensis)
Mai Men Dong (Radix Ophiopogonis Japonici)
Gou Qi Zi (Fructus Lycii)
Du Zhong (Cortex Eucommiae Ulmoidis)
Niu Xi (Radix Achyranthis Bidentatae)
Chao Shan Yao (Rhizoma Dioscoreae Oppositae, stir-fried)
Chao Qian Shi (Semen Euryales Ferocis, stir-fried)
Tu Si Zi (Semen Cuscutae)
Wu Wei Zi (Fructus Schisandrae)

Suo Yang (Herba Cynomorii Songarici)
Rou Cong Rong (Herba Cistanches Deserticolae)
Bu Gu Zhi (Fructus Psoraleae Corylifoliae)
Ba Ji Tian (Radix Morindae Officinalis)
Hu Lu Ba (Semen Trigonellae Foeni-graeci)
Xu Duan (Radix Dipsaci)
Fu Pen Zi (Fructus Rubi Chingii)
Chu Shi Zi (Fructus Broussonetiae)
Qiu Shi‡ (Depositum Praeparatum Hominis Urinae)
Chen Pi (Pericarpium Citri Reticulatae)
Hua Jiao (Pericarpium Zanthoxyli)
Chen Xiang (Lignum Aquilariae Resinatum)
Xiao Hui Xiang (Fructus Foeniculi Vulgaris)
Da Qing Yan‡ (Halitum)
Source: *Jing Yue Quan Shu* [The Complete Works of Zhang Jingyue]

Ren Shen Gu Ben Wan (Ginseng Pill for Consolidating the Root)

Ren Shen (Radix Ginseng)
Tian Men Dong (Radix Asparagi Cochinchinensis)
Mai Men Dong (Radix Ophiopogonis Japonici)
Sheng Di Huang (Radix Rehmanniae Glutinosae)
Shu Di Huang (Radix Rehmanniae Glutinosae Conquita)
Source: *Yi Fang Ji Jie* [Collection of Prescriptions with Notes]

Ren Shen Gui Pi Wan (Ginseng Pill for Restoring the Spleen)

Ren Shen (Radix Ginseng)
Sha Ren (Fructus Amomi)
Zhi Ke (Fructus Citri Aurantii)
Gan Cao (Radix Glycyrrhizae)
Shan Yao (Rhizoma Dioscoreae Oppositae)
Mu Xiang* (Radix Aucklandiae Lappae)
Yi Yi Ren (Semen Coicis Lachryma-jobi)
Shan Zha (Fructus Crataegi)
Bai Zhu (Rhizoma Atractylodis Macrocephalae)
Gu Ya (Fructus Setariae Italicae Germinatus)
Bai Bian Dou (Semen Dolichoris Lablab)
Qian Shi (Semen Euryales Ferocis)
Lian Zi (Semen Nelumbinis Nuciferae)
Chen Pi (Pericarpium Citri Reticulatae)
Qing Pi (Pericarpium Citri Reticulatae Viride)
Dang Gui (Radix Angelicae Sinensis)
Shen Qu (Massa Fermentata)
Source: *Jing Yue Quan Shu* [The Complete Works of Zhang Jingyue]

Ren Shen Jian Pi Wan (Ginseng Pill for Fortifying the Spleen)

Ren Shen (Radix Ginseng)
Cao Dou Kou (Semen Alpiniae Katsumadai)
Zhi Ke (Fructus Citri Aurantii)
Gan Cao (Radix Glycyrrhizae)
Shan Yao (Rhizoma Dioscoreae Oppositae)
Mu Xiang* (Radix Aucklandiae Lappae)
Yi Yi Ren (Semen Coicis Lachryma-jobi)
Shan Zha (Fructus Crataegi)
Bai Zhu (Rhizoma Atractylodis Macrocephalae)
Gu Ya (Fructus Setariae Italicae Germinatus)

Bai Bian Dou (Semen Dolichoris Lablab)
Qian Shi (Semen Euryales Ferocis)
Lian Zi (Semen Nelumbinis Nuciferae)
Chen Pi (Pericarpium Citri Reticulatae)
Qing Pi (Pericarpium Citri Reticulatae Viride)
Dang Gui (Radix Angelicae Sinensis)
Shen Qu (Massa Fermentata)
Source: *Jing Yue Quan Shu* [The Complete Works of Zhang Jingyue]

San Huang Wan (Three Yellows Pill)

Huang Lian (Rhizoma Coptidis)
Huang Qin (Radix Scutellariae Baicalensis)
Da Huang (Radix et Rhizoma Rhei)
Source: *Zhu Ren Kang Lin Chuang Jing Yan Ji* [A Collection of Zhu Renkang's Clinical Experiences]

San Jie Ling (Efficacious Remedy for Dissipating Nodules)

Feng Xiang Zhi (Resina Liquidambaris)
Zhi Cao Wu* (Radix Aconiti Kusnezoffii, mix-fried with honey)
Wu Ling Zhi‡ (Excrementum Trogopteri)
Di Long‡ (Lumbricus)
Mu Bie Zi (Semen Momordicae Cochinchinensis)
Ru Xiang (Gummi Olibanum)
Mo Yao (Myrrha)
Dang Gui (Radix Angelicae Sinensis)
Xiang Mo‡ (Atramentum)
Shi Chang Pu (Rhizoma Acori Graminei)
Source: *Wai Ke Zheng Zong* [An Orthodox Manual of External Diseases]

San Miao Wan (Mysterious Three Pill)

Huang Bai (Cortex Phellodendri)
Cang Zhu (Rhizoma Atractylodis)
Chuan Niu Xi (Radix Achyranthis Bidentatae)
Source: *Yi Xue Zheng Zhuan* [Orthodox Medical Problems]

Sang Ju Yin (Mulberry Leaf and Chrysanthemum Beverage)

Sang Ye (Folium Mori Albae)
Ju Hua (Flos Chrysanthemi Morifolii)
Jie Geng (Radix Platycodi Grandiflori)
Lian Qiao (Fructus Forsythiae Suspensae)
Xing Ren (Semen Pruni Armeniacae)
Bo He (Herba Menthae Haplocalycis)
Gan Cao (Radix Glycyrrhizae)
Lu Gen (Rhizoma Phragmitis Communis)
Source: *Wen Bing Tiao Bian* [Treatise on the Identification of Warm Diseases]

Sha Shen Mai Dong Yin (Adenophora and Ophiopogon Beverage)

Bei Sha Shen (Radix Glehniae Littoralis)
Mai Men Dong (Radix Ophiopogonis Japonici)
Yu Zhu (Rhizoma Polygonati Odorati)
Tian Hua Fen (Radix Trichosanthis)
Sang Ye (Folium Mori Albae)
Gan Cao (Radix Glycyrrhizae)
Bai Bian Dou (Semen Dolichoris Lablab)
Source: *Wen Bing Tiao Bian* [Treatise on the Identification of Warm Diseases]

Shen Ling Bai Zhu Wan **(Ginseng, Poria and White Atractylodes Pill)**
Lian Zi (Semen Nelumbinis Nuciferae)
Yi Yi Ren (Semen Coicis Lachryma-jobi)
Sha Ren (Fructus Amomi)
Jie Geng (Radix Platycodi Grandiflori)
Bai Bian Dou (Semen Dolichoris Lablab)
Fu Ling (Sclerotium Poriae Cocos)
Ren Shen (Radix Ginseng)
Gan Cao (Radix Glycyrrhizae)
Bai Zhu (Rhizoma Atractylodis Macrocephalae)
Shan Yao (Rhizoma Dioscoreae Oppositae)
Source: *Tai Ping Hui Min He Ji Ju Fang* [Prescriptions from the Peaceful Benevolent Dispensary]

Shen Qi Wan **(Kidney Qi Pill)**
Gan Di Huang (Radix Rehmanniae Glutinosae Exsiccata)
Shan Yao (Rhizoma Dioscoreae Oppositae)
Shan Zhu Yu (Fructus Corni Officinalis)
Ze Xie (Rhizoma Alismatis Orientalis)
Fu Ling (Sclerotium Poriae Cocos)
Mu Dan Pi (Cortex Moutan Radicis)
Gui Zhi (Ramulus Cinnamomi Cassiae)
Fu Zi* (Radix Lateralis Aconiti Carmichaeli Praeparata)
Source: *Jin Kui Yao Lue* [Synopsis of Prescriptions from the Golden Cabinet]

Shen Xiao Tuo Li San **(Wondrous Effect Powder for Drawing Out Toxins from the Interior)**
Ren Dong Teng (Caulis Lonicerae Japonicae)
Huang Qin (Radix Scutellariae Baicalensis)
Dang Gui (Radix Angelicae Sinensis)
Gan Cao (Radix Glycyrrhizae)
Source: *Tai Ping Hui Min He Ji Ju Fang* [Prescriptions from the Peaceful Benevolent Dispensary]

Sheng Fa Wan **(Generating Hair Pill)**
Dang Shen (Radix Codonopsitis Pilosulae)
Bai Zhu (Rhizoma Atractylodis Macrocephalae)
Shu Di Huang (Radix Rehmanniae Glutinosae Conquita)
Bai Zi Ren (Semen Biotae Orientalis)
He Shou Wu (Radix Polygoni Multiflori)
Tu Si Zi (Semen Cuscutae)
Fu Ling (Sclerotium Poriae Cocos)
Chuan Xiong (Rhizoma Ligustici Chuanxiong)
Gan Cao (Radix Glycyrrhizae)
Source: Empirical formula

Sheng Ma He Qi Yin **(Bugbane Beverage for Harmonizing Qi)**
Gan Jiang (Rhizoma Zingiberis Officinalis)
Chao Zhi Ke (Fructus Citri Aurantii)
Ge Gen (Radix Puerariae)
Cang Zhu (Rhizoma Atractylodis)
Jie Geng (Radix Platycodi Grandiflori)
Sheng Ma (Rhizoma Cimicifugae)
Dang Gui (Radix Angelicae Sinensis)
Fa Ban Xia (Rhizoma Pinelliae Ternatae Praeparata)
Fu Ling (Sclerotium Poriae Cocos)
Bai Zhi (Radix Angelicae Dahuricae)
Chen Pi (Pericarpium Citri Reticulatae)

Gan Cao (Radix Glycyrrhizae)
Bai Shao (Radix Paeoniae Lactiflorae)
Da Huang (Radix et Rhizoma Rhei)
Source: *Tai Ping Hui Min He Ji Ju Fang* [Prescriptions from the Peaceful Benevolent Dispensary]

Sheng Xue Run Fu Yin **(Beverage for Generating Blood and Moistening the Skin)**
Dang Gui Shen (Corpus Radicis Angelicae Sinensis)
Sheng Di Huang (Radix Rehmanniae Glutinosae)
Shu Di Huang (Radix Rehmanniae Glutinosae Conquita)
Huang Qi (Radix Astragali seu Hedysari)
Tian Men Dong (Radix Asparagi Cochinchinensis)
Mai Men Dong (Radix Ophiopogonis Japonici)
Wu Wei Zi (Fructus Schisandrae)
Huang Qin (Radix Scutellariae Baicalensis)
Gua Lou Ren (Semen Trichosanthis)
Tao Ren (Semen Persicae)
Hong Hua (Flos Carthami Tinctorii)
Sheng Ma (Rhizoma Cimicifugae)
Source: *Yi Xue Zheng Zhuan* [Orthodox Medical Problems]

Shi Quan Da Bu Tang [Wan] **(Perfect Major Supplementation Decoction [Pill])**
Dang Gui (Radix Angelicae Sinensis)
Chuan Xiong (Rhizoma Ligustici Chuanxiong)
Bai Shao (Radix Paeoniae Lactiflorae)
Shu Di Huang (Radix Rehmanniae Glutinosae Conquita)
Dang Shen (Radix Codonopsitis Pilosulae)
Bai Zhu (Rhizoma Atractylodis Macrocephalae)
Zhi Gan Cao (Radix Glycyrrhizae, mix-fried with honey)
Fu Ling (Sclerotium Poriae Cocos)
Huang Qi (Radix Astragali seu Hedysari)
Rou Gui (Cortex Cinnamomi Cassiae)
Sheng Jiang (Rhizoma Zingiberis Officinalis Recens)
Da Zao (Fructus Ziziphi Jujubae)
Source: *Tai Ping Hui Min He Ji Ju Fang* [Prescriptions from the Peaceful Benevolent Dispensary]

Shi Xiao San **(Sudden Smile Powder)**
Chao Pu Huang (Pollen Typhae, stir-fried)
Wu Ling Zhi‡ (Excrementum Trogopteri)
Source: *Tai Ping Hui Min He Ji Ju Fang* [Prescriptions from the Peaceful Benevolent Dispensary]

Shou Wu Wan **(Fleeceflower Root Pill)**
He Shou Wu (Radix Polygoni Multiflori)
Source: *Wai Ke Zheng Zong* [An Orthodox Manual of External Diseases]

Shu Feng Qing Re Tang **(Decoction for Dredging Wind and Clearing Heat)**
Ku Shen (Radix Sophorae Flavescentis)
Zao Jiao (Fructus Gleditsiae Sinensis)
Zao Jiao Ci (Spina Gleditsiae Sinensis)
Chao Quan Xie‡ (Buthus Martensi, stir-fried)
Fang Feng (Radix Ledebouriellae Divaricatae)
Jing Jie Sui (Spica Schizonepetae Tenuifoliae)
Jin Yin Hua (Flos Lonicerae)
Chao Chan Tui‡ (Periostracum Cicadae, stir-fried)
Source: *Yi Zong Jin Jian* [The Golden Mirror of Medicine]

Si Jun Zi Tang (Four Gentlemen Decoction)
Dang Shen (Radix Codonopsitis Pilosulae)
Bai Zhu (Rhizoma Atractylodis Macrocephalae)
Fu Ling (Sclerotium Poriae Cocos)
Zhi Gan Cao (Radix Glycyrrhizae, mix-fried with honey)
Source: *Tai Ping Hui Min He Ji Ju Fang* [Prescriptions from the Peaceful Benevolent Dispensary]

Si Miao Tang [San] (Mysterious Four Decoction [Powder])
Huang Bai (Cortex Phellodendri)
Yi Yi Ren (Semen Coicis Lachryma-jobi)
Cang Zhu (Rhizoma Atractylodis)
Huai Niu Xi (Radix Achyranthis Bidentatae)
Source: *Wai Ke Jing Yao* [Essence of Diagnosis and Treatment of External Diseases]

Si Wu Tang (Four Agents Decoction)
Dang Gui (Radix Angelicae Sinensis)
Chuan Xiong (Rhizoma Ligustici Chuanxiong)
Bai Shao (Radix Paeoniae Lactiflorae)
Shu Di Huang (Radix Rehmanniae Glutinosae Conquita)
Source: *Tai Ping Hui Min He Ji Ju Fang* [Prescriptions from the Peaceful Benevolent Dispensary]

Si Zhi Xiang Fu Wan (Quadruply Processed Cyperus Pill)
Chao Xiang Fu (Rhizoma Cyperi Rotundi, stir-fried)
Dang Gui (Radix Angelicae Sinensis)
Chuan Xiong (Rhizoma Ligustici Chuanxiong)
Chao Bai Shao (Radix Paeoniae Lactiflorae, stir-fried)
Shu Di Huang (Radix Rehmanniae Glutinosae Conquita)
Bai Zhu (Rhizoma Atractylodis Macrocephalae)
Chen Pi (Pericarpium Citri Reticulatae)
Ze Lan (Herba Lycopi Lucidi)
Huang Bai (Cortex Phellodendri)
Chao Gan Cao (Radix Glycyrrhizae, stir-fried)
Source: *Zhang Zhi Li Pi Fu Bing Lin Chuang Jing Yan Ji Yao* [A Collection of Zhang Zhili's Clinical Experiences in the Treatment of Skin Diseases]

Tao Hong Si Wu Tang [Wan] (Peach Kernel and Safflower Four Agents Decoction [Pill])
Dang Gui (Radix Angelicae Sinensis)
Bai Shao (Radix Paeoniae Lactiflorae)
Shu Di Huang (Radix Rehmanniae Glutinosae Conquita)
Chuan Xiong (Rhizoma Ligustici Chuanxiong)
Tao Ren (Semen Persicae)
Hong Hua (Flos Carthami Tinctorii)
Source: *Tai Ping Hui Min He Ji Ju Fang* [Prescriptions from the Peaceful Benevolent Dispensary]

Tian Ma Gou Teng Yin (Gastrodia and Uncaria Beverage)
*Tian Ma** (Rhizoma Gastrodiae Elatae)
Gou Teng (Ramulus Uncariae cum Uncis)
Shi Jue Ming‡ (Concha Haliotidis)
Zhi Zi (Fructus Gardeniae Jasminoidis)
Huang Qin (Radix Scutellariae Baicalensis)
Chuan Niu Xi (Radix Achyranthis Bidentatae)
Du Zhong (Cortex Eucommiae Ulmoidis)
Yi Mu Cao (Herba Leonuri Hetcrophylli)
Sang Ji Sheng (Ramulus Loranthi)
Ye Jiao Teng (Caulis Polygoni Multiflori)
Fu Shen (Sclerotium Poriae Cocos cum Ligno Hospite)
Source: *Za Bing Zheng Zhi Xin Yi* [New Explanations for Patterns and Treatment of Miscellaneous Diseases]

Tong Jing Zhu Yu Tang (Decoction for Freeing the Channels and Expelling Blood Stasis)
Tao Ren (Semen Persicae)
Hong Hua (Flos Carthami Tinctorii)
*Chuan Shan Jia** (Squama Manitis Pentadactylae)
Zao Jiao Ci (Spina Gleditsiae Sinensis)
Lian Qiao (Fructus Forsythiae Suspensae)
Di Long‡ (Lumbricus)
Chai Hu (Radix Bupleuri)
Ru Xiang (Gummi Olibanum)
Source: *Yi Lin Gai Cuo* [Corrections of the Errors in Medical Works]

Tu Huai Yin (Glabrous Green Briar and Pagoda Tree Flower Beverage)
Tu Fu Ling (Rhizoma Smilacis Glabrae)
Huai Hua (Flos Sophorae Japonicae)
Gan Cao (Radix Glycyrrhizae)
Source: *Zhao Bing Nan Lin Chuang Jing Yan Ji* [A Collection of Zhao Bingnan's Clinical Experiences]

Tu Ling Yin Chen Tang (Glabrous Green Briar and Oriental Wormwood Decoction)
Tu Fu Ling (Rhizoma Smilacis Glabrae)
Yin Chen Hao (Herba Artemisiae Scopariae)
Bai Xian Pi (Cortex Dictamni Dasycarpi Radicis)
Ku Shen (Radix Sophorae Flavescentis)
Long Dan Cao (Radix Gentianae Scabrae)
Huang Qin (Radix Scutellariae Baicalensis)
Che Qian Zi (Semen Plantaginis)
Ze Xie (Rhizoma Alismatis Orientalis)
Mu Dan Pi (Cortex Moutan Radicis)
Chao Zhi Zi (Fructus Gardeniae Jasminoidis, stir-fried)
Source: Empirical formula

Tuo Li Wen Zhong Tang (Decoction for Drawing Toxins from the Interior and Warming the Middle)
Bai Zhu (Rhizoma Atractylodis Macrocephalae)
*Mu Xiang** (Radix Aucklandiae Lappae)
Ding Xiang (Flos Caryophylli)
Ren Shen (Radix Ginseng)
Yi Zhi Ren (Fructus Alpiniae Oxyphyllae)
Pao Jiang (Rhizoma Zingiberis Officinalis Praeparata)
Fa Ban Xia (Rhizoma Pinelliae Ternatae Praeparata)
Chen Pi (Pericarpium Citri Reticulatae)
Qiang Huo (Rhizoma et Radix Notopterygii)
Bai Dou Kou (Fructus Amomi Kravanh)
Gan Cao (Radix Glycyrrhizae)
*Fu Zi** (Radix Lateralis Aconiti Carmichaeli Praeparata)
Fu Ling (Sclerotium Poriae Cocos)
Sheng Jiang (Rhizoma Zingiberis Officinalis Recens)
Da Zao (Fructus Ziziphi Jujubae)
Source: *Yang Yi Da Quan* [The Complete Book of External Diseases]

Note: In those countries where internal use of *Fu Zi** (Radix Lateralis Aconiti Carmichaeli Praeparata) is not permitted, *Rou Gui* (Cortex Cinnamomi Cassiae) may be substituted.

Tuo Min Wan Er Hao (Desensitization Pill No. 2)
Chan Tui‡ (Periostracum Cicadae)
Bai Ji Li (Fructus Tribuli Terrestris)
Source: Empirical formula

Tuo Min Wan Yi Hao (Desensitization Pill No. 1)
Jiao Chan Tui‡ (Periostracum Cicadae, scorch-fried)
Source: Empirical formula

Wang Shi Bao Chi Wan (Master Wang's Red Pill for Protecting Infants)
Da Huang (Radix et Rhizoma Rhei)
Huang Lian (Rhizoma Coptidis)
Zhi Nan Zing (Rhizoma Arisaematis Praeparata)
Chuan Bei Mu (Bulbus Fritillariae Cirrhosae)
Source: Empirical formula from Wang Mianzhi

Wu Mei Wan (Black Plum Pill)
Wu Mei (Fructus Pruni Mume)
*Xi Xin** (Herba cum Radice Asari)
*Pao Fu Zi** (Radix Lateralis Aconiti Carmichaeli Praeparata, blast-fried)
Gui Zhi (Ramulus Cinnamomi Cassiae)
Dang Shen (Radix Codonopsitis Pilosulae)
Huang Bai (Cortex Phellodendri)
Gan Jiang (Rhizoma Zingiberis Officinalis)
Huang Lian (Rhizoma Coptidis)
Dang Gui (Radix Angelicae Sinensis)
Hua Jiao (Pericarpium Zanthoxyli)
Source: *Shang Han Lun* [On Cold Damage]

Wu She Pian (Black-Tail Snake Tablet)
Wu Shao She‡ (Zaocys Dhumnades)
Source: Empirical formula

Wu She Zhi Yang Wan (Black-Tail Snake Pill for Alleviating Itching)
Wu Shao She‡ (Zaocys Dhumnades)
Ku Shen (Radix Sophorae Flavescentis)
Cang Zhu (Rhizoma Atractylodis)
Dang Gui (Radix Angelicae Sinensis)
She Chuang Zi (Fructus Cnidii Monnieri)
Mu Dan Pi (Cortex Moutan Radicis)
Fang Feng (Radix Ledebouriellae Divaricatae)
Ren Gong Niu Huang‡ (Calculus Bovis Syntheticus)
Source: *Quan Guo Zhong Yao Cheng Yao Chu Fang Ji* [National Collection of Chinese Herbal Patent Medicines]

Wu Shen Tang (Five Spirits Decoction)
Fu Ling (Sclerotium Poriae Cocos)
Jin Yin Hua (Flos Lonicerae)
Niu Xi (Radix Achyranthis Bidentatae)
Zi Hua Di Ding (Herba Violae Yedoensitis)
Che Qian Zi (Semen Plantaginis)
Source: *Wai Ke Zhen Quan* [True Notes on External Diseases]

Wu Wei Xiao Du Yin (Five-Ingredient Beverage for Dispersing Toxicity)
Jin Yin Hua (Flos Lonicerae)

Ye Ju Hua (Flos Chrysanthemi Indici)
Pu Gong Ying (Herba Taraxaci cum Radice)
Zi Hua Di Ding (Herba Violae Yedoensitis)
Tian Kui Zi (Tuber Semiaquilegiae)
Source: *Yi Zong Jin Jian* [The Golden Mirror of Medicine]

Xi Huang Xing Xiao Wan (Western Bovine Bezoar Awakening and Dispersing Pill)
Niu Huang‡ (Calculus Bovis)
*She Xiang** (Secretio Moschi)
Ru Xiang (Gummi Olibanum)
Mo Yao (Myrrha)
Huang Mi Fan (Semen Setariae Conquitum)
Source: *Wai Ke Zheng Zhi Quan Sheng Ji* [A Life-Saving Manual of the Diagnosis and Treatment of External Diseases]

Xi Jiao Di Huang Tang [Wan] (Rhinoceros Horn and Rehmannia Decoction [Pill])
Shui Niu Jiao‡ (Cornu Bubali)
Sheng Di Huang (Radix Rehmanniae Glutinosae)
Chi Shao (Radix Paeoniae Rubra)
Mu Dan Pi (Cortex Moutan Radicis)
Source: *Qian Jin Yao Fang* [Prescriptions Worth a Thousand Gold Pieces for Emergencies]

Xi Jiao Sheng Ma Tang (Rhinoceros and Bugbane Decoction)
Shui Niu Jiao‡ (Cornu Bubali)
Sheng Ma (Rhizoma Cimicifugae)
Fang Feng (Radix Ledebouriellae Divaricatae)
Qiang Huo (Rhizoma et Radix Notopterygii)
Chuan Xiong (Rhizoma Ligustici Chuanxiong)
*Fu Zi** (Radix Lateralis Aconiti Carmichaeli Praeparata)
Bai Zhi (Radix Angelicae Dahuricae)
Huang Qin (Radix Scutellariae Baicalensis)
Gan Cao (Radix Glycyrrhizae)
Source: *Ben Shi Fang* [Original Prescriptions]
Note: In those countries where internal use of *Fu Zi** (Radix Lateralis Aconiti Carmichaeli Praeparata) is not permitted, *Fu Pen Zi* (Fructus Rubi Chingii) may be substituted.

Xiang Bei Yang Rong Tang (Cyperus and Fritillaria Decoction for Nourishing Ying Qi)
Chao Bai Zhu (Rhizoma Atractylodis Macrocephalae, stir-fried)
Ren Shen (Radix Ginseng)
Fu Ling (Sclerotium Poriae Cocos)
Chen Pi (Pericarpium Citri Reticulatae)
Shu Di Huang (Radix Rehmanniae Glutinosae Conquita)
Chuan Xiong (Rhizoma Ligustici Chuanxiong)
Dang Gui (Radix Angelicae Sinensis)
Bei Mu (Bulbus Fritillariae)
Chao Xiang Fu (Rhizoma Cyperi Rotundi, stir-fried)
Chao Bai Shao (Radix Paeoniae Lactiflorae, stir-fried)
Jie Geng (Radix Platycodi Grandiflori)
Gan Cao (Radix Glycyrrhizae)
Source: *Yi Zong Jin Jian* [The Golden Mirror of Medicine]

Xiang Ju Dan (Tangerine Peel and Cyperus Special Pill)
Fu Ling (Sclerotium Poriae Cocos)
Chen Pi (Pericarpium Citri Reticulatae)
Xiang Fu (Rhizoma Cyperi Rotundi)

Bai Zhu (Rhizoma Atractylodis Macrocephalae)
Fa Ban Xia (Rhizoma Pinelliae Ternatae Praeparata)
Chao Shan Yao (Rhizoma Dioscoreae Oppositae, stir-fried)
Lian Zi (Semen Nelumbinis Nuciferae)
Chao Bai Bian Dou (Semen Dolichoris Lablab, stir-fried)
Zhi Shi (Fructus Immaturus Citri Aurantii)
Chao Yi Yi Ren (Semen Coicis Lachryma-jobi, stir-fried)
Hou Po (Cortex Magnoliae Officinalis)
Jiao Shan Zha (Fructus Crataegi, scorch-fried)
Jiao Shen Qu (Massa Fermentata, scorch-fried)
Jiao Mai Ya (Fructus Hordei Vulgaris Germinatus, scorch-fried)
Sha Ren (Fructus Amomi)
Ze Xie (Rhizoma Alismatis Orientalis)
Gan Cao (Radix Glycyrrhizae)
Mu Xiang* (Radix Aucklandiae Lappae)
Source: *Zui Xin Fang Ji Shou Ce* [A New Handbook of Chinese Materia Medica Formulae]

Xiang Lian Wan (Aucklandia and Coptis Pill)
Mu Xiang* (Radix Aucklandia Lappae)
Huang Lian (Rhizoma Coptidis), stir-fried with *Wu Zhu Yu* (Fructus Evodiae Rutaecarpae)
Source: *Tai Ping Hui Min He Ji Ju Fang* [Prescriptions from the Peaceful Benevolent Dispensary]

Xiao Bai Du Gao (Minor Toxicity-Vanquishing Syrup)
Da Huang (Radix et Rhizoma Rhei)
Huang Bai (Cortex Phellodendri)
Chi Shao (Radix Paeoniae Rubra)
Pu Gong Ying (Herba Taraxaci cum Radice)
Chen Pi (Pericarpium Citri Reticulatae)
Mu Bie Zi (Semen Momordicae Cochinchinensis)
Jin Yin Hua (Flos Lonicerae)
Ru Xiang (Gummi Olibanum)
Gan Cao (Radix Glycyrrhizae)
Dang Gui (Radix Angelicae Sinensis)
Bai Zhi (Radix Angelicae Dahuricae)
Tian Hua Fen (Radix Trichosanthis)
Source: *Zhao Bing Nan Lin Chuang Jing Yan Ji* [A Collection of Zhao Bingnan's Clinical Experiences]

Xiao Chai Hu Tang (Minor Bupleurum Decoction)
Chai Hu (Radix Bupleuri)
Huang Qin (Radix Scutellariae Baicalensis)
Dang Shen (Radix Codonopsitis Pilosulae)
Fa Ban Xia (Rhizoma Pinelliae Ternatae Praeparata)
Zhi Gan Cao (Radix Glycyrrhizae, mix-fried with honey)
Sheng Jiang (Rhizoma Zingiberis Officinalis Recens)
Da Zao (Fructus Ziziphi Jujubae)
Source: *Shang Han Lun* [On Cold Damage]

Xiao Er Jian Fu Tang Jiang (Syrup for Fortifying Children's Skin)
Jin Yin Hua (Flos Lonicerae)
Zhi Zi (Fructus Gardeniae Jasminoidis)
Bai Xian Pi (Cortex Dictamni Dasycarpi Radicis)
Dan Zhu Ye (Herba Lophatheri Gracilis)
Deng Xin Cao (Medulla Junci Effusi)
Jiao Mai Ya (Fructus Hordei Vulgaris Germinatus, scorch-fried)
Di Gu Pi (Cortex Lycii Radicis)
Lü Dou Yi (Testa Phaseoli Radiati)

Source: *Zhang Zhi Li Pi Fu Bing Yi An Xuan Cui* [A Collection of Zhang Zhili's Skin Disease Cases]

Xiao Feng San (Powder for Dispersing Wind)
Dang Gui (Radix Angelicae Sinensis)
Sheng Di Huang (Radix Rehmanniae Glutinosae)
Fang Feng (Radix Ledebouriellae Divaricatae)
Chan Tui‡ (Periostracum Cicadae)
Zhi Mu (Rhizoma Anemarrhenae Asphodeloidis)
Ku Shen (Radix Sophorae Flavescentis)
Hei Zhi Ma (Semen Sesami Indici)
Jing Jie (Herba Schizonepetae Tenuifoliae)
Cang Zhu (Rhizoma Atractylodis)
Niu Bang Zi [Fructus Arctii Lappae]
Shi Gao‡ (Gypsum Fibrosum)
Gan Cao (Radix Glycyrrhizae)
Mu Tong* (Caulis Mutong)
Source: *Yi Zong Jin Jian* [The Golden Mirror of Medicine]
Note: In those countries where it is illegal to include *Mu Tong** (Caulis Mutong) in a prescription, *Tong Cao* (Medulla Tetrapanacis Papyriferi) will normally be substituted.

Xiao Li Wan (Dispersing Scrofula Pill)
Xia Ku Cao (Spica Prunellae Vulgaris)
Hai Zao (Herba Sargassi)
Hai Piao Xiao‡ (Os Sepiae seu Sepiellae)
Huang Qin (Radix Scutellariae Baicalensis)
Zhi Ke (Fructus Citri Aurantii)
Source: Empirical formula

Xiao Yao San [Wan] (Free Wanderer Powder [Pill])
Chai Hu (Radix Bupleuri)
Dang Gui (Radix Angelicae Sinensis)
Bai Shao (Radix Paeoniae Lactiflorae)
Bai Zhu (Rhizoma Atractylodis Macrocephalae)
Fu Ling (Sclerotium Poriae Cocos)
Gan Cao (Radix Glycyrrhizae)
Bo He (Herba Menthae Haplocalycis)
Sheng Jiang (Rhizoma Zingiberis Officinalis Recens)
Source: *Tai Ping Hui Min He Ji Ju Fang* [Prescriptions from the Peaceful Benevolent Dispensary]

Xie Gan Tang (Decoction for Draining the Liver)
Chai Hu (Radix Bupleuri)
Qin Pi (Cortex Fraxini)
Xi Xin* (Herba cum Radice Asari)
Zhi Zi (Fructus Gardeniae Jasminoidis)
Sheng Ma (Rhizoma Cimicifugae)
Rui Ren (Semen Prinsepiae)
Jue Ming Zi (Semen Cassiae)
Source: *San Yin Fang* [Formulae for the Three Categories of Etiological Factors]

Xie Huang San (Yellow-Draining Powder)
Huo Xiang (Herba Agastaches seu Pogostemi)
Zhi Zi (Fructus Gardeniae Jasminoidis)
Shi Gao‡ (Gypsum Fibrosum)
Gan Cao (Radix Glycyrrhizae)
Fang Feng (Radix Ledebouriellae Divaricatae)
Source: *Xiao Er Yao Zheng Zhi Jue* [Key to the Treatment of Children's Diseases]

Xin Liu Wei Pian (New Six-Ingredient Tablet)
Sheng Di Huang (Radix Rehmanniae Glutinosae)
Shan Yao (Radix Dioscoreae Oppositae)
Nü Zhen Zi (Fructus Ligustri Lucidi)
Fu Ling (Sclerotium Poriae Cocos)
Chi Shao (Radix Paeoniae Rubra)
Ze Xie (Rhizoma Alismatis Orientalis)
Source: Empirical formula

Xing Xiao Wan (Awakening and Dispersing Pill)
Ru Xiang (Gummi Olibanum)
Mo Yao (Myrrha)
*She Xiang** (Secretio Moschi)
*Xiong Jing** (Realgar Lucidum)
Source: *Wai Ke Zheng Zhi Quan Sheng Ji* [A Life-Saving Manual of the Diagnosis and Treatment of External Diseases]

Xiong Huang Jie Du San (Realgar Powder for Relieving Toxicity)
*Xiong Huang** (Realgar)
Han Shui Shi ‡ (Calcitum)
Ming Fan ‡ (Alumen)
Source: *Zheng Zhi Zhun Sheng* [Standards of Diagnosis and Treatment]

Xue Fu Zhu Yu Tang (Decoction for Expelling Stasis from the House of Blood)
Dang Gui (Radix Angelicae Sinensis)
Sheng Di Huang (Radix Rehmanniae Glutinosae)
Tao Ren (Semen Persicae)
Hong Hua (Flos Carthami Tinctorii)
Zhi Ke (Fructus Citri Aurantii)
Chi Shao (Radix Paeoniae Rubra)
Chai Hu (Radix Bupleuri)
Gan Cao (Radix Glycyrrhizae)
Jie Geng (Radix Platycodi Grandiflori)
Chuan Xiong (Rhizoma Ligustici Chuanxiong)
Huai Niu Xi (Radix Achyranthis Bidentatae)
Source: *Yi Lin Gai Cuo* [Corrections of the Errors in Medical Works]

Yang Du Sheng Ma Tang (Bugbane Decoction for Yang Toxins)
Sheng Ma (Rhizoma Cimicifugae)
Shui Niu Jiao Fen ‡ (Cornu Bubali, powdered)
She Gan (Rhizoma Belamcandae Chinensis)
Huang Qin (Radix Scutellariae Baicalensis)
Ren Shen (Radix Ginseng)
Gan Cao (Radix Glycyrrhizae)
Source: *Sheng Ji Zong Lu* [General Collection for Holy Relief]

Yang He Tang (Harmonious Yang Decoction)
Shu Di Huang (Radix Rehmanniae Glutinosae Conquita)
Rou Gui (Cortex Cinnamomi Cassiae)
*Ma Huang** (Herba Ephedrae)
Lu Jiao Jiao ‡ (Gelatinum Cornu Cervi)
Bai Jie Zi (Semen Sinapis Albae)
Pao Jiang (Rhizoma Zingiberis Officinalis Praeparata)
Gan Cao (Radix Glycyrrhizae)
Source: *Wai Ke Zheng Zhi Quan Sheng Ji* [A Life-Saving Manual of the Diagnosis and Treatment of External Diseases]

Yang Wei Tang (Nourishing the Stomach Decoction)
Hou Po (Cortex Magnoliae Officinalis)
Cang Zhu (Rhizoma Atractylodis)
Fa Ban Xia (Rhizoma Pinelliae Ternatae Praeparata)
Huo Xiang (Herba Agastaches seu Pogostemi)
Cao Guo (Fructus Amomi Tsaoko)
Ren Shen (Radix Ginseng)
Fu Ling (Sclerotium Poriae Cocos)
Gan Cao (Radix Glycyrrhizae)
Ju Hong (Pars Rubra Epicarpii Citri Erythrocarpae)
Sheng Jiang (Rhizoma Zingiberis Officinalis Recens)
Wu Mei (Fructus Pruni Mume)
Source: *Zheng Zhi Zhun Sheng* [Standards of Diagnosis and Treatment]

Ye Ju Bai Du Tang (Wild Chrysanthemum Decoction for Vanquishing Toxicity)
Ye Ju Hua (Flos Chrysanthemi Morifolii)
Xuan Shen (Radix Scrophulariae Ningpoensis)
Lian Qiao (Fructus Forsythiae Suspensae)
Zi Hua Di Ding (Herba Violae Yedoensitis)
Jin Yin Hua (Flos Lonicerae)
Pu Gong Ying (Herba Taraxaci cum Radice)
Zhe Bei Mu (Bulbus Fritillariae)
Gan Cao (Radix Glycyrrhizae)
Source: Empirical formula

Ye Qiang Wei Lu (Multiflora Rose Distillate)
Qiang Wei Hua (Flos Rosae Multiflorae)
The herb is steamed to produce 2500ml of distillate for every 500g of the dried material (also used as a mouthwash).
Source: Empirical formula

Yi Ma Er Zhi Wan (Black Sesame Double Supreme Pill)
Hei Zhi Ma (Semen Sesami Indici)
Nü Zhen Zi (Fructus Ligustri Lucidi)
Han Lian Cao (Herba Ecliptae Prostratae)
Zhi Shou Wu (Radix Polygoni Multiflori Praeparata)
Ce Bai Ye (Cacumen Biotae Orientalis)
Gou Qi Zi (Fructus Lycii)
Sheng Di Huang (Radix Rehmanniae Glutinosae)
Shu Di Huang (Radix Rehmanniae Glutinosae Conquita)
Huang Jing (Rhizoma Polygonati)
Source: *Zhao Bing Nan Lin Chuang Jing Yun Ji* [A Collection of Zhao Bingnan's Clinical Experiences]

Yi Shen Rong Fa Wan (Pill for Boosting the Kidneys and Nourishing the Hair)
Shu Di Huang (Radix Rehmanniae Glutinosae Conquita)
Zhi Shou Wu (Radix Polygoni Multiflori Praeparata)
Bu Gu Zhi (Fructus Psoraleae Corylifoliae)
Tu Si Zi (Semen Cuscutae)
Gu Sui Bu (Rhizoma Drynariae)
Chuan Xiong (Rhizoma Ligustici Chuanxiong)
Zhi Huang Qi (Radix Astragali seu Hedysari, mix-fried with honey)
Zi He Che ‡ (Placenta Hominis)
Huang Jing (Rhizoma Polygonati)
Dang Shen (Radix Codonopsitis Pilosulae)
Chen Pi (Pericarpium Citri Reticulatae)
Chao Bai Zhu (Rhizoma Atractylodis Macrocephalae, stir-fried)

Fu Ling (Sclerotium Poriae Cocos)
Zhi Gan Cao (Radix Glycyrrhizae, mix-fried with honey)
Feng Mi‡ (Mel)
Source: Empirical formula

Yin Chen Hao Tang (Oriental Wormwood Decoction)
Yin Chen Hao (Herba Artemisiae Scopariae)
Zhi Zi (Fructus Gardeniae Jasminoidis)
Da Huang (Radix et Rhizoma Rhei)
Source: *Shang Han Lun* [On Cold Damage]

Yin Hua Tang (Honeysuckle Decoction)
Jin Yin Hua (Flos Lonicerae)
Huang Qin (Radix Scutellariae Baicalensis)
Dang Gui (Radix Angelicae Sinensis)
Gan Cao (Radix Glycyrrhizae)
Gou Qi Ye (Folium Lycii)
Source: *Zhu Lin Si Nü Ke Quan Shu* [Complete Gynecology from Zhulin Temple]

Yin Le Wan (Psoriasis Happiness Pill)
Dang Gui (Radix Angelicae Sinensis)
Dan Shen (Radix Salviae Miltiorrhizae)
Ji Xue Teng (Caulis Spatholobi)
Ye Jiao Teng (Caulis Polygoni Multiflori)
Mu Dan Pi (Cortex Moutan Radicis)
Da Qing Ye (Folium Isatidis seu Baphicacanthi)
Chi Shao (Radix Paeoniae Rubra)
Bai Shao (Radix Paeoniae Lactiflorae)
San Leng (Rhizoma Sparganii Stoloniferi)
E Zhu (Rhizoma Curcumae)
Bai Hua She She Cao (Herba Hedyotidis Diffusae)
Tu Fu Ling (Rhizoma Smilacis Glabrae)
Feng Fang‡ (Nidus Vespae)
Bai Xian Pi (Cortex Dictamni Dasycarpi Radicis)
Ku Shen (Radix Sophorae Flavescentis)
Source: Empirical formula

Yin Qiao San (Honeysuckle and Forsythia Powder)
Jin Yin Hua (Flos Lonicerae)
Lian Qiao (Fructus Forsythiae Suspensae)
Jie Geng (Radix Platycodi Grandiflori)
Niu Bang Zi (Fructus Arctii Lappae)
Gan Cao (Radix Glycyrrhizae)
Dan Zhu Ye (Herba Lophatheri Gracilis)
Jing Jie (Herba Schizonepetae Tenuifoliae)
Dan Dou Chi (Semen Sojae Praeparatum)
Bo He (Herba Menthae Haplocalycis)
Lu Gen (Rhizoma Phragmitis Communis)
Source: *Wen Bing Tiao Bian* [Treatise on the Identification of Warm Diseases]

Yu Ping Feng San (Jade Screen Powder)
Huang Qin (Radix Scutellariae Baicalensis)
Bai Zhu (Rhizoma Atractylodis Macrocephalae)
Fang Feng (Radix Ledebouriellae Divaricatae)
Source: *Shi Yi De Xiao Fang* [Effective Formulae Handed Down for Generations]

Yu Quan San (Jade Spring Powder)
Shui Niu Jiao† (Cornu Bubali)
Chuan Xiong (Rhizoma Ligustici Chuanxiong)

Huang Lian (Rhizoma Coptidis)
Bing Pian (Borneolum)
Source: *Zheng Zhi Zhun Sheng* [Standards of Diagnosis and Treatment]

Zeng Ye Jie Du Tang (Decoction for Increasing Body Fluids and Relieving Toxicity)
Pu Gong Ying (Herba Taraxaci cum Radice)
Xuan Shen (Radix Scrophulariae Ningpoensis)
Jin Yin Hua (Flos Lonicerae)
Lian Qiao (Fructus Forsythiae Suspensae)
Mai Men Dong (Radix Ophiopogonis Japonici)
Sheng Di Huang (Radix Rehmanniae Glutinosae)
Gan Cao (Radix Glycyrrhizae)
Source: Empirical formula

Zeng Ye Tang (Decoction for Increasing Body Fluids)
Xuan Shen (Radix Scrophulariae Ningpoensis)
Mai Men Dong (Radix Ophiopogonis Japonici)
Sheng Di Huang (Radix Rehmanniae Glutinosae)
Source: *Wen Bing Tiao Bian* [Treatise on the Identification of Warm Diseases]

Zhi Bai Di Huang Tang [Wan] (Anemarrhena, Phellodendron and Rehmannia Decoction [Pill])
Shu Di Huang (Radix Rehmanniae Glutinosae Conquita)
Shan Zhu Yu (Fructus Corni Officinalis)
Shan Yao (Rhizoma Dioscoreae Oppositae)
Zhi Mu (Rhizoma Anemarrhenae Asphodeloidis)
Huang Bai (Cortex Phellodendri)
Mu Dan Pi (Cortex Moutan Radicis)
Fu Ling (Sclerotium Poriae Cocos)
Ze Xie (Rhizoma Alismatis Orientalis)
Source: *Yi Zong Jin Jian* [The Golden Mirror of Medicine]

Zhi Zi Qin Hua Wan (Gardenia, Scutellaria and Trichosanthes Root Pill)
Zhi Zi (Fructus Gardeniae Jasminoidis)
Huang Qin (Radix Scutellariae Baicalensis)
Jiu Da Huang (Radix et Rhizoma Rhei, mix-fried with wine)
Huang Bai (Cortex Phellodendri)
Tian Hua Fen (Radix Trichosanthis)
Zhi Mu (Rhizoma Anemarrhenae Asphodeloidis)
Huang Lian (Rhizoma Coptidis)
Source: *He Jian Liu Shu* [He Jian's Works]

Zi Yin Chu Shi Tang (Decoction for Enriching Yin and Eliminating Dampness)
Sheng Di Huang (Radix Rehmanniae Glutinosae)
Xuan Shen (Radix Scrophulariae Ningpoensis)
Dang Gui (Radix Angelicae Sinensis)
Dan Shen (Radix Salviae Miltiorrhizae)
Fu Ling (Sclerotium Poriae Cocos)
Ze Xie (Rhizoma Alismatis Orientalis)
Bai Xian Pi (Cortex Dictamni Dasycarpi Radicis)
She Chuang Zi (Fructus Cnidii Monnieri)
Source: *Zhu Ren Kang Lin Chuang Jing Yan Ji* [A Collection of Zhu Renkang's Clinical Experiences]

Zi Yin Yang Yin Tang (Decoction for Enriching and Nourishing Yin)
Dang Gui (Radix Angelicae Sinensis)

Sheng Di Huang (Radix Rehmanniae Glutinosae)
Chuan Xiong (Rhizoma Ligustici Chuanxiong)
Bai Shao (Radix Paeoniae Lactiflorae)
Bei Sha Shen (Radix Glehniae Littoralis)
Xuan Shen (Radix Scrophulariae Ningpoensis)
Bai Xian Pi (Cortex Dictamni Dasycarpi Radicis)
Ku Shen (Radix Sophorae Flavescentis)
Source: Empirical formula

Zuo Gui Yin (Restoring the Left [Kidney Yin] Beverage)
Shu Di Huang (Radix Rehmanniae Glutinosae Conquita)

Shan Yao (Rhizoma Dioscoreae Oppositae)
Gou Qi Zi (Fructus Lycii)
Shan Zhu Yu (Fructus Corni Officinalis)
Niu Xi (Radix Achyranthis Bidentatae)
Tu Si Zi (Semen Cuscutae)
Lu Jiao Jiao‡ (Gelatinum Cornu Cervi)
Gui Ban Jiao* (Gelatinum Plastri Testudinis)
Source: *Jing Yue Quan Shu* [The Complete Works of Zhang Jingyue]

Note

Animal, insect and mineral materia medica are marked with the symbol ‡; materia medica whose use may be restricted in certain countries are marked with the symbol *. Please refer to the author's preface for further details.

TCM external formulae used in the treatment of skin disorders

This appendix lists the ingredients of external applications referred to by name only in the text. Preparation methods are also included where appropriate; where powder preparations are involved, unless otherwise indicated, the ingredients are ground together to produce a fine powder. Some of these external applications are available through materia medica suppliers; others require preparation by the practitioner.

A small number of the external formulae listed below may contain ingredients whose use may not be permitted in certain countries outside China (marked with *). Where possible, alternatives for these preparations have been suggested in the text. However, in certain instances, notably in case histories and modern clinical experience reports, the original formulae have also been retained to give practitioners an insight into the way the particular condition involved would be treated in China.

Practitioners should always check the contents of any patent medicines or other commercially available preparations to ensure that they comply with the legal requirements of the country in which they practice.

Ba Hen Ruan Hua Gao (Softening Scar Paste)
Zinc oxide ‡ 500g
Gelatin 500g
Glycerin 500g
Wu Bei Zi ‡ (Galla Rhois Chinensis) 750g
Wu Gong ‡ (Scolopendra Subspinipes) 10 pieces
Bing Pian (Borneolum) 50g
Zhang Nao (Camphora) 50g
Water 500-1000ml
Preparation: Mix the zinc oxide ‡, gelatin and glycerin with water to prepare a zinc oxide ointment; grind the materia medica into a fine powder and add to the ointment to produce a thick paste.
Source: *Xin Yi Yao Xue Za Zhi* [New Medicine and Pharmacology Journal]

Ba Jia Gao (Nail-Removing Plaster)
Bi Ma Zi (Semen Ricini) 45g
She Tui ‡ (Exuviae Serpentis) 15g
Tian Nan Xing (Rhizoma Arisaematis) 45g
Hua Jiao (Pericarpium Zanthoxyli) 30g
Da Feng Zi (Semen Hydnocarpi) 30g
*Chuan Wu** (Radix Aconiti Carmichaeli) 18g
Wu Mei (Fructus Pruni Mume) 30g
Zao Jiao (Fructus Gleditsiae Sinensis) 45g
Di Fu Zi (Fructus Kochiae Scopariae) 30g
Xing Ren (Semen Pruni Armeniacae) 30g
Wei Ling Xian (Radix Clematidis) 30g
Feng Xian Zi (Semen Impatientis Balsaminae) 120g
Qian Jin Zi (Semen Euphorbiae Lathyridis) 45g
Wu Jia Pi (Cortex Acanthopanacis Gracilistyli Radicis) 45g
Jiang Can ‡ (Bombyx Batryticatus) 30g
*Cao Wu** (Radix Aconiti Kusnezoffii) 18g
Feng Xian Hua (Flos Impatientis Balsaminae) 60g
Di Gu Pi (Cortex Lycii Radicis) 45g
Xiang You (Oleum Sesami Seminis) 1500ml
Nao Sha ‡ (Sal Ammoniacum) 60g
Qian Dan ‡ (Minium) 60g
Preparation: Fry all the materia medica with the exception of the last two in the sesame oil until they turn black and the concentrated oil no longer adheres to the fingers. Then add *Qian Dan* ‡ (Minium) and *Nao Sha* ‡ (Sal Ammoniacum) to the oil to produce the plaster.
Source: *Zhong Yi Wai Ke Xue* [External Diseases in Traditional Chinese Medicine, Zhu Renkang]

Bai Bu Ding (Stemona Root Tincture)
Bai Bu (Radix Stemonae) 180g
75% Alcohol 360ml
Preparation: Grind *Bai Bu* (Radix Stemonae) into a powder and soak the powder in the alcohol for seven days. After filtration, the liquid is stored for use.
Source: *Zhao Bing Nan Lin Chuang Jing Yan Ji* [A Collection of Zhao Bingnan's Clinical Experiences]
Note: This preparation is also known as *Bai Bu Jiu* (Stemona Wine).

Bai Xie Feng Ding (Seborrhea Tincture)
She Chuang Zi (Fructus Cnidii Monnieri) 40g
Ku Shen (Radix Sophorae Flavescentis) 40g
Tu Jin Pi (Cortex Pseudolaricis) 20g
Bo He Nao (Menthol) 10g
Preparation: Grind the herbs into a coarse powder and soak them in 80ml of 75% alcohol for 6 hours. An extract of the herbs is then obtained through percolation with 920ml of 75% alcohol; this procedure is repeated until a tincture of 1,000ml is obtained. The menthol is added to the tincture at the end.
Source: *Zhong Yi Wai Ke Lin Chuang Shou Ce* [A Clinical Handbook of External Diseases in Chinese Medicine]

Bai Zhi Shui Xi Ji (White Angelica Root Wash Preparation)
Bai Zhi (Radix Angelicae Dahuricae) 60g
Hou Po (Cortex Magnoliae Officinalis) 30g
Man Jing Zi (Fructus Viticis) 15g

Preparation: Soak the herbs in 1000ml of cold water for 30 minutes, then bring to the boil and decoct for 20 minutes. Remove the residue and allow the decoction to cool to luke-warm before using as an external wash.
Source: Empirical formula from the author's hospital

Ban Mao Cu Jin Ji (Mylabris Vinegar Steep Preparation)
Quan Xie‡ (Buthus Martensi) 16 pieces
Ban Mao‡ (Mylabris) 12 pieces
Po Xiao‡ (Mirabilitum Non-Purum) 12g
Wu Mei (Fructus Pruni Mume) 30g
Mi Cu (Acetum Oryzae) 500ml
Preparation: Steep the materia medica in the vinegar for 7 days. Filter off the liquid, which is then ready for use. Do not use on severely inflamed skin or wounds.
Source: *Zhang Zhi Li Pi Fu Bing Yi An Xuan Cui* [A Collection of Zhang Zhili's Skin Disease Cases]

Bing Huang San (Borneol, Cat-Tail Pollen and Phellodendron Powder)
Bing Pian (Borneolum) 0.9g
Huang Bai (Cortex Phellodendri) 6g
Pu Huang (Pollen Typhae) 6g
Ren Zhong Bai‡ (Sedimentum Urinae Hominis) 3g
Gan Cao (Radix Glycyrrhizae) 6g
Qing Dai (Indigo Naturalis) 1.5g
Po Xiao‡ (Mirabilitum Non-Purum) 1.5g
Peng Sha‡ (Borax) 1.5g
Huang Lian (Rhizoma Coptidis) 6g
Bo He (Herba Menthae Haplocalycis) 6g
Ku Fan‡ (Alumen Praeparatum) 0.5g
Source: *Yan Hou Jing Yan Mi Chuan* [Secret Empirical Prescriptions in the Treatment of Throat Diseases]

Bing Liu San (Borneol and Sulfur Powder)
Liu Huang‡ (Sulphur) 9g
Zhang Nao (Camphor) 6g
Chuan Jiao (Pericarpium Zanthoxyli) 6g
Ming Fan‡ (Alumen) 6g
Source: *Wai Ke Zheng Zong* [An Orthodox Manual of External Diseases]

Bing Pian Lu Gan Shi Xi Ji (Borneol and Calamine Wash Preparation)
Bing Pian (Borneolum) 1g
Lu Gan Shi‡ (Calamina) 15g
Zinc oxide‡ 10g
Glycerin 5ml
Preparation: Mix the ingredients with enough water to produce 100ml of solution.
Source: *Zhang Zhi Li Pi Fu Bing Yi An Xuan Cui* [A Collection of Zhang Zhili's Skin Disease Cases]

Bing Shi San (Borneol and Gypsum Powder)
Duan Shi Gao‡ (Gypsum Fibrosum Calcinatum) 30g
Bing Pian (Borneolum) 0.6g
Preparation: Grind the ingredients into a very fine powder (the finer the better) and mix them thoroughly, store in an airtight jar and seal firmly. Apply the powder to the affected area and cover with a paste, cream or ointment if required.
Source: Empirical formula from the author's hospital

Bo Jie Tang (Peppermint and Schizonepeta Decoction)
Bo He (Herba Menthae Haplocalycis) 30g
Jing Jie (Herba Schizonepetae Tenuifoliae) 30g
Ku Shen (Radix Sophorae Flavescentis) 30g
Preparation: Soak the herbs in 1000ml of water for 30 minutes, then boil for 20 minutes. Use lukewarm as an external wash.
Source: *Wai Ke Mi Lu* [Secret Records of External Diseases]

Cang Fu Shui Xi Ji (Atractylodes and Broom Cypress Wash Preparation)
Cang Er Zi (Fructus Xanthii Sibirici) 15g
Di Fu Zi (Fructus Kochiae Scopariae) 15g
Tu Jin Pi (Cortex Pseudolaricis) 15g
She Chuang Zi (Fructus Cnidii Monnieri) 15g
Ku Shen (Radix Sophorae Flavescentis) 15g
Bai Bu (Radix Stemonae) 15g
Ku Fan‡ (Alumen Praeparatum) 6g
Preparation: Place the materia medica in 1000ml of cold water and boil until 500ml of concentrated decoction remains. Filter off the decoction for application as an external wash.
Source: *Zhang Zhi Li Pi Fu Bing Lin Chuang Jing Yan Ji Yao* [A Collection of Zhang Zhili's Clinical Experiences in the Treatment of Skin Diseases]

Cang Wu Cuo Yao (Xanthium and Clamshell Massage Preparation)
Cang Er Zi (Fructus Xanthii Sibirici) 60g
Chu Tao Ye (Folium Broussonetiae) 60g
Wei Ling Xian (Radix Clematidis) 60g
Ding Xiang (Flos Caryophylli) 60g
Hai Piao Xiao‡ (Os Sepiae seu Sepiellae) 120g
Water 4000-5000ml
Preparation: Grind the herbs into a coarse powder and add to the water with *Hai Piao Xiao*‡ (Os Sepiae seu Sepiellae). Bring to the boil and simmer for two hours. Then take out *Hai Piao Xiao*‡ (Os Sepiae seu Sepiellae) and use to rub the lesion gently. Application of an ointment such as *Huang Lian Ruan Gao* (Coptis Ointment) after the massage increases the effectiveness of the treatment.
Source: Empirical formula

Chong He Gao (Harmonious Flow Paste)
Chao Zi Jing Pi (Cortex Cercis, stir-fried) 300g
Du Huo (Radix Angelicae Pubescentis) 180g
Chi Shao (Radix Paeoniae Rubra) 120g
Bai Zhi (Radix Angelicae Dahuricae) 60g
Shi Chang Pu (Rhizoma Acori Graminei) 90g
Preparation: Grind the ingredients to a fine powder and mix to a paste with Vaseline® in a ratio of 1:4.
Source: *Wai Ke Zheng Zong* [An Orthodox Manual of External Diseases]

Chong He San (Harmonious Flow Powder)
Chao Zi Jing Pi (Cortex Cercis, stir-fried) 300g
Du Huo (Radix Angelicae Pubescentis) 180g
Chi Shao (Radix Paeoniae Rubra) 120g
Bai Zhi (Radix Angelicae Dahuricae) 60g
Shi Chang Pu (Rhizoma Acori Graminei) 90g
Source: *Wai Ke Zheng Zong* [An Orthodox Manual of External Diseases]

Cong Bai Tang (Scallion Decoction)
Cong Bai (Bulbus Allii Fistulosi) 20g
Chen Pi (Pericarpium Citri Reticulatae) 20g
Dong Kui Zi (Semen Malvae Verticillatae) 40g
Preparation: Steep the ingredients in 1000ml of water for 30 minutes, then boil for 20 minutes. Use the decoction as a soak when warm.
Source: *Quan Sheng Zhi Mi Fang* [A Guide to Secret Prescriptions for a Lifetime]

Cu Pao Fang (Vinegar Soak Formula)
Jing Jie (Herba Schizonepetae Tenuifoliae) 18g
Fang Feng (Radix Ledebouriellae Divaricatae) 18g
Hong Hua (Flos Carthami Tinctorii) 18g
Di Gu Pi (Cortex Lycii Radicis) 18g
Zao Jiao (Fructus Gleditsiae Sinensis) 30g
Da Feng Zi (Semen Hydnocarpi) 30g
Ming Fan‡ (Alumen) 18g
Mi Cu (Acetum Oryzae) 1500ml
Preparation: Soak the materia medica in the rice vinegar for 3-5 days; remove the residue and the liquid is ready for use.
Source: *Zhu Ren Kang Lin Chuang Jing Yan Ji* [A Collection of Zhu Renkang's Clinical Experiences]

Cuo Chuang Xi Ji (Acne Wash Preparation)
Liu Huang‡ (Sulphur) 6g
Zhang Nao (Camphora) 10g
Xi Huang Qi Jiao (Gummi Tragacanthi) 1g
Lime water‡ 100ml
Preparation: Grind the dry ingredients to a powder and mix thoroughly in the lime water. Wash the affected area with warm water before applying the lotion.
Source: *Zhong Yi Wai Ke Xue* [External Diseases in Traditional Chinese Medicine, Zhu Renkang]

Da Huang San (Rhubarb Powder)
Da Huang (Radix et Rhizoma Rhei)
Cang Zhu (Rhizoma Atractylodis)
Huang Bai (Cortex Phellodendri)
Preparation: Grind equal quantities of the ingredients to a fine powder and mix thoroughly.
Source: *Zhong Yi Pi Fu Ke Zhen Liao Xue* [Diagnosis and Treatment of Skin Diseases with Chinese Medicine]

Dan Huang You (Egg Yolk Oil)
Hen's eggs‡ 10-15
Preparation: Hard-boil the eggs and allow them to cool. Separate the yokes and cook over a low heat in a wok with one teaspoonful of vegetable oil until black egg yolk oil gradually separates.
Source: Empirical formula

Dang Gui Gao (Chinese Angelica Root Paste)
Dang Gui (Radix Angelicae Sinensis) 200g
Xiang You (Oleum Sesami Seminis) 500ml
Huang La‡ (Cera Aurea) 20g
Preparation: Fry *Dang Gui* (Radix Angelicae Sinensis) in the sesame oil until it turns dark yellow. Remove the residue and add the wax to the warm oil to produce a paste.
Source: *Zhong Yi Wai Ke Xue* [External Diseases in Traditional Chinese Medicine, Zhu Renkang]

Di Hu Hu (Sanguisorba and Giant Knotweed Paste)
Di Yu (Radix Sanguisorbae Officinalis)
Hu Zhang (Radix et Rhizoma Polygoni Cuspidati)
Preparation: Grind equal quantities of the ingredients into a fine powder and mix with Vaseline® in the ratio of 1:3 to produce a 25% paste.
Source: Empirical formula

Di Hu San (Sanguisorba and Giant Knotweed Powder)
Di Yu (Radix Sanguisorbae Officinalis)
Hu Zhang (Radix et Rhizoma Polygoni Cuspidati)
Preparation: Grind equal quantities of the ingredients into a fine powder and mix thoroughly.
Source: Empirical formula

Di Long Pian (Earthworm Tablet)
Di Long‡ (Lumbricus)
Preparation: Grind *Di Long*‡ (Lumbricus) into a powder to make tablets with a vehicle. Each tablet consists of *Di Long* (Lumbricus) 0.3g.
Source: Empirical formula

Di Yu Shi Fu Tang (Sanguisorba Wet Compress Decoction)
Di Yu (Radix Sanguisorbae Officinalis) 30g
Ce Bai Ye (Cacumen Biotae Orientalis) 30g
Ma Chi Xian (Herba Portulacae Oleraceae) 30g
Preparation: Soak the herbs in 800ml of water for 30 minutes and then boil for 20 minutes. Remove the residue and use the liquid as a wash or wet compress.
Source: Empirical formula

Dian Dao San (Reversal Powder)
Da Huang (Radix et Rhizoma Rhei)
Liu Huang‡ (Sulphur)
Preparation: Grind equal quantities of the ingredients into a fine powder and mix thoroughly.
Source: *Yi Zong Jin Jian* [The Golden Mirror of Medicine]

Dian Dao San Xi Ji (Reversal Powder Wash Preparation)
Da Huang (Radix et Rhizoma Rhei) 7.5g
Liu Huang‡ (Sulphur) 7.5g
Hua Shi‡ (Talcum) 10g
Preparation: Grind *Da Huang* (Radix et Rhizoma Rhei) and *Liu Huang*‡ (Sulphur) into a fine powder and mix thoroughly. Add 100ml of water to *Hua Shi*‡ (Talcum) and shake until the solution is clear, then add to the powdered ingredients.
Source: *Zhong Yi Wai Ke Xue* [External Diseases in Traditional Chinese Medicine, Zhu Renkang]

Ding Gui San (Clove and Cinnamon Powder)
Ding Xiang (Flos Caryophylli)
Rou Gui (Cortex Cinnamomi Cassiae)
Preparation: Grind equal quantities of the ingredients into a fine powder and mix thoroughly.
Source: *Wai Ke Chuan Xin Ji* [Inherited Secrets of External Diseases]

Dong Chong Xia Cao Jiu (Cordyceps Wine)
Dong Chong Xia Cao‡ (Cordyceps Sinensis) 60g
75% Alcohol 250ml
Preparation: Soak *Dong Chong Xia Cao*‡ (Cordyceps Sinensis) in alcohol for 7 days.

Source: *Zhao Bing Nan Lin Chuang Jing Yan Ji* [A Collection of Zhao Bingnan's Clinical Experiences]

Dong Chuang Gao (Frostbite Paste)
Feng Mi ‡ (Mel) 50%
Zhu Zhi ‡ (Adeps Suis) 30%
Zhang Nao (Camphora) 20%
Preparation: Grind *Zhang Nao* (Camphora) to a fine powder and mix well with the lard and honey to produce a paste (percentages refer to weight).
Source: *Zhong Yi Wai Ke Xue* [External Diseases in Traditional Chinese Medicine, Zhu Renkang]

Dong Fan San (Minium and Alum Powder)
Qian Dan ‡ (Minium)
Ming Fan ‡ (Alumen)
Preparation: Grind equal quantities of the ingredients into a powder.
Source: *Zhong Yi Wai Ke Xue* [External Diseases in Traditional Chinese Medicine, Zhu Renkang]

Dong Fang Yi Hao Yao Gao (Oriental Medicated Plaster No. 1)
Mao Zhu (Rhizoma Atractylodis Maoshanense) 30g
Huang Bai (Cortex Phellodendri) 30g
Han Fang Ji * (Radix Stephaniae Tetrandrae) 30g
Mu Gua (Fructus Chaenomelis) 30g
Yan Hu Suo (Rhizoma Corydalis Yanhusuo) 30g
Yu Jin (Radix Curcumae) 30g
Sheng Di Yu (Radix Sanguisorbae Officinalis Recens) 30g
Bai Ji (Rhizoma Bletillae Striatae) 60g
Duan Shi Gao ‡ (Gypsum Fibrosum Calcinatum) 240g
Lu Gan Shi ‡ (Calamina) 240g
Bing Pian (Borneolum) 3g
Xiang You (Oleum Sesami Seminis) 1000g
Preparation: Soak the first eight materia medica in the sesame oil for 24 hours and boil over a low heat for 2-2.5 hours or until the herbs turn dark yellow. Remove the residue and filter off the oil. Heat the filtered oil over a low heat for another 2-2.5 hours or until a drop of oil forms a pearl in water. While the oil is still very hot, add finely powdered *Duan Shi Gao* ‡ (Gypsum Fibrosum Calcinatum) and *Lu Gan Shi* ‡ (Calamina), stirring all the time while adding. Boil for 2-2.5 hours. After the mixture cools down, add *Bing Pian* (Borneolum) and stir until smooth.
Source: *Shi Yong Zhong Yi Wai Ke Xue* [Practical Treatment of External Diseases with Traditional Chinese Medicine]

Du Jiao Lian Gao (Giant Typhonium Paste)
Bai Fu Zi (Rhizoma Typhonii Gigantei) 45g
Bai Zhi (Radix Angelicae Dahuricae) 45g
Zao Jiao (Fructus Gleditsiae Sinensis) 45g
Fang Ji * (Radix Stephaniae Tetrandrae) 45g
Lian Qiao (Fructus Forsythiae Suspensae) 45g
Chuan Shan Jia * (Squama Manitis Pentadactylae) 45g
Jin Yin Hua (Flos Lonicerae) 45g
Dang Gui (Radix Angelicae Sinensis) 45g
Hai Tong Pi (Cortex Erythrinae) 45g
Sheng Nan Xing (Rhizoma Arisaematis Crudum) 45g
Su Mu (Lignum Sappan) 45g
Ci Wei Pi ‡ (Pellis Erinacei) 45g
Hai Dai (Herba Zosterae Marinae) 45g

Huo Ma Ren (Semen Cannabis Sativae) 45g
Xue Yu Tan ‡ (Crinis Carbonisatus Hominis) 45g
Xi Xian Cao (Herba Siegesbeckiae) 45g
Gan Chan ‡ (Bufo Siccus) 3 pieces
Ru Xiang (Gummi Olibanum) 36g
Mo Yao (Myrrha) 36g
Xiang You (Oleum Sesami Seminis) 6000ml
Preparation: Grind all the dry ingredients to a fine powder and mix to a paste with the sesame oil.
Source: *Zhong Yi Wai Ke Xue* [External Diseases in Traditional Chinese Medicine, Zhu Renkang]
Note: *Du Jiao Lian* is an alternative name for *Bai Fu Zi*.

Du Sheng Gao (Single Garlic Paste)
Da Suan (Herba Allii Sativi) whole head
Preparation: Pound the head of garlic into a paste, leave to dry in the sun and store in a jar for use in winter.
Source: *Wai Ke Zheng Zong* [An Orthodox Manual of External Diseases]

E Huang San (Light Yellow Powder)
Lü Dou Fen (Semen Phaseoli Radiati, powdered) 30g
Duan Shi Gao ‡ (Gypsum Fibrosum) 15g
Huang Bai (Cortex Phellodendri) 9g
Qing Fen * (Calomelas) 6g
Source: *Wai Ke Zheng Zong* [An Orthodox Manual of External Diseases]

E Kou San (Goose-Mouth Sore Powder)
Han Shui Shi ‡ (Calcitum) 3g
Huang Lian (Rhizoma Coptidis) 3g
Qing Dai (Indigo Naturalis) 2g
Peng Sha ‡ (Borax) 0.1g
Bing Pian (Borneolum) 0.5g
Source: *Zhang Zhi Li Pi Fu Bing Lin Chuang Jing Yan Ji Yao* [A Collection of Zhang Zhili's Clinical Experiences in the Treatment of Skin Diseases]

E Zhang Feng Jin Pao Ji (Soak Preparation for Goose-Foot Wind)
Da Feng Zi (Semen Hydnocarpi) 9g
Yan Gao (Depositum Pipae) 9g
Hua Jiao (Pericarpium Zanthoxyli) 9g
Wu Jia Pi (Cortex Acanthopanacis Gracilistyli Radicis) 9g
Zao Jiao (Fructus Gleditsiae Sinensis) 5g
Di Gu Pi (Cortex Lycii Radicis) 9g
She Tui ‡ (Exuviae Serpentis) one piece
Ming Fan ‡ (Alumen) 12g
Xian Feng Xian Hua (Flos Impatientis Balsaminae Recens) 9g
Preparation: Soak the ingredients in vinegar for one day. Remove the residue and soak the affected area in the liquid.
Source: Empirical formula of Shanghai College of TCM

E Zhang Feng Xuan Yao Shui (Goose-Foot Wind Tinea Lotion)
Bai Bu (Radix Stemonae) 125g
She Chang Zi (Fructus Cnidii Monnieri) 125g
Da Feng Zi (Semen Hydnocarpi) 125g
Tu Jin Pi (Cortex Pseudolaricis) 250g
Tou Gu Cao (Herba Speranskiae seu Impatientis) 125g
Hua Jiao (Pericarpium Zanthoxyli) 125g

Ban Mao ‡ (Mylabris) 3g
Fang Feng (Radix Ledebouriellae Divaricatae) 50g
Wu Zhu Yu (Fructus Evodiae Rutaecarpae) 50g
Dang Gui (Radix Angelicae Sinensis) 100g
Ce Bai Ye (Cacumen Biotae Orientalis) 100g
Chan Tui ‡ (Periostracum Cicadae) 75g
Mi Cu (Acetum Oryzae) 1000ml
Preparation: Soak the herbs in the vinegar for one day. Remove the residue and apply the liquid to the affected area.
Source: *Zhong Yi Wai Ke Xue* [External Diseases in Traditional Chinese Medicine, Zhu Renkang]

E Zhang Feng Zhi Yang Fen (Powder for Alleviating Goose-Foot Wind Itching)
Zhang Nao (Camphora) 6g
Peng Sha ‡ (Borax) 30g
Ku Fan ‡ (Alumen Praeparatum) 30g
Bing Pian (Borneolum) 6g
Xiong Huang * (Realgar) 20g
Source: *Zhong Yi Wai Ke Xue* [External Diseases in Traditional Chinese Medicine, Zhu Renkang]

Er Bai San (Two Whites Powder)
Bai Shi Zhi ‡ (Kaolin) 9g
Bai Lian (Radix Ampelopsis Japonicae) 9g
Xing Ren (Semen Pruni Armeniacae) 9g
Preparation: Grind the ingredients to a fine powder and mix thoroughly. This powder is often mixed with egg white for application.
Source: *Zhao Bing Nan Lin Chuang Jing Yan Ji* [A Collection of Zhao Bingnan's Clinical Experiences]

Er Fan San (Alum and Melanterite Powder)
Bai Fan ‡ (Alumen) 36g
Zao Fan ‡ (Melanteritum) 36g
Er Cha (Pasta Acaciae seu Uncariae) 15g
Ce Bai Ye (Cacumen Biotae Orientalis) 250g
Source: *Wai Ke Da Cheng* [A Compendium of External Diseases]

Fei Chuang Gao (Fat Sore Paste)
Ma Qian Zi * (Semen Nux-Vomicae) 18g
Dang Gui (Radix Angelicac Sinensis) 15g
Li Lu (Radix et Rhizoma Veratri) 15g
Huang Bai (Cortex Phellodendri) 9g
Ku Shen (Radix Sophorae Flavescentis) 9g
Xing Ren (Semen Pruni Armeniacae) 9g
Lang Du (Radix Euphorbiae Fischerianae) 9g
Bai Fu Zi (Rhizoma Typhonii Gigantei) 9g
Yu Dan ‡ (Vesica Fellea Piscis) 2 pieces
Xiang You (Oleum Sesami Seminis) 500ml
Huang La ‡ (Cera Aurea) 3.5g
Preparation: Stir fry the dry ingredients in the sesame oil until dark brown, then remove the residue. Melt the wax thoroughly in the oil, then filter to produce a paste to be stored in an airtight jar.
Source: *Yi Zong Jin Jian* [The Golden Mirror of Medicine]

Fei Zi Fen (Miliaria Powder)
Hua Shi ‡ (Talcum) 30g
Lu Gan Shi ‡ (Calamina) 15g
Huang Bai (Cortex Phellodendri) 6g

Bo He (Herba Menthae Haplocalycis) 3g
Bing Pian (Borneolum) 3g
Source: *Zhang Zhi Li Pi Fu Bing Yi An Xuan Cui* [A Collection of Zhang Zhili's Skin Disease Cases]

Feng Fang Gao (Hornet Nest Paste)
Feng Fang ‡ (Nidus Vespae) 30g
She Tui ‡ (Exuviae Serpentis) 30g
Xuan Shen (Radix Scrophulariae Ningpoensis) 50g
She Chuang Zi (Fructus Cnidii Monnieri) 30g
Huang Qin (Radix Scutellariae Baicalensis) 30g
Xing Ren (Semen Pruni Armeniacae) 30g
Xue Yu ‡ (Crinis Hominis) 10g
Xiang You (Oleum Sesami Seminis) 500ml
Mi La ‡ (Cera) 3.5g
Preparation: Stir fry the dry ingredients in the sesame oil until dark brown, then remove the residue. Melt the wax thoroughly in the oil, then filter to produce a paste to be stored in an airtight jar.
Source: *Zheng Zhi Zhun Sheng* [Standards of Diagnosis and Treatment]

Fu Fang Tu Jin Pi Ding (Compound Golden Larch Bark Tincture)
Tu Jin Pi (Cortex Pseudolaricis) 10g
80% Alcohol 100ml
Benzoic acid 12g
Salicylic acid 6g
75% Alcohol 100ml
Preparation: Grind *Tu Jin Pi* (Cortex Pseudolaricis) to a coarse powder and soak it in the 80% alcohol for 24 hours. Remove the residue and filter off the tincture. Dissolve the benzoic and salicylic acids in 30ml of 75% alcohol, then mix in the tincture before adding the rest of the alcohol.
Source: *Zhong Yi Wai Ke Xue* [External Diseases in Traditional Chinese Medicine, Zhu Renkang]

Fu Long Gan San (Oven Earth Powder)
Zao Xin Tu (Terra Flava Usta)
Source: *Wai Ke Qi Xuan* [Revelations of the Mystery of External Diseases]

Fu Ping Cu (Duckweed Vinegar Preparation)
Fang Feng (Radix Ledebouriellae Divaricatae) 10g
Jing Jie (Herba Schizonepetae Tenuifoliae) 10g
Sheng Chuan Wu * (Radix Aconiti Carmichaeli Cruda) 10g
Sheng Cao Wu * (Radix Aconiti Kusnezoffii Cruda) 10g
Wei Ling Xian (Radix Clematidis) 10g
Qiang Huo (Rhizoma et Radix Notopterygii) 10g
Du Huo (Radix Angelicae Pubescentis) 10g
Ya Zao (Fructus Parvus Gleditsiae Sinensis) 10g
Fu Ping (Herba Spirodelae Polyrrhizae) 12-15g
Jiang Can ‡ (Bombyx Batryticatus) 12-15g
Huang Jing (Rhizoma Polygonati) 12-15g
Xian Feng Xian (Herba Impatientis Balsaminae Recens) one stalk, with the root removed
Chen Cu (Acetum Vetum) 1000ml
Preparation: Soak the ingredients in the vinegar for 24 hours. Cook the mixture over a very low heat until boiling. Remove the residue and store the preparation in an airtight container.
Source: Empirical formula from the author's hospital

***Fu Rong Gao* (Cotton Rose Flower Paste)**
Huang Bai (Cortex Phellodendri) 10g
Huang Qin (Radix Scutellariae Baicalensis) 10g
Huang Lian (Rhizoma Coptidis) 10g
Da Huang (Radix et Rhizoma Rhei) 10g
Fu Rong Ye (Folium Hibisci Mutabilis) 10g
Ze Lan (Herba Lycopi Lucidi) 10g
Preparation: Grind the ingredients to a fine powder and mix with Vaseline® to obtain a 20 percent paste.
Source: *Zhao Bing Nan Lin Chuang Jing Yan Ji* [A Collection of Zhao Bingnan's Clinical Experiences]

***Fu Yang San* (Skin Ulcer Powder)**
Available only from the Pharmaceutical Factory of Nanjing University

***Gan Cao You* (Licorice Oil)**
Gan Cao (Radix Glycyrrhizae) 10g
Vegetable oil 100ml
Preparation: Soak *Gan Cao* (Radix Glycyrrhizae) in the oil for 24 hours, then cook over a low heat until the herb turns dark yellow. Remove the residue and retain the oil.
Source: *Zhang Zhi Li Pi Fu Bing Yi An Xuan Cui* [A Collection of Zhang Zhili's Skin Disease Cases]

***Gan Ge Shui Xi Ji* (Kudzu Vine Root Wash Preparation)**
See *Ge Gen Shui Xi Ji* (Kudzu Vine Root Wash Preparation)

***Gan Lan San* (Chinese Olive Powder)**
Chao Gan Lan (Fructus Canarii Albi, stir-fried) 10g
Ren Zhong Huang‡ (Radix Glycyrrhizae cum Excremento Hominis Praeparatum) 2g
Source: Empirical formula

***Gan Shi San* (Calamine Powder)**
Lu Gan Shi‡ (Calamina) 30g
Shi Jue Ming‡ (Concha Haliotidis) 30g
Duan Long Gu‡ (Os Draconis Calcinatum) 30g
Shi Gao‡ (Gypsum Fibrosum) 60g
Song Hua Fen (Pollen Pini) 60g
Ku Fan‡ (Alumen Praeparatum) 15g
Bing Pian (Borneolum) 6g
Source: *Zhong Yi Pi Fu Bing Ke Lin Chuang Shou Ce* [A Clinical Manual of Dermatology in Chinese Medicine]

***Ge Gen Shui Xi Ji* (Kudzu Vine Root Wash Preparation)**
Ge Gen (Radix Puerariae) 30g
Ming Fan‡ (Alumen) 15g
Preparation: Decoct the ingredients in 500ml of water for 20 minutes, then use the decoction as a wash for the affected areas.
Source: *Yang Yi Da Quan* [The Complete Book of External Diseases]

***Gou Ji Shui Xi Ji* (Cibot Wash Preparation)**
Gou Ji (Rhizoma Cibotii Barometz) 30g
Chen Pi (Pericarpium Citri Reticulatae) 30g
*Xi Xin** (Herba cum Radice Asari) 15g
Xiang Fu (Rhizoma Cyperi Rotundi) 15g
Preparation: Decoct the ingredients in 700ml of water and boil down to make 500ml of decoction, which is used to soak the affected area for 10-15 minutes two or three times a day.
Source: Empirical formula

***Gu Yue Fen* (Ancient Moon Powder)**
Hu Jiao (Fructus Piperis)
Source: Empirical formula

***Gui Ban San* (Tortoise Plastron Powder)**
*Gui Ban** (Plastrum Testudinis) 620g
Huang Lian (Rhizoma Coptidis) 30g
*Hong Fen** (Hydrogyrum Oxidatum Crudum Rubrum) 15g
Bing Pian (Borneolum) 3g
Source: *Zhang Zhi Li Pi Fu Bing Lin Chuang Jing Yan Ji Yao* [A Collection of Zhang Zhili's Clinical Experiences in the Treatment of Skin Diseases]

***Gui Zhi Ban Mao Ding* (Cinnamon Twig and Mylabris Tincture)**
Gui Zhi (Ramulus Cinnamomi Cassiae) 12g
Gan Jiang (Rhizoma Zingiberis Officinalis) 10g
Chuan Xiong (Rhizoma Ligustici Chuanxiong) 5g
Ban Mao‡ (Mylabris) 3g
50% Alcohol 85-100ml
Glycerin 1 teaspoon
Preparation: Grind the materia medica into a coarse powder and steep in the alcohol for 7-10 days. Filter off the liquid and mix with the glycerin. Store in an airtight container.
Source: Empirical formula

***Han Ban Ca Ji* (Sweat Macules Rub Preparation)**
*Mi Tuo Seng** (Lithargyrum) 30g
Liu Huang‡ (Sulphur) 30g
Bai Fu Zi (Rhizoma Typhonii Gigantei) 15g
Preparation: Grind the ingredients into a fine powder. The powder is then mixed to a paste with vinegar and applied to the affected area with a cucumber stalk or cotton wool wrapped in gauze.
Source: *Zhu Ren Kang Lin Chuang Jing Yan Ji* [A Collection of Zhu Renkang's Clinical Experiences]

***Hei Bu Yao Gao* (Black Cloth Medicated Paste)**
Lao Hei Cu (Acetum Atrum Vetum) 2500ml
Wu Bei Zi‡ (Galla Rhois Chinensis) 840g
Wu Gong‡ (Scolopendra Subspinipes) 10 pieces
Bing Pian (Borneolum) 3g
Feng Mi‡ (Mel) 180g
Preparation: Grind *Wu Bei Zi*‡ (Galla Rhois Chinensis), *Wu Gong*‡ (Scolopendra Subspinipes) and *Bing Pian* (Borneolum) separately to a powder. Boil the black vinegar in a clay pot for 30 minutes. Then add the honey to the pot and boil for a while, gradually adding the powdered *Wu Bei Zi*‡ (Galla Rhois Chinensis), always stirring in the same direction. After the vinegar solution has been concentrated to a paste by boiling over a gentle heat, add the powdered *Wu Gong*‡ (Scolopendra Subspinipes) and *Bing Pian* (Borneolum) to the paste, stirring all the time. The paste should be black, shiny and soft and must be stored in glass or porcelain containers, not in metal containers.
Source: *Zhao Bing Nan Lin Chuang Jing Yan Ji* [A Collection of Zhao Bingnan's Clinical Experiences]

***Hei Dou Liu You Ruan Gao* (Black Soybean and Vaseline® Ointment)**
5% *Hei Dou You* (Black Soybean Oil)
15% Zinc oxide‡

Preparation: Mix the ingredients with Vaseline® to produce 5-10% ointment.
Source: *Zhao Bing Nan Lin Chuang Jing Yan Ji* [A Collection of Zhao Bingnan's Clinical Experiences]

Hei Se Ba Gao Gun (Black Medicated Plaster Stick)
Paste ingredients
Tu Da Huang (Radix Rumicis Madaio) 60g
Da Feng Zi (Semen Hydnocarpi) 60g
Bai Bu (Radix Stemonae) 60g
Zao Jiao Ci (Spina Gleditsiae Sinensis) 60g
Feng Xian Hua (Flos Impatientis Balsaminae) 30g
Yang Chi Chu Hua (Flos Azaleae Sinensis) 30g
Tou Gu Cao (Herba Speranskiae seu Impatientis) 30g
*Ma Qian Zi** (Semen Nux-Vomicae) 30g
Xing Ren (Semen Pruni Armeniacae) 30g
Bai Guo (Semen Ginkgo Bilobae) 30g
Feng Fang (Radix Ledebouriellae Divaricatae) 30g
Ku Shen (Radix Sophorae Flavescentis) 30g
*Chuan Shan Jia** (Squama Manitis Pentadactylae) 15g
*Chuan Wu** (Radix Aconiti Carmichaeli) 15g
*Cao Wu** (Radix Aconiti Kusnezoffii) 15g
Quan Xie‡ (Buthus Martensi) 15g
Ban Mao‡ (Mylabris) 15g
Wu Gong‡ (Scolopendra Subspinipes) 15 pieces
Xiang You (Oleum Sesami Seminis) 4000ml
Tong You (Oleum Aleuritis Seminis) 1000ml

Medicinal powder ingredients
Bai Ji (Rhizoma Bletillae Striatae) 30g
Teng Huang (Resina Garciniae) 15g
*Qing Fen** (Calomelas) 15g
Nao Sha‡ (Sal Ammoniacum) 9g

Other ingredients
Qian Dan‡ (Minium) 300g
Song Xiang (Resina Pini) 60g

Preparation: Steep the materia medica for the paste in an iron pot with the sesame and tung oils, then fry over a gentle heat until the ingredients turn dark yellow. Remove the residue and heat the medicinal oil to a temperature of 240°C. Mix *Qian Dan*† (Minium), *Song Xiang* (Resina Pini) and 90g of the medicinal powder with 500ml of the medicinal oil to produce the plaster stick.
Source: *Zhang Zhi Li Pi Fu Bing Lin Chuang Jing Yan Ji Yao* [A Collection of Zhang Zhili's Clinical Experiences in the Treatment of Skin Diseases]

Hong Ling Jiu (Red Spirit Wine)
Dang Gui (Radix Angelicae Sinensis) 60g
Hong Hua (Flos Carthami Tinctorii) 30g
Hua Jiao (Pericarpium Zanthoxyli) 30g
Rou Gui (Cortex Cinnamomi Cassiae) 60g
Zhang Nao (Camphora) 1.5g
*Xi Xin** (Herba cum Radice Asari) 15g
Gan Jiang (Rhizoma Zingiberis Officinalis) 30g
Preparation: Soak the herbs in 1000ml of 95% alcohol for seven days.
Source: *Zhong Yi Wai Ke Xue* [External Diseases in Traditional Chinese Medicine, Zhu Renkang]

Hu Po Er Wu Hu Gao (Two Blacks Paste with Amber)
Wu Bei Zi‡ (Galla Rhois Chinensis) 45g
Hu Po‡ (Succinum) 15g
*Cao Wu** (Radix Aconiti Kusnezoffii) 15g
*Chuan Wu** (Radix Aconiti Carmichaeli) 15g
Han Shui Shi‡ (Calcitum) 6g
Bing Pian (Borneolum) 6g
Preparation: Grind the materia medica into a fine powder and mix with Vaseline® to produce a 25-30% paste.
Source: Empirical formula

Hua Du Gao (Transforming Toxicity Paste)
Huang Bai (Cortex Phellodendri) 60g
Ru Xiang (Gummi Olibanum) 60g
Mo Yao (Myrrha) 60g
Chan Tui‡ (Periostracum Cicadae) 30g
Quan Xie‡ (Buthus Martensi) 30g
Dang Gui (Radix Angelicae Sinensis) 120g
Bai Zhi (Radix Angelicae Dahuricae) 60g
Sheng Di Huang (Radix Rehmanniae Glutinosae) 120g
Hong Hua (Flos Carthami Tinctorii) 60g
She Tui‡ (Exuviae Serpentis) 30g
Xue Yu‡ (Crinis Hominis) 30g
Wu Gong‡ (Scolopendra Subspinipes) 30g
Bi Ma Zi (Semen Ricini) 30g
*Ma Qian Zi** (Semen Nux-Vomicae) 30g
Chi Shao (Radix Paeoniae Rubra) 120g
Preparation: Grind the materia medica into a fine powder. Add Vaseline® 80g to every 20g of powder and mix to a paste.
Source: *Meng He Si Jia Yi An* [Meng He's Case Studies from Four Families]

Hua Du San (Powder for Transforming Toxicity)
Huang Lian (Rhizoma Coptidis) 60g
Ru Xiang (Gummi Olibanum) 60g
Mo Yao (Myrrha) 60g
Chuan Bei Mu (Bulbus Fritillariae Cirrhosae) 60g
Tian Hua Fen (Radix Trichosanthis) 120g
Da Huang (Radix et Rhizoma Rhei) 120g
Chi Shao (Radix Paeoniae Rubra) 120g
*Xiong Huang** (Realgar) 60g
Gan Cao (Radix Glycyrrhizae) 45g
Niu Huang‡ (Calculus Bovis) 12g
Bing Pian (Borneolum) 15g
Source: *Zhao Bing Nan Lin Chuang Jing Yan Ji* [A Collection of Zhao Bingnan's Clinical Experiences]

Hua Du San Gao (Powder Paste for Transforming Toxicity)
Hua Du San (Powder for Transforming Toxicity) 20g
Vaseline® 80g
Preparation: Mix the ingredients thoroughly.
Source: *Zhao Bing Nan Lin Chuang Jing Yan Ji* [A Collection of Zhao Bingnan's Clinical Experiences]

Hua Jiao You (Chinese Prickly Ash Oil)
Hua Jiao (Pericarpium Zanthoxyli) 9g
Xiang You (Oleum Sesami Seminis) 500ml
Preparation: Put the sesame oil in a bronze pot, bring to the boil, then remove from the heat. Add *Hua Jiao* (Pericarpium

Zanthoxyli) and allow the oil to cool. Then remove *Hua Jiao* (Pericarpium Zanthoxyli) and retain the medicinal oil.
Source: Empirical formula

Hua Rui Shi San (Ophicalcite Powder)
Hua Rui Shi ‡ (Ophicalcitum) 30g
Peng Sha ‡ (Borax) 10g
Ku Fan ‡ (Alumen Praeparatum) 20g
Hua Shi ‡ (Talcum) 40g
Source: Empirical formula

Huang Ai You (Coptis and Mugwort Leaf Oil)
Huang Lian (Rhizoma Coptidis) 30g
Ai Ye (Folium Artemisiae Argyi) 5g
Vegetable oil 20ml
Preparation: Grind *Huang Lian* (Rhizoma Coptidis) into a fine powder. Mix with some of the vegetable oil and smear around a bowl, which is then placed above smoldering *Ai Ye* (Folium Artemisiae Argyi) and smoked until the *Huang Lian* (Rhizoma Coptidis) turns brownish-black. Remove the *Huang Lian* (Rhizoma Coptidis), mix with the rest of the vegetable oil and store in a sealed jar.
Source: Empirical formula

Huang Ding Shui Xi Ji (Siberian Solomonseal and Cloves Wash Preparation)
Huang Jing (Rhizoma Polygonati) 30g
Ding Xiang (Flos Caryophylli) 30g
Ming Fan ‡ (Alumen) 10g
Preparation: Decoct the ingredients in 700ml of water and boil down to 500ml of a decoction, which can be used as a wet compress or soak.
Source: Empirical formula

Huang Jing Shui Xi Ji (Siberian Solomonseal Wash Preparation)
Huo Xiang (Herba Agastaches seu Pogostemi) 20g
Huang Jing (Rhizoma Polygonati) 20g
Da Huang (Radix et Rhizoma Rhei) 10g
Zao Fan ‡ (Melanteritum) 20g
Xu Chang Qing (Radix Cynanchi Paniculati) 20g
Preparation: Soak the ingredients in 1000ml of water, then boil for 20-30 minutes and use when warm.
Source: *Zhong Yi Wai Ke Xue* [External Diseases in Traditional Chinese Medicine, Zhu Renkang]

Huang Lian Gan Ru Gao (Coptis, Calamine and Frankincense Paste)
Huang Lian Fen (Rhizoma Coptidis, powdered) 30g
Ru Xiang Fen (Gummi Olibanum, powdered) 30g
Lu Gan Shi ‡ (Calamina) 60g
Qu Shi Yao Gao (Medicated Paste for Dispelling Dampness) 210g
Preparation: Mix the powdered ingredients to a paste with *Qu Shi Yao Gao* (Medicated Paste for Dispelling Dampness) or Vaseline®.
Source: *Zhao Bing Nan Lin Chuang Jing Yan Ji* [A Collection of Zhao Bingnan's Clinical Experiences]

Huang Lian Ruan Gao (Coptis Ointment)
Huang Lian Mian (Rhizoma Coptidis, finely powdered) 30g
Qu Shi Yao Gao (Medicated Paste for Dispelling Dampness) 270g

Preparation: Mix the ingredients together to form a smooth paste. Vaseline® may be used instead of *Qu Shi Yao Gao* (Medicated Paste for Dispelling Dampness).
Source: *Zhao Bing Nan Lin Chuang Jing Yan Ji* [A Collection of Zhao Bingnan's Clinical Experiences]

Huang Lian Ye (Coptis Lotion)
Huang Lian (Rhizoma Coptidis) 30g
Bing Pian (Borneolum) 0.3g
Boric acid ‡ 4g
Preparation: Grind *Huang Lian* (Rhizoma Coptidis) into a coarse powder and soak in 100ml of distilled water for 48 hours. Strain off the water into a container and steam in a double boiler for 30 minutes. Add more distilled water to bring the liquid up to 100ml. Add the boric acid while the liquid is still hot and make sure that it dissolves completely. Once the liquid has become cold, add *Bing Pian* (Borneolum).
Source: Empirical formula

Huang Lian You (Coptis Oil)
Huang Lian Su Pian (Berberine Tablet) 2g
Xiang You (Oleum Sesami Seminis) 100ml
Preparation: Grind the tablets into a powder, add to the sesame oil and mix thoroughly.
Source: Empirical formula

Huang Ling Dan (Yellow Spirit Special Pill)
Da Huang (Radix et Rhizoma Rhei) 36g
Huang Bai (Cortex Phellodendri) 9g
Hu Huang Lian (Rhizoma Picrorhizae Scrophulariiflorae) 18g
Shi Gao ‡ (Gypsum Fibrosum) 18g
Source: *Nei Wai Yan Fang Mi Chuan* [Complete Secret Prescriptions in Internal and External Diseases]

Hui Yang Xun Yao (Yang-Returning Fuming Preparation)
Rou Gui (Cortex Cinnamomi Cassiae) 10g
Pao Jiang (Rhizoma Zingiberis Officinalis Praeparata) 10g
Ren Shen Lu (Rhizoma Ginseng) 10g
Chuan Xiong (Rhizoma Ligustici Chuanxiong) 10g
Dang Gui (Radix Angelicae Sinensis) 10g
Bai Jie Zi (Semen Sinapis Albae) 30g
Ai Ye (Folium Artemisiae Argyi) 30g
Bai Lian (Radix Ampelopsis Japonicae) 15g
Huang Qin (Radix Scutellariae Baicalensis) 15g
Preparation: Grind the ingredients into a powder and wrap them in paper (similar to a moxa cone). Light the paper and fume the affected area.
Source: *Zhang Zhi Li Pi Fu Bing Yi An Xuan Cui* [A Collection of Zhang Zhili's Skin Disease Cases]

Huo Huang Jin Ji Tang (Agastache/Patchouli and Siberian Solomonseal Soak Preparation)
Huo Xiang (Herba Agastaches seu Pogostemi) 20g
Huang Jing (Rhizoma Polygonati) 20g
Da Huang (Radix et Rhizoma Rhei) 20g
Zao Fan ‡ (Melanteritum) 10g
Cu (Acetum) 500ml
Preparation: Soak the materia medica in the vinegar for seven days. Remove the residue and use the preparation as a soak.
Source: *Zhong Yi Wai Ke Xue* [External Diseases in Chinese Medicine, Xu Zhiyin]

Huo Xiang Jin Pao Ji (Agastache/Patchouli Soak Preparation)

Huo Xiang (Herba Agastaches seu Pogostemi) 20g
Huang Jing (Rhizoma Polygonati) 20g
Da Huang (Radix et Rhizoma Rhei) 20g
Ming Fan‡ (Alumen) 1.5g
Cu (Acetum) 500ml
Preparation: Soak the materia medica in the vinegar for seven days. Remove the residue and use the preparation as a soak.
Source: *Zhong Yi Wai Ke Xue* [External Diseases in Chinese Medicine, Xu Zhiyin]

Ji Yan Gao Er Hao (Corn Plaster No. 2)

Wu Mei (Fructus Pruni Mume)
Bu Gu Zhi (Fructus Psoraleae Corylifoliae)
Qian Dan‡ (Minium)
Salicylic acid
Novocaine
Sodium salicylate‡
Source: *Zhong Yi Wai Ke Xue* [External Diseases in Traditional Chinese Medicine, Zhu Renkang]

Ji Yan Gao Yi Hao (Corn Plaster No. 1)

Qian Dan‡ (Minium)
Salicylic acid
Benzocaine
White sugar
Source: *Zhong Yi Wai Ke Xue* [External Diseases in Traditional Chinese Medicine, Zhu Renkang]

Ji Yan San (Corn Powder)

Salicylic acid 50g
Qian Dan‡ (Minium) 3g
Benzocaine 2g
Cane sugar 2g
Preparation: Grind the ingredients together to produce a powder, which is normally mixed to a thick paste with 75% alcohol before application to the corns.
Source: *Zhong Yi Wai Ke Xue* [External Diseases in Traditional Chinese Medicine, Zhu Renkang]

Jiao Ai Tang (Prickly Ash and Mugwort Decoction)

Hua Jiao (Pericarpium Zanthoxyli) 15g
Ai Ye (Folium Artemisiae Argyi) 15g
Hong Hua (Flos Carthami Tinctorii) 15g
Gui Zhi (Ramulus Cinnamomi Cassiae) 15g
Tou Gu Cao (Herba Speranskiae seu Impatientis) 30g
Wang Bu Liu Xing (Semen Vaccariae Segetalis) 30g
Preparation: Soak the ingredients in 800ml of water for 30 minutes, then boil for 20 minutes. Allow the decoction to cool before applying to the affected areas as a wet compress or soak.
Source: Empirical formula

Jie Du Dan (Special Pill for Relieving Toxicity)

Qing Dai (Indigo Naturalis) 6g
Huang Bai (Cortex Phellodendri) 6g
Duan Shi Gao‡ (Gypsum Fibrosum Calcinatum) 6g
Source: *Yao Lian Qi Mi* [Explanation of the Secrets of Medicine]

Jin Huang Gao (Golden Yellow Paste)

Da Huang (Radix et Rhizoma Rhei) 250g
Huang Bai (Cortex Phellodendri) 250g
Jiang Huang (Rhizoma Curcumae Longae) 250g
Bai Zhi (Radix Angelicae Dahuricae) 250g
Tian Nan Xing (Rhizoma Arisaematis) 100g
Chen Pi (Pericarpium Citri Reticulatae) 100g
Cang Zhu (Rhizoma Atractylodis) 100g
Hou Po (Cortex Magnoliae Officinalis) 100g
Gan Cao (Radix Glycyrrhizae) 100g
Tian Hua Fen (Radix Trichosanthis) 500g
Preparation: Grind the ingredients together into a fine powder, which is mixed with Vaseline® in a ratio of 1:4.
Source: Empirical formula, based on *Wai Ke Zheng Zong* [An Orthodox Manual of External Diseases]

Kang Fu Ying Gao (Healthy Skin Plaster)

Da Feng Zi (Semen Hydnocarpi) 30g
*Ma Qian Zi** (Semen Nux-Vomicae) 30g
Xing Ren (Semen Pruni Armeniacae) 30g
*Chuan Wu** (Radix Aconiti Carmichaeli) 15g
*Cao Wu** (Radix Aconiti Kusnezoffii) 15g
Quan Xie‡ (Buthus Martensi) 15g
Ban Mao‡ (Mylabris) 15g
Wu Gong‡ (Scolopendra Subspinipes) 15g
Nao Sha‡ (Sal Ammoniacum) 15g
Xiang You (Oleum Sesami Seminis) 750 ml
Preparation: Deep-fry the ingredients in the sesame oil until charred. Remove the residue, then simmer until sticky (where a drop of oil takes on the shape of a pearl when dropped in cold water). Soak in cold water to remove the Fire Toxins. Add a sufficient amount of *Qian Dan*‡ (Minium) to produce a paste when mixed.
Source: Empirical formula

Kou Gan San (Mouth Gan Powder)

Feng Huang Yi‡ (Membrana Ovi Galli) 3g
Gan Lan He (Endocarpium et Semen Canarii Albi) 3g
Er Cha (Pasta Acaciae seu Uncariae) 2g
Bing Pian (Borneolum) 0.5g
Source: *Dang Dai Zhong Yao Wai Zhi Shi Ke Bai Bing Qian Fang* [Current TCM External Treatments of Hundreds of External Diseases With Thousands of Formulae]

Ku Fan Fen (Prepared Alum Powder)

Ku Fan‡ (Alumen Praeparatum)
Preparation: Grind an appropriate amount to a powder and apply to the affected area.
Source: *Zhong Yi Pi Fu Ke Zhen Liao Xue* [Diagnosis and Treatment of Skin Diseases with Chinese Medicine]

Ku Lian Pi Gao (Chinaberry Bark Paste)

Ku Lian Pi (Cortex Meliae Radicis) 60g
Zhu Zhi‡ (Adeps Suis) 240g
Preparation: Peel the skin from *Ku Lian Pi* (Cortex Meliae Radicis) and stir-fry until brown but not charred. Grind the herb to a fine powder and mix to a paste with the pork lard in a ratio of 1:4.
Source: *Zhu Ren Kang Lin Chuang Jing Yan Ji* [A Collection of Zhu Renkang's Clinical Experiences]

Ku Shen Gao (Flavescent Sophora Root Paste)

Ku Shen (Radix Sophorae Flavescentis)
Vaseline®

Preparation: Grind the herb into a powder and mix to a paste with Vaseline® in a ratio of 1:4.
Source: *Zhao Bing Nan Lin Chuang Jing Yan Ji* [A Collection of Zhao Bingnan's Clinical Experiences]

Ku Shen Jiu (Flavescent Sophora Root Wine)
Ku Shen (Radix Sophorae Flavescentis) 310g
Bai Bu (Radix Stemonae) 90g
Ye Ju Hua (Flos Chrysanthemi Indici) 90g
Feng Yan Cao (Fructus Ailanthi Altissimae) 90g
Zhang Nao (Camphora) 125g
75% Alcohol 5000ml
Preparation: Soak the first four ingredients in the alcohol for seven days. Remove the residue and add *Zhang Nao* (Camphora).
Source: *Zhu Ren Kang Lin Chuang Jing Yan Ji* [A Collection of Zhu Renkang's Clinical Experiences]

Ku Shen Tang (Flavescent Sophora Root Decoction)
Ku Shen (Radix Sophorae Flavescentis) 30g
Di Yu (Radix Sanguisorbae Officinalis) 10g
Huang Lian (Rhizoma Coptidis) 10g
Wang Bu Liu Xing (Semen Vaccariae Segetalis) 10g
Du Huo (Radix Angelicae Pubescentis) 10g
Ai Ye (Folium Artemisiae Argyi) 10g
Dan Zhu Ye (Herba Lophatheri Gracilis) 15g
Preparation: Soak the herbs in 1000ml of water for 30 minutes then boil for 20 minutes. Allow to cool somewhat before use.
Source: *Qian Jin Yao Fang* [Prescriptions Worth a Thousand Gold Pieces for Emergencies]

Lang Du Gao (Euphorbia Paste)
Lang Du (Radix Euphorbiae Fischerianae) 90g
*Bing Lang** (Semen Arecae Catechu) 90g
Hua Jiao (Pericarpium Zanthoxyli) 90g
She Chuang Zi (Fructus Cnidii Monnieri) 90g
Da Feng Zi (Semen Hydnocarpi) 90g
Liu Huang‡ (Sulphur) 90g
Wu Bei Zi‡ (Galla Rhois Chinensis) 90g
Po Xiao‡ (Mirabilitum Non-Purum) 90g
Huang La‡ (Cera Aurea) 250g
Zhu Dan‡ (Vesica Fellea Suis) 10 pieces
Xiang You (Oleum Sesami Seminis) 1300ml
Preparation: Grind the first seven ingredients separately into a powder. Gradually add *Po Xiao*‡ (Mirabilitum Non-Purum) into the hot sesame oil, then add *Huang La*‡ (Cera Aurea), *Zhu Dan*‡ (Vesica Fellea Suis) and the powdered ingredients one after another to produce a paste.
Source: *Yi Zong Jin Jian* [The Golden Mirror of Medicine]

Leng Shui Dan (Cold Water Special Pill)
Huang Lian (Rhizoma Coptidis) 6g
Bai Zhi (Radix Angelicae Dahuricae) 6g
Zi Cao (Radix Arnebiae seu Lithospermi) 6g
Zhang Nao (Camphora) 6g
Huang La‡ (Cera Aurea) 250g
Xiang You (Oleum Sesami Seminis) 180ml
Preparation: Deep-fry the first three herbs in the sesame oil until charred. Remove the residue, then add *Zhang Nao* (Camphora) and *Huang La*‡ (Cera Aurea) and mix evenly; allow to cool before application.
Source: Empirical formula

Li Lu Gao (Veratrum Root Paste)
Li Lu (Radix et Rhizoma Veratri) 20g
Liu Huang‡ (Sulphur) 20g
Vaseline® 100g
Preparation: Grind the dry ingredients into a powder and mix to a paste with Vaseline®.
Source: *Zhong Yi Pi Fu Bing Ke Lin Chuang Shou Ce* [A Clinical Manual of Dermatology in Chinese Medicine]

Ling Yi Gao (Miraculous Difference Ointment)
Yu Jin (Radix Curcumae) 20g
Gan Cao (Radix Glycyrrhizae) 20g
Sheng Di Huang (Radix Rehmanniae Glutinosae) 20g
Zhu Zhi‡ (Adeps Suis)
Preparation: Stir-fry *Yu Jin* (Radix Curcumae) and *Gan Cao* (Radix Glycyrrhizae) until brown but not charred, then grind to a fine powder with *Sheng Di Huang* (Radix Rehmanniae Glutinosae). Mix to a paste with the pork lard in a ratio of 1:4.
Source: *Wai Ke Da Cheng* [A Compendium of External Diseases]

Liu Huang Ruan Gao (Sulfur Ointment)
Liu Huang‡ (Sulphur) 5-10g
Vaseline® 90-95g
Preparation: Grind *Liu Huang* (Sulphur) to a powder and mix into a paste with Vaseline®.
Source: *Zhong Yi Wai Ke Lin Chuang Shou Ce* [A Clinical Handbook of External Diseases in Chinese Medicine]

Liu Lei Xi Ji (Sulfur and Resorcinol Wash Preparation)
Liu Huang‡ (Sulphur)
Resorcinol
Zinc oxide‡
Water
Source: *Zhang Zhi Li Pi Fu Bing Yi An Xuan Cui* [A Collection of Zhang Zhili's Skin Disease Cases]
Note: In most countries, this will be a prescription-only medicine.

Liu Yi San (Six-to-One Powder)
Hua Shi‡ (Talcum) 180g
Gan Cao (Radix Glycyrrhizae) 30g
Source: *Shang Han Zhi Ge* [A Direct Guide to Cold Damage]

Long Dan Cao Shui Xi Ji (Chinese Gentian Wash Preparation)
Long Dan Cao (Radix Gentianae Scabrae) 30g
Long Kui (Herba Solani Nigri) 15g
Preparation: Add the herbs to 1000ml of water and boil down to a concentrated decoction of 300ml. Remove the residue and use the decoction for a wash or compress.
Source: Empirical formula

Lou Lu Tang (Globethistle Root Decoction)
Lou Lu (Radix Rhapontici seu Echinopsis) 6g
Lian Qiao (Fructus Forsythiae Suspensae) 6g
Bai Lian (Radix Ampelopsis Japonicae) 6g
Mang Xiao‡ (Mirabilitum) 6g
Gan Cao (Radix Glycyrrhizae) 6g
Da Huang (Radix et Rhizoma Rhei) 30g
Sheng Ma (Rhizoma Cimicifugae) 9g
Zhi Shi (Fructus Immaturus Citri Aurantii) 9g
*Ma Huang** (Herba Ephedrae) 9g

Huang Qin (Radix Scutellariae Baicalensis) 9g
Preparation: Soak the ingredients in 1000ml of water for 30 minutes, then boil for 20 minutes and drain off the liquid for use when lukewarm.
Source: *Wai Ke Jing Yi* [The Essence of External Diseases]

Lu Hu Xi Ji (Calamine and Giant Knotweed Wash Preparation)
Lu Gan Shi ‡ (Calamina) 10g
Hu Zhang Fen (Radix et Rhizoma Polygoni Cuspidati, powdered) 5g
Bo He Nao (Menthol) 1g
Preparation: Add the ingredients to 100ml of distilled water and 30ml of glycerin and shake to mix.
Source: Empirical formula

Lu Hui Ru Ji (Aloe Cream)
*Xian Lu Hui** (Herba Aloes Recens) 45g
Eucalyptus oil 4.5g
Gum arabic 10g
Preparation: Wash *Xian Lu Hui** (Herba Aloes Recens) and pound it to produce a juice. Gradually add the gum arabic while stirring continuously until the solution becomes milky, then add the eucalyptus oil and mix thoroughly.
Source: Empirical formula

Lu Lu Tong Shui Xi Ji (Sweetgum Fruit Wash Preparation)
Lu Lu Tong (Fructus Liquidambaris) 60g
Cang Zhu (Rhizoma Atractylodis) 60g
Bai Bu (Radix Stemonae) 15g
Ai Ye (Folium Artemisiae Argyi) 15g
Ku Fan ‡ (Alumen Praeparatum) 15g
Preparation: Add the ingredients to 1500ml of water and boil down to make 800ml of decoction.
Source: Empirical formula

Lü Liu Ding (Chloramphenicol Salicylate Tincture)
Chloramphenicol 1g
Salicylic acid 2g
75% Alcohol 100ml
Source: *Zhang Zhi Li Pi Fu Bing Lin Chuang Jing Yan Ji Yao* [A Collection of Zhang Zhili's Clinical Experiences in the Treatment of Skin Diseases]
Note: In most countries, this will be a prescription-only medicine.

Lü Pao San (Green Robe Powder)
Bo He (Herba Menthae Haplocalycis) 15g
Qing Dai (Indigo Naturalis) 6.5g
Peng Sha ‡ (Borax) 6.5g
Er Cha (Pasta Acaciae seu Uncariae) 9g
Gan Cao (Radix Glycyrrhizae) 9g
Huang Bai (Cortex Phellodendri) 3g
Tong Lü ‡ (Robigo Aeris) 3g
Bing Pian (Borneolum) 3g
Xuan Ming Fen ‡ (Mirabilitum Depuratum) 6g
Bai Cao Shuang (Fuligo Herbarum Ustarum) 6g
Jing Jie (Herba Schizonepetae Tenuifoliae) 15g
Source: *Zhi Zhen Quan Shu* [A Complete Volume of the Treatment of Rashes]

Lü Yun Gao (Green Cloud Paste)
Huang Lian (Rhizoma Coptidis) 3g
Da Huang (Radix et Rhizoma Rhei) 3g

Huang Qin (Radix Scutellariae Baicalensis) 3g
Xuan Shen (Radix Scrophulariae Ningpoensis) 3g
Huang Bai (Cortex Phellodendri) 3g
*Ma Qian Zi** (Semen Nux-Vomicae) 3g
Xiang You (Oleum Sesami Seminis) 50ml
Song Xiang (Resina Pini) 250g
Zhu Dan ‡ (Vesica Fellea Suis) 3 pieces
Tong Lü ‡ (Robigo Aeris) 9g
Preparation: Grind the first six ingredients into a powder and cook in the sesame oil until dark brown. Remove the residue, add *Song Xiang* (Resina Pini) and continue cooking until a paste is produced. Soak the paste in cold water until it turns golden. Then heat again with *Zhu Dan* ‡ (Vesica Fellea Suis) and *Tong Lü* ‡ (Robigo Aeris). Allow the mixture to cool before covering with vinegar and steeping overnight. Remove the residue before use.
Source: *Yi Xue Zheng Zhuan* [Orthodox Medical Problems]

Ma Chi Xian Shui Xi Ji (Purslane Wash Preparation)
Ma Chi Xian (Herba Portulacae Oleraceae) 30g
Preparation: Boil the herb for 20 minutes in 1000ml of water and allow to cool before use.
Source: *Zhao Bing Nan Lin Chuang Jing Yan Ji* [A Collection of Zhao Bingnan's Clinical Experiences]

Mao Yan Cao Gao (Crescent Euphorbia Paste)
Mao Yan Cao (Herba Euphorbiae Lunulatae)
Xiang You (Oleum Sesami Seminis)
Preparation: Grind *Mao Yan Cao* (Herba Euphorbiae Lunulatae) into a fine powder and mix to a paste with the sesame oil.
Source: *Bian Min Tu Zuan* [A Handy Illustrated Edition]

Miao Tie San (Wondrous Adhering Powder)
Liu Huang Mo ‡ (Sulphur, powdered)
Qiao Mai Mian (Farina Fagopyri)
Bai Mian Fen (Farina Tritici)
Preparation: Mix the ingredients in the proportion of 2:1:1 and add sufficient water to allow the mixture to adhere together thickly. Dry in the wind. Grind the mixture to a powder before application.
Source: *Wai Ke Zheng Zong* [An Orthodox Manual of External Diseases]

Mie Xuan Zhi Shi Fen (Powder for Eliminating Tinea and Alleviating Dampness)
Liu Huang ‡ (Sulphur) 20g
Zhang Nao (Camphora) 2g
Wu Zhu Yu (Fructus Evodiae Rutaecarpae) 10g
Hai Piao Xiao ‡ (Os Sepiae seu Sepiellae) 20g
Source: *Zhong Yi Wai Ke Xue* [External Diseases in Traditional Chinese Medicine, Zhu Renkang]

Mo Feng Gao (Fashionable Paste)
*Ma Huang** (Herba Ephedrae) 15g
Qiang Huo (Rhizoma et Radix Notopterygii) 9g
Sheng Ma (Rhizoma Cimicifugae) 6g
Fang Feng (Radix Ledebouriellae Divaricatae) 6g
Dang Gui Shen (Corpus Radicis Angelicae Sinensis) 3g
Bai Ji (Rhizoma Bletillae Striatae) 3g
Bai Tan Xiang (Lignum Santali Albi) 1.5g
Xiang You (Oleum Sesami Seminis) 250ml
Huang La ‡ (Cera Aurea) 20g

Preparation: Soak the materia medica in the sesame oil for three days and then fry over a gentle heat until the herbs turn dark yellow. Remove the residue, add the wax and heat again until it has melted completely. Allow the liquid to cool to produce a paste
Source: *Yi Zong Jin Jian* [The Golden Mirror of Medicine]

Mu Fan Dan (Oyster, Alum and Minium Powder)
Mu Li Fen ‡ (Concha Ostreae, powdered) 30g
Qian Dan ‡ (Minium) 5g
Ku Fan ‡ (Alumen Praeparatum) 10g
Source: *Lei Zheng Zhi Cai* [Treatment of Classified Patterns]

Pi Yan Xi Ji (Dermatitis Wash Preparation)
Sheng Di Huang (Radix Rehmanniae Glutinosae) 30g
Mu Dan Pi (Cortex Moutan Radicis) 9g
Chi Shao (Radix Paeoniae Rubra) 9g
Zhi Mu (Rhizoma Anemarrhenae Asphodeloidis) 9g
Shi Gao ‡ (Gypsum Fibrosum) 30g
Jin Yin Hua (Flos Lonicerae) 9g
Lian Qiao (Fructus Forsythiae Suspensae) 9g
Dan Zhu Ye (Herba Lophatheri Gracilis) 9g
Gan Cao (Radix Glycyrrhizae) 9g
Preparation: Add the ingredients to 800ml of water and boil until 500ml of decoction is left for use as a wash.
Source: *Zhu Ren Kang Lin Chuang Jing Yan Ji* [A Collection of Zhu Renkang's Clinical Experiences]

Pi Zhi Gao (Skin Grease)
Qing Dai (Indigo Naturalis) 6g
Huang Bai (Cortex Phellodendri) 6g
Duan Shi Gao ‡ (Gypsum Fibrosum Calcinatum) 60g
Yan Jiao ‡ (Fuligo Oleacea Coriarii) 60g
Preparation: Grind the ingredients into a fine powder and mix to a paste with Vaseline® 500g.
Source: *Zhu Ren Kang Lin Chuang Jing Yan Ji* [A Collection of Zhu Renkang's Clinical Experiences]

Pian Zhi Gao (Callus Plaster)
Sheng Shi Gao ‡ (Gypsum Fibrosum Crudum)
Zhang Nao Fen (Camphora, powdered)
Sodium ‡
Hard soap
Source: *Zhong Yi Wai Ke Xue* [External Diseases in Traditional Chinese Medicine, Zhu Renkang]

Pu Ji Dan (Universal Salvation Special Pill)
Zhi Da Huang (Radix et Rhizoma Rhei, mix-fried with honey) 5g
Sheng Da Huang (Radix et Rhizoma Rhei Crudae) 15g
Jiang Can ‡ (Bombyx Batryticatus) 30g
Preparation: Grind the ingredients into a powder and mix with ginger juice (*Sheng Jiang Zhi*, Succus Rhizomatis Zingiberis Officinalis Recens) to make 6g pills.
Source: *Xian Nian Ji* [A Collection Held by Immortals]

Pu Lian Gao (Universal Coptis Paste)
Huang Qin (Radix Scutellariae Baicalensis) 10g
Huang Bai (Cortex Phellodendri) 10g
Vaseline® 80g
Preparation: Grind the herbs into a powder and mix with Vaseline®.

Source: *Zhang Zhi Li Pi Fu Bing Lin Chuang Jing Yan Ji Yao* [A Collection of Zhang Zhili's Clinical Experiences in the Treatment of Skin Diseases]
Note: This paste is also known as *Qin Bai Gao* (Scutellaria and Phellodendron Paste)

Pu Xuan Shui (Universal Tinea Lotion)
Sheng Di Yu (Radix Sanguisorbae Officinalis Recens) 50g
Chuan Lian Zi (Fructus Meliae Toosendan) 50g
Tu Jin Pi (Cortex Pseudolaricis) 95g
Ban Mao ‡ (Mylabris) 1.5g
Preparation: Grind the first three ingredients to a powder and wrap *Ban Mao* ‡ (Mylabris) in a piece of gauze. Steep all the ingredients in 1000ml of 75% alcohol in a sealed container for two weeks. Remove the residue and store the tincture.
Source: *Zhu Ren Kang Lin Chuang Jing Yan Ji* [A Collection of Zhu Renkang's Clinical Experiences]

Qin Bai Gao (Scutellaria and Phellodendron Paste)
See *Pu Lian Gao* (Universal Coptis Paste)

Qing Bai San (Green-White Powder)
Qing Dai (Indigo Naturalis) 30g
Hai Piao Xiao ‡ (Os Sepiae seu Sepiellae) 90g
Duan Shi Gao ‡ (Gypsum Fibrosum Calcinatum) 370g
Bing Pian (Borneolum) 3g
Preparation: Grind *Qing Dai* (Indigo Naturalis) first, then add *Hai Piao Xiao* ‡ (Os Sepiae seu Sepiellae) to the mortar and grind them together. Finally add *Duan Shi Gao* ‡ (Gypsum Fibrosum Calcinatum) and *Bing Pian* (Borneolum) and grind again to produce the powder.
Source: *Zhu Ren Kang Lin Chuang Jing Yan Ji* [A Collection of Zhu Renkang's Clinical Experiences]

Qing Chui Kou San (Indigo Mouth Insufflation Powder)
Duan Shi Gao ‡ (Gypsum Fibrosum Calcinatum) 9g
Duan Ren Zhong Bai ‡ (Sedimentum Hominis Urinae Calcinatum) 9g
Qing Dai (Indigo Naturalis) 3g
Bing Pian (Borneolum) 3g
Bo He (Herba Menthae Haplocalycis) 1.5g
Huang Lian (Rhizoma Coptidis) 1.5g
Huang Bai (Cortex Phellodendri) 2g
Duan Peng Sha ‡ (Borax Calcinatum) 18g
Preparation: Grind *Duan Shi Gao* ‡ (Gypsum Fibrosum Calcinatum), *Duan Ren Zhong Bai* ‡ (Sedimentum Hominis Urinae Calcinatum) and *Qing Dai* (Indigo Naturalis) separately to a fine powder and mix well. Sprinkle water over the mixture and grind again until no noise can be heard during grinding. Dry the powder in the sun and grind again before mixing thoroughly with a fine powder of the other five ingredients.
Source: *Zhong Yi Wai Ke Xue* [External Diseases in Traditional Chinese Medicine, Zhu Renkang]

Qing Dai Gao (Indigo Paste)
Qing Dai San (Indigo Powder) 75g
Vaseline®
Preparation: Melt the Vaseline® over a low heat and allow to cool. Add *Qing Dai San* (Indigo Powder) to the Vaseline® in a proportion of 1:4 and mix well.
Source: *Zhong Yi Wai Ke Lin Chuang Shou Ce* [A Clinical Handbook of External Diseases in Chinese Medicine]

Qing Dai San (Indigo Powder)
Qing Dai (Indigo Naturalis) 60g
Shi Gao ‡ (Gypsum Fibrosum) 120g
Hua Shi ‡ (Talcum) 120g
Huang Bai (Cortex Phellodendri) 60g
Source: *Zhong Yi Wai Ke Jiang Yi* [Teaching Materials for External Diseases in Chinese Medicine]

Qing Guo Shui Xi Ji (Chinese Olive Wash Preparation)
Zang Qing Guo (Fructus Immaturus Terminaliae Chebulae) 9-15g
Mu Zei (Herba Equiseti Hiemalis) 9g
Jin Lian Hua (Flos Trollii) 6g
Preparation: Decoct the herbs in 1000ml of water and boil down until a concentrated solution of 250ml remains.
Source: *Zhong Yi Pi Fu Ke Zhen Liao Xue* [Diagnosis and Treatment of Skin Diseases with Chinese Medicine]

Qing Liang Fei Zi Fen (Cool Clearing Miliaria Powder)
Liu Yi San (Six-To-One Powder) 30g
Ku Fan ‡ (Alumen Praeparatum) 3g
Bing Pian (Borneolum) 3g
Bai Zhi (Radix Angelicae Dahuricae) 10g
Gan Song (Radix Nardostachydis) 6g
Preparation: Grind the ingredients into a fine powder, wrap in gauze and apply to the affected area two or three times a day.
Source: Empirical formula

Qing Liang Fen (Cool Clearing Powder)
Liu Yi San (Six-To-One Powder) 120g
Bing Pian (Borneolum) 12g
Preparation: Grind *Bing Pian* (Borneolum) into a fine powder, mix well with *Liu Yi San* (Six-To-One Powder) and store in a jar.
Source: Empirical formula

Qing Liang Gao (Cool Clearing Paste)
Dang Gui (Radix Angelicae Sinensis) 30g
Zi Cao (Radix Arnebiae seu Lithospermi) 6g
Da Huang Mian (Radix et Rhizoma Rhei, finely powdered) 4.5g
Huang La ‡ (Cera Aurea) 120-180g
Xiang You (Oleum Sesami Seminis) 300ml
Preparation: Soak *Dang Gui* (Radix Angelicae Sinensis) and *Zi Cao* (Radix Arnebiae seu Lithospermi) in the sesame oil for three days and then fry over a gentle heat until the herbs turn dark yellow. Remove the residue, add the wax and melt in the hot oil. Allow the oil to cool before adding powdered *Da Huang* (Radix et Rhizoma Rhei), stirring continuously to produce a paste.
Source: *Zhao Bing Nan Lin Chuang Jing Yan Ji* [A Collection of Zhao Bingnan's Clinical Experiences]

Qing Ye San (Indigo Fluid Powder)
Qing Dai (Indigo Naturalis)
Pu Xiao ‡ (Mirabilitum Non-Purum)
Bing Pian (Borneolum)
Preparation: Grind equal amounts of the materia medica into a powder.
Source: *Zheng Zhi Zhun Sheng* [Standards of Diagnosis and Treatment]

Qu Du Yao Fen (Medicated Powder for Eliminating Toxins)
Ma Chi Xian (Herba Portulacae Oleraceae) 30g
Bo He (Herba Menthae Haplocalycis) 3g

Hong Hua (Flos Carthami Tinctorii) 3g
Da Huang (Radix et Rhizoma Rhei) 3g
Xiong Huang * (Realgar) 3g
Zi Hua Di Ding (Herba Violae Yedoensitis) 30g
Bai Jiang Cao (Herba Patriniae cum Radice) 30g
Chi Shao (Radix Paeoniae Rubra) 24g
Shi Gao ‡ (Gypsum Fibrosum) 24g
Lü Dou Fen (Semen Phaseoli Radiati, powdered) 45g
Bai Ji (Rhizoma Bletillae Striatae) 6g
Xue Jie (Resina Draconis) 6g
Bing Pian (Borneolum) 3g
Source: *Zhao Bing Nan Lin Chuang Jing Yan Ji* [A Collection of Zhao Bingnan's Clinical Experiences]

Qu Shi San (Powder for Dispelling Dampness)
Da Huang Mian (Radix et Rhizoma Rhei, finely powdered) 30g
Huang Qin Mian (Radix Scutellariae Baicalensis, finely powdered) 30g
Han Shui Shi Mian ‡ (Calcitum, finely powdered) 30g
Qing Dai (Indigo Naturalis) 3g
Source: *Zhang Zhi Li Pi Fu Bing Yi An Xuan Cui* [A Collection of Zhang Zhili's Skin Disease Cases]

Qu Shi Yao Gao (Medicated Paste for Dispelling Dampness)
Ku Shen (Radix Sophorae Flavescentis) 120g
Bo He (Herba Menthae Haplocalycis) 90g
Bai Zhi (Radix Angelicae Dahuricae) 90g
Fang Feng (Radix Ledebouriellae Divaricatae) 60g
Jing Jie Sui (Spica Schizonepetae Tenuifoliae) 120g
Lian Qiao (Fructus Forsythiae Suspensae) 120g
Cang Zhu (Rhizoma Atractylodis) 90g
Da Huang (Radix et Rhizoma Rhei) 90g
He Shi Cao (Herba Carpesii) 90g
Wei Ling Xian (Radix Clematidis) 120g
Bai Xian Pi (Radix Dictamni Dasycarpi Radicis) 150g
Wu Bei Zi ‡ (Galla Rhois Chinensis) 150g
Da Feng Zi (Semen Hydnocarpi) 300g
Qing Dai (Indigo Naturalis) 18g
Bai La ‡ (Cera Alba) 3600g
Xiang You (Oleum Sesami Seminis) 10 liters
Preparation: Grind all the dry ingredients except *Qing Dai* (Indigo Naturalis) to a powder and steep in the oil for 24 hours. Then cook over a mild heat until the ingredients are a dark yellow color. Filter off the oil and add the wax; for every 500ml of the medicated oil, add 90g of wax in winter, 120g in spring and autumn, and 150g in summer. Finally add 1.5g of *Qing Dai* (Indigo Naturalis) for every 500ml of medicated oil and mix to a paste.
Source: *Zhao Bing Nan Lin Chuang Jing Yan Ji* [A Collection of Zhao Bingnan's Clinical Experiences]

Rou Ci San (Flesh Thorn Powder)
Ming Fan ‡ (Alumen) 30g
Ya Dan Zi (Fructus Bruceae Javanicae) 30g
Copper sulfate ‡ 30g
Source: *Beng Bu Fang* [Empirical Formulae from Bengbu College]

Ru Bing San (Ice-Like Powder)
Po Xiao ‡ (Mirabilitum Non-Purum) 150g
Han Shui Shi ‡ (Calcitum) 90g

Ge Fen‡ (Concha Meretricis seu Cyclinae Pulverata) 90g
Bai Zhi (Radix Angelicae Dahuricae) 30g
Zhang Nao (Camphora) 3g
Preparation: Grind the first four ingredients together to produce a powder, then add *Zhang Nao* (Camphora) to the mixture and grind again.
Source: *Zheng Zhi Zhun Sheng* [Standards of Diagnosis and Treatment]

Ru Yi Jin Huang San (Agreeable Golden Yellow Powder)
Tian Hua Fen (Radix Trichosanthis) 48g
Huang Bai (Cortex Phellodendri) 48g
Da Huang (Radix et Rhizoma Rhei) 48g
Jiang Huang (Rhizoma Curcumae Longae) 48g
Bai Zhi (Radix Angelicae Dahuricae) 30g
Hou Po (Cortex Magnoliae Officinalis) 18g
Chen Pi (Pericarpium Citri Reticulatae) 18g
Gan Cao (Radix Glycyrrhizae)18g
Cang Zhu (Rhizoma Atractylodis) 10g
Sheng Nan Xing (Rhizoma Arisaematis Crudum) 18g
Source: *Zhang Zhi Li Pi Fu Bing Lin Chuang Jing Yan Ji Yao* [A Collection of Zhang Zhili's Clinical Experiences in the Treatment of Skin Diseases]

Run Ji Gao (Flesh-Moistening Paste)
Xiang You (Oleum Sesami Seminis) 120g
Dang Gui (Radix Angelicae Sinensis) 15g
Zi Cao (Radix Arnebiae seu Lithospermi) 3g
Huang La‡ (Cera Aurea) 15g
Preparation: Soak *Dang Gui* (Radix Angelicae Sinensis) and *Zi Cao* (Radix Arnebiae seu Lithospermi) in the oil for two days, then fry over a gentle heat until the herbs are charred. Remove them from the oil and add *Huang La*‡ (Cera Aurea). Melt it in the hot oil, stirring constantly to produce a paste as the mixture gradually cools.
Source: *Wai Ke Zheng Zong* [An Orthodox Manual of External Diseases]

San Huang Xi Ji (Three Yellows Wash Preparation)
Da Huang (Radix et Rhizoma Rhei)
Huang Bai (Cortex Phellodendri)
Huang Qin (Radix Scutellariae Baicalensis)
Ku Shen (Radix Sophorae Flavescentis)
Preparation: Grind equal amounts of the herbs into a powder, 10-15g of which is suspended in 100ml of distilled water and 1ml of phenol. The preparation should be shaken before use.
Source: *Shi Yong Zhong Yi Wai Ke Xue* [Practical Treatment of External Diseases with Traditional Chinese Medicine]

San Miao San (Mysterious Three Powder)
Huang Bai (Cortex Phellodendri)
Cang Zhu (Rhizoma Atractylodis)
*Bing Lang** (Semen Arecae Catechu)
Preparation: Grind the herbs into a powder in the proportions of 2:2:1.
Source: *Yi Zong Jin Jian* [The Golden Mirror of Medicine]

San Shi Shui (Three Stones Lotion)
Lu Gan Shi‡ (Calamina) 90g
Shu Shi Gao‡ (Gypsum Fibrosum Conquitum) 90g
Chi Shi Zhi‡ (Halloysitum Rubrum) 90g

Bing Pian (Borneolum) 9g
Glycerin 150ml
Preparation: Grind the materia medica into a powder. Prepare a suspension with 1000ml of distilled water and then add the glycerin. Shake the lotion before application.
Source: *Zhu Ren Kang Lin Chuang Jing Yan Ji* [A Collection of Zhu Renkang's Clinical Experiences]

San Xiang Gao (Three Fragrances Paste)
Ru Xiang (Gummi Olibanum)
Song Xiang (Resina Pini)
Xiang You (Oleum Sesami Seminis)
Preparation: Grind equal amounts of *Ru Xiang* (Gummi Olibanum) and *Song Xiang* (Resina Pini) into a fine powder and then mix to a paste with the sesame oil.
Source: *Shou Shi Bao Yuan* [Safeguarding the Origins of Longevity]

Sang Bai Pi Shui Xi Ji (White Mulberry Root Bark Wash Preparation)
Sang Bai Pi (Cortex Mori Albae Radicis) 30g
Wu Bei Zi‡ (Galla Rhois Chinensis) 15g
Qing Xiang Zi (Semen Celosiae Argenteae) 60g
Preparation: Add the materia medica to 1000ml of water and boil down to 750ml of a concentrated decoction for use as an external wash.
Source: Empirical formula

Shan Dou Gen Shui Xi Ji (Subprostrate Sophora Root Wash Preparation)
Shan Dou Gen (Radix Sophorae Tonkinensis) 30g
Sang Bai Pi (Cortex Mori Albae Radicis) 15g
Man Jing Zi (Fructus Viticis) 15g
Wu Bei Zi‡ (Galla Rhois Chinensis) 15g
Hou Po (Cortex Magnoliae Officinalis) 12g
Preparation: Add the materia medica to 1500ml of water and boil down to make 500ml of a concentrated decoction for use as a wash or soak.
Source: Empirical formula

Shan Dou Gen You Ji (Subprostrate Sophora Root Oil Preparation)
Shan Dou Gen (Radix Sophorae Tonkinensis) 15g
Zhang Nao You (Oleum Camphorae) 5ml
Zhi Wu You (Oleum Vegetale) 100ml
Preparation: Fry *Shan Dou Gen* (Radix Sophorae Tonkinensis) in the vegetable oil over a low heat until dark yellow. Remove the residue, add in *Zhang Nao You* (Oleum Camphorae) and mix well.
Source: Empirical formula

She Chuang Zi Xi Ji (Cnidium Fruit Wash Preparation)
Wei Ling Xian (Radix Clematidis) 15g
She Chuang Zi (Fructus Cnidii Monnieri) 15g
Dang Gui Wei (Extremitas Radicis Angelicae Sinensis) 15g
Tu Da Huang (Radix Rumicis Madaio) 15g
Ku Shen (Radix Sophorae Flavescentis) 15g
Suo Sha Ke (Pericarpium Amomi) 9g
Lao Cong Tou (Bulbus Allii Fistulosi Vetus) 7 pieces
Preparation: Grind the ingredients into a powder, wrap in a gauze cloth and place on *Sang Zhi* (Ramulus Mori Albae) twigs in a pot of water. Boil the water and collect the distillate.

Alternatively, the ingredients may also be boiled in water to produce a decoction.
Source: *Yi Zong Jin Jian* [The Golden Mirror of Medicine]

Sheng Fa Ding (Generating Hair Tincture)
Ban Mao‡ (Mylabris) 2 pieces
Bai Bu Ding (Stemona Root Tincture) 100ml
Preparation: Soak *Ban Mao* (Mylabris) in *Bai Bu Ding* (Stemona Root Tincture) for seven days.
Source: *Zhang Zhi Li Pi Fu Bing Lin Chuang Jing Yan Ji Yao* [A Collection of Zhang Zhili's Clinical Experiences in the Treatment of Skin Diseases]

Sheng Ji Bai Yu Gao (White Jade Paste for Generating Flesh)
Shi Gao‡ (Gypsum Fibrosum) 90% by weight
Lu Gan Shi‡ (Calamina) 10% by weight
Preparation: Soak *Shi Gao*‡ (Gypsum Fibrosum) in urine for half a year, then rinse regularly in tap water for two months before calcining and grinding into a fine powder. After mixing with *Lu Gan Shi*‡ (Calamina) and a small amount of sesame oil, an ointment can be produced with Vaseline® in a ratio of 3:7.
Source: *Zhong Yi Wai Ke Jiang Yi* [Teaching Materials for External Diseases in Chinese Medicine]

Shi Du Gao (Damp Toxin Paste)
Qing Dai (Indigo Naturalis) 150g
Huang Bai Fen (Cortex Phellodendri, powdered) 310g
Duan Shi Gao‡ (Gypsum Fibrosum Calcinatum, powdered) 310g
Lu Gan Shi‡ (Calamina, powdered) 180g
Wu Bei Zi‡ (Galla Rhois Chinensis, powdered) 90g
Preparation: Mix *Qing Dai* (Indigo Naturalis) and powdered *Huang Bai* (Cortex Phellodendri) together first, then add the other three powdered ingredients and combine thoroughly. Finally, mix with Vaseline® to produce a 30% ointment.
Source: *Zhu Ren Kang Lin Chuang Jing Yan Ji* [A Collection of Zhu Renkang's Clinical Experiences]

Shi Liu Pi Shui Xi Ji (Pomegranate Rind Wash Preparation)
*Shi Liu Pi** (Pericarpium Punicae Granati) 30g
Wu Bei Zi‡ (Galla Rhois Chinensis) 30g
Wei Ling Xian (Radix Clematidis) 15g
Chen Pi (Pericarpium Citri Reticulatae) 15g
Preparation: Soak the ingredients in 800ml of water for 30 minutes and then boil for 20 minutes. Remove the residue and allow the decoction to cool before use for a wet compress.
Source: *Zhong Yi Pi Fu Ke Zhen Liao Xue* [Diagnosis and Treatment of Dermatological Disorders in Chinese Medicine]

Shi Zhen Fen (Eczema Powder)
Duan Shi Gao‡ (Gypsum Fibrosum Calcinatum, powdered) 310g
Ku Fan‡ (Alumen Praeparatum) 150g
Bai Zhi (Radix Angelicae Dahuricae) 60g
Bing Pian (Borneolum) 15g
Preparation: Grind *Bing Pian* (Borneolum) and *Bai Zhi* (Radix Angelicae Dahuricae) together first, then add the other materia medica and grind them all together to produce the powder.
Source: *Zhu Ren Kang Lin Chuang Jing Yan Ji* [A Collection of Zhu Renkang's Clinical Experiences]

Shi Zhen Yi Hao Gao (No. 1 Eczema Paste)
Qing Dai (Indigo Naturalis) 60g

Huang Bai (Cortex Phellodendri) 60g
Zinc oxide‡ 620g
Duan Shi Gao‡ (Gypsum Fibrosum Calcinatum) 620g
Xiang You (Oleum Sesami Seminis) 620ml
Vaseline® 930g
Preparation: Grind the first four ingredients to a fine powder and mix with Vaseline® and the sesame oil to produce a paste.
Source: *Zhu Ren Kang Lin Chuang Jing Yan Ji* [A Collection of Zhu Renkang's Clinical Experiences]

Shou Gan Sheng Ji Yao Fen (Medicated Powder for Promoting Contraction and Generating Flesh)
Ru Xiang Mian (Gummi Olibanum, finely powdered) 30g
Mo Yao Mian (Myrrha, finely powdered) 30g
Hu Po Mian‡ (Succinum, finely powdered) 6g
Xue Jie Mian (Resina Draconis, finely powdered) 12g
Er Cha Mian (Pasta Acaciae seu Uncariae, finely powdered) 15g
Lu Gan Shi‡ (Calamina) 20g
Source: *Zhao Bing Nan Lin Chuang Jing Yan Ji* [A Collection of Zhao Bingnan's Clinical Experiences]

Shui Jing Gao (Crystal Paste)
Nuo Mi (Semen Oryzae Glutinosae) 100g
15 % Potassium hydroxide‡ 250ml
Preparation: Soak the glutinous rice in the potassium hydroxide solution for 24 hours. Remove the rice and pound into a transparent paste.
Source: *Zhu Ren Kang Lin Chuang Jing Yan Ji* [A Collection of Zhu Renkang's Clinical Experiences]

Shui Yang Suan Ruan Gao (Salicylic Acid Ointment)
Salicylic acid
Vaseline®
Preparation: Mix an appropriate amount of salicylic acid with Vaseline® to produce a 2-10% ointment, depending on requirements.
Source: *Zhang Zhi Li Pi Fu Bing Yi An Xuan Cui* [A Collection of Zhang Zhili's Skin Disease Cases]
Note: In some countries, this ointment may only be available through pharmacies.

Si Huang Gao (Four Yellows Paste)
Huang Qin (Radix Scutellariae Baicalensis) 30g
Huang Bai (Cortex Phellodendri) 30g
Huang Lian (Rhizoma Coptidis) 30g
Tu Da Huang (Radix Rumicis Madaio) 30g
Ze Lan (Herba Lycopi Lucidi) 30g
Huang La‡ (Cera Aurea) 125g
Xiang You (Oleum Sesami Seminis) 250ml
Preparation: Melt the wax in the sesame oil in a pot over a moderate heat. Grind the other ingredients to a powder and stir into the oil after removing the pot from the heat.
Source: *Zhu Ren Kang Lin Chuang Jing Yan Ji* [A Collection of Zhu Renkang's Clinical Experiences]

Tang Shang Gao (Scald Paste)
Di Yu Mian (Radix Sanguisorbae Officinalis, finely powdered) 18g
Ru Xiang Fen (Gummi Olibanum, powdered) 12g
Vaseline® 120g
Preparation: Combine the two powdered herbs and mix to a paste with Vaseline®.

Source: *Zhao Bing Nan Lin Chuang Jing Yan Ji* [A Collection of Zhao Bingnan's Clinical Experiences]

Tao Ye Xi Ji (Paper Mulberry Leaf Wash Preparation)
Chu Tao Ye (Folium Broussonetiae) 100g
Water 1000ml
Source: *Zhang Zhi Li Pi Fu Bing Lin Chuang Jing Yan Ji Yao* [A Collection of Zhang Zhili's Clinical Experiences in the Treatment of Skin Diseases]

Tie Gu San Gao (Iron Hoop Powder Paste)
Sheng Nan Xing (Rhizoma Arisaematis Crudum)
Sheng Ban Xia (Rhizoma Pinelliae Ternatae)
Sheng Chuan Wu* (Radix Aconiti Carmichaeli Cruda)
Bai Ji (Rhizoma Bletillae Striatae)
Bai Lian (Radix Ampelopsis Japonicae)
Bai Zhi (Radix Angelicae Dahuricae)
Bei Mu (Bulbus Fritillariae)
Bo He (Herba Menthae Haplocalycis)
Huang Bai (Cortex Phellodendri)
Da Huang (Radix et Rhizoma Rhei)
Jiang Huang (Rhizoma Curcumae Longae)
Huang Qin (Radix Scutellariae Baicalensis)
Ya Zao (Fructus Parvus Gleditsiae Sinensis)
Jing Jie Sui (Spica Schizonepetae Tenuifoliae)
Preparation: Grind equal amounts of the ingredients into a very fine powder. Add *Feng Mi‡* (Mel) 60g to every 30g of the medicinal powder and mix smoothly to produce the paste.
Source: *Zhang Zhi Li Pi Fu Bing Lin Chuang Jing Yan Ji Yao* [A Collection of Zhang Zhili's Clinical Experiences in the Treatment of Skin Diseases]

Tou Gu Cao Shui Xi Ji (Speranskia Wash Preparation)
Tou Gu Cao (Herba Speranskiae seu Impatientis) 30g
Ce Bai Ye (Cacumen Biotae Orientalis) 30g
Zao Jiao (Fructus Gleditsiae Sinensis) 15g
Ming Fan‡ (Alumen) 15g
Peng Sha‡ (Borax) 30g
Sodium bicarbonate‡ 30g
Preparation: Decoct the first four ingredients in 2000ml of water for 20 minutes, remove the residue and then add *Peng Sha‡* (Borax) and sodium bicarbonate‡. Use warm to wash the hair.
Source: *Zhang Zhi Li Pi Fu Bing Yi An Xuan Cui* [A Collection of Zhang Zhili's Skin Disease Cases]

Tu Chuang Gao (Bald Sore Paste)
Zi Cao (Radix Arnebiae seu Lithospermi) 60g
Bai Bu (Radix Stemonae) 125g
Xiang You (Oleum Sesami Seminis) 370ml
Po Xiao‡ (Mirabilitum Non-Purum) 50g
Liu Huang‡ (Sulphur) 15g
Zhang Nao (Camphora) 6g
Huang La‡ (Cera Aurea) 60g
Preparation: Pour the sesame oil into a bronze pot, add *Bai Bu* (Radix Stemonae) and *Zi Cao* (Radix Arnebiae seu Lithospermi) and stir-fry until the herbs turn dark yellow. Remove the pot from the heat, then gradually add in *Po Xiao‡* (Mirabilitum Non-Purum), followed by *Liu Huang‡* (Sulphur) and *Zhang Nao* (Camphora) and mix in smoothly. Finally, melt the wax in the mixture to produce the paste.

Source: *Zhu Ren Kang Lin Chuang Jing Yan Ji* [A Collection of Zhu Renkang's Clinical Experiences]

Tu Da Huang Gao (Madaio Dock Root Paste)
Liu Huang‡ (Sulphur) 72g
Ming Fan‡ (Alumen) 36g
Hua Jiao (Pericarpium Zanthoxyli) 18g
Preparation: Grind the ingredients into a powder and mix to a paste with the juice extracted from *Tu Da Huang* (Radix Rumicis Madaio).
Source: *Wai Ke Zheng Zong* [An Orthodox Manual of External Diseases]

Tu Jin Pi Bai Bu Ding (Golden Larch Bark and Stemona Root Tincture)
Tu Jin Pi (Cortex Pseudolaricis) 180g
Bai Bu (Radix Stemonae) 20g
Wu Mei (Fructus Pruni Mume) 20g
Zhang Nao (Camphor) 10g
Bing Pian (Borneolum) 3g
75% Alcohol 700ml
Preparation: Steep the ingredients in the alcohol for seven days, remove the residue and the tincture is ready for use.
Source: *Zhao Bing Nan Lin Chuang Jing Yan Ji* [A Collection of Zhao Bingnan's Clinical Experiences]

Tu Jin Pi Ding (Golden Larch Bark Tincture)
Tu Jin Pi (Cortex Pseudolaricis) 180g
75% Alcohol 500ml
Preparation: Steep the ingredients in the alcohol for seven days.
Source: *Zhang Zhi Li Pi Fu Bing Lin Chuang Jing Yan Ji Yao* [A Collection of Zhang Zhili's Clinical Experiences in the Treatment of Skin Diseases]

Tu Jin Pi San (Golden Larch Bark Powder)
Tu Jin Pi (Cortex Pseudolaricis)
Source: *Wai Ke Zheng Zong* [An Orthodox Manual of External Diseases]

Tuo Se Ba Gao Gun (Decolorizing Medicated Plaster Stick)
Hei Se Ba Gao Gun (Black Medicated Plaster Stick) 500g
Qing Fen* (Calomelas) 420g
Qian Dan‡ (Minium) 60g
Song Xiang (Resina Pini) 60g
Medicinal powder ingredients
Bai Ji (Rhizoma Bletillae Striatae) 30g
Teng Huang (Resina Garciniae) 15g
Qing Fen* (Calomelas) 15g
Nao Sha‡ (Sal Ammoniacum) 9g
Preparation: Prepare the medicinal oil as for *Hei Se Ba Gao Gun* (Black Medicated Plaster Stick). Mix *Qing Fen** (Calomelas), *Qian Dan‡* (Minium), *Song Xiang* (Resina Pini), and 60g of the medicinal powder with 500ml of the medicinal oil to produce the plaster stick.
Source: *Zhang Zhi Li Pi Fu Bing Yi An Xuan Cui* [A Collection of Zhang Zhili's Skin Disease Cases]

Wu Mei Gao (Black Plum Paste)
Wu Mei (Fructus Pruni Mume) 30g
Granulated sugar 9g
Water 50ml
Cu (Acetum) 15ml

Preparation: Dissolve the sugar in the water, then add *Wu Mei* (Fructus Pruni Mume) and steep for 24 hours. Remove *Wu Mei* (Fructus Pruni Mume), add the vinegar and mix thoroughly before application to the affected area.
Source: *Zhong Yi Wai Ke Lin Chuang Shou Ce* [A Clinical Handbook of External Diseases in Chinese Medicine]

Wu Mei Shui Xi Ji (Black Plum Wash Preparation)
Wu Mei (Fructus Pruni Mume) 15g
Can Sha ‡ (Excrementum Bombycis Mori) 10g
Wu Zhu Yu (Fructus Evodiae Rutaecarpae) 10g
Ming Fan ‡ (Alumen) 10g
Preparation: Decoct the herbs in 1000-1500ml of water and boil down to make 500-800ml of a concentrated decoction for use as a wash or wet compress.
Source: Empirical formula

Wu Shi Gao (Five-Stone Paste)
Qing Dai (Indigo Naturalis) 9g
Huang Bai (Cortex Phellodendri) 9g
Ku Fan ‡ (Alumen Praeparatum) 9g
Ge Fen ‡ (Concha Meretricis seu Cyclinae Pulverata) 60g
Duan Shi Gao ‡ (Gypsum Fibrosum Calcinatum) 90g
Hua Shi ‡ (Talcum) 12g
Lu Gan Shi ‡ (Calamina) 60g
Vaseline® 370g
Xiang You (Oleum Sesami Seminis) 250ml
Preparation: Grind the dry ingredients into a powder and mix to a paste with the Vaseline® and sesame oil.
Source: *Zhu Ren Kang Lin Chuang Jing Yan Ji* [A Collection of Zhu Renkang's Clinical Experiences]

Wu Yun Gao (Black Cloud Paste)
Song Xiang (Resina Pini) 60g
Liu Huang ‡ (Sulphur) 30g
Preparation: Grind the ingredients to a powder and mix to a paste with *Xiang You* (Oleum Sesami Seminis).
Source: *Yi Zong Jin Jian* [The Golden Mirror of Medicine]

Xi Gua Shuang (Watermelon Frost)
See page 49.

Xi Gua Shuang Pen Ji (Watermelon Frost Spray Preparation)
Xi Gua Shuang (Praeparatio Mirabiliti et Citrulli)
Huang Lian (Rhizoma Coptidis)
Huang Qin (Radix Scutellariae Baicalensis)
Huang Bai (Cortex Phellodendri)
Zhe Bei Mu (Bulbus Fritillariae Thunbergii)
She Gan (Rhizoma Belamcandae Chinensis)
Shan Dou Gen (Radix Sophorae Tonkinensis)
Bing Pian (Borneolum)
Source: Empirical prescription

Xi Lei San (Tin-Like Powder)
Xi Gua Shuang (Praeparatio Mirabiliti et Citrulli) 6g
Peng Sha ‡ (Borax) 6g
Han Shui Shi ‡ (Calcitum) 9g
Qing Dai (Indigo Naturalis) 18g
Bing Pian (Borneolum) 1.5g
Zhen Zhu ‡ (Margarita) 9g
Nao Sha ‡ (Sal Ammoniacum) 6g
Niu Huang ‡ (Calculus Bovis) 2.4g

Source: *Wen Re Jing Wei* [A Compendium on Epidemic Febrile Diseases]

Xi Shi Xin Ba Gao (Dilute Plaster Preparation)
Hei Se Ba Gao Gun (Black Medicated Plaster Stick) 500g
Qian Dan ‡ (Minium) 30g
Qing Fen ‡ (Calomelas) 210g
Song Xiang (Resina Pini) 60g
Medicinal powder ingredients
Bai Ji (Rhizoma Bletillae Striatae) 30g
Teng Huang (Resina Garciniae) 15g
Qing Fen * (Calomelas) 15g
Nao Sha ‡ (Sal Ammoniacum) 9g
Preparation: Prepare the medicinal oil as for *Hei Se Ba Gao Gun* (Black Medicated Plaster Stick). Mix *Qing Fen* * (Calomelas), *Qian Dan* ‡ (Minium), *Song Xiang* (Resina Pini), and 30g of the medicinal powder with 500ml of the medicinal oil to produce the plaster stick.
Source: *Zhang Zhi Li Pi Fu Bing Lin Chuang Jing Yan Ji Yao* [A Collection of Zhang Zhili's Clinical Experiences in the Treatment of Skin Diseases]

Xi Xuan Fang (Tinea Wash Formula)
Ku Shen (Radix Sophorae Flavescentis)
Li Lu (Radix et Rhizoma Veratri)
Cao Wu * (Radix Aconiti Kusnezoffii)
Po Xiao ‡ (Mirabilitum Non-Purum)
Gui Zhi (Ramulus Cinnamomi Cassiae)
Preparation: Decoct equal quantities of the ingredients in 1500ml of water for 20 minutes, remove the residue and use the decoction as a wash.
Source: *Wai Ke Zheng Zong* [An Orthodox Manual of External Diseases]

Xia Ku Cao Gao (Prunella Paste)
Xia Ku Cao (Spica Prunellae Vulgaris)
Preparation: Pound the herb to a paste and infuse in a little warm water.
Source: *Zheng Zhi Zhun Sheng* [Standards of Diagnosis and Treatment]

Xiang Mu Shui Xi Ji (Cyperus and Scouring Rush Herb Wash Preparation)
Mu Zei (Herba Equiseti Hiemalis) 30g
Xiang Fu (Rhizoma Cyperi Rotundi) 30g
Di Fu Zi (Fructus Kochiae Scopariae) 30g
Xi Xin * (Herba cum Radice Asari) 9g
Preparation: Decoct the herbs in 1000ml of water for 20 minutes, remove the residue and retain the decoction for use as a wash or wet compress.
Source: Empirical formula

Xiao Yan Gao (Paste for Dispersing Inflammation)
Ru Yi Jin Huang San (Agreeable Golden Yellow Powder) 25-30g
Vaseline® 75-80g
Preparation: Melt the Vaseline® over a low heat, slowly add *Ru Yi Jin Huang San* (Agreeable Golden Yellow Powder), mix smoothly and allow to cool.
Source: Empirical formula

Xin San Miao San (New Mysterious Three Powder)
Huang Bai Mian (Cortex Phellodendri, finely powdered) 300g

Qing Dai Mian (Indigo Naturalis, finely powdered) 30g
Han Shui Shi Mian‡ (Calcitum, finely powdered) 150g
Preparation: Grind the ingredients into a powder and sprinkle over the lesions or mix to a paste with vegetable oil.
Source: *Zhao Bing Nan Lin Chuang Jing Yan Ji* [A Collection of Zhao Bingnan's Clinical Experiences]

Xin Wu Yu Gao (New Five-Jade Paste)
Qu Shi San (Powder for Dispelling Dampness) 1560g
Liu Huang‡ (Sulphur, powdered) 150g
Wu Bei Zi‡ (Galla Rhois Chinensis, powdered) 150g
*Qing Fen** (Calomelas) 150g
Jin Huang Gao (Golden Yellow Paste) 2200-2500g
Preparation: Mix the powdered ingredients into *Jin Huang Gao* (Golden Yellow Paste). If the mixture is too dry, add a little *Xiang You* (Oleum Sesami Seminis) to produce a softer paste.
Source: *Zhu Ren Kang Lin Chuang Jing Yan Ji* [A Collection of Zhu Renkang's Clinical Experiences]

Xing Ren Gao (Apricot Kernel Paste)
Yang Zhi‡ (Adeps Ovis) 500g
Dang Gui (Radix Angelicae Sinensis) 50g
Xing Ren (Semen Pruni Armeniacae) 50g
Bai Zhi (Radix Angelicae Dahuricae) 50g
Chuan Xiong (Rhizoma Ligustici Chuanxiong) 50g
Preparation: Grind the herbs into powder and mix with *Yang Zhi*‡ (Adeps Ovis). Steam to produce a paste.
Source: *Pu Ji Fang* [Prescriptions for Universal Relief]

Xing Ren Xi Fang (Apricot Kernel Wash Formula)
Xing Ren (Semen Pruni Armeniacae) 30g
Preparation: Add *Xing Ren* (Semen Pruni Armeniacae) to 300ml of water, bring to the boil and boil down until 100ml of concentrated liquid remains.
Source: *Sheng Ji Zong Lu* [General Collection for Holy Relief]

Xiong Huang Jie Du San Ding Ji (Realgar Powder Tincture Preparation for Relieving Toxicity)
*Xiong Huang** (Realgar) 30g
Han Shui Shi‡ (Calcitum) 30g
Ming Fan‡ (Alumen) 120g
75% Alcohol 100ml
Preparation: Grind the ingredients together to produce a powder, then soak in the 75% alcohol solution for seven days.
Source: *Zhao Bing Nan Lin Chuang Jing Yan Ji* [A Collection of Zhao Bingnan's Clinical Experiences]

Xu Shi Yue Fu San (Xu's Powder for Improving the Skin)
Dong Gua Ren (Semen Benincasae Hispidae) 30g
Shan Yao (Rhizoma Dioscoreae Oppositae) 30g
Lü Dou Fen (Semen Phaseoli Radiati, powdered) 30g
Fu Ling (Sclerotium Poriae Cocos) 12g
Jiang Can‡ (Bombyx Batryticatus) 10g
Chuan Xiong (Rhizoma Ligustici Chuanxiong) 5g
Preparation: Grind the ingredients into a very fine powder.
Source: Empirical formula

Xuan Jiu (Wine Preparation for Tinea)
Tu Jin Pi (Cortex Pseudolaricis) 100g
Tian Nan Xing (Rhizoma Arisaematis) 50g
*Bing Lang** (Semen Arecae Catechu) 50g
Zhang Nao (Camphora) 50g

Mu Zei (Herba Equiseti Hiemalis) 100g
Ban Mao‡ (Mylabris) 50g
Chan Su‡ (Venenum Bufonis) 20g
75% Alcohol 1500ml
Preparation: Soak the materia medica in the alcohol for 15-30 days, then remove the residue and store the medicated wine.
Source: *Wai Ke Zheng Zhi Quan Sheng Ji* [A Life-Saving Manual of the Diagnosis and Treatment of External Diseases]

Xuan Yao Shui Er Hao (No. 2 Medicated Lotion for Tinea)
Tu Jin Pi (Cortex Pseudolaricis) 1250g
Qian Jin Zi (Semen Euphorbiae Lathyridis) 6g
Ban Mao‡ (Mylabris) 12g, wrapped
Gao Liang Jiu (Spiritus Sorghi) 5000ml
Preparation: Soak the materia medica in the sorghum liquor for 15-30 days, then remove the residue and store the lotion.
Source: *Zhu Ren Kang Lin Chuang Jing Yan Ji* [A Collection of Zhu Renkang's Clinical Experiences]

Xuan Yao Shui San Hao (No. 3 Medicated Lotion for Tinea)
Tu Jin Pi (Cortex Pseudolaricis) 72g
Bai Bu (Radix Stemonae) 18g
Bai Ji (Rhizoma Bletillae Striatae) 9g
Zhang Nao (Camphora) 9g
Ban Mao‡ (Mylabris) 3g
Gao Liang Jiu (Spiritus Sorghi) 2500ml
Preparation: Soak the materia medica in the sorghum liquor for 15-30 days, then remove the residue and store the lotion.
Source: *Zui Xin Zhong Cheng Yao Shou Ce* [A Manual of Current TCM Patent Medicines]

Yan Kao San (Buttock-Submerging Sore Powder)
Liu Yi San (Six-To-One Powder)
Ku Fan‡ (Alumen Praeparatum)
Chi Shi Zhi‡ (Halloysitum Rubrum)
Huang Bai (Cortex Phellodendri)
Bing Pian (Borneolum)
Source: *Zhong Yi Wai Ke Xue* [External Diseases in Traditional Chinese Medicine, Zhu Renkang]

Yang He Jie Ning Gao (Harmonious Yang Decongealing Plaster)
Xian Niu Bang (Herba et Radix Arctii Lappae Recens) 1500g
Xian Bai Feng Xian Geng (Caulis Impatientis Balsaminae Recens) 120g
Chuan Xiong (Rhizoma Ligustici Chuanxiong) 120g
*Fu Zi** (Radix Lateralis Aconiti Carmichaeli Praeparata) 60g
Gui Zhi (Ramulus Cinnamomi Cassiae) 60g
Da Huang (Radix et Rhizoma Rhei) 60g
Dang Gui (Radix Angelicae Sinensis) 60g
Rou Gui (Cortex Cinnamomi Cassiae) 60g
*Cao Wu** (Radix Aconiti Kusnezoffii) 60g
Di Long‡ (Lumbricus) 60g
Jiang Can‡ (Bombyx Batryticatus) 60g
Chi Shao (Radix Paeoniae Rubra) 60g
Bai Zhi (Radix Angelicae Dahuricae) 60g
Bai Ji (Rhizoma Bletillae Striatae) 60g
Ru Xiang (Gummi Olibanum) 60g
Mo Yao (Myrrha) 60g
Xu Duan (Radix Dipsaci) 30g
Fang Feng (Radix Ledebouriellae Divaricatae) 30g

Jing Jie (Herba Schizonepetae Tenuifoliae) 30g
Wu Ling Zhi‡ (Excrementum Trogopteri) 30g
Mu Xiang* (Radix Aucklandiae Lappae) 30g
Xiang Yuan (Fructus Citri Medicae seu Wilsonii) 30g
Chen Pi (Pericarpium Citri Reticulatae) 30g
Su He Xiang (Styrax Liquidus) 120ml
She Xiang* (Secretio Moschi) 30g
Cai Zi You (Oleum Brassicae Napi Seminis) 5000ml
Preparation: Fry *Xian Niu Bang* (Herba et Radix Arctii Lappae Recens) and *Xian Bai Feng Xian Geng* (Caulis Impatientis Balsaminae Recens) in the rapeseed (colza) oil until they turn dark yellow; remove the residue and retain the oil. On the next day, fry all the other ingredients in the oil except *Ru Xiang* (Gummi Olibanum), *Mo Yao* (Myrrha), *She Xiang** (Secretio Moschi), and *Su He Xiang* (Styrax Liquidus), adding *Qian Dan* (Minium) 350g for each 500ml of the oil. Once the warm paste no longer adheres to the finger after the pot is removed from the heat, *Ru Xiang* (Gummi Olibanum), *Mo Yao* (Myrrha), *She Xiang** (Secretio Moschi), and *Su He Xiang* (Styrax Liquidus) can be stirred into the thin paste. Store the paste for two weeks before use.
Source: *Wai Ke Zheng Zong* [An Orthodox Manual of External Diseases]

Yang Ti Gen Jiu (Curled Dock Root Wine)
Yang Ti Gen (Radix Rumicis Crispi) 180g
75% Alcohol 500ml
Preparation: Pound *Yang Ti Gen* (Radix Rumicis Crispi) to a pulp and steep in the alcohol for one week. Filter off the residue and use the liquid.
Source: *Zhao Bing Nan Lin Chuang Jing Yan Ji* [A Collection of Zhao Bingnan's Clinical Experiences]

Yang Ti Gen San (Curled Dock Root Powder)
Ku Fan‡ (Alumen Praeparatum) 30g
Tu Da Huang (Radix Rumicis Madaio) 120g
Source: *Yi Zong Jin Jian* [The Golden Mirror of Medicine]

Yang Yin Sheng Ji San (Powder for Nourishing Yin and Generating Flesh)
Xiong Huang* (Realgar) 2g
Qing Dai (Indigo Naturalis) 2g
Gan Cao (Radix Glycyrrhizae) 2g
Bing Pian (Borneolum) 2g
Niu Huang‡ (Calculus Bovis) 1g
Huang Bai (Cortex Phellodendri) 1g
Long Dan Cao (Radix Gentianae Scabrae) 1g
Source: Empirical formula from Beijing Medical University Stomatology Hospital

Yin Hua Gan Cao Ye (Honeysuckle and Licorice Lotion)
Jin Yin Hua (Flos Lonicerae) 20g
Xia Ku Cao (Spica Prunellae Vulgaris) 20g
Gan Cao (Radix Glycyrrhizae) 10g
Preparation: Decoct the herbs for 20 minutes in 500ml of water to prepare the lotion.
Source: *Zhong Hua Kou Qiang Za Zhi* [Chinese Journal of Stomatology]

Yin Xuan Yao Shui Yi Hao (No. 1 Medicated Lotion for Genital Region Tinea)
Bai Ji (Rhizoma Bletillae Striatae) 60g

Bing Lang* (Semen Arecae Catechu) 60g
Tu Jin Pi (Cortex Pseudolaricis) 120g
Da Feng Zi (Semen Hydnocarpi) 60g
Bai Bu (Radix Stemonae) 100g
Ban Mao‡ (Mylabris) 50g
Bai Jiu (Spiritus Granorum Incolor) 1500ml
Preparation: Soak the materia medica in *Bai Jiu* (Spiritus Granorum Incolor) for 15-30 days, then remove the residue and store the medicated lotion.
Source: *Zhong Yi Wai Ke Xue* [External Diseases in Traditional Chinese Medicine, Zhu Renkang]

Yin Xuan You (Genital Region Tinea Oil)
Song Mao (Folium Pini) 50g
Zhang Nao (Camphora) 20g
Zhi Wu You (Oleum Vegetale) 250ml
Preparation: Stir-fry *Song Mao* (Folium Pini) in the vegetable oil until dark brown. Remove the residue and melt *Zhang Nao* (Camphora) in the oil.
Source: *Zhong Yi Wai Ke Xue* [External Diseases in Traditional Chinese Medicine, Zhu Renkang]

You Xi Fang (Wart Wash Formula)
Ma Chi Xian (Herba Portulacae Oleraceae) 60g
Feng Fang‡ (Nidus Vespae) 9g
Chen Pi (Pericarpium Citri Reticulatae) 15g
Cang Zhu (Rhizoma Atractylodis) 15g
Xi Xin* (Herba cum Radice Asari) 9g
She Chuang Zi (Fructus Cnidii Monnieri) 9g
Ku Shen (Radix Sophorae Flavescentis) 15g
Preparation: Soak the ingredients in 1000ml of water for 30 minutes and then decoct for 20 minutes. Remove the residue and use the medicinal lotion as a wash.
Source: *Zhu Ren Kang Lin Chuang Jing Yan Ji* [A Collection of Zhu Renkang's Clinical Experiences]

Yu Ji Gao (Jade Flesh Paste)
Preparation: Mix *Yu Ji San* (Jade Flesh Powder) to a paste with Vaseline® in the proportion of 1:4.

Yu Ji San (Jade Flesh Powder)
Lü Dou (Semen Phaseoli Radiati) 250g
Hua Shi‡ (Talcum) 6g
Bai Zhi (Radix Angelicae Dahuricae) 6g
Bai Fu Zi (Rhizoma Typhonii Gigantei) 6g
Source: *Wai Ke Zheng Zong* [An Orthodox Manual of External Diseases]

Yu Lu Gao (Jade Dew Ointment)
Fu Rong Ye (Folium Hibisci Mutabilis) 60g
Vaseline® 310g
Preparation: Grind the dried leaves of *Fu Rong Ye* (Hibisci Mutabilis Folium) to a fine powder and mix to an ointment-like consistency with Vaseline®.
Source: *Zhu Ren Kang Lin Chuang Jing Yan Ji* [A Collection of Zhu Renkang's Clinical Experiences]

Yu Lu San (Jade Dew Powder)
Fu Rong Ye (Folium Hibisci Mutabilis)
Preparation: Grind the dried leaves to a fine powder, which is normally applied with *Yin Hua Gan Cao Ye* (Honeysuckle and Licorice Lotion) and honey or vegetable oil.

Source: *Yao Lian Qi Mi* [Initiation into the Secrets of the Medicine Cabinet]

Yu Rong San (Jade Countenance Powder)
Bai Qian Niu (Semen Album Pharbitidis) 30g
Bai Lian (Radix Ampelopsis Japonicae) 30g
*Xi Xin** (Herba cum Radice Asari) 30g
Gan Song (Radix Nardostachydis) 30g
Cornstarch 30g
Bai Ge Fen‡ (Excrementum Columbae) 30g
Bai Ji (Rhizoma Bletillae Striatae) 30g
Bai Lian Rui (Stamen Ampelopsis Japonicae) 30g
Bai Zhi (Radix Angelicae Dahuricae) 30g
Bai Zhu (Rhizoma Atractylodis Macrocephalae) 30g
Jiang Can‡ (Bombyx Batryticatus) 30g
Fu Ling (Sclerotium Poriae Cocos) 30g
Jing Jie (Herba Schizonepetae Tenuifoliae) 15g
Du Huo (Radix Angelicae Pubescentis) 15g
Qiang Huo (Rhizoma et Radix Notopterygii) 15g
Bai Fu Zi (Rhizoma Typhonii Gigantei) 30g
Ying Tiao Bai‡ (Excrementum Album Aquilae) 30g
Bai Bian Dou (Semen Dolichoris Lablab) 30g
Fang Feng (Radix Ledebouriellae Divaricatae) 15g
Bai Ding Xiang‡ (Excrementum Passeris) 30g
Source: *Yi Zong Jin Jian* [The Golden Mirror of Medicine]

Yuan Hua Shui Xi Ji (Genkwa Wash Preparation)
Yuan Hua (Flos Daphnes Genkwa) 15g
Hua Jiao (Pericarpium Zanthoxyli) 15g
Huang Bai (Cortex Phellodendri) 30g
Ku Shen (Radix Sophorae Flavescentis) 30g
Preparation: Decoct the herbs for 20 minutes in 1500ml of water. Remove the residue and use the preparation as a wash.
Source: *Zhang Zhi Li Pi Fu Bing Lin Chuang Jing Yan Ji Yao* [A Collection of Zhang Zhili's Clinical Experiences in the Treatment of Skin Diseases]

Yue Shi San (Borax Powder)
Peng Sha‡ (Borax)
Source: Empirical formula

Zhen Jun Miao Tie San (True Gentleman's Wondrous Powder for External Application)
Liu Huang‡ (Sulphur)
Qiao Mai Mian (Farina Fagopyri)
Bai Mian Fen (Farina Tritici)
Source: *Wai Ke Zheng Zong* [An Orthodox Manual of External Diseases]

Zheng Hong Hua You (Regular Safflower Oil)
Bai Zhang You (White Camphor Oil)
Gui Ye You (Myrcene)
Gui Quan You (Cinnamic Alcohol)
Song Jie You (Turpentine Oil)
Dong Qing You (Wintergreen Oil)
Bai You (White Oil)
Source: Empirical formula

Zhi Hou Tang (Decoction for Treating Warts)
Shu Di Huang (Radix Rehmanniae Glutinosae Conquita) 30g
He Shou Wu (Radix Polygoni Multiflori) 15g

Du Zhong (Cortex Eucommiae Ulmoidis) 6g
Bai Shao (Radix Paeoniae Lactiflorae) 15g
Chi Shao (Radix Paeoniae Rubra) 15g
Tao Ren (Semen Persicae) 10g
Hong Hua (Flos Carthami Tinctorii) 10g
Mu Dan Pi (Cortex Moutan Radicis) 10g
Chi Xiao Dou (Semen Phaseoli Calcarati) 15g
Bai Zhu (Rhizoma Atractylodis Macrocephalae) 10g
Niu Xi (Radix Achyranthis Bidentatae) 10g
*Chuan Shan Jia** (Squama Manitis Pentadactylae) 6g
Preparation: Cook the materia medica in 1000ml of water for 20 minutes and boil down to make 750ml of a decoction for use as a soak.
Source: *Zhong Yi Wai Ke Xue* [External Diseases in Traditional Chinese Medicine, Zhu Renkang]

Zhi Yang Fen (Powder for Alleviating Itching)
Song Hua Fen (Pollen Pini) 500g
Bo He (Herba Menthae Haplocalycis) 10g
She Chuang Zi (Fructus Cnidii Monnieri) 20g
Ming Fan‡ (Alumen) 10g
Bing Pian (Borneolum) 2g
Source: *Zhong Yi Wai Ke Xue* [External Diseases in Traditional Chinese Medicine, Zhu Renkang]

Zhi Yang Gao (Paste for Alleviating Itching)
Zhi Yang Fen (Powder for Alleviating Itching) 20g
Vaseline® 80g
Preparation: Mix *Zhi Yang Fen* (Powder for Alleviating Itching) to a paste with the Vaseline®.
Source: *Zhong Yi Wai Ke Xue* [External Diseases in Traditional Chinese Medicine, Zhu Renkang]

Zhi Yang Xi Fang Yi Hao (No. 1 Wash Formula for Alleviating Itching)
Xi Xian Cao (Herba Siegesbeckiae) 30g
Ku Shen (Radix Sophorae Flavescentis) 30g
Di Fu Zi (Fructus Kochiae Scopariae) 15g
Ming Fan‡ (Alumen) 9g
Preparation: Decoct the materia medica in 1000ml of water for 20 minutes to obtain 750ml of liquid. Allow to cool somewhat and use warm an external wash for 15 minutes twice a day.
Source: *Zhong Yi Wai Ke Xue* [External Diseases in Traditional Chinese Medicine, Zhu Renkang]

Zhi Yi Xi Fang (Seborrhea Wash Formula)
Cang Er Zi (Fructus Xanthii Sibirici) 30g
Wang Bu Liu Xing (Semen Vaccariae Segetalis) 30g
Ku Shen (Radix Sophorae Flavescentis) 15g
Ming Fan‡ (Alumen) 9g
Preparation: Soak the materia medica in 800ml of water for 30 minutes, then boil for 20 minutes. Remove the residue and use as a wash for the scalp.
Source: *Zhu Ren Kang Lin Chuang Jing Yan Ji* [A Collection of Zhu Renkang's Clinical Experiences]

Zhi Zhu Hua You (Yellow Azalea Flower Oil)
Nao Yang Hua (Flos Rhododendri Mollis) 200g
Huang La‡ (Cera Aurea) 2g
Zhi Wu You (Oleum Vegetale) 500ml

Preparation: Fry *Nao Yang Hua* (Flos Rhododendri Mollis) in the vegetable oil until dark brown, then remove the residue, add *Huang La*‡ (Cera Aurea) and allow to cool before use.
Source: *Yi Zong Jin Jian* [The Golden Mirror of Medicine]
Note: *Zhi Zhu Hua* is an alternative name for *Nao Yang Hua*.

Zhu Huang San (Pearl and Bezoar Powder)
Zhen Zhu‡ (Margarita)
Niu Huang‡ (Calculus Bovis)
Preparation: Grind equal amounts of the materia medica into a fine powder and mix thoroughly.
Source: *Quan Guo Zhong Yao Cheng Yao Chu Fang Ji* [National Collection of Chinese Herbal Patent Medicines]

Zi Cao You (Gromwell Root Oil)
Zi Cao (Radix Arnebiae seu Lithospermi) 100g
Huang Bai (Cortex Phellodendri) 50g
Xiang You (Oleum Sesami Seminis) 450ml
Preparation: Fry the herbs in the sesame oil until dark yellow, then remove the residue and filter off the oil.
Source: Empirical formula

Zi Lian Gao (Gromwell Root and Coptis Paste)
Zi Cao (Radix Arnebiae seu Lithospermi) 30g
Huang Lian Fen (Rhizoma Coptidis, powdered) 15g
Xiang You (Oleum Sesami Seminis) 1000ml
Huang La‡ (Cera Aurea) as required
Preparation: Fry *Zi Cao* (Radix Arnebiae seu Lithospermi) in the sesame oil over a low heat until it burns. Mix in the powdered *Huang Lian* (Rhizoma Coptidis) and add the yellow wax, stirring to ensure even distribution so that a paste will be produced when the mixture cools down.
Source: Empirical formula

Zi Se Xiao Zhong Fen (Purple Powder for Dispersing Swelling)
Zi Cao (Radix Arnebiae seu Lithospermi) 15g
Sheng Ma (Rhizoma Cimicifugae) 30g
*Guan Zhong** (Rhizoma Dryopteris Crassirhizomae) 6g
Chi Shao (Radix Paeoniae Rubra) 30g
Zi Jing Pi (Cortex Cercis) 15g
Dang Gui (Radix Angelicae Sinensis) 60g
Fang Feng (Radix Ledebouriellae Divaricatae) 15g
Bai Zhi (Radix Angelicae Dahuricae) 60g
Hong Hua (Flos Carthami Tinctorii) 15g
Qiang Huo (Rhizoma et Radix Notopterygii) 15g
Jing Jie Sui (Spica Schizonepetae Tenuifoliae) 15g
Jing Jie (Herba Schizonepetae Tenuifoliae) 15g
Er Cha (Pasta Acaciae seu Uncariae) 15g
Shen Qu (Massa Fermentata) 15g
Source: *Zhao Bing Nan Lin Chuang Jing Yan Ji* [A Collection of Zhao Bingnan's Clinical Experiences]

Zi Se Xiao Zhong Gao (Purple Paste for Dispersing Swelling)
Zi Se Xiao Zhong Fen (Purple Powder for Dispersing Swelling) 120g
Xue Jie Hua (Flos Daemonoropsis Draconis) 3g
Shan Nai (Rhizoma Kaempferiae) 6g
Ru Xiang (Gummi Olibanum) 12g
Mo Yao (Myrrha) 12g
Preparation: Combine *Zi Se Xiao Zhong Fen* (Purple Powder for Dispersing Swelling) with a powder made from the other four ingredients, then mix to a paste with 120g of Vaseline®.
Source: *Zhao Bing Nan Lin Chuang Jing Yan Ji* [A Collection of Zhao Bingnan's Clinical Experiences]

Note

Animal, insect and mineral materia medica are marked with the symbol ‡; materia medica whose use may be restricted in certain countries are marked with the symbol *. Please refer to the author's preface for further details.

Bibliography

Classical works

Bao Ying Cuo Yao [Essentials for the Care of Infants], Xue Kai, 1556.

Bei Ji Qian Jin Yao Fang, see *Qian Jin Yao Fang*.

Ben Cao Gang Mu [A Compendium of Materia Medica], Li Shizhen, 1590.

Ben Shi Fang [Original Prescriptions], Xu Shuwei, 12th century.

Bian Zheng Lu [Pattern Identification Records], Chen Shiduo, 1687.

Chi Shui Xuan Zhu [Red Water and Mysterious Pearl], Sun Yikui, 1584.

Chuang Yang Jing Yan Quan Shu [A Complete Manual of Experience in the Treatment of Sores], Dou Hanqing, 1569.

Dan Xi Shou Jing [Danxi's Handy Mirror], Zhu Danxi, 1350.

Dan Xi Xin Fa [Danxi's Experiential Therapy], Zhu Danxi (revised by Cheng Yun, 1481).

Dong Tian Ao Zhi (Wai Ke Mi Lu) [Secret Records of External Diseases], Chen Shiduo, 1694.

Dong Yuan Shi Shu [Li Dongyuan's Ten Works], Li Dongyuan, 1529.

Dou Zhen Xin Fa [Experiences in Treating Pox and Papules], Wan Quan, 1568.

Feng Shi Jin Nang Mi Lu [Feng's Secret Records of the Best Counsels], Feng Zhaozhang, 1702.

Fu Ren Liang Fang [Best Prescriptions for Women], Chen Ziming, 1237.

Gu Jin Tu Shu Ji Cheng Yi Bu Quan Lu [Complete Medical Works of the Library Collection, Ancient and Modern], Jiang Tingxi, 1723.

He Jian Liu Shu [He Jian's Works], Liu Wansu (1120-1200).

Huang Di Nei Jing [The Yellow Emperor's Classic of Internal Medicine], Warring States period.

Huang Di Nei Jing Su Wen Zhu [Notes on Simple Questions from the Yellow Emperor's Classic of Internal Medicine], Wang Bing, Tang.

Jin Kui Yao Lue [Synopsis of Prescriptions from the Golden Cabinet], Zhang Zhongjing (Zhang Ji), Eastern Han, part of *Shang Han Za Bing Lun* [Treatise on Miscellaneous Cold Diseases].

Jing Yue Quan Shu [The Complete Works of Zhang Jingyue], Zhang Jiebin (Zhang Jingyue), 1624.

Lei Zheng Zhi Cai [Treatment of Classified Patterns], Lin Peiqin, 1839.

Lin Zheng Zhi Nan Yi An: Yang Ke [Case History Guide to Clinical Symptoms: Skin Diseases], Ye Gui, 1766.

Ling Shu [The Miraculous Pivot], part of *Huang Di Nei Jing* [The Yellow Emperor's Internal Classic], Warring States period.

Liu Juan Zi Gui Yi Fang [Liu Juanzi's Remedies Left Behind by Ghosts], Gong Qingxuan, Southern Qi dynasty (479-502).

Ma Zhen Ji Cheng [Collected Abstracts on Measles], Zhu Chufen, 1824.

Meng He Si Jia Yi An [Meng He's Case Studies from Four Families], Meng He, 1726

Nan Jing [Classic on Medical Problems], Qin or Western Han (exact date unknown).

Nei Ke Zhai Yao [A Digest of Internal Medicine], Xue Lizhai, c. 1540.

Nei Wai Shang Bian Huo Lun [Discussion on Difficult Problems Related to Internal and External Damage], Li Gao, 1247.

Pi Wei Lun [A Treatise on the Spleen and Stomach], Li Gao, 1249.

Pu Ji Fang [Prescriptions for Universal Relief], Teng Hong, 1406.

Qian Jin Yao Fang [Prescriptions Worth a Thousand Gold Pieces for Emergencies], Sun Simiao, 682.

Qian Jin Yi Fang [A Supplement to Prescriptions Worth a Thousand Gold Pieces for Emergencies], Sun Simiao, 682.

Quan Sheng Zhi Mi Fang [A Guide to Secret Prescriptions for a Lifetime], Wang Kuang, 12th century.

Ru Men Shi Qin [Confucians' Duties to Their Parents], Zhang Congzheng, 1228.

Rui Zhu Tang Jing Yan Fang [Rui Zhutang's Empirical Formulae], Shatu Musu, 1326.

San Yin Fang [Formulae for the Three Categories of Etiological Factors], Chen Wuze, 1174.

Shang Han Lun [On Cold Damage], Zhang Zhongjing (Zhang Ji), Eastern Han, part of *Shang Han Za Bing Lun* [Treatise on Miscellaneous Cold Diseases].

Shang Han Za Bing Lun [Treatise on Miscellaneous Cold Diseases], Zhang Zhongjing (Zhang Ji), Eastern Han.

She Sheng Zong Yao [A Summary of Secret Prescriptions for Preserving Health], Ming Hongji, 1905 (revised edition).

Shen She Zun Sheng Shu [Master Shen's Book on the Importance of Respecting Life], Shen Jin'ao, 1773.

Sheng Ji Zong Lu [General Collection for Holy Relief], anon., 1111-1117.

Shi Shi Mi Lu [Secret Records of the Stone Chamber], Chen Shiduo, 1687.

Shi Yi De Xiao Fang [Effective Formulae Handed Down for Generations], Wei Yilin, 1345.

Shou Shi Bao Yuan [Safeguarding the Origins of Longevity], Gong Tingxian, 16th century.

Su Wen [Simple Questions], part of *Huang Di Nei Jing* [The Yellow Emperor's Internal Classic], Warring States period.

Tai Ping Hui Min He Ji Ju Fang [Prescriptions from the Peaceful Benevolent Dispensary], Bureau of Imperial Physicians [Song dynasty], 1078-1085.

Tai Ping Sheng Hui Fang [Peaceful Holy Benevolent Prescriptions], Wang Huaiyin, 992.

Wai Ke Bai Xiao Quan Shu [A Compendium of Effective Treatments for External Diseases], Gong Juyuan (date unknown).

Wai Ke Chuan Xin Ji [Inherited Secrets of External Diseases], Ma Peizhi, Qing (exact date unknown).

Wai Ke Da Cheng [A Compendium of External Diseases], Qi Kun, 1665.

Wai Ke Jing Yao [Essence of Diagnosis and Treatment of External Diseases], Chen Ziming, 1263.

Wai Ke Jing Yi [The Essence of External Diseases], Qi Dezhi, 1335.

Wai Ke Li Li [Theory and Case Reports on External Diseases], Wang Ji, 1531.

Wai Ke Mi Lu, see *Dong Tian Ao Zhi (Wai Ke Mi Lu)* [Secret Records of External Diseases].

Wai Ke Qi Xuan [Revelations of the Mystery of External Diseases], Shen Douyuan, 1604.

Wai Ke Shu Yao [Essentials of External Diseases], Xue Jizhuan, 1571.

Wai Ke Tu Shuo [Illustrated Explanations of External Diseases], Gao Wenjin, 1834.

Wai Ke Wen Da [Questions and Answers in External Diseases], Gao Qiyun, 1517.

Wai Ke Yi An Hui Bian [A Collection of Case Histories Relating to External Diseases], Yu Jinghe, 1894.

Wai Ke Zhen Quan [True Notes on External Diseases], Zou Yue, 1838.

Wai Ke Zheng Zhi Quan Sheng Ji [A Life-Saving Manual of the Diagnosis and Treatment of External Diseases], Wang Weide, 1740.

Wai Ke Zheng Zhi Quan Shu: Bai Bi [A Compendium of External Symptoms and Treatment: White Crust], Xu Kechang, 1831.

Wai Ke Zheng Zong [An Orthodox Manual of External Diseases], Chen Shigong, 1617.

Wai Tai Mi Yao [Secrets of a Frontier Official], Wang Tao, 752.

Wen Bing Tiao Bian [Treatise on the Identification of Warm Diseases], Wu Tang, 1798.

Wen Re Jing Wei [A Compendium on Epidemic Febrile Diseases], Wang Mengying, 1852.

Wu Shi Er Bing Fang [Prescriptions for the Fifty-Two Diseases], Ma Wangdui Tomb Collection Classification Group (found in 1973, but date of publication unknown).

Xian Nian Ji [A Collection Held by Immortals], Li Wenbing, Qing (exact date unknown).

Xiao Er Wei Sheng Zong Wei Lun Fang: Pao Zhen Lun [General Discussion on Children's Hygiene: Herpes], author unknown, 15th century.

Xiao Er Yao Zheng Zhi Jue [Key to the Treatment of Children's Diseases], Qian Yi, 1119.

Xiao Zhu Fu Ren Liang Fang [Proof and Explanation of Woman's Formulae], Xue Ji (1486-1558).

Xue Shi Yi An [Xue Ji's Casebook], Xue Ji, 1573.

Xue Zheng Lun [A Treatise on Blood Patterns], Tang Rongchuan, 1884.

Yan Hou Jing Yan Mi Chuan [Secret Empirical Prescriptions in the Treatment of Throat Diseases], Cheng Yongpei, Qing (revised edition, original author unknown).

Yang Ke Gang Yao [A Summary of External Diseases], Zhang Shouyi, 1917.

Yang Ke Xin De Ji [A Collection of Experiences in the Treatment of Sores], Gao Bingjun, 1805.

Yang Ke Xun Cui [Essential Collection for the Treatment of Sores], Chen Wenzhi, 1628.

Yang Yi Da Quan [The Complete Book of External Diseases], Gu Shicheng, 1760.

Yao Dui [Compatibility of Medicines], Xu Zhicai (493-572).

Yi Fang Ji Jie [Collection of Prescriptions with Notes], Wang Ang, 1682.

Yi Ji: Za Bing Lei Fang [Medical Works: Prescriptions for Various Categories of Miscellaneous Diseases], Dong Xiyuan, 1777.

Yi Lin Gai Cuo [Corrections of the Errors in Medical Works], Wang Qingren, 1830.

Yi Men Fa Lu [Laws of Medicine], Yu Chang, 1658.

Yi Shu [Medical Records], Cheng Wenyou, 1826.

Yi Xue Liu Yao [Six Essentials of Medical Criteria], Zhang Sanxi, 1585.

Yi Xue Ru Men [Elementary Medicine], Li Chan, 1575.

Yi Xue Xin Wu [An Understanding of Medicine], Cheng Guopeng, 1732.

Yi Xue Zheng Zhuan [Orthodox Medical Problems], Yu Tuan, 1515.

Yi Xue Zhong Zhong Can Xi Lu [Records of Traditional Chinese and Western Medicine Used in Combination], Zhang Xichun, 1918-1934.

Yi Zhen Yi De [An Understanding of Epidemic Diseases with Eruptions], Yu Shiyu, 1785.

Yi Zong Bi Du [Required Readings for Medical Professionals], Li Zhongzi, 1637.

Yi Zong Jin Jian [The Golden Mirror of Medicine], Wu Qian, 1742.

You You Ji Cheng [A Complete Work on Pediatrics], Chen Fuzheng, 1750.

You You Xin Shu [A New Book of Pediatrics], Liu Fang, 1132.

Za Bing Yuan Liu Xi Zhu [Enlightenment of the Origins of Miscellaneous Diseases], Shen Jin'ao, 1773.

Zhang Shi Yi Tong [Zhang Lu's Understanding of Medicine], Zhang Lu, 1695.

Zhen Jiu Da Quan [The Complete Book of Acupuncture], Xu Feng, 1439.

Zheng Yin Mai Zhi [On the Pulse and Treatment of Signs and Symptoms], Qin Jingming, 1706.

Zheng Zhi Zhun Sheng [Standards of Diagnosis and Treatment], Wang Kentang, 1602.

Zhou Hou Bei Ji Fang [A Handbook of Prescriptions for Emergencies], Ge Hong, Western Jin.

Zhu Bing Yuan Hou Lun [A General Treatise on the Causes and Symptoms of Diseases], Chao Yuanfang, 610.

Zhu Lin Si Nü Ke Quan Shu [Complete Gynecology from Zhulin Temple], Jing Guan, 1771.

Modern works

An Jiafeng and Zhang Fan, *Zhang Zhi Li Pi Fu Bing Yi An Xuan Cui* [A Collection of Zhang Zhili's Skin Disease Cases], Beijing: People's Medical Publishing House, 1994.

Beijing Hospital of Traditional Chinese Medicine, *Zhao Bing Nan Lin Chuang Jing Yan Ji* [A Collection of Zhao Bingnan's Clinical Experiences], Beijing: People's Medical Publishing House, 1975.

Braun-Falco O., Plewig, G., Wolff, H.H., and Burgdorf, W.H.C., *Dermatology* (2nd ed.), Berlin: Springer Verlag, 1999.

Champion, R.H., Burton, J.L., Burns, D.A., and Breathnach, S.M. (eds.), *Textbook of Dermatology* (6th ed.), Oxford: Blackwell Science, 1998.

Chang Qing, *Dang Dai Zhong Yao Wai Zhi Shi Ke Bai Bing Qian Fang* [Current TCM External Treatments of Hundreds of External Diseases With Thousands of Formulae] Beijing: Traditional Chinese Medicine Classic Book Publishing House, 1998.

Chen Keji, *Ci Xi Guang Xu Yi Fang Xuan Yi* [Selective Explanation of Ci Xi and Guang Xu's Medical Prescriptions], Beijing: China Book Publishing House, 1981.

Chen Sicheng, *Mei Chuang Mi Lu* [Secret Prescriptions for Fungus and Sores], Beijing: Beijing Academic Publishing House, 1994.

Chen Zesen, *Ming Yi Te Se Jing Yan Jing Hua* [Quintessence of the Distinctive Experiences of Eminent Doctors], Shanghai: Shanghai TCM University Press, 1987.

Cheng Qiusheng, *Pi Fu Bing Zhong Yi Xi Zhi Liao Fa* [TCM External Washes in the Treatment of Skin Diseases], Xi'an: Northwest University Press, 1993.

Dai Qiusun, *Shi Yong Zhen Jiu Zhi Liao Xue* [Practical Acupuncture Treatment], Beijing: People's Medical Publishing House, 2000.

Ding Ganren, *Ding Gan Ren Yi An* [Ding Ganren's Case Histories], Shanghai: Shanghai Science and Technology Publishing House, 1960.

Editorial Committee of the Dictionary of Traditional Chinese Medicine, *Jian Ming Zhong Yi Ci Dian* [A Concise Dictionary of Traditional Chinese Medicine], Beijing: People's Medical Publishing House, 1980.

External Disease Department of Shanghai College of Traditional Chinese Medicine, *Zhong Yi Wai Ke Jiang Yi* [Teaching Materials for External Diseases in Chinese Medicine], Shanghai: Shanghai Science and Technology Publishing House, 1964.

External Disease Department of Shanghai College of Traditional Chinese Medicine, *Zhong Yi Wai Ke Lin Chuang Shou Ce* [A Clinical Handbook of External Diseases in Chinese Medicine], Shanghai: Shanghai Science and Technology Publishing House, 1966.

Fan Weihong, *Zui Xin Fang Ji Shou Ce* [A New Handbook of Chinese Materia Medica Formulae], Zhengzhou: Henan Science and Technology Publishing House, 1998.

Gu Bohua, *Shi Yong Zhong Yi Wai Ke Xue* [Practical Treatment of External Diseases with Traditional Chinese Medicine], Shanghai: Shanghai Science and Technology Publishing House, 1985.

Gu Bohua, *Wai Ke Jing Yan Xuan* [Selected Experiences in the Treatment of External Diseases], Shanghai: Shanghai People's Publishing House, 1977.

Guan Fen, *Shi Yong Zhong Yi Pi Fu Bing Xue* [Practical Dermatology in Traditional Chinese Medicine], Lanzhou: Gansu People's Publishing House, 1981.

Habif, Thomas P., Campbell, James L., Quitadamo, Mark J., and Zug, Kathryn A., *Skin Disease: Diagnosis and Treatment*, St. Louis: Mosby, 2001.

Hu Ximing (ed.), *Zhong Guo Zhong Yi Mi Fang Da Quan* [A Compendium of Secret Prescriptions of Traditional Chinese Medicine], Shanghai: Wen Hui Publishing House, 1991.

Hunter J.A.A., Savin, J.A. and Dahl, M.V., *Clinical Dermatology* (3rd ed.), Oxford, Blackwell Science, 2002.

Li Bojian, *Pi Fu Ke Yi Lan* [Key to the Understanding of Skin Diseases], Beijing: Traditional Chinese Medicine Publishing House, 1989.

Li Jingwei and Deng Tietao (eds.), *Zhong Yi Da Ci Dian* [A Dictionary of Chinese Medicine], Beijing: People's Medical Publishing House, 1998.

Li Lin, *Niu Pi Xuan Zhong Yi Liao Fa* [Treatment of Psoriasis with Traditional Chinese Medicine], Beijing: Traditional Chinese Medicine Publishing House, 1989.

Liu Furen, *Shi Yong Pi Fu Bing Xue* [Practical Dermatology], Beijing: People's Medical Publishing House, 1984.

Lü Yaoqing, *Zhong Guo Ren Pi Fu Bing Tu Pu* [Atlas of Chinese Skin Diseases], Taiwan: Current Medical Journal Publishing House, 1984.

Luo Yutian, *Zhong Yi Wai Ke Lin Zheng Ji Yao* [Principles of Chinese Medicine in the Treatment of External Disease According to Patterns], Chengdu: Sichuan Science and Technology Publishing House, 1987.

Pei Zhengxue, *Xue Zheng Lun Ping Shi* [Assessment and Explanation of *A Treatise on Blood Patterns*], Beijing: People's Medical Publishing House, 1980.

Pharmacopoeia Commission of The People's Republic of China, *Zhong Hua Ren Ming Gong He Guo Yao Dian* [Pharmacopoeia of the People's Republic of China], Beijing: Chemical Industry Press, 2000.

Shan Shujian and Chen Zihua, *Gu Jin Ming Yi Lin Zheng Jin Jian: Wai Ke Juan* [The Golden Mirror of Clinical Practice of Famous Doctors Ancient and Modern: External Diseases], Beijing: Traditional Chinese Medicine Publishing House, 1999.

Shan Zhengao, *Shi Yong Zhong Cheng Yao Shou Ce* [A Compilation of Chinese Herbal Patent Medicines], Beijing: People's Military Medicine Publishing House, 1998.

Shi Xuemin, *Shi Xue Min Zhen Jiu Lin Zheng Ji Yan* [Collection of Shi Xuemin's Clinical Experiences in Acupuncture and Moxibustion], Tianjin: Tianjin Science and Technology Publishing House, 1998.

Shi Yuguang and Shan Shujian (eds.), *Dang Dai Ming Yi Lin Zheng Jing Hua: Pi Fu Bing Zhuan Ji* [A Selection of Clinical Experiences of Famous Contemporary Practitioners: Skin Disease Specialists], Beijing: Traditional Chinese Medicine Publishing House, 1992.

Song Zhaoyou, *Zhong Yi Pi Fu Bing Ke Lin Chuang Shou Ce* [A Clinical Manual of Dermatology in Chinese Medicine], Beijing: People's Medical Publishing House, 1996.

State Bureau of Technical Supervision, *National Acupuncture Points Standard: Acupuncture Points Schedule*, Beijing: State Standardization Press, 1990.

Tan Xinhua, *Zhong Yi Wai Ke Xue* [External Diseases in Traditional Chinese Medicine], Beijing: People's Medical Publishing House, 1999.

Tian Conghuo, *Zhen Jiu Yi Xue Yan Ji* [A Collection of Experiences in Acupuncture], Beijing: Beijing Science and Technology Publishing House, 1985.

Traditional Chinese Medicine Research Academy: Beijing Guang'anmen Hospital, *Zhu Ren Kang Lin Chuang Jing Yan Ji* [A Collection of Zhu Renkang's Clinical Experiences], Beijing: People's Medical Publishing House, 1979.

Wang Baofang, *Cuo Chuang* [Acne], Singapore Medicine and Health Publishing House, 1998.

Wang Yuxi (ed.), *Shi Yong Zhong Yi Wai Ke Fang Ji Da Ci Dian* [Dictionary of Practical TCM Formulae for External Treatment], Beijing: Traditional Chinese Medicine Publishing House, 1993.

Xiang Ping, *Nan Jing Zhong Yi Yao Da Xue Zhong Yi Xue Jia Zhuan Ji* [Collected Experiences of TCM Experts from Nanjing University of TCM], Beijing: People's Medical Publishing House, 1999.

Xie Yuanming, *Tou Fa De Zhong Yi Fang Zhi* [Prevention and Treatment of Hair Loss with Traditional Chinese Medicine], Xi'an: Shaanxi Science and Technology Publishing House, 1988.

Xu Fusong, *Xu Lü He Wai Ke Yi An Yi Hua Ji* [A Collection of Xu Lühe's Medical Records and Notes on External Diseases], Beijing: China Science and Technology Publishing House, 1986.

Xu Li and Wang Wei, *Chinese Materia Medica: Combinations and Applications*, London: Donica Publishing, 2002.

Xu Rongzhai, *Chong Ding Tong Su Shang Han Lun* [Simplified Revision of *On Cold Damage*], Beijing: New Medicine Book Publishing Company, 1956.

Xu Yihou, *Pi Fu Bing Zhong Yi Zhen Liao Xue* [Diagnosis and Treatment of Skin Diseases in Traditional Chinese Medicine], Beijing: People's Medical Publishing House, 1997.

Xu Yihou, *Pi Fu Ke Zhen Jiu Zhi Liao Xue* [Acupuncture in the Treatment of Skin Diseases], Beijing: Beijing Science and Technology Publishing House, 1994.

Xu Yihou, *Shan Cang Gui Wai Ke Jing Yan Ji* [A Collection of Shan Canggui's Experiences in Treating External Diseases], Wuhan: Hubei Science and Technology Publishing House, 1984.

Xu Yihou, *Shou Zu Pi Fu Bing Fang Zhi* [Treatment of Skin Disorders of the Hands and Feet], Beijing: People's Medical Publishing House, 1991.

Xu Yihou, *Xu Yi Hou Pi Fu Bing Lin Chuang Jing Yan Ji Yao* [A Summary of Xu Yihou's Clinical Experiences in the Treatment of Skin Diseases], Beijing: China Medical Science and Technology Publishing House, 1998.

Xu Zhiyin, *Zhong Yi Wai Ke Xue* [External Diseases in Chinese Medicine], Nanjing: Southeast University Press, 1998.

Yang Sishu, *Zhong Yi Lin Chuang Da Quan* [Clinical Compendium of Traditional Chinese Medicine], Beijing: Beijing Science and Technology Publishing House, 1991.

Zhang Hong, *Zui Xin Zhong Cheng Yao Shou Ce* [A Manual of Current TCM Patent Medicines], Shenyang: Liaoning Science and Technology Publishing House, 1998.

Zhang Manhua et al., *Zhong Yi Pi Fu Bing Xue Jing Hua* [Essentials of Dermatology in Traditional Chinese Medicine], Guangzhou: Guangdong Higher Education Publishing House, 1988.

Zhang Shanlei, *Yang Ke Gang Yao* [Essentials for the Treatment of Sores], Shanghai: Shanghai Health Publishing House, 1958.

Zhang Zhili, *Zhang Zhi Li Pi Fu Bing Lin Chuang Jing Yan Ji Yao* [A Collection of Zhang Zhili's Clinical Experiences in the Treatment of Skin Diseases], Beijing: People's Medical Publishing House, 2001.

Zhao Bian, *Lin Chuang Pi Fu Bing Xue* [Clinical Dermatology], Nanjing: Jiangsu Science and Technology Publishing House, 1989.

Zhao Jinduo, *Zhong Yi Zheng Chuang Jian Bie Zhen Duan Xue* [Diagnosis and Differentiation of Symptoms with Traditional Chinese Medicine], Beijing: People's Medical Publishing House, 1993.

Zhu Renkang, *Zhong Yi Wai Ke Xue* [External Diseases in Traditional Chinese Medicine], Beijing: People's Medical Publishing House, 1987.

Zhu Yeqing, *Chang Yong Zhong Cao Yao Bu Liang Fan Ying Ji Qi Fang Zhi* [Adverse Effects Induced by Commonly Used Chinese Materia Medica and Their Prevention and Treatment], Shanghai: Shanghai Medical University Press, 1998.

Zhuang Guokang, *Chuang Yang Wai Yong Ben Cao* [External Application of Herbs in the Treatment of Sores], Beijing: People's Medical Publishing House, 1982.

Zou Wufeng, *Wai Ke Zhen Quan* [The Truth About External Diseases], Shanghai New Knowledge Publishing House, 1965.

Index